Clinical Considerations in School-based Health

Robert P. Olympia • Jodi Brady-Olympia
Editors

Clinical Considerations in School-based Health

An Evidence-Based Guide for Physicians, Advanced practice providers and School nurses

Springer

Editors
Robert P. Olympia
Department of Emergency Medicine
and Pediatrics
Penn State College of Medicine
Attending Physician
Hershey, PA, USA

Division of Pediatric Emergency Medicine
Department of Emergency Medicine
Penn State Milton S. Hershey
Medical Center
Hershey, PA, USA

Jodi Brady-Olympia
Department of Pediatrics Penn State
College of Medicine Attending Physician
Division of Adolescent Medicine
Department of Pediatrics, Penn State
Children's Hospital
Hershey, PA, USA

ISBN 978-3-031-85764-5 ISBN 978-3-031-85765-2 (eBook)
https://doi.org/10.1007/978-3-031-85765-2

This Springer imprint is published by the registered company Springer Nature Switzerland AG
The registered company address is: Gewerbestrasse 11, 6330 Cham, Switzerland

Preface

> Children are not a distraction from more important work. They are the most important work. —C.S. Lewis

As pediatricians, my wife and I have dedicated our lives to maintaining the physical and mental health and well-being of children and adolescents. Our professions became passions early in our careers as school-based health encompassed both our clinical and academic paths. For me it started on September 11, 2001 when, as a Pediatric Emergency Medicine physician in New York City, I was inspired by the tragedy to ensure that schools in the United States were prepared to deal with emergencies, disasters, and mass casualty incidents. For my wife, her passion for school-based health developed as an Adolescent Medicine pediatrician working at the Milton Hershey School, a private boarding school in central Pennsylvania. Unfortunately, school-based health became a personal journey when our youngest daughter, Madelyn, was diagnosed with severe food allergies. In our pursuit of a safe learning environment for our daughter, we learned first-hand the challenges that school nurses/staff and school districts have in optimizing the health and well-being of their students.

School nurses are often undervalued and underappreciated in our society, often working in difficult circumstances with less than optimal resources. This book is dedicated to you—on behalf of the lives that you have affected and protected and advocated for, we (including the Olympia family) thank you. You are appreciated and loved, and my wife and I will continue to support and advocate for you, your students, and your profession.

> Education is the kindling of a flame, not the filling of a vessel —Socrates

During our careers, my wife and I have had the tremendous opportunity to interact with and educate school nurses. Whether it was giving lectures at the National Association of School Nurses (NASN) or Pennsylvania Association of School Nurses and Practitioners (PASNAP) annual meetings, writing evidence-based articles for the *NASN School Nurse* series "School Nurses on the Front Lines of Medicine," training school nurses in STOP THE BLEED or Basic Life Support, or publishing research on topics such as emergency and disaster preparedness, sports medicine/concussions, and mental and behavioral health, we feel that the education of school nurses and school providers is of utmost importance to the health and well-being of children and adolescents.

Through *Clinical Considerations in School-Based Health*, we wanted to share our passion for school-based health with our readers and inspire them to optimize the care provided to their students. This book will provide school-based health practitioners a comprehensive, "go-to" resource to access evidence-based recommendations for the assessment/screening, triage, initial stabilization, and treatment, and recognition of acute and chronic conditions and disease processes often seen in students. It aims to utilize modern methods of learning to improve retention and implementation, such as algorithms, mnemonics, case studies, tables, and lists. Authors have been recruited, both regionally and nationally, with expertise in school-based health, general pediatrics, developmental pediatrics, subspecialty pediatrics, mental and behavioral health, infectious diseases, sports medicine, emergency medicine, and adolescent medicine. We hope that the knowledge you gain by reading this book "kindles your flame" to optimize the care you provide to your students. Thank you for the opportunity.

Hershey, PA, USA Robert P. Olympia

Acknowledgments

To our children, Abigail Riley and Madelyn Bailey. We are so lucky and blessed to be your mommy and daddy. You inspire us every day to be the best people we can be. You have taught us about teamwork and friendship, about sacrifice and the relentless pursuit of goals, about overcoming obstacles with honesty and grace, about forgiveness and selfless love, about patience and listening, and about making an impact on our world, faithfully taking one day at a time while walking in the footsteps of our Jesus Christ. There is nothing better than viewing the world through your eyes, and we feel complete because you both are part of our world. We are so proud of the young women you have become, and look forward to the future, but never forget, you will always be our babies. Keep learning and shooting for the stars, and strive to make an impact with everything you do. We love you to the moon and back!

Don't just fly, soar. —Dumbo

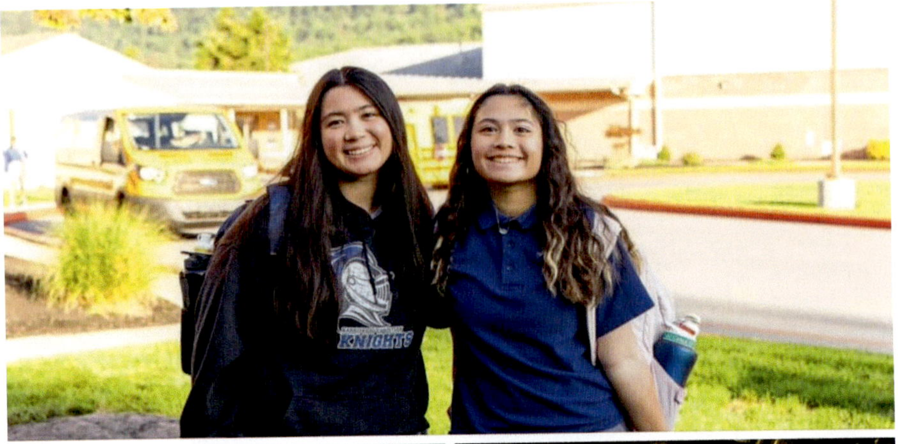

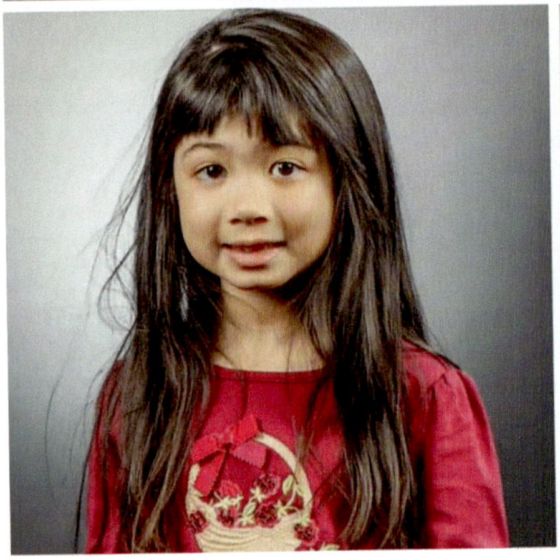

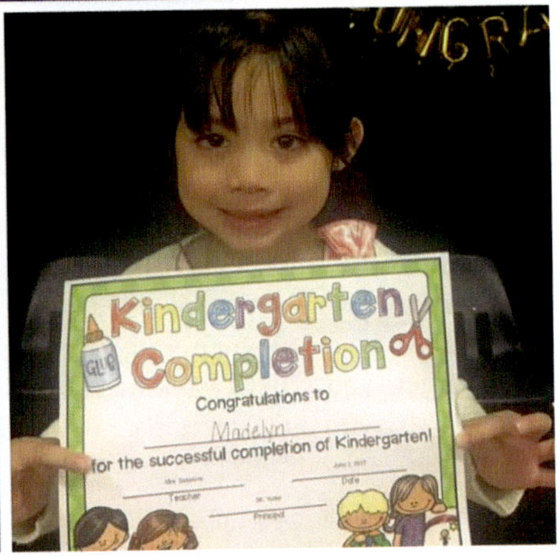

Robert

To my wife, Jodi, my Little Love and "Mo Chuisle" (my blood, my pulse), for supporting me with an unconditional love and for allowing me to pursue my professional and personal dreams. Any success in my life is because of you, and your belief in me has allowed me to overcome any obstacle in life. We make a pretty awesome team, in life and love (25th year anniversary in May 2025), as parents, as colleagues at the Penn State Children's Hospital, and as co-editors on *Clinical Considerations in School-Based Health.* Here's to another 25 years LL, much love and appreciation.

To my parents (Manuel and Delia), my grandparents (Manuel, Avelina, Teofilo, Gliceria), Coco, my sisters (Patricia, Catherine, Nicole, Lauren), my brothers (Rob, Mark, Matthew, Andy), Grant, Isabel, Gracie, Sienna, Drew, Moriah, Quinn, and Theo, Bob and Nancy Brady, and extended family from all over the world. Thank you for your unwavering love and support, and for being amazing role models. I hope that I have made you proud!

To teachers and mentors who have made the most impact in my life and career: Jeannette Otley (Ursuline Academy), Lex Meginniss (Saint Edmond's Academy), Louis LoBosco (Archmere Academy), Jodi Mindell (Saint Joseph's University), Dr. Magdy Attia (Jefferson Medical College), Dr. Steven Selbst (DuPont Hospital for Children), and Drs. Waseem Hafeez and Jeff Avner (Children's Hospital at Montefiore). Thank you for cultivating my love of life-long learning, helping me to find my passions in life, teaching me that education extends beyond the classroom, and emphasizing the need to "pay it forward" and educate and mentor our future.

To Lady, who always greets me with a lick on the cheek, no matter what time I come home and whatever my mood is.

All our dreams can come true, if we have the courage to pursue them. —Walt Disney

Jodi

To my husband, Bob, thank you for allowing me to pursue my dreams and encouraging me to do things beyond my comfort zone. Thank you for your love and support and for all that you do for me and our family. Thank you for being an example of what it means to be an excellent doctor, teacher, mentor, and partner in life. You have taught me so much as we continue to grow in our relationship together. You inspire me to work harder and not give up.

To my parents (Bob and Nancy) for always believing in me and encouraging me to dream big and supporting me with your love and your time. To my sister and brother and their families, Nicole and Andy, Sienna, Drew and Moriah and Matthew and Lauren, Quinn and Theo for always being there for me and encouraging me throughout my life. To my extended family, Lolo and Lola and Coco, Teena, Rob, Isabel and Grace, Patsy, Mark and Grant, thank you for welcoming me into your family. My life is blessed by all your love and support.

To my mentors, colleagues, residents, and students who have contributed to this book with their time, encouragement, and knowledge. I have learned so much from you all and appreciate all you do.

Contents

Part V Managing a Student with Mental and Behavioral Health Disorders

Contributors

Elizabeth M. Alderman The Children's Hospital at Montefiore, Bronx, NY, USA

Ermal Aliu Penn State Children's Hospital, Hershey, PA, USA

Natalie Allen, MD Penn State Health Milton S Hershey Medical Center, Hershey, PA, USA

Joseph Andrie Penn State Milton S. Hershey Medical Center, Hershey, PA, USA

Elizabeth W. Barnhardt, DO, MAEd Assistant Professor of Pediatrics, Division of Developmental and Behavioral Pediatrics, Nationwide Children's Hospital/ The Ohio State University, Columbus, OH, USA

Amy Barnhorst University of California Davis, Bullet Points Project, Davis, CA, USA

Sophie Baron Penn State Children's Hospital, Hershey, PA, USA

Joshua Belfer Perelman School of Medicine, University of Pennsylvania, Philadelphia, PA, USA

Ellen M. Benitah Bulbarelli Jefferson Einstein Philadelphia Hospital, Philadelphia, PA, USA

Einstein Healthcare Network, Philadelphia, PA, USA

Apurva Bhatt Stanford University, Stanford, CA, USA

Bridgett Bilenski, MSN, RN, NCSN North Allegheny School District, Pittsburgh, PA, USA

Greta L. S. Bires Einstein Healthcare Network, Philadelphia, PA, USA

Jeffrey Birnbaum Children's Hospital Los Angeles, Los Angeles, CA, USA

Ramnarine Boodoo Penn State Hershey Medical Center, Hershey, PA, USA

Alana Hughes Boone Children's National Hospital, Richmond, VA, USA

Jodi Brady-Olympia Department of Pediatrics Penn State, College of Medicine Attending Physician, Division of Adolescent Medicine, Department of Pediatrics, Penn State Children's Hospital, Hershey, PA, USA

Makenna Brezitski Penn State Milton S. Hershey Medical Center, Hershey, PA, USA

William Bruno Penn State Health Hershey Medical Center, Hershey, PA, USA

Kimberly Burbank, MD Wake Forest University School of Medicine, Winston-Salem, NC, USA

Jessica F. Butts Penn State Hershey Medical Center, Hershey, PA, USA

Debra Byler Penn State Children's Hospital, Hershey, PA, USA

Jeffrey Campbell Boston Medical Center, Boston, MA, USA

Alissa Cerny, MD All Star Pediatrics, Exton, PA, USA

Keanna Chang, MD Maria Fareri Children's Hospital at Westchester Medical Center, Valhalla, NY, USA

Paige Chardavoyne Medical College of Wisconsin, Milwaukee, WI, USA

Nungshitombi Chongtham Penn State Hershey Medical Center, Hershey, PA, USA

Avani Chopra Penn State College of Medicine, Hershey, PA, USA

Douglas Comeau Boston College, Chestnut Hill, MA, USA

Catherine Considine, BSN, RN, CPHON Dana-Farber Cancer Institute, Boston, MA, USA

Mina Cunningham, MD St. Louis University Southwest IL Family Medicine, O'Fallon, IL, USA

Matthew Demarest Los Angeles General Medical Center, Los Angeles, CA, USA

Matthew Donahue Nebraska Department of Health and Human Services, Lincoln, NE, USA

Amy A. Dooley Penn State Children's Hospital, Hershey, PA, USA

Katharine Doughty, APN Nationwide Children's Hospital, Columbus, OH, USA

Diana Dur Great Valley School District, Malvern, PA, USA

Ashley Ebersole, MD, MS Nationwide Children's Hospital, Columbus, OH, USA

Zhanna Elberg University at Buffalo Jacobs School of Medicine and Biomedical Sciences, Buffalo, NY, USA

Adesuwa Emovon Pennsylvania State University College of Medicine, Hershey, PA, USA

Lindsay Ercole UPMC Children's Hospital of Pittsburgh, Pittsburgh, PA, USA

Jennifer M. Dunnick Division of Pediatric Emergency Medicine, Duke University Hospital, Durham, NC, USA

Joseph A. Gehrz Naval Medical Center San Diego, San Diego, CA, USA

S. Rosie Gellman Psych for Tykes and Teens, LLC, Louisville, CO, USA

Sarah Ghattas Nemours Children's Health, Jacksonville, FL, USA

Joshua Glasser Penn State Hershey Medical Center, Hershey, PA, USA

Melinda Graybill-Barrett Commonwealth University of Pennsylvania, Bloomsburg, PA, USA

Estelle Anh-Thu Green Boston Children's Hospital, Boston, MA, USA

Aliza Grossberg, MD, MPH New York University Grossman School of Medicine, New York, NY, USA

Neha Gupta, MD George Washington University Hospital, Washington, DC, USA

Rochelle Haas Nemours Children's Health, Delaware Campus, Wilmington, DE, USA

Timothy Hahn Penn State Hershey Medical Center, Hershey, PA, USA

Paul Haidet, MD, MPH The Pennsylvania State University College of Medicine, Hershey, PA, USA

Laurie Seidel Halmo University of Colorado School of Medicine, Aurora, CO, USA

Selena Hariharan University of Cincinnati College of Medicine, Cincinnati, OH, USA

Josiah Harmes Penn State Health Children's Hospital, Hershey, PA, USA

Stephanie Harvison Penn State Hershey Medical Center, Hershey, PA, USA

Christopher Collin Hayes Penn State Children's Hospital, Hershey, PA, USA

Isabel Hendrickson Johns Hopkins All Children's Hospital, St. Petersburg, FL, USA

Christina Hermann Penn State College of Medicine, Hershey, PA, USA

Sixtine Valdelièvre Herold Boston Children's Hospital, Boston, MA, USA

Ryunosuke Hisatomi LSU Health Science Center Shreveport, Shreveport, LA, USA

Katherine Hole Johns Hopkins All Children's Hospital, St. Petersburg, FL, USA

Catherine M. Huber, MD Nationwide Children's Hospital, Columbus, OH, USA

Lina Huerta-Saenz, Dr. Division of Pediatric Endocrinology and Diabetes, Penn State Health Children's Hospital, Penn State College of Medicine, Hershey, PA, USA

Kathryn Italia, MD Downingtown, PA, USA

Khalida Itriyeva Cohen Children's Medical Center, Zucker School of Medicine at Hofstra/Northwell, Hempstead, NY, USA

Sneha Jadhav Johns Hopkins School of Medicine, Baltimore, MD, USA

Banku Jairath Penn State Health Milton S. Hershey Medical Center, Hershey, PA, USA

Janice Joseph Lehigh Valley Reilly Children's Hospital, Allentown, PA, USA

Ashley Kane Penn State Health Milton S. Hershey Medical Center, Hershey, PA, USA

Ashlyn Katz The Brooklyn Hospital Center, Brooklyn, NY, USA

Leah Kaye Penn State College of Medicine, Hershey, PA, USA

Jack Keeley Wake Forest Baptist Medical Center, Winston-Salem, NC, USA

Deborah Kees-Folts Penn State Hershey Medical School, Hershey, PA, USA

Lori Kelley, MSN, RN, NCSN North Allegheny School District, Pittsburgh, PA, USA

Tara Kelly Penn State Hershey Medical Center, Hershey, PA, USA

Anum Khan UW Health Swedish American Hospital, Rockford, IL, USA

Masrur Khan NYU Langone Health, New York, NY, USA

Christina Kim Boston College, Chestnut Hill, MA, USA

Robin Kingston Penn State Children's Hospital, Hershey, PA, USA

Fiana Klein North Shore Child and Family Guidance Center, Plainview, NY, USA

Brianna Koehnke The Milton S. Hershey Medical Center, Hershey, PA, USA

Andrew Kung Penn State Hershey Medical Center, Hershey, PA, USA

Jasmin Gange Lagman Penn State Hershey Medical Center, Hershey, PA, USA

Bradley Lauck University of North Carolina School of Medicine, Chapel Hill, NC, USA

Caroline Hayley Lee Penn State College of Medicine, Hershey, PA, USA

Timothy Lequang Penn State College of Medicine, Hershey, PA, USA

Thejasvi N. Lingamchetty Penn State Hershey Medical Center, Hershey, PA, USA

Patrick Lin Lehigh Valley Reilly Children's Hospital, Allentown, PA, USA

Laura Lintner Wake Forest Baptist Medical Center, Winston-Salem, NC, USA

Jeff Lubin Penn State Milton S. Hershey Medical Center, Hershey, PA, USA

Christy Lucas, MD Dana-Farber Cancer Institute/Boston Children's Cancer and Blood Disorders Center, Boston, MA, USA

Kristen Lutzkanin Penn State Children's Hospital, Hershey, PA, USA

Kelly M. Lynch Penn State Hershey Medical Center, Hershey, PA, USA

Gayatra Mainali Penn State Children's Hospital, Hershey, PA, USA

MaryAnn Mansour, MD, MPH NYU Grossman School of Medicine, New York, NY, USA

Manvita Mareboina Penn State Hershey Medical Center, Hershey, PA, USA

Danae Massengill Rocky Mountain Poison and Drug Safety, Denver Health and Hospital Authority, Denver, CO, USA

Kimberly Matthews Penn State Health Children's Hospital, Hershey, PA, USA

Richard E. Mattison Penn State Hershey Medical School, Hershey, PA, USA

Corey McBrayer Penn State Health Medical Center, Hershey, PA, USA

James M. McCluskey III The University of Nebraska Medical Center, Omaha, NE, USA

Hallie McGrew UPMC Children's Hospital of Pittsburgh, Pittsburgh, PA, USA

Lauren A. McNickle Penn State Hershey Medical Center, Department of Emergency Medicine, Division of Pediatric Emergency Medicine, Hershey, PA, USA

Sarah Meyers Boston Medical Center, Boston, MA, USA

Theodore Miller Penn State College of Medicine, Hershey, PA, USA

Lauren Misik Fellow, Developmental and Behavioral Pediatrics, Nationwide Children's Hospital, Columbus, OH, USA

Anisha Mittal, MD, M.Ed The Pennsylvania State University College of Medicine, Hershey, PA, USA

Pankhuri Mohan Penn State Hershey Medical School, Hershey, PA, USA

Pritish Mondal Penn State Hershey Medical Center, Hershey, PA, USA

Kiran Mullur Wake Forest University School of Medicine, Winston-Salem, NC, USA

Connor Murray Johns Hopkins All Children's Hospital, St. Petersburg, FL, USA

Beverly L. Nazarian UMass Memorial Children's Medical Center/UMass Chan Medical School, Worcester, MA, USA

Chris Nelson Wake Forest University School of Medicine, Winston-Salem, NC, USA

Thuy Ngo Johns Hopkins All Children's Hospital, St. Petersburg, FL, USA

Lorie-Mae Nicolas Penn State Children's Hospital, Hershey, PA, USA

Dieudonne Nonga Nationwide Children's Hospital, Columbus, OH, USA

Ariel Tassy Nunez Northwell, New Hyde Park, NY, USA

Abigail Olympia Messiah University, Mechanicsburg, PA, USA

Madelyn Olympia Harrisburg Christian School, Harrisburg, PA, USA

Robert P. Olympia Department of Emergency Medicine and Pediatrics, Penn State College of Medicine Attending Physician, Hershey, PA, USA

Division of Pediatric Emergency Medicine, Department of Emergency Medicine, Penn State Milton S. Hershey Medical Center, Hershey, PA, USA

Michael Osterholt University of Nebraska Medical Center, Omaha, NE, USA

Laura Owens Nemours Children's Health, Wilmington, DE, USA

Vlad Panaitescu University of Florida-Jacksonville, Jacksonville, FL, USA

John Park, MD Maria Fareri Children's Hospital at Westchester Medical Center, Valhalla, NY, USA

Rohan Patel, MD Assistant Professor of Pediatrics, Division of General Pediatrics and Adolescent Medicine, Unviersity of North Carolina at Chapel Hill, Chapel Hill, NC, USA

Meenal Pathak Penn State Health, Hershey, PA, USA

Sita Paudel Penn State Children's Hospital, Hershey, PA, USA

Elena Petkovska University of Cincinnati College of Medicine, Cincinnati, OH, USA

Julia E. Potter Mass General for Children/Harvard Medical School, Boston, MA, USA

Natasha Ramsey Montefiore Medical Group, Bronx, NY, USA

Sundeep Singh Randhawa, MD Assistant Professor of Child & Adolescent Psychiatry, RUSH University Medical Center, Chicago, IL, USA

Nikhil Rao Oregon Health and Sciences University, Portland, OR, USA

Carla Reale Jefferson Einstein Philadelphia Hospital, Philadelphia, PA, USA

Leighton Reed Johns Hopkins All Children's Hospital, St. Petersburg, FL, USA

Paige Reese Penn State Hershey Medical Center, Hershey, PA, USA

Kristen Reilly, MD, MSW Division of Adolescent and Transition Medicine, Cincinnati Children's Hospital Medical Center, Cincinnati, OH, USA

Andrea Riley Children's Nebraska, Omaha, NE, USA

Timothy P. Roach Penn State Milton S. Hershey Medical Center, Hershey, PA, USA

Nicholas A. Roberts Naval Medical Center San Diego, San Diego, CA, USA

Rosemary Claire Roden Penn State Children's Hospital, Hershey, PA, USA

Natalie Ronshaugen Children's Nebraska, Omaha, NE, USA

Angela Ropka Penn State Hershey Medical Center, Hershey, PA, USA

Emily Rose Los Angeles General Medical Center, Los Angeles, CA, USA
Keck School of Medicine of USC, Los Angeles, CA, USA

Rachel Rothstein Children's Hospital of Philadelphia, Philadelphia, PA, USA

Sheryl Ryan Penn State Health Medical Center, Hershey, PA, USA

Raul E. Sanchez Division of Gastroenterology, Hepatology, and Nutrition, Nationwide Children's Hospital, Columbus, OH, USA

Stephen Sandelich Penn State Hershey Medical Center, Hershey, PA, USA

Jessica Santucci Penn State College of Medicine, Hershey, PA, USA

Nandini Sarkar Penn State College of Medicine, Hershey, PA, USA

Alice I. Sato The University of Nebraska Medical Center, Omaha, NE, USA

Marc E. Schaefer Penn State Health Children's Hospital, Hershey, PA, USA

Sandra Schumacher Boston Children's Hospital, Boston, MA, USA

Marie E. Schwalbe Penn State Hershey Medical Center, Hershey, PA, USA

Kari N. Schweiger Penn State Hershey Medical Center, Hershey, PA, USA

Joseph Schwob, DO Maria Fareri Children's Hospital at Westchester Medical Center, Valhalla, NY, USA

Kara K. Seaton Children's Minnesota, Minneapolis, MN, USA

Peter H. Seidenberg LSU Health Shreveport School of Medicine, Shreveport, LA, USA

Natalie Seminario, MD Bright Futures Psychiatry for Kids and Teens, LLC, Jupiter, Florida, USA

Maya Sevrin Moorestown Friends School, Moorestown, NJ, USA

Caroline Shank Cohen Children's Medical Center, Hempstead, NY, USA

Eileen Shieh Nemours Children's Health, Jacksonville, FL, USA

Jennifer Kosoy Shook Penn State Children's Hospital, Hershey, PA, USA

Matthew Silvis Penn State Health, Hershey, PA, USA

Gayle M. Smink Penn State Hershey Medical Center, Hershey, PA, USA

Neil Sparks Wake Forest University School of Medicine, Winston-Salem, NC, USA

Alexis Steefel Penn State Hershey Medical Center, Hershey, PA, USA

Ashley K. Sturts Penn State Hershey Medical Center, Hershey, PA, USA

Marlliny Sullivan SUNY Upstate Medical University, Syracuse, NY, USA

Adam Michael Sunday The Milton S. Hershey Medical Center, Hershey, PA, USA

Jeremy Swisher, MD Wake Forest University School of Medicine, Winston-Salem, NC, USA

Jill Sylvester University of North Carolina School of Medicine, Chapel Hill, NC, USA

Ee Tein Tay NYU Langone Health, New York, NY, USA

Khoon-Yen Tay Children's Hospital of Philadelphia, Philadelphia, PA, USA

Rebecca V. Taylor, MD, MA Duke University School of Medicine, Durham, NC, USA

Jaclyn Tencer Penn State Children's Hospital, Hershey, PA, USA

Robert T. Tisherman Duke University Hospital, Durham, NC, USA

Kanani E. Titchen University of California San Diego, San Diego, CA, USA

Rady Children's Health, San Diego, CA, USA

Robert D. Tunks Penn State Children's Hospital, Hershey, PA, USA

Kyle Tuohy, MD, MS Department of Neurosurgery, Penn State Hershey Medical Center, Hershey, PA, USA

Matthew Turner Penn State Milton S. Hershey Medical Center, Hershey, PA, USA

Ulrick Vieux Hackensack University Medical Center, Hackensack, NJ, USA

Olivia Waldron Penn State College of Medicine, Hershey, PA, USA

Matthew Waldrop Wake Forest University School of Medicine, Winston-Salem, NC, USA

Charles Webb LSU Health Science Center Shreveport, Shreveport, LA, USA

Rebecca Wilding Nemours Children's Health, Wilmington, DE, USA

Andrew Wilkinson LSU Health Shreveport School of Medicine, Shreveport, LA, USA

Andrew Yeich Penn State College of Medicine, Hershey, PA, USA

Lydia Younger Penn State Children's Hospital, Hershey, PA, USA

Elizabeth Zorovich University of Florida-Jacksonville, Jacksonville, FL, USA

Part I
General Concepts in School-Based Health

Chapter 1
History of School-Based Health and School-Based Health Clinics

Matthew Turner

90% of US children attend publicly funded schools, making them a valuable place to provide healthcare [1]. School-based health clinics (SBHCs)—consisting of a health care facility located on-site, staffed by trained healthcare providers, and able to provide primary and preventative care [2]—have been shown to improve both the educational and health outcomes of students [3]. More than 70% of students in schools with SBHCs are either racial or ethnic minorities, making SBHCs an important part of addressing health disparities within these populations [2]. With the significant expansion of SBHCs in recent decades, they have become an essential component of providing healthcare to the general population [2]. To appreciate the utility of SBHCs, it is important to review the history that led to their development.

The early days of school-based health were largely focused on preventing the spread of infectious diseases. Healthcare largely consisted of routine inspections, often done by teams of physicians hired to inspect children for an hour a day [4]. Guidelines such as the "rule of exclusion" mandated by the New York City Board of Health simply sent sick students home without any treatment during which these students often played with other children, further spreading the disease [2]. As a result, student absenteeism rates were often shockingly high [2]. Follow-up was typically limited to written recommendations, an ineffective means of communication due to the era's high rates of illiteracy and poverty [4]. The New York City Board of Education reported that that this program did nothing to reduce the spread of disease [4].

The standard of care began to gradually change with the end of the nineteenth century and the dawn of the twentieth. In 1891, Dr. Malcom Morris recommended that nurses perform inspections of English elementary schools rather than physicians—within 6 years the London School Nurses Society began to regularly visit

M. Turner (✉)
Penn State Milton S. Hershey Medical Center, Hershey, PA, USA
e-mail: mturner7@pennstatehealth.psu.edu

R. P. Olympia, J. Brady-Olympia (eds.), *Clinical Considerations in School-based Health*, https://doi.org/10.1007/978-3-031-85765-2_1

impoverished schools in the city [4]. Several years later, the NYC Board of Health approached Lillian Wald for any recommendations [4]. Wald was already a famous figure within American nursing and the wider Progressive movement, known to city officials as "That Damned Nurse Troublemaker" for her popular campaigns advocating for public health [5]. Wald proposed that a fellow nurse named Lina Rogers work for a single month as a school nurse—if the Board were satisfied with Rogers' results, they would pay for her salary and supplies [4]. The Board agreed to these terms, and in October 1902 Rogers began to visit children in 4 New York City schools. Instead of relying on often-misunderstood written communication, she went into the community to instruct family members face-to-face on appropriate care and follow-up [4]. She also practiced educational activities regarding dental, hearing, and vision screenings [4]. By the end of the month, her results were so significant that the Board hired her as the "first municipally sponsored school nurse" [4]. Within 1 year, Rogers and 12 other school nurses reduced New York City's absenteeism rate by nearly 90% [2]. Rogers moved back to Canada in 1913, where she developed another successful school nursing program [4] (Fig. 1.1).

For the next several decades, school nurses followed Rogers' example and were employed by municipal health departments [7]. Although Rogers did introduce some educational aspects to school-based health [4], the focus remained on the

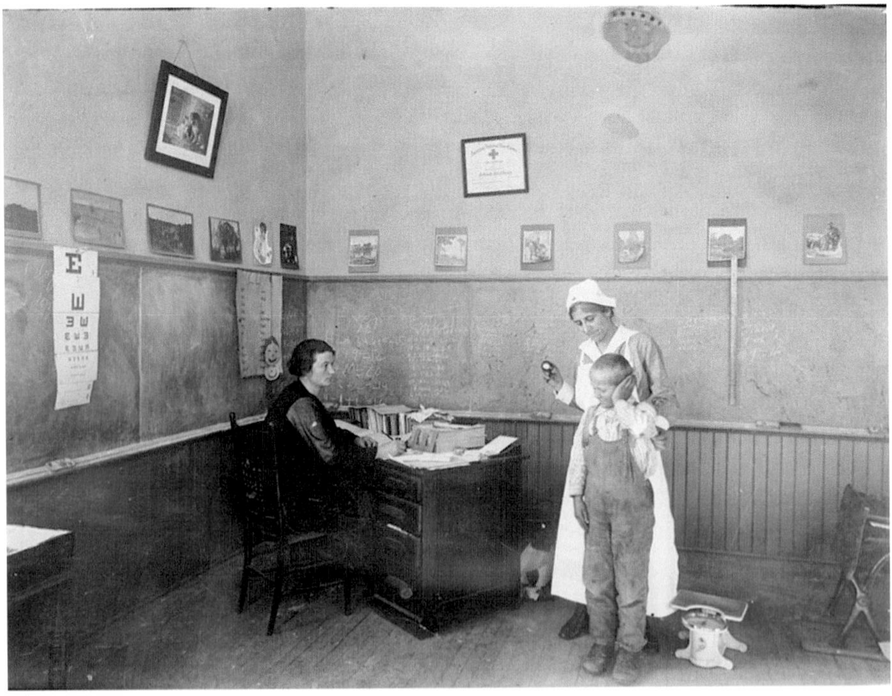

Fig. 1.1 A photograph of school-based nursing screening in the early twentieth century. In this image, a nurse screens a young boy's hearing by having him listen to the ticking of a watch [6]

largest threat to public health at the time: prevention and treatment of infectious disease [7]. However, as the threat from infectious diseases waned, by the 1950s, school-based healthcare began to transition toward a greater emphasis on screening and education, both for students and for faculty [7].

As the 1960s dawned, the United States experienced a significant shortage of pediatricians and other primary health care providers [2], due to an explosion in available specialty residencies due to the GI Bill following World War II [8] an increased demand for healthcare resources following significant advances in medical technology [9], and the 1965 Medicare Act [10]. The "doctor shortage" was a source of great public anxiety [9]. In response, Nursing Professor Loretta C. Ford and Dr. Henry K. Silver, a pediatrician, founded the first Nurse Practitioner (NP) program at the University of Colorado in 1965 [10]. NP programs quickly spread across the country, and in 1973, the National Association of Pediatric Nurse Practitioners was founded [10]. The first physician assistant (PA) program, largely made up of former combat medics from the Vietnam War, was initiated at Duke University during this timeframe as well [11].

Pediatric nurse practitioners (PNP), along with PAs, quickly became an integral aspect of school-based healthcare and remain the majority of providers to this day [2]. As these professions spread, so too did the idea of the SBHC. Dr. Phillip J. Porter began to open "neighborhood health centers" in Cambridge, Massachusetts, staffed primarily by PNPs, while similar programs opened in Dallas and St. Paul [2]. The need for SBHCs to focus on adolescent health became more visible in as the post-war baby boom exploded the 15–24 year age group throughout the 1960s and 1970s [12]. Given this, the St. Paul SBHC was largely focused on family planning and teenage pregnancy prevention and support. The clinic claimed to reduce pregnancy rates by 40% in the school's student body [13], generating headlines across the nation and helping to trigger a pivot toward reproductive healthcare for adolescents [2]. The 1975 Education for All Handicapped Children Act (EHA) acted as a further incentive as a federal requirement that disabled children have services available at school [7].

Teenage pregnancy would remain a priority for SBHCs for years afterwards. In 1985, the Center for Population Options—an organization focused on reducing adolescent pregnancy—reported that there were 31 SBHCs. 3 years later, a repeat census found that there were 120 SBHCs, primarily in high schools [13]. Despite some initial controversy regarding this early focus on reproductive health and parental rights, SBHCs continued to rapidly spread [14]. A great deal of this growth was due to a number of national foundations, including the National Healthy Children Program and the School-Based Adolescent Health Care Program [2].

A shift to comprehensive medical care in SBHCs grew throughout the 1980s, with a number developing expanded mental health programs [12]. The pace of SBHC expansion accelerated in the 1990s, due to an increasing number of private investments by organizations such as the Robert Wood Johnson Foundation and the W.K. Kellogg Foundation [2]. A number of state governments began to fund the creation of new SBHCs as well, with further support from the Federal Medicaid and State Children's Health Insurance Programs (SCHIP) [2]. In 1990, the US government amended the EHA into the Individuals with Disabilities Education Act (IDEA), a more thorough piece of legislation that corrected for many of the loopholes and limited eligibility of the earlier EHA legislation. Under IDEA, children with disabilities were required to go to school, with school systems required to provide individualized care and individualized health plans, thus further incentivizing SBHC development [7]. By 1998, the number of SBHCs had swollen to 1135, with more representation in middle and elementary schools and funding from 38 state governments [13].

In the first two decades of the 2000s, federal expansion of the primary care safety net through programs such as the Affordable Care Act (ACA) significantly increased the number of SBHCs available [13]. Guidelines such as the Healthy People 2020 Objectives, released by the US Department of Health and Human Services in 2010, have further emphasized school-based healthcare [7]. Although the number of states directly funding SBHCs has decreased, state funding has increased from $61.9 million in 1998–1999 to over $90 million in 2016–2017 [13]. Advocacy organizations such as the School-Based Health Alliance have also played a significant role in the proliferation of SBHCs across the nation [13]; other organizations that support SBHCs include the American Academy of Pediatrics and the Centers for Disease Control and Prevention (CDC) [14]. The pace of expansion has continued; from 2011 to 2019, the number of SBHCs increased by 20% to well over 2000 [14].

In the current day, the complex history of SBHCs is best reflected in their multiple streams of funding, including private sources, state and federal governments, schools, and partner organizations [14]. Their importance in the US healthcare system has grown with each passing decade [2], and their effectiveness in improving both health and educational outcomes has been proven [3]. Providers in SBHCs should be aware of this impressive history, and appreciate the decades of progress it has taken to reach this point.

Extra Credit Points

1. SBHCs have a long history that stretches back to the Progressive Era.
2. SBHCs have evolved into their current form over many decades.
3. Due to their history, SBHCs often have multiple sources of funding.
4. SBHCs have been steadily growing in number for over 40 years.

References

1. Richardson JW, Juszczak LJ. Schools as sites for health-care delivery. Public Health Rep. 2008;123(6):692–4.
2. Keeton V, Soleimanpour S, Brindis CD. School-based health centers in an era of health care reform: building on history. Curr Probl Pediatr Adolesc Health Care. 2012;42(6):132–56.
3. Knopf JA, Finnie RK, Peng Y, Hahn RA, Truman BI, Vernon-Smiley M, Johnson VC, Johnson RL, Fielding JE, Muntaner C, Hunt PC. School-based health centers to advance health equity: a community guide systematic review. Am J Prev Med. 2016;51(1):114–26.
4. Schumacher C. Lina Rogers: a pioneer in school nursing. J Sch Nurs. 2002;18(5):247–9.
5. Clare C, Lillian D. Wald: progressive activist. New York: The City University of New York; 1989.

6. *The small boy's hearing is proven fit when he hears the tick of the Red Cross Nurse's watch. School Nursing*. 5 x 7 in glass negative. Photograph given to the Library of Congress by the American National Red Cross on 9 December 1919. Image obtained from the American Library of Congress at https://www.loc.gov/pictures/item/2017670751/. The American National Red Cross Collection includes negatives and prints made by the staff of the organization, as well as materials collected by them, dating ca. 1880s-1950. The American National Red Cross gave the collection to the Library of Congress in 1944, placing no restrictions on their use, as documented at https://www.loc.gov/rr/print/res/717_anrc.html.
7. Conelius J. Overview of school-based health and primary care settings. In: Mager DR, Conelius J, editors. Population health for nurses: improving community outcomes. New York: Springer; 2021.
8. Dalen JE, Ryan KJ, Alpert JS. Where have the generalists gone? They became specialists, then subspecialists. Am J Med. 2017;130(7):766–8.
9. Wright D, Flis N, Gupta M. The 'Brain Drain' of physicians: historical antecedents to an ethical debate, c. 1960–79. Philos Ethics Humanit Med. 2008;3:24.
10. Brennan C. Tracing the history of the nurse practitioner profession in 2020, the year of the nurse. J Pediatr Health Care. 2020;34(2):83–4.
11. Holt N. "Confusion's masterpiece": the development of the physician assistant profession. Bull Hist Med. 1998;72(2):246–78.
12. Flaherty LT, Weist MD, Warner BS. School-based mental health services in the United States: history, current models and needs. Community Ment Health J. 1996;32(1):341–52.
13. Love HE, Schlitt J, Soleimanpour S, Panchal N, Behr C. Twenty years of school-based health care growth and expansion. Health Aff. 2019;38(5):755–64.
14. Arenson M, Hudson PJ, Lee N, Lai B. The evidence on school-based health centers: a review. Global Pediatr Health. 2019;6(1):2333794X19828745.

Chapter 2
The Role of School Physician

Beverly L. Nazarian and Julia E. Potter

2.1 Why Have a School Physician?

"Healthier children learn better; and, reciprocally, more educated adults lead healthier, more productive, wealthier, and longer lives" [1]. School physicians serve a key role in the network of health professionals who work with schools, charged with promoting the health of students. One key concept illustrating the importance of school health is that healthy students attend school more regularly. Students who are absent from school due to chronic physical and mental health conditions miss valuable instructional time and are less likely to graduate, which in turn impacts access to higher education and employment.

The concept of a physician working closely with a school system has a long, rich history [2]. Involvement of physicians in school health began over a century ago, initially prompted by the need to mitigate infectious disease outbreaks in schools and later to screen for physical conditions. Typically, the school physician role was filled by a general practitioner who had minimal pediatric training. The school physician role has evolved over time to be more consultative, supporting nursing leaders and school districts to address the primary, chronic health care, and social-emotional needs of students.

The shift from school physician as a public health role to that of an individual practitioner or consultant occurred during the early part of the twentieth century. Prior to World War I, school health was focused on medical inspection, hygiene, and

B. L. Nazarian
UMass Memorial Children's Medical Center/UMass Chan Medical School, Worcester, MA, USA
e-mail: beverly.nazarian@umassmemorial.org

J. E. Potter (✉)
Mass General for Children/Harvard Medical School, Boston, MA, USA
e-mail: jepotter@mgh.harvard.edu

R. P. Olympia, J. Brady-Olympia (eds.), *Clinical Considerations in School-based Health*, https://doi.org/10.1007/978-3-031-85765-2_2

health instruction. However, the war revealed problems related to poverty and poor health of US school children and helped to shift thinking about the goals of school health programs [3]. In addition, the American Academy of Pediatrics (AAP) was founded in 1930 and the AAP Committee on School Health was established soon after. This committee was tasked with determining the AAP's early policies related to school health. Such policies addressed health and illness management in school, the importance of child's education, and the role of the pediatrician in the school setting. Prior to involvement of the AAP in school health, pediatricians had little representation among the population of physicians serving schools, and there was little communication between physicians working in schools and pediatricians in the community [4].

Defining the current role of a school physician proves challenging, as there is a lack of consensus about what the role entails. For instance, there are no national policies or laws pertaining to school physicians. The 2013 AAP Policy Statement, "Role of the School Physician" (reaffirmed in 2019) seeks to shed light and provide guidance on the role of school physician [5]. In this statement, the AAP Council on School Health defines the role of a school physician broadly, as "*any physician who serves in any capacity for a school district, such as, but not limited to, an advisor, consultant, medical director, volunteer, team physician, medical inspector, or district physician*". In a 2016 policy statement, the AAP advocates "for a minimum of 1 full-time professional school nurse in every school with medical oversight from a school physician in every school district" [6]. The American Medical Association echoes this recommendation, recommending that health services in schools be supervised by a physician [7].

The role of the school physician has been described as having nine critical functions: administration and planning, liaison to community physicians, direct service, clinical consultation, policy consultation, health education, public relations, advocacy and systems development consultation [8]. Some examples within each of these functions are included below (Table 2.1).

2.2 Who Serves in the Role?

There are limited data on the presence and number of school physicians in individual states and districts. While some states (Massachusetts, Connecticut) have legislation requiring school physician oversight, many have no such requirement. Ideally, the school physician role is filled by a pediatrician or family medicine physician with expertise in children and adolescents. The school physician may be employed by the school, compensated as a consultant, or in some cases, serve in a volunteer capacity. Sometimes a physician from the local board of health may serve in this role.

Even if there is no formal school physician role in a district, partnerships between schools and community physicians are essential. The Whole School/Whole Community/Whole Child model promoted by the Centers for Disease Control

Table 2.1 Functions of the School Physician

Administration and planning
Meets regularly with health services leadership to determine health priorities for the school year
Liaison to community MDs
Communicates with local pediatricians about students with special health care needs or about services the overlap between the school and the medical home
Direct service
Conducts physicals or sports preparticipation exams
Clinical consultation
Serves as a resource to school nurses for case consultation, such as in the setting of a clinical need or infectious disease outbreak
Policy consultation
Participates in development or review of school health policies, i.e. infectious disease response, attendance, medication administration
Health education
Provides professional development to nurses, educates students and community members on health topics
Public relations
Communicates with community members/media on relevant health topics as needed
Advocacy and systems development consultation
Advocates for needed resources, works with policy makers at the local and state levels

emphasizes the connection between health and school achievement and the need for collaboration between schools and communities [9]. It broadens the concept of school health to include ten components: health services, nutrition, physical education/activity, health education, community involvement, family engagement, employee wellness, physical environment, social and emotional environment, and counseling/social services (Fig. 2.1). Each of these components have been shown to positively influence both student health and educational achievement [1, 10]. The model places the child/student at the center and emphasizes family engagement and connection to the community.

2.3 Day-to-Day Responsibilities

Most school physicians work primarily in collaboration with a school nurse and/or school nurse leader, meeting with them regularly, typically at least monthly. While the school nurse is the face of school health within the school building, the capacity of nurses to care for students in school is enhanced by collaboration with a physician.

The day-to-day role for the school physician may include some or all of the following:

- Review and sign standing orders for over-the-counter medications and for emergency medications available on an as-needed basis (i.e. albuterol, epinephrine).

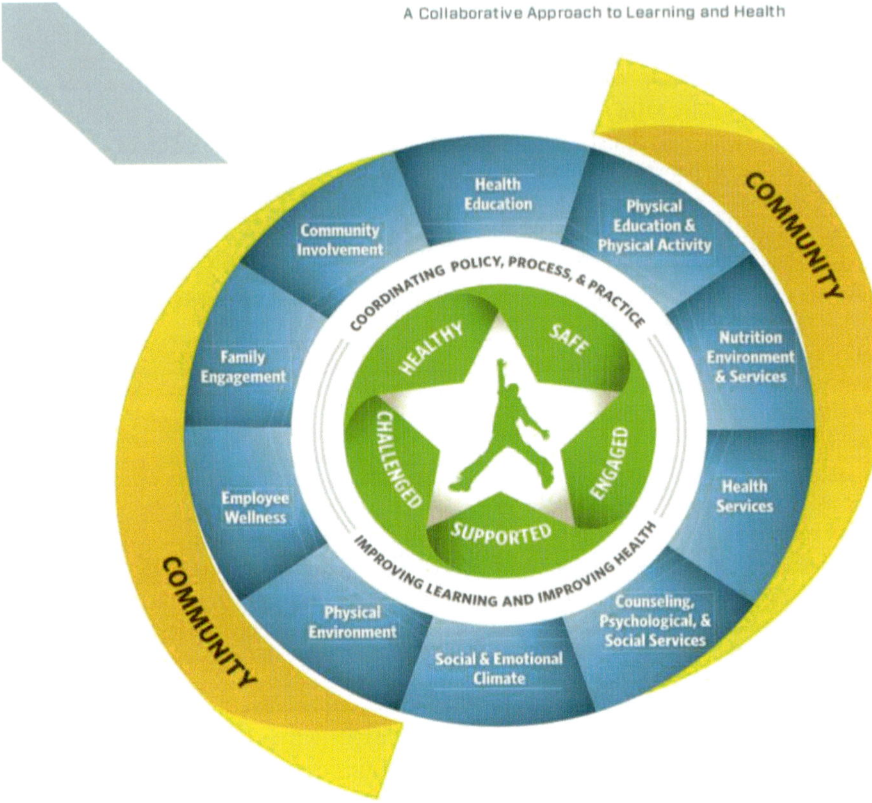

Fig. 2.1 The Whole School/Whole Community/Whole Child Model

- Review and provide input on processes and policies: e.g. absences, medication administration, emergency response, naloxone administration.
- Assist in management of infectious disease outbreaks, often in collaboration with public health entities (i.e. reviewing communication to families and identifying at risk students who have been exposed).
- Participate in school health advisory councils, which often include representation from nursing, other departments within the school, students, families and community partners.
- Liaison with local health care providers regarding the individual health and educational needs of students.
- Consult regarding children with special health care needs (i.e. reviewing the need for a 1:1 or shared nurse for tracheostomy care, gastrostomy feeding, or other skilled needs).
- Meet with school nurses in the district to hear their concerns, provide updates, and offer professional development.

- Advocate for school health staffing (need for nurse in every school) and other resources such as supplies (automated external defibrillators, naloxone, and bag-valve-mask) and school-based vaccine clinics.
- Connect learners (nursing and medical students/residents) with schools, both to volunteer and to expose them to the role of school nurses

School health needs are in constant flux. Below are case examples that illustrate the potential contribution of a school physician to school health and how the school physician can collaborate with school nurses.

Case 1 A 10 year-old student has come to the nursing office with wheezing 5 times in the last 2 weeks. He has an albuterol inhaler at school but does not have a spacer. The school nurse is concerned that his asthma is not well controlled. The school nurse reaches out to the student's pediatrician, but is unable to connect.

School physician role

It can be challenging for school nurses to reach community physicians by phone. The school physician often has relationships with local pediatricians and can serve as a liaison to pediatricians and other specialty providers about the need to provide medication orders/authorization for asthma inhalers to be used in school. The school physician can additionally:

- Educate primary care providers (PCPs) about the need for signed medication orders to allow nurses to administer albuterol in school.
- Suggest controller medications be provided/administered in schools for students with poor asthma control and when home administration is problematic.
- Suggest that PCPs prescribe an additional inhaler and spacer for school use.
- Provide asthma education for school nurses.
- Create a policy for a standing albuterol order to be delivered in school.
- Advocate to stock spacers in school nursing offices for teaching or for students lacking a spacer.
- Increase awareness of the impact of allergens on asthma and the importance of school ventilation.
- Promote flu vaccine clinics in the schools.

Case 2 Two siblings who attend the same elementary school present to a local emergency department with signs and symptoms of chickenpox. Further conversation with the family and the department of public health indicates that these are confirmed cases of chickenpox (varicella). Although the large, urban school district where the students attend school has a policy requiring documentation of mandatory childhood immunizations prior to school entry, there are other students residing at the same shelter and attending school who do not have documented varicella vaccination. The department of public health policy on varicella requires that unvaccinated students be vaccinated within 5 days of exposure or be excluded from school for days 8–21 post-exposure.

School physician role

Infectious disease outbreaks in schools require a coordinated response and clear communication with school leaders, parents, and community stakeholders. A school physician can serve a critical role in crafting a message and providing a voice of expertise, often in conjunction with a state or local department of public health. In addition, a school physician can:

- Help to coordinate vaccination for unvaccinated students at their medical home or local community health center, or to organize a school-based vaccine clinic.
- Communicate with worried parents and provide health information about the disease, including incubation period, symptoms, diagnosis, and treatment strategies.
- Work with school leaders to enact public health policies, such as response to infectious disease outbreaks, and school exclusion for lack of immunization.

Case 3 Twenty students present to the school nurse over the course of the week for itchy, red eyes. It is pollen season, and these symptoms are preventing students from being actively engaged in classroom learning, and there is little the nurses can offer to help. Teachers are worried that students have "pink eye" and are contagious. Pollen covers everything outside, but the classroom is too warm to keep the windows closed, as there is no air-conditioning in the building. There is a standing order available for diphenhydramine, but nurses express hesitancy providing oral medication that can make students drowsy.

School physician role

Over the counter medications can be a mainstay of in school acute symptom management, but they require a physician order for administration in school. Administration of medications such as acetaminophen, ibuprofen, diphenhydramine, or cetirizine can help keep kids in school in the event of acute discomfort due to a known, benign condition. A standing order signed by the school physician in addition to signed parent/guardian permission allows nurses to be able to administer medications in school. The school physician can:

- Create a new standing order for a non-sedating antihistamine (i.e. cetirizine).
- Deliver a professional development talk on management of allergic conjunctivitis.
- Advocate for provision of air conditioners in school to help prevent asthma and allergy exacerbation.
- Collaborate with area pediatricians to provide preventive care for allergic conjunctivitis, including providing medication orders for antihistamine eye drops when indicated.

Case 4 A 16 year-old student collapses on the floor of her school building, so the school nurse is called and rushes to the scene. The student is conscious but looks pale, drowsy and has slow, shallow breathing. Heart rate is normal, O_2 sat is normal, and BP is unable to be obtained. The nurse hears from a student's friends that they were vaping an unknown substance in the bathroom.

The nurse rushes to get the school's naloxone supply to have on hand. 911 is called and emergency responders arrive within 15 min.

School physician role

A key role of the school physician is helping to ensure that procedures are in place in the event of an in-school medical emergency, such as altered mental status or respiratory arrest. School nurses are often the only health professionals in the building and rely on protocols, training, and access to necessary equipment to be able to intervene prior to the arrival of emergency responders. School physicians also can:

- Advocate for and coordinate emergency response training through simulation, training in basic life support, and case practice.
- Help to standardize access to emergency equipment, such as oxygen saturation detectors and bag valve masks.
- Create a standing order and policy for the delivery of naloxone for suspected opioid overdose.
- Educate the local school community about the importance of automated external defibrillators in schools, availability of naloxone, and access to epinephrine in the event of anaphylaxis.

Extra Credit Points

1. School physicians can support community physicians by providing them with information about school requirements (immunizations, physicals, and other screenings) and partnering with them on the specific needs of students with chronic health conditions.
2. School physicians can educate community physicians about the rights of students with health conditions and disabilities.
3. School physicians may collaborate with schools on issues like chronic absenteeism that require a community approach and have a significant impact on school performance.
4. In districts without a school physician, school nurses are well-served to establish partnerships with community physicians in order to open lines of communication and to collaborate on the care of students with specific health care needs.

References

1. Kolbe LJ. School health as a strategy to improve both public health and education. Annu Rev Public Health. 2019;40:443–63.
2. Institute of Medicine (US). Committee on comprehensive school health programs in grades K-12. In: Allensworth D, Lawson E, Nicholson L, et al., editors. Schools and health: our Nation's investment. Washington, DC: National Academies Press (US); 1997.
3. Mitchell HH. School medical service in perspective. Pediatrics. 1965;35(6):1011–20.
4. School Health Services. Pediatrics. 1953;12(3S):16–8. http://publications.aap.org/pediatrics/article-pdf/12/3S/16/890277/16.pdf. Accessed 17 May 2024.

5. Council on School Health, DiLaura Devore C, Wheeler LSM, Allison M, Ancona R, Barnett S, et al. AAP 2013 policy statement (reaffirmed 2019): role of the school physician. Pediatrics. 2013;131(1):178–82.
6. COUNCIL ON SCHOOL HEALTH, Holmes BW, Sheetz A, Allison M, Ancona R, Attisha E, Beers N, et al. Role of the school nurse in providing health services. Pediatrics. 2016;137(6):e20160852.
7. American Medical Association. Policy statement H-60.991: providing medical services through school-based health programs. Chicago, IL: American Medical Association; 2012.
8. Template for Massachusetts: the role and responsibilities of the school physician. Accessed 17 May 2024.
9. Guest Editor: Hunt H. Special Supplement on Whole School, Whole Community, Whole Child. Center for Disease Prevention. J Sch Health. 2015;85(11):729–823.
10. Michael SL, Merlo CL, Basch CE, Wentzel KR, Wechsler H. Critical connections: health and academics. J Sch Health. 2015;85(11):740–58.

Chapter 3
Role of the School Nurse

Melinda Graybill-Barrett

School nurses seek to provide evidence-based, student-focused care through collaboration with the interprofessional school health services team. School nurses are a central figure in coordinating activities, policies, and programs that support student health, wellness, and a safe learning environment. The National Association of School Nurses (NASN) has developed a School Nursing Practice Framework™, hereafter referred to as the Framework™, that serves as a guide for the school nurse roles and responsibilities in the areas of care coordination, leadership, quality improvement, and community and public health [1]. Figure 3.1 illustrates how the school nurse incorporates School Nurse Scope and Standards of Practice and the four key areas mentioned earlier to provide a holistic approach to caring for the student, family, and school community. School nurse scope and standards of practice are embedded in and align with the Framework's™ key principles [2]. Although not an exhaustive list, school nurse competencies include assessment, diagnosis, planning, implementation, ethical considerations, advocacy, scholarly inquiry, and leadership. Beyond providing direct care, school nurses are capable and competent community health leaders and public policy change makers [3]. Members of the interprofessional team, both within the school and among community providers, can draw upon and collaborate with school nurses in the areas of care coordination, leadership, quality improvement, and community and public health (Table 3.1).

Social determinants of health (SDOH) are the non-medical factors that influence health and are the conditions where people work, grow, and live [4]. These include socioeconomic status, education, housing, food insecurity, man-made conflict, and access to health care. Additionally, the World Health Organization reports that SDOH can have greater impact on health than health care itself or lifestyle choices [4]. School nurses are well-positioned to assess and evaluate impact of SDOH on

M. Graybill-Barrett (✉)
Commonwealth University of Pennsylvania, Bloomsburg, PA, USA
e-mail: mbarrett@commonwealthu.edu

R. P. Olympia, J. Brady-Olympia (eds.), *Clinical Considerations in School-based Health*, https://doi.org/10.1007/978-3-031-85765-2_3

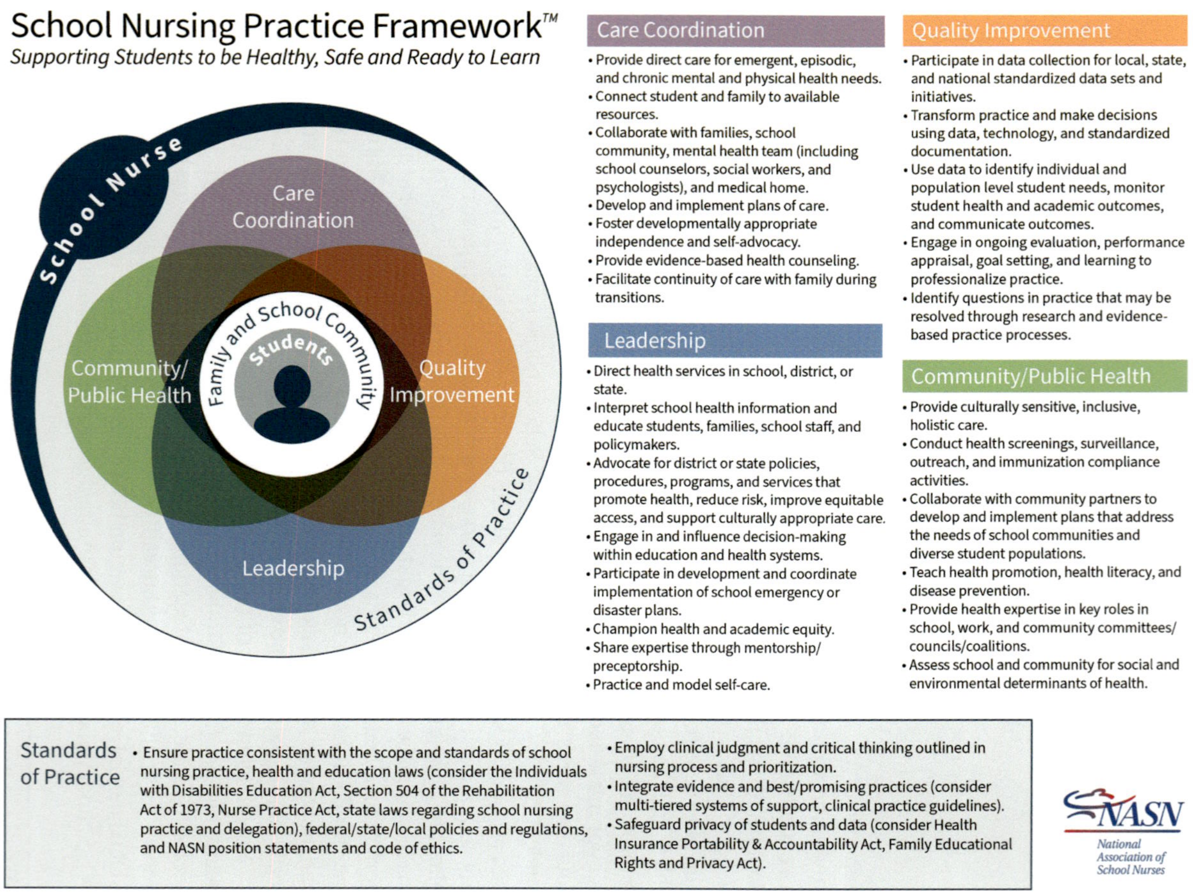

Fig. 3.1 School Nursing Practice Framework ™. (Re-printed with permission by the National Association of School Nurses)

Table 3.1 School Nursing Practice Framework™ roles and responsibilities

	Roles and responsibilities
Care coordination	– Direct care provider – Link to community resources – Create, implement, and evaluate individualized plans of care – Provide individuals, families, communities and members of the interprofessional team with evidence-based information needed to make informed decisions – Support self-advocacy skills
Leadership	– Interpret and share health information with students, families, administrators, and policymakers – Involvement in disaster prevention, planning, mitigation, and recovery – Advocacy for local, state, and federal policies that support health promotion, access to care, and equity for students and school nursing – Consider utilizing (I)SBAR (identify, situation, background, assessment, recommendation) approach when speaking with policymakers – Share expertise through mentorship
Quality improvement	– Utilize data, technology, and review of emerging evidence to drive practice decisions – Develop and take part in research projects to advance professional school nursing practice and health promotion – Integrate lifelong learning into professional practice goals – Practice routine self-reflection of strengths and areas to improve
Community and public health	– Incorporate levels of prevention: primary, secondary, and tertiary into practice – Collaborate and take part in community assessment of health needs and priorities of school-age and diverse populations – Assess social determinants of health, impact, and take part in developing solutions

the physical, mental, emotional, and social health of school-age populations in their care (Table 3.2). They can capitalize on strengths in areas of advocacy, leadership, and collaboration to take an upstream approach to addressing social factors which in turn, improve health outcomes and reduce inequities.

School nurse roles and responsibilities as outlined in the Framework™ encompass all levels of prevention. The overlapping domains of care coordination, leadership, quality improvement, and community and public health highlight primary, secondary, and tertiary levels of prevention that can be carried out at the individual (student), family, community, state, and federal levels (Table 3.3). As part of a community and public health approach to school nursing, emphasis is placed on taking an upstream approach that focuses on health promotion and prevention efforts.

The school nurse role of advocacy for local, state, and federal policies supports health promotion, access to care, and equity for students and the school nursing profession. Key facilitators to effective advocacy are understanding the process of policy creation and having an organized approach to communicating with decision-makers [5]. Consider utilizing (I)SBAR (identify, situation, background, assessment, recommendation) approach when speaking with policymakers [6] (Table 3.4).

Table 3.2 School nurse role in addressing social determinants of health: Case examples

Social determinants of health	Case examples
Early identification and intervention for health problems	**Case 1**: School nurses collaborate with local undergraduate and graduate nursing programs to have nursing students help with screenings early in the school year so referrals can be made expediently. Screenings may include: vision, hearing, dental, height, weight, scoliosis, blood pressure, physical exam. **Case 2**: A local health system is conducting a community assessment and seeks input from the school nurse about areas of need with school-age populations. As a result, the school district has access to the report that contains data on health and social needs of the community and a comprehensive listing of referral sources for housing, food, education, transportation, and free or reduced cost access to health care
Food insecurity	**Case 1**: After several elementary school age students report lacking food in their homes over weekends and holiday breaks, the school nurse collaborates with the Parent Teacher Organization (PTO) to start a back-pack program. Each Friday, students can pick up a back pack full of easy to prepare foods and fresh fruits. **Case 2**: Nurses in both rural and urban school districts join forces with teachers and local community businesses to start a community garden program. Students take part in planning, maintenance, and harvest of healthy foods. Education about healthy food, physical activity, and community service are integrated into the gardening program.
Access to health care	**Case 1**: The school nurse reaches out to the state Medicaid and Children's Health Insurance Program offices to obtain materials to send home with first day of school packets. The school social worker and guidance counselor support this effort by helping families complete applications for health insurance and other forms of assistance. **Case 2**: The school nurse joins other members of the state school nurse's association for their annual Day on the Hill where meetings with state level legislators are arranged. The nurses prepare succinct talking points and real-life examples of how to improve the health of school-age populations. They discuss policy to improve access to essential health services, support care of diverse populations, and advocate for lowering of the school nurse to student ratio.
Management of chronic illness and disability	**Case 1**: Families caring for students with chronic illnesses such as diabetes, asthma, ADD/ADHD, cystic fibrosis, muscular dystrophy, and spinal cord injuries face challenges with obtaining medical equipment such as wheelchairs, hospital beds, medications, respite care, and transportation. The impact of long-term chronic illness can take many forms: parental loss of work time, social isolation, and economic strain. The nurse supports families by openly communicating and creating relationships with health care providers to obtain necessary care and supplies, social services to ensure coordination of home and community-based care, and school staff to create individualized health plans. **Case 2**: The school nurse needs to be knowledgeable about state and federal policies that protect students with health conditions and disabilities. The nurse will advocate for an Individualized Education Program (IEP) or 504 Service Agreement to ensure that appropriate accommodations are in place for students with disabilities or serious health conditions.

Table 3.3 School nurse role in prevention

Primary prevention	Secondary prevention	Tertiary prevention
Health promotion and prevention education and programming: healthy eating, exercise, coping, hydration	Screenings: vision, hearing, height, weight, blood pressure, mental health	Care of acute and episodic illness and injury
Immunizations: stay current on state immunization requirements, educate parents, students, and the community about importance of immunizations in preventing serious illness, and refer to immunization clinics in the community	Collecting and monitoring data: facilitates early intervention, program, and policy development to prevent or address issues with housing, food, poverty, transportation, language barrier	Referral to treatment

Table 3.4 Use (I)SBAR to effectively and efficiently communicate with policy/change makers

(Identify)	– State who you are – Share your name, where you work or live, and who you represent
Situation	– Share a concise statement of the problem – What is going on now – Succinctly describe the issue you are addressing
Background	Pertinent and brief information related to the situation – What has happened – Put a human face on your request, tell a story
Assessment	– Analysis and consideration of options – What you found or think is going on – Contributing factors such as SDOH
Recommendation	– Recommend action – What do you want to happen or be done – Share a fact sheet that includes your contact information

Nurses are often familiar with this approach to sharing assessment information with colleagues and therefore may support confidence when speaking with policy and change makers.

Case Example: (I)SBAR Ava who has worked as a school nurse in both rural and urban school districts over the past decade has noted an increase in acuity of health problems among school-age populations, safety issues created when a school lacks a dedicated registered nurse on site, and challenges with recruitment and retention of school nurses. As a member of her state school nurse association, Ava, has scheduled an in person visit with her Congressional representative as part of their annual Day on the Hill. In preparing for the visit, Ava is utilizing an (I)SBAR approach to communicating her rationale behind asking for support of legislation that has recently been proposed to support placement of more licensed registered nurses in elementary and secondary schools.

(I) Hello Representative Jones. My name is Ava McGrath and I live and have worked as a school nurse in your congressional district for the past 10 years. I appreciate you taking the time to meet with me.

(S) Health and learning are connected and that's why I'm concerned about the fact that not all schools in our region have a licensed registered nurse in each building.

(B) Students are in school every day with serious health concerns including diabetes, asthma, and life-threatening allergies with the National Center for Education Statistics reporting that 14% of public school children have special health care needs [7]. Considering the critical role nurses play in managing these health conditions, it is very concerning that about 26% of schools in the United States go without any school nurse coverage [8]. For example, an elementary school-age student recently had a serious asthma attack and the school nurse was able to quickly assess the student and provide immediate treatment. Typically, there's not a nurse assigned to that building every day. The outcome might have been vastly and tragically different had the nurse not been there to act.

(A) Additionally, for many, the school nurse is often the sole health care provider for the growing number of children that are living in poverty and uninsured. Health care happens in schools and the school nurse is there to care for and manage acute and chronic illness and injury, carry out health screenings, and connect families to community resources.

(R) I'm asking for your support of House Bill 305 which authorizes grant programs to assist local educational agencies with ensuring that each elementary and secondary school has at least one registered nurse on staff. The bill goes even farther by supporting recruitment and hiring of school nurses. I appreciate you taking the time to speak with me and hope you will support this valuable legislation that seeks to eliminate health inequities while supporting the health and academic success of today's school-age populations. Here's my business card with contact information. I look forward to seeing progress on this important policy.

Extra Credit Points

School Nurses:

1. Assess and address social determinants of health by connecting to community resources, accessing health care, educating, and empowering families.
2. Provide specialized health services: diabetes management including insulin pumps, tube feedings, medication administration.
3. Drive health promotion and prevention efforts for students, families, and the community through policy development and implementation at the school, district, local, state, and national levels.
4. Are often the only health care professional interacting with students on a routine basis and therefore serve as a valuable source of assessment and referral information for primary care and emergent care providers.
5. Are community health leaders and policy changemakers at the school district, community, state, and federal levels.
6. Integrate all levels of prevention into the roles and responsibilities outlined in the School Nursing Practice Framework™ with a focus on primary health promotion and prevention.

References

1. National Association of School Nurses. School Nursing Practice Framework™. 2024. https://www.nasn.org/nasn-resources/framework.
2. National Association of School Nurses. School nursing: scope and standards of practice. 4th ed. Silver Spring, MD: NASN; 2022.
3. Rankine J, Goldberg L, Miller E, et al. School nurse perspectives on addressing chronic absenteeism. J Sch Nurs. 2023;39(6):296–505.
4. World Health Organization. Social determinants of health. 2024. https://www.who.int/health-topics/social-determinants-of-health#tab=tab_1.
5. Jurns C. Policy advocacy motivators and barriers: research results and applications. Online J Issues Nurs. 2019;24(3):1–13. https://doi.org/10.3912/OJIN.Vol24No03PPT63.
6. Jurns C. Using SBAR to communicate with policymakers. Online J Issues Nurs. 2019;24(1):1–7. https://doi.org/10.3912/OJIN.Vol24No01PPT47.
7. National Center for Education Statistics. Students with disabilities. Condition of Education. U.S. Department of Education, Institute of Education Sciences. 2022. https://nces.ed.gov/programs/coe/indicator/cgg/students-with-disabilities.
8. Willgerodt MA, Brock DM, Maughan EM. Public school nursing practice in the United States. J Sch Nurs. 2018;34(3):232–44.

Chapter 4
Emergency Preparedness

Robert P. Olympia

Case 1 You are a school nurse that covers several elementary, middle, and high schools in your district. You have been asked to review your school district's medical emergency response plan (MERP) after a student in a neighboring district died from a severe head injury sustained during gym class. It was determined that signs of severe head injury and increased intracranial pressure were not recognized by school staff immediately, that the student had an associated seizure lasting 20 min and interventions to support ABCDEs (airway/breathing/circulation/disability/exposure) were not instituted appropriately, and that there was a delay in contacting local Emergency Medical Services (EMS) due to a lack of a communication device in the bathroom where the seizure occurred. How should you approach the review of your school district's emergency response plan?

Since children spend a significant proportion of their day in school, pediatric emergencies, such as acute illness, the exacerbation of chronic medical conditions, mental health crisis, and accidental injuries, may occur. Studies have shown that the most common emergencies encountered by school nurses include extremity sprains/strains/fractures, shortness of breath, seizures, head/neck injuries, lacerations, mental health crisis, abdominal pain, syncope, and anaphylaxis [1].

National recommendations have been published to guide school leaders and their communities towards optimal emergency preparedness, and include general medical emergencies, as well as specific medical emergencies, such as anaphylaxis, asthma, cardiac arrest, head injuries, and seizures (Table 4.1). Test your school's

R. P. Olympia (✉)
Department of Emergency Medicine and Pediatrics, Penn State College of Medicine
Attending Physician, Hershey, PA, USA

Division of Pediatric Emergency Medicine, Department of Emergency Medicine, Penn State Milton S. Hershey Medical Center, Hershey, PA, USA
e-mail: rolympia@hmc.psu.edu

R. P. Olympia, J. Brady-Olympia (eds.), *Clinical Considerations in School-based Health*, https://doi.org/10.1007/978-3-031-85765-2_4

Table 4.1 National recommendations for school emergency preparedness

Medical or traumatic conditions	Recommendation resources
General medical emergencies—Medical emergency response plan (MERP)	American Academy of Pediatrics [2]
Anaphylaxis	American Academy of Pediatrics [3] National Association of School Nurses [4]
Asthma	American Academy of Pediatrics [2]
Sudden cardiac arrest—Cardiac emergency response plan (CERP)	American Academy of Pediatrics [2] American Heart Association [5] National Association of School Nurses [6]
Head injuries	American Academy of Pediatrics [2] National Association of School Nurses [7]
Seizures	American Academy of Pediatrics [2, 8]

Table 4.2 Checklist for general emergency preparedness

Emergency preparedness	Check YES or NO
My school has a written Medical Emergency Response plan (MERP)	
My MERP is practiced at least once a year	
My MERP has algorithms to distinguish minor injuries and illnesses from emergencies that require EMS activation	
My school has established relationships with local EMS to develop emergency response procedures	
My school has efficient communication network linking all parts of the school campus, including playgrounds and athletic fields (cellular phones, walkie-talkies, intercoms, public address systems, etc.)	
My school has a written MERP specific to children with special needs (cerebral palsy, epilepsy, tracheostomy tubes, gastric tubes, ventriculo-peritoneal shunts, etc.)	
Have you activated your MERP in the past year	
If you have activated your MERP in the past year, was quality improvement and assurance strategies implemented following the event	

current state of emergency preparedness by utilizing the checklist for general emergencies (Table 4.2) and cardiac, respiratory, and other medical emergencies (Table 4.3) as delineated by the American Academy of Pediatrics (AAP), National Association of School Nurses (NASN), and American Heart Association (AHA). An efficient and effective Medical emergency response plan (MERP), including those specific to cardiac and respiratory emergencies, would improve the

Table 4.3 Checklist for cardiac, respiratory, and other medical emergencies

Cardiac emergencies	Check YES or NO
My school has a MERP specific to cardiac emergencies (CERP)	
My CERP is practiced at least once a year	
My school has an AED strategically located on campus to deliver shock within 3 min of collapse	
EMS is integrated with my CERP	
I have utilized an AED during the previous year for a student	
I have utilized an AED during the previous year for an adult	
I have activated my CERP in the previous year	
If you have utilized your CERP in the past year, was quality improvement and assurance strategies implemented following the event	
Respiratory emergencies	
Does your school require students with life-threatening food/environmental allergies to carry a self-injectable epinephrine pen on their person	
Does your school have a self-injectable epinephrine device in your office should the student misplaces their device or requires an additional dose	
Does your school district and/or state allows you to have and administer an unassigned self-injectable device for general use in students who does not have a previously diagnosed environmental or food allergy	
Have you administered a self-injectable epinephrine device to a student with an unknown food/environmental allergy for a severe allergic reaction in the past year	
Has your state has adopted a stock albuterol policy (school can administer a single inhaler containing albuterol to anyone, whether they have a diagnosis of asthma or allergies, who experiences respiratory distress)	
Have you administered albuterol to a student with respiratory distress but does not have a history of asthma or allergies in the past year	
Other medical emergencies	
Does your school have an emergency preparedness and response plan for students with opioid related overdose	
Does your school have accommodation and assimilation guidelines/protocols to assist students when returning to school after a concussion (allowing rest breaks during the day, allowing additional time for assignments, limiting computer time, wearing sunglasses, avoiding noisy areas, shortening the school day, etc.)	

assessment, triage, and management of ill and injured children and facilitate transfer of these children to an acute care facility by EMS.

The commitment of an entire community is required to improve the preparedness of schools to deal with life-threatening illness and injury:

1. School and community physicians should assist in the planning, development, training, implementation, and review of school emergency response plans; work with school staff, EMS personnel, law enforcement, social workers, and counselors to ensure optimal preparedness; assist school nurses with implementing IHP, ECP, IEP and 504 plans for students with chronic medical conditions (Chap.

37); train school staff in basic life support, first aid, automated external defibrillator (AED) use, and emergency medication administration; provide guidelines and recommendations on the contents of the emergency kit and supplies; oversee school emergency drills; work collaboratively with district's school health services and advocate for the health and wellbeing of students [2].
2. School nurses should lead the development of plans for responding to emergencies, act as liaisons between health care professionals and the community, spearhead educational initiatives for school staff and students, and provide efficient, effective, and evidence-based care to students with acute illness and injuries, and children with chronic medical conditions [9].
3. Lastly, emergency physicians and EMS should be involved in the development and organization of systems for the effective recognition, stabilization, and transport of life-threatening emergencies that occur in schools. In addition, they should identify strategies to manage, prevent, and overcome barriers associated with emergency preparedness, and advocate through local legislation for the implementation of school health emergency systems, for improvement in school nurse staffing ratios, for the immediate availability of emergency medications, supplies, and equipment in schools, and for school administration and staff training [10].

Case 2 An 8-year girl, Brynn, is found unresponsive and pulseless on the school playground. Classmates say that Brynn was standing on the top of the monkey bars, fell forward and her chest hit the slide below. There is no school nurse or physician on campus. A school aide who is nearby is not trained in basic life support (BLS) or cardiopulmonary resuscitation (CPR), nor does she know how to use an AED that is brought over by the school administrative secretary (who also does not know BLS, CPR, or how to use an AED). EMS arrives 20 min later, Brynn receives defibrillation for ventricular fibrillation secondary to commotio cordis, is stabilized at the local emergency department (ED), but dies several days later in the pediatric intensive care unit due to cerebral edema and hypoxic encephalopathy. How could the outcome have been different?

One important barrier to the preparedness of schools to respond to life and limb threatening emergencies in children occurs when there is not a school nurse or school physician present on campus. Therefore, in schools that do not have a full-time school nurse or school physician, efforts should be made to establish, practice, and optimize a MERP/CERP, to increase the training of teachers and administrative staff to perform BLS, CPR, and the utilization of an AED, and to educate school staff on the recognition of common pediatric emergencies (such as respiratory distress, seizures, altered mental status, anaphylaxis) and institute the ABCDE's of stabilization. Studies have even shown that older high school students have the capabilities to recognize cardiac emergencies, institute CPR, and utilize an AED effectively. Test your school's current state of emergency preparedness by utilizing the checklist for the training of school nurses and staff (Table 4.4) as delineated by the AAP, NASN, and AHA [2–8, 11].

Table 4.4 Training and education of school nurses and staff

		Check YES or NO
Certified in Basic Life Support	School nurses	
	Teachers	
	Coaches	
	Administrative staff	
	Students	
Certified in Cardiopulmonary Resuscitation (CPR)	School nurses	
	Teachers	
	Coaches	
	Administrative staff	
	Students	
Are you or your school trained in STOP the BLEED		
Are you trained in the administration of a self-injectable epinephrine device		
Are you trained in the recognition of symptoms and immediate treatment of a student who has sustained a concussion		
Are you trained in the recognition of symptoms and immediate treatment of a student with an opioid related overdose		

Case 3 You are the school physician in a small, rural high school. You are summoned to the school cafeteria by an overhead announcement. Upon your arrival, you encounter a chaotic scene. You quickly find out that 16 year old A.J., who has no significant medical history, is having an allergic reaction to an unknown food substance. He is pale, having difficulty speaking and breathing, with swollen face and lips. His vital signs reveal a heart rate of 136 beats per minute, respiratory rate of 10 breaths per minute, and an oxygen saturation of 78% on room air. On auscultation of his lungs, you cannot hear breath sounds. He proceeds to vomiting. You promptly activate your school's MERP, and are notified that it will take approximately 20–30 min for EMS to arrive to your school. The closest ED is approximately 20 min away. What should you do?

Shortness of breath and anaphylaxis are two common emergencies reported in schools [1]. In addition to the recognition of airway compromise and respiratory distress, and the stabilization of the ABCs (airway/breathing/circulation), the administration of life-saving medications may improve the morbidity and mortality of students experiencing these disease processes. Implementation of "stock" albuterol and epinephrine autoinjector protocols (for students without a history of reactive airway disease, asthma, or anaphylaxis, but who are exhibiting symptoms consistent with these disease processes) has been advocated by the AAP [2, 12] and has been implemented in several states. The availability of "stock" medications is of utmost importance, especially in schools where EMS and the nearest ED are not conveniently located or in schools that do not staff a fulltime school nurse or physician. In addition to "stock" medications, supplemental oxygen which would benefit students with respiratory distress, seizures, anaphylaxis, altered mental status, overdose, cardiac arrest, and other life-threatening emergencies should be widely available in schools. If schools in the United States can successfully implement AED programs for pediatric cardiac arrest (the least common emergency reported by school nurses [1]), then we as a health profession should advocate for the allocation of resources dedicated to "stock" medications and supplemental oxygen to limit morbidity and mortality associated with common and other life-threatening emergencies. Intramuscular epinephrine, albuterol, oxygen, and intravenous fluids were administered to A.J. upon EMS arrival, but he succumbed to anaphylaxis and died at his local ED (Fig. 4.1).

Test your school's current state of emergency preparedness by utilizing the checklist for recommended emergency medications, supplies, and equipment (Table 4.5) as delineated by the AAP, NASN, and AHA [2–8, 13].

Extra Credit Points

1. The most common emergencies encountered by school nurses include extremity sprains/strains/fractures, shortness of breath, seizures, head/neck injuries, lacerations, mental health crisis, abdominal pain, syncope, and anaphylaxis.
2. National recommendations by the AAP, NASN, and AHA have been published to guide school leaders and their communities towards optimal emergency pre-

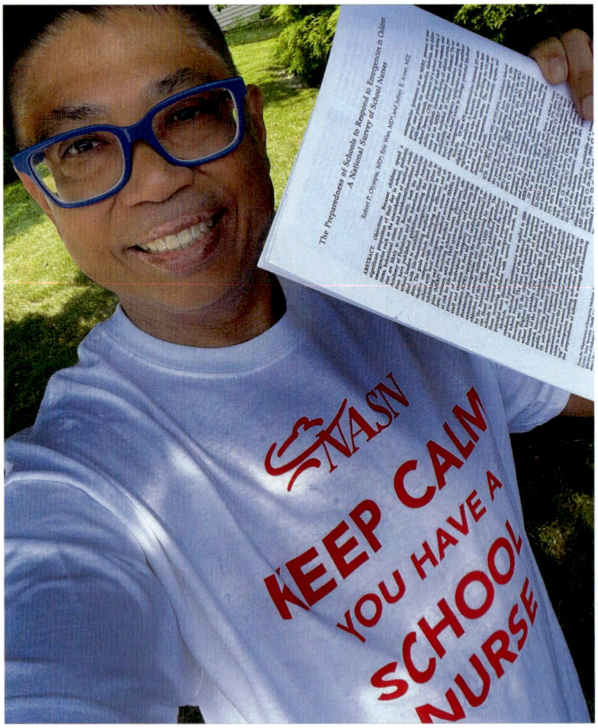

Fig. 4.1 Emergency preparedness begins with our heroes … our school nurses, who have dedicated their lives to the health and wellbeing of our children. Thank you!

Table 4.5 Checklist for the immediate availability of medications, supplies, and equipment

	Check YES or NO
Suction device	
Self-inflating resuscitation device and appropriately-sized masks (bag-valve-mask)	
Oxygen source	
Albuterol inhalers with spacers (stock)	
Albuterol nebulizers (stock)	
Epinephrine pen (stock)	
CPR one-way resuscitation mask	
Stethoscope	
C-spine immobilizer	
Glucose monitoring device	
Extremity splints	
Blunt scissors	
Stop the Bleed or other bleeding control kits for life threatening hemorrhage	
Combat application tourniquet	
Combat gauze	
Trauma shears	
Naloxone for opioid overdose	
Personal protective equipment: face shields or eye protection (other than glasses)	
Personal protective equipment: surgical masks	
Personal protective equipment: N95 or other respirators	
Personal protective equipment: face shields or eye protection	
Personal protective equipment: disposable gowns	
Personal protective equipment: disposable gloves	

paredness, and include general medical emergencies, as well as specific medical emergencies, such as anaphylaxis, asthma, cardiac arrest, head injuries, and seizures.

3. The commitment of an entire community is required to improve the preparedness of schools to deal with life-threatening illness and injury.
4. In schools that do not have a fulltime school nurse or school physician, efforts should be made to establish, practice, and optimize a MERP/CERP, to increase the training of teachers and administrative staff to perform BLS, CPR, and the utilization of an AED, and to educate school staff on the recognition of common pediatric emergencies (such as respiratory distress, seizures, altered mental status, anaphylaxis) and institute the ABCDE's of stabilization.
5. We as a health profession should advocate for the allocation of resources dedicated to "stock" medications and supplemental oxygen to limit morbidity and mortality associated with common and other life-threatening emergencies.

References

1. Olympia RP, Wan E, Avner JR. The preparedness of schools to respond to emergencies in children: a national survey of school nurses. Pediatrics. 2005;116(6):e738–45.
2. Gereige RS, Gross T, Jastaniah E, et al. Individual medical emergencies occurring at school. Pediatrics. 2022;150(1):e2022057987.
3. Sicherer SH, Mahr T, American Academy of Pediatrics Section on Allergy and Immunology. Management of food allergy in the school setting. Pediatrics. 2010;126(6):1232–9.
4. National Association of School Nurses. "Allergies and Anaphylaxis". https://www.nasn.org/nasn-resources/resources-by-topic/allergies-anaphylaxis. Accessed 13 Jul 2024.
5. American Heart Association. "Cardiac Emergency Response Plan". https://cpr.heart.org/en/training-programs/cardiac-emergency-response-plan-cerp. Accessed 13 Jul 2024.
6. Rose K, Goble M, Berger S, et al. Cardiac emergency response planning for schools: a policy statement. NASN Sch Nurse. 2016;31(5):263–70.
7. National Association of School Nurses. NASN position statement: concussions—the role of the school nurse. NASN Sch Nurse. 2017;32(1):59–60.
8. Harman AL, Devore C, Section on Neurology, American Academy of Pediatrics. Rescue medicine for epilepsy in education settings. Pediatrics. 2016;137(1):e20153876.
9. American Academy of Pediatrics, Council on School Health. Role of the school nurse in providing school health services. Pediatrics. 2016;137(6):e20160852.
10. American College of Emergency Physicians. "The Role of Emergency Physicians in the Care of Children". 2019. https://www.acep.org/patient-care/policy-statements/the-role-of-emergency-physicians-in-the-care-of-children. Accessed 13 Jul 2024.
11. Callahan JM, Fuchs SM, Committee on Pediatric Emergency Medicine. Advocating for life support training of children, parents, caregivers, school personnel, and the public. Pediatrics. 2018;141(6):e20180704.
12. Pappalardo AA, Gerald LB. Let them breathe: a plea to pediatricians to advocate for stock inhaler policies at school. Pediatrics. 2019;144(1):e20182857.
13. National Association of School Nurses. Emergency equipment and supplies in the school setting—issue brief. NASN Sch Nurse. 2012;27(3):172–5.

Chapter 5
Disaster Preparedness and STOP THE BLEED®

Rachel Rothstein and Khoon-Yen Tay

Case 1 You witness a school bus traveling at a high speed crash into the school brick wall. You call 911 and activate emergency medical services (EMS). You inspect the scene to ensure there are no additional threats to safety before entering the bus. You identify three children with injuries. Sam is awake and alert, with a superficial 2 cm laceration to her left knee with scant bleeding. Jack is awake, alert, and screaming, with a 4 cm laceration over his abdomen and visible blood on the front of his shirt. Sarah is pale, diaphoretic, and light-headed, with a deep 8 cm laceration to her right thigh and visible blood on her pants, as well as pooled on the floor below her leg. What are your next steps until EMS arrival?

Accidental and non-accidental trauma can occur in schools when least expected. Therefore, school-based health providers must equip themselves ahead of time with systematic approaches to disaster preparedness and trauma management. Chapter 23 discusses two approaches to trauma more broadly, including the "Pediatric Assessment Triangle" and the "ABCDE Approach." For penetrating trauma specifically, providers can employ an additional ABCD approach (Table 5.1).

The first step of this approach is to **a**lert 911. Activating EMS provides additional skilled hands, resources, and the ability to transport to definitive care if ultimately needed. Before intervening, the provider must **a**ssess the scene for threats to safety. Providers are unable to help others if they sustain a personal injury. If available, apply gloves for personal protection. In cases of accidental direct contact with blood, clean the skin with a disinfectant and contact a health provider for further instructions. If victims are at risk of further injury in their current environment,

R. Rothstein (✉) · K.-Y. Tay
Children's Hospital of Philadelphia, Philadelphia, PA, USA
e-mail: rothsteirl@chop.edu; tayk@chop.edu

R. P. Olympia, J. Brady-Olympia (eds.), *Clinical Considerations in School-based Health*, https://doi.org/10.1007/978-3-031-85765-2_5

Table 5.1 ABCD Approach to Penetrating Trauma

A:	**A**lert/**A**ssess	– Alert 911 to activate EMS – Assess the scene for additional threats to safety – Assess injury acuity using the "Pediatric Assessment Triangle"
B:	**B**leeding	– Identify the presence of a bleeding injury – Remove clothing at the site of injury – Assess the location and severity of bleeding
C:	**C**ompression	– Apply steady pressure directly to the wound – Utilize wound packing and tourniquets if applicable
D:	**D**isposition	– Transport to definitive care if needed

Adapted from: Erdman et al. (2019); American College of Surgeons (2019), [1]

Table 5.2 Signs of Life-Threatening Hemorrhage

The 6 P's:	• **P**ulsatile bleeding • **P**ersistent steady bleeding • **P**ooling blood on the ground • **P**rofusely blood-soaked clothing • **P**eripheral amputation • **P**rogression to shock (Table 5.3)

Adapted from: Erdman et al. (2019); American College of Surgeons (2019); [1]

move them to safety if able. If multiple victims are present, use the "Pediatric Assessment Triangle" (Chap. 23) to rapidly **a**ssess for visual and auditory clues to triage injury severity and prioritize care.

Next, the provider must identify the presence of penetrating trauma causing **b**leeding and assess for signs of life-threatening bleeding (Table 5.2) and hemorrhagic shock (Table 5.3). Victims of penetrating trauma with evidence of life-threatening bleeding or hemorrhagic shock should be prioritized for hemorrhage control and transfer to an appropriate facility. Exposure is important to making this assessment. Remove clothing at the site of injury to better assess the location and severity of the injury, and to reduce interference when intervening. Leave impaled objects in place, as they may be maintaining a degree of hemostasis and their removal may exacerbate bleeding.

After visualizing the wound, the provider can attempt hemorrhage control by **c**ompression in three ways, depending on the location and size of the wound: (1) Direct pressure, (2) Wound packing, and/or (3) Tourniquet application. Providers should first start with application of direct pressure, by placing cloth, gauze, or a gloved hand on the site, straightening the arms, and shifting body weight over the injury (Fig. 5.1a). If bleeding control measures, such as wound packing or tourniquets, are unavailable or not appropriate, the provider should continue to apply direct pressure until EMS arrives, even if suspecting hemostasis. Large deep wounds may additionally benefit from wound packing with hemostatic gauze, regular gauze, or cloth (Fig. 5.1b), to internally compress bleeding vessels. Hemostatic gauze contains agents that accelerate blood clotting and is therefore preferred, if available, to regular gauze or cloth for wound packing. After packing the wound, the provider should leave the packing in place and re-apply direct pressure until EMS arrival. Do not lift pressure or remove packing to check if the wound has stopped bleeding.

Table 5.3 Signs of Hemorrhagic Shock

Vital sign changes	*Tachycardia (heart rate, BPM)* • Infant (1–12 months): >180 • Toddler (1–2 years): >140 • Preschooler (3–5 years): >120 • School-aged (6–9 years): >118 • Adolescent (>9 years): >100	*Hypotension (systolic, mmHg)* • Infant: <72 • Toddler: <86 • Preschooler: <89 • School-aged: <97 • Adolescent: <110
Abnormal breathing	• Tachypnea or respiratory distress (compensatory respiratory alkalosis) • Loss of airway or respiratory drive (secondary to poor brain perfusion)	
Poor perfusion	• Weak thready pulses • Delayed capillary refill (>2 s) • Pallor or dusky skin • Cool extremities • Altered mental status (E.g. confusion, difficulty arousing, unconscious)	

Adapted from: Erdman et al. (2019); [2]

For extremity injuries, the provider should promptly apply a standard commercial limb tourniquet if available. Tourniquets are not appropriate for penetrating trauma to the head, neck, shoulders, chest, abdomen, pelvis, and hips, and should not be applied directly to joints, such as the elbows, wrists, knees or ankles. Current literature *does not* support improvised tourniquets (E.g. Belts, strips of cloth, or clothing), as their application may not achieve hemostasis and may delay equally, if not more efficacious, strategies such as direct steady pressure [3, 4]. The Committee on Tactical Combat Casualty Care guidelines recommend a number of commercially available tourniquets, including the Combat Application Tourniquet (CAT) displayed in Fig. 5.1c [3–5].

The provider should apply the tourniquet 2–3 in. proximal to the injury. Fasten the self-adhering band as tight as possible (such that two fingers cannot pass underneath) and rotate the windlass rod until bleeding stops. Secure the windlass rod into the windlass clip and reinforce with the windlass strap. If able, write the time on the windlass strap, so that EMS knows the total duration of tourniquet application. If not able, note the time of tourniquet application for EMS documentation. If bleeding continues despite maximal tightening and securing, apply a second tourniquet proximal to the initial tourniquet, while leaving the initial tourniquet in place. For children with smaller limbs, if tourniquet application does not achieve hemostasis, continue to apply pressure.

Once successfully applied, the tourniquet should remain in place until definitive care at a hospital. A correctly applied tourniquet will cause the victim significant discomfort in their extremity; However, providers should not loosen or remove the tourniquet under any circumstances, including concern for limb ischemia. Previous literature demonstrates that tourniquets rarely cause ischemia if applied for less than 2 h [3, 6]. Furthermore, the benefits of tourniquet application for hemorrhage control, prevention of shock, and improvement in prehospital survival outweigh the risk of limb ischemia. Effective tourniquet placement requires training. Less than one-in-four laypersons with no prior training can correctly apply a tourniquet [7]. Table 5.4 highlights common pitfalls of tourniquet application.

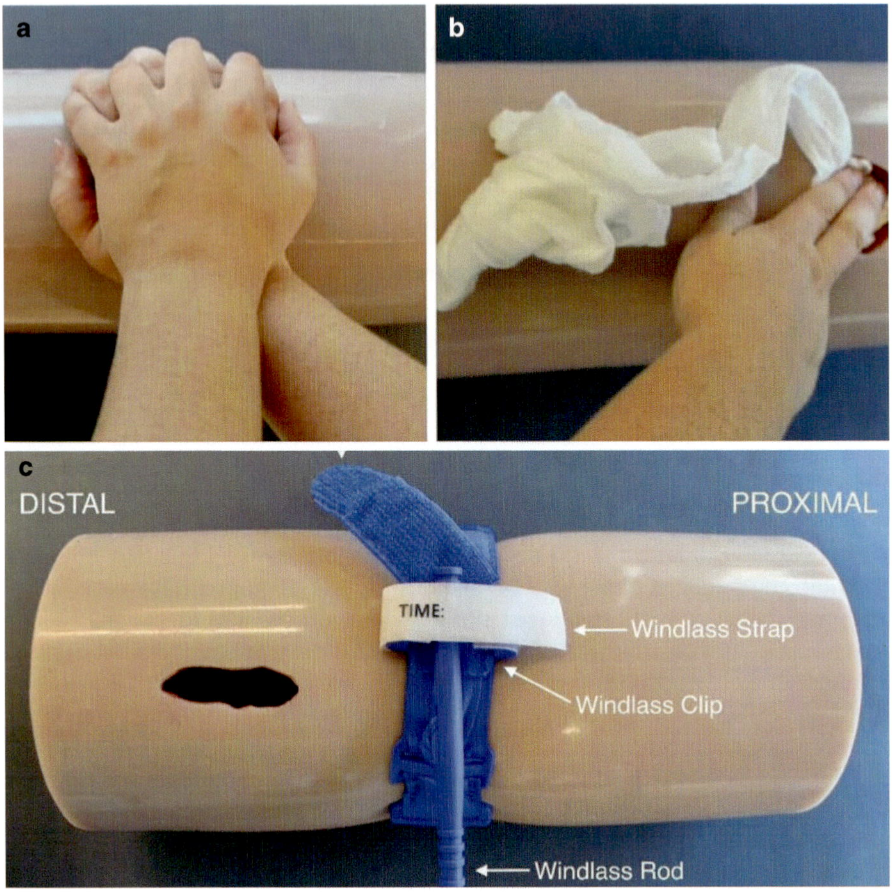

Fig. 5.1 Effective Application of (**a**) Direct Pressure, (**b**) Wound Packing, and (**c**) Limb Tourniquet

Table 5.4 Common Pitfalls of Tourniquet Application

- Lack of access to an effective commercial tourniquet
- Failure to apply a tourniquet when warranted (E.g. life-threatening bleeding)
- Failure to apply a tourniquet promptly and in a timely manor
- Application of a tourniquet when not warranted (E.g. minor bleeding)
- Application of a tourniquet more than 2–3 in. proximal to the wound
- Failure to tighten the tourniquet enough to achieve hemostasis
- Failure to apply a second tourniquet when warranted
- Inappropriately removing the tourniquet once hemostasis is achieved
- Loosening the tourniquet periodically to prevent ischemic injury

Adapted from: Erdman et al. (2019); Ross et al. (2018); Holcomb et al. (2015) [1]

5.1 Case Conclusion

You appropriately triage: (1) Sam's injury is non-life threatening, (2) Jack's injury is more severe and could become life-threatening, but he is currently hemodynamically stable, and (3) Sarah's injury is life-threatening, with signs of hemorrhagic shock (Tables 5.2 and 5.3). You and your colleagues apply direct pressure on each child's wounds. You instruct the principal to obtain a bleeding control kit. You pack Sarah's thigh wound, apply a tourniquet 2–3 in. proximally, tighten until you achieve hemostasis and mark the time on her tourniquet. Recognizing a tourniquet is not appropriate based on the location of injury, you pack Jack's abdominal wound and reapply direct pressure. You prioritize Sarah in the first ambulance and Jack in the second. Your colleagues, students, and families are grateful for your ability to recognize and acutely stabilize life-threatening hemorrhage and ask how they can learn these skills. Additionally, the impressed board is requesting that you review the school district's disaster preparedness plans for compliance with current national standards and recommendations.

Created by the American College of Surgeons, STOP THE BLEED® is a national campaign that seeks to teach lay bystanders life-saving hemorrhage control skills, including direct pressure application, wound packing, and tourniquet application [4]. With appropriate education, bystanders (including students) are: (1) Capable of recognizing life-threatening hemorrhage, (2) Willing and comfortable to intervene, and (3) Able to correctly employ hemorrhage control skills [8–10]. STOP THE BLEED® courses are typically free of charge, easily accessible in the community, welcome to all ages and skill levels, and last less than 90 min. Alternatively, school health providers can arrange to bring the STOP THE BLEED® course directly to their schools [11]. The lecture portion of STOP THE BLEED® is also available online for free. School health providers can purchase tourniquets, wound packing materials or comprehensive bleeding control kits (which include an instructional booklet, tourniquet(s), hemostatic gauze, gloves, and other supplies) through STOP THE BLEED®. For more information on STOP THE BLEED®, visit the resources in Table 5.5.

Table 5.5 STOP THE BLEED® Resources

Resource	Link
To register for a local course	https://cms.bleedingcontrol.org/class/search
To organize a course at your school	stopthebleed@facs.org
To access the free online course	https://www.stopthebleed.org/training/online-course/
To become an instructor	https://cms.bleedingcontrol.org/applicant/create
To purchase hemorrhage supplies	https://www.bleedingkits.org/all-products.html
To download free instructional posters	https://www.stopthebleed.org/resources-poster-booklet/

Case 2 You are the school physician responsible for five schools in your district. You are asked to develop a Medical Emergency Response Plan to respond to mass casualty incidents, coordinating each school with their local EMS and emergency department. Furthermore, you are asked to review the current state of disaster preparedness associated with school shootings in your district (including "lockdown" procedures, locked entrances and exits, and crisis teams with clearly identified roles during a disaster), as well as ensuring an educational STOP THE BLEED® program at these schools and the availability of bleeding control kits. How would you start?

Children are uniquely vulnerable when disasters occur, due to risk factors such as: (1) Reliance on adults for instruction and/or maintenance of basic needs, (2) Lack of physical ability and/or resources to escape danger, (3) Inability to recognize, or curiosity to approach, hazards, (4) Altruistic desires to help others, at the expense of endangering oneself, (5) Exaggerated emotional responses, (6) Impulsive decision-making, and (7) Physiologically increased propensity for illness and injury [12]. Given these vulnerabilities, and the continued threat of firearm-related and other emergencies, it is critical that schools follow the six steps (Table 5.6) to develop comprehensive disaster preparedness plans [13]. Visit the references below for resources on disaster preparedness planning for schools and families [12], emergency supplies and equipment for schools [14], and psychosocial support for children following crises [12, 15].

Extra Credit Points

1. Employ the **ABCD** approach to penetrating trauma and hemorrhage control: **A**lert/**A**ssess, **B**leeding, **C**ompression, and **D**isposition (Table 5.1).
2. Recognize the **6P's** of life-threatening hemorrhage: **P**ulsatile bleeding, **P**ersistent steady bleeding, **P**ooling blood on ground, **P**rofusely blood-soaked clothing, **P**eripheral amputation, and **P**rogression to shock.
3. Signs of hemorrhagic shock include tachycardia, hypotension, abnormal breathing, altered mental status, and poor distal perfusion (Table 5.3).
4. For extremity injuries, apply a tourniquet 2–3 in. proximal to the wound and tighten until hemostasis is achieved. If bleeding continues, apply a second tourniquet proximal to the initial, while leaving the initial in place. Once achieving hemostasis, do not remove bleeding control measures to mediate patient discomfort or ischemia.
5. The six steps of disaster preparedness planning are: (1) Form a Collaborative Planning Team, (2) Understand the Situation, (3) Determine Goals and Objectives, (4) Plan Development, (5) Plan Preparation, Review and Approval, and (6) Plan Implementation and Maintenance (Table 5.6).

Table 5.6 Six Steps of Disaster Preparedness Planning

(1) "Form a Collaborative Planning Team" • Create a team of key community and school stakeholders ([13], p. 6) • Form a shared understanding of stakeholders' vocabulary, command structure, and culture • Outline each stakeholders' roles and responsibilities • Establish regularly scheduled meetings amongst stakeholders
(2) "Understand the Situation" • Identify potential threats/hazards via local, state, and federal agencies ([13], p. 7) • Use assessments ([13], p. 9) to determine the risks posed by and vulnerabilities to the above • Categorize the above as low, medium, or high risk; consider probability of occurrence, impact, warning time, duration, and downstream effects ([13], p. 12)
(3) "Determine Goals and Objectives" • Determine which of the above potential threats/hazards to address • Develop three *goals* (desired outcomes before, during and after) per threat/hazard • Develop *objectives* (specific measurable actions to achieve the above goals) • Identify *functions* (overlapping objectives that apply to multiple threats/hazards) • Develop three goals and objectives (before, during and after) per function
(4) "Plan Development (Identifying Courses of Action)" • Enact scenarios, determine response time, and identify decision points for each threat/hazard • Consider the questions posed by [13] (p. 15) to develop potential courses of action • Compare potential courses of action (E.g. costs/benefits, alignment with goals/objectives) • Determine the preferred course(s) of action with which to proceed • Identify available and needed resources necessary to execute course(s) of action
(5) "Plan Preparation, Review and Approval" • Formulate a plan, including three sections: (1) Basic plan, (2) Functional Annexes, (3) Threat- and Hazard-Specific Annexes ([13], p. 18 and 23–36) • Review adequacy, feasibility, acceptability, completeness, and compliance with stakeholders • Obtain leadership approval of plan; disseminate to necessary and authorized parties
(6) "Plan Implementation and Maintenance" • Train stakeholders on the plan and their roles ([13], p. 20) • Practice the plan using drills and/or tabletop, functional, and full-scale exercises ([13], p. 21) • Continually review, revise, and maintain the plan

Adapted from: Guide for Developing High-Quality School Emergency Operations Plans (2013)

References

1. Holcomb JB, Butler FK, Rhee P. Hemorrhage control devices: tourniquets and hemostatic dressings. J Spec Oper Med. 2015;15(4):153–6.
2. America Heart Association. Pediatric Advanced Life Support Digital Reference Card. 2020. https://shopcpr.heart.org/pals-digital-reference-card. Accessed 1 Jun 2024.
3. Erdman MO, Chardavoyne P, Olympia RP. School nurses on the front lines of medicine: the approach to a student with severe traumatic bleeding. NASN Sch Nurse. 2019;34(5):280–6.
4. American College of Surgeons. STOP THE BLEED® Course. 2019. https://www.stopthebleed.org/media/omalhrif/lay-public-stop-the-bleed-presentation-pdf.pdf. Accessed 1 Jun 2024.
5. Committee on tactical combat casualty care. Recommended Devices & Adjuncts. 2021. https://learning-media.allogy.com/api/v1/pdf/c1e1c696-c61d-43ae-bb6d-16dcd1cb7ff2/contents. Accessed 1 Jun 2024.
6. Holcomb JB, Dorlac WC, Drew BG, et al. Rethinking limb tourniquet conversion in the prehospital environment. J Trauma Acute Care Surg. 2023;95(6):e54–60.
7. Ross EM, Mapp JG, Redman TT, Brown DJ, Kharod CU, Wampler DA. The tourniquet gap: a pilot study of the intuitive placement of three tourniquet types by laypersons. J Emerg Med. 2018;54(3):307–14.
8. Goolsby C, Rojas LE, Rodzik RH, Gausche-Hill M, Neal MD, Levy MJ. High-school students can stop the bleed: a randomized, controlled educational trial. Acad Pediatr. 2021;21(2):321–8.
9. McCarty JC, Caterson EJ, Chaudhary MA, et al. Can they stop the bleed? Evaluation of tourniquet application by individuals with varying levels of prior self-reported training. Injury. 2019;50(1):10–5.
10. Goolsby C, Schuler K, Rodzik R, et al. The fast VIP (first aid for severe trauma "virtual" in-person) educational study. West J Emerg Med. 2021;22(4):951–7.
11. STOP THE BLEED® Info. Stop the Bleed. 2024. https://www.stopthebleed.org/frequently-asked-questions/. Accessed 1 Jun 2024.
12. Disaster and emergency preparedness in schools. American Academy of Pediatrics. 2022. https://www.aap.org/en/patient-care/school-health/disaster-and-emergency-preparedness-in-schools/. Accessed 22 Jul 2024.
13. Guide for developing high-quality school emergency operations plans. Readiness and Emergency Management for Schools. 2013. https://rems.ed.gov/docs/School_Guide_508C.pdf. Accessed 22 Jul 2024.
14. Strouse D, MacFarland S, Shannon R, Bland-Slaffey J. Emergency resources, equipment and supplies list for schools. Silver Spring, MD: National Association of School Nurses; 2020. https://higherlogicdownload.s3.amazonaws.com/NASN/8575d1b7-94ad-45ab-808e-d45019cc5c08/UploadedImages/PDFs/Textbook/Comprehensive_Text_Chapter_39.pdf. Accessed 22 Jul 2024.
15. National Center for School Crisis and Bereavement. 2024. https://www.schoolcrisiscenter.org/. Accessed 22 Jul 2024.

Chapter 6
Gun Violence Prevention

Apurva Bhatt, Jeffrey Birnbaum, and Amy Barnhorst

Case 1 Stephanie is a 6 year old female who was referred to the school nurse due to falling asleep in class multiple times interfering with her ability to actively participate. Upon asking if everything is okay at home, she shares that she is scared of being shot. She shares that her older brother was shot a few days ago and she is afraid that the same will happen to her. You contact her parents who state that they are not sure how best to support her. They disclose they recently purchased a firearm for protection.

6.1 Screening for Firearms

Firearms are now the leading cause of death in children with over 2000 children killed annually [1, 2]. For every fatal firearm-related injury, there are 2–3 non-fatal injuries [3]. 40% of children live in a household with firearms [4]. With both firearms access and injuries continuing to rise, it is no longer a safe assumption that school-aged children are not personally affected by firearm violence. Schools are increasingly faced with the challenge of confronting firearm-related issues. It is more important than ever for pediatric healthcare providers to engage in discussions

A. Bhatt (✉)
Stanford University, Stanford, CA, USA
e-mail: apbhatt@stanford.edu

J. Birnbaum
Children's Hospital Los Angeles, Los Angeles, CA, USA
e-mail: jrbirnbaum@chla.usc.edu

A. Barnhorst
University of California Davis, Bullet Points Project, Davis, CA, USA
e-mail: abarnhorst@ucdavis.edu

R. P. Olympia, J. Brady-Olympia (eds.), *Clinical Considerations in School-based Health*, https://doi.org/10.1007/978-3-031-85765-2_6

with their patients and their families about access to firearms given the disproportionate risk they pose to children's health.

It may seem straightforward on how to approach a conversation about firearms. However, it can actually be quite challenging to open a productive dialogue with a family, especially without a long-standing relationship. Rather than asking *"Do you own a firearm?"* a more productive opening line may be *"How do you keep your child safe from firearms?"*

The latter question does two things well that are important to highlight. First, it provides the background as to why you are asking. Second, it works to lessen the divide between gun owners and non-gun owners by making the safe assumption that a child has a high likelihood of entering into a home, primary residence or otherwise, with a firearm.

Many gun owners have experienced perceived judgment concerning their decision to own a firearm, especially in locations where their children spend time. Gun owners may be cautious to enter a conversation without clear goals and direction. By focusing on childhood safety, you are providing context and reassurance to a family on why you, as a school-based medical provider, are asking about firearms. It may also be helpful to take this one step further to normalize the inquiry in the setting of injury prevention. Adding an opening such as *"firearms are the number one cause of injury-related death in children, which is why I ask all our student's families about firearms."* may be better received.

Now that you have successfully broached the topic of firearm access, how can you best counsel a family on how to keep their child safe from harm?

6.2 Safe Storage

The best way to prevent firearm injury is to remove firearms from the home [5]. However, this is not always the best starting point to engage with families who own firearms. The decision to own a firearm is complex and often rooted in increasing personal safety [6]. Furthermore, with 40% of households in the United States containing at least one firearm, children are at risk of encountering firearms even if there are none in their primary residence [7]. There are three things that gun owners can do to decrease the risk of unintentional injury to children.

The tenants of firearm safe storage include ensuring a firearm is **UN**loaded, **SE**parate from its **A**mmunition, and **L**ocked up. You may use the mnemonic **UNSEAL** to remember this. Common locking devices include cable locks, trigger locks, and gun safes.

Of course preventing firearm violence is the ideal, but often healthcare providers are tasked with responding to children who have already been affected by exposure to gun violence.

6.3 Toxic Stress

Firearm violence is a common cause of toxic stress in children, which is defined as strong, frequent, or prolonged activation of stress response systems. The consequences of toxic stress include cognitive impairment and increased mental health disorders, such as anxiety, depression, and post-traumatic stress disorder [8]. Toxic stress has also been linked to medical diseases due to its association with chronic inflammation, elevated blood pressure, and obesity [9].

Children who are exposed to firearm violence directly through a family member or indirectly through their community have increased healthcare utilization [8]. Increasing vigilance for firearm-related stress can help address mental and physical health issues early before they become more challenging.

Back to the Case 1 In speaking with Stephanie's parents, you frame your discussion around the shared goal of safety from future firearm injury or death and discuss safe storage options. They agree to keep the newly purchased firearm in a biometric safe, inaccessible to the children in the home.

Case 2 Jordan is a 12-year-old male referred by his teacher after submitting homework with an erased drawing depicting suicide themes. Over the past year, Jordan has become more withdrawn and irritable, with his grades dropping from Bs to Ds and Fs. His parents' contentious divorce, finalized recently, has significantly impacted him, and he meets weekly with the school counselor but has no external mental health support. During your meeting, Jordan exhibits poor eye contact and admits to persistent sadness, low energy, a lack of interest in activities he once enjoyed, and feelings of hopelessness. He also reports passive suicidal thoughts with no plan last occurring 3 days ago. He denies current suicidal or self-harm thoughts or plans, and denies plans to harm others. What are your next steps?

6.4 Lethal Means Counseling for High-Risk Students

Follow your school's suicide safety protocol, including screening for suicide risk using an evidence-based tool. If your school or school district does not have a protocol or policy for suicide prevention, consider resources from the American Foundation for Suicide Prevention [10] and HEARD Alliance [11].

When asking about access to lethal means, ***always*** ask about access to firearms in addition to other lethal means (medications, poisons, sharps, ropes, etc.). Jordan shares his father has several firearms at home, including one that is unlocked and loaded in a bedroom dresser. Given Jordan's recent thoughts of suicide and given that he lives in a home with firearms, you recognize Jordan is at elevated risk of suicide by firearm. Jordan's parents are called to the school to discuss next steps. As you are discussing your concerns about Jordan's suicide risk, you begin providing evidence-based firearm safety counseling to prevent suicide by firearm. This can be done using The BulletPoints Project 3A's framework (Table 6.1, Fig. 6.1).

Back to the Case 2 In speaking with Jordan and his parents, you share your concern for Jordan's risk of suicide by firearm and collaborate on a safety plan, emphasizing the shared goal of Jordan's safety and wellbeing. Jordan's father agrees to lock up all firearms in the home until Jordan is feeling better. Jordan's mother agrees to talk with Jordan's grandfather about locking up his hunting rifles (located in a shed on his property) given Jordan spends time with him after school a few days a week. They also agree to bring him to a local mental health crisis center or emergency department for a mental health evaluation for depression.

Extra Credit Points

1. Children are likely to encounter firearms, even if not present in their primary home.
2. Firearms are now the leading cause of death of children living in the USA, and exposure to firearm violence can contribute to toxic stress in childhood.
3. Discussing the principles of firearm safe storage can help provide tangible steps for parents to increase their child's safety from firearm injury or death.
4. When screening for suicide risk, always assess access to lethal means including firearms, and provide firearm safety counseling for at-risk students and their families. Using a collaborative approach, emphasize secure storage and reducing access to firearms during periods of elevated risk.
5. Educate caregivers on safe storage laws, potential legal consequences, and consider options such as temporary transfer of firearms or civil protection orders to ensure safety.

Table 6.1 The BulletPoints Project 3 A's Framework to provide counseling on firearms

Approach
• *Be Informed*: Know why people own firearms and how to store them safely. Also know your state's gun laws and local policies, including your school district's policy related to guns, including secure storage policies. Learn more about your state's policies regarding firearms at the Giffords Law Center: https://giffords.org/lawcenter/gun-laws/
– *Language matters*. Consider using the below phrases when offering this type of counseling:
"Secure storage" or "safe storage" when talking about storage (rather than "gun safety")
"Reducing access" when talking about making guns inaccessible to those who should not have access
Emphasize the "temporary" and "voluntary" nature when talking about options for removing guns out of the home "during times of crisis or risk"
When possible, use terms like "voluntary and collaborative"
Politics has no place in these conversations. If political views emerge, redirect the conversation toward the shared goal of safety and reducing risk
• *Be Respectful*: Respect an individual's decision to own firearms and recognize that firearm ownership may be an important part of their sense of safety and/or their identity
• *Focus on Harm reduction*: Your role is to keep students and others as safe and healthy as possible. Reducing some risk is better than not reducing any risk
• *Be Individualized*: find an individualized solution that works for your student and their family

(continued)

Table 6.1 (continued)

Assess

- Assess for risk factors for firearm-related injury or death:
  - Guns that are kept in a way that is easily accessible to children and at-risk individuals
  - Children living in a home with firearms
  - History of prior suicide attempts
  - History of impulsivity, depression, cognitive impairments, bipolar disorder, schizophrenia spectrum disorders (more commonly self-inflicted firearm injury or death)
  - Substance use
  - History of violence, trauma, or bullying (victimization or perpetration)
- *Assess for the presence of ideations or threats*
  - Certain situations are always considered higher risk:
    If a student has thoughts about harming themselves or someone else or has made threats to hurt themselves or someone else
- *Assess for access to guns*
  - If risk factors and/or thoughts of self- or other-directed harm are present, it's time to assess the individual's access to firearms. *Remember, it's important to bring up firearm access in the context of risk and safety*
  - Assess for access to guns at all homes that the student spends time in
- *Assess for willingness to collaborate*
  - If a student is at risk of firearm-related injury or death and has access to firearms, assessing their and their parent/caregiver's ability and willingness to collaborate on a plan for their safety will inform your choice of intervention
  - Whenever possible, take a collaborative approach and work with the student and their loved ones to find out what will work best for them
  - If the student or caregiver is unwilling or unable to collaborate, involuntary actions may be warranted to prevent harm

Act

Your choice of interventions will depend upon the student's risk level, type of risk present, and the student and family's willingness to collaborate

- *Safe storage*: When there are children living in the home, regardless of risk level or type of risk, recommending safe storage of ALL firearms is *always* an appropriate recommendation
- *Educate on Safe Storage Laws and Child Access Prevention Laws*: Ensure that caregivers understand your state laws and potential legal consequences of not storing firearms safely when there is a child or at-risk individual living in the home
- *Temporary Transfer*: Consider temporary transfer of firearms when removing firearms from the home is the safest option and the family is willing to collaborate. Depending on state law, firearms can be temporarily transferred to a family member or other trusted person, law enforcement, or some gun ranges or gun stores
- *Mental health hold*: If a student needs mental health treatment, consider a mental health hold. Note that this does not automatically restrict the student's access to firearms after discharge, so families should be reminded about safe firearm storage before discharge and on an ongoing basis afterwards. Note that depending on state laws, a student who had been placed on a mental health hold may still be able to purchase or acquire firearms later in life
- *Civil protection orders*: These are court orders that can remove firearms from individuals who are a danger to themselves or others. There are several types (extreme risk protection orders, gun violence restraining orders). Depending on your state's legal process, these can be initiated by law enforcement or family members

Adapted from the BulletPoints Project [12]

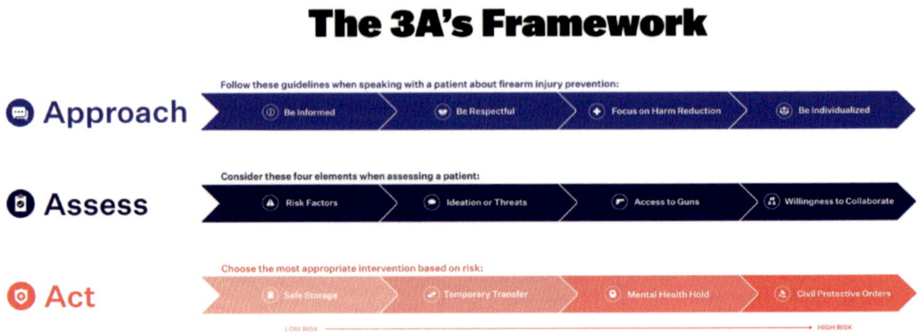

Fig. 6.1 BulletPoints Project 3 A's Framework to provide counseling on firearms

References

1. Lee LK, Douglas K, Hemenway D. Crossing Lines—a change in the leading cause of death among U.S. Children. N Engl J Med. 2022;386(16):1485–7. https://doi.org/10.1056/NEJMp2200169.
2. Gramlich J. Gun deaths among U.S. children and teens rose 50% in two years. Pew Research Center. 2023. https://www.pewresearch.org/short-reads/2023/04/06/gun-deaths-among-us-kids-rose-50-percent-in-two-years/. Accessed 29 May 2024.
3. Naik-Mathuria BJ, Cain CM, Alore EA, Chen L, Pompeii LA. Defining the full spectrum of pediatric firearm injury and death in the United States: it is even worse than we think. Ann Surg. 2023;278(1):10–6. https://doi.org/10.1097/SLA.0000000000005833.
4. Miller M, Azrael D. Firearm storage in US households with children: findings from the 2021 National Firearm Survey. JAMA Netw Open. 2022;5(2):e2148823. Published 2022 Feb 1. https://doi.org/10.1001/jamanetworkopen.2021.48823.
5. Farah MM, Simon HK, Kellermann AL. Firearms in the home: parental perceptions. Pediatrics. 1999;104(5 Pt 1):1059–63. https://doi.org/10.1542/peds.104.5.1059.
6. Ye GF, Thatipamala P, Siegel M. Assessment of reasons for ownership and attitudes about policies among firearm owners with and without children. JAMA Netw Open. 2022;5(1):e2142995. Published 2022 Jan 4. https://doi.org/10.1001/jamanetworkopen.2021.42995.
7. Parker K, Horowitz JM, Igielnik R, Oliphant JB, Brown A. America's complex relationship with guns. Pew Research Center. 2017. https://www.pewresearch.org/social-trends/2017/06/22/americas-complex-relationship-with-guns/. Accessed 29 May 2024.
8. Vasan A, Mitchell HK, Fein JA, Buckler DG, Wiebe DJ, South EC. Association of Neighborhood Gun Violence with Mental Health-Related Pediatric Emergency Department Utilization. JAMA Pediatr. 2021;175(12):1244–51. https://doi.org/10.1001/jamapediatrics.2021.3512.
9. Holloway K, Cahill G, Tieu T, Njoroge W. Reviewing the literature on the impact of gun violence on early childhood development. Curr Psychiatry Rep. 2023;25(7):273–81. https://doi.org/10.1007/s11920-023-01428-6.
10. Bring suicide prevention to your school. American Foundation for Suicide Prevention. n.d. https://afsp.org/bring-suicide-prevention-to-your-school/. Accessed 30 May 2024.
11. HEARD Alliance Homepage—HEARD Alliance. HEARD Alliance—Health Care Alliance for Response to Adolescent Depression; HEARD Alliance. 2016. https://www.heardalliance.org/.
12. Bulletpointsproject.org. https://www.bulletpointsproject.org/how-to-counsel/. Accessed 30 May 2024.

Chapter 7
School-Based Screening: Asthma, Dental, Vision, Hearing, Obesity and Scoliosis

Lori Kelley and Bridgett Bilenski

Case **School Nurse Betty works in an underserved rural school district. 98% of her students qualify for the free and reduced lunch programs. The primary employer in the small town is a steel mill, making noise and air pollution a concern. Approximately 60% of her rural community uses well water, which does not contain fluoride. Because of the remote nature of her community, many students have difficulty accessing health care and do not have a medical home. In addition, Betty feels that the limited state-mandated screenings are inadequate to meet the needs of this underserved community. How should she proceed?**

When exploring a school based screening program, there are many factors that should be considered, including the "*School Nursing Practice Framework*" [1], *School Nursing: Scope and Standards of Practice* [2], district policies, state and federal regulations, and effectiveness and benefit to the school community. With state mandates differing, school health providers should assess whether the mandated screenings adequately meet the needs of their school community. Further consideration should be given to:

- Are the mandated screening programs adequate to meet student/community needs?
- Do the students within the school community have regular access to a medical home?
- Are there frequently occurring health conditions within the community that are left undiagnosed?
- Do these conditions have a high potential to impact learning and overall wellness? [3]

L. Kelley (✉) · B. Bilenski
North Allegheny School District, Pittsburgh, PA, USA
e-mail: lkelley@northallegheny.org; bbilenski@northallegheny.org

R. P. Olympia, J. Brady-Olympia (eds.), *Clinical Considerations in School-based Health*, https://doi.org/10.1007/978-3-031-85765-2_7

School health providers must also evaluate the effectiveness of the existing screening program. The American Academy of Pediatrics lists 8 aspects of an effective screening program. These aspects can be remembered with the mnemonic Do The Select Screening Troubles Ruin a Child's Progress (Table 7.1). Table 7.2 describes school screening recommendations and considerations.

It is not recommended that mass asthma screenings be completed in school. However, it is vital that school nurses complete health histories to monitor for students that have been diagnosed with asthma by their healthcare provider [3]. Additional support to the school community by nurses can include referring students that exhibit possible symptoms of asthma to the appropriate medical providers, cultivate collaborative relationships with community providers to best support students diagnosed with asthma, assist in eliminating asthma triggers in the school environment, and provide continuing education to the school community [22].

7.1 Case Conclusion

Betty knows that obesity and vision screenings are required every year for every student, but there are no requirements for other screenings. She is concerned about the health impacts of the local steel mill and the lack of fluoride in the water. Betty gets an updated health history from every student annually and closely monitors the students with a history of asthma. She has utilized the scope and standards of practice, the "School *Nursing Practice Framework*," and monitors district statistics, knowing the impacts of dental disease and hearing loss on attendance and school achievement. School nurse Betty presents the data and information to her school administration and gains their support to add an every other year dental school screening program. She also gains support for a hearing screening program that

Table 7.1 Considerations for determining the screenings appropriate for a school community [3]

	Considerations
Do	**Disease:** Does the disease have a high occurrence of undiagnosed cases in the population, resulting in adverse educational outcomes?
The	**Treatment:** Is there effective treatment readily available? Can the school nurse provide resources for those unable to access the needed health care?
Select	**Screening Test:** Is the test specific, brief and easy to perform?
Screening	**Screener:** Is the screener well trained? How will the training be conducted?
Troubles	**Target Population:** Which students are the targeted disease most likely to impact?
Ruin a	**Referral and Treatment:** Does the school have a referral process that results in effective treatment? Do at least 90% of the referrals get returned, as recommended by the AAP?
Child's	**Cost/Benefit Ratio:** Do the benefits outway the costs associated with the screening program?
Progress	**Program Maintenance:** Is the screening program regularly evaluated utilizing the data? Is there meaningful training for the available screening teams?

Table 7.2 School screening recommendations and considerations

Screening program	Impact on health and learning	Common screening procedures	Recommendations and considerations for referrals	Resources available
Dental	13.3% of children and adolescents aged 6–19 years have untreated dental caries in their permanent teeth [5] Numbers are much higher for students living in poverty [4]	Coordinated by the school nurse in collaboration with a dentist, or hygienist, depending on policy, regulation and availability [6] Include dental health education in screening program [6]	Implement a procedure for communicating the need for dental interventions with families Provide resources for students to access care when dental referrals are necessary Develop a process for connecting students with a dental home [4]	Medicaid programs; Children's Health Insurance Program (CHIP); Partnerships with local dentists or mobile dental clinics health departments; American Academy of Pediatric Dentistry; My Children's Teeth [6, 7]
Vision	41 states require some sort of vision screening for school aged children [8] National guidelines provided by the American Academy of Pediatrics and Bright Futures, recommend children have annual eye exams beginning at age 3 to 6 years, then again every 2 years, during the well child visits [9] There are recommendations to continue to monitor a child in the odd years for any difficulties [9]	Assessment of the student's medical history for any conditions that may place the student at risk for vision issues [10] Two screening methods available for the school setting include opto-type based screening for visual acuity and instrument based screening to determine refractive error and the possibility of adverse eye conditions [10] Screening methods should include screening for distance visual acuity, near visual acuity, color vision deficiency screening, and stereoacuity [10]	Refer any student with results greater than 20/32 in either eye, for distance or near visual acuity screening [11]	Medicaid programs CHIP NASN VSP Eyes of Hope (NASN 2024) Local Lions Club Consider Partnerships with local optometrist

(continued)

Table 7.2 (continued)

Screening program	Impact on health and learning	Common screening procedures	Recommendations and considerations for referrals	Resources available
Hearing	Hearing loss impacts communication and language acquisition, which can lead to significant difficulties with school achievement [15]	Recommended when a child enters school, at ages 6, 8 and 10 years, once in middle school, once in high school [12] Coordinate with the school nurse, the school speech therapist and/or the school audiologist Minimize background noise and distractions Properly maintain equipment, including annual calibrations [13] Incorporate hearing loss prevention education [12]	Use the preferred screening test, the pure tone audiometric sweep test [14] Conduct for 1000, 2000 and 4000 Hz Conduct at 20 decibels in ideal conditions With a lack of ideal conditions, including the presence of ambient noise, screening at 25 decibels is acceptable [14] Re-screen if a student is unable to hear the required tones during a sweep test before referring Consider using a pure tone threshold test for the re-screening process [16]	Cultivate collaborative relationships with community providers CHIP/Medicaid School Audiologists
Obesity	Obese school children have higher absentee rates and increased difficulties with social emotional skills while at school [17]. Obesity/BMI screening is mandated in many states [18] Evidence that school-based BMI screenings are beneficial is lacking [18]	Involve parents early in the planning process [18] Ensure privacy [18] Use well maintained accurate equipment [18] Evaluate the program periodically for effectiveness [17]	Institute an effective follow-up or referral process Send an explanation of the result along with appropriate follow-up actions needed to all parents [17] Never utilize BMI results to evaluate the performance of teachers or students in the Physical Education Program [17, 18]	Partner with Food Services in preventative nutrition Collaborate with health and physical education teachers, for lifestyle based prevention education Coordinate with local food banks to increase access to fresh fruits and vegetables

(continued)

Table 7.2 (continued)

Screening program	Impact on health and learning	Common screening procedures	Recommendations and considerations for referrals	Resources available
Scoliosis	Lateral curvature and twisting of the spine that involves the coronal, sagittal, and axial planes [19] Classified by etiology and includes congenital, idiopathic, and neuromuscular [19] Affects 2–3% of the adolescent population and affects females more than the males, with idiopathic scoliosis comprising approximately 80% of cases [19]	Provide privacy for the student and screen on an individual basis A visual assessment of the spine is performed, as the student stands in front of the screeners, for asymmetries in the shoulders, scapulae, hips, and waist. Students are then asked to bend for the forward bend test, while measuring with a scoliometer [20]	Any scoliometer reading equal to or greater than seven degrees requires further medical evaluation with radiography [21] Confidentiality and sensitivity should be exercised when sharing the information with the student or family	Medicaid programs CHIP Cultivate collaborative relationships with community providers

follows CDC recommendations for pure tone audiometric sweep tests to be done in kindergarten, second, fourth, seventh and eleventh grades. She partners with a local dentist that is able to bill Medicaid to provide corrective services for the students found to have dental caries. Additionally, the closest children's hospital, which is a 90 min drive away, has agreed to send a provider twice a year to consult on students failing hearing screenings.

Extra Credit Points

1. Know the federal, state, and local regulations and mandates related to school health screenings.
2. Know any applicable professional policies and guidance.
3. Advocate and collaborate with school administrators to gain support from the school community for a comprehensive screening program.
4. Assess your school community for additional health needs.
5. Create a robust, culturally sensitive referral process, utilizing a network of resources for students who have difficulty accessing health care.

References

1. School Nursing Practice Framework. School Nursing Practice Framework-National Association of School Nurses. https://www.nasn.org/nasn-resources/framework. Accessed 1 May 2024.
2. School nursing: scope and standards of practice. National Association of School Nurses; 2022.
3. Wheeler LSM, Barbot O. Chapter 3. Health services. Section 1: Guidance for school-based screenings. In: School health: policy and practice. 7th ed. Elk Grove Village, IL: American Academy of Pediatrics; 2016. p. 35–45.
4. Dental Caries (Tooth Decay). National Institute of Dental and Craniofacial Research, U.S. Department of Health and Human Services. www.nidcr.nih.gov/research/data-statistics/dental-caries#:~:text=Dental%20caries%20(tooth%20decay)%20remains,remain%20among%20some%20population%20groups. Accessed 28 Feb 2024.
5. State dental screening Laws for children: examining the ... Children's Dental Project, American Dental Partners Foundation. 2019. www.astdd.org/docs/state-dental-screening-laws-for-children-examining-the-trend-and_-impact-an-update-to-the-2008-report.pdf.
6. Oral Health in Schools. Home. American Academy of Pediatrics. 2022. www.aap.org/en/patient-care/school-health/oral-health-in-schools/#:~:text=AAP%20Oral%20Health%20and%20Education,referral%20relationships%20with%20dental%20professionals.&text=The%20Smiles%20For%20Life%20curriculum,oral%20health%20into%20primary%20care.
7. MCT: Resources for Parents. MCT | Resources for Parents. American Pediatric Dentists. www.mychildrensteeth.org/resources-for-parents/. Accessed 29 Feb 2024.
8. Wahl MD, et al. A comprehensive review of state vision screening mandates for schoolchildren in the United States. Optom Vis Sci. 2021;98(5):490–9. https://doi.org/10.1097/opx.0000000000001686.
9. Recommendations for preventive pediatric health care. American Academy & Bright Futures. 2023. https://downloads.aap.org/AAP/PDF/periodicity_schedule.pdf. Accessed 23 Feb 2024.
10. Nottingham Chaplin PK, Baldonado K, Hutchinson A, Moore B. Vision and eye health. NASN Sch Nurse. 2015;30(3):154–60. https://doi.org/10.1177/1942602x15581054.
11. Member Resources. Member Resources—American Association for Pediatric Ophthalmology and Strabismus. aapos.org/members/vision-screening-guidelines#:~:text=Refer%20children%20who%20cannot%20read,not%20reading%20at%20grade%20level. Accessed 19 Feb 2024.
12. Promoting Hearing Health in Schools. Centers for Disease Control and Prevention, Centers for Disease Control and Prevention. 2015. www.cdc.gov/healthyschools/noise/promoting.htm.
13. Seekhar D, Beiler JS, Schaefe EW, Henning A, Dillon JF, Czarnecki B, Zalewski TR. Certified school nurse perspectives on state-mandated hearing screens. J Sch Health. 2016;86(8):612–9.
14. American Academy of Audiology Clinical Practice Guidelines: clinical practice guidelines. American Academy of Audiology. 2011.
15. Guidelines for Audiology Service Provision in and for Schools. American Speech-Language-Hearing Association, American Speech-Language-Hearing Association. www.asha.org/policy/gl2002-00005/. Accessed 29 Feb 2024.
16. Mandated School Health Programs. Department of Health. 2022. www.health.pa.gov/topics/school/Pages/Mandated-School-Health-Programs.aspx.
17. Kowalski AE, Hartung SQ. Are body mass index screening programs in schools enough? Body mass index notification, follow-up, and school nurse role. NASN Sch Nurse. 2018;34(4):223–7. https://doi.org/10.1177/1942602x18814771.

18. Centers for Disease Control and Prevention. Body mass index (BMI) measurement in schools. Centers for Disease Control and Prevention. 2022. https://www.cdc.gov/healthyschools/obesity/bmi/bmi_measurement_schools.htm.
19. Scaturro D, et al. Adolescent idiopathic scoliosis screening: could a school-based assessment protocol be useful for an early diagnosis? J Back Musculoskelet Rehabil. 2021;34(2):301–6. https://doi.org/10.3233/bmr-200215.
20. Pennsylvania School Health Procedures: Conducting Scoliosis Screening. 2022.
21. Grossman DC, et al. Screening for adolescent idiopathic scoliosis. JAMA. 2018;319(2):165. https://doi.org/10.1001/jama.2017.19342.
22. Managing Asthma: A Guide For Schools. National Heart, Lung, and Blood Institute, National Asthma Education and Prevention Program (NAEPP). 2014. www.nhlbi.nih.gov/files/docs/resources/lung/NACI_ManagingAsthma-508%20FINAL.pdf. Accessed 28 Feb 2024.

Chapter 8
Immunizations

Alice I. Sato and Matthew Donahue

Immunizations, specifically school-age immunizations, are responsible for some of the greatest public health successes of all time. In addition to the complete eradication of smallpox from the world, school-age immunizations have enabled and sustained the eradication of two poliovirus strains and the elimination of endemic polio from United States, as well as the elimination of endemic measles and rubella from the Unites States. High immunization rates have led to dramatic reductions in other vaccine-preventable diseases (VPDs) as well. However, a disease may be reintroduced by an individual infected abroad and spread to susceptible persons, making maintenance of population immunity by vaccination an ongoing public health imperative.

8.1 Impact of School-Age Immunizations on Public Health

School-age immunization requirements in the United States originated in the 1850s with compulsory smallpox vaccination prior to kindergarten entry in Massachusetts. While many additional states enforced similar requirements by the 1900s, a nationally coordinated vaccine initiative for children involving local, state, and federal governments gained momentum in 1955 after Dr. Jonas Salk's poliovirus vaccine became fully licensed. In the years leading up to a licensed vaccine (1951–1954), polio caused an average of 16,316 cases of paralysis and 1879 deaths per year in the United States, mostly among children [1]. Following vaccine availability, incidence

A. I. Sato (✉)
The University of Nebraska Medical Center, Omaha, NE, USA
e-mail: alice.sato@unmc.edu

M. Donahue
Nebraska Department of Health and Human Services, Lincoln, NE, USA

R. P. Olympia, J. Brady-Olympia (eds.), *Clinical Considerations in School-based Health*, https://doi.org/10.1007/978-3-031-85765-2_8

declined to less than 100 cases of paralysis per year in the 1960s [2], with the last locally acquired case documented in 1979 [1]. Despite the elimination of endemic polio transmission in the United States, school-age polio immunization remains as important as ever to ensure children and communities are safeguarded against polio importations into the United States from the global community as a case of paralytic polio in an unvaccinated Rockland County, New York young adult in August 2022 clearly demonstrated [3].

Case 1 An 11 year old unvaccinated (due to religious exemptions) child is sent to the nurse's office by his teacher for a runny nose, cough, and watery redness of his eyes. He is found to have a fever of 102 so he is sent home with advice to seek medical care. The next day, the county health department calls to inform you that he is suspected to have measles, acquired from his visiting unvaccinated cousins who had been abroad.

Measles elimination in the United States, through school-age immunizations, is similarly impactful. Measles is highly communicable and spread through airborne transmission, with more than a 90% attack rate among unimmune close contacts. While measles was encountered frequently prior to the arrival of licensed vaccine in 1963 (90% of children estimated to be infected by 15 years of age) [4], it had serious health impacts: 1 in 5 unvaccinated patients with measles required hospitalization; 1 out of every 1000 children infected developed encephalitis; and 1–3 out of every 1000 children infected died [5]. In the years leading up to a licensed vaccine (1958–1962), public health authorities identified an average of 503,282 measles cases (true estimates of 3–4 million per year prior to vaccine) and 432 measles-related deaths per year [1]. Following the arrival of measles vaccine, measles incidence declined by more than 95% and endemic measles transmission was declared eliminated from the United States in 2000. Measles outbreaks in the United States today are characterized by measles importations from the global community and transmission among under-vaccinated communities [6]. For January 1-May 23, 2024, there were 142 cases of measles in the US reported in 21 jurisdictions [7]. Only 5% of cases were fully immunized. More than half required hospitalization for isolation or management of measles complications. One dose of MMR remains 93% effective, and two doses 97% effective at preventing measles [7].

Case 1 Resolution You quickly review your school's vaccination data and work with the health department to generate a list of high-risk contacts who need to be excluded and those who should be offered vaccination or screened by their health provider for prophylaxis. You also collaborate on family and community notification letters in appropriate languages and help provide community education on the disease and its risks, especially for those at high risk of severe disease. You support your health department in connecting families with social and educational supports needed, particularly for those who require extended quarantine and school exclusion.

8.2 Herd Immunity and Outbreak Prevention

School-age immunizations not only prevent illness and school absences in individual students, they can also support "herd immunity" which affords widespread protection from disease and outbreaks to whole communities. Individuals can become immune through either vaccination or through infection. Herd immunity is typically defined as the threshold of collective immunity, as a proportion of the population, that results in overall reduction of disease transmission in that community, and accordingly indirectly benefits those who are not immune [8]. Herd immunity is a critical tool in reducing disease in communities because not everyone can get vaccinated, such as those who are immunocompromised, taking chemotherapy, living with HIV, too young to receive vaccines, unable to access vaccines, or refuse vaccines.

Herd immunity threshold estimates are different for each disease and are based on the speed at which different diseases can be transmitted between people (the basic reproductive rate.) Generally, to prevent transmission in a community, 95% or 80% of individuals in that community must be immune to measles or polio, respectively [9]. Recent measles outbreaks have been able to propagate due at least in part by communities falling below this estimated herd immunity threshold.

8.3 Immunization Basics

Although vaccines may be designed using different approaches, all recommended vaccines help train the immune system to defend against a disease without the harms that come from a full-blown infection with that pathogen. Immunization results in specific immunity via antibodies and/or specialized lymphocytes that recognize bits of the pathogen or infected host cells. For contagious infections (spread from person to person), immunization can help prevent spread to others by blocking infection or decreasing the amount of pathogen produced that could spread to others. A few vaccines recommended for US children (e.g. Measles-Mumps-Rubella, Varicella, Rotavirus) are live-attenuated vaccines, meaning that they are weakened, so do not cause disease in the small doses given; the immune response to the attenuated strain is nearly identical to that produced by natural infection (*aka* infection induced immunity). However, live vaccines may pose a health threat to persons with compromised immune systems so these persons may be exempted if risk of that specific vaccination exceeds its benefit. In some situations, so-called passive immunity is provided by giving the person antibody-containing products (such as monoclonal antibody preparation or pooled immunoglobulins from blood donors) that bind to the pathogen and may neutralize and/or help with immune system clearance of the pathogen.

The majority of vaccines are non-live or non-replicating vaccines. These vaccines (examples in parentheses) include inactivated or "killed" bacterial or viruses (inactivated polio), subunit (hepatitis B), protein-polysaccharide conjugate (*Haemophilus influenzae* type b), toxoid-based (tetanus), or mRNA vaccines (COVID-19). These vaccines generally require more doses than live vaccines to establish immunity, and booster doses to maintain it. However, they are safe for immunocompromised individuals to receive. Some vaccines, such as seasonal influenza and COVID-19, require updated vaccines to cover currently circulating strains or serotypes of the pathogens.

All recommended vaccines have undergone extensive pre-approval safety and efficacy testing. Multiple vaccine safety systems, such as the Vaccine Adverse Event Reporting System (VAERS) and the Vaccine Safety Datalink (VSD), provide ongoing monitoring and proactive searches of vaccine-related data [10]. Vaccine recommendations are ultimately made by the CDC's independent Advisory Committee on Immunization Practices (ACIP), a group of medical and public health experts who recommend ages when vaccines should be administered, number of doses and timing, precautions and contraindications for use [11]. The immunization schedules are updated annually and available online [12] or as the "CDC Vaccines Schedules" free app [13]. Versions in English or Spanish designed for parents are also available [14].

Additional vaccines are in development. With newer vaccine technologies, including mRNA platforms and more rapid development techniques for protein subunit vaccines, interest in vaccine development for regionally relevant diseases (e.g. Lyme disease, dengue virus), common diseases with latency (e.g. EBV), diarrheal diseases (e.g. norovirus, Shigella) or potential emerging or reemerging diseases (e.g. tuberculosis, novel influenza viruses) has grown. However, such vaccines are unlikely to be required for school attendance, at least in the near term.

8.4 The Role of School Nurses and School Based Health Centers

Schools are required to collect and report immunization compliance data, perform communicable disease surveillance, and work to improve the number of students receiving required immunizations. School immunization records must be maintained, and an immunization information system (IIS) can provide an accessible and searchable file for each student. Whatever system is used, school nurses need to be able to rapidly identify students and staff susceptible to disease due to lack of immunization so that notification of families and school administrators of who needs to be excluded following exposure to an infected person can be done in a timely manner. Sharing of school vaccination coverage data with local and state public health officials as allowable by law also helps identify communities in need of increased support to meet vaccination goals.

Some states support vaccination registries which may be particularly helpful for determining vaccination status of children whose families have incomplete records, who have received care in multiple locations or jurisdictions, who have moved school districts, or have housing insecurity or other challenges. Students may have also received vaccinations in other countries. The Minnesota Department of Health offers the VaxRef form to help families enter vaccination information in some select languages [15]. The New Mexico Department of Health has prepared a helpful guide to disease, vaccine and related terms in 33 languages and a list of international trade names of common vaccines [16]. Vaccine doses received abroad are acceptable if schedules and doses are compatible with the US ACIP recommendations [17]. Determination of the validity and acceptability of international vaccines should be conducted with the school medical advisor and/or patient's personal medical provider, and when in doubt the prior immunizations should be disregarded and catch-up immunization performed instead [17].

Case 2 Your school in the last school year had to delay the entry of many kindergartners due to incomplete vaccination that failed to meet the minimum requirements set by state law. Feedback from families highlighted a lack of understanding of the requirements prior to the school year start date and lack of access to medical care or understanding of where to receive low cost or free immunizations. You discuss your concerns with the school medical advisor and local health department.

Despite the recent decrease in immunization, the Healthy People 2030 target of 95% routine kindergarten vaccination coverage [18] by ensuring vaccination of all kindergartners without a documented exemption remains achievable. The CDC has developed the "Let's RISE [Routine Immunizations on Schedule for Everyone]" campaign and associated toolkits to support actionable strategies to get all Americans on track for recommended vaccines [19]. Schools are recognized as one of key pillars along with health departments, health care professionals, and other partners for this work. Schools can provide information on vaccines, communicate the importance of vaccination, and guide and support families to make sure their students are appropriately vaccinated. Summer communications are recommended to allow for catch-up vaccination so that students are ready for entry at the next school year. Importantly, schools can help connect students with vaccination services. School-located vaccination events, school-based health clinics, or immunization services provided by the local health department (either off campus or with mobile support to bring vaccination to the school) can reduce barriers to students receiving needed immunizations. Schools can help connect students and families to providers at community health centers or local pharmacies as well. School-located vaccine clinics (SLVs) have offered both routine and seasonal influenza vaccinations for decades, meaningfully lowering the rates of infection and illness due to vaccine preventable diseases (VPDs). School nurses can provide leadership and collaborate with community partners and stakeholders on the logistics of SLVs and unite school administrators and educators in support. School nurses engaged in personal outreach efforts (e.g. phone calls with families) increase participation in SLVs and improve community perceptions of vaccination. Resources to support SLVs are available online from the Association of Immunization Managers [20].

Case 2 Resolution With support from your school administration and local health department, you are able to send out communications over the summer to families about the vaccine requirements. You are able to post information in other public areas, including libraries and WIC offices. You organize a community event that includes additional information and the public health department provides a free mobile clinic to assist with vaccination.

8.5 Public Health Law and School-Age Immunizations

Challenges to school-age immunization requirements have persisted alongside those requirements since their original inception for smallpox immunizations [21]. In 1905, the United States Supreme Court upheld the authority of states to pass and enforce immunization requirements in order to support common welfare [22]. The United States Supreme Court further supported school-age immunization requirements through city ordinance in 1922 [23]. Despite a long history of legal challenges, all 50 states have legislation requiring school-age immunizations [24]. Most states' laws apply to both public and private schools, and several states include homeschools as well [25, 26]. Although specifics and exemptions vary by state, most require four common vaccines (DTaP, polio, MMR, varicella) for kindergarten enrollment. The number of required doses may also vary; for example, Nebraska only requires 3 doses of polio vaccine and DTaP, while most states require 4 and 5 doses respectively. Many states additionally require meningococcal vaccine and/or TdaP booster for middle school entry. In the 2022–2023 school year, 28 states allowed for provisional enrollment or grace period status for kindergartners to attend school while on a catch-up vaccine schedule. Exemptions themselves pose a risk to children and communities. Across the US, children with an exemption (medical or non-medical) increased from 2.6% during the 2021–2022 school year to 3.0% in the 2022–2023 school year [27], not only the highest exemption rate on record but with the increase solely attributable to an increase in non-medical exemptions from 2.3% to 2.8%. Concerningly, increases in exemptions occurred in 40 states and D.C., and in 10 states the exemption rate exceeds 5%, making it virtually impossible to achieve the 95% MMR coverage goal. Nonetheless, the goal remains to achieve as high a rate of immunization of students, staff and families as possible.

Extra Credit Points

1. Vaccines have improved the lives of Americans by preventing disease, serious complications, and spread of infection to other people.
2. There is a concerning decrease in immunization rates amongst children.
3. School nurses have an important role in identifying children in need of, advocating for, and administering of vaccines.

References

1. CDC. Impact of Vaccines Universally Recommended for Children—United States, 1990–1998. MMWR Morb Mortal Wkly Rep. 1999;48(12):243–8.
2. CDC. Pinkbook: Poliomyelitis. 2023. www.cdc.gov/vaccines/pubs/pinkbook/polio.html.
3. CDC Newsroom. United States confirmed as country with circulating vaccine-derived poliovirus. 2022. www.cdc.gov/media/releases/2022/s0913-polio.html.
4. CDC. Pinkbook: Measles. 2022. www.cdc.gov/vaccines/pubs/pinkbook/meas.html.
5. CDC. Measles symptoms and complications. Measles (Rubeola). www.cdc.gov/measles/signs-symptoms/index.html.
6. Mathis AD. Measles—United States, January 1, 2020–March 28, 2024. MMWR Morb Mortal Wkly Rep. 2024;73:295–300. https://doi.org/10.15585/mmwr.mm7314a1.
7. CDC. Measles cases and outbreaks. Measles (Rubeola). www.cdc.gov/measles/data-research/index.html.
8. Bullen M, Heriot GS, Jamrozik E. Herd immunity, vaccination and moral obligation. J Med Ethics. 2023;49(9):636–41. https://doi.org/10.1136/jme-2022-108485.
9. The relationship between vaccines and herd immunity. Columbia University Mailman School of Public Health. www.publichealth.columbia.edu/news/relationship-between-vaccines-herd-immunity.
10. CDC. Vaccine safety monitoring. 2024. www.cdc.gov/vaccinesafety/ensuringsafety/monitoring/index.html.
11. Understanding the ACIP and how vaccine recommendations are made in the US. 2022. www.youtube.com/watch?v=WWf4xVw1-PE.
12. CDC. Help your patients stay up-to-date. Centers for Disease Control and Prevention. www.cdc.gov/vaccines/schedules/hcp/index.html.
13. CDC. Vaccine schedules App. www.cdc.gov/vaccines/schedules/hcp/schedule-app.html.
14. CDC. Vaccine schedules for parents. www.cdc.gov/vaccines/parents/schedules/index.html.
15. VaxRef Form—MN Dept. of Health. https://forms.web.health.state.mn.us/es/form/vaxref.
16. Foreign language terms. www.nmhealth.org/publication/view/help/453/.
17. CDC. Immunizations. Immigrant and refugee health. www.cdc.gov/immigrant-refugee-health/hcp/domestic-guidance/immunizations.html.
18. Maintain the vaccination coverage level of 2 doses of the MMR vaccine for children in kindergarten—IID-04—healthy People 2030. https://health.gov/healthypeople/objectives-and-data/browse-objectives/vaccination/maintain-vaccination-coverage-level-2-doses-mmr-vaccine-children-kindergarten-iid-04.
19. CDC. Routine immunizations on schedule for everyone (RISE). www.cdc.gov/vaccines/partners/routine-immunizations-lets-rise.html.
20. Association of Immunization Managers. School-located vaccination clinics toolkit. www.immunizationmanagers.org/resources-toolkits/slv-toolkit/.
21. Smith PJ, Wood D, Darden PM. Highlights of historical events leading to National Surveillance of vaccination coverage in the United States. Public Health Rep. 2011;126(Suppl 2):3–12.
22. Jacobson v. Massachusetts, 197 U.S. 11 1905. Justia Law. https://supreme.justia.com/cases/federal/us/197/11/.
23. Zucht v. King, 260 U.S. 174 (1922). Justia Law. https://supreme.justia.com/cases/federal/us/260/174/.
24. The development of the immunization schedule. https://historyofvaccines.org/getting-vaccinated/vaccines-children/development-immunization-schedule.

25. Seither R. Coverage with selected vaccines and exemption from school vaccine requirements among children in kindergarten—United States, 2022–23 school year. MMWR Morb Mortal Wkly Rep. 2023;72:1217. https://doi.org/10.15585/mmwr.mm7245a2.
26. CDC. State School Immunization Requirements and Vaccine Exemption Laws. https://www.cdc.gov/phlp/docs/school-vaccinations.pdf.
27. CDC. SchoolVaxView Interactive School Vaccination Coverage. www.cdc.gov/vaccines/imz-managers/coverage/schoolvaxview/data-reports/index.html.

Chapter 9
Health Education for Students

Diana Dur

Case 1 **You are asked to put together a presentation that will help kindergarten students gain familiarity with the school nurse, demonstrate the type of care available in the nurse's office, and ease the fear of needing treatment during the school day. What kind of presentation would you propose?**

Case 2 **A 13-year-old student comes to the nurse's office with an itchy head. Upon examining her head, the nurse discovers numerous live lice and nits. What forms of education should the nurse be preparing and who is the target audience?**

Case 3 **The administrative team is gearing up for all the events that come with spring in high school such as proms, graduation, dances, etc. The team has tasked you, the school nurse, to help them along with counselors and teachers to put together a safety event. The goal of the event is to demonstrate the importance of safe, responsible actions that teens should take as well as making them aware of the consequences of unsafe irresponsible choices. Topics will include drinking under age, driving under the influence, and drug use. What type of event could you put together that is appropriate for this age group?**

School nurses themselves often debate their role in health education of students. Discussions vary from enthusiasm to provide education, to hesitancy due to school hierarchy, to uncertainty that it is even an expectation of the role of a school nurse. The National Association of School Nurse's (NASN) has published a position statement advocating for health education in schools while fully supporting the school nurse to collaborate with the other members of the school team in the delivery of health education [1]. NASN further obligates school nurses with the duty of

D. Dur (✉)
Great Valley School District, Malvern, PA, USA

R. P. Olympia, J. Brady-Olympia (eds.), *Clinical Considerations in School-based Health*, https://doi.org/10.1007/978-3-031-85765-2_9

ensuring that the health education provided is evidence-based while also considering laws and regulations that guide the planning and implementation processes [1]. Working with other members of the school team, school nurses use the Framework for twenty-first Century School Nursing Practice™ to influence health education for students whether it be in the health office, classroom, or community [1]. The School Nursing Practice Framework published by NASN includes four practice principles for school nurses two of which mention health education of students [2]. Health education of students fall under both the leadership practice principle as well as the community/public health practice principle [2].

9.1 Health Literacy

School nurses promote health literacy in the students they support at school by creating relationships built on trust [2]. Health literacy is defined as a person's capability of discovering and applying health information to make choices and take actions on issues regarding their health [3]. One of the most important focuses on Health literacy is to not only comprehend information related to health but to utilize services and skills based on knowledge rather than what is acceptable [3]. Informed decision making can help make more knowledgeable and self-advocating healthcare consumers [4]. School nurses are a routine part of the school environment with open doors that welcome children anytime they are sought out [4]. This relationship is one where students are able to help school aged children become comfortable with healthcare professionals and practice control over their health and wellness [4]. Healthcare anxiety is not only a barrier to health literacy but also to seeking medical attention, however school nurses are poised to combat health care anxiety by reinforcing the desire of health professionals to help [4].

9.2 One on One

Health education often comes in the one on one setting during routine health visits. Nurses teach students about normal body functions and share tips for routine first aid and self-care.

School nurses help students understand complex medical diagnoses and help them understand how to navigate their diagnosis on a daily basis.

9.3 Classroom

For school nurses who teach a health education class to a group of students they must be familiar with course designs, developing a syllabus, grading, and instruction methods. Health education can take the form of classroom instruction depending on state requirements. Some states require a teaching license to teach a class full of students. For example, Pennsylvania Department of Education states, "A person holding a valid and active Pennsylvania teaching certificate in the area of Health and Physical Education K-12 is qualified to teach all health and physical education courses in grades K-12" [5]. Detailed age appropriate academic standards have been defined by PDE as well and have been broken down by school setting in Table 9.1 [6].

School nurses should plan their health education curriculum depending on the presence of official school board voted health curriculums [7]. If no specific health

Table 9.1 Health Standards by School Setting

	Elementary school	Middle school	High school
Health concepts	I.D. Stages of growth	Analyze nutritional concepts	Evaluate factors that impact growth and development into adulthood (acute/chronic illness, relationships, career choices)
	I.D. Major body systems (digestive, musculoskeletal, circulatory, etc.)	Describe factors that influence adolescent drug use	Evaluate issue that arise related to use/nonuse of drugs (laws, impact, psychology of addiction, etc.)
Living healthy	I.D environmental factors that influence health (pollutions, temperatures, insects, etc.)	Decision making theory on making health choices along with the influence of social media on health	Evaluate products that impact adult health and what influences/impacts the health choices of adults
	Personal hygiene practices that promote health	Explore environmental factors that influence health (indoor pollution, chemicals, etc.)	Explore environmental factors and community health (public health policy, recreational activities)
Safety and Injury Prevention	Learn safe and unsafe actions at home and school	Explain and apply safe actions in home, school, and community	Explore laws and consequences of unsafe actions (Mock DUI)
	Conflict awareness	Strategies to avoid and solve conflict and violence	Understand the impact of violence on the individual and the community
Physical activity	Engage in physical activity	Engage in physical activity	Engage in physical activity
	Know positive effects of exercise	Identify ways to monitor response to physical exercise (BP and HR monitoring)	Analyze how physical activity affects adult health

curriculum has been previously adopted by the school district the school nurse may move forward with exploring state adopted health education standards that outline specific learning goals broken down by grade level to guide lesson planning [7]. The Centers for Disease Control and Prevention (CDC) after much research has advised that health curriculums should account for obtainment of knowledge and skill while acknowledging the influence of "attitudes, norms, and beliefs" on learning [8]. These lessons can be demonstrative forms of teaching such as handwashing lessons while visiting the classroom or interactive games that reinforce content [7]. The effective school nurse should develop lessons that teach content while keeping students engaged and allowing room for demonstration of learning and feedback [7].

9.4 Bulletin Boards

Nurses also provide health education through bulletin boards that can cover a variety of topics from nutrition and physical activity to raising awareness about seizures and allergies (Fig. 9.1). The boards are a way to reach a larger number of students than the one on one discussions. Visually attractive boards capture attention and relay small amounts of information to student that pass by [7]. Boards are helpful

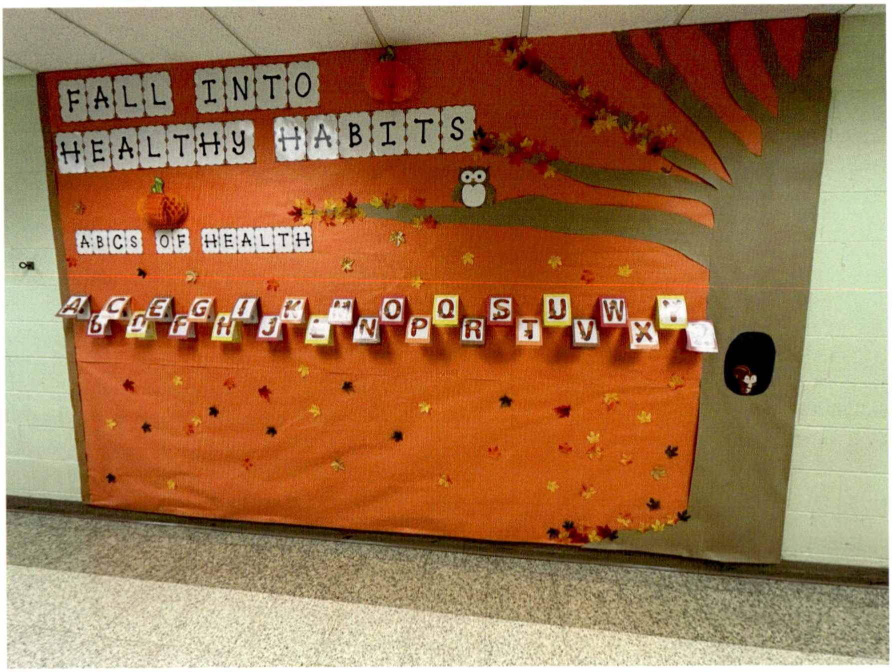

Fig. 9.1 A bulletin board provides health education to many students who walk through the hallway

for the school nurse with limited free time to devote to specific student education opportunities [7].

9.5 Newsletters

Newsletters and articles in both student and parent focused publications and emails are also tools that can be used to provide health education to students [7]. Preparing topics on a regular basis can provide tips for staying well or overcoming illness [7]. This form of communication also allows for electronic sources and activities to be shared with families to review or engage their student with.

9.6 Virtual Lessons

The time during the school day is a limitation reported by many school nurses. Virtual classroom lessons help the school nurse provide health education without leaving the health office. Examples of virtual lessons include video recordings of lessons on health education made by the school nurse that classroom teachers play for the class [7]. Another option is virtual meetings that allow nurses to interact with students in real time from a location other than the classroom. This type of set up could allow nurses to interreact with multiple classrooms simultaneously, making it time effective.

9.7 Programs and Outside Collaboration

School nurses will also collaborate with outside programs for health education. Some groups will bring in health education programs on specific topics such as dental health. Other groups may bring in physical challenges that work specifically within the physical education class such as turkey trots. Sometimes there may be assemblies and other whole school initiatives like health fairs to deliver health education like dental education and bicycle safety [9]. In these situations, the school nurse is using their leadership and networking skills to bring these programs to their students rather than directly providing the education to students themselves.

9.8 Barriers/Considerations/Limitations

Time is one of the biggest obstacles to providing health education for school nurses who are also responsible for data collection for the state, record keeping, charting, health screening, and daily care for all students. Nurses report not having enough time in the day to complete all of their tasks. Language barriers are another limitation in providing health education due to the need for school nurse to translate documents and lessons as needed which takes more valuable time but is necessary to effectively reach all students. Budgets are another thing that nurses need to consider when providing health education. Utilizing outside resources may incur costs that need to be appropriately budgeted, some school health budgets do not have room for these services [9]. Collaborating with other community members to identify free services may be feasible but will require the school nurse to find time to network and build relationships for the endeavors to be successful.

9.9 The Future of Student Health Education

Since 2020 schools made major changes to the delivery models for education moving to more online and electronic forms of delivery [10]. Since the return to the classroom many of these new technologies remain present in the learning setting as an adjunct to tradition classroom interactions and these may help shape the future of school health education for students. Some school districts have moved toward offering telehealth visits in the school-based health center and schools such as cyber charter schools have always relied on virtual services [10]. While these services might not be the future of all health education in the public school setting it does offer some insight into what the future of school health education might look like for the school nurse. In the virtual health offices, the school nurse can send electronic forms of education, and integrate other apps to help students create actionable steps to meet their individualized health plan goals. This could be adapted to all types of school settings [10].

Social media may also play a role in health education for students. Patients use the internet and social media to find answers to health questions and health professionals are increasing their presence on social networking sites [11]. Typical social media use related to health education are to change behavior, learning how to prevent or manage disease, and learning more through blogs, discussion boards, and app based social media [11]. Positive results of online/ social media health interactions include learning new information and skills while on the go and improved communication with providers [11]. Problems with social media, especially in teens, include further isolation, exposure to possible cyber bullying, and reinforcing addictive behaviors [11]. Balancing the positive and negative aspects of social media is a challenge but virtual health offices, school nurse websites like Greater Commonwealth Virtual School, and even TikTok™ pages run by school nurses, such as @mrs.palo, offer a new way of offering student health education to students in the online space.

9.10 Case Resolution

Case 1 The school nurse could plan a classroom visit for an in-person lesson or prepare a prerecorded video that could be shown by the classroom teacher. The nurse would introduce themselves and explain the types of care they provide from cleaning injuries and applying Band-Aids to reviewing treatment options for common kindergarten illness complaints. A recorded presentation allows the nurse to provide a brief tour of the office and health office procedures. A handwashing lesson may also be a helpful topic that reinforces personal hygiene practices.

Case 2 School District policy may influence the procedure in which health education will be provided. The student will be the first person that the nurse will educate. Compassionate and one on one age appropriate education will help the student understand what is happening and how it is treated. Education for a student of this age can verbal or written and parents should be included. Other classmates might have itching symptoms that will be sent to the nurse for assessment. Based on findings the nurse will provide education to that student while maintaining the confidentiality of the first student. School district policy will also dictate what information, if any, is sent home to families for an incidence of lice in school. The nurse may also have lice information on the district-based website that can referenced or in the school board documents.

Case 3 For the high school age group presentations are a way to reach a large student body with information regarding health and safety. Mock crash presentations can raise the awareness of driver safety and safe decision making while showing students the potential outcomes of unsafe decisions in a controlled environment. The school-based team may also choose to work with other outside organizations, such as Mothers Against Drunk Driving (MADD) that bring in speakers or virtual presentations about age specific topics that help high school student better understand safety and legal/societal consequences of unsafe actions.

Extra Credit Points

1. School Nurses provided health education in a variety of settings including classrooms, the health office, and virtual.
2. Newsletters, billboards, classroom curriculum, video, websites, programs and one on one conversations allow nurse to provided health education to students.
3. As social media use increases this may be a new way to provide students with health education.

References

1. National Association of School Nurses. Position Statement: Comprehensive Health Education in Schools. NASN Sch Nurse. 2022;38(3):155–6. https://doi.org/10.1177/1942602X221124671.
2. Tanner A, Griffin R, Stanislo K, Hinkley T, Walsh C, Clark E, Graf K, La Point R, D'Souza-Vazirani D. A contemporary framework update for today's school nursing landscape: introducing the school nursing practice framework™. NASN Sch Nurse. 2024;39(3):140–7. https://doi.org/10.1177/1942602X241241092.
3. What is Health Literacy? Centers for Disease Control Update. 2023. https://www.cdc.gov/healthliteracy/learn/index.html. Accessed 20 Apr 2024.
4. School nurses play vital role in developing children's health literacy. Penn State Pro Wellness. 2023. https://prowellness.childrens.pennstatehealth.org/school-nurses-play-vital-role-in-developing-childrens-health-literacy/. Accessed 21 Mar 2024.
5. Health and Physical Education. Pennsylvania Department of Education. https://www.education.pa.gov/Teachers%20%20Administrators/Curriculum/HealthPhysicalEd/Pages/default.aspx#:~:text=Certification,courses%20in%20grades%20K%2D12. Accessed 21 Mar 2024.
6. Academic Standards for Health, Safety, and Physical Education. Pennsylvania Department of Education. https://www.stateboard.education.pa.gov/Documents/Regulations%20and%20Statements/State%20Academic%20Standards/SandyHealth.pdf. Accessed 14 Jun 2024.
7. Galemore C. Health education—it's elementary, or not? NASN Sch Nurse. 2023;38(3):108–11. https://doi.org/10.1177/1942602X231164811.
8. Johns J, Moyer M. The attitudes, beliefs, and norms framework: a tool for selecting student-centered, theory-informed affective learning objectives in health education. J Health Educ Teach. 2018;9(1):14–26.
9. Lineberry M, Whitney E, Nolan M. The role of school nurses, challenges, and reactions to delegation legislation: a qualitative approach. J Sch Nurs. 2018;34(3):222–31. https://doi.org/10.1177/1059840517741526.
10. Marrapese B, Gormley J, Deschene K. Reimagining school nursing: lessons learned from a virtual school nurse. NASN Sch Nurse. 2021;36(4):218–25. https://doi.org/10.1177/1942602X21996432.
11. Giustini D, Ali S, Fraser M, Kamel BM. Effective uses of social media in public health and medicine: a systematic review of systematic reviews. Online J Public Health Inform. 2018;10(2):e215. https://doi.org/10.5210/ojphi.v10i2.8270.

Chapter 10
Research and Scholarship in School-Based Health

Robert P. Olympia and Christina Hermann

Case 1 **You are a school-based physician. You have been approached by several colleagues in your state requesting that you collaborate on a multi-institutional research study. The study examines factors that contribute to the increasing number of students being referred to local emergency departments for asthma exacerbations during the past year, and whether adopting a statewide stock albuterol policy would decrease the number of referrals. You have never conducted clinical research, and wonder if participating in this study may be beneficial to your career.**

A career in academic medicine involves *demonstrating scholarship, gaining knowledge, and providing education. Demonstrating scholarship* involves imparting knowledge that results from study and research in a particular field and the dissemination of this knowledge, thus becoming an expert in a particular field. *Knowledge* is the sum or range of what is perceived, discovered, and learned over time, therefore practicing "life-long learning". Providing education is the act of imparting knowledge and skill to another person/group or to cause to learn by example or experience, thus becoming a teacher and mentor. Reasons to participate in research and scholarship are listed in Table 10.1.

R. P. Olympia (✉)
Department of Emergency Medicine and Pediatrics, Penn State College of Medicine
Attending Physician, Hershey, PA, USA

Division of Pediatric Emergency Medicine, Department of Emergency Medicine, Penn State
Milton S. Hershey Medical Center, Hershey, PA, USA
e-mail: rolympia@hmc.psu.edu

C. Hermann
Penn State College of Medicine, Hershey, PA, USA

R. P. Olympia, J. Brady-Olympia (eds.), *Clinical Considerations in School-based Health*, https://doi.org/10.1007/978-3-031-85765-2_10

Table 10.1 Why should you care about research and scholarship?

Networking	Whether it is collaborating with colleagues on multi-institutional research projects, participating on panel discussions, or networking with providers at scientific assemblies or conferences who share the same passions that you do, participating in research and education can open doors to other scholarship opportunities
Financial gain	Institutions may incentivize scholarship disseminated, provide payment for lectures given, or reimburse registration fees and travel expenses for the dissemination of knowledge
Travel opportunities	Scientific assemblies and conferences are often in large cities or exotic locations, which adds to the allure of presenting research or giving lectures
Advancing your career	Broadening your curriculum vitae through involvement in research, education and other forms of scholarship may advance your career and open opportunities in administration, leadership, or academia, both regionally and nationally
Climbing the academic ladder	The goal of any academic physician is climbing the academic ladder, from Clinical Instructor to Assistant Professor to Associate Professor and ultimately Professor. Performance expectations increase as you advance in academic rank, developing mastery and independence in your field, increasing scholarly accomplishments, growing your regional and national reputation, and demonstrating professional leadership One of the criteria for promotion involves achieving professional excellence in the area of "Research and Creative Accomplishments", which includes evidence of scholarship such as (a) publications [peer-reviewed journal articles, book chapters, review articles, case reports, or becoming a book or journal editors], (b) research projects [completed, current, planned, internal and external grants obtained], and (c) other creative products (e.g., educational methods or computer software developed; inventions; clinical guidelines disseminated)

10.1 Pearls from a Scholarship Enthusiast

10.1.1 Find Your Passion, Seek Out Your Niche

Do you remember why you chose school-based health as a career? Allow this passion to motivate your career in academia and guide your research, education and scholarship. Research can be fun and rewarding as long as it aligns with your interests and fits within the construct of your career goals and work-life balance. Passions and priorities may shift during your career and life, so continuously performing self-reflection to determine your passions is the most important step to becoming a successful academic healthcare provider.

10.1.2 Be Innovative and Strive for Greatness in Your Scholarship

If you select "hot topics" for research and lectures, and projects that are innovative, interesting, or impactful, your audience will be excited to hear about your scholarship, and subsequently disseminate the knowledge you provided to others. Find out what research has been published in the past (Table 10.2), and take the initiative to develop innovative ideas for future scholarship based on deficiencies in the evidence. Go to scientific assemblies and conferences, hear what ground breaking research is being presented or what lecture topics create the most buzz, and be inspired to build on that scholarship. Be the academician and educator that the world wants to hear about.

10.1.3 Not All Scholarship Is Research

Not everyone is inspired to participate in hypothesis driven research. It can be time consuming and exhausting. Scholarship can include writing chapters for medical textbooks, case reports or review articles, developing podcasts to disseminate knowledge, or participating in quality improvement projects to elevate the health of students at your school.

Table 10.2 Most common topics reported in a bibliometric analysis of school-based research articles, 2014–2024[a] [1]

Topics	Number of publications	Percentage of total publications in the sample (n = 953)
Physical activity and nutrition	344	36%
Health promotion/health education	236	25%
Mental health	176	19%
Obesity	145	15%
Substance use	117	12%
Socioeconomic status/minorities	64	7%
Violence (includes abuse and bullying)	54	6%
Home environment/parents	50	5%
Reproductive health	45	5%
Academic performance	42	4%
Oral health	32	3%
Wellness	31	3%
Hygiene	27	3%

[a]A bibliometric analysis of 953 articles published from 2014 to 2024 resulting from a PubMed search of keyword terms "School Health Services" and "School Mental Health Services"

10.1.4 Surround Yourself with Greatness

Find advisors and mentors that will guide you not only through your career in academia, but also with life. During the planning stages for research, surround yourself with experts in the field (both regionally and nationally, and might involve "strategic stalking"—utilizing medical literature or Google searches to contact and develop relationships with colleagues who have conducted research or lectured on your research topic) and a research team (medical librarian, biostatistician, ethicist, Human Subject Protection Office member, etc.). Teamwork makes the dream work.

10.1.5 Keep Lecturing and Writing, Become a Scholar

Seek out educational opportunities—lectures at your institution may turn into Grand Rounds regionally, and then expert panels nationally. Turn lectures into review articles or book chapters, turn clinical questions into research ideas, turn quality improvement ideas into scholarship. Lectureships and publications will increase your reputation, and in turn lead to multicenter research collaborations, opportunities to serve within your specialty, and means to improve the care of children globally. A laptop, pen/paper, and thinking outside the box will be your best friend.

Case 2 You are a school-based physician with a passion for emergency and disaster preparedness. You have recently completed a questionnaire-based study examining the current state of emergency and disaster preparedness of schools in the United States and would like to disseminate your results. What steps should you take to demonstrate scholarship?

With the assistance of a research mentor, you have successfully collected and analyzed data to answer your research question. You have organized piles of data spreadsheets and have met with your biostatistician, so what do you do next? It's time to create the impact that you hoped for with the research you have conducted, but before you do that, here are some questions you want to think about before you decide how to disseminate your results:

Who is your audience? Who will benefit the most from the research you have conducted? Is it your students, or the physicians, school nurses, and school-health providers who care for students worldwide? Is it school staff and administrators, athletic trainers, or coaches? Is it policy makers or specific organizations/society leadership? Is it the general public? Defining your audience is an important first step to determine the most effective method of research dissemination.

What do you want your audience to learn from your research? It is likely that once your research project is completed, you will feel overwhelmed with the amount of data you have collected. Step back and think about your hypothesis, your primary and secondary outcomes, and the data that you have collected that supports or rejects your hypothesis. Now select 2–3 main points/conclusions you want your audience to take away from hearing or reading about your research. This simplifies your results and conclusions, and allows your audience to remember and disseminate the results of your study.

Are there any aspects of your research that will make it difficult to disseminate? Every study faces aspects that may make dissemination difficult. Recognizing these obstacles and addressing their effect on your conclusion is an important step before you disseminate your results. These include study design limitations, obtaining negative or equivocal results, results that contradict previously published data, and types of bias, including information bias, selection bias, and confounding bias.

10.2 Methods of Research Dissemination

Now that you have answered the questions above, it is time to consider methods of research dissemination. The most common methods include:

1. Publication of your research in a peer-reviewed journal.
2. Presentation of your research at a national and/or regional scientific assembly.
3. Non-traditional forms of research dissemination.

10.2.1 Publication of Your Research in a Peer-Reviewed Journal

Find a journal that will target your chosen audience, that will create the most "buzz" and reach the most people, and that will create impact within a reasonable amount of time. Aspects to consider when choosing an appropriate journal include audience, impact factor, traditional subscription journals vs. open access journals, and indexing.

(a) *Audience*: Most peer-reviewed journals target a particular audience/specialty or are sponsored by a specific society/membership (such as the American Academy of Pediatrics' *Pediatrics* or the National Association of School Nurses' *The Journal of School Nursing*). Consider your audience when choosing a peer-reviewed journal to submit to. Table 10.3 lists some possible journals for submission of school-based original research or case reports.

(b) *Impact factor:* A journal's impact factor for a particular year is calculated by the total number of times articles in the journal were cited during the previous 2 years divided by the total number of citable articles in the journal during those 2 years. In most fields, an impact factor of 10 or greater is considered an excellent score while 3 is considered good, but it is important to remember that these impact factors vary across disciplines. If you want your research to reach the

Table 10.3 Possible journals and their 2023 impact factors for school-based research and case reports

General medical journals	2023 Impact factor
The Lancet	98.4
The New England Journal of Medicine	96.2
BMJ	93.6
JAMA	63.1
JAMA Network Open	13.8
General pediatrics journals	
JAMA Pediatrics	26.1
Pediatrics	8.0
Archives of Disease in Childhood	4.3
The Journal of Pediatrics	3.9
Pediatric Research	3.1
Frontiers in Pediatrics	2.1
BMC Pediatrics	2.0
School-based health journals	
Journal of School Health	1.8
Journal of School Nursing	1.5
Miscellaneous[a]	
BMC Public Health	3.5
Trials	2.0
BMJ Open	2.9
International Journal of Environmental Research and Public Health	N/A
Public Library of Science One	2.9
International Journal of Behavioral Nutrition and Physical Activity	5.6
Prevention Science	3.0
Contemporary Clinical Trials	2.0
Nutrients	4.8
Journal of Adolescent Health	6.1
American Journal of Preventive Medicine	4.3
Implementation Science	8.8
Case reports	
American Journal of Case Reports	1.0
Journal of Medical Case Reports	0.9
Clinical Medicine Insights	0.8
Clinical Case Reports	0.6
Oxford Medical Case Reports	0.5
Journal of Pediatric Surgical Case Reports	0.2
BMJ Case Reports	N/A

[a]A bibliometric analysis of 953 articles published from 2014 to 2024 resulting from a PubMed search of keyword terms "School Health Services" and "School Mental Health Services" [1]. The journals under "Miscellaneous" are listed in descending order based on frequency articles in the sample were cited in each particular journal

most people, consider a journal with a higher impact factor. Examples of journal impact factors reported in 2023 can be found in Table 10.3.

(c) *Traditional subscription journals vs. open access journals*: There are benefits and disadvantages to traditional subscription and open access journals (Table 10.4). Hybrid journals are fundamentally subscription journals that offer authors the option of making their articles open access. In this model, the author can publish using the traditional model where it's free for the author but not free for the reader, or the author can publish using an open access model where the author pays and it's free for the reader.

(d) *Indexing*: In order for research to be impactful and discoverable, researchers must consider indexing of journals. There are several indexing options that journals can pursue, from general search engines to discipline-specific databases (Table 10.5). Journals go through an extensive process to be included, or indexed, in reputable bibliographic databases. Once a journal is indexed by a database, it is immediately available to all users of that database. Researchers should consider indexing when deciding on which journal to submit to, as each index type varies in their reach and impact, and offers different levels of detail, from article titles, abstracts, and references to full article files.

Table 10.4 Traditional subscription vs. open access journals

Traditional subscription journals	Open access journals
1. Individuals or institutions (university or company libraries) pay subscription charges to have access to the journal's content, so therefore, due to financial constraints, access to your article may be limited or non-existent 2. Authors can publish their article for free 3. The journal owns the copyright to the publication, so the author cannot freely distribute their own article or legally publish it on your own web page. Some exceptions include distribution of a PDF version after an embargo period or distribution of a different version of the article, such as a pre-publication version 4. Subscription journals are more familiar to the medical community 5. Rejection rates are higher compared with open access journals	1. Articles are freely and permanently available online, so anyone, anywhere can read it and distribute it 2. Journals are less familiar to the medical community and, in general, have lower impact factors 3. Often the author will receive 3–10 times more readers than traditional subscription journals 4. Articles are free to the reader, and therefore the journals often have a higher citation rate 5. Authors pay an article processing charge (APC) to publish their article. APC range from \$1000 to \$10,000, and average \$2800–\$3000 6. Authors retain the copyright and are made available under a Creative Commons license. Readers may use the article in any way they would like to, as long as they attribute the authors of that article 7. Rejection rates are lower compared with traditional subscription journals 8. Several open access journals may be considered "predatory" or fraudulent, as they do not provide the same quality assurance and services delivered by reputable journals

Table 10.5 Types of indexing

Index type	Examples	Features
General search engines	Google Bing	Easily accessible to medical professionals and the general public Any journal can be added to general search engines
Scholarly search engines	Google Scholar Microsoft Academic	Ensures the websites they index are from academic sources
General and discipline-specific scholarly indexing databases	Ulrichsweb Directory of Open Access Journals (DOAJ) Scopus (Elsevier) Web of Science (Institute for Scientific Information) Academic Search (EBSCO) PubMed (National Center for Biotechnology Information) IJIFACTOR EMBASE	Covers all or multiple disciplines and/or discipline-specific databases

10.2.2 Presentation of Your Research at a National and/or Regional Scientific Assembly

Another form of research dissemination are presentations given at a national and/or regional scientific assemblies. Choosing a scientific assembly to submit your abstract to resembles the initial process involved with choosing a journal (determining the audience, defining 2–3 main points/conclusions, identifying limitations and biases). Table 10.6 lists several scientific assemblies that features pediatrics and school-based health, but also consider subspecialty conferences based on your research or case report topic.

10.2.3 Non-Traditional Forms of Research Dissemination

In addition to publications and presentations, there are various forms of non-traditional methods of research dissemination, summarized below (Table 10.7). Before you utilize these methods of dissemination, check with your publisher (if your research is published in a traditional subscription journal), since copyright policies may limit the method or format that your research is disseminated.

Based on my 25 years as an academic physician, here are 10 pearls when it comes to research dissemination (Table 10.8).

Table 10.6 Scientific assemblies that feature pediatrics and school-based health research

Scientific assembly	Topic	Time of the year
Pediatric Academic Societies (PAS) meeting	General Pediatrics, Pediatric subspecialties, School-based Health	Spring
American Academy of Pediatrics (AAP) National Conference and Exhibition	General Pediatrics, Pediatric subspecialties, School-based Health	Fall
School-based Health Alliance	School health providers and nurses	Summer
National Association of School Nurses	School nurses	Summer
Society for Adolescent Health and Medicine (SAHM)	Pediatrics and Adolescent Medicine	Spring
American College of Emergency Physicians (ACEP) Annual Conference	Emergency Medicine and urgent care medicine	Fall
Society for Academic Emergency Medicine (SAEM) Annual Conference	Emergency Medicine and urgent care medicine	Spring

Table 10.7 Non-traditional forms of research dissemination [2]

Dissemination method	Examples	Comments
Workshops and seminars	Scientific assemblies, Webinars, TED talks, science festivals, science slams, road shows	Success of dissemination is associated with knowing the motivation of the learners, building upon the audience's previous experiences, matching the learning approach with the audience background and diversity, and actively involving the learners
News media	Newspapers, television, radio, online newsletters and magazine	News stories that are likely to gain attention are associated with the seriousness of the problem, human interest in the form of a personal story, local angle for a national or state headline, timeliness, conflict or controversy
Social media	Twitter, LinkedIn, Facebook, Personal blogs	Associated with more downloads and eventual citations Following people and organizations with similar interest increases dissemination Use appropriate hashtags to reach relevant audiences Altmetrics—describes the number of times a scholarly item is mentioned in social media
Issue or policy briefs	Infographics, research summary document, science comics	A summary of research information usually enhanced with data visualization (charts, tables, pictures)
E-mail lists and distribution		Compile a mailing list that includes funders, your community, other researchers, medical organizations and societies, journalists, politicians, policymakers, and practitioners
Audiovisual clips	YouTube, Vimeo, Vine clips	Often picked up by general search engines Keep clips brief (less than 4 min) Add clips to your Twitter and Facebook accounts
Post to Wikipedia		Well indexed and optimized for search engines Widely used and accessible

Table 10.8 Olympia's pearls for research dissemination

1	Read and follow the Instructions for Authors provide by each journal carefully. One of the first things that reviewers do, even before they read your manuscript, is assure that the Instructions for Authors are abided by. You may have an innovative and impactful study, but if you are not careful enough to follow the Instructions for Authors, then reviewers may question the validity of your results, and decide on rejection
2	Often I write the Results section first. Choose the 2–3 major points you want the audience to focus on, decide how to present these 2–3 major points (text, table, figure), and then decide which of the other data points you have collected adds to your main conclusion. Not every data point you collect needs to be in the manuscript. Simplicity is key
3	If you have the time, I would recommend submitting your manuscript to a journal with a wide circulation and high impact factor, even if you think rejection is inevitable. Although the acceptance rate is lower than other journals with lower impact factors, rejections are usually accompanied by suggestions from editors/reviewers that, if used to revise your manuscript, result in a better product. Publication decisions are usually decided by a selected few, and you never know what their opinion would be unless you submit your manuscript. You did the work, now shoot for the stars
4	When choosing a journal to submit to, look through a few years of published studies in that journal to determine if your manuscript would be a good fit, in style and research topic
5	Before I submit a manuscript, a typically give it a few weeks to "rest". I usually have colleagues, medical students/residents, biostatisticians, English majors, and unbiased reviewers, who are unaware of the study, read and review the manuscript for content and grammar. Incorporate their suggestions, perform a final review, and hit the "submit" button
6	Although several scientific assemblies have virtual options for poster presentations, the era of having rows and rows of posters pinned onto bulletin boards in a huge convention hall still exist. The key is attracting the horde of audience members to your comparatively small poster, to educate and disseminate. There are two types of poster presenters: The "quiet type" who stands to the side of the poster, available to answer questions, or the "salesman", who will walk up to anyone who will listen and start telling you about their research. There is no right or wrong way of poster presenting, but find what you are comfortable with and go with it
7	When developing a poster, I use the 5 foot rule. If you are standing 5 feet away from the poster, you should be able to easily read the text, tables, and figures on the poster. If you can't read it, then there is potentially too much information on the poster. Also, bullet points often work better than full paragraphs, and usually no more than 2–3 tables/figures per poster
8	For both oral and poster presentations, make note of comments, suggestions, and questions from audience members. Incorporate these into your manuscript, as often journal reviewers, and those who think similarly, may be the ones judging the fate of your manuscript submission
9	As most audience members will only have a few minutes to read your poster or listen to your oral presentation, make copies of your abstract to hand out, with your name and contact information on them. Consider handing out business cards. This allows them to read about your research in a less stressful environment, to contact you if they have any questions, and to potentially create networks and relationships for future research, mentoring, jobs, etc
10	Feel free to submit an abstract to multiple scientific assemblies, both nationally and regionally, and to various specialty and subspecialty conferences. Only a handful of scientific assemblies will discourage or disallow multiple presentations. The goal is to disseminate your research to as many people as possible, and very few medical professionals are able to attend every scientific assembly

Case 3 You are a school nurse who has been asked to be a speaker at your state's Association of School Nurses and Practitioners annual meeting. You have given a few lectures to the community on injury prevention and to your school staff on the recognition of brain concussions, but have never addressed an audience to this scale. Where do you start?

Although giving a lecture in front of a large audience may be anxiety provoking, consider it as an opportunity to educate and inspire, and to be impactful. Whether it is to advance your career by building up your curriculum vitae, or to undergo the academic promotion process, or ultimately improve the care of children and adolescents in the school setting, educational opportunities such as providing lectures/seminars/courses, supervising research, or mentoring medical and nursing colleagues and learners is vital to becoming an academic healthcare provider.

I often utilize mnemonics while teaching, whether it be at the bedside, formal lectures, written chapters, or published research. "IGNITE" is a mnemonic that may be helpful when considering educational and mentoring opportunities (Table 10.9).

My role as a researcher and educator has factored into a significant portion of my career. I become overwhelmed with pride when I think about the thousands of children that have been affected by the impact I have made on my learners through formal education, mentorship, role modeling, and research. The pride I feel ignites a passion in me to become the best researcher and educator that I can be for my learners and for my patients. My wish is that your journey into education and scholarship is as rewarding as it has been for me during my career (Fig. 10.1).

Extra Credit Points

1. A career in academic medicine involves demonstrating scholarship, gaining knowledge, and providing education. Demonstrating scholarship involves imparting knowledge that results from study and research in a particular field and the dissemination of this knowledge, thus becoming an expert in a particular field.
2. Research can be fun and rewarding as long as it aligns with your interests and fits within the construct of your career goals and work-life balance. Self-reflection to determine your passions is the first step to becoming a successful academic healthcare provider.
3. Methods of research dissemination include publication of your research in a peer-reviewed journal, presentation of your research at a national and/or regional scientific assembly, and non-traditional forms of research dissemination.
4. IGNITE" is a mnemonic that may be helpful when considering educational and mentoring opportunities.

Table 10.9 IGNITE mnemonic for education

"I" is Ignite	One of my favorite quotes is by Socrates: "Education is the kindling of a flame, and not the filling of a vessel." Our job is to ignite passion in our learners, to make them feel the importance of the education that we provide, and to realize the impact that education will have on their patients. My learners will likely utilize the lessons I provide if they feel the passion emanating from the words that come from my mouth or the thoughts I translate on paper. Choose a lecture topic that you are passionate about, and kindle your audience's flame
"G" is Guidance	I believe that the education of learners does not stop after the lecture ends or after the research is published. Mentorship is nurtured over time and careers, and requires effort and constant communication. I believe that part of my job as an educator and mentor is to assist my learners realize their own passions, developing their own career and scholarship paths, so that they may inspire, impact, and ignite others. Allow this educational opportunity to lead to the potential mentorship of audience members and hopefully lead to additional teaching opportunities
"N" is Noteworthy	I often choose lecture or research topics based on what may be considered timely or debatable, or "hot topics". I believe fostering conversation among learners leads to discovery and scholarship. I challenge myself and my learners to educate based on what may be considered interesting, unique, or noticeable
"I" is Imitation	We are constantly being watched by our learners. Education is not only the medical facts or evidence we provide, but how we demonstrate leadership, professionalism, and communication. Being an educator involves being a role model, and I strive to be a physician and educator that my learners can look up to
"T" is Techniques	Utilize both traditional (lectures, panel discussions, journal clubs, etc.) and non-traditional methods of education and retention, such as gamification, simulation/virtual reality, flipped classroom learning, case-based learning, infographics, mnemonics, tables/algorithms, podcasts, and instructional videos. The retention of information by your audience will hopefully lead to imitation, both in the clinical and educational realm
"E" is Evidence	To be a teacher, one must always continue to be a learner, keeping up with the medical literature. Education based on the evidence and research leads to physicians and healthcare providers who provide competent, compassionate, and cutting-edge care. One of my personal goals as an academic physician is to not only educate learners, but to inspire them to become lifelong learners and educators themselves

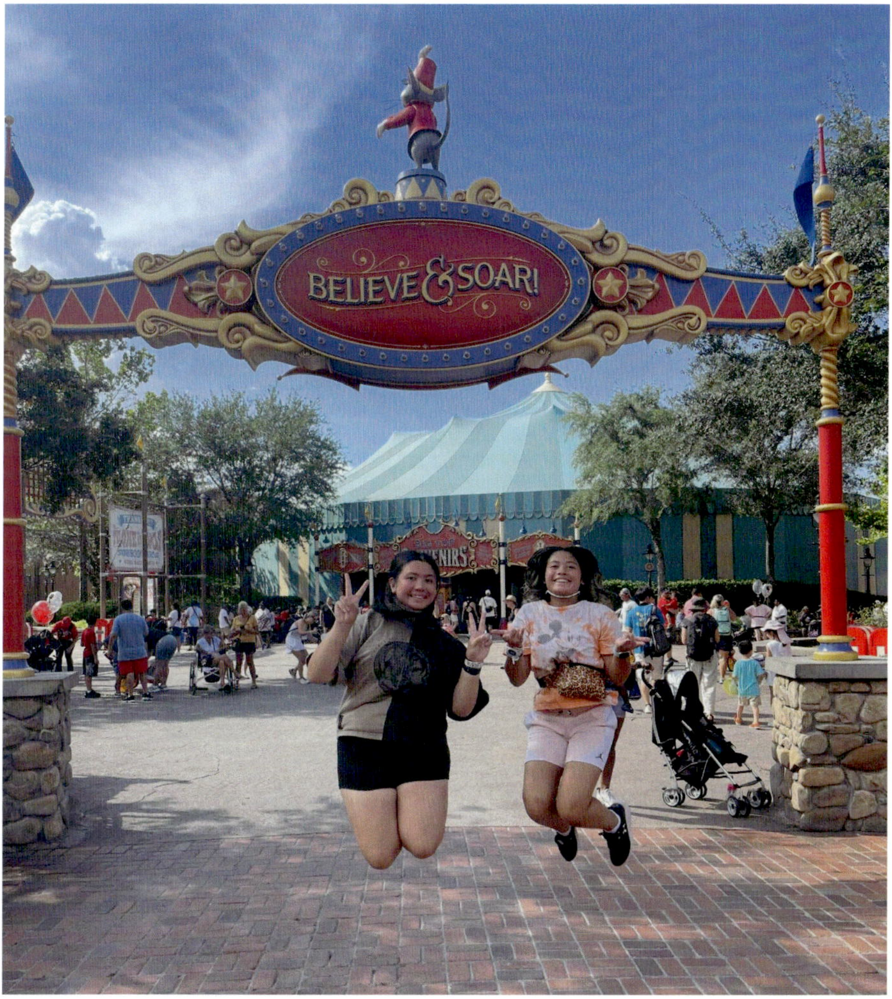

Fig. 10.1 "Don't just fly, soar."—Dumbo

References

1. Hermann C, Olympia RP. Publishing trends on the Topic of School Based Health from the 2014 to 2024: a bibliometric analysis (in progress).
2. Brownson RC, Eyler AA, Harris JK, et al. Getting the word out: new approaches for disseminating public health science. J Public Health Manag Pract. 2018;24(2):102–11.

Chapter 11
Telemedicine and School-Based Health

Neha Gupta and Adesuwa Emovon

Telehealth is the use of digital information and communication technologies to access healthcare services remotely. There are several delivery methods of telehealth, including video conferencing, audio only (telephone), secure messaging or chat, remote patient monitoring, and store and forward technology (such as sharing imaging). It can be utilized for primary care consultations, specialist consultations, mental health services, chronic disease management, health education, prescription and management, and health staff education. Telehealth has significantly grown, particularly during COVID-19 pandemic, and has been rapidly integrated into healthcare settings [1]. The use of telehealth in schools allows increased access to care especially for rural and underserved populations and increased convenience for parents who may require time off of work or for transportation arrangement for a child's medical appointment. It also facilitates continuity of care with regular check-ups and follow ups, especially for chronic conditions, special health needs, and medication checks. A major benefit is reducing absenteeism, allowing students to received care at school, perhaps during lunch breaks or between classes [1].

You are a school nurse working in a school-based health clinic on a busy Tuesday morning. During your first hour, ten students have presented to your clinic with a variety of chief complaints. After performing an initial history and physical examination, you have decided that these students could benefit from the supplementation of telehealth. Students presenting with various chief complaints are detailed in Table 11.1 with the unique opportunities and benefits of telehealth utilization in Table 11.2.

N. Gupta (✉)
George Washington University Hospital, Washington, DC, USA

A. Emovon
Pennsylvania State University College of Medicine, Hershey, PA, USA
e-mail: aemovon@pennstatehealth.psu.edu

R. P. Olympia, J. Brady-Olympia (eds.), *Clinical Considerations in School-based Health*, https://doi.org/10.1007/978-3-031-85765-2_11

Table 11.1 Student presentations to the school nurse's office

1. Emilia is 9 year old that presents with sore throat, fever, and body aches. She started feeling symptoms when she got to school this morning, but she has been progressively worsening. She now has a fever of 101 F, erythematous pharynx with exudates, and lymphadenopathy
2. Mateo is a 12 year old with a history of asthma that presents after gym class with wheezing throughout on auscultation of his lungs, tachypnea, and oxygen saturation of 91%
3. Rahul is a 15 year old who presents with a sudden severe headache with nausea. The pain is more intense than any headache he has experienced before. But he has no neurological deficits or fever. No loss of consciousness, seizures, difficulty speaking or ambulating. He does have a history of headaches. There is a local urgent care that does have a CT scan
4. Kai is a 12 year old who has been struggling with anxiety and depression for several months. One day during class, they become visibly distressed, started crying uncontrollably and express thoughts of self-harm to the teacher. You are called but you have no full-time mental health professional on staff
5. Alejandro is a 13 year old who lives in a sustained a concussion during a soccer game 2 weeks ago. He has been cleared to return to school part-time but is still having headaches, difficulty concentrating, sensitivity to light and noise. He and his family live in a rural area, 4 h from the nearest pediatric concussion specialist
6. Kwame is a 10 year old with type 1 diabetes. Her endocrinologist is 2 h away. She uses a continuous glucose monitor (CGM) to track her blood sugar levels
7. Amara is a 15 year old who has been having difficulty concentrating, zoning out in class and missing instructions. Her desk and backpack are messy and she forgets materials for class. She has been turning all of his assignments in late. The parents notice she daydreams at home and her frequently easily distracted
8. Zara is a 12 year old with epilepsy who takes medications mid-day while at school. She also has her emergency rescue medications at the nurse's office. She last had a seizure at school a month ago
9. Yuki is a 9 year old seems uncomfortable, fatigued and has a reddish-purple rash over the lower extremities and buttocks. There is also some swelling of the ankles. She has a decreased appetite and a low grade fever of 38 °C
10. Mia is a 5 year old girl who presents with a severe headache of sudden onset. She has no history of headaches. She has some neck stiffness

Table 11.2 Opportunities and benefits of Telehealth utilization

1. For immediate medical attention allows students to receive care more efficiently for common illnesses without having to leave school for care or wait long periods of time at a hospital or urgent care. Instead of recommending that this child make an appointment with their pediatrician, they can do the COVID or strep throat tests and be connected with a healthcare provider via secure video conferencing for prescription of medications that parents can pick up at a pharmacy
2. A school nurse could set up an online video to an emergency room pediatrician and use a digital stethoscope to allow the pediatrician to listen to the patient's lungs remotely. The pediatrician can confirm the diagnosis of asthma exacerbation, direct the school team to administer albuterol, and write a prescription for additional albuterol for the parents to pick up. All 50 states and the District of Columbia have laws that allow students with asthma to self-carry and self-administer personal inhalers. However, as of 2024, 17 states have laws or state guidelines that allow schools to stock albuterol for students. Consultation to a provider who can prescribe albuterol would decrease the gap of time that a child may have to be without treatment
3. For triage to differentiate the need to go to an urgent care or an emergency department. Given the sudden and severe onset, a triaging physician may suggest an emergency department to rule out serious conditions such as meningitis, aneurysm, tumor, and stroke. If the conversation provides some reassurance that it is not life-threatening but still requires medical intervention, such as migraines, they may suggest to be treated in an Urgent Care to be evaluated and treated more quickly. In this specific scenario, the school nurse and telehealth provider would want to collect additional information such as exact intensity and characteristic of headache, accompanying symptoms (vision changes, weakness, difficulty speaking, numbness), how quickly symptoms development, past medical history, etc.
4. For immediate assessment with a licensed mental health professional, one who specializes in child and adolescent psychiatry. This professional will be able to evaluate risk of self-harm, provide immediate crisis counseling, and develop a safety plan. Parents can even be involved in the telehealth session and provide them with guidance to best support their child. If a psychiatrist is required to prescribe medications or adjust the ones currently being taken, they can be consulted via telehealth. Several other benefits may also be possible including follow-up virtual sessions while at school to ensure continuity, resource coordination, and education for teachers
5. For regular check ins with a concussion specialist to assess symptoms and cognitive function while at school. His return-to-learn plan based on his progress could be regularly altered and recommendations for academic accommodations can be given directly to the school staff. Given that he is in a rural area, telehealth would allow this child to avoid the long car trip which may aggravate symptoms, could have more regular check-ins, and have more multidisciplinary support by connecting professionals from several areas
6. Her endocrinologist could access her CGM date in real-time, allowing quick adjustments to her insulin regimen if required. She could have brief video consultations with a multidisciplinary diabetes care team during lunch or free periods, which would minimize time away from class. In the event that she has symptoms of hyperglycemia, a care team could be quickly consulted via telehealth to avoid unnecessary trip to the ED or even recommend an ER visit if there is concern for diabetic ketoacidosis requiring intervention

(continued)

Table 11.2 (continued)

7. If there is no mental health professional, this child would benefit from a telehealth session to help with a diagnosis of ADHD. He would benefit from regular check-ins to assess symptoms, behavior, and possible medication effectiveness if appropriate. A mobile app can also be used to track daily tasks and moods that his care team can see to make telehealth sessions more effective
8. Epilepsy needs frequent management and re-evaluation. While schools nurses regularly see children with epilepsy, it would be helpful to have frequent check ins with the child's neurologist, especially if any medications need to be adjusted. A clear action should be developed and shared with school staff via telehealth training sessions. In the event that this child does have a seizure, staff can quickly connect with the neurologist for immediate guidance if needed
9. After isolating this student, you assess the rash and are unsure what the cause of this rash is. It doesn't appear to look like chickenpox or even rash from a tick bite. You want additional opinion so you do a telehealth consultation. You are able to show the rash to a physician over video, who asks you to press on the rash and show that it is non-blanching. The physician recommends lab work to rule out diagnosis, especially to look at blood counts. The student is sent to the Emergency Department for evaluation. Workup is consistent with Henoch Schonlein Purpura
10. To differentiate the need to go to an urgent care or an emergency department. Given the sudden and severe onset, a triaging physician may suggest an emergency department to rule out serious conditions such as meningitis, aneurysm, tumor, and stroke. If the conversation provides some reassurance that it is not life-threatening but still requires medical intervention, such as migraines, they may suggest to be treated in an Urgent Care to be evaluated and treated more quickly. In this specific scenario, the school nurse and telehealth provider would want to collect additional information such as exact intensity and characteristic of headache, accompanying symptoms (vision changes, weakness, difficulty speaking, numbness), how quickly symptoms development, past medical history, etc.

11.1 Equity in Telehealth

The use of telehealth in schools allows increased access to care especially for rural and underserved populations and increased convenience for parents who may require time off of work or for transportation arrangements for a child's medical appointment. It also facilitates continuity of care with regular checkups and follow ups, especially for chronic conditions, special health needs, and medication checks. A major benefit is reducing absenteeism, allowing students to receive care at school, perhaps during lunch breaks or between classes [1]. Telehealth services do not replace the school nurse. School nurses should be up to date with modern technology to support and enhance clinical practice. Their involvement is crucial in the utilization of telehealth in the school setting.

For example, in the United States, asthma affects 10% of school aged children. However, there is a significant burden of asthma on children in high-risk communities, low-income and minority children. They experience significantly higher prevalence that is double the national average. Chronically uncontrolled symptoms and acute illness are linked to school and work absenteeism for both students and their caregivers. Thus, these children are at risk for having poorer academic performance achievement gaps leading to downstream consequences in education such as risky-health behaviors, compromised health status, and reduced longevity [2, 3]. For children in rural communities, they experience similar challenges including rural tailored interventions, lack of transportation, and/or financial constraints due to travel which shifts the burden to emergency care services [4].

According to the Behavioral Risk Factor Surveillance Child Asthma Call survey, one of the modifiable factors for absenteeism was inability to connect with a provider or asthma specialist. Telehealth exclusive school-based health centers provide access to care at a fixed site on a school campus and providers are remotely available at a distinct site location. School-based Health Centers serve a majority of low-income communities and schools that qualify for Title 1 programs. Thus, telehealth integration is key for both urban at-risk populations and rural regions especially [5].

Current initiatives including traditional SBHC that utilize some form of telehealth and telehealth exclusive programs center around students from rural communities that experience primary care shortages, schools in low-income communities that qualify for Title 1 funding, and in elementary school settings. Most of the state's telehealth exclusive School-Based Health Centers are sponsored by medical centers and hospitals with most located in the southern part of the United States including Texas, North Carolina, and South Carolina.

11.2 Challenges of Telehealth

Telehealth does offer the ability to provide necessary medical care to families who historically have barriers to in-person care. However, the pandemic did highlight the rapid uptake of new technology does come with additional challenges in implementation and can amplify health disparities. Digital redlining is a modern-day manifestation of historical redlining due to disinvestment in broadband infrastructure that has affected people of color, low-income, and rural communities disproportionately. As a result, widespread utilization of technology does worsen disparities in access to critical health information, medical care, and digital literacy.

Digital literacy is defined at ease, comfort, and skill to access technology [6]. The unfamiliarity with technology creates apprehension and distrust regarding data security and privacy issues. This is particularly important when considering communities that historically have had distrust in healthcare systems. Therefore, it is crucial to explore avenues of maintaining trust within the community when implementing new technologies [7].

There is still low stakeholder engagement of telehealth services by healthcare providers which limits confidence built in telehealth systems, restricts opportunities for adequate training, and negatively impacts adoption rates and awareness of benefits. Mental health professionals are leading the way with about 85% of psychiatrists using telehealth modalities (e.g. videoconferencing and telephone) for diagnosing/treating patients and chronic disease management even prior to the pandemic. Although primary care providers did utilize telehealth modalities at high rates (79%), utilization did different across subspecialties. Pediatricians were less likely to provide care by telephone compared to general interest and family medicine practitioners (64% compared to about 74%). They were also less likely to provide services for chronic disease management and preventive care [8].

Lastly, the lack of consistent policies for reimbursement through private payers and state-based Medicaid organizations hinders the implementation and sustainability of telehealth programs. Thus, school programs may face challenges in continuing to offer services without a diversified source of funding [9].

11.3 Reimbursement

In the Spring of 2020, the Centers for Medicare & Medicaid Services (CMS) public health emergency status enabled increased flexibility in reimbursement policies for telehealth visits, permitting schools and homes to qualify as originating sites across all 50 states. While some states have permanently adopted these public health emergency reimbursement policies, restrictions and regulations on type of services and eligible providers continue to vary across states. In addition, during the COVID-19 pandemic, temporary waivers allowed healthcare providers to get reimbursed for audio-only virtual visits helped mitigate lack of broadband access for individuals who not have the necessary technology to support video calls [10]. Moving forward, states and insurance companies need to make adjustment to their reimbursement policies to allow for telehealth accessibility and utilization thereby maximizing potential health benefits [11].

The future of telehealth implementation in schools is promising and has several key directions as detailed throughout this chapter. As technologies continue to advance, schools are likely to see more sophisticated technologies that may incorporate artificial intelligence and machine learning to enhance patient monitoring, provide more individualized delivery of care, and create more seamless triaging processes. Implementation of an effective telehealth program requires a multidisciplinary team of stakeholders including communication with school district leaders, local health departments, local providers, students, and their family.

Extra Credit Points

1. Telehealth providers should be trained in telehealth triage including protocols.
2. Integration with EHRs to access patient history and other relevant clinical information. Telehealth providers should remain in regular contact with the patient's primary physician and any relevant specialty care.
3. Incorporate new data points: videos, messages, and images into patient's medical record. This allows the data to be actionable and protected.
4. Improve continuity of care by continuing to monitor patient after telehealth encounter.
5. Standardize social determinants of health screening tools that account for digital literacy and broadband assessment to effectively communicate with patients.

6. Ensure a trusted relationships between school nurse and external provider as school nurse are the first-line in facilitating primary care.
7. Personnel involved in telehealth programs within school based health centers should be well-informed on Family Educational Rights and Privacy Acts (FERPA) and HIPAA. School nurses typically act as telepresenters in this setting and clinical care provided through primary care providers are governed differently.
8. With the growth of undocumented youth in public schools, telehealth programs should offer tailored responses to both cultural and health care needs.
9. Ensure adequate patient confidentiality through additional privacy measures at home and school-based set-ups including managing the caregiver's involvement.

References

1. Curfman AL, Hackell JM, Herendeen NE, Alexander JJ, Marcin JP, Moskowitz WB, Bodnar CEF, Simon HK, McSwain SD, Section on Telehealth Care, Committee on Practice and Ambulatory Medicine, Committee on Pediatric Workforce. Telehealth: improving access to and quality of pediatric health care. Pediatrics. 2021;148(3):e2021053129. https://doi.org/10.1542/peds.2021-053129.
2. Perry TT, Turner JH. School-based telemedicine for asthma management. J Allergy Clin Immunol Pract. 2019;7(8):2524–32. https://doi.org/10.1016/j.jaip.2019.08.009.
3. Knopf JA, Finnie RK, Peng Y, et al. School-based health centers to advance health equity: a community guide systematic review. Am J Prev Med. 2016;51(1):114–26. https://doi.org/10.1016/j.amepre.2016.01.009.
4. Mayfield CA, Priem JS, Effinger T, McGinnis S, Grinton P. School-based telemedicine and reduced avoidable emergency care among rural pediatric patients. Telemed J E Health. 2023;29:1819–27.
5. Love H, Panchal N, Schlitt J, Behr C, Soleimanpour S. The use of telehealth in school-based health centers. Glob Pediatr Health. 2019;6:2333794X19884194. PMID: 31692723; PMCID: PMC6811756. https://doi.org/10.1177/2333794X19884194.
6. Wang ML, Gago CM, Rodriguez K. Digital redlining—the invisible structural determinant of health. JAMA. 2024;331(15):1267–8. https://doi.org/10.1001/jama.2024.1628.
7. Shaw RJ. Access to technology and digital literacy as determinants of health and health care. Creat Nurs. 2023;29(3):258–63. https://doi.org/10.1177/10784535231211682.
8. Kane CK. Policy research perspectives: telehealth in 2020: survey data show widespread use across Most physician specialties and for a variety of functions. Chicago, IL: American Medical Association; 2021. https://www.ama-assn.org/system/files/2020-prp-telehealth.pdf.
9. Garber K, Wells E, Hale KC, King K. Connecting kids to care: developing a school-based telehealth program. J Nurse Pract. 2021;17(3):273–8. ISSN 1555-4155. https://doi.org/10.1016/j.nurpra.2020.12.024.
10. Harris Y, Tutty M, Mishra V, Goldwater J, Lloyd S. Future of health: advancing the appropriate use of telehealth within medical specialties. Chicago, IL: American Medical Association; 2022. https://www.ama-assn.org/system/files/future-health-telehealth-use.pdf. Accessed 10 Jan 2024.
11. Center for Connected Health Policy. State Telehealth Laws and Reimbursement policies report: fall 2023. Sacramento, CA: Center for Connected Health Policy; 2023. https://www.cchpca.org/resources/state-telehealth-laws-and-reimbursement-policies-report-fall-2023-2. Accessed 3 Aug 2024.

Chapter 12
Urgent Care Medicine and School-Based Health

Robert P. Olympia

You are a school nurse working in a school-based health clinic on a busy Monday morning. During your first hour, 10 students have presented to your clinic with a variety of chief complaints (Table 12.1). After performing an initial history and physical examination, you have decided that each student needs a higher level of care. You contact each student's parent or guardian for pick up. You are familiar with an urgent care center (UCC) located 5 miles away from the school that recently opened. Should the students be evaluated in an UCC or your local Emergency Department (ED)?

The growth of the Urgent Care Medicine (UCM) industry over the past few decades can be attributed to the general population's need to seek convenient, high quality, low cost care, in response to overcrowding in emergency departments (ED) and limited hours and physician shortages in primary care physician offices. Urgent care centers (UCCs) provide services such as (1) a medical examination, diagnosis and treatment for non-life or -limb threatening illnesses and injuries that are within the capability of an UCC which accepts unscheduled, walk-in patients seeking medical attention during all posted hours of operation and is supported by on-site evaluation services, including radiology and laboratory services; and (2) any further medical examination, procedure, and treatment to the extent they are within the capabilities of the staff and facilities available at the UCC.

Some fun facts regarding UCCs [1]: As of July 2023, there are approximately 14,382 UCCs in the United States (US), 8% are pediatric patient specific. Over 78%

R. P. Olympia (✉)
Department of Emergency Medicine and Pediatrics, Penn State College of Medicine
Attending Physician, Hershey, PA, USA

Division of Pediatric Emergency Medicine, Department of Emergency Medicine, Penn State
Milton S. Hershey Medical Center, Hershey, PA, USA
e-mail: rolympia@hmc.psu.edu

R. P. Olympia, J. Brady-Olympia (eds.), *Clinical Considerations in School-based Health*, https://doi.org/10.1007/978-3-031-85765-2_12

Table 12.1 Ten Student Presentations: Urgent care center or Emergency Department?

Case #1: Grant is a 7-year-old presenting with a sore throat and headache. He demonstrates no signs of dehydration or altered mental status. You notice that he has a fever of 104.5 degrees Fahrenheit. He has no difficulty breathing or swallowing, has no neck stiffness, and is able to speak in full sentences
Case #2: Patty is a 15-year-old presenting with abdominal pain that started this morning. She has no fever, sore throat, cough, vomiting, or diarrhea. Her abdominal pain is generalized. She is able to jump up and down in your office without discomfort. She does admit to mild discomfort when she urinates
Case #3: Madelyn is a 13-year-old with a history of food allergies and asthma who presents with difficulty catching her breath after volleyball practice. She does not complain of lightheadedness, difficulty swallowing or abdominal pain, and she has no hives. Her symptoms improve after four puffs of her albuterol inhaler, but she continues to cough. She is able to speak in full sentences and has no evidence of respiratory distress (tachypnea, grunting, or intercostal retractions)
Case #4: Isabel is a 9-year-old that presents with a painful rash on her right leg. 4 days ago she slipped and fell during a cross country meet, sustaining a large abrasion to her right calf. Since then the abrasion has become painful, swollen (3 × 4 cm), and productive of purulent discharge. She has no fever, is able to ambulate with mild pain, but you notice red streaking extending to her right hip
Case #5: Jodi is a 17-year-old with a history of seizures who "passed out" during music class. She skipped breakfast this morning and pulled an "all-nighter" studying for midterms. Her classmates, who caught her before she hit the ground, did not witness any convulsions. She has no alteration of her mental status, no amnesia, and her neurologic examination is normal. She feels better after drinking some orange juice. She denies chest pain, shortness of breath, palpitations, or headache associated with the event
Case #6: Catherine is a 5-year-old who presents with 2 episodes of watery non-bloody diarrhea. She had one episode of vomiting before getting on the bus this morning. She has no fever and no abdominal pain. She is alert, her eyes are not sunken, her tongue is slightly dry, and her capillary refill is brisk. You notice a maculopapular erythematous rash on her trunk
Case #7: Grace is a 12-year-old presenting with a swollen right ankle after she twisted it during basketball practice. Her ankle is neurovascularly intact, but she cannot bear weight. She has a moderate amount of swelling on the lateral aspect of her ankle
Case #8: Rob is a 10-year-old who presents with right ear pain and fever. His pinna is not displaced and he does not have pain over the mastoid. While you complete is examination, he begins to have a left-sided nose bleed that persists for 10 min despite pressure
Case #9: Abigail is a 16-year-old presenting with a 1 cm laceration to her forehead after she tripped during musical rehearsal and hit her head on the floor. She did not lose consciousness and she reports no amnesia to the event. Her bleeding is well-controlled with pressure, and her neurologic examination is normal
Case #10: Mark is an 8-year-old who presents with fever, runny nose, and bilateral leg pain. He is awake and follows commands, and there is no evidence of respiratory distress. He is able to bear weight and walk around your office slowly. His capillary refill is 4–5 s, but his eyes are not sunken and his mucous membranes are moist

of the US population lives within a 10-min drive of an UCC. UCCs have reported a median patient volume of 40 patients per day (206 million patient visits per year for non-emergent cases), increasing during late fall and winter. 52.8% of UCCs are affiliated with hospital-based systems. The presence of UCCs in the community have decreased ED visits by 17.2%. Services potentially provided by UCCs can be found in Table 12.2.

Table 12.2 Services often offered in urgent care centers

Appropriate chief complaints [2]	Initial assessment and management of chief complaints listed on the "URGENT CARES" infographic (Fig. 12.1) [and likely not chief complaints listed on the "STOP AT AN ER STAT" infographic (Fig. 12.2)]
Providers	The majority of UCCs employ family medicine and emergency medicine trained physicians, as well as other licensed healthcare professionals (physician assistants, nurse practitioners, registered nurses, and radiology technicians) UCCs may also employ pediatric specific providers (pediatricians and pediatric emergency medicine specialists)
Diagnostic testing	On-site laboratory testing: complete blood counts, comprehensive metabolic profiles, diabetic testing (Hemoglobin A1c), urine pregnancy, urinalysis, rapid strep and throat cultures, rapid viral testing, Tuberculosis testing, drug screens, and Sexually Transmitted Infection (STI) testing On-site radiologic testing: X-rays, ultrasonography, CT scans
Additional services	Electrocardiogram Intravenous fluids Oral, intravenous, and nebulized medications Active and passive immunizations Procedural sedation and analgesia Reduction/casting/splinting of an extremity fracture or dislocation or sprains Laceration repair Incision and drainage Foreign body removal Management of epistaxis Adolescent pelvic examinations On-site radiology and laboratory technologists Telehealth consultation Mental health services Primary care and preventative care visits Sport and employment physical examinations Initial stabilization of adult and pediatric patients who may present with life-threatening medical or traumatic complaints and transfer of these critically ill or injured patients to an ED via Emergency Medical Services

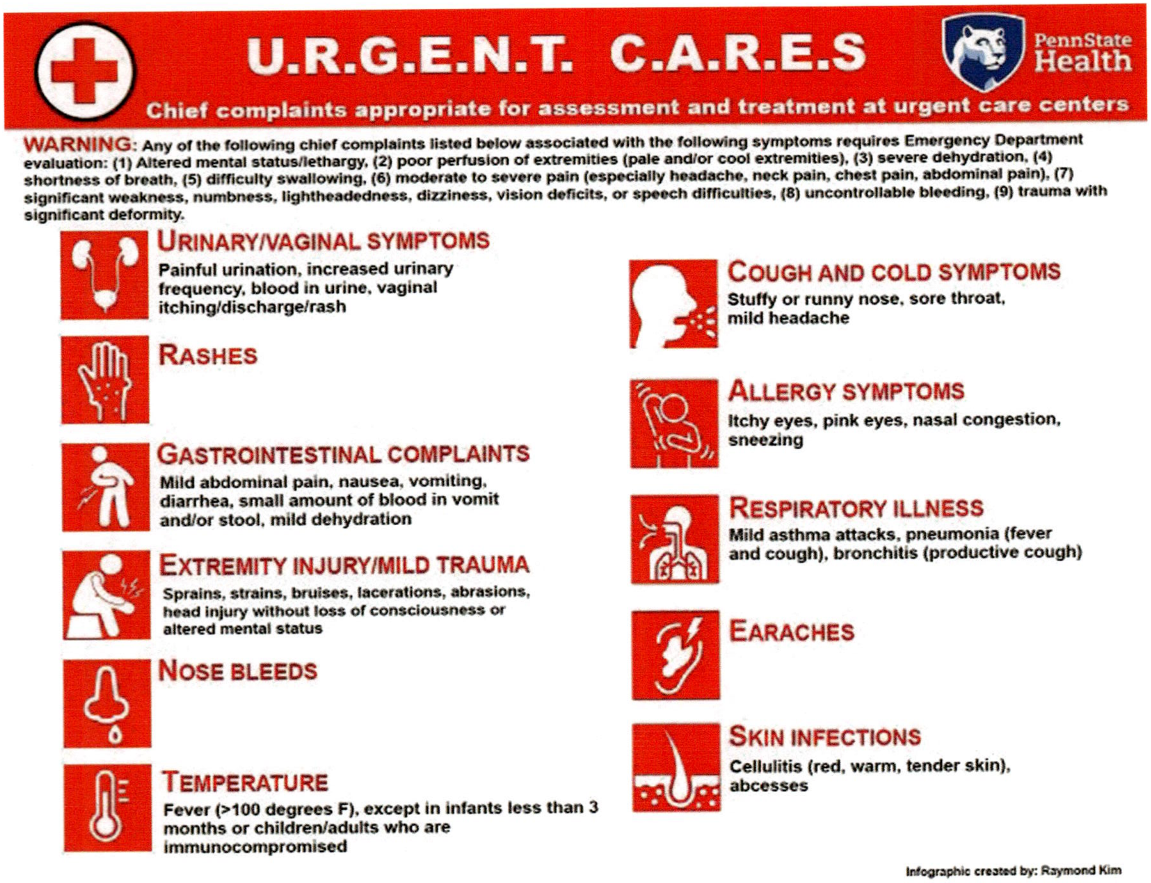

Fig. 12.1 Mnemonic used to classify chief complaints as urgent [2]

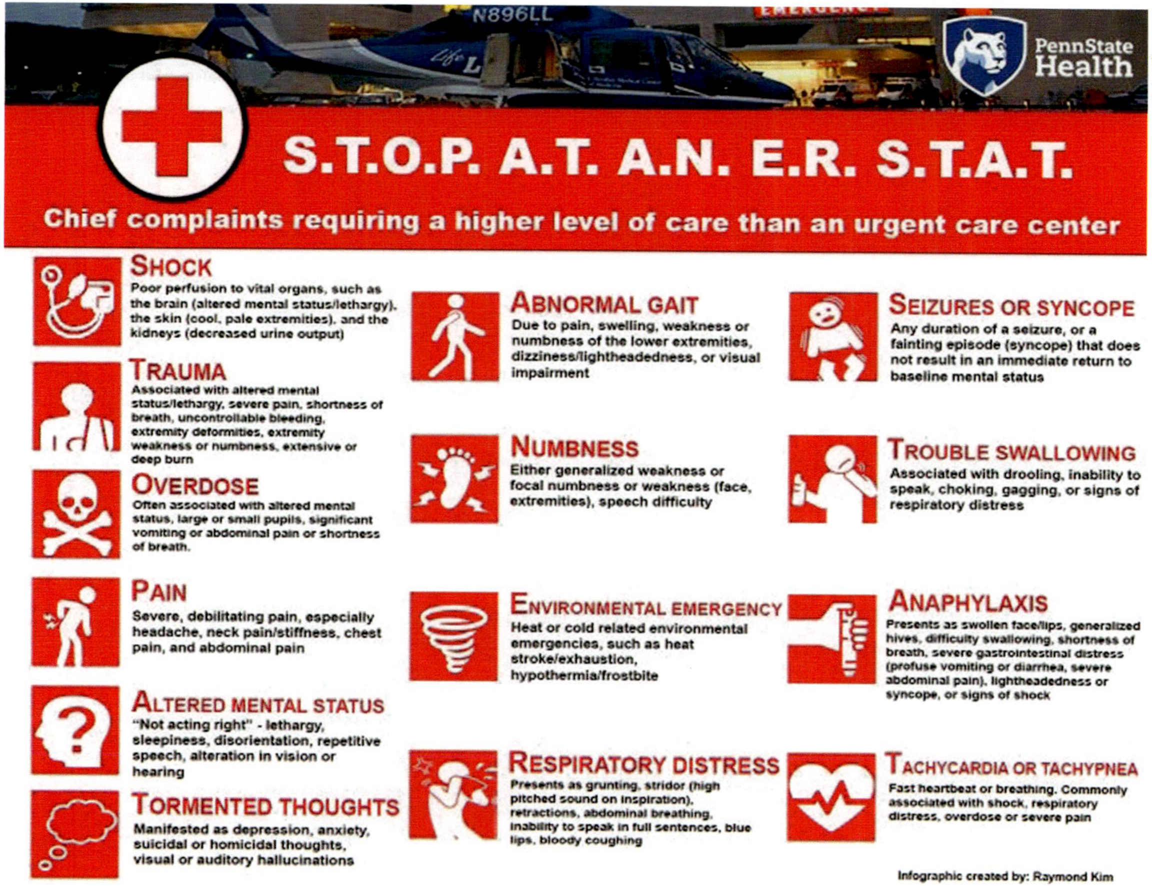

Fig. 12.2 Mnemonic used to classify chief complaints as emergent [2]

12.1 Case Conclusions

Each of your 10 students may be referred to your local UCC based on the mnemonic (URGENT CARES), although the following table lists "red flags" that would require emergent ED transfers.

Student Case and likely diagnosis	Reasons for ED transfer via EMS
Case #1: Grant is a 7-year-old presenting with a sore throat, headache, and fever Likely diagnosis: viral illness/pharyngitis, strep pharyngitis Urgent care resource: rapid strep testing, oral antibiotic if positive	– Difficulty swallowing or decreased range of motion of his neck (retropharyngeal/neck abscess) – Signs of meningitis (Kernig and Brudzinski signs) – Depressed mental status (meningitis or significant dehydration) *Referral to an ED should not be based solely on the height of the fever (unless immunocompromised)*
Case #2: Patty is a 15-year-old presenting with generalized abdominal pain and dysuria Likely diagnosis: functional abdominal pain, constipation, urinary tract infection Urgent care resource: re-evaluation of abdominal pain, X-ray of abdomen, urinalysis and urine culture, oral antibiotics if positive	– Inability to jump up and down without pain or significant right lower quadrant abdominal pain (appendicitis or ovarian process) – Blood seen in the urine (renal stone) – Signs of significant dehydration – Concern for pregnancy
Case #3: Madelyn is a 13-year-old with resolving shortness of breath after albuterol treatments and persistent cough Likely diagnosis: mild asthma exacerbation Urgent care resource: reassessment of shortness of breath, additional albuterol treatments, oral steroids	– Signs of anaphylaxis (involvement of cardiovascular, respiratory, gastrointestinal, and/or skin/mucous membrane organ systems) – Signs of respiratory distress or central cyanosis
Case #4: Isabel is a 9-year-old that presents with a painful rash on her right leg with red streaking Likely diagnosis: cellulitis with lymphangitis, abscess Urgent care resource: ultrasonography to determine abscess, incision and drainage if abscess, oral antibiotics for cellulitis	– Evidence of sepsis or septic shock (organ hypoperfusion) – Concern for extremity fracture – Pain out of proportion to your examination (necrotizing fasciitis) *Lymphangitis does not necessarily need intravenous antibiotics or hospitalization*
Case #5: Jodi is a 17-year-old with a history of seizures who "passed out" Likely diagnosis: syncope due to hypoglycemia Urgent care resource: reassessment of mental status, point-of-care blood glucose, electrocardiogram, intravenous fluids for mild to moderate dehydration	– Syncope during physical activity, or associated with chest pain, shortness of breath, palpitations, seizure activity – Concern for seizure – Concern for significant head trauma (altered mental status, signs of basilar skull fracture, history of loss of consciousness, significant vomiting, severe headache) – Concern for cervical spine injury – Abnormal neurologic examination – Significant dehydration – Concern for intoxication or overdose/exposure

(continued)

Student Case and likely diagnosis	Reasons for ED transfer via EMS
Case #6: Catherine is a 5-year-old who presents with vomiting and diarrhea, and a maculopapular erythematous rash on her trunk Likely diagnosis: viral gastroenteritis with viral exanthem, mild dehydration Urgent care resource: point-of-care blood glucose, zofran and oral trial, intravenous fluids for mild dehydration if oral trial fails	– Significant dehydration – Significant abdominal pain (concern for appendicitis or bacterial enteritis) – Fever and bloody diarrhea – Petechiae and/or purpura (concern for meningococcemia) *Most urinary tract infections and pyelonephritis can be diagnosed and treated in the urgent care setting*
Case #7: Grace is a 12-year-old presenting with a swollen right ankle after she twisted it during basketball practice Likely diagnosis: ankle sprain Urgent care resource: X-ray of ankle, splinting for sprain or minor fracture	– Concern for dislocation – Concern for open fracture – Significant deformity – Concern for neurovascular compromise
Case #8: Rob is a 10-year-old who presents with right ear pain, fever, and epistaxis. Likely diagnosis: viral upper respiratory with epistaxis, otitis media Urgent care resource: oral antibiotics for an otitis media, nasal packing for persistent epistaxis	– Concern for mastoiditis (ear pinna displaced, pain or erythema posterior to the ear) – Prolonged epistaxis despite pressure – Signs of hypovolemic shock due to blood loss
Case #9: Abigail is a 16-year-old presenting with a 1 centimeter laceration to her forehead due to a head injury Likely diagnosis: facial contusion and laceration Urgent care resource: reassessment of neurologic status, laceration repair	– Concern for significant head trauma (altered mental status, signs of basilar skull fracture, history of loss of consciousness, significant vomiting, severe headache) – Prolonged or significant blood loss (concern for hypovolemic shock) – Abnormal neurologic examination
Case #10: Mark is an 8-year-old who presents with fever, runny nose, bilateral leg pain and prolonged capillary refill Likely diagnosis: viral upper respiratory distress with myositis, mild dehydration Urgent care resource: point-of-care blood glucose, respiratory viral panel, intravenous fluids for failed oral trial	– Altered mental status – Significant dehydration – Shortness of breath – Unable to ambulate (concern for myositis and rhabodomyolysis)

Extra Credit Points

1. Urgent care centers are increasing in numbers throughout the US, and their ability to provide convenient, high quality, low cost care, in response to overcrowding in EDs and limited hours and physician shortages in primary care physician offices, makes their services valuable within a health care system.
2. Get to know the UCC in your community, and become familiar with the services they offer, specifically associated with pediatric patients, and their ability to stabilize critically ill and injured pediatric patients for transfer to an ED via EMS [3].

References

1. Urgent Care Association. Urgent Care Industry White Paper: The essential nature of the urgent care in the healthcare ecosystem post-COVID-19. 2023. https://urgentcareassociation.org/wp-content/uploads/2023-Urgent-Care-Industry-White-Paper.pdf. Accessed 7 Mar 2024.
2. Rothstein R, Zhen K, Kim RY, et al. Acuity—appropriate triage of chief complaints found on urgent care center organization websites. Am J Emerg Med. 2021;43:276–80.
3. Rothstein R, Zhen K, Olympia RP. School nurses on the front lines of medicine: when you Don't need to "STOP AT AN ER STAT!"—the role of urgent care centers in the management of students with nonemergent chief complaints. NASN Sch Nurse. 2020;35(1):24–9.

Chapter 13
Diversity, Equity, and Inclusion

Ariel Tassy Nunez

Case 1 **A 16-year-old Black female presents to a school-based health center inquiring about Plan B. During the history she anxiously explains to the doctor (who also happens to be Black) that she had sex last night without a condom and needs Plan B. At the end of the encounter, she is provided with appropriate anticipatory guidance and the medication. She looks relieved. She says to the doctor, "The last time I came in for Plan B the doctor told me that I should be on birth control since I always forget to use a condom. I felt like I was being judged. I'm just glad to finally speak to a doctor who looks like me and doesn't judge me."**

Diversity is defined as having a varied representation of a population [1]. Diversity can refer to racial, ethnic, or gender diversity, as well as religion, age, disability status, education, geography, socioeconomic status, life experiences, and so on. Diversity in the workplace has several important benefits including increasing perspective, creativity, engagement, and perceived value [2]. In healthcare, these benefits are especially significant, as diversity in medicine has been shown to not only improve patient experiences but also positively impact health outcomes, and reduce health disparities.

Health disparity is defined as differences in healthcare utilization and health outcomes [3]. Health disparities exist in every field in medicine. For example, studies have shown that Black and Hispanic adolescents, independent of socioeconomic status, receive fewer primary care and mental health visits than their White counterparts [4]. Disparities such as these are rooted in historically unjust social constructs. Since their inception in 1967, school-based health centers have worked to reduce health disparities. Establishing clinics within schools, drastically increased students' access to necessary and comprehensive care.

A. T. Nunez (✉)
Northwell, New Hyde Park, NY, USA
e-mail: anunez17@northwell.edu

R. P. Olympia, J. Brady-Olympia (eds.), *Clinical Considerations in School-based Health*, https://doi.org/10.1007/978-3-031-85765-2_13

Today school-based health centers can continue to target health disparities by increasing the diversity of the providers and staff who care for the students. Studies have shown that physician-patient racial concordance can improve health outcomes. For example, physician-patient racial concordance is associated with decreased morbidity among Black newborns, increased medication adherence, and overall improvement in communication [5, 6]. This is especially important to consider in the vulnerable adolescent population, who we want to feel comfortable disclosing personal and sensitive information to their medical team. Other forms of diversity, such as sexual orientation, gender identity, and ability/disability status, are also important to have represented in school-based health centers. Valuing diversity in schools can improve students' confidence, and even improve overall health by lowering cardiometabolic health risks [7].

Strategies to increase diversity in healthcare include targeted recruitment, pipeline and STEM (science, tech, engineering, and mathematics) enrichment programs, and college support and mentoring for minority students. Providers at school-based health centers should consider their patients and students as potential future healthcare professionals and strive to serve as role-models and mentors whenever possible.

Training on cultural humility and social determinants of health are needed for all healthcare professionals, including those who care for children and adolescents in school-based health centers. Trainings should be mandatory, structured, and comprehensive. Institutions may choose to develop individualized sessions with a focus on subjects that they may have a particular need for. Needs assessment surveys are helpful in identifying gaps in knowledge and topics that require more attention. Interactive workshops and seminars that incorporate adult learning principles such as case-based discussions, are preferred. Feedback from sessions should be collected, and the overall efficacy of the programs formally evaluated (for example by using pre/post knowledge tests). Trainings like this, especially when completed during formative years, can improve the quality-of-care providers deliver to patients of all backgrounds and life experiences [8].

Case 2 A 17-year-old male presents to a school-based health center. He tells the doctor he received a letter stating that he is not allowed to return to school until his vaccines are up-to-date. You review his vaccine records which show he is past due for the meningitis booster. As part of your history taking, you ask him when he last saw his pediatrician. He says she does not remember when and that both of his parents work long hours and it's hard for him to get to the doctor.

Health equity can be defined as the principle that all people have a fair and just opportunity to be healthy [9]. The Robert Wood Johnson Foundation provides the following explanation of health equity: "The attainment of health equity requires removing obstacles to health, such as poverty, discrimination, and their consequences, including powerlessness and lack of access to good job with fair pay, quality education and housing, safe environments, and health care" [9]. School-based health centers are an excellent example of the pursuit of true health equity. Not only do school-based health centers provide access to essential healthcare to a vulnerable population, but they have also been shown to improve both health-related and educational outcomes in the students that they serve [10]. Importantly, school-based health centers are associated with decreased emergency department use and hospital admissions, decreased asthma morbidity, and increased contraceptive use among females [10]. When it comes to educational outcomes-students at schools with school-based health centers have higher grade point averages, and lower suspension and noncompletion rates [10].

While school-based health centers are strong drivers of health equity, it is still important to ensure that the medical providers and processes that make up school-based health centers work in a way that continues to address systemic barriers and challenges to health equity. This can be done by looking at social determinants of health. Social determinants of health are "the conditions and the environments where people are born, live, learn, work, play, and worship", that affect health risk and outcomes" [11]. Standardized screenings for social determinants of health should be in place at all school-based health centers. Examples of such tools are provided in Table 13.1 below. Providers at school-based health centers should be well-educated on what clinical information they should be seeking to better understand students' life and environmental circumstances. This may mean increasing social determinants of health training, and ensuring there is a process in place for feedback and assessment of these trainings.

Additionally, it is imperative that when screening for social determinants of health, there are proper resources in place to be able to address all and any positive screenings. It is not enough to understand where there may be a need, school-based health centers must have the capacity to address these needs in real time, ideally with the partnership of experienced social workers and resources such as reputable community-based organizations [12].

Case 3 A 13-year-old female is seen in a school-based health center with a chief complaint of abdominal pain. The patient's preferred language is Spanish. The provider goes into the room and begins to take a history. Initially the provider assumes that the patient may be exaggerating her symptoms or misunderstanding them due to the language barrier. During the encounter the provider recognizes this bias in real-time, and with the help of an interpreter is able to ask clarifying questions to obtain a better history. At the end of the encounter, the provider reviews the diagnosis of constipation, and checks for understanding using the teach-back method. The provider also finds a handout of high-fiber foods in Spanish to provide to the patient.

Inclusion is defined by Collins Dictionary as the "act of making a person a part of a group or collection". Inclusion in medicine has been conceptualized as "a set of social processes that influence an individual's access to information and sense of belonging" [13]. When we think about inclusion in school-based health centers, it's important to first address the issue of implicit bias. Implicit bias refers to "unconscious mental processes that lead to associations and reactions that are automatic and without intention" [14]. Simply put, implicit biases are unconscious judgements we make about people or a group of people that are typically based on stereotypes

Table 13.1 Standardized screenings for social determinants of health

Screening tool	Link
Pediatric ACEs and Related Life Events Screener	https://cblcc.acf.hhs.gov/wp-content/uploads/PEARLS-Handouts-English.pdf
AAFP Social Needs Screening Tool	https://www.aafp.org/dam/AAFP/documents/patient_care/everyone_project/hops19-physician-form-sdoh.pdf
The Accountable Health Communities Health-Related Social Needs Screening Tool	https://www.cms.gov/priorities/innovation/files/worksheets/ahcm-screeningtool.pdf
Upstream Risks Screening Tool and Guide	https://www.aamc.org/system/files/c/2/442878-chahandout1.pdf

or preconceived notions. Implicit bias is also sometimes called unconscious bias for this reason. Implicit bias is different from explicit bias. Explicit biases are preferences, beliefs, and attitudes that we have about other people that we are *consciously* aware of. Table 13.2 below shows examples of explicit versus implicit biases.

Implicit bias has been shown to play a significant role in how certain groups of people are treated in healthcare settings. For example, studies have shown that higher levels of implicit bias among health care providers is associated with disparities in treatment recommendations, pain management, and even empathy [15]. This is particularly important to consider in the care of adolescent patients in school-based health centers, an already vulnerable and often underserved population.

Providers' implicit biases can affect their perception or understanding of their patient based on factors such as race, ethnicity, gender, sexual orientation, or socio-economic status, etc. This can in-turn lead to differences in how that patient is cared for and ultimately impact treatment recommendations. Importantly, the language and tone a healthcare provider uses can be influenced by their implicit biases as well. Offensive language and tone can lead to misunderstanding, discomfort, and emotional or physical distress for the patient. Eliminating implicit bias entirely is a challenging goal due to the unconscious and deeply rooted nature of the systemic issues that lead to these biases. However, there are several strategies that can be used to shine light on our implicit biases and mitigate their downstream effects, specifically in terms of patient care.

The first strategy in addressing implicit bias is creating a sense of acknowledgement and awareness of the importance of understanding our own specific implicit biases and the potential underlying reasons why they may exist. This can be done by instituting regular mandatory implicit bias training for all providers and staff at school-based health centers. The training should include general education on implicit bias, but also an opportunity to assess individual implicit biases such as the Harvard Implicit Association Test [16]. Another strategy to help mitigate bias is to create structural change. One example is creating standardized protocols and guidelines that reduce variability and thus bias in clinical decision making. Creating standardized processes and relying on evidence-based medicine helps to ensure that treatment plans do not rely on any explicit or implicit feelings or attitudes held by any one provider.

Table 13.2 Examples of explicit versus implicit biases

Explicit bias	Implicit bias
"I don't treat patients from that racial group because they are always non-compliant with treatment plans"	Spending less time with patients of certain racial group because you may unintentionally assume they are not going to be compliant with your recommendations anyway
"I don't want to hire a woman for the position because they don't take their work seriously"	Not asking a woman back for second interview because you assume she does not seem like someone who prioritizes her career
"Gay men are always flamboyant"	Assuming heterosexuality or homosexuality based off someone's personality or demeanor

Inclusion and implicit bias are intertwined and closely related. By creating inclusive environments, we provide opportunity for people from different perspectives and backgrounds to create connections. These connections can help us challenge any stereotypes, assumptions, or prejudices we may hold. This is called counter-stereotyping and is another important mitigator of implicit bias [17]. By finding ways to implement these strategies at school-based health centers, we are working to build more inclusive environments for our patients, where they can feel a true sense of belonging.

Extra Credit Points

1. School-based health centers are an important paradigm for reducing health disparities among adolescents.
2. Creating diverse and inclusive school-based health centers can positively impact student health and education outcomes.
3. Addressing social determinants of health in this population is an essential component of the work towards achieving health equity.

References

1. Clayborne EP, Martin DR, Goett RR, Chandrasekaran EB, McGreevy J. Diversity PIPELINES: The rationale to recruit and support minority physicians. J Am Coll Emerg Physicians Open. 2021;2(1):e12343. Published 2021 Jan 2. https://doi.org/10.1002/emp2.12343.
2. Miller J. Council post: the power of diversity and inclusion: driving innovation and success. Forbes. https://www.forbes.com/sites/forbesbusinesscouncil/2023/08/16/the-power-of-diversity-and-inclusion-driving-innovation-and-success/?sh=1eb2df32505d. Accessed 31 May 2024.
3. Riley WJ. Health disparities: gaps in access, quality and affordability of medical care. Trans Am Clin Climatol Assoc. 2012;123:167–74.
4. Elster A, Jarosik J, VanGeest J, Fleming M. Racial and ethnic disparities in health care for adolescents: a systematic review of the literature. Arch Pediatr Adolesc Med. 2003;157(9):867–74. https://doi.org/10.1001/archpedi.157.9.867.
5. Greenwood BN, Hardeman RR, Huang L, Sojourner A. Physician–patient racial concordance and disparities in birthing mortality for newborns. Proc Natl Acad Sci. 2020;117(35):21194–200. https://doi.org/10.1073/pnas.1913405117.
6. Thornton RL, Powe NR, Roter D, Cooper LA. Patient-physician social concordance, medical visit communication and patients' perceptions of health care quality. Patient Educ Couns. 2011;85(3):e201–8. https://doi.org/10.1016/j.pec.2011.07.015.
7. Levine CS, Markus HR, Austin MK, Chen E, Miller GE. Students of color show health advantages when they attend schools that emphasize the value of diversity. Proc Natl Acad Sci. 2019;116(13):6013–8. https://doi.org/10.1073/pnas.1812068116.
8. Wilbur K, Snyder C, Essary AC, Reddy S, Will KK. Developing workforce diversity in the health professions: a social justice perspective. Health Prof Educ. 2020;6(2):222–9. https://doi.org/10.1016/j.hpe.2020.01.002.
9. Robert Wood Johnson Foundation. What is health equity? Princeton, NJ: RWJF; 2017. https://www.rwjf.org/en/insights/our-research/2017/05/what-is-health-equity-.html.
10. Knopf JA, Finnie RKC, Peng Y, et al. School-based health centers to advance health equity: a community guide systematic review. Am J Prev Med. 2016;51(1):114–26. https://doi.org/10.1016/j.amepre.2016.01.009.

11. Healthy People 2030. Social determinants of health. Healthy people 2030. 2020. https://health.gov/healthypeople/priority-areas/social-determinants-health.
12. Houlihan J, Leffler S. Assessing and addressing social determinants of health. Prim Care Clin Off Pract. 2019;46(4):561–74. https://doi.org/10.1016/j.pop.2019.07.013.
13. Person SD, Jordan CG, Allison JJ, Fink Ogawa LM, Castillo-Page L, Conrad S, Nivet MA, Plummer DL. Measuring diversity and inclusion in Academic Medicine: the diversity engagement survey. Acad Med. 2015;90(12):1675–83. https://doi.org/10.1097/ACM.0000000000000921.
14. Vela MB, Erondu AI, Smith NA, Peek ME, Woodruff JN, Chin MH. Eliminating explicit and implicit biases in health care: evidence and research needs. Annu Rev Public Health. 2022;43:477–501. https://doi.org/10.1146/annurev-publhealth-052620-103528.
15. Maina IW, Belton TD, Ginzberg S, Singh A, Johnson TJ. A decade of studying implicit racial/ethnic bias in healthcare providers using the implicit association test. Soc Sci Med. 2018;199(199):219–29. https://doi.org/10.1016/j.socscimed.2017.05.009.
16. Project Implicit. Implicit association test. Harvard. 2011. https://implicit.harvard.edu/implicit/takeatest.html.
17. *8 STRATEGIES to REDUCE/INTERRUPT IMPLICIT BIAS STRATEGY # 1-Increase Your Awareness*. https://communityactionpartnership.com/wp-content/uploads/2018/05/CAP8strategies.pdf.

Part II
Understanding and Supporting Your Students

Chapter 14
Normal Growth and Development: Elementary School Students

Banku Jairath

Elementary school age children are made of constantly changing individuals. Hence, a knowledge of normal growth and developmental changes is necessary for the providers to identify any deviation in growth and development (Table 14.1). You are a school-based physician spending your Saturday morning conducting well-child visits for your students:

Case 1 Graham is a 6-year-old student with no significant past medical history, and his parents ask you what normal motor physical skills are for his age?

Fundamental motor skills being developed at his age are- running, galloping, jumping, hopping, skipping, throwing, catching, striking, kicking [1].

Case 2 Patricia is a 10-year-old student with a history of asthma. Her mother is concerned that she is taller than most of the boys in her grade and she has also noticed some breast budding. Is this normal?

Discuss physical development with your students and their parents, and tell them the approximate time they should expect accelerated growth. For girls, this may occur at ages 9 to 11 years, and typically 1 to 2 years before the onset of menarche. For boys, this may not occur until about age 12 years or older [1]. Thelarche is the first sign of puberty in girls and totally normal at her age. Reassurance and education should be provided to Patricia and her mother.

Case 3 Greg is an 8-year-old student with a history of autism. His father is concerned about his weight, which has increased significantly over the school year. You notice that his BMI is above the 95th percentile. Is this a concern?

B. Jairath (✉)
Penn State Health Milton S. Hershey Medical Center, Hershey, PA, USA
e-mail: bjairath@pennstatehealth.psu.edu

R. P. Olympia, J. Brady-Olympia (eds.), *Clinical Considerations in School-based Health*, https://doi.org/10.1007/978-3-031-85765-2_14

Table 14.1 Normal motor, cognitive, emotional, and social development in elementary school aged children

	Motor	Cognitive	Emotional/social	Red flags
Kindergarten-1st grade (5–6 years)	• Draws a person with at least 8 parts • Run, skip, jump and climb • Use safety scissors easily • Write letters numbers • More coordinated in activities	• Starts to grasp the concept of time • Can follow a series of at least three step commands	• Starts to understand feelings of others with some help from teachers and parents	• Significant loss of skills • Cannot differentiate between real and pretend • Vision problems • Unable to complete complex fine motor tasks (e.g., writing)
2nd and 3rd grade (7–8 years)	• Better at complex moving skills-zizag running • Good pencil hold, better writing letter formation skills	• Able to solve complex addition and subtraction problems • Starts to enjoy reading	• More interest in organized sports • Starts to show interest in certain subjects, hobbies and activities • Able to better express their feelings	• School avoidance • Daytime wetting • Problems concentrating • Excessive tantrums • Aggressive behavior
4th and 5th grade (9–11 years)	• Improved handwriting • Better at using variety of tools	• Organized, logical thinking • Increased attention span • Able to solve complex problems	• Forms strong and complex friendships • More independent	• Persistent withdrawal • Isolation from peers • Trouble following multi-step instructions • Bullying

Emphasize that achieving and maintaining a healthy weight is best accomplished through healthy eating behaviors and regular physical activity [1]. Healthy nutrition and physical activity help contribute towards developing all round physical and mental health of the child. Healthy weight, appropriate food intake, adequate calcium, water instead of soda, adequate physical activity in organized sports, limits on screen times, all help contribute towards normal healthy growth of the child. Encourage children, especially those who are overweight, to limit sedentary behaviors (e.g., watching television and videotapes, playing computer games) to 1 to 2 h a day.

14.1 Physical Growth

Usual physical growth is the pattern of change in height and weight as assessed with established values for the population. These values should always be interpreted within the context of genetic potential with an emphasis on growth velocity (change of measurement over time) as opposed to utilizing one single measurement [2]. It is vital to understand typical growth patterns to help recognize pathologic deviations. School age children grow in predictable patterns which typically include pulsatile episodes of rapid growth (growth spurts) followed by periods of no measurable growth [3].

Growth evaluation should start with taking a history, including evaluation of weight and length. Child's past medical history and dietary history should be the core. A thorough review of systems focusing on signs and symptoms of systemic disease as well as family history including parental height, parental growth patterns, and birth history along with maternal history is important [4].

Following history, evaluation of growth percentiles for age and sex including proportionality is the next step in evaluation. If a measurement deviates from normal percentile range and/or from the individuals' prior growth trajectory, measurements should first be repeated. Measurements should be plotted on known and validated growth charts. The CDC growth chart is typically used for elementary school age children. This growth chart is based on the growth of children in the United States from 1963 to 1994 and was then updated and reviewed in 2000 to include a more ethnically diverse population as well as more breastfed infants [5]. There are also certain populations with known altered patterns of growth where alternative growth charts may be used, including Down syndrome (Trisomy 21), Turner syndrome, Williams syndrome, Achondroplasia, and Prader-Willi syndrome.

14.2 Motor Development

Motor development is broadly divided into gross motor and fine motor skills. Gross motor development describes the process by which children gain the ability to move around their world independently and purposefully [6]. Fine motor development describes the process of gaining the use of the arms and hands to manipulate the environment for purposes of self-help, play, and work [6]. As elementary students become older, they develop motor skills, like kicking, catching, and throwing and then over time learn more complex activities, like dancing, shooting a basketball, or playing the piano.

14.3 Socioemotional Development

Elementary school aged children become more independent, develop self-esteem, have more social interactions outside of the household, and have the ability to manage and resolve conflicts [1].

Students who fall outside the normal growth and development for age and sex should be referred to a pediatric specialist (Table 14.2).

Extra Credit Points

1. School performance is an efficient marker of child's development and achievements across all developmental realms during middle childhood.
2. Nutrition and physical activity dictates both their mental and physical well-being.
3. Consider referrals to pediatric subspecialists (medical and psychiatric) when growth and development fall outside the norm for age and sex.

Table 14.2 Referrals for growth and development deviations from the norm

Concerns	Screening and referral recommended	Associated chapter
Behavioral concerns pertaining to anxiety/depression	Screening questionnaires, referral to behavioral therapy and if needed, a Psychiatry referral	Anxiety (Chap. 68) Depression (Chap. 74)
Hearing concerns	Hearing screen, if abnormal, audiology referral	Chap. 87
Vision issues	Vision screen, if abnormal ophthalmology referral	Chap. 87
Learning disabilities Attention concerns	Psychological and educational assessments may need IEP at school Vanderbilt assessment for ADHD	Learning disability (Chap. 80) Attention concerns (Chap. 66)
Speech delay	Intermediate Unit referral for Speech therapy	Chapter 85
Motor delays, handwriting issues	Intermediate Unit referral for physical and occupational therapy	Not applicable
Short stature	Bone age, laboratory testing, Endocrinology referral	Not applicable
BMI falling below the 5th percentile	Laboratory testing, Gastroenterology referral	Chap. 75
BMI trending above the 95th percentile	Laboratory testing, weight management clinic referral	Chap. 62

References

1. Hagan JF, Shaw JS, Duncan PM. Bright futures: guidelines for health supervision of infants, children, and adolescents. Washington, DC: American Academy of Pediatrics; 2017.
2. Lifshitz F, Cervantes CD. Short stature. In: Pediatric Endocrinology, vol. 25. New York: Marcel Dekker; 1996. p. 25–31.
3. Thalange NK, Foster PJ, Gill MS, Price DA, Clayton PE. Model of normal prepubertal growth. Arch Dis Child. 1996;75(5):427–31.
4. Rao P, Vander Schaaf EB, Steiner MJ, Perry M. Normal child growth and development; 2023. p. 295–309.
5. Grummer-Strawn LM, et al. Use of World Health Organization and CDC growth charts for children aged 0–59 months in the United States. MMWR Recomm Rep. 2010;59:1–15.
6. Gerber RJ, Wilks T, Erdie-Lalena C. Developmental milestones 3: social-emotional development. Pediatr Rev. 2011;32(12):533–6.

Chapter 15
Effective Communication with Elementary School Students

Josiah Harmes and Hallie McGrew

Case 1 **Anthony, a 7-year-old student, was playing on the monkey bars. Anthony, following a dare from his classmate, was attempting to skip two monkey bars and fell. He lands on his left arm and strikes his head. Anthony is crying complaining of significant pain in his arm, head, and neck pain as he enters the nurse's office. How do you respond and prepare him knowing that he will need further treatment?**

Case 2 **Julia is a 9-year-old female who was in art class painting when she trips and falls landing on a wooden easel. Julia comes to the health clinic holding a cloth on her leg crying and saying her leg hurts. When you remove the towel, you see a deep 6-centimeter laceration on her leg. How do you approach this situation to help Julia stay calm while treating her?**

Case 3 **Kerian is a 10-year-old male who was running around in the Gym class when he started having a difficult time breathing. He comes to the nurse's office complaining of chest tightness and difficulty breathing. You notice that he is having a difficult time speaking, that he is wheezing, and looks like he is starting to panic. How do you help Kerian stay calm while he is getting scared because he cannot breathe?**

Picture this: you are in a foreign country, and you unexpectedly become extremely sick. You are rushed to a local hospital where no one speaks your language, and they appear to be practicing some kind of alternative medicine. You are trying to tell

J. Harmes (✉)
Penn State Health Children's Hospital, Hershey, PA, USA
e-mail: Jharmes1@pennstatehealth.psu.edu

H. McGrew
UPMC Children's Hospital of Pittsburgh, Pittsburgh, PA, USA
e-mail: mcgrewhn@upmc.edu

R. P. Olympia, J. Brady-Olympia (eds.), *Clinical Considerations in School-based Health*, https://doi.org/10.1007/978-3-031-85765-2_15

them that you are uncomfortable and what they are doing is not helping, but they don't understand you and you are too weak to fight them. You lay there, terrified. What is happening to you? Will you ever be okay again? The only words they say that you understand are, "You're okay, you're okay." But you do not feel okay.

The situation described is how many young children feel during their first visit to a school nurses' office or school-based clinic to see a physician. They are told by strangers, "We are just trying to help you," but everything is uncomfortable or hurts. At home, when these kids are sick or get hurt, they usually receive comfort from a caregiver who genuinely makes them feel better. However, that is not always the case when entering a nurses' office or school-based clinic. They are poked and prodded, given medicine that tastes bad or even makes them feel sick, they are told not to eat before procedures that are already super scary, strangers touch and move injuries that hurt, and the list goes on and on. What medical professionals see as "helping" young children feel as "hurting." Professionals must learn to speak the "child's language" to earn the child's trust and truly be able to provide the care needed to help the child.

15.1 Age-Appropriate Language Choice Within the Context of Development

While it at first may seem like a simple everyday task, numerous parts of communication are necessary for accurate transmission of what is meant. We say hi, we shake hands, and we introduce ourselves. Is this it? Is it just the words we say? It would not be surprising if you answered no, because you are correct, there is more to communication. Communication can be complicated between adults, yet there are further layers of complexity when discussing communication between adults and elementary-aged children. For instance, it is important to note that elementary-aged children may be unable to understand the long-term nature of sickness or illness. At this age, children's memory works more in the short term. They do not have the abstract thought to realize that some illnesses and sicknesses last longer, the cause of their illness, or even that medicine that might make them feel sick is helping them. Furthermore, we must remind them that they did not cause the sickness as elementary-aged children occasionally think that they caused the illness [1]. What we communicate builds the therapeutic relationship that then allows us to help them.

When working with elementary-aged children what word choice are we using? Are we using language that they understand and relate to? The normal language that we use in adult-to-adult conversations makes sense to us, and we may not think about it, but it can have another meaning for children. For instance, describing a blood pressure cuff feels like a "hug" may make them confused as when it happens and gets really tight? Hugs are not supposed to be this tight. Instead try describing it like: "It is going to feel like a big squeeze and if you stay still, it will stop squeezing your arm faster." Examples that you use need to be concrete, like the example provided above. Try to explain a new concept by relating it to something they already understand. The following are a few examples of ways to explain medical terminology in an age-appropriate way:

- An Emergency Room is a place where we go to get help and feel better when we are sick. There are many people there to help you feel better.
- An Ambulance is a vehicle such as a truck that quickly takes you to the emergency room.
- A neck brace goes around your neck to keep it still while the doctors make sure your neck is not hurt.
- Vital signs tell us how you are breathing, how your heart is beating and your temperature.
- An IV is a medicine straw that gives your body medicine and gives your body a drink.
- A CT scan, X-ray, or MRI are big picture machines that take pictures of you to see what is happening, and just like another picture it does not hurt or touch you.
- Stitches are string Band-Aids.
- NPO means you are not allowed to eat or drink for a while before a procedure or until we figure out why you are not feeling well.
- A nasal cannula is a small tube that sits at your nose to give you more oxygen.

Try your best to relate what you explain to things they know and understand, and if they are giving you blank looks then change up the example [1]. Children learn by touching and seeing things, and if it is safe and appropriate use some of the medical supplies as props. Let them feel the stethoscope, the blood pressure cuff, and other things to help them learn and clear up misconceptions. Many children and adults do not realize that once an IV is in the needle is removed and all that is left is the catheter that works like a little straw. Children often see the hospital environment as painful and scary, so communicating when things will not hurt and proving it helps build trust. It is important to be honest with them, but being honest does not mean we have to be blunt with the information. We take time to explain it so that they can process and understand; allowing them to work with us instead of against us. By using age-appropriate language, we help children participate in their care and further encourage them to be compliant and confident patients (Fig. 15.1).

15.2 Connecting with the Patient

Building rapport with patients is always an essential piece of a healthcare professional's role. Rapport building is the process of building a trusting and honest relationship that enables us to understand and better care for those in our care. It is crucial to understand a child's way of thinking in order to understand their feelings and how to best meet their emotional and psychosocial needs. When rapport is built, it helps the patient trust which causes them to be more compliant and honest with healthcare providers. Children notice a lot even when adults do not think they do. Be sure to include the child in conversation by utilizing child-friendly phrases and asking them questions directly when possible. If a child seems apprehensive, drop

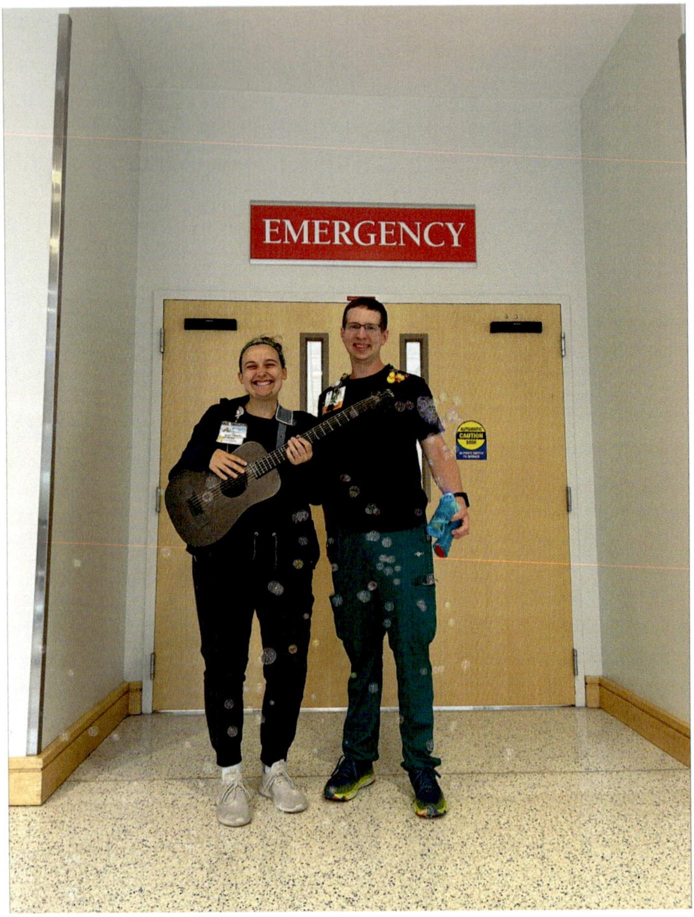

Fig. 15.1 Facilitating communication with children in our emergency department at Penn State Children's Hospital include the expertise of Child Life Specialist (Josiah Harmes) and Music Therapy (Tara Kelly)

the medical talk for a couple of minutes to build rapport. It can help to be aware of popular shows, movies, or toys for that age group. (i.e. "Do you like Paw Patrol? My favorite pup is Rubble.") By adding in this simple interaction, it shows the child that you can understand them, so maybe they can trust you. It can also be helpful to know this information for distraction purposes later on. If a child needs some type of procedure or test done later, it is helpful for a child to have something else to focus on than the test or procedure. When a child is focused on distraction, because they are paying less attention to what is happening, and they are more likely to remain still. You can facilitate distraction with a video or movie on a phone or tablet, a look and find book, bubbles, fidgets, and other things. This is also a way that you can give them a choice and help them feel involved in their care.

However, despite our best efforts some children do not want to talk to us. This situation must be handled carefully because if we try to force the conversation it just makes children interact less. It is important to be respectful of when a child wants to speak and does not. What does their non-verbal behavior indicate to us? Do you see a confused look, a fearful look, a sad look, or an upset look? If so, then adjust what you are doing and saying to help them feel more comfortable. Also, just because a child does not seem to be paying attention it does not mean that they aren't paying attention. Children pick up many things when we assume they would not be listening. The best thing is to be patient with children and try to coax them into interacting.

Next, are you talking with the child or at them? Sometimes it is easy to just talk at children rather than ensuring the child's understanding and talking with them [2]. Include the child in the conversation by asking them questions when possible or utilizing developmentally appropriate language. Change your conversations from talking AT a child to talking WITH them. Furthermore, it is easy to just engage with the parents and let them speak for their children. We often look at children's caregivers when communicating with children because a child may be shy or may not want to talk to us. We then communicate and engage with the parents instead of the child. However, we must not forget to engage with the patient or child and ensure their understanding. It is helpful to continue to engage with the child and use language that includes them [1] such as "Anna, what hurts?" instead of saying to the caregiver, "Where does Anna hurt?" This also encourages them to continue to speak up and be involved in their care. If a patient has a question or concern about their care, it must be addressed and explained not just brushed away just because they are a child [3]. It is their body, and they live with what is happening. As providers we want them to share with us how they are feeling and what is happening. If we do not take what the patient says seriously, it discourages them from talking with us in the future and then we could lose their trust, jeopardizing their willingness to work with us.

While every child is different and it takes different things to build rapport with each one, it is helpful and important to build rapport. Building rapport is an excellent way to make the healthcare experience a positive experience. It is important to try to make the interactions positive as it takes just one traumatic experience to make a child scared and less likely to cooperate and engage with medical staff. After traumatic experiences, it takes many good experiences to overcome the traumatic ones. Children are much easier to treat when we encourage and allow them to cooperate with us.

Seven quick and easy changes you can implement now to increase your communication with school-aged patients:

1. **Utilize positive reinforcement instead of bribing the patient**: A simple way of doing this is to remember to avoid "if/then" statements. Instead of saying "If you do this, then you can have a prize." Try saying "Remember, when this is all done, I will get you that toy you wanted." It is a very slight change, but by removing "if/then" statements, you reduce anxiety. Promises made as a bribe can add stress to the situation for the child. For instance, if the child feels too scared to get a shot and you try using bribery, it may feel impossible for them to get the

thing they want, resulting in added stress. By changing the wording, it reminds them that they will be getting the fun thing after the difficult task is done without relying on their performance. It becomes reassuring and comforting instead of stressful.

2. **Give options versus asking yes/no questions:** When a child is in a stressful situation and is asked yes/no questions they tend to answer "no." (Ex: The doctor asks, "Can I listen to your heart? The patient responds, "No.") When this happens the provider is faced with having to walk away and respect the patient's "No," or break the patient's trust. The problem with this is the thing being asked of the patient is not an option at all. It's typically something the doctor or nurse NEEDS to do. When the patient answers "No," and the professional proceeds anyway, they are increasing the chance of medical-related trauma and only making future encounters more difficult and more stressful for the patient. What if instead of asking, "Can I listen to your heart?" the doctor had said, "Would you like me to listen to your heart or look at your ears first?" These are two things that need to be done, but this way, the doctor increases the patient's sense of autonomy without breaking his/her trust.
3. **Reframe negative statements into positive ones:** During procedures, it is easy to look at a squirming child and say things like, "Don't move!" or "Don't touch that!" Instead, try saying, "It is your job to hold still." Then, you can even add in options of what they can do like, "It's okay to cry and you can watch a show or squeeze your mom's hands if you need to." You cannot assume that when you tell a child what *not* to do, that they can come up with what they *can* do on their own. It may seem obvious to an adult to think, "If I'm told not to move, maybe I can hold on to the arms of the chair to hold myself still." But for a child, moving may feel like the only option and by telling them not to do that, they might not know what else to do.
4. **Show the patient medical equipment first instead of starting right into an exam:** Even though we know that stethoscopes and otoscopes don't cause any pain, a child seeing one for the first time doesn't. By showing the child the equipment, letting them touch it, and even performing quick evaluations on caregivers for the child to see, you can earn their trust and cooperation. This is the same for all medical equipment.
5. **Praise specific actions instead of saying "Good Job"**: Whenever conducting a procedure, you may think it is comforting to say, "Good Job," to a patient. For instance, if a doctor is putting sutures in a child's arm and there are nurses helping to hold the patient's arm still, it is common for the provider to say "Good job" over and over to the patient. It may be well-intentioned, but it is actually not helpful. If the child is crying or yelling and hearing "Good job," it will seem empty and ingenuine. On the flip side a child may be fully cooperating, but hearing "Good job," may still seem empty and ingenuine because in their mind, they aren't doing anything to warrant a "Good job." Instead, try praising specific actions, "Good job *holding still*, it makes this so much safer and easier for all of us." If a kid is crying or upset you can say, "Good job *telling me how you feel.*"

6. **Do not just stand over them while talking to them:** When you enter the room, do you stand and tower above them or physically get down to their level [4]? Elementary students are often smaller and shorter than you and it can be intimidating to them to have someone they do not know towering over them [4]. When they are intimidated or scared, children will be less likely to engage. Is there a chair or stool you can sit on? Can you put one knee on the ground while talking with them? This shows that you want to meet them where they are, facilitating trust. We can then use this trust while caring for patients to accomplish our jobs easier and faster.
7. **Do not just say, "it's okay":** It is easy as an adult to hear a child crying and immediately try to make it stop. While this is well-intentioned, crying is not always bad, crying is a form of coping too. If a child is crying during a procedure, resist saying, "It's okay," because, to them, it probably doesn't feel "okay." Instead try saying, "You are safe." Or "We are helping you." However, don't expect this to necessarily stop the crying. Instead, create a safe space for tears. Try telling them, "It's okay to cry." Or "We know this makes you upset, but it is something we have to do to help you get better." This makes a room more comforting and safer even in scary moments.

15.3 Case Conclusions

1. First, you remind Anthony that he is safe and that the staff are calling his parents, and until they come you will be with him. You maintain a calm voice while explaining and talking to him through everything you are doing. While you wait for his parents or for transport to a medical facility you distract him through conversation or maybe watching something on your phone so that he stays calm while remaining still.
2. First, you get down to Julia's level and introduce yourself. While you talk with her and her parents you explain that the cut needs stitches and they are like string band aids. You explain that you will numb it so that she does not feel it. You then offer her the choice of distraction while you fix up her cut.
3. First, you tell Kerian calmly not to worry about talking and that you just want him to focus on his breathing while you take care of him. You focus on talking calmly as your nervousness or anxiety could make Kerian more nervous. You focus on explaining things to him and not just what you are doing but how it can help him as well.

Extra Credit Points

1. What can you say instead of "Good Job?"
2. What do you do when you hear a child crying and a nurse just saying, "You're ok."
3. You ask a patient to listen to their heart and look in their ears and they say no. What do you do and how could you have avoided this?

References

1. Damm L, Leiss U, Habeler U, Ehrich J. Improving care through better communication: continuing the debate. J Pediatr. 2015;167(2):501–2.e5. https://doi.org/10.1016/j.jpeds.2015.05.040.
2. Levetown M. Communicating with children and families: from everyday interactions to skill in conveying distressing information. Pediatrics. 2008;121(5):e1441–60. https://doi.org/10.1542/peds.2008-0565.
3. Lee T, Lin EC, Lin HC. Communication skills utilized by physicians in the pediatric outpatient setting. BMC Health Serv Res. 2022;22(1):993. https://doi.org/10.1186/s12913-022-08385-5.
4. Bell J, Condren M. Communication strategies for empowering and protecting children. J Pediatr Pharmacol Ther. 2016;21(2):176–84. https://doi.org/10.5863/1551-6776-21.2.176.

Chapter 16
Normal Growth and Development: Middle School Students

Natalie Allen

Most middle schools in the United States include sixth, seventh, and eighth grades. These schools often serve children as young as 11 years and as old as 15 years. During this time, children go through significant developmental changes including physical growth, pubertal development, and cognitive and social skills development. Growth and development occur at each child's own pace with a wide range of appropriate development and developmental stages among peers.

16.1 Physical Development

Girls typically begin pubertal development between 8 and 13 years, initially starting with breast development and pubic hair with the average age of onset of menses being 12 years and typically occurring between 10 and 14 years [1]. Boys may begin pubertal development between 9 and 14 years with most boys beginning around age 12 years. Thus the pubertal stage of children during this time is highly variable as is their physical growth with prepubertal children growing at a typical childhood rate around 5–6 cm/year and their pubertal peers undergoing growth spurts with growth rates of ~9–12 cm/year [2].

N. Allen (✉)
Penn State Health Milton S Hershey Medical Center, Hershey, PA, USA
e-mail: Nallen4@pennstatehealth.psu.edu

R. P. Olympia, J. Brady-Olympia (eds.), *Clinical Considerations in School-based Health*, https://doi.org/10.1007/978-3-031-85765-2_16

16.2 Cognitive Development

The middle school years (ages 11–15 years) are a time when rapid cognitive development is underway. Similar to physical development, children move through at their own pace. In this phase of development, adolescents are often concerned about the present and not necessarily the long term with shorter term implications of decision-making at the forefront. The ability to think abstractly and take alternative perspectives into account is developing throughout this period as well as expansion of intellectual interests. Often rules and fairness are very concrete particularly if they feel they are not being treated fairly. This phase of development may coincide with increased risk-taking behaviors as individuals do not yet fully understand behaviors with possible negative consequences. Often children may have a sense of invincibility, thinking that 'this can't happen to me' [3].

16.3 Emotional and Social Development

Adolescents go through profound emotional and social changes during the middle school years. They begin to grapple with formation of their identity and values. Peer relationships during this time increase in importance and there is often a strong desire for acceptance. Individuals may have heightened emotions with changing moods and increased sensitivity. Pressure to conform with peers and to be attractive or desirable is often significant during this phase of development and can lead to risk taking or maladaptive behaviors. Alongside these developments, curiosity about romantic relationships emerges, and a growing need for independence manifests as they strive for autonomy and decision-making power [3]. These developments can lead to increased conflict in peer and family relationships.

Case 1 Paul is a 13-year-old eighth grader who competes on the wrestling team. It is noted that on his school physical form, he is nearly the same height as on his prior physical form last year. He notes that given his size, he feels he must stay in the lowest weight bracket to be able to compete well for the team. He does not have facial hair or voice change. On review of his BMI, he is at the 2%ile.

Childhood growth is a multifactorial process reflecting familial genetics, nutritional status, overall health, appropriate hormone production, and pubertal timing. Prepubertal children typically grow at a rate of approximately 5–6 cm/year. They will often have a brief slow-down in rate of growth prior to the pubertal growth spurt with girls and boys growing at approximately 8–11 cm/year and 9–12 cm/year respectively [2]. Growth rates taper off as adolescents approach completion of pubertal and adult height attainment.

In a prepubertal child, lack of height gain in the last year would be cause for additional evaluation. Height gain should be taken in context with weight gain during an evaluation to assess for possible causes of growth failure. Continued or advancing weight gain may suggest an endocrine cause for poor growth including hypothyroidism, growth hormone deficiency, or Cushing syndrome (endogenous or iatrogenic). When weight loss or poor weight gain precedes lack of height gain, chronic medical conditions and inadequate nutritional status are more likely. Medical conditions following this pattern are broad, including inflammatory bowel disease, celiac disease, chronic kidney disease, and eating disorder among others [2, 4]. In this situation, once weight gain resumes, height growth typically recovers as shown in Fig. 16.1.

Case 2 Emily is an eighth grade female who is 14 years old and has been seen in the counseling office for repeated frustrations about her lack of physical development. On review of her physical forms and appearance, it is noted that she is very small for age at less than the 1%ile for height and has no signs of breast development. She reports that she is upset and frustrated that her peers have mostly started their menses and she has yet to have any signs of puberty. She notes that there has been some bullying in her class due to her small size and lack of development.

In females, the first sign of central puberty is breast development typically occurring between 8 and 12 years; in males, central puberty begins with testicular enlargement between 9 and 14 years. Delayed puberty in girls is classified with lack of breast development by 13 years or lack of menses by 16 years. In males, delayed puberty is lack of testicular enlargement by age 15 years [1]. Delayed puberty is thought to occur in roughly 3% of children with the vast majority of cases secondary to Constitutional Delay of Growth and Puberty (CDGP). Delayed puberty is important to recognize as it can cause emotional distress and may indicate an underlying etiology with broad health implications.

While CDGP is the leading cause of delay, chronic illness may also contribute including cystic fibrosis, kidney disease, sickle cell disease, and others. Additional causes include hypogonadism at the level of the pituitary or gonad. Genetic diagnoses including Klinefelter syndrome, Turner syndrome, and Kallman syndrome are also possible causes of delayed puberty [1]. It would be important to recognize delayed pubertal development to prompt evaluation with the child's primary care provider or pediatrician. Definitions of early, on time, and delayed pubertal development are shown in Table 16.1.

16.4 Case Conclusions

Case 1 Paul was referred back to his primary care physician with concerns about poor growth and malnutrition. The outpatient pediatrician completed an evaluation for poor weight and height gain with initial labs including complete blood count, comprehensive metabolic panel, sedimentation rate, and celiac screening which returned normal. After further discussion, Paul reported extreme dietary restriction

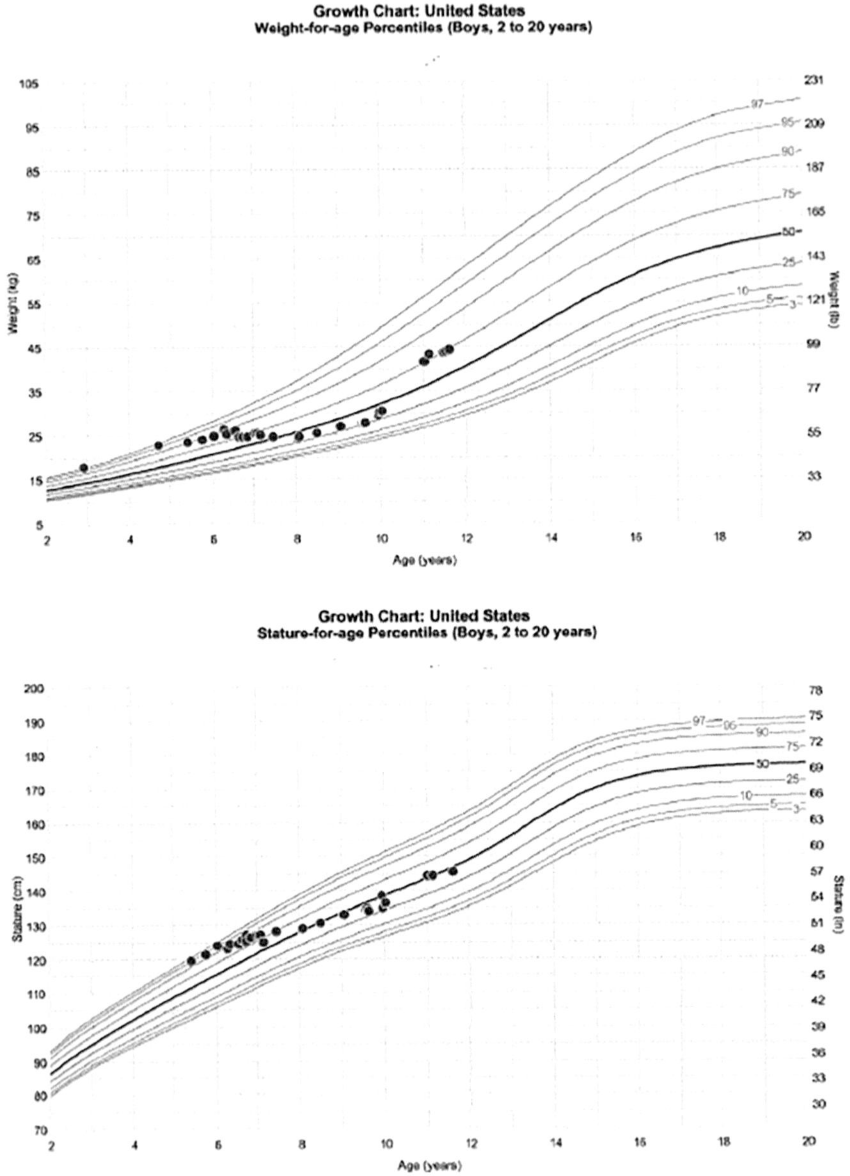

Fig. 16.1 Growth chart depicting poor weight gain leading to height growth failure with subsequent recovery

Table 16.1 Appropriate timing of pubertal development in boys and girls

Puberty	Early	On time	Delayed
Girls	Breast development before 8 years	Breast development starts between 8 and 12 years Menarche between 10 and 14 years	No breast development by 13 years No menarche by 16 years
Boys	Testicular enlargement before 9 years	Testicular enlargement between 9 and 14 years	No testicular enlargement by 15 years

Table 16.2 Associated findings of Turner syndrome and recommended screenings

Associated finding	Screening recommended
Cardiac findings • Coarctation of the aorta • Bicuspid aortic valve • Risk of aortic dissection	Echocardiogram and/or cardiac MRI Referral to cardiology
Malformations of the kidney	Renal ultrasound
Hearing loss	Audiology evaluation every 5 years
Ocular issues	Ophthalmology referral
Learning disabilities	Psychological and educational assessments

and some food purging behaviors. The primary pediatrician referred Paul for further outpatient treatment with an eating disorder clinic.

Case 2 Emily was referred back to her primary care physician with concerns of poor growth and lack of pubertal development. The outpatient pediatrician confirmed the school provider's concerns with pubertal exam showing Sexual Maturity Rating (SMR) I for breast development, indicating prepubertal status for this child. Laboratory evaluation was initiated with luteinizing hormone (LH), follicle stimulating hormone (FSH), estradiol, thyroid stimulating hormone, free T4, and karyotype showing elevated LH and FSH along with 45, X karyotype [5]. Emily was appropriately screened for conditions associated with Turner syndrome (Table 16.2) and initiated on pubertal induction with estrogen medication [5].

Extra Credit Points

1. Middle school is characterized by significant physical, cognitive, emotional, and social development in children. School-based medical providers have the benefit of frequently interacting with students and must understand the range of typical development to identify possible concerns that should be addressed (Table 16.3).
2. Lack of height growth or BMI less than the 5%ile should warrant referral back to the student's primary care provider.
3. Social withdrawal and bullying behaviors call for further evaluation of a student's emotional and social development and well-being.

Table 16.3 Development in middle school age children

	Physical	Cognitive	Emotional/social
6th grade (11–13 years)	± Puberty signs Growth at 5 cm/year or more ***Lack of vertical growth***	Concerned with fairness Short-term thinking Expanding interests	Seeking social acceptance Focus on self Impulsivity
7th grade (12–14 years)	± Puberty signs Growth at 5 cm/year or more ***Lack of vertical growth***	Feelings of invincibility Evolving self-expression Development of ideals Questioning beliefs	Developing identity Friendships very important Desire for independence
8th grade (13–15 years)	+ puberty signs Growth variable ***Lack of pubertal development in girls***	Developing organization Developing operational thinking Experimental risk-taking ***Lack of academic independence***	Peer pressure increases Testing rules and authority Struggling with identity Desire for autonomy
Red flags (11–15 years)	***BMI less than 5%ile***	***Trouble following multi-step instructions***	***Persistent withdrawal*** ***Isolation from peers*** ***Bullying behaviors***

Appropriate physical, cognitive, emotional, and social development by age is noted with 'red flags' for further assessment in italics

References

1. Wolf RM, Long D. Pubertal development. Pediatr Rev. 2016;37(7):292–300. https://doi.org/10.1542/pir.2015-0065. PMID: 27368360.
2. Braun LR, Marino R. Disorders of growth and stature. Pediatr Rev. 2017;38(7):293–304. https://doi.org/10.1542/pir.2016-0178.
3. Sanders RA. Adolescent psychosocial, social, and cognitive development. Pediatr Rev. 2013;34(8):354–9. https://doi-org.ezaccess.libraries.psu.edu/10.1542/pir.34-8-354
4. Hornberger LL, Lane MA, Committee on Adolescence. Identification and management of eating disorders in children and adolescents. Pediatrics. 2021;147(1):e2020040279. https://doi.org/10.1542/peds.2020-040279. Epub 2020 Dec 21. PMID: 33386343.
5. Shankar RK, Backeljauw PF. Current best practice in the management of Turner syndrome. Ther Adv Endocrinol Metab. 2018;9(1):33–40. https://doi.org/10.1177/2042018817746291. Epub 2017 Dec 18. PMID: 29344338; PMCID: PMC5761955.

Chapter 17
Effective Communication with Middle School Students

Josiah Harmes and Hallie McGrew

Case 1 **Alexandra is a 13-year-old female who comes into the nurse's office complaining of sharp pain in her head and nausea. Alexandra comments that her symptoms get worse when she moves or there are bright lights. A friend told her that it might be a brain tumor, and Alexandra is worried because she also read on her phone that it might be a brain tumor. How do you help Alexandra to calm down?**

Case 2 **Aiden is a 12-year-old male who threw up while sitting in math class. Aidan comes into the school-based clinic, and he says that he started having pain this morning before school around the center of his abdomen. Now Aiden now complains of sharp pain and points to the right side of his abdomen. How are you going to prepare Aiden and let him know what is happening?**

Case 3 **Olivia is an 11-year-old female who fell while running in gym class. Olivia has a small laceration on her right forearm. Olivia comes into the clinic crying and upset that she doesn't want stitches or needles. What can you do to help Olivia both?**

J. Harmes (✉)
Penn State Health Children's Hospital, Hershey, PA, USA
e-mail: Jharmes1@pennstatehealth.psu.edu

H. McGrew
UPMC Children's Hospital of Pittsburgh, Pittsburgh, PA, USA
e-mail: mcgrewhn@upmc.edu

R. P. Olympia, J. Brady-Olympia (eds.), *Clinical Considerations in School-based Health*, https://doi.org/10.1007/978-3-031-85765-2_17

17.1 Age-Appropriate Language Choice Within the Context of Development

The ability to communicate effectively with middle school students and families, while it may seem straightforward, is multifaceted. As is true for all communication, what works for one person may not work for another. What a patient says dictates our response. Just as communication changes based on an individual, communication needs for middle school students varies from elementary school students and adolescent school students. Middle-school aged students are a small group of individuals who do not quite fall in the scope of elementary-school aged students but are also not quite in the scope of adolescent aged students. Think of this age group as a spectrum, depending on the individual they may lean more toward an elementary mindset or an adolescent one. This population requires extra attention because many factors other than age play into where on the spectrum your patient lands.

Middle school students tend to think logically and in a concrete manner [1]. As they get closer to adolescence they start to develop more abstract thought, but primarily during this age range they benefit from logical information with concrete examples. Additionally, middle-school-aged patients better understand the long term and short-term nature of sickness and injuries than younger patients [1]. This then allows them to be more involved in care, with assistance from their caregivers. It is also during this time that they begin to realize that medical professionals are trying to help them. Yet despite this knowledge, if middle-school-aged patients are getting a painful procedure, they will need support remembering why they are experiencing this and what they need to do to help the healthcare team. It is because of their greater understanding that medical staff are trying to help them that, as healthcare professionals, we must work as a team and collaborate with the patient to accomplish the goal of medical treatment. As their development is progressing, middle school age patients are beginning to understand more hypothetical and abstract situations [2]. They do not fully understand hypothetical and abstract situations like adolescents or adults, but they are beginning to understand, and it is this beginning to understand that can be utilized. For instance:

An eleven-year-old patient came in for surgery and needed an IV placed for anesthesia. As a Child Life Specialist, it is my job to assess a patient's understanding and provide psychosocial support during procedures to maximize the potential for success. Prior to meeting the patient, I spoke with the nurse who stated, "He's fine! I'm sure he will have no problem letting us place his IV. He has been very easy-going and in good spirits all morning." I went in to meet the patient and the nurse was right, he was very easy to talk to, confident about his upcoming procedure and post-op, but as we discussed his upcoming IV placement, I noticed he started getting quiet and avoiding eye contact. The nurse then came into the room to begin setting up and the patient began to cry and held his arms to not allow the nurse to look for an IV. He kept saying, "I don't want a shot!" This is when I took a moment to explain the reasons for getting an IV, what every step of the process would be like, and discussed coping mechanisms with him. He calmed down, and cooperated through the whole process with reminders from me on what was happening next, as well as, guided deep breathing for coping.

Was the nurse wrong in her assessment? Not necessarily, but the way he presented at the beginning of their interaction reminded her of an adolescent patient who would have a greater capacity for abstract thinking. An adolescent patient would have a large enough grasp on the "why" that they would not need the support that much younger patients require. Yet, because this middle-school aged child has some ability to understand these things, with the right support, they can still be successful. To help middle-school-aged patients we will need to spend more time explaining. Relating the more abstract or hypothetical concepts to concrete examples, allowing more time for processing and encouraging questions from the patients can increase understanding and cooperation [3]. As an example, a 12-year-old female came into the ER because she got bit by an animal. At first, the patient did not want the rabies injections because there would be multiple shots. We could have been inclined to just hold the patient down kicking and screaming. But we helped the 12-year-old patient understand that without the treatment they would get sick and that there were more long-term effects from not getting the treatment than from the short-term discomfort. Instead of just holding her down, traumatizing her and making her scared of hospitals and medical providers, the patient was given the support and care she needed to understand. This granted the medical staff the ability to quickly and safely administer the medical treatment with a cooperative patient rather than a moving patient who had to be restrained.

Even though middle-school-age patients are better able to understand the language of adults, care must still be taken to explain what we mean without being too abstract. For example, a good way to help middle-school-age patients understand anesthesia is by saying, "anesthesia is a medicine that makes you fall asleep and when they stop giving it to you, then you will wake up. Have you ever fallen asleep in the car and when you wake up you have arrived? This is what happens with anesthesia." Examples like this allow middle school students to relate anesthesia to something that they already know and understand. With new medical procedures, try to relate them to things that they know and understand. Here are a few other examples:

- The Emergency Room is a place where you go to get help and when you are sick or injured. There are many people in the Emergency Room to help you feel better.
- An Ambulance is a vehicle such as a truck that quickly takes you to the emergency room.
- A neck brace goes around your neck to keep it still while the doctors make sure your neck is not hurt.
- Vital signs tell us how you are breathing, how your heart is beating, and your temperature.
- An IV is a medicine straw that lets us take some blood to test and give you medicine to help you feel better.
- A CT scan, X-ray, or MRI are cameras that take pictures of you. Like a camera on your phone, but these cameras take pictures of what is inside of you. And just like regular cameras they do not hurt or touch you.
- Stitches are like shoelaces to close your cut.

- NPO means no eating or drinking either before a procedure or until we figure out how to help you feel better. Because eating before certain medicines can make you sicker.
- A nasal cannula is a small tube that sits at your nose to give you more oxygen which helps you breathe.

Relating what is unknown to what is known gives middle-school-aged patients the opportunity to become familiar with the potential unknown and stressful environment. It also allows the opportunity to partner with the patients and help them help us. It enables them to know not only what to expect, but we can also tell them what they can do to help us help them.

17.2 Connecting with the Patient

Just as it is important to adapt our language choices to development and age, it is just as important to build a relationship with the patients that we care for [4]. This relationship helps patients be honest and trust us as medical providers with information that they may not share with anyone else. An effective way to connect with a child is to focus on something they like. What are some popular bands, what are some recent video games, and what is a popular sport/sports team? All of these can open the door to building a relationship with the patients that then allows us to care for them. If you don't know or understand who or what something is, ask. Don't fake that you know it, because they can tell. If they realize that you are faking, then they will be less likely to get engaged and share. Also, by asking, it can start a conversation that you can turn to medicine and their care.

Next, are your conversations one-sided or two-sided? Sometimes there is a tendency to just talk at children rather than taking the time to ensure the child understands what is happening and why it is happening [4]. Make sure you are talking with them rather than talking at them. Do you prefer being talked at or talked with? Being talked at sends a vastly different message than being talked with. Talking with patients invites the patient to take part in their care. Patients who are cooperative and honest with us are more likely to seek help when they need it. Part of talking with middle-school-aged patients is ensuring that you are including them and not just talking with their parents [1]. Middle-school-aged patients know their bodies and what is going on, even if they do not fully understand what is happening. It is important to get the parents' input and feedback, yet it is vital that we let the patient communicate what is happening to them. Middle-school-aged children benefit from the opportunity to engage with the medical staff to better understand what is currently happening and what is going to happen [3]. For example, an 11-year-old female came into the ER because she had high blood sugar. The medical staff had to quickly do two IVs to help the patient. The first thing I did when engaging with this child was to kneel to get down to her level while talking with her. Then the patient and I talked about the IVs to help her understand how it works and the importance of them for her care. We talked about how with IVs there is a small needle, but that the needle does not stay in her arm. Then we went over the fact that her job was just to stay still and breathe, we were able to do this in the time that it took the nurses to get their supplies and get set up. The patient did an amazing job with both IVs, and we made sure the patient knew she did great. The patient then verbalized that she did not like needles, and I was honest that few people like IVs, but they are important to help us feel better. We were able to help the 11-year-old patient understand the situation and how she could help rather than just spewing information without any regard for the patient's comprehension. The other important topic that this example highlights is the level at which you are speaking to the patient. By getting down to the patient's level it is less intimidating or scary to them than standing over them helping them feel more comfortable and encouraging them to engage [2]. You can do this by kneeling or sitting on a chair or stool which shows that you want to meet them where they are. Meeting children where they are builds trust and allows them to participate in their care. Engaging them and working with them makes the care less stressful and faster as a cooperating middle-school-aged patient is much easier to work with than an uncooperative one. Additionally, the patient receives better holistic care.

Four quick and easy changes you can implement now to increase your communication with middle-school-aged patients:

1. **Don't talk to the patient like they are a young child:** Nothing will make a middle-school-age patient shutdown faster than using "baby talk" or talking at them like they are a small child. They have enough understanding of things going on that they want to be talked to with respect. Remain compassionate but avoid using a high-pitched "baby-talk" voice or acting like the child cannot understand. Take the time to explain things to them and allow them to ask questions that exhibit their understanding.
2. **Don't assume the child understands what you are talking about:** Talk to them with respect, but remember they are still young and have had a lot less life experience than you. They might not know what anesthesia, an IV, or even a vein is. Ask them what they understand, but do not be condescending. If you are getting ready to place an IV and they have never had one, start with the basics. "Do you know what a vein is?" Starting with the most basic piece of information allows you to build concrete information that the child can understand. "An IV is a small straw that goes in your vein so we can draw blood to run tests or give you medicine that gets through your body faster than swallowing it."
3. **Ask for the child's opinion:** When making plans for treatment, don't just ask the parents for input. Ask the patient, "How do you feel about this?" or "What are your thoughts about this plan?" rather than just telling them the plan. You may get insight into their feelings or even their misunderstandings, which will allow you the opportunity to provide needed clarification and earn their respect.
4. **Get to know your patients:** Find out at least one thing they like and talk to them about it. If you have knowledge on this topic, talk to them about it. If you do not, ask them about it. Utilize active listening skills to display care.

17.3 Case Conclusions

1. Talk with Alexandria to figure out what her symptoms are and remind her that it is probably a headache or migraine and when she asks questions treat her questions seriously. Remind her the importance of not just believing what she reads on her phone about medicine and that it is better to talk with her parents and a healthcare provider when she is sick or has concerns.
2. Talk to Aiden and let him know that you are going to try to help figure out what is going on. Explain what you are doing and let him know that if there is anything he does not understand, he can ask about it so you can do your best to answer it. After doing tests and finding some answers, talk with him about his diagnosis/what you think is making him sick. Do not talk down to him, like a young child, or over him, straight to the parent. Furthermore, if he will need to be transported to a hospital, let him know what to expect so that he knows.
3. Introducing yourself and talk with Olivia to get to know her and let her know that you can be trusted and are going to work with her to figure this out. Letting her know that we will take it one step at a time. Once you figure out what the best way to fix it is, talk to Olivia and make a plan for how you want to work together to fix it whether it will be stitches, Dermabond, or something else.

Extra Credit Points

1. Your patient has a laceration to their leg, and you can use stitches or Dermabond. Parents do not care which one. How can you involve the patient in this decision?
2. How did you get this booboo? How can you rephrase this in an age-appropriate way.
3. You say that you are going to get their vitals, assuming that they will know what you mean. How do you respond to their confused/blank look on their face while treating them in a developmentally appropriate way?

References

1. Damm L, Leiss U, Habeler U, Ehrich J. Improving care through better communication: continuing the debate. J Pediatr. 2015;167(2):501–2.e5. https://doi.org/10.1016/j.jpeds.2015.05.040.
2. Bell J, Condren M. Communication strategies for empowering and protecting children. J Pediatr Pharmacol Ther. 2016;21(2):176–84. https://doi.org/10.5863/1551-6776-21.2.176.
3. Lee T, Lin EC, Lin HC. Communication skills utilized by physicians in the pediatric outpatient setting. BMC Health Serv Res. 2022;22(1):993. https://doi.org/10.1186/s12913-022-08385-5.
4. Levetown M. Communicating with children and families: from everyday interactions to skill in conveying distressing information. Pediatrics. 2008;121(5):e1441–60. https://doi.org/10.1542/peds.2008-0565.

Chapter 18
Normal Growth and Development: High School Students

Estelle Anh-Thu Green and Rosemary Claire Roden

The high school years are a pivotal time for teenagers, as it marks the transition from childhood and adulthood. During this period, adolescents undergo significant physical (Table 18.1), as well as cognitive and psychosocial developmental milestones (Tables 18.2, 18.3, and 18.4). Although the pace at which these individual changes occur may vary, the timing and sequence of these changes relative to one another are predictable. The wide range of normal processes through these developmental milestones is affected by genetics, chronic conditions, and psychosocial environment [1]. In this chapter, we explore the normal growth and development of high school students and how it influences their emotions, thoughts, and interactions with the world around them.

The high school period is a crucial time that bridges the gap between childhood and adulthood. Adolescents experience unique transitions and transformations during this period which encompass the early, middle, and late stages of adolescence. These changes include physiological, cognitive, and psychosocial developments that may shape their identities and future. By understanding these developmental milestones, caregivers and educators offer essential support and guidance to adolescents during their high school years (Table 18.5).

E. A.-T. Green
Boston Children's Hospital, Boston, MA, USA
e-mail: estelle.green@childrens.harvard.edu

R. C. Roden (✉)
Penn State Children's Hospital, Hershey, PA, USA
e-mail: rroden@pennstatehealth.psu.edu

R. P. Olympia, J. Brady-Olympia (eds.), *Clinical Considerations in School-based Health*, https://doi.org/10.1007/978-3-031-85765-2_18

Table 18.1 Average physiological development in adolescent boys and girls [1–3]

	Boys	Girls
Early	Testicular enlargement (ages 10.5–15 years) Sperm production (spermarche/semenarche) Increasing scrotum pigmentation Penile growth (ages 11.5–14 years) Pubarche (ages 12–14 years) Growth spurt (begins at age 11.5 years)	Breast bud development (thelarche, ages 10–13.5 years) Pubic hair development (pubarche, ages 11–13 years) First period (menarche, ages 10–15 years) Anovulatory/irregular menstrual cycles (due to immature hypothalamic-pituitary-ovarian axis) Enlargement of ovaries, uterus, labia, and clitoris Thickening of endometrium and vaginal mucosa Growth spurt (begins at age 10 years)
Middle	Increase in lean body mass (strength spurt) Vocal instability (cracking) Deepening of voice Peak height velocity (age 13.5 years) Development of acne and body odor	Increased proportion of body fat Peak height velocity (age 12 years) Development of acne and body odor
Late	Growth completed (ends at 15.5 years)	Growth completed (ends at 14 years)

Table 18.2 Cognitive and psychological development early adolescents [4, 5]

Domains of development	Key changes
Psychological	Concrete thinking Mood swings and intense emotions Perception of the world primarily from own perspective (egocentrism) Constant feeling of being judged by others (imaginary audience) Belief feelings and experiences are unique from others (personal fable) Strong sense of absolute and unquestionable right vs. wrong Moral principles derived from authority figures Rule conformation to avoid punishment
Psychosocial	Desire for independence and privacy from parental authority Exploration of parental boundaries Rejection of parental advice and involvement Strong same-sex peers and peer group identification Intense non-romantic friendships Increased sexual awareness Experimentation with gender and sexuality

Table 18.3 Cognitive and psychosocial development of middle adolescents [4, 5]

Domains of development	Key changes
Psychological	Abstract thinking Capacity to consider other's needs, feelings, and perspectives Sense of invulnerability Moral principles influenced by desire to fit in
Psychosocial	Continued separation from parental authority Decreased interest in family activities Peak parent-child conflict Search for alternative role models beyond immediate family Increased importance of peers and power of peer pressure Risk-taking behaviors Concern about attractiveness and desirability to others Interest in dating and sexual intimacy Short and intense romantic relationship Value sexual attraction over emotional intimacy

Table 18.4 Cognitive and psychosocial development of late adolescents [4, 5]

Domains of development	Key changes
Psychological	Operational thinking Future orientation Stronger sense of self Ability to compromise, set long-term goals, and delay gratification Development of personal morals and values Refinement of interests, moral, religious, and sexual values
Psychosocial	Transition to "adult-adult" relationship with parents Less vulnerable to peer influence Prioritization of personal qualities over physical characteristics in relationships Preparation for further education, career advancement, and family planning

Table 18.5 Case presentations: normal or abnormal growth and development of high school students?

	Case description	Abnormal or normal?	Rationale
Case 1: Why are my period irregular?	A 13-year-old girl is concerned about her irregular period. She had her menarche at 12 years old. Her period are sometimes irregular with up to 3 months in between	This is normal development. Nothing to do	Immaturity of the hypothalamic-pituitary-ovarian (HPO) axis can cause anovulatory cycles or irregular bleeding in nonpregnant adolescents the first 1–2 years after menarche
Case 2: What is this mass?	A 14-year-old boy is worried about developing breasts. He noticed a lump growing behind his right nipple a couple of months ago. His physical exam is consistent with Tanner stage 4	This is normal pubertal timing. Nothing to do	Pubertal gynecomastia is a physiologic enlargement of the glandular breast tissue that occurs in over 50% of male adolescent. It peaks during mid-puberty and typically resolves within 1–3 years

(continued)

Table 18.5 (continued)

	Case description	Abnormal or normal?	Rationale
Case 3: Can you make decisions?	A 15-year-old girl gets straight As in her math class but forgets to clean her room. Her parents are worried that she is not mature enough to remember daily medication	Trial of daily medication, if indicated, with parental support is appropriate	The ability to remember to do homework in the school domain is not related to the ability to remember daily medicine or daily chores, as these are different domains
Case 4: What is that smell?	A 14-year-old boy you teach has started to outgrow his clothes in the last few months, and does not seem to notice increased body odor	This is normal pubertal timing. Nothing to do	At age 14, most males are experiencing their fastest rate of height growth and the effect of testosterone on the skin, including increased body odor, oiliness, and acne
Case 5: Trying to be healthy	A 15 year old boy has his height and weight taken as part of his school's health program. He has lost 30 lb in the last year, and gone from the 90th percentile for BMI to the 50th. He reports eating 3 meals a day, and is a competitive baseball player, track athlete, and golfer	This is abnormal weight loss. This boy should be evaluated for excessive weight loss due to medical or behavioral cause	While the boy had an elevated BMI previously, this degree of weight loss is alarming due to crossing many height percentiles. Males are often delayed in diagnosis of eating disorder, as are individuals who are at elevated weight before onset of symptoms
Case 6: I get winded sometimes	A 15 year old girl is a competitive middle-distance runner with her track team and is generally healthy. One day during practice, she becomes unconscious and collapses while running. She makes a quick recovery, and states she felt well, just a bit short of breath	This is abnormal and may represent several severe problems	This young person should be referred for emergency services, as her episode may represent cardiac problems, seizure, electrolyte imbalance, or any number of other concerns
Case 7: Angry teenagers	A 14 year old girl who was previously doing well in school has recently started to struggle with her grades. Her parents note that he is irritable, slamming doors, and spending most of her time in her room. She is eating less and seems tired. She changed schools 6 months ago. Her parents would like to have her tested for drugs	This is abnormal. Refer to mental health or counseling services	This young woman may be struggling with depression, anxiety, or learning disability and should be evaluated by psychiatry or psychology services. While drugs may be a cause of behavior changes, drug screening should never be done without patient assent

(continued)

Table 18.5 (continued)

	Case description	Abnormal or normal?	Rationale
Case 8: Newest fashions	A 15 year old boy recently started wearing eyeliner and nail polish to school. He has been asking his parents to take him clothes shopping and has been wearing mostly black. He is letting his hair grow out. His parents are concerned that he is using drugs or is depressed	This is normal adolescent behavior, there is nothing to do	It is normal for mid-adolescent teenagers to "try out" various types of self-expression, including changing friends, activities, appearance including clothes and makeup, and interests
Case 9: What about friends?	A 16 year old girl gets good grades in school, but doesn't have many friends. She is an avid student of math and hopes to be an engineer. She has a strict routine when she is at home for her hygiene, eating, and activity schedules and gets upset when it is disrupted. She has an encyclopedic knowledge of her favorite fiction series. She struggles with group work at school. Her parents worry about her social development	This may be abnormal, and evaluation is recommended	This young woman is very rigid with her routines, habits, and interests, and this appears to interfere with her ability to make social relationships, though it is unclear if she is bothered by this. She should be evaluated by developmental pediatrics or psychiatry for autism
Case 10: What are we waiting for?	A 17-year-old girl used to be of average height compared to her classmates, and now she is the shortest. She has not had her period. She started to have breast buds in fifth grade	This is abnormal pubertal timing. Evaluate potential causes for delayed puberty	At age 17, most girls have started to have periods and have had their height growth spurt. Periods usually start not more than 4 years after breast growth. This is not normal development

Extra Credit Points

1. Pubertal development involves the development of secondary sex characteristics, growth in stature, gaining the ability to reproduce, and changes in body systems.
2. Cognitive development includes the transition from concrete thinking to abstract thinking and formal operational thinking.
3. Psychosocial development varies greatly depending on an individual's unique living situation and experiences.
4. Cognitive and psychosocial changes can occur in any order and can occur at different rates in different parts of life.

5. Teens who drop percentiles on their BMI growth curve, even from elevated to "normal" ranges, should be evaluated for eating disorders or abnormal weight loss
6. Girls who have not had breast development by age 14 or no periods by age 15 and boys who have not started a growth spurt by age 15 should be evaluated for delayed puberty.
7. Changes in grades, hygiene, and/or overall functioning should prompt a referral to the primary care provider or behavioral health.

References

1. Chulani VL, Gordon LP. Adolescent growth and development. Prim Care Clin Off Pract. 2014;41(3):465–87. https://doi.org/10.1016/j.pop.2014.05.002.
2. Wood CL, Lane LC, Cheetham T. Puberty: normal physiology (brief overview). Best Pract Res Clin Endocrinol Metab. 2019;33(3):101265. https://doi.org/10.1016/j.beem.2019.03.001.
3. Tanner JM, Whitehouse RH. Growth at adolescence. 2nd ed. Springfield, IL: Blackwell Scientific Publications; 1962.
4. Sanders RA. Adolescent psychosocial, social, and cognitive development. Pediatr Rev. 2013;34(8):354–9. https://doi.org/10.1542/pir.34.8.354.
5. Tulloch T, Kaufman M. Adolescent sexuality. Pediatr Rev. 2013;34(1):29–37; quiz 38. https://doi.org/10.1542/pir.34-1-29.

Chapter 19
Effective Communication with High School Students

Natasha Ramsey and Elizabeth M. Alderman

Case 1 **Jan is a 14 year old cis girl who has been having dysmenorrhea which causes her to miss school often. She came to the school SBHC for a heat pack and medicine for her cramps. You bring her into the private exam room to assess her. You review her chart and see that she has been seen several times for painful menstrual cramps. You provide her ibuprofen and discuss some methods for menstrual management including birth control. She is interested and wants to know more. You remind her of the confidentiality policies in your state and gather more history about her menstrual cycle and sexual activity. She denies being sexually active and is interested in starting the pill. You review any contraindications and provide her thorough instructions about the pill including a handout she can review later. She asks you call her mother and share the information with her so she can help remind her to take her medicine every day.**

Case 1: Key Lessons Reviewing confidentiality, gathering a sexual history, providing age and developmentally appropriate information and counseling, partnering with the student and parent, partnering with the school.

Case 2 **Billy is a 16 year old cis male who comes to the SBHC because he has a bad cough. After reviewing confidentiality related to substance use, on further history you find out that he is vaping daily. Vaping has cost him a lot of money and has gotten him in trouble with his parents and the school administration because he sometimes brings it to school. Upon examination you notice some**

N. Ramsey (✉)
Montefiore Medical Group, Bronx, NY, USA
e-mail: naramsey@montefiore.org

E. M. Alderman
The Children's Hospital at Montefiore, Bronx, NY, USA
e-mail: ealderma@montefiore.org

R. P. Olympia, J. Brady-Olympia (eds.), *Clinical Considerations in School-based Health*, https://doi.org/10.1007/978-3-031-85765-2_19

wheezing and administer albuterol. Billy informs you that he sometimes uses albuterol prior to going for a run, which he hasn't been doing as often. You explain to Billy the consequences of vaping and acknowledge it can be difficult to quit and validate Billy's feelings. You help Billy identify that running is very important to him and that he would like to get back to. You identify that he was pre-contemplative and is now contemplating cutting down on vaping so that he can start running again. You partner with Billy to come up with a plan to cut down and provide information about nicotine replacement. You schedule Billy to follow up in 2 weeks.

Case 2: Key Lessons Reviewing confidentiality, substance use, providing age and developmentally appropriate information and counseling, partnering with the student, motivational interviewing.

Why is effective communication with adolescents so important for quality health care?

Effective communication is the cornerstone of quality care for adolescents. Adolescents are a unique population with unique needs, and exploring and understanding those needs helps to facilitate care. Adolescents are often misunderstood by providers and non-medical professionals can struggle to communicate with them at times. They are sensitive to verbal and non-verbal communication as well as the physical environment. If there are communication challenges, real or perceived, adolescents may not seek services or advocate for the services they need. A primary goal is to protect patients from harm through risk reduction and promotion of protective factors. Effective communication and maintaining confidentiality are necessary for achieving these goals.

Health care being provided in a school-based setting provides significant benefits. Because the SBHC is in the school environment and community, the SBHC can often times feel like a safe space for youth. School-based health centers (SBHCs) are where children and adolescents spend a lot of their time, so scheduling and transportation barriers are minimized. SBHCs increase adolescents' use of health care services, particularly for sexual health issues, substance use problems, and mental health concerns, by providing convenient and confidential care in an adolescent friendly and familiar setting [1]. Adolescents may have several medical, mental health and social concerns that may require multiple visits as well as establishing trust to address. Being in a school setting allows for easy access for youth in their own environment. Communication with adolescents can be more thorough and effective because visits can be broken down into multiple visits. Counseling and education can occur at one visit, information can be sent home for the parent or guardian to review, and treatment can be initiated at another visit. The school-based setting is a unique environment given patients are a part of the school community. There may be specific challenges to assuring confidentiality. Because they are in school, adolescents may feel that information might be shared with school personnel or that teachers know about appointments because they may need to leave class. Also, other students and other school staff may see the student utilizing the SBHC. It is also critical to incorporate parents, when appropriate, given students are seeking care independently. Despite these challenges, the school-based setting is an excellent environment to foster effective communication and create an adolescent friendly environment.

19.1 Setting the Stage: Creating an Adolescent Friendly Environment

Creating an adolescent friendly environment goes beyond just the verbal communication between the adolescent and the provider. The physical environment is also important. Presenting the SBHC as a safe space starts with the location and signage. Is it in the basement or the very top floor of the school building? Is it an easy to find location with clear signage? Does the SBHC have bright vibrant and welcoming colors, posters and decor that are adolescent friendly and are relatable to adolescents? Involving adolescents in the design can be helpful in ensuring a youth friendly environment. Services provided in the SBHC should be clearly displayed, including confidential care and that services are free or at no cost to students. Clear policies regarding accessing care should be communicated such as requiring a pass from the teacher and the hours the SBHC, the types of providers and their names. Walk-in and drop-in appointments should be available. Information for other SBHC sites should be provided for emergencies and for holiday and summer breaks. Is there a window that exposes patients and potentially breaches their confidentiality to other students? To mitigate these concerns there should be clear distinctions between the waiting areas from clinical areas. SBHC areas should be soundproof to protect other students from hearing other patients' information. If possible, restrooms should be available in the SBHC for students to provide specimen samples and not have to go in the public restrooms. The provider should have counseling and examination areas to discuss sensitive topics with adolescents that provide visual and auditory privacy. Other health care staff or students should not hear the conversation or see who is in the visit. Materials and handouts available should be youth friendly, youth specific, appropriate literacy levels, and appropriate for adolescent development. Social media can be used as a tool for effective communication and to market services in the SBHC. Reputable social media resources can be provided to students to learn more about health-related topics. Engaging youth in the development of a marketing strategy can help with community outreach as well.

Beyond the physical environment, the interactions with staff are critical to creating an adolescent friendly environment [2]. Culturally competent care is provided, meaning all care is respectful of each adolescent's culture, race, ethnicity, religion, language, community values, educational level, sex, gender, and sexual orientation. For example, a disabled student should be offered reproductive health services the same as their able-bodied counterparts. Some students and parents may require interpreter services and those should be offered and available to all students. Students should be assisted with referrals such as scheduling outside appointments, coordinating transportation to appointments at other SBHCs and education about navigating insurance, etc. The health center environment and staff should leave adolescent patients feeling respected and engaged in their health care. Not only is the provider responsible for fostering an adolescent friendly environment but also the ancillary staff such as the front desk and health educators need to contribute to this culture. Ongoing trainings should be done and new personnel will need orientation. At the front desk or check-in area as much as possible, assuring privacy is key. Using a piece of paper for students to write what services they are interested in or having a prepared template with common services provided (i.e. STI testing, emergency contraception) that students can simply point to can help maintain confidentiality regarding sensitive services they are seeking. Ensuring confidentiality is critical to ensuring an adolescent friendly space where students feel free and safe to ask questions and be honest which fosters an environment for effective communication. Feedback from students can identify if the SBHC is adolescent friendly as well as utilizing some online tools [3].

19.2 Setting the Stage: Confidentiality and Privacy

Ensuring confidentiality and privacy are critical for creating an adolescent friendly environment where effective communication can take place. Confidentiality laws vary by state so being familiar with state laws regarding sexual health, mental health, substance use is important and should be communicated to patients, parents and school administration both written and verbally. Providers should also be aware of The Family Educational Rights and Privacy Act (FERPA), a Federal law that protects the privacy of student education records. FERPA gives parents certain rights with respect to their children's education records. These rights transfer to the student when he or she reaches the age of 18 or attends a school beyond the high school level [4]. Although they are in a school setting, if they enter a SBHC that is run by a health care organization, not the school, itself, they are in SBHC space and Health Insurance Portability and Accountability Act (HIPPA) should be enforced. An adolescent's health information cannot be shared with anyone—including parents or guardians—without the adolescent's written permission, unless required by law or if the health care provider is concerned the adolescent might harm him or herself or someone else. SBHC staff members should also not discuss adolescents' information in common office spaces. Medical records are kept secure and accessible only to select health care staff, such as through locked files or password-protected electronic medical records. Sometimes students may be escorted to the SBHC by school staff. Best practices are important not to discuss medical history and perform exams with school staff present and that the adolescents' health information should not be shared with school staff. Special considerations can be made on a case-by-case basis, i.e. discussion with the school therapist for mental health referrals. In some cases, disposition planning such as the student being discharged to home may require communication with the school staff, but this should be done by providing only the information that is necessary and should be communicated to the student prior to discussion with the school administration. Communication with the parents is also recommended to facilitate disposition planning. Creating an adolescent friendly space in the SBHC that upholds the confidentiality of the students is the foundation for effective communication [5].

19.3 Tools for Communication: Adolescent Development

Understanding adolescent development and how to communicate depending on adolescent stage are part of the building blocks for effective communication. Communicating effectively and respectfully with adolescents requires an understanding of their developmental stage and the challenges they face. Adolescent development typically encompasses several stages, each characterized by unique physical, cognitive, social, and emotional changes (Table 19.1).

Regardless of the developmental stage, it's important to maintain open and honest communication, show empathy, and respect their individuality. Building a trusting relationship based on mutual respect lays the foundation for effective communication with adolescents at any stage of development [6].

Table 19.1 Adolescent development stages

Stage	Tips for communication
Early adolescence (11–14 years)	Be patient and provide support as they navigate these rapid changes Avoid using complex language or jargon Keep your communication simple and straightforward Clearly communicate expectations and boundaries while allowing room for exploration and autonomy Encourage them to express their opinions and make their own decisions within safe limits
Middle adolescence (15–17 years)	Respect their developing independence Offer guidance and support without being overly controlling Help them navigate challenges and make informed decisions Discuss consequences Encourage critical thinking Be available for conversations and offer your support without judgment
Late adolescence (18–21 years)	Acknowledge their transition into adulthood and autonomy Discuss future plans Encourage them to take responsibility for their actions and make decisions independently Offer mentorship and guidance as they navigate the transition into adulthood Respect their opinions

19.4 Tools for Communication: Psychosocial Interviewing HEADSSS and SHADESS Frameworks

The American Academy of Pediatrics (AAP) recommends use of a psychosocial assessment for screening such as the HEADSSS and SHADESS frameworks [7, 8]. Both the HEADSSS and SHADESS frameworks are structured approaches used in healthcare settings to assess various aspects of adolescent health and well-being. They are great tools for effective communication with adolescents. Introduce the concept of the psychosocial interview, normalize it as a routine thing done for every student and review the confidentiality policies before starting questioning. "I am asking you these routine questions to identify if you have any concerns and find ways to help support you." Start with less sensitive topics, give a trigger warning before transitioning into the more sensitive questions "Next I am going to ask you some routine questions about sexual health. Your answers are confidential meaning I can't discuss what you tell me with anyone including your parents unless you give your consent or unless you want to hurt yourself, someone else, or someone is hurting you" (Table 19.2).

Table 19.2 HEADSSS vs SHADESSS psychosocial interview

HEADSSS	SHADESS
Home environment: Assessing the adolescent's living situation, family dynamics, and stressors at home	Strengths: Identifying the adolescent's strengths, resources, and positive coping mechanisms
Education and employment: Evaluating the adolescent's educational status, involvement in school, and employment	Home and environment: Assessing the home environment, family relationships, and living conditions
Activities and peer relationships: Examining the adolescent's social life, including friendships, hobbies, and peer groups	Activities and peer relationships: Examining the adolescent's social life, including friendships, hobbies, and social support networks
Drugs and alcohol: Assessing substance use behaviors, including alcohol, tobacco, and illicit drug use	Drugs: Evaluating substance use behaviors, including alcohol, tobacco, and drug use Education, employment, and eating: Addressing educational status, involvement in school or work, and eating habits
Sexuality: Addressing sexual health, including sexual activity, orientation, and contraceptive use	Sexuality and suicide: Assessing sexual health, sexual orientation, and mental health concerns such as suicide and depression
Suicide and depression: Evaluating mental health concerns such as depression, anxiety, and suicidal ideation	Sexuality and suicide: Assessing sexual health, sexual orientation, and mental health concerns such as suicide and depression
Safety: Identifying safety concerns and risk factors impacting the adolescent's well-being	Safety: Identifying safety concerns, including exposure to violence, bullying, or risky behaviors

19.5 Tools for Communication: Motivational Interviewing

Use of motivational interviewing for adolescents has been shown to decrease risky sexual behaviors, help prevent unplanned pregnancy, increase physical activity levels, and decrease substance use. Motivational interviewing (MI) is a collaborative, goal-oriented communication approach particularly effective with adolescents. MI can also help with provider burnout. In the stages of change model, the pediatrician facilitates change by matching counseling strategy to patient readiness. The Stages of Change model, also known as the Transtheoretical Model (TTM), is a framework for understanding the process of intentional behavior change. It was developed by James Prochaska and Carlo DiClemente in the late 1970s and is widely used in health psychology and behavior modification programs [9]. The model outlines stages through which individuals progress when changing a behavior (Table 19.3).

Understanding these stages helps healthcare providers, counselors, and others tailor their interventions to match the individual's readiness for change, thereby increasing the likelihood of successful and sustained behavior change.

Table 19.3 The transtheoretical model (TTM)

Precontemplation	Individuals are not yet considering change. They may be unaware of the need for change or believe that the behavior is not problematic. Often, they resist change and may feel demoralized by past unsuccessful attempts to alter the behavior
Contemplation	Individuals are aware of the need for change and are considering it but have not yet committed to taking action. They weigh the pros and cons of changing and often experience ambivalence. This stage can last a long time as individuals resolve their mixed feelings about change
Preparation	Individuals intend to take action soon, usually within the next month. They start making small steps toward change and develop a plan of action. This stage involves gathering information and resources, setting goals, and building confidence in their ability to change
Action	Individuals actively implement their plan and make observable changes in their behavior. This stage requires considerable time and energy as new behaviors are practiced and old patterns are disrupted. Support and reinforcement are crucial during this stage to maintain motivation
Maintenance	Individuals work to sustain the new behavior over the long term. They focus on preventing relapse and consolidating the gains achieved during the action stage. Maintenance can last from 6 months to several years, depending on the behavior and individual circumstances
Termination	For some behaviors, this stage represents the ultimate goal, where the individual has complete confidence that they will not return to their old behaviors. The new behavior is fully integrated into their lifestyle, and there is no temptation to relapse. However, for many behaviors, individuals remain in the maintenance stage indefinitely
Relapse	Relapse can occur at any stage, where individuals revert to their previous behavior. This is considered a normal part of the change process, and individuals can re-enter the stages of change at any point to continue their progress

19.6 Partnership with Caregivers and School Administration

While maintaining confidentiality is imperative for communication with adolescents, involvement of parents and caregivers may also improve health outcomes. Best practices are to involve the caregivers as supportive participants in the student's health care whenever appropriate and possible. For younger adolescents or those with complex medical problems, caregiver involvement can assist with adherence etc. Best practices are to call parents after encounters, especially if medications are provided or referrals are placed. For more sensitive topics, getting permission from patients to discuss care with parents is critical. Providing information for parents to review such as visit summaries can also facilitate communication.

A positive relationship with the school administration is necessary for a successful SBHC. This relationship can be fostered through attending school events such as parent/caregiver teacher nights, fundraisers, open houses, school board meetings, athletic events, and other extracurricular events. Provide an annual teacher and staff orientation to your SBHC. Creating and maintaining positive relations between your SBHC and school can be challenging. There can be frequent school staff and administration turnover, varied understanding of the services provided by the SBHC, and concern about students missing class for appointments. Also, the importance of maintaining confidentiality can be hard to express to professionals outside the health field. But strong partnerships between the school and SBHC are critical to the program's success and longevity (Fig. 19.1).

Extra Credit Points

1. Creating an adolescent friendly environment goes beyond just the verbal communication between the adolescent and the provider
2. Ensuring confidentiality and privacy are critical for creating an adolescent friendly environment where effective communication can take place.
3. Understanding adolescent development and how to communicate depending on adolescent stage are part of the building blocks for effective communication.
4. Psychosocial assessment for screening such as the HEADSSS and SHADESS frameworks and motivational interviewing are great tools for optimizing the health care visit with adolescents.

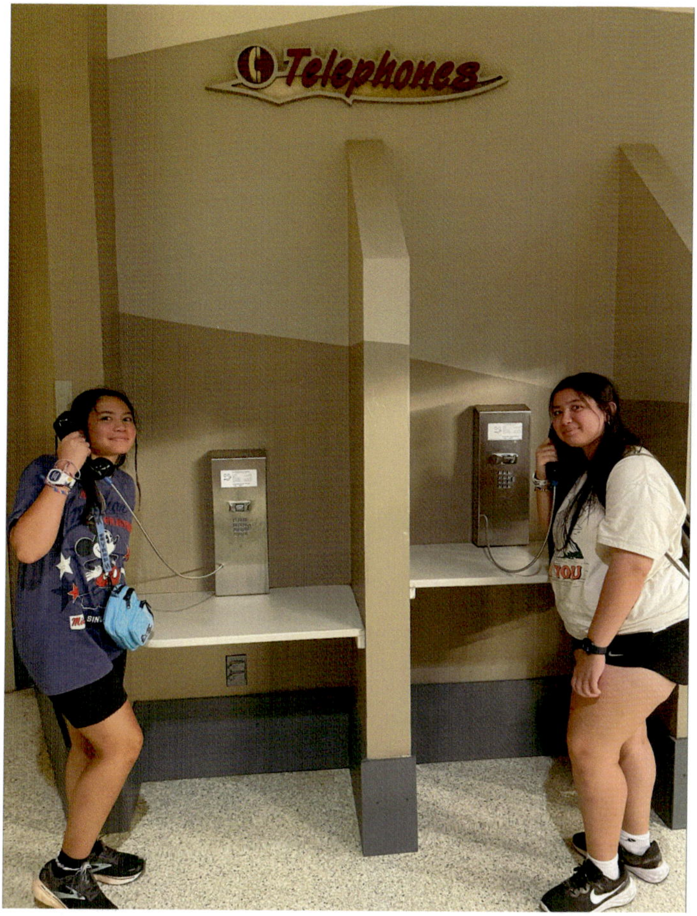

Fig. 19.1 Modern day adolescents communicating with ancient devices

References

1. Lear JG, Barnwell EA, Behrens D, Goldsmith MF, Kaye C. School-based health centers and pediatric practice. Pediatrics. 2012;129(2):387–93. https://publications.aap.org/pediatrics/article/129/2/387/32611/School-Based-Health-Centers-and-Pediatric-Practice.
2. Adolescent Health Initiative. Youth-friendly services starter guide. University of Michigan Health System; 2023. https://www.michiganmedicine.org/sites/default/files/2024-04/youth-friendly-services-starter-guide.pdf.
3. Healthy Teen Network. Youth-friendly services assessment. Healthy Teen Network. http://www.healthyteennetwork.org/resources/youth-friendly-services-assessment
4. U.S. Department of Education and U.S. Department of Health and Human Services. Joint Guidance on the Application of the Family Educational Rights and Privacy Act (FERPA) and the Health Insurance Portability and Accountability Act of 1996 (HIPAA) to Student Health Records. 2019. https://studentprivacy.ed.gov/sites/default/files/resource_document/file/2019%20HIPAA%20FERPA%20Joint%20Guidance%20508.pdf.

5. Chung RJ, Lee JB, Hackell JM, Alderman EM, Committee on Adolescence, Committee on Practice & Ambulatory Medicine. Confidentiality in the care of adolescents: policy statement. Pediatrics. 2024;153(5):e2024066326. https://doi.org/10.1542/peds.2024-066326.
6. American Academy of Child and Adolescent Psychiatry. Provider-youth communication: improving practice with LGBTQIA+ youth. https://www.aacap.org/App_Themes/AACAP/Docs/member_resources/SOGIIC/Provider-Youth-Comm.pdf. Accessed 28 Jun 2024.
7. American Academy of Pediatrics. Bright futures adolescence tools. https://www.aap.org/en/practice-management/bright-futures/bright-futures-materials-and-tools/bright-futures-tool-and-resource-kit/bright-futures-adolescence-tools/. Accessed 28 Jun 2024.
8. American Academy of Pediatrics. Chapter 32: Gender and sexual development. In: Hagan JF, Shaw JS, Duncan PM, editors. Bright futures: guidelines for health supervision of infants, children, and adolescents. 4th ed. Elk Grove Village, IL: American Academy of Pediatrics; 2017. p. 611–23. https://www.aap.org/contentassets/0e45de0366d54ec38fbfcb72382a0c6c/rt2e_ch32_sahm.pdf. Accessed 28 Jun 2024.
9. Norcross JC, Krebs PM, Prochaska JO. Stages of change†. J Clin Psychol. 2011;67:143–54. https://doi.org/10.1002/jclp.20758.

Chapter 20
Promoting Wellness and Balance Among Students

Anisha Mittal and Paul Haidet

Case 1 A school provider recognizes an increased number of fights and violence in a school. She traces the fights to bullying, cyberbullying, and increased drug use. She wonders how she might improve wellness in the student body.

The health of school-aged students is multifaceted, including both physical and mental wellbeing. The demands of school can sometimes be difficult for students to manage, contributing to declining health in individuals, as well as the student body as a whole. The school provider is often the first person who can recognize students' various needs and intervene, through both clinical and non-traditional methods. This chapter takes a population health-based approach to the issue, using key principles to direct implementation of wellness initiatives that could help to improve the overall health of a student body.

20.1 Population Health-Based Definition of Wellness

Population health is a field that focuses on the health outcomes of groups as opposed to individuals. As defined by Kindig and colleagues, "These populations are often geographic regions, such as nations or communities, but they can also be other groups, such as employees, ethnic groups, disabled persons, or prisoners. In addition, many determinants of health, such as medical care systems, the social environment, and the physical environment, have their biological impact on individuals in part at a population level" [1].

For our purposes in this chapter, we consider the population of interest to be the student body at a school. In so doing, we suggest that school health personnel direct

A. Mittal (✉) · P. Haidet
The Pennsylvania State University College of Medicine, Hershey, PA, USA
e-mail: phaidet@pennstatehealth.psu.edu

R. P. Olympia, J. Brady-Olympia (eds.), *Clinical Considerations in School-based Health*, https://doi.org/10.1007/978-3-031-85765-2_20

part of their attention toward wellness outcomes, and the determinants of such outcomes that can realistically be impacted from activities directed by the school's health office. We therefore focus upon wellness and balance, two outcomes that are dependent on primarily school-driven social determinants of health, such as stress, the social environment, quality of education, and safety within a school. A population health-based definition of wellness focuses on optimal health for the mind, body, and community [2] of students. Case 1 provides an example of a school-driven health problem, with examples of how to apply population health-based principles to guide wellness initiative development later in the chapter.

20.2 Four Key Population Health Based Principles to Guide Wellness Initiatives in a Student Body

There are four key population health-based principles that can be helpful in guiding the development and implementation of any wellness initiative at a school. These principles were derived from the state of Vermont's "Five Principles for Improving Population Health" and are reformulations of those principles to be relevant to a student population [3]. We realize that the scope and application of the principles at a particular school will be dependent upon available resources, time and effort of health personnel, and potential partnerships with teachers, administrators, and other interested individuals. Ideally, a population health-directed initiative aimed at student wellness would be a concerted effort, supported by administration, operationalized and planned by a broadly represented group of dedicated individuals, and coordinated and/or led by the student health office(s).

20.2.1 Use Population-Level Clinical Data to Track Wellness of the Student Body

School providers are busy meeting the clinical demands of scores of students each day. One way to track the wellness of a student body is via the use of population-level student clinical data. Problems can be identified using the clinic as a resource, performing health record audits to track patterns across the student body. Wellness issues may include, but are not limited to, a number of students who may feel stressed, unsafe in the school environment, alone without much socialization, or physically unwell. In a sense, the student health clinic becomes an important sampling point for the kinds of health issues that are prevalent among the student body. Other offices, such as the student counseling office and principal's offices, could similarly track outcomes determined to be of importance to student wellness. Once a major problem or theme across the student body is identified, wellness initiatives can be created and targeted toward addressing the problem. In addition to chart and record audits, targeted issues could be queried via questionnaires administered in the waiting room of the student health offices. Although the specific questionnaire administered would depend on the targeted issue(s) a school health office would like to focus on, the following population health mnemonic can be used to drive a questionnaire once a focus is decided upon:

The five W's:

1. Who: The person or population of interest
2. What: Definition of the health event or area of interest
3. When: The time frame of evaluation via the questionnaire
4. Where: The place the health event occurs
5. Why: The causes, risk factors, and modes of transmission of the health event

Again, the purpose of such questionnaires would be to get a sampling of the student body with respect to generic student wellness issues such as stress level, safety, and social interactions, or they could be targeted toward particular areas identified through chart and record audits. The essence of this first principle is that, before embarking on any wellness initiative, gathering data at a population level can provide critical insights on the nature of the issue to be addressed, and can provide an ongoing evidence base for tracking any wellness-based initiative's success.

20.2.2 Focus on Wellness Interventions at Both Individual and Schoolwide Levels

While wellness starts at the individual level, individuals can collectively be well or unwell at the population, or student body, level. In general, providers may promote wellness among the student body through presentations to students (including inviting speakers from the community), health education in the classroom, health fairs, and others. While these are the typical things that come to mind when thinking about student wellness, some other, less common, activities may be equally powerful. These can include developing partnerships and collaborations with other departments in the school (such as the arts teachers, music teachers, dance and theater instructors, physical education instructors, etc.) to develop new offerings and programs aimed at student wellness. These could include creative and interactive initiatives, such as health-education focused games and outings.

Providers may also consider simple and practical ideas to improve student wellness inside a provider's waiting room and clinical space, as well as throughout the school (Table 20.1).

Although school providers focus primarily on clinical activities due to the constraints of their role and time limitations, the importance of non-clinical wellness initiatives such as the ones outlined above cannot be underscored. Design strategies for implementing interventions are provided under the fourth principle below.

Table 20.1 Ideas to improve wellness inside a provider's waiting room, clinical space, and school

Waiting room	• Have student-friendly, calming background music playing in the school provider's clinic • Offer basic but safe art supplies for students to use. This includes coloring books, drawing paper and crayons, and activity books • Offer brain games, including puzzle books or small jigsaw puzzles • Have magazines or short picture books (for younger students) available in the school provider's waiting room
Clinical office	• Like the waiting room, offer background music • Design the office space to be bright and cheerful, with student-friendly educational posters or pictures on the walls
School	• Provide a student lounge with activities to de-stress, including games and musical instruments such as a keyboard • Add colors and photos in school hallways, and infographics on walls of classrooms, cafeterias, gyms, etc.

20.2.3 Address School-Based Contributors to Health Outcomes

School-based contributors to health outcomes, or school-based social determinants of health, must be evaluated in order to identify priorities and target actions. Examples of school-based contributors to health outcomes include: school stress, student safety, social environment, quality of education, school nutrition, and more [4]. These various school-based contributors must be considered when identifying a problem area and implementing a wellness initiative to combat that problem.

Once a specific area of focus is identified, a wellness initiative should be tailored toward that area. For example, if a provider believes that a high school student population seems to be emotionally unwell without an outlet away from school stressors, the provider might consider advocating for a school-wide intervention such as an activity fair to present extracurricular opportunities such as sports and arts programs that students can become involved with. Table 20.2 lists some examples of wellness initiatives that can be considered to improve school-based contributors to health outcomes.

20.2.4 Engage Partners Across School Departments and the Community to Promote Wellness

On a larger scale, school health providers can extend their influence to include various school departments and community agencies. Implementing wellness initiatives with such partners can create connectedness amongst the school community. Providers are often busy meeting the clinical demands of students, so involving other school departments and community partners will also make the implementation of large-scale initiatives more feasible. As presented earlier, the example of holding an activity fair for a student body may involve collaboration with various school departments such as music, arts, and physical education. Community

Table 20.2 Examples of wellness initiatives that can be used to improve school-based contributors to health outcomes

School-based contributor	Wellness initiative
School stress	• Activity fair to present extracurricular options such as sports and arts programs that can be used as an outlet to reduce stress • Alternatively, present a brochure to students that lists available extracurricular options • Teach students basic coping methods, including breathing techniques, meditation, and stretches
Student safety	• Talk therapy: Allow students time to talk to trusted adults to express concerns • Students can join trusted peer support groups to have discussions with their peers and become involved in a supportive network
Social environment	• Encourage extracurricular activity participation, which allows the formation of a strong social network • Consider implementing a buddy system based on shared student interests, which may help promote a positive social environment
Quality of education	• Regularly assess student feedback and concerns regarding their education through anonymous surveys • Through educational assessments and talks with educators, identify students who may benefit from additional assistance such as mentoring or tutoring • Establish a peer mentorship program at your school, to enable students to help one another
School nutrition	• Survey students on their favorite healthy nutrition options, and encourage the cafeteria to provide some of those options • Encourage school administration to consider free or reduced lunch prices for students in need • Invite nutritional experts to present food nutrition education to students

partners for an activity fair could include local recreation centers, YMCAs, Boys and Girls Clubs, and other organizations which may provide opportunities for student wellness. Table 20.3 presents some examples of collaborative ideas with various departments and community resources.

Case 1 Conclusion The provider uses the four population health-based principles to guide the development of a wellness initiative to improve the school violence and school safety:

1. ***Use population-level clinical data to track wellness of the student body***: The provider administers an anonymous survey to a sample of students to assess their safety, fears, perception of violence in the school, and any underlying contributors to feeling unsafe.
2. ***Focus on wellness interventions at both individual and schoolwide levels***: The provider believes that select students may benefit from individual support as well as promoting schoolwide wellness to help overcome the overall problem.
3. ***Address school-based contributors to health outcomes***: The provider decides to send out an email to students in order to encourage affected students to sign up for peer support groups in which students may have discussions with one another,

Table 20.3 Collaborative ideas to promote wellness in students

Department/ community resources (if available)	Ideas for collaboration
Counseling	• Work with counselors and social workers to identify students who may be struggling with balance • Gather information on potential barriers to success (mental health, family environment, drugs, alcohol, etc.)
Music	• Work with the music department to not only increase participation in the school band and other optional music activities, but also encourage participation by all students through required music instruction or the potential for after-school/summer music camps • Inquire about the possibility of music therapy for students who may benefit, either through the music department or a trained music therapist
Art, theater, or dance	• Very similar to the collaboration with the music department, work with these departments to encourage student participation and activities outside of the formal curriculum • Ideas include arts and crafts workshops, dance classes, or theater/drama camps • Work with drama instructors and social studies teachers to implement workshops on improv, communication, and civic awareness
Library	• Work with the library to encourage literary involvement, reading, journaling, and creative writing as a wellness outlet for students
Administration	• Work with school administration to advocate for and gain approval for new creative initiatives for students • One idea is advocating for "Fun Fridays" where educators and/or community volunteers could lead simple 30-min creative activities for students, something for students to look forward to each week • Administration can help to advocate for resources that may not be available (e.g., music/arts programs, organized sports, title IX programs, etc.)
Local Health Department	• Ask the local health department about resources and handouts for students • Invite them for a school health fair, presentation for students, or other creative initiative
Local recreation centers, YMCA, Boys and Girls Club	• Ask about opportunities for student wellness, including sports programs, after-school activities, and summer camps and how to best facilitate these opportunities for a student body • Invite these organizations to be a part of a school activity fair during which students can learn about extracurricular opportunities
Community volunteers	• Community volunteers often bring expertise in areas outside of a school provider's day-to-day job, including the following: Career planning, financial planning, time management, multitasking, creating goals, mentorship, study techniques, work-life balance, stress reduction and coping skills, exercise and nutrition, social media safety, and much more • Invite healthcare volunteers to assist with health fairs and presentations • Invite volunteers in other fields such as music, dance, or the arts to plan non-clinical wellness activities

which is a form of talk therapy, and become involved in a supportive network. At a schoolwide level, the provider seeks experts who may be able to educate students on bullying, safe internet use to prevent cyberbullying, and drug safety.

4. ***Engage partners across school departments and the community to promote wellness***: Bringing in school and outside experts to give informational talks to students is an example of a collaborative idea. The provider also encourages school counselors to identify and work with students who might be especially affected by the increased violence

Overall, utilizing the four key population health-based principles, providers may identify a target problem and work with school and community partners to develop and implement an individual or school-wide wellness initiative.

20.3 A Model for Designing Arts-Based Interventions Aimed at Promoting Wellness

Case 2 A high school in a suburban area has seen an uptick in fights and altercations about an upcoming local election, in which two ideologically-opposed candidates have been advertising widely via social media and other outlets. The school health office is asked to partner with the school music department to develop a school assembly that aims to promote understanding and dialogue among the student body. The music teaching staff suggests building the assembly around the use of a musical track "Get Into My Groove" by the band Incognito (album: No Time Like the Future, Talkin' Loud Records, 538 947-2). The music teachers think the lyrics of the song speak for themselves, but request help from the school health office to design an assembly that might have maximum impact in promoting students taking a thoughtful approach to talking with each other about politically sensitive topics.

In this final section, we use a model from the medical education literature to focus on the design of educational interventions, such as school assemblies, sessions within courses, etc., to maximize the effect of such interventions upon student reflection and behavior change. While this model focuses on the arts, it has equal relevance for a variety of educational experiences beyond the arts, including sports and physical education, group wellness activities such as yoga or tai chi, or experiences off site such as field trips (Fig. 20.1 [5]). In the model, any educational intervention begins with an *experience*, which is represented by the first two boxes (qualities of the arts and engagement with the arts). Such experiences are critical triggers for engaging students both with the topic at hand, and with each other. For example, if a field trip to an art museum is planned as a wellness activity to help students focus on the role of social interactions in promoting community, then the pictures chosen to observe as a group should be relevant and representational of the topic of social interactions and community (box 1: qualities of the arts), and should

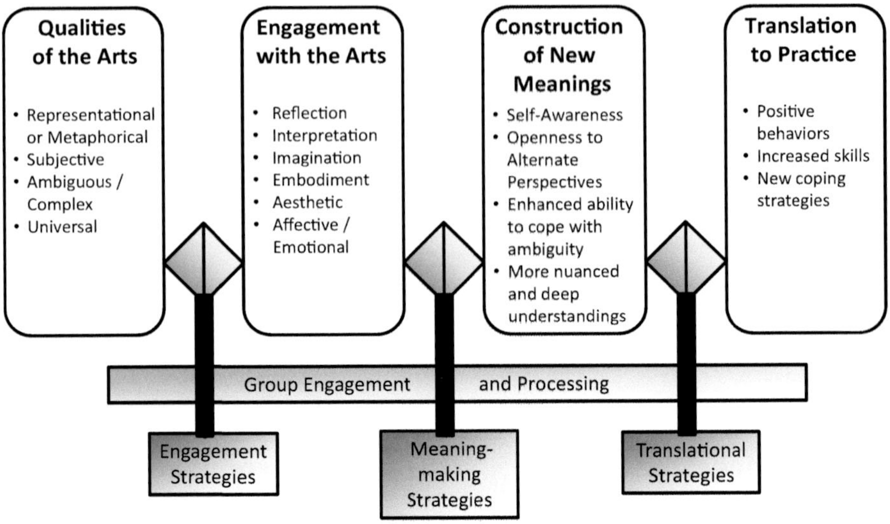

Fig. 20.1 A model to maximize the power of experiences in education. (Adapted from Haidet et al. [5])

be accessible and engaging to students (box 2: engagement with the arts). The initial experience provides the entrée into the topic and fosters collaboration with each other. It is here that partnerships with arts and music teachers, physical education instructors, etc. can be critical to ensure that the experience is topical, relevant, and engaging for students.

Unfortunately, many educational interventions stop with the experience itself, assuming that the desired outcomes will come, after a good experience. They won't, without further activities intended to help students process the experience and translate it to their daily lives as students. These are represented by the next two boxes in the figure (construction of new meanings and translation to practice). These activities usually involve some form of reflection on the part of students, either individually or in groups (construction of new meanings). Such reflective activities could include reflective writing, think aloud exercises, or small group discussions, and are prompted by carefully written questions intended to help students construct their own personal meanings from the experience that has just happened. For example, the website Art History Kids has a number of examples using art to create the construction of new meanings. In the example of the art museum and social interactions and community above, if the students viewed Keith Harring's painting "untitled", the website suggests the following questions to stimulate construction of new meanings:

- Why did the artist decide to stylize all the people to look the same?
- When are we individuals, and when do we blend into the group as a whole?
- What is political/social activism? [6]

Finally, perhaps the most important step is to have students develop a plan for how they will think and act when they re-engage in their daily lives (translation to practice). Construction of new meanings, when it happens, needs to be contextualized and connected to a plan for sustainable action in the real world. This is where translational strategies come in and provide a critical capstone to any educational intervention that is based upon an experience. We often have students write down a concrete plan for one thing they will do this afternoon, tomorrow, next week, and onward based upon what has happened in the session. We ask students to put their written plan in their locker, on their nightstand, or somewhere they will consistently see it as a reminder of their new meaning, and as an aid to translating the lessons learned to their own health and wellbeing.

Case 2 Conclusion The health provider uses the three "movement points" in the model (engagement, meaning making, and translation) to help the music directors to design the 1-h assembly:

1. ***The piece of art used should foster ENGAGEMENT:*** The track in question was released in 1999, approximately 7 years before most 2024 high school seniors were born. This could be an advantage if most students have not heard the track before, fostering everyone experiencing it for the first time, or it could be a disadvantage if the music is heard as dated and not relevant to today's musical tastes. It would be advantageous to engage several students on the design team to listen to the music and advise on how modern students will "hear" the track, and plan for the way the track will be presented to the students.
2. ***After the experience, student activities should aim at creating MEANING:*** The experience of listening alone will not necessarily create new meanings in the minds of students if they have not done extra mental processing of that experience. For example, the track lyrics pose the question "How ya gonna change the world when ya haven't got the love?" One activity might be to have students discuss in small groups (simultaneously in the assembly hall) the prompt: "What is the nature of LOVE in this lyric, and what, if anything, does it have to do with political discourse?" After students have discussed in small groups, the assembly teachers could foster a discussion among the whole assembly, harvesting lessons learned from the student body itself. The teachers could take the assembly students through several iterations of discussion, prompted by various lines from the song's lyrics.
3. ***Once meanings have been created, activities should focus on students TRANSLATING lessons learned to their daily lives***: If the preceding large group discussions have generated useful and relevant dialogue, the students will need to walk away with concrete ideas for how they can translate these new meanings into action in their daily lives. One activity might be to have each student write an "exit ticket" about one big idea that they want to try out this week, and put that idea into a note on their phone with a reminder set to ping them later in the week.

As a school health professional, it is easy to be focused entirely on the health of individual patients, who come to you with real and pressing problems that need to be solved immediately. Such activities are reactive, and responsive to problems as they occur. While this is a critical role, school providers are also ideally positioned to be proactive, coordinating efforts that can have effects on the wellbeing of the entire population of students. Using the principles of population health outlined in this chapter can aid in the planning and organization of such efforts. Additionally, the principles of educational design can maximize the power of individual events to promote wellness. Partnering with students, teachers, and administration can make the workload manageable, and can help reap wellness benefits, for individual students and for the student body as a whole.

Extra Credit Points

1. School providers should consider students' emotional and mental health needs that extend beyond traditional clinical medicine.
2. Providers can utilize the four population health-based principles to track wellness and implement individual and school-wide wellness initiatives with departmental and community engagement.
3. The conceptual model discussed in this chapter can guide the development of both arts-based and other educational interventions aimed at promoting wellness in school students.

References

1. Kindig D, Stoddart G. What is population Health? Am J Public Health. 2003;93(3):380–3. https://doi.org/10.2105/ajph.93.3.380.
2. Population Health. Wellsource. Published 2020. https://www.wellsource.com/population-health/#:~:text=Population%20health%20that%20focuses%20on. Accessed 18 May 2024.
3. Five principles for improving population health; 2017. https://www.healthvermont.gov/sites/default/files/documents/2017/01/SYST_5%20Principles%20for%20PH%20Improvement.pdf. Accessed 18 May 2024.
4. Huang KY, Cheng S, Theise R. School contexts as social determinants of child health: current practices and implications for future public health practice. Public Health Rep. 2013;128(6_suppl 3):21–8. https://doi.org/10.1177/00333549131286s304.
5. Haidet P, Jarecke J, Adams NE, et al. A guiding framework to maximise the power of the arts in medical education: a systematic review and metasynthesis. Med Educ. 2016;50(3):320–31. https://doi.org/10.1111/medu.12925.
6. Art History Lessons: Exploring the idea of community through famous paintings. Art History Kids. Published 11 Oct 2016. https://www.arthistorykids.com/blog/2016/10/10/art-history-lessons-exploring-the-idea-of-community-in-famous-paintings.

Chapter 21
Supporting Your Students Dealing with Grief

Natalie Seminario

Case 1 **Esteban is an 8-year-old male whose father was diagnosed with cancer 6 months ago. When he shared this with his teacher Ms. Sosa, Esteban and his parents met with Ms. Sosa and together devised a system to take quiet time breaks for Esteban. By quietly putting a box of tissues on his desk, Esteban excused himself at any time he felt overwhelmed in class and Ms. Sosa would periodically check in with him. Through the duration of his father's treatment, Esteban continued to excel academically, attend school, and interact appropriately with his peers and school staff. While Esteban had been open about what he was going through, he had not shared with anyone that his father passed away last night. Esteban was found by a passing teacher alone crying in a bathroom stall with his pants wet with urine and taken to the school nurse. What is your approach?**

Grief stemming from bereavement has significant short and long-term implications on a child's well-being. Childhood bereavement could result in poor health outcomes including psychiatric morbidities, substance abuse, heart disease, chronic inflammation, and cognitive decline. Additionally, mental health status prior to and immediately after a parent's death along with caregiver functioning impact the level of functional impairment in a bereaved child [1, 2]. With the Covid-19 pandemic leaving an estimated 10.5 million children bereaved of their parents and caregivers and 70–80% of schools with a bereaved child at one time, it is important for school systems to be aware and prepared to assist with bereavement and grief for any student [1, 3–5]. Schools have the unique opportunity to not only mitigate grief, considered an adverse childhood experience (ACE), but to also promote positive childhood experiences (PCE) by way of creating a consistently safe open environment for students and their caregivers. Positive outcomes from childhood grief depend on the support the child receives and can result in a positive trajectory for adult flourishment [1] (Table 21.1).

N. Seminario (✉)
Bright Futures Psychiatry for Kids and Teens, LLC, Jupiter, Florida, USA

R. P. Olympia, J. Brady-Olympia (eds.), *Clinical Considerations in School-based Health*, https://doi.org/10.1007/978-3-031-85765-2_21

Table 21.1 Examples of adverse childhood experiences and positive childhood experiences [1]

ACE	PCE
Emotional neglect Household violence Sexual abuse Community violence Emotional abuse Family mental illness Incarcerated household member Physical abuse Family substance abuse Physical neglect Bullying	Ability to verbalize feelings with family Family support through difficult times Feeling safe and protected at home by an adult Harmonious family relationships Fair treatment at school Sense of belonging at school Friend support Having at least 2 nonparent adults who took a genuine interest in you Receive support, encouragement, or affirmation

When working with a child experiencing grief, consider that reactions and needs will vary and depend greatly on the age and developmental stage of the bereaved child [6]. Children with normal grief may temporarily become sad, angry, fearful, restless, withdrawn, regress to an earlier developmental stage (e.g. potty training), and may also have difficulties with expressing emotions, appetite, sleep, concentration, learning, and academic performance [6, 7].

The school nurse's initial approach of this child should include immediately creating a safe space along with offering him immediate basic needs of hygiene, clean clothing, food, water, and comfort. Secondly, it is important to contact his caregiver to confirm the loss and communicate any personal or cultural preferences on how to share the news with others. These first steps of respecting the family's wishes, addressing the child's needs, and acknowledging their family's loss help foster a positive and supportive relationship with the child and their caregiver. Supportive school and home environments welcome safe, supported, healthy grieving that will give the bereaved child the greatest opportunity for a PCE and help mitigate potential negative outcomes.

As of 2024, there are no federally mandated national guidelines specifically requiring states to train school staff on grief management for children. Policies, rules, and legislation will vary by state, county, state education departments, and school district, however, training, education, and resources are made available by certain federal agencies and national professional organizations (Table 21.2). By preparing the school staff, administrators, school counselors, teachers, and classmates, schools are able to effectively help a bereaved child feel safe and comfortable in the classroom. Administration, teachers, and staff should always first confirm the loss and communicate the news in a way that is comfortable for the bereaved family by asking what they wish to publicly share as well as considering their cultural preferences. School staff and teachers should review basic information about grief and loss, prepare staff to answer students' questions about death honestly and directly to avoid confusion, review signs of normal vs unhealthy grief reaction (Table 21.3), review how to identify when to ask for help, identify who can help with escalation of care, and discuss protocols to keep the classroom a safe place.

Table 21.2 List of reputable agencies and organizations for resources, training, guidelines, and best practices

Department of Education
National Institute of Mental Health
American School Counselor Association (ASCA)
National Alliance for Grieving Children (NAGC)
National Center for School Crisis and Bereavement
National Child Traumatic Stress Network
Child Bereavement Center
Dougy Center for Grieving Children and Families
Canadian Virtual Hospice (Canada)
The Childhood Bereavement Network (UK)
The Australian Center for Grief and Bereavement (Australia)

Table 21.3 Examples of healthy and unhealthy grief [8, 9]

Healthy Grief Reactions	Unhealthy Grief Reactions
Emotional disturbance	Persistent anxieties
Regression	Hopes of reunion or desire to die
Denial	Persistent blame and guilt
Decreased appetite	Patterns of overactivity with aggressive and destructive outbursts
Difficulty sleeping	Compulsive caregiving and self-reliance
Decreased ability to concentrate	Euphoria with depersonalization and identification symptoms
Increased sadness	Unwillingness or inability to speak about the deceased parent
Social withdrawal	Exaggerated clinging to the surviving parent
Anger	Expression of only positive or only negative feelings about the deceased
Poor daily functioning	Prolonged dysfunction in school
Reactions to birthdays, holidays, anniversaries of the death	New stealing or illegal acts

Within the classroom, give the bereaved child's classmates time to meaningfully prepare for their classmate's return by reviewing what grief can look like, sharing their past grief experiences and what they felt was helpful that they could do for their bereaved classmate, discussing practical ways to support their classmate during this time, and answering any general questions about death directly and honestly and as well as about the current situation within the family's comfort level [10].

Additionally, it is important for the school staff, administrators, school counselors, and teachers to be aware and mindful of the appropriate time to refer a student to a higher level of care. While certain behaviors may not be directly due to grief, the school's consistent contact with their bereaved student will be important in contributing what is baseline and functional for that individual child at school. With any immediate safety concerns, it would be most prudent for the child to be directly referred to an emergency department for evaluation. For less emergent concerns, teachers and staff may also refer students to the school counselor, school psychologist, or school social worker. Per the National Association of School Psychologists, data shows that there is a shortage of school psychologists in the US. Despite schools having at least one school psychologist on staff though, this may not necessarily a dedicated full-time one nor meet the recommended student to psychologist ratio of 1:500 [11]. In the event a school does not have access to mental health resources at school, students should be directed to their pediatrician who will be able to assist with their care as well as connect them with the appropriate referrals and resources.

Case 2 Luna, a 13-year-old female with asthma and ADHD, has recently moved with her family and started seventh grade at a new school in a new town halfway through the academic school year. She had issues while at her previous school where she was absent for almost two to three times per week following the loss of a friend at a mall shooting 3 months ago. Her new teachers were not aware of Luna's recent traumatic loss of a friend. The school notifies her mother who shares that Luna has been withdrawn, avoiding crowded spaces, and refusing to speak about the incident. In addition to poor academic performance and absences, her teachers have noted poor hygiene, excessive social isolation, low mood, low motivation and have been concerned about her recent excessive time in the bathroom. Luna's teachers feel she needs more help and are not sure how to best help her. What is your approach?

Between 10–30% of children who experience a traumatic event will develop chronic psychological disorders, including Post Traumatic Stress Disorder (PTSD) and those with prior psychiatric disorders are at higher risk for poor outcomes including substance use, suicide, and school failures [1, 12]. Trauma reactions are unique for each child with different traumatic experiences; however, persistent, and extreme reactions need to be monitored and treated promptly in order to prevent development of chronic pathology [9]. Teacher interventions in the classroom have been associated with successful reduction in traumatized children's psychological reactions to trauma. With the significant amount of time teachers spend with their students, they have frequent opportunities to support, monitor symptoms, identify obstacles, and advocate for more specialized care when necessary [12]. Supporting the teachers is supporting the students thus promoting positive outcomes. Teachers can be shown support with specialized training to better understand and manage ACEs, trauma, and child bereavement, opportunities to practice how to discuss death with students, periodic reviews of normal and abnormal signs and behaviors, designated person to assist with struggling students in need of referrals for escalation of care (typically a school counselor), sharing resources and different levels of support available for students (Table 21.4), and emotional support from their school and colleagues for the emotional weight of the traumas they experience second hand [1, 9, 12]. The effects of traumatic events may present immediately after the trauma and can be long lasting and monitoring for inappropriate behavioral reactions can change the trajectory of a child's life [1, 12].

Table 21.4 Levels of School Support [8, 13]

Level of School Support	Support System Participants
1. General, caring, supportive relationships at school	Parents, teachers, friends, community
2. Psychoeducational interventions such as individual or Group Counseling Within or outside the school	Facilitated by teachers Care from trained mental health staff school psychologist, school counselors, social workers If these resources are unavailable at school, refer to the child's pediatrician
3. Therapeutic interventions Commonly outside of the school environment	Care from highly specialized trained professionals Psychiatrists, clinical psychologists, marriage and family therapists, LCSW, school psychologist

21.1 Case Conclusions

1. This case started with a high stress moment for Esteban, as well as for the teacher who found him and the school nurse tasked with managing the next important steps in a bereaved child's initial grief. The teacher properly supported the child in a kind and gentle manner by removing him from a stressful situation and getting appropriate help. The school nurse appropriately prioritized comfort and care for Esteban during a time of heightened distress. Her next move was to reach out the family who were appreciative for her sympathy and for her kindness, support, and attention to Esteban's needs. The nurse clarified the family's wishes and proceeded to alert administration and staff. In Esteban's case, his father's death was not unexpected, he had been open with his teacher and classmates, and already felt well supported in the classroom. The school nurse alerted his teacher about the situation and she proceeded to prepare the class by way of discussion, role playing, sharing previous experiences, and answering questions with open, honest, concrete answers. As the nurse offered Esteban a snack and drink while he had some quiet time in her office, she continued with the school's crisis plan which she was familiar with because it was reviewed a month ago at a staff meeting. The school nurse next gingerly investigated whether it was safe to bring Esteban back into his classroom of 16 kids. She was able to quietly assess that Esteban's reaction was normal and made a note to regularly check on him to monitor for any prolonged or intense symptomatology and his teacher for any signs of additional support needs. Esteban returned to the classroom and felt relief to be in a comfortable, safe place. Esteban missed his father and at times acted out, had temporary regressed behaviors, and had a poor appetite. While his grief fluctuated over the next few months, his teacher was flexible with his academic expectations and continued to watch the progression of grief in the event he needed more support from the school psychologist. The school staff knew his behaviors were normal and fortunately Esteban was given the space and support he needed to feel better and his academic performance, attendance, and motivation all returned to baseline. Esteban's ability to heal and return to a healthy level of functioning also protected him from experiencing ACE's from this trauma.

2. The teachers have observed and correctly identified Luna to have unhealthy and inappropriate behaviors following a traumatic loss. With good communication with Luna's family, they share their concerns for Luna with her mother and also gather more information confirming their concerns to seek more specialized care for Luna. Luna's mother had concerns about her isolating and avoidance behaviors but was unsure if it was normal teenage behaviors. Because Luna's teachers periodically review normal and abnormal grief signs, they were able to teach and reassure mom thus initiating timely care for Luna. This case illuminates the importance of training for all school staff including teachers about the variety of normal grief behaviors and trauma reactions, prolonged and intense unhealthy behaviors, when to seek more specialized care, and the different levels of support available. The teachers escalated concerns about Luna and with the help of the school psychologist, Luna starts therapy and is referred to her pediatrician for evaluation and medication management. With the escalation of support from her pediatrician and therapist, Luna begins to consistently attend school. While cautious about the possible need of more specialized care, Luna's teachers observe consistent improvements in her academic performance and efforts, and through consistent communication with Luna's mother are kept updated on her progress at home. Luna may have had a traumatic experience, but with the help of her teachers, the school psychologist, her pediatrician, and her classmates, she has gradually started to feel better and joined the choir and swim team.

Extra Credit Points

1. Grief looks different for everyone. Finding the right support can be difficult as a child's response can be unpredictable. Consider differences in age, developmental stage, cultural norms, previous life experiences, emotional health before the loss, family and social environment, and individual capacity to understand and cope with stress.
2. It's common, healthy, and normal to be sad after a loss.
3. Be flexible and patient with your grieving students' timeline. Reset academic expectations
4. It's important to train school staff to differentiate normal grief from complicated grief to better identify which students need more specialized help.
5. When speaking to children about death, be mindful of their age and developmental stage. When answering questions children may have about events related to a death, be reassuring, do not lie, and speak directly and concretely as children may misunderstand and misinterpret figures of speech.

References

1. Linder L, Lunardini M, Zimmerman H. Supporting childhood bereavement through school-based grief group. OMEGA J Death Dying. 2022;89(2):741–58. https://doi.org/10.1177/00302228221082756.
2. Peng A, Qiu X, Ji S, et al. The impact of childhood parental loss on risk for depression and anxiety in adulthood: a community-based study in Southwest China. J Affect Disord. 2022;298:104–9. https://doi.org/10.1016/j.jad.2021.10.093.
3. National Association of School Psychologists. Addressing grief: tips for teachers and administrators. Published 2015. https://www.nasponline.org/resources-and-publications/resources-and-podcasts/school-safety-and-crisis/mental-health-resources/addressing-grief/addressing-grief-tips-for-teachers-and-administrators. Accessed 28 Apr 2024.
4. McManus E, Paul S. Addressing the bereavement needs of children in school: an evaluation of bereavement training for school communities. Improv Sch. 2019;22(1):72–85. https://doi.org/10.1177/1365480219825540.
5. Hillis S, N'konzi JPN, Msemburi W, et al. Orphanhood and caregiver loss among children based on new global excess COVID-19 death estimates. JAMA Pediatr. 2022;176(11):1145–8. https://doi.org/10.1001/jamapediatrics.2022.3157.
6. Osterweis M, Solomon F, Green M. Bereavement during childhood and adolescence. Bereavement—NCBI Bookshelf. Published 1984. https://www.ncbi.nlm.nih.gov/books/NBK217849/#:~:text=People%20who%20interact%20with%20recently. Accessed 24 Apr 2024.
7. McGlauflin H. Helping children grieve at school. Prof Sch Couns. 1988;1(5):46–9. http://www.jstor.org/stable/42731870.
8. Graydon KS, Jimerson SR, Fisher ES, National Association of School Psychologists. Death and grief in the family: providing support at school. 2010. Accessed 26 Apr 2024. https://starstoolkit.org/sites/default/files/_files/Death%20and%20Grief%20in%20the%20Family.pdf?utm_source=textcortex&utm_medium=zenochat.
9. Frei-Landau R. Who should support grieving children in school? Applying Winnicott's viewpoint to conceptualize the dyadic roles of teachers and school mental-health professionals in the context of pediatric grief. Front Psych. 2023;14:1290967. https://doi.org/10.3389/fpsyt.2023.1290967. PMID: 38025458; PMCID: PMC10657861.
10. Dougy Center. Dougy Center for grieving children & families | Portland, OR. https://www.dougy.org/resource-articles/when-death-impacts-your-school. Published 12 Nov 2020. Accessed 14 Apr 2024. https://www.dougy.org/resource-articles/when-death-impacts-your-school.
11. National Association of School Psychologists. State Shortages Data Dashboard. National Association of School Psychologists (NASP). Accessed 17 Jul 2024. https://www.nasponline.org/about-school-psychology/state-shortages-data-dashboard.
12. Alisic E. Teachers' perspectives on providing support to children after trauma: a qualitative study. Sch Psychol Q. 2012;27(1):51–9. https://doi.org/10.1037/a0028590.
13. Alvis L, Zhang N, Sandler IN, Kaplow JB. Developmental manifestations of grief in children and adolescents: caregivers as key grief facilitators. J Child Adolesc Trauma. 2022;16(2):447–57. https://doi.org/10.1007/s40653-021-00435-0.

Chapter 22
Adverse Childhood Experiences

S. Rosie Gellman

Case 1 Landon is a 7-year-old male sent by his first-grade teacher to the school nurse's office to calm down following disruptive behavior including throwing chairs during class. The school has placed multiple phone calls to his mother since the start of the school year due to escalating behavior concerns including emotional outbursts and verbal aggression towards peers. He has also been struggling academically, having already repeated kindergarten, and is now behind in reading. He is known to live in a single parent household with five school-aged siblings, in which they often face food insecurity and frequently present in weathered shoes and clothes. What is your approach?

The Center for Disease Control (CDC) defines ACEs as preventable, potentially traumatic events that occur in childhood (0–17 years), including aspects of the child's environment that can undermine their sense of safety, stability, and bonding (Table 22.1) [1]. ACEs can affect a child's brain development, stress response, and immune system and likely occur secondary to high levels of stress hormones in childhood [1, 2]. Children with ACEs are known to have poorer outcomes in terms of chronic medical conditions, disorders of learning and development, substance use problems, formation of healthy relationships, educational outcomes, and job potential, with these effects persisting into adulthood (Table 22.2) [1, 3–5]. In recent data, fewer than 47.7% of school-aged children meet basic criteria for flourishing [6]. In the school setting, this may present as failure to meet academic milestones, learning or developmental disabilities, problems with behavior and emotional regulation in the classroom or with peers including noted sadness or worry, poor school engagement, frequent visits to the nurse for somatic or physical health concerns such as asthma or abdominal pain, and poor or worsening overall physical health.

S. R. Gellman (✉)
Psych for Tykes and Teens, LLC, Louisville, CO, USA
e-mail: DrGellman@psychfortykesandteens.com

R. P. Olympia, J. Brady-Olympia (eds.), *Clinical Considerations in School-based Health*, https://doi.org/10.1007/978-3-031-85765-2_22

Table 22.1 List of ACEs as defined by the CDC-Kaiser Study

Abuse	• Emotional abuse • Physical abuse • Sexual abuse
Household challenges	• Mother treated violently • Substance abuse in the household • Mental illness in the household • Parental separation or divorce • Incarcerated household member
Neglect	• Emotional neglect • Physical neglect

Table 22.2 Adverse effects secondary to ACEs exposure

Injury	• Traumatic brain injury • Fractures • Burns
Mental and behavioral health	• Depression • Anxiety • Suicide • Post-traumatic stress disorder • Poor self-esteem • Aggression • Mood dysregulation • Developmental delays • Learning disabilities • Neurodevelopmental disorders
Maternal health	• Unintended pregnancy • Pregnancy complications • Fetal death
Infectious disease	• Human immunodeficiency virus • Sexually transmitted infections
Chronic disease	• Cancer • Diabetes • Heart disease • Obesity • Asthma • Kidney disease • Chronic obstructive pulmonary disease • Stroke
Risky behaviors	• Alcohol and drug abuse • Unsafe sex
Opportunities	• Education • Occupation • Income • Relationships

The evaluation of this child should initially include ensuring safety in the current and home environments. After safety is addressed, evaluation for potential ACEs contributing to his present condition and struggles in school would help ensure that he is provided appropriate referrals, further evaluation, and resources, including medical evaluation for underlying medical problems, mental and behavioral health referrals, neuropsychological including educational testing, and community resources for issues such as respite childcare and food security in the home.

Case 2 Katie, a 12-year-old female with obesity and asthma, is caught vaping tobacco in bathroom. The school notifies her grandmother, her custodian for the past 8 years after removal from her mother's custody for domestic violence in the home. She is currently failing most of her classes, and teachers have noted some social isolation and low mood. What is your approach?

Those that experience ACEs have a greater risk for mental health disorders, including substance use suicide, as well as school failure, and are also less likely to have access to mental health services [2, 4].

According to the National Survey of Children's Health conducted in 2011–2012, 52% of adults reported experiencing no ACEs, 25% experienced 1 ACE, and 23% experienced 2 or more ACEs during their upbringing. Strikingly, one in six adults reported being exposed to 4 or more ACEs [6]. The impact of ACEs also appears to be cumulative, with those exposed to more ACEs facing poorer overall outcomes [3]. Risk factors for exposure to ACEs include certain racial and ethnic groups including black, Hispanic, or multiracial, those with less than a high school education, those with annual income less than $15,000, those who were unemployed or unable to work, female gender, and those identifying as gay/lesbian or bisexual [1, 7].

In this child, a safety assessment should be done for the current and home environment and include assessment for dangerous substance abuse as well as potential for increased suicidality. Her medical conditions should also be assessed for stability (e.g. confirm no acute asthma exacerbations secondary to the vaping). This child should be referred to appropriate treatment resources including primary care for physical health to manage her chronic conditions and regular follow up, mental and behavioral health to assess and treat mood and substance use concerns, and potential educational evaluation for investigations into school failure. Her caregiver should also be given community resources and education to assist with needs and struggles in the home setting. Potential recommended and evidence-based prevention strategies in line with the National Association of School Nursing (NASN) initiatives of providing care in accordance with the Whole School, Whole Community, Whole Child model are summarized in Table 22.3 [1, 8–10].

22.1 Case Conclusion

1. Safety assessment is conducted with Landon and his mother, and both report feeling safe at home with no concerns for abuse. The nurse screens for ACEs and detects that Landon has been exposed to 4 ACEs throughout his life. The nurse refers to primary care to ensure that he will be followed up closely for existing

Table 22.3 Evidence-based prevention and care plan strategies for ACEs in the school-setting

Education-based	• Universal ACEs and trauma-informed education for school staff • Caregiver education about ACEs, stresses in the home, prevention and intervention strategies (consider teaching sessions and written handouts) • Caregiver education on parenting skills and family relationship approaches (consider teaching sessions and written handouts) • Caregiver education on local resources (e.g. financial assistance, food banks, respite childcare, etc.) • Teaching skills to students to manage stress and education on healthy lifestyle and risk-taking behaviors • Social worker or case manager within the school to help with teaching sessions and case management
Community-based resources	• After school or mentoring programs • Extracurricular activities
Accommodations within school	• Educational testing and interventions including 504 and IEP plans • Scheduled visits to counselor or nurse • Regular conferences with parents and caregivers • Additional tutoring • Implement school-based health centers when available • Encourage family engagement in the school setting
Care coordination	• Primary care physician • Mental and behavioral health providers • Developmental therapists and services
Screening	• Consider universal screening for risk factors for ACEs and stresses in the home at time of enrollment • Start in young children (e.g. ages 0–5 years) • Safety assessments on any child with concern and referral if needed

and emerging medical concerns, weight, and general welfare. The nurse provides resources for the after-care program in the school for Landon and his siblings, as well as resources for community mentoring and behavior health. The school conducts further neuropsychological testing. Landon is found to have dyslexia and Attention Deficit Hyperactivity Disorder (ADHD), and an education plan is arranged for appropriate accommodations. Landon starts therapy in the community and attends scheduled, frequent check-ins at school counselor. His mother receives resources for community assistance, and his she acquires assistance from a local food bank and respite care with a tie in to a local organization. Landon's behavior and academic success improve over the course of a few months.

2. The nurse conducts a safety assessment with Katie which yields no abuse or safety concerns. Katie denies any thoughts of hurting herself or others. The nurse also checks Katie's respiratory status and finds no signs of acute asthma exacerbation. Katie reports vaping began recently to deal with some of her depression and loneliness. The nurse screen for ACEs and finds Katie has had exposure to 4 ACEs. The nurse places a referral to her primary care physician to discuss vap-

ing and behavioral health care, as well as for asthma assessment. The nurse also provides Katie some education and age-appropriate handouts about the dangers of substance use and vaping. Katie is scheduled for frequent visits with the school counselor, and she starts to see a therapist in the community. The school schedules a conference with her grandmother, during which she receives education and handouts on parenting skills and relationship building at home, healthy lifestyle choices, and community resources for additional help. Katie joins the school volleyball team, which helps her form friendships and encourages physical activity to aid in healthy lifestyle. Katie starts afterschool tutoring, and her grades start to improve.

Extra Credit Points

1. ACEs can lead to lasting negative outcomes on a child's physical, mental and behavioral health, educational attainment, relationship-building, and future career success.
2. Over 60% of children experience at least one ACE, with many exposed to more, making screening and intervention critical to ensure optimal child well-being and development into adulthood. Consider ACEs screening for any child who is presenting with concerns, including behavioral, emotional, physical, educational, etc., since multiple domains may be affected.
3. Consider safety concerns and evaluation when an ACE is detected.
4. Consider universal screening for risk factors at time of enrollment, as well as frequent student and family engagement in the school and community settings to help with prevention and early intervention.
5. Collaborative care with the community resources and outside care providers can be beneficial in caring for children exposed to ACEs.

References

1. Center for Disease Control and Prevention. Preventing adverse childhood experiences (ACEs): leveraging the best available evidence. Atlanta, GA: Centers for Disease Control and Prevention; 2019.
2. Larson S, Chapman S, Spetz J, Brindis CD. Chronic childhood trauma, mental health, academic achievement, and school-based health center mental health services. J Sch Health. 2017;87(9):675–86. https://doi.org/10.1111/josh.12541. PMID: 28766317.
3. Felitti VJ, Anda RF, Nordenberg D, et al. Relationship of childhood abuse and household dysfunction to many of the leading causes of death in adults. The Adverse Childhood Experiences (ACE) Study. Am J Prev Med. 1998;14(4):245–58.
4. Loveday SL, Hall T, Constable L, et al. Screening for adverse childhood experiences in children: a systematic review. Pediatrics. 2022;149(2):e2021051884.
5. Centers for Disease Control and Prevention. Youth risk behavioral surveillance survey—United States, 2019. Morb Mortal Wkly Rep. 2020;69(1). US Department of Health and Human Services. https://www.cdc.gov/mmwr/volumes/69/su/pdfs/su6901-H.pdf.
6. Health Resources and Services Administration, Maternal and Child Health Bureau. Data Resource Center for Child & Adolescent Health: a project of the child and adolescent health

measurement initiative. National Survey of Children's Health (NSCH), Interactive Data Query; 2016. https://www.childhealthdata.org/browse/survey.
7. Merrick MT, Ford DC, Porta KA, et al. Prevalence of adverse childhood experiences from the 2011-2014 behavior risk factors surveillance system in 23 states. JAMA Pediatr. 2018;172(11):1038–44. https://doi.org/10.1001/jamapediatrics.2018.2537.
8. National Association of School Nurses. Framework for 21st Century School Nursing Practice™: clarifications and updated definitions. NASN Sch Nurse. 2020;35(4):225–33. https://doi.org/10.1177/1942602x20928372.
9. Dubowitz H, Finkelhor D, Zolotor A, Kleven J, Davis N. Addressing adverse childhood experiences in primary care: challenges and considerations. Pediatrics. 2022;149(4):e2021052641. https://doi.org/10.1542/peds.2021-052641. PMID: 35362065; PMCID: PMC9405315.
10. Parker C. ACE awareness in school nursing—becoming a trauma-informed service. Br J Child Health. 2022;3(1):39–43. https://doi.org/10.12968/chhe.2022.3.1.39.

Part III
The Sick Student: An Initial Approach for the School Nurse

Chapter 23
The Pediatric Assessment Triangle: Initial Assessment and Triage

Robert P. Olympia

Case 1 **Twelve year old Asher comes to your office with complaints of difficulty breathing, chest pain, palpitations, and dizziness. His lips appear "blue" and he has intercostal retractions and grunting. His vital signs are: Heart Rate (HR) 126 beats per minute, Respiratory rate (RR) 38 breaths per minute, Blood pressure (BP) 128/76.**

Case 2 **Ten year old Alyson was found slumped over her desk during class. She recently had nasal packing placed 24 h ago for a prolonged nose bleed. She appears very weak and responds slowly to your voice. She is unsure of where she is. She proceeds to vomit. Her vital signs: HR 160 beats per minute, RR 24 breaths per minute, BP 80/45. Capillary refill is prolonged (>5 s) with cool extremities and a weak, thready pulse.**

Case 3 **You are summoned to the high school gymnasium. There you find Jennifer, a 16 year old student, pale, motionless and unresponsive. Her HR is 50 beats per minute and her RR is 10 breaths per minute. You see vomitus in her mouth, and she has snoring shallow respirations. Her pulse is weak and thready.**

School nurses are often faced with making critical decisions when evaluating an acutely ill or injured student. An organized method of assessment should include the following steps:

R. P. Olympia (✉)
Department of Emergency Medicine and Pediatrics, Penn State College of Medicine
Attending Physician, Hershey, PA, USA

Division of Pediatric Emergency Medicine, Department of Emergency Medicine, Penn State
Milton S. Hershey Medical Center, Hershey, PA, USA
e-mail: rolympia@hmc.psu.edu

R. P. Olympia, J. Brady-Olympia (eds.), *Clinical Considerations in School-based Health*, https://doi.org/10.1007/978-3-031-85765-2_23

Table 23.1 The Pediatric Assessment Triangle (appearance, work of breathing, circulation to the skin) [1]

Appearance	Tone Interactiveness Consolability Look/gaze Speech/cry
Work of Breathing	Abnormal breath sounds (stridor/grunting) Abnormal positioning (tripoding) Retractions Nasal flaring
Circulation to the skin	Pallor Mottling Cyanosis

- Application of the Pediatric Assessment Triangle (PAT)
- Interpretation of vital signs
- Utilization of the ABCDE approach—Airway, Breathing, Circulation, Disability, and Exposure
- Implementation of the SAMPLE mnemonic
- Determination of disposition

The Pediatric Assessment Triangle (PAT), developed as a tool to standardize the initial assessment of acutely ill or injured children, examines *Appearance, Work of Breathing, and Circulation to the Skin* (Table 23.1) [1]. The PAT is intended to rapidly assess the child using only visual and auditory clues without any equipment, and should take no more than 30 s. *Appearance* reflects the adequacy of ventilation, oxygenation, and brain perfusion. *Work of Breathing* is a more accurate indicator of oxygenation and ventilation than respiratory rate or auscultation. *Circulation to the skin* is an assessment of cardiac output and perfusion of vital organs. Following the initial assessment, a student's severity of illness can be categorized as "sick" (0 of 3), "sicker" (1 of 3), or "sickest" (2–3 of 3) based on the involvement of Appearance, Work of Breathing, and Circulation to the Skin. Furthermore, based on which on the 3 components are involved, a physiologic diagnosis can be assigned (Table 23.2). The PAT has been shown to be effectively utilized in the prehospital setting [1] and by nurse triage [2].

Following the application of the PAT to determine severity and pathophysiological derangement, vital signs should be obtained and the ABCDE approach utilized [3]. In regards to vital signs, absolute values are not as important as determining whether there are abnormalities (high or low), except in the case of hypotension or hypoxia (Table 23.3). Keep in mind that interventions associated with the ABCDE approach may be limited by the availability of equipment and medications (Table 23.4), so rapid activation of Emergency Medical Services (EMS) is of

Table 23.2 Physiologic diagnosis based on components of the Pediatric Assessment Triangle [1]

	Appearance	Work of Breathing	Circulation to skin
Respiratory distress	Normal	Abnormal	Normal
Respiratory failure	Abnormal	Abnormal	Normal or abnormal
Compensated shock	Normal	Normal or abnormal	Abnormal
Decompensated shock	Abnormal	Normal or abnormal	Abnormal
Central nervous or metabolic dysfunction	Abnormal	Normal	Normal
Cardiopulmonary failure	Abnormal	Abnormal	Abnormal

Table 23.3 Differential diagnosis based on the assessment of vital signs

	High	Low
Temperature	Infection Environmental (heat related illness) Toxic exposure	Infection Environmental (cold related illness) Toxic exposure
Heart rate	Fever Pain or anxiety Dehydration Shock Primary cardiac (tachydysrhythmias, myocarditis, etc.) Toxic exposures	Normal for an adolescent or athlete Primary cardiac (bradydysrhythmias, heart block, etc.) Toxic exposures Eating disorders Increased intracranial pressure
Respiratory rate	Fever Pain or anxiety Primary respiratory (asthma, pneumonia, anaphylaxis, etc.) Dehydration Increased intracranial pressure Toxic exposures	Impending respiratory failure Toxic exposures
Blood pressure Minimum systolic BP: 70 + 2 (age in years) for children aged 4–8 years < 90 for children greater than 9 years of age	Pain or anxiety Primary renal problem Early shock Increased intracranial pressure Toxic exposures	Decompensated shock Toxic exposures
Pulse oximetry (<90%)		Primary respiratory Congenital and acquired heart disease Toxic exposures

Table 23.4 Airway, breathing, circulation, disability, and exposure (ABCDE approach)

	Assessment	Interventions
Airway	Is the student able to speak to you? If not, is the airway open? – What do you hear? (snoring, stridor, secretions or vomitus in the oral cavity) – What do you feel? (air movement) – Tripoding? (upper airway obstruction)	Clearing of secretions and/or vomitus after turning the student to their side and wiping away the obstruction (without entering the oral cavity) Head tilt and chin lift to maximize the airway
Alignment (in event of trauma)	For suspected head/neck injury or in an unconscious student, always consider a cervical spine injury	Maintain in-line cervical spine immobilization with a collar or an assistant's hand/arms Utilize jaw thrust to maximize the airway
Breathing	Do you see chest rise? Is there fast or slow breathing? Is there central cyanosis (lips/face/chest)? Are there signs of respiratory distress? – Inability to speak in full sentences – Grunting – Intercostal retractions – Abdominal breathing Is there wheezing, rales or crackles on auscultation?	Provide rescue breaths If available: – Oxygen by face mask – Albuterol – Epinephrine autoinjector If not available, activation of Emergency Medical Services (EMS) is of utmost importance to administer these respiratory medications and oxygen
Circulation	Is there mottling or a pale color of the skin? Are the extremities cool or clammy? What is the central capillary refill (best performed on the trunk or abdomen, and not the extremities/hands)? Are the pulses weak and thready, or strong and bounding (indicative of shock)? Are there signs of dehydration: – A sleepy or lethargic student – Sunken eyes or lack of tears – Dry mucous membranes – Prolonged capillary refill	Intravenous fluids are necessary, so activation of Emergency Medical Services (EMS) is of utmost importance
Disability	Don't worry about a Glasgow Coma Score, utilize "AVPU"—is the student: – Alert – Responsive to verbal stimuli – Responsive to painful stimuli (sternal rub) – Unresponsive Pupillary size and response	Stabilize the ABCs above Consider the "AEIOU-TIPS" mnemonic for a student with depressed mental status (Table 23.5) and stabilize appropriately [4]
Exposure	Is there a concern for a heat or cold related illness or injury? Is there concern for a toxic exposure?	If warm, cool down with cold compresses, ice bags to axilla/groin, and fans directed toward the student If cold, provide warmth with blankets

Table 23.5 Differential diagnosis for a student with depressed mental status ("AEIOU-TIPS" mnemonic)

A	Anoxia or hypoxia
E	Epilepsy (active seizure or post-ictal period)
I	Insufficient glucose
O	Overdose or toxic exposure
U	Uremia, hepatic encephalopathy, electrolyte abnormalities
T	Trauma (head, or other trauma leading to hypoxia or blood loss)
I	Infection (meningitis or encephalitis) or inflammation (vasculitis)
P	Psychogenic (a diagnosis of exclusion)
S	Shock (lack of perfusion to the end organs) or syncope

Table 23.6 SAMPLE mnemonic

S	Signs and symptoms
A	Allergies
M	Medications
P	Past medical, psychiatric, and surgical history
L	Life situation (social history)
E	Events leading up to or following the present illness or injury

paramount importance. Implementing the SAMPLE mnemonic (Table 23.6) may involve accessing the student's medical information form, asking the student directly, or in the case of a student who may have altered mental status, questioning school staff or classmates who may have witnessed the event, or events leading up to or following the event.

Based on the application of the Pediatric Assessment Triangle, the interpretation of vital signs, the utilization of the ABCDE approach, and the implementation of the SAMPLE mnemonic, the student's disposition may include EMS activation to the ED (Table 23.7) [5], referral to an urgent care center (See Chap. 12) or primary care provider, or return to the classroom (Fig. 23.1).

Table 23.7 Scenarios that require EMS activation to the ED

• "Sick", "Sicker", or "Sickest" on the PAT
• Inability to speak or speak in full sentences
• Evidence of upper airway obstruction—gagging, drooling, gurgling respirations, stridor, "tripod" positioning
• Significant lips, tongue, or facial swelling
• Central cyanosis
• Evidence of lower airway disease—grunting, nasal flaring, intercostal retractions, tachypnea
• Decreased aeration on lung auscultation associated with wheezing, crackles, or rhonchi
• Evidence of anaphylaxis
• Depressed mental status
• Significant vision or hearing deficits
• Cushing's triad (hypertension, bradycardia, abnormal respirations)
• Evidence of shock (poor perfusion of end organs) or severe dehydration
• Syncope during physical activity, or associated with chest pain, shortness of breath, palpitations, seizure activity
• Seizures
• Concern for congestive heart failure (tachycardia, tachypnea, hepatosplenomegaly)
• Significant head, chest, abdominal, groin or extremity pain
• Weakness or numbness of the extremities
• Ingestion, toxic exposure, or inhalational injury
• Significant trauma to head, face, cervical spine, chest, abdomen and/or extremities
• Significant bleeding despite pressure

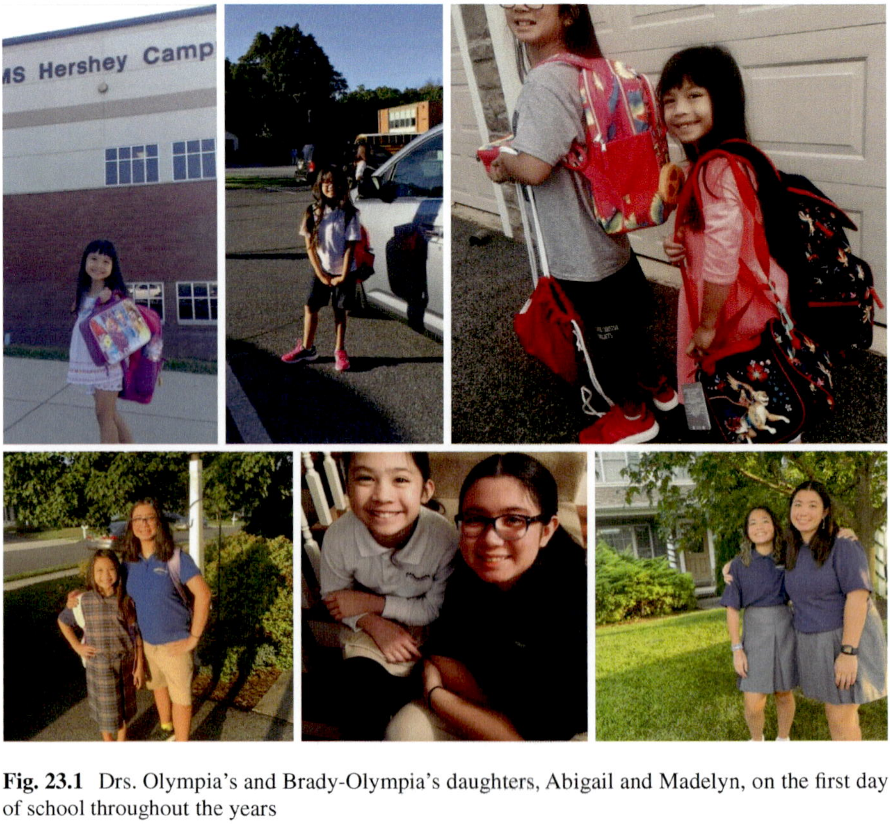

Fig. 23.1 Drs. Olympia's and Brady-Olympia's daughters, Abigail and Madelyn, on the first day of school throughout the years

Case resolution utilizing a stepwise approach

	Case 1	Case 2	Case 3
Pediatric Assessment Triangle	Sicker (2/3): Work of breathing Circulation of skin	Sicker (2/3): Appearance Circulation of skin	Sickest (3/3): Appearance Work of breathing Circulation of skin
Vital signs	Tachycardia Tachypnea	Tachycardia Hypotension	Bradycardia Decreased RR
ABCDE approach	Speaking in short phrases Retractions and grunting Circulation appropriate Alert Albuterol MDI administered	Able to speak No evidence of respiratory distress Poor circulation Responds to verbal stimuli Concern for shock, EMS activated	Vomitus in mouth and snoring respirations Shallow respirations Poor circulation Unresponsive Concern for opiate overdose, you provide head tilt chin lift and cervical spine immobilization, and administer Naloxone
Sample	S: Chest pain, difficulty breathing, palpitations, dizziness A: NKDA M: Seasonal allergy and asthma medications P: Seasonal allergies and asthma L: No smokers in home E: Symptoms started during gym class	S: Disoriented, vomited A: NKDA M: No medications P: No past medical history L: Unknown E: Nasal packing 24 h ago for epistaxis	S: Vomited A: Unknown M: Unknown P: Unknown L: Has been suspended several times in the past year for violent behavior E: Unknown
Disposition	EMS activated to the ED for assumed asthma attack	EMS activated to the ED for suspected shock, likely septic shock syndrome	Responds to verbal stimuli following Naloxone, EMS activated to the ED

ED Emergency Department, *EMS* Emergency Medical Services, *MDI* Meter dose inhaler, *NKDA* No Known Drug Allergies, *RR* respiratory rate

Extra Credit Points

1. The Pediatric Assessment Triangle evaluates appearance, work of breathing, and circulation to the skin to determine severity of illness/injury and pathophysiologic diagnosis, in less than 30 s.
2. The absolute values of vital signs are not as important as to whether they are abnormal (high or low), except for blood pressure (hypotension) and pulse oximetry (hypoxia).
3. Most arrests in children are respiratory in origin, and not cardiac, so maximize the airway (clear secretions/vomitus, apply appropriate positioning utilizing either head tilt-chin lift or jaw thrust/cervical spine immobilization) and support breathing (providing rescue breaths if necessary, and administer oxygen/albuterol/epinephrine if available).
4. Remember AVPU and AEIOU-TIPS in the students with depressed mental status.
5. Contact EMS as soon as possible once the decision is made to transport a child to the ED.

References

1. Dieckmann RA, Brownstein D, Gausche-Hill M. The Pediatric Assessment Triangle: a novel approach for the rapid evaluation of children. Pediatr Emer Care. 2010;26:312–5.
2. Horeczko T, Enriquez B, McGrath NE, et al. The Pediatric Assessment Triangle: accuracy of its application by nurses in the triage of children. J Emerg Nurs. 2013;39(2):182–9.
3. Thim T, Krarup NHV, Grove EL, et al. Initial assessment and treatment with the Airway, Breathing, Circulation, Disability, Exposure (ABCDE) approach. Int J Gen Med. 2012;5:117–21.
4. Patterson K, Brady J, Olympia RP. School nurses on the front lines of medicine: uppers and downers: the approach to the student with altered mental status. NASN Sch Nurse. 2017;32(6):350–5.
5. Loaec M, Olympia RP. School nurses on the front lines of medicine: take a BREATH: the approach to a student with respiratory distress. NASN Sch Nurse. 2018;33(1):29–35.

Chapter 24
Altered Mental Status

Lydia Younger

The initial assessment of the student with altered mental status should start with application of the Pediatric Assessment Triangle (appearance, work of breathing, and circulation to the skin), the interpretation of vital signs, the utilization of the ABCDE approach (airway, breathing, circulation, disability, and exposure), the implementation of the SAMPLE mnemonic, and determination of disposition (Chap. 23). In a student with altered mental status, determination of the "AVPU" status (whether the child is alert, responsive to verbal stimuli, responsive to painful stimuli, or is unresponsive) will help guide differential diagnosis and disposition. For a student with depressed mental status, remember the AEIOU-TIPS mnemonic [1] (Table 24.1).

The term "altered mental status" can include both delirium and psychosis - differentiating between the two can be helpful to guide the evaluation (Table 24.2). Both delirium and psychosis can present with agitation or restlessness, disorientation, unusual thoughts, poor concentration, and hallucinations. Delirium is typically caused by an underlying medical process, while psychosis is caused by psychiatric disease [2].

As noted in the table, abnormal vital signs (for instance, the presence of a fever and tachycardia) might suggest an underlying medical etiology for the delirium. In addition, delineating between visual and auditory hallucinations may also help differentiate between delirium (more commonly visual and tactile) and psychosis (more commonly auditory). Considering a patient's prior psychiatric history can be a helpful clue, although it is important to remember that an acute medical condition causing delirium can be present in a patient with a prior history of mental health disorders. Level of consciousness is another helpful distinction—somnolence or lethargy are more suggestive of delirium caused by a medical condition, while being alert is more suggestive of psychosis. Psychosis can be caused by bipolar disorder,

L. Younger (✉)
Penn State Children's Hospital, Hershey, PA, USA
e-mail: lyounger@pennstatehealth.psu.edu

R. P. Olympia, J. Brady-Olympia (eds.), *Clinical Considerations in School-based Health*, https://doi.org/10.1007/978-3-031-85765-2_24

Table 24.1 Differential diagnosis for depressed mental status: the "AEIOU-TIPS" mnemonic

A	Anoxia or hypoxia
E	Epilepsy (active seizure or post-ictal period)
I	Insufficient glucose
O	Overdose or toxic exposure
U	Uremia, hepatic encephalopathy, electrolyte abnormalities
T	Trauma (head, or other trauma leading to hypoxia or blood loss)
I	Infection (meningitis or encephalitis) or inflammation (vasculitis)
P	Psychogenic (a diagnosis of exclusion)
S	Shock (lack of perfusion to the end organs) or syncope

Table 24.2 Difference between delirium and acute psychosis

	Delirium	Acute psychosis
Onset	Acute	Acute
Vital signs	Often abnormal	Often normal
Prior psychiatric history	Uncommon	Common
Course	Fluctuating	Stable
Level of consciousness	Depressed	Usually alert
Hallucinations	Visual, or visual and auditory	Primarily auditory
Orientation	Abnormal	Normal
Concentration	Usually impaired	Occasionally impaired
Speech	Pressured, slow, possibly incoherent	Usually coherent
Course	Typically resolves	Responds to treatment, can be recurrent

Table 24.3 Differential diagnosis of delirium: the "DELIRIOUS" mnemonic

D	Drugs/withdrawal (alcohol, anesthetics, anticholinergics, hallucinogens, psychostimulants, narcotics, sedative/hypnotics, ecstasy, inhalants, PCP)
E	Endocrinopathies (adrenal, thyroid, or parathyroid disease, hyper/hypoglycemia)
L	Lytes (electrolyte abnormalities, hepatic or renal dysfunction)
I	Infection (encephalitis, meningitis, urinary tract infection, pneumonia, sepsis)
R	Rising temperature/heat stroke
I	Insufficient oxygen (hypoxia)
O	Oncology (primary tumors and metastases)
U	Unavailable vitamins (vitamin B12, folate, niacin, thiamine)
S	Stoke and other central nervous system disorders (hemorrhage, head trauma, seizures, vasculitis)

depression with psychotic features, psychotic disorders, schizoaffective disorder, and schizophrenia. The DELIRIOUS mnemonic (Table 24.3) can help organize the differential diagnosis for delirium.

Here are some cases to illustrate the approach to a student with altered mental status:

Case 1 You are asked to evaluate a 6-year-old boy who has been complaining of intermittent abdominal pain all day. He then proceeds to have several episodes of dark green emesis and becomes tired and less responsive. When you assess him, he appears sleepy and pale, but responds to your voice. Pupils are 3 mm and reactive bilaterally. Vital signs show a heart rate 148, respiratory rate 24, temperature 37.6 °C, pulse oximetry 97%, and blood pressure 94/62.

Using the assessment skills discussed earlier in this scenario, he is responsive to verbal stimuli, has equal and reactive pupils, vital signs are notable for tachycardia for age, and he appears pale. The abdominal pain and bilious emesis are suggestive of intussusception. Ileocolic intussusception is a surgical emergency that presents with severe intermittent abdominal pain and vomiting. The vomiting can be bilious since the obstruction occurs between the small and large intestine at the ileocecal valve. The obstruction occurs because the small intestine telescopes into the large intestine and becomes fixed. Children can present with lethargy between the episodes of pain. A less common, but classically described symptom of intussusception is "currant jelly" stool—this is a bloody stool caused by tissue edema and vascular congestion. This is a late finding which develops due to bowel wall ischemia. This condition typically occurs in infants and toddlers, however when it occurs in older children, it is typically a result of mesenteric lymphadenopathy or bowel wall edema associated with gastroenteritis [3]. Intussusception is diagnosed using an abdominal ultrasound. First line treatment for an ileocolic intussusception without intestinal perforation is an air enema, which uses pneumatic pressure to reduce the telescoping of the bowel. This child should be sent to an emergency department for evaluation with an abdominal ultrasound [4].

Case 2 You are asked to evaluate a 7-year-old girl for lethargy. She responds to touch, but is lethargic. She appears pale with equal and reactive pupils. Her vitals are: heart rate 136, respiratory rate 36, temperature 37.4 °C, pulse oximetry 98%, and blood pressure 84/56. She had cough, congestion, and fatigue earlier in the day and then had several episodes of vomiting before becoming lethargic. Her capillary refill is delayed at 3–4 seconds and she has decreased tone. You obtain a point of care glucose and it is 42. In her medical forms, you see that she was recently diagnosed with type 1 diabetes.

Hypoglycemia can be a presenting symptom of a wide variety of conditions and is a common cause of altered mental status. If the child has known diabetes and uses insulin, it may be due to excessive exogenous insulin administration or inadequate oral intake. If the child is sick with a viral illness, it may be related to poor oral intake. Management of children with diabetes is discussed in further detail in Chap. 46. In children without diabetes, a normal glucose level is typically greater than 70. If the child is awake and alert enough to drink, they should consume 15 g of carbohydrates, which is equivalent to about 4 ounces of juice. If they are not alert enough to drink, then they should immediately be evaluated by emergency medical services and transported to the emergency department. Children with diabetes will likely also be prescribed glucagon, which could be used in a situation where they are unable to eat or drink. If the child is able to drink, a repeat blood sugar should be obtained after oral intake in order to ensure that it has improved to greater than 70. Any child with hypoglycemia less than 50 should be evaluated by a medical provider in order to determine the etiology of the hypoglycemia [5]. The child in our scenario requires immediate attention and administration of her rescue glucagon. She should be transported to an emergency department in order to obtain lab work and likely be resuscitated with IV fluids and dextrose.

A less common etiology of altered mental status and hypoglycemia are inborn errors of metabolism [6]. These are relatively uncommon in the population as a whole, but they are a serious and potentially life-threatening condition resulting from buildup of toxic byproducts from the metabolic processes in the body. Hypoglycemia and altered mental status can be the first presenting symptoms of these conditions, often triggered by an otherwise relatively mild infection or physiologic stress. Once children are diagnosed with an inborn error of metabolism, they will typically have a "sick plan" which will likely include prompt emergency department evaluation in times of illness in order to check electrolytes and monitor glucose.

Case 3 A 9-year-old male is brought to the nurse's office at school due to fatigue. He is alert and eyes are spontaneously open, but he does appear tired and pale. Pupils are equal, round, reactive, and approximately 3 mm bilaterally. His vitals are: heart rate 136, respiratory rate 42, temperature 37.8, and pulse oximetry of 86%. He has a tight dry cough and is in respiratory distress with subcostal and intercostal retractions, decreased aeration bilaterally, and inspiratory and expiratory wheezing. His capillary refill is about 3 s. Reviewing his chart, he has reported a history of asthma and eczema and he has a prescription for an albuterol inhaler.

Hypoxia is a common cause of altered mental status. If hypoxia and respiratory distress are profound and untreated, they can progress to respiratory arrest and ultimately cardiac arrest. It is crucial to identify and treat respiratory distress early. In this scenario, the child's wheezing and past medical history suggest that he is experiencing an acute asthma exacerbation. Given that he is in respiratory distress and hypoxic, he should be evaluated in the emergency department immediately. Administering his prescribed albuterol inhaler while awaiting emergency medical services can help decrease his work of breathing and hopefully improve the hypoxia as well. Ultimately, he will require steroids and frequent albuterol treatments in order to manage this exacerbation [7].

Case 4 You are asked to evaluate a 14-year-old female who is lethargic after being struck in the head with a softball. She did not pass out and initially seemed a little dazed, but was responding appropriately. However, then she quickly progressed to being quite lethargic. She has vomited once. On your assessment, she is responsive to calling her name loudly and to painful stimuli. Her pupils are slow to respond, but equal bilaterally. She appears pale. Vital signs are: heart rate 52, respiratory rate is irregular and varies between 16 and

24, temperature 36.7 °C, pulse oximetry 98%, and blood pressure 142/54. Her respiratory rate is variable, but she does not have labored breathing and is maintaining her airway with no signs of sonorous respirations. She has a large hematoma over the right temporal area.

Traumatic brain injury describes a wide variety of conditions, ranging from a concussion to a life-threatening intracranial hemorrhage. Severe headache, lethargy, neurologic deficits, and vomiting are concerning symptoms of a serious head injury. A late sign of serious intracranial injury is decorticate and decerebrate posturing. Decorticate posturing is when the arms are flexed (think "arms to the CORE"), back and head are arched, legs are in extension, and toes are in plantar flexion. Decerebrate posturing involves the extremities being held in an extended position with head and back arched and toes in plantar flexion. Both types of posturing indicate severe brain injury [8]. In this scenario, the child's lethargy, vomiting, and slow pupillary reaction are concerning. In addition, her vital signs are displaying Cushing's triad, which consists of bradycardia, irregular respirations, and widened pulse pressure (increased systolic blood pressure and decreased diastolic blood pressure) [9]. Cushing's triad results from increased intracranial pressure and is an ominous sign. This vital sign trend can also be seen with any cause of increased intracranial pressure like an intracranial mass or hydrocephalus due to shunt failure in a child with a ventriculoperitoneal or ventriculoatrial shunt. The child in this scenario should be transported to the nearest emergency department and have a head CT completed emergently.

Case 5 A 6-year-old male is brought to your office due to fever. The teacher notes that he has seemed tired all day and has reported having a headache. Then this afternoon he started to become more lethargic and was talking about seeing purple spiders crawling on the ceiling. In your office, he appears pale and lethargic. Pupils are equal, round, and reactive to light bilaterally. Vital signs are: temperature 39.6 °C, heart rate 146, respiratory rate 36, pulse oximetry 98%, and blood pressure 84/46. His capillary refill is 3–4 s.

This child is showing signs of sepsis and likely encephalitis given the presence of headache and confusion. He is experiencing hypoperfusion, as evidenced by his delayed capillary refill. Although his blood pressure is preserved at the moment, hypotension can be a late sign of sepsis so it is important for him to be emergently evaluated in an emergency department in order to undergo laboratory testing and to receive antibiotics. Sepsis is one of the leading causes of morbidity and mortality for children, which is why it is important to be vigilant for the early warning signs of sepsis such as altered mental status, tachycardia and delayed capillary refill and to refer to the emergency department for prompt evaluation [10]. In this specific scenario, the presence of visual hallucinations and lethargy are suggestive of delirium, likely related to an underlying encephalitis.

Case 6 A 17-year-old male is brought for evaluation after becoming agitated at a school dance. His friends report that he was speaking very quickly and was talking about seeing green aliens. Pupils are equal, round, and reactive to light. Vital signs are: temperature 38.2 °C, heart rate 146, respiratory rate 26, blood

pressure 156/92, and pulse oximetry 98% on room air. He appears flushed and diaphoretic and is agitated with pressured speech. He is redirectable, but constantly fidgeting. He asks for water and quickly drinks a whole cup when it is offered to him.

This teenager is exhibiting signs of delirium. His vital signs hold clues with hyperthermia, tachycardia, and hypertension, suggestive of a stimulant or serotonergic overdose. He is flushed but is also sweaty, which would point away from an anticholinergic overdose. Agitation, pressured speech, and hallucinations can be seen with serotonergic, anticholinergic, and stimulant overdoses. In this situation, this teenager ingested MDMA ("ecstasy") for the first time at the school dance, triggering his delirium. Excessive thirst can be seen with MDMA overdose. Severe effects of MDMA ingestion include arrhythmias, seizures, intracranial hemorrhage, and rhabdomyolysis [11]. He should be evaluated in the emergency department to rule out heat stroke or other infectious etiologies.

Case 7 A 16-year-old female is brought to the office due to trouble breathing in gym class. She shares that this year she has noticed a lot of changes—she feels warm all the time, often feels that her heart is racing, feels more anxious, and has lost 10 pounds since the start of the school year, even though she insists she has not changed her eating or exercise habits. She is visibly anxious and agitated in your office, with a temperature of 39.4 °C, heart rate 156, respiratory rate 28, blood pressure 96/68, and pulse oximetry 100% on room air. She is flushed and her hands are trembling. Pupils are equal, round, and reactive to light. You notice some swelling around her neck. Her speech is tangential, talking about things that you know are not true, such as worrying about planning her sixth birthday party.

This child is presenting with an interesting constellation of palpitations, anxiety, and weight loss and has abnormal vital signs with fever, significant tachycardia, and hypotension. While the presence of anxiety associated with weight loss might be a sign of psychiatric etiology or an eating disorder, the presence of fever points away from those diagnoses. This child is showing signs of hyperthyroidism and thyrotoxicosis. The most common cause of hyperthyroidism is Graves' disease, which is an autoimmune process causing the thyroid to overproduce thyroid hormones. Thyrotoxicosis can present with heart failure, lethargy, and severely altered mental status with psychosis. She requires evaluation in the emergency department for laboratory testing, hemodynamic support, and endocrinology consultation [12].

Case 8 A 17-year-old male with a history of depression and ADHD is brought to your office due to unusual behaviors. His classmates have noticed that he seems to be talking to himself a lot. His personal hygiene has worsened in the last few weeks as well. Today he was talking to some classmates about how people are watching them through video cameras in the hand sanitizer dispensers. His vitals are: temperature 37.6 °C, heart rate 78, respiratory rate 16, blood pressure 118/76, and pulse oximetry 100% on room air. He appears withdrawn. He reports hearing whispers and seeing dark shadows while sitting in

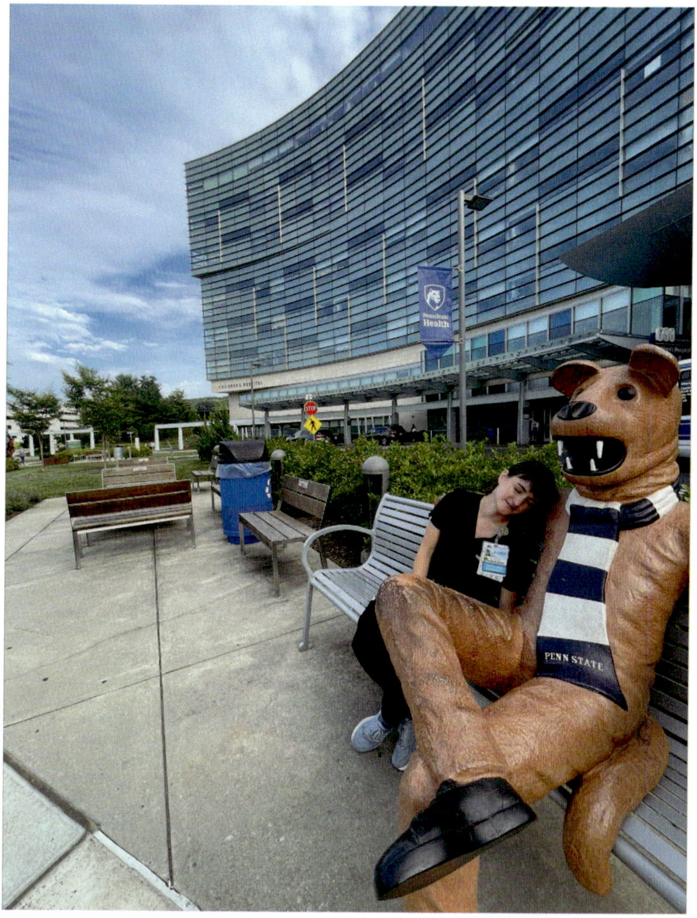

Fig. 24.1 Unresponsive … or just dreaming?

class. He expresses fear that the hand sanitizer dispenser on your desk is recording the conversation.

This child is presenting with psychosis. He has age appropriate vital signs. His symptoms of anxiety, social withdrawal, poor personal hygiene, and both visual and auditory hallucinations are suggestive of early onset schizophrenia (i.e. onset before 18 years old). Onset in males is typically earlier than females. This is a complex psychiatric diagnosis and requires specialty evaluation by a psychiatrist and will require a multidisciplinary team to manage his symptoms [13].

Altered mental status can be a challenging symptom to evaluate, particularly outside of the hospital environment. During the initial evaluation, keep in mind that delirium and psychosis can both present with altered mental status. An extensive work up including laboratory studies and imaging is often necessary in order to complete a thorough evaluation for the underlying etiology of a change in mental status (Fig. 24.1).

Extra Credit Points

1. Start the evaluation for altered mental status using the AVPU, ABCDE, and SAMPLE mnemonics, as well as a full set of vital signs and measuring a point of care glucose.
2. Differentiating between delirium (typically caused by a medical condition) and psychosis (typically caused by a psychiatric condition) can help guide the evaluation and differential diagnosis. Vital signs, level of consciousness, and the presence and type of hallucinations can be helpful initial clues.
3. Assessment for the underlying cause of altered mental status (refer to AEIOU-TIPS and DELIRIOUS mnemonics for differential diagnosis) often requires evaluation in the emergency department and a thorough work up including labs and imaging studies.

References

1. Henry K. Altered mental status. Society for Academic Emergency Medicine. https://www.saem.org/about-saem/academies-interest-groups-affiliates2/cdem/for-students/online-education/peds-em-curriculum/approach-to/altered-mental-status. Accessed 4 Jun 2024.
2. Huang J. Delirium. Merck Manual Professional Edition. Feb 2023. https://www.merckmanuals.com/professional/neurologic-disorders/delirium-and-dementia/delirium. Accessed 24 Jul 2024.
3. Mandeville K, Chien M, Willyerd FA, et al. Intussusception: clinical presentations and imaging characteristics. Pediatr Emerg Care. 2012;28(9):842–4. https://doi.org/10.1097/PEC.0b013e318267a75e.
4. Ramachandran P. Intussusception. In: Puri P, Höllwarth M, editors. Pediatric surgery. Berlin: Springer; 2009. p. 485–90.
5. Lord K, De Leon-Crutchlow D. Approach to hypoglycemia in infants and children. UpToDate. https://www.uptodate.com/contents/approach-to-hypoglycemia-in-infants-and-children?search=hypoglycemia&source=search_result&selectedTitle=2~150&usage_type=default&display_rank=2#H2724462568. Accessed 4 Jun 2024.
6. Schrier Vergano S. Inborn errors of metabolism: becoming ready for rare. Pediatr Rev. 2022;43(7):371–83. https://doi.org/10.1542/pir.2022-005088.
7. Pollart SM, Compton RM, Elward KS. Management of acute asthma exacerbations. Am Fam Physician. 2011;84(1):40–7.
8. Knight J, Decker L. Decerebrate and decorticate posturing. In: StatPearls [Internet]. Treasure Island (FL): StatPearls Publishing; 2024.
9. Dinallo S, Waseem M. Cushing reflex. In: StatPearls [Internet]. Treasure Island (FL): StatPearls Publishing; 2024.
10. Miranda M, Nadel S. Pediatric sepsis: a summary of current definitions and management recommendations. Curr Pediatr Rep. 2023;11(2):29–39. https://doi.org/10.1007/s40124-023-00286-3.
11. Figurasin R, Lee VR, Maguire NJ. 3,4-Methylenedioxymethamphetamine (MDMA) toxicity. [Updated 2024 Jan 17]. In: StatPearls [Internet]. Treasure Island (FL): StatPearls Publishing; 2024. https://www.ncbi.nlm.nih.gov/books/NBK538482/.
12. Kravets I. Hyperthyroidism: diagnosis and treatment. Am Fam Physician. 2016;93(5):363–70. https://www.aafp.org/pubs/afp/issues/2016/0301/p363.html.
13. Grover S, Avasthi A. Clinical practice guidelines for the management of schizophrenia in children and adolescents. Indian J Psychiatry. 2019;61(Suppl 2):277–93. https://doi.org/10.4103/psychiatry.IndianJPsychiatry_556_18.

Chapter 25
Ingestions, Exposures, and Overdoses

Danae Massengill and Laurie Seidel Halmo

Case 1 **Alex is a 12-year-old female who is brought to the school nurse after her friends received a text message where she stated she wanted to end her life. She appears tearful and refuses to disclose what medications she took. Her vitals are notable for a heart rate (HR) 115 beats per minute, respiratory rate (RR) 30, and blood pressure (BP) of 119/78. How would you approach this patient?**

Case 2 **Caleb is a 5-year-old male who is found near a closet where cleaning supplies are kept, sitting next to an open bottle of bleach. He is taken to the nurse's office where you notice that his shirt appears damp, but he is well-appearing and smiling. His vitals are age appropriate with a HR 110 beats per minute, RR 22, BP 95/55, and an oxygen saturation of 98% on room air. He does not exhibit any oral erythema, vomiting, drooling or difficulty breathing. How would you approach this patient?**

For the past decade, poison control centers have consistently received >2,000,000 calls annually regarding reported human exposures with pediatric cases representing >50% of those calls. Within the pediatric population specifically, there is a bimodal distribution with peaks in exposures occurring in children <6 years old and adolescents >12 years old [1]. The majority of reported exposures occur at a residence (either the child's own or another's), but exposures also occur at schools, in public spaces, and in other locations [1]. Because not all exposures are immediately

D. Massengill (✉)
Rocky Mountain Poison and Drug Safety, Denver Health and Hospital Authority, Denver, CO, USA
e-mail: danae.massengill@rmpds.org

L. S. Halmo
University of Colorado School of Medicine, Aurora, CO, USA
e-mail: Laurie.Halmo@childrenscolorado.org

R. P. Olympia, J. Brady-Olympia (eds.), *Clinical Considerations in School-based Health*, https://doi.org/10.1007/978-3-031-85765-2_25

clinically apparent, many exposures that occurred in the child's home become clinically apparent later, during the school day. Thus, recognition of presentation, identification of intent, and proper triage in school-based settings is imperative.

Among pediatric exploratory ingestions, the most commonly reported exposures are household cleaning substances, analgesics, cosmetics/personal care products, dietary supplements, and foreign bodies. While most of these accidental ingestions are generally lower-risk, there are certain higher-risk exposures to recognize [2, 3] (Table 25.1).

Among adolescent ingestions, the most commonly reported exposures in suicidal ingestions are analgesics, antidepressants, atypical antipsychotics, and antihistamines [4]. Of the pharmaceutical agents implicated in adolescent fatalities, the most common are analgesics, antidepressants, stimulants and street drugs (Table 25.2), antihistamines and cardiovascular drugs [1, 5]. Notably, many of these medications are readily available over-the-counter (e.g., analgesics) or are prescribed to the adolescent directly (e.g., antidepressants).

With regards to expected outcomes, pediatric exploratory ingestions often have a lower morbidity and mortality when compared to intentional ingestions where

Table 25.1 Pediatric exploratory ingestions[a]

Higher-risk exposures	Generally lower-risk exposures[b]
Prescription or illicit xenobiotics (i.e., opioids, sedative-hypnotics, antidiabetic agents, cardiovascular agents)	Hand soaps and lotions
Ethanol	Crayons, plain drawing chalk
Liquid nicotine products (typically intended for use in electronic cigarettes/vape devices)	Graphite pencils, ballpoint pen ink
Magnets, if >1 ingested	Hand sanitizer, perfume, deodorants, mouthwash[c]
Oil of wintergreen	
Button batteries	Candles
Camphor oils	Modeling dough compound[d]
Hydrocarbons (often found in fuels, some cleaning products)	Watercolor paints
High concentration hydrogen peroxide (>10%)	Putty, slime, kinetic sand
Caustic substances (often found in cleaners, detergents)	Glue
Expanding polymer compounds (i.e., water beads)	Glitter
Foreign body with potential for airway compromise	Clay
	Sunscreen[e]
	Toothpaste
	Lip balm
	Silica packets

[a] Not a comprehensive list

[b] Many of these can become higher-risk exposures if large quantities are ingested, such as in an intentional exposure. Certain products in these categories may also be higher-risk, even in small-volume exploratory exposures. As such, all exposures should prompt a call to the poison control center for specific guidance

[c] Some products may contain ethanol

[d] Some compounds contain large concentrations of table salt, which if ingested can lead to toxicity

[e] Some products may contain salicylates

Table 25.2 Common and emerging substances of abuse

Substance	Clinical effects
Ethanol	Sedative-hypnotic toxidrome
Stimulants (i.e., methamphetamine, prescription amphetamines, cocaine)	Sympathomimetic toxidrome
Synthetic cathinones ("bath salts"), prescribed cathinones such as bupropion	Sympathomimetic-like toxidrome
Kratom	Opioid and stimulant-like effects
Opioids and synthetic opioids (i.e. oxycodone, illicitly manufactured fentanyl, nitazenes)	Opioid toxidrome
Tianeptine	Euphoria, opioid-like effects
Xylazine	Sedative-hypnotic toxidrome; sometimes mixed with opioids producing an overlapping toxidrome
Benzodiazepines and synthetic benzodiazepines (i.e., etizolam, flubromazolam)	Sedative-hypnotic toxidrome
Cannabinoids and synthetic cannabinoids (i.e., K2, spice)	Euphoria, anxiety, paranoia, confusion
Hallucinogens (i.e, MDMA, ketamine, LSD, NBOMe, psilocybin)	Hallucinations, anxiety, paranoia, potential for serotonin syndrome
Over the counter cough and cold products (particularly containing dextromethorphan and/or diphenhydramine)	Euphoria, hallucinations, agitation, confusion

Table 25.3 "MVPs" ingestion assessment mnemonic

	Assessment/physical exam findings
Mental status	Depressed, delirium, agitation, normal
Vital signs	HR, RR, BP, temperature
Pupils	Miosis, mydriasis, normal
Skin	Flushed, diaphoretic, dry

recreational use (to get "high"), self-harm or suicide are the objective [2]. As such, triage often reflects age, overall intent, substance ingested (if known) and hemodynamic assessment.

The approach to the poisoned patient can be challenging as oftentimes the exposure is unknown. Recognizing common ingestion trends, physical exam findings utilizing the "MVPs" mnemonic (Table 25.3), toxidromes (Table 25.4), and historical clues can be helpful in identifying/narrowing the differential diagnosis. It is important to understand that many patients present with only a partial toxidrome or without a toxidrome at all, and some exposures can be asymptomatic initially despite the potential for significant harm (Table 25.5). While an in-depth review of substances of abuse is beyond the scope of this chapter, being aware of emerging substance use trends and associated clinical presentations can also be of clinical importance when approaching an intoxicated patient [5] (Table 25.2). Lastly, speaking to specially trained medical professionals through your local Poison Control Center is a readily available, free resource that should be utilized with any exposure

Table 25.4 Common toxidromes

Toxidrome	Exposure examples	Vitals	Physical exam findings	Pre-hospital intervention/disposition[a]
Anticholinergic	Diphenhydramine, atropine, scopolamine, jimson weed	HR: ↑ RR: –/↑ BP: –/↑ Temp: –/↑	Mental status: Delirium, agitation Pupils: Mydriasis Skin: Dry Other(s): Flushed skin, urinary retention ("red as a beet, dry as a bone, blind as a bat, mad as a hatter, hot as a hare, full as a flask" mnemonic)	Emergency Department
Cholinergic	Organophosphates (found in some pesticides)	HR: –/↓ RR: –/↓ BP: –/↓ Temp: –	Mental status: Normal to depressed Pupils: Miosis Skin: Diaphoresis Other(s): Diarrhea, urination, bradycardia, bronchorrhea, emesis, lacrimation, lethargy, salivation (DUMBBELLS mnemonic)	Emergency Department
Nicotine	Cigarettes, nicotine-containing e-cigarette refills, nicotine patches, nicotine gum, hookah	HR: ↑ RR: –/↑ BP: ↑ Temp: –	Mental status: Anxiety, agitation Pupils: Miosis Skin: Diaphoresis Other(s): Nausea, vomiting, pallor, diarrhea, salivation Late presentation (>30 min—4 h) can present with apnea, bradycardia, hypotension and weakness	Emergency Department

(continued)

Table 25.4 (continued)

Toxidrome	Exposure examples	Vitals	Physical exam findings	Pre-hospital intervention/ disposition[a]
Sympatho-mimetic	Cocaine, stimulant medications (e.g., methylphenidate), caffeine	HR: ↑ RR: ↑ BP: ↑ Temp: –/↑	Mental status: Agitation Pupils: Mydriasis Skin: Diaphoresis	Emergency Department
Opioid	Fentanyl, oxycodone, methadone	HR: ↓ RR: ↓ BP: ↓ Temp: –/↓	Mental status: Depressed Pupils: Miosis Skin: –	Administration of naloxone for respiratory depression and transfer to Emergency Department; see Chap. 67 for a more in-depth review of opioid toxicity
Sedative-hypnotic	Benzodiazepines, ethanol	HR: –/↓ RR: –/↓ BP: –/↓ Temp: –	Mental status: Depressed Pupils: –/miosis Skin: –	Emergency Department
Serotonin syndrome	SSRI, SNRI, monoamine oxidase inhibitors	HR: ↑ RR:—/↑ BP: ↑ Temp: –/↑	Mental status: Agitation Pupils: Mydriasis or no change Skin: Diaphoresis Other(s): Tremulous, clonus, hyperreflexia	Emergency Department

Key: ↑ = increase, ↓ = decrease, – = no change
[a]Poison Control should be called with all ingestions, available 24/7 at 1-800-222-1222

to assist with risk assessment and triage (available 24 h a day, 7 days a week via phone (1-800-222-1222)).

In summary, patients with low-risk exploratory ingestions who are asymptomatic and well appearing with age-appropriate vitals can often be medically cleared to return to school. Those with a high-risk exploratory or recreational ingestion, any symptoms, vital sign abnormalities, or any ingestion with a self-harm or suicidal intent (even if asymptomatic) should be referred to the emergency department for a full assessment.

Table 25.5 Common ingestions/exposures without a toxidrome

Exposure	Exposure examples	Notable features/ physical exam findings	Intervention/disposition[a]
Analgesics	Acetaminophen, ibuprofen, naproxen, aspirin	Nausea, vomiting, tachypnea, but often can be asymptomatic early in course	Emergency Department
Neuropsychiatric medications	Antiepileptics, antipsychotics	Nausea, vomiting, CNS alterations	Emergency Department
Iron	Ferrous sulfate, prenatal vitamins	Nausea, vomiting, diarrhea	Emergency Department if symptomatic, or known ingestion >20 mg/kg elemental iron[b]
Carbon monoxide	Car exhaust, gas powered space heaters, camp stoves, generators	Non-specific symptoms, often mimics flu-like illness	Emergency Department if symptomatic
Hydrocarbons	Chemical solvents, camphor oil, gasoline, kerosene	Chemical pneumonitis (can be delayed), CNS alterations	Emergency Department for evaluation and chest x-ray
Caustics	Bleach, sodium hydroxide or potassium hydroxide (lye)	Oral burns, drooling, dysphagia, stridor, abdominal pain, and/or vomiting	Emergency Department for large volume dilute bleach ingestions (>40 mL or 5 mL/kg), any high concentration bleach product (>6% hypochlorite), or if symptomatic regardless of amount/concentration ingested. Small volumes of dilute bleach ingestions can return to school if asymptomatic.
FRIONs, coolants	Malfunctioning heating/cooling systems	–	Return to school if asymptomatic
Methanol, ethylene glycol, diethylene glycol	Antifreeze, chafing fluid, windshield wiper fluid	Nausea, vomiting, CNS alterations, anion gap metabolic acidosis	Emergency Department
Methemoglobin inducers	Sodium nitrate/ nitrite, amyl nitrite ("poppers")	Cyanosis that doesn't respond to supplemental oxygen	Emergency Department

(continued)

Table 25.5 (continued)

Exposure	Exposure examples	Notable features/ physical exam findings	Intervention/disposition[a]
Accidental double dose medication	–		Emergency Department if symptomatic or higher risk medication, such as insulin, sulfonylureas, cardiovascular medications or bupropion [6]
Foreign body	Coin, nail, button battery, rock, magnet, expanding polymer compounds (e.g., water beads)	Often times asymptomatic early in course	Emergency Department if symptomatic, or for any ingested sharp object, button battery, or multiple magnets. Ingestions of expanding polymer compounds or their insertion into ears or nose should also be seen in the Emergency Department

[a] Poison Control should be called with all ingestions, available 24/7 at 1-800-222-1222
[b] Iron preparations are typically labelled with a total dose and an elemental iron dose (e.g., Ferrous sulfate 325 mg, elemental iron 65 mg)

25.1 Case Resolutions

Case 1 Alex is transferred to the local emergency due to both her vital sign abnormalities and suicide attempt. She subsequently becomes more agitated and her labs are notable for a 4-h acetaminophen concentration of 185 μg/mL. She is admitted to the hospital where she requires benzodiazepines for agitation and n-acetylcysteine for a toxic acetaminophen concentration. Following clinical improvement, she discloses that she drank a bottle of an over-the-counter cough and cold combination product containing acetaminophen, diphenhydramine, doxylamine and dextromethorphan in an attempt to die by suicide. Following medical clearance, she is transferred to inpatient psychiatry for ongoing mental health support and care coordination.

Case 2 Caleb remains in the nurse's office while you gather more information requested from the Poison Control Center about his ingestion. You identify that Caleb was found sitting next to a bleach bottle that contains <6% sodium hypochlorite (a dilute, household bleach solution). Poison Control informs you that the evidence suggests children who have accidentally ingested small amounts of household bleach and are asymptomatic do not require medical assessment [7]. Thus, Caleb does not need to go to the emergency department and can return to school.

Extra Credit Points

1. Pediatric ingestions are a significant cause of morbidity and mortality that tend to occur in a bimodal distribution among children <6 years old and adolescents >12 years old

2. Oftentimes the specific agent(s) ingested are unknown, a patient's exam does not fit a classic toxidrome, or the patient is initially asymptomatic; however, these features do not imply safety nor a lack of concern. Many of these patients will still require emergency department evaluation
3. Any patient with symptoms, high-risk ingestion/exposure, and/or suicide attempt (even if asymptomatic) should be referred to the local emergency department
4. The Poison Control Center is a free resource available 24/7 via phone (1-800-222-1222) that should be called with any ingestion, exposure, or overdose concern

References

1. Gummin DD, Mowry JB, Beuhler MC, et al. 2022 Annual report of the National Poison Data System® (NPDS) from America's Poison Centers®: 40th annual report. Clin Toxicol (Phila). 2023;61(10):717–939. https://doi.org/10.1080/15563650.2023.2268981.
2. Sheridan DC, Hughes A, Horowitz BZ. Pediatric ingestions: new high-risk household hazards. Pediatr Rev. 2021;42(1):2–10. https://doi.org/10.1542/pir.2019-0309.
3. Olson K, Wu A, Blanc P, et al. Poisoning and drug overdose. 8th ed. McGraw-Hill Education/Medical; 2022.
4. Sheridan DC, Hendrickson RG, Lin AL, Fu R, Horowitz BZ. Adolescent suicidal ingestion: national trends over a decade. J Adolesc Health. 2017;60(2):191–5. https://doi.org/10.1016/j.jadohealth.2016.09.012.
5. Drug Enforcement Administration, U.S. Department of Justice. Drugs of abuse: a DEA resource guide. DEA.gov. Published Dec 2022. https://www.dea.gov/sites/default/files/2022-12/2022_DOA_eBook_File_Final.pdf. Accessed 13 May 2024.
6. Correia MS, Whitehead E, Cantrell FL, Lasoff DR, Minns AB. A 10-year review of single medication double-dose ingestions in the nation's largest poison control system. Clin Toxicol (Phila). 2019;57(1):31–5. https://doi.org/10.1080/15563650.2018.1493205.
7. Slaughter RJ, Watts M, Vale JA, Grieve JR, Schep LJ. The clinical toxicology of sodium hypochlorite. Clin Toxicol (Phila). 2019;57(5):303–11. https://doi.org/10.1080/15563650.2018.1543889.

Chapter 26
Cough and Shortness of Breath

Timothy P. Roach and Amy A. Dooley

Case 1 **An 11 year old female comes to your office for issues with difficulty breathing, cough, and fever. She says she has felt this way for several days, however today is the worst. She is fatigued, pale, and uncomfortable in appearance. Her heart rate is 140, respiratory rate is 40, and her blood pressure is 116/78. She has a fever of 102.4 °F. Her work of breathing is increased, crackles are auscultated on exam, and her mucus membranes appear dry.**

Case 2 **An 8 year old male was sent to your office by the teacher for frequent, loud barky cough that is interrupting class. You recognize him as a student that has visited you twice over the last 3 days for congestion and cough though he otherwise appeared well. He complains of sore throat. His heart rate is 120, respiratory rate is 24, and blood pressure is 106/70. He is afebrile.**

Case 3 **A 6 year old male comes to your office with new, sudden onset of cough shortly after the end of indoor recess. The aid was concerned about the child after seeing several children playing with a toy containing several small pieces and running around the classroom, noting he had trouble catching his breath. His heart rate is 130, respiratory rate of 36, and blood pressure 96/72. He is afebrile. In the office he has a recurring cough, appears uncomfortable, and complains of chest pain.**

Cough is one of the most common pediatric complaints and has a myriad of causes, many of which are benign, though some can be life-threatening if not

T. P. Roach
Penn State Milton S. Hershey Medical Center, Hershey, PA, USA
e-mail: troach@pennstatehealth.psu.edu

A. A. Dooley (✉)
Penn State Children's Hospital, Hershey, PA, USA
e-mail: adooley@pennstatehealth.psu.edu

R. P. Olympia, J. Brady-Olympia (eds.), *Clinical Considerations in School-based Health*, https://doi.org/10.1007/978-3-031-85765-2_26

assessed and treated quickly. Some of the more common causes, basic treatment, and disposition are listed in Table 26.1.

Cough may also be a common exacerbating symptom of several chronic medical conditions, such as asthma, chronic lung disease, congenital heart disease, impaired airway clearance, bronchiectasis, or cystic fibrosis. Primary assessment, and evaluation of the child's work of breathing and oxygen saturation, if available, are paramount for correct triage to appropriate resources. Initial assessment, including respiratory examination and vital signs, is discussed in Chap. 23. Fever and anxiety, when present, often contribute to not only vital sign changes such as tachycardia and tachypnea, but increased work of breathing as well.

Elucidating a relevant history when appropriate can help decide appropriate treatment as well. Common examples would be food allergies, anaphylaxis, and atopic dermatitis. Children complaining of cough, chest discomfort, respiratory distress, or wheezing with an underlying a diagnosis of asthma should have rescue medication, such as albuterol, administered. When available, hypoxemic children

Table 26.1 "PAROXYSMS" mnemonic for cough in school age children, signs/symptoms, treatment, disposition

	Examples	Treatment	Disposition
P: Pneumonia/ pertussis	Bacterial, viral infection	Antibiotic therapy, symptomatic care	PCP, urgent care, ED depending on severity
A: Airway obstruction	Croup, anaphylaxis	Corticosteroids, racemic epinephrine, IM epinephrine	Urgent care or ED based on croup severity, ED for anaphylaxis
R: Reactive airway disease	Asthma exacerbation	Albuterol, systemic corticosteroids	PCP, urgent care, ED depending on severity
O: Objects	Coins, toys	Position of comfort, supplemental oxygen, avoidance of irritating/ invasive procedures when able	ED
X: refluX	Irritation from stomach acid reflux	Antacid, histamine-2 receptor blocker, proton pump inhibitor	PCP
Y: Yrritants (irritants)	Smoking, vaping, noxious fumes/ gases	Supplemental oxygen	Urgent care, ED
S: Sinusitis	Viral, bacterial	Symptomatic, antibiotic for bacterial etiology	PCP
M: Mental	Psychogenic	Behavior modification	PCP
S: Seizure/motor tics	Vocal cord dysfunction, focal epilepsy	Speech therapy for VCD, anti-epileptic drug therapy for epilepsy	PCP

ED Emergency Department, *IM* intramuscular, *PCP* Primary Care Physician, *VCD* Vocal cord dysfunction

should have supplemental oxygen applied quickly. Children should also be allowed to maintain a position of comfort when permissible, as this is often their way of using accessory muscles to aid their work of breathing. Presence of mucus and presence of color is poorly correlated with underlying cause. Relatively invasive and irritating procedures such as oral/ear temperature measurements, blood pressure measurements, ear/mouth exams should be weighed against their benefit in evaluation.

A thorough respiratory examination often helps triage treatment and gauge effectiveness of interventions. With severe signs of respiratory distress, such as severe tachypnea, air hunger, tripoding, choking, or cyanosis, prompt emergency response via Emergency Medical Services (EMS) is warranted [1]. Prompt recognition of the child's inability to oxygenate or ventilate (exhale CO_2) is life-saving. Absence of severe signs of distress should lead the school staff to differentiate concerning upper airway from lower airway signs, as well as symptoms consistent with an acute versus chronic cause. Cyanosis, particularly when centrally located, is a late sign of respiratory distress and EMS response is indicated [1]. These children are often referred for ancillary testing as indicated, such as imaging and lab evaluation.

Contributing history, such as current medication use, often helps with triage of appropriate intervention. If the child admits to several days of antibiotic use or frequent rescue doses of albuterol, appropriate support can often be rendered. Blood-tinged sputum, or hemoptysis, is often a sign of lower respiratory tract involvement and can often present with pneumonia, bronchitis, or foreign-body aspiration [2]. Signs of shortness of breath due to upper airway obstruction or disease include hoarseness, stridor, barking cough, or preference for the "sniffing position" (neck flexion with head extension) [2]. Paroxysms of cough, and audible "whoop" can signify pertussis (whooping cough). Signs of lower airway pathology include retractions, prolonged expiratory phase of respiration, grunting, rhonchi, and wheezing or rales (crackles) by auscultation [3]. Several common respiratory exam findings are described in detail in Table 26.2. Frequent nighttime cough without other signs and symptoms of illness is commonly due to untreated/undertreated asthma. It is

Table 26.2 Common respiratory exam findings

Stridor	Continuous, high-pitched sound classically on inspiration and is caused by narrowing of the upper airway or trachea (ex: croup)
Crackles (rales)	Inconsistent, "popping" open of smaller airways or alveoli by auscultation from air entry as a result of displacement of pathologic fluid on inspiration; present in conditions such as pneumonia or that cause pulmonary edema
Rhonchi	Continuous, "bubbling" during inspiration and expiration and represent movement of fluid in the larger airways commonly found in URIs, or mild asthma exacerbations. May improve with cough, unlike other airway pathologic sounds on auscultation
Wheezing	Continuous, caused by vibration and movement of air through narrowed smaller airways heard on auscultation (ex: asthma)
Grunting	Consistent, expiratory sound of exhalation against a partially closed glottis, indicating lower airway disease

Adapted from Kliegman et al. [3]

important to note that cough commonly persists for several weeks after treatment depending on the underlying cause, such as bacterial/viral pneumonia or viral upper respiratory infections or acute asthma exacerbations.

Frequent clinical reassessments, as well as changes in the respiratory examination, can also help determine the need for further treatment. Further decline in respiratory status, such as in the presence of depressed mental status, is a sign of impending respiratory failure [4]. Likewise, should work of breathing resolve with treatment, such as resolution of wheezing and tachypnea with albuterol in a child known to have asthma, return to class and activity may be appropriate. Mild cough symptoms and associated discomfort can often be treated with over-the-counter cough medications or lozenges, though with variable results and use should be cautioned in younger children due to concerns for ineffectiveness or aspiration respectively.

26.1 Case Resolution

Case 1 This 11 year old child should be triaged to an immediate response, with 911 being the most appropriate due to significant respiratory distress and dehydration. She was evaluated and treated for bacterial pneumonia, which is consistent with her fever, tachypnea, increased work of breathing, and abnormal breath sounds. Treatment of her fever and respiratory support as able are appropriate until EMS arrival.

Case 2 Signs and symptoms of this 8 year old are most consistent with croup. He exhibits no respiratory distress. You treat his sore throat with an oral pain reliever such as acetaminophen, which also helps the cough, and notify his parents about the possibility of this illness, recommending follow-up with their primary care physician.

Case 3 This 6 year old child, with sudden onset respiratory distress and cough, most likely aspirated a foreign body. EMS should be notified and evaluation sought at the nearest hospital. This patient should be kept in a position of comfort and monitored continuously until EMS arrives. Multiple chest radiograph views (especially the use of bilateral lateral decubitus imaging to reveal “ball valving” for foreign bodies that completely occlude and right or left mainstem bronchus) can help elucidate location and cause.

Extra Credit Points

1. The causes of cough and shortness of breath (“PAROXYSMS” mnemonic) are varied and can be dependent on age and situation. History plays a significant role in ascertaining the underlying cause and degree of treatment needed.
2. Patients with underlying medical conditions, such as asthma, should have a low-threshold for obtaining treatment in the office, such as their rescue inhalers. In

patients with severe distress, treatment should not be withheld pending EMS or parent arrival.
3. Clinical appearance of the child, as well as presence of fever and severe symptoms, is perhaps the largest factor in determining necessary initial treatment and vital in appropriate triage.
4. Some signs and symptoms associated with cough and shortness of breathing requiring emergent evaluation in an emergency department include:

   - altered mental status
   - signs of severe respiratory distress—grunting, head bobbing, intercostal retractions, abdominal breathing
   - central cyanosis
   - stridor
   - tripoding
   - anaphylaxis
   - severe dehydration
   - unable to speak in complete sentences due to respiratory effort

References

1. Bachur RG, Shaw KN. In: Chamberlain J, Lavelle J, Nagler J, Shook JE, editors. Fleisher & Ludwig's textbook of pediatric emergency medicine. 8th ed. Wolters Kluwer Health; 2020.
2. Hoffman RJ, Wang VJ, Scarfone R, Godambe S, Nagler J. Fleisher & Ludwig's 5-minute pediatric emergency medicine consult. Lippincott Williams & Wilkins; 2019.
3. Kliegman RM, Toth H, Bordini BJ, Basel D, editors. Nelson pediatric symptom-based diagnosis: common diseases and their mimics. 2nd ed. Elsevier—Health Sciences Division; 2022.
4. Brown CA, Sakles JC, Mick NW, editors. The Walls manual of emergency airway management. 5th ed. Lippincott Williams and Wilkins; 2017.

Chapter 27
Vomiting, Diarrhea, and Dehydration

Connor Murray and Thuy Ngo

Case 1 **On a hot summer day in the first week back to school in August, 12-year-old Deb comes to your office at the direction of the PE teacher after she asked to sit out during the timed mile run during fitness assessment testing. She shares that during the third lap around the track she began feeling dizzy, thirsty, hot, and overall unwell. She was pulled to the side and allowed to sit in the shade where she began to drink a bottle of water. On arrival to your office, she looks overall well. You note perspiration on face and shirt, and slight facial flushing of her cheeks. Her vital signs are temperature 99.6, heart rate 100 beats per minute, respiratory rate 22 breaths per minute, blood pressure 110/80. Her capillary refill time of 2 s. The remainder of her exam is without concern.**

Case 2 **Eight-year-old Sean is sent to your office after complaining of nausea and generalized abdominal discomfort. At first glance, he appears mildly uncomfortable, with facial pallor, holding his belly. He reports an episode of emesis on the way from class to nurse office and has a second episode of emesis shortly after arrival. You observe non-bloody, non-bilious, and non-projectile emesis that is clear/yellow tinged in color. His vitals are temperature 100.9, heart rate 105 beats per minute, respiratory rate 20 breaths per minute, blood pressure 100/70, and capillary refill between 2–3 s. His exam is significant for tactile warmth, but he is nontender to palpation of his abdomen and remainder of exam is normal. Following the exam, he rushes to use the restroom and reports loose, watery, brown stool.**

C. Murray (✉) · T. Ngo
Johns Hopkins All Children's Hospital, St. Petersburg, FL, USA
e-mail: connor.murray@jhmi.edu; thuy.ngo@jhmi.edu

R. P. Olympia, J. Brady-Olympia (eds.), *Clinical Considerations in School-based Health*, https://doi.org/10.1007/978-3-031-85765-2_27

Case 3 Fourteen-year-old Jasper arrives in your office shortly after lunch period. He reports warmth, loss of appetite, nausea, lower abdominal pain, and one episode of emesis prior to arrival. Immediately you notice he appears somewhat uncomfortable and grimaces as he sits down in the chair. He informs you that he ate only a small dinner last night and this morning he struggled to eat a few bites of banana and sips of orange juice due to stomachache. Throughout the morning, he became increasingly uncomfortable and warm. His stomach pain continued to progress, stating it has become sharper and has increased intensity. He points to his belly button when asked to localize where the pain is most intense. He reports he has had no interest in food or drink since this morning and was unable to even look at food in the cafeteria during lunch. His vitals are as follows: temperature 101.3, heart rate 117 beats per minute, respiratory rate 19 breaths per minute, blood pressure 105/80, and capillary refill between 2–3 s. He appears uncomfortable when going from seated to laying position for the exam. He also demonstrates significant tenderness on palpation of the lower abdomen.

Pause for a moment, consider the following for each of the above scenarios:

- What are the initial steps in the evaluation of these patients?
- Are any of these children dehydrated, if so to what degree?
- What are the common causes of these presenting symptoms?
- Do any of these children exhibit symptoms that necessitate urgent/emergent medical attention?
- Could any of these patients potentially remain at school? If not, when might they be eligible to return?

Vomiting and diarrhea are common symptoms in a myriad of pediatric illnesses. Both can lead to and/or worsen dehydration. Globally, diarrheal illness still accounts for a sizable proportion of pediatric mortality. In resource abundant countries, especially since the adoption of rotavirus vaccines into routine immunization schedule and attention to the sanitation of and access to safe drinking water, the mortality has significant improved. Despite this, morbidity and the burden of illness remains significant [1, 2].

The evaluation of pediatric patients with concerns of vomiting, diarrhea, or dehydration should initially begin with the pediatric assessment triangle, utilization of the ABCDE approach (Airway, Breathing, Circulation, Disability, Exposure), obtaining and interpretation of vital signs, and implementation of the SAMPLE mnemonic (Signs & symptoms, Allergies, Medications, Past Medical History, and Events). Because diarrhea and vomiting are common symptoms of pediatric illness, it is especially important to investigate potential causes, and rule out conditions that would require emergent medical attention or preclude them from the educational setting.

27.1 Dehydration [3–5]

In a 2015 study from the Harvard T.H. Chan School of Public Health, researchers found the prevalence of inadequate hydration in more than half (54%) of the 4000+ children aged 6–16 studied as determined by increased urine osmolality. Assessment of the patient's fluid status is important to determine presence/degree of dehydration. Dehydration occurs when there is an imbalance between fluid intake and fluid losses causing the body to be at a fluid deficit. During illness, fluid needs will be higher as diarrhea and vomiting increase fluid losses, while fever and tachypnea when present will also increase insensible fluid loss.

Review the signs and symptoms of dehydration (Table 27.1). It is more important to consider the whole patient and utilize multiple exam findings to make your assessment rather than a single finding alone—as some measures like urine output are less sensitive than others, especially in isolation. Please note using a central capillary refill (chest or abdomen) is more reliable than peripheral refill (fingers, toes, hands), especially in students with fever, dehydration.

Initiate oral rehydration with water or low osmolarity solutions including unsweetened coconut water, broths/soups, or oral rehydration solutions, which are commercially available in premixed formulations (i.e. Pedialyte, Gastrolyte). Low osmolarity solutions have a slight benefit over water alone as the sodium content helps to facilitate extraintestinal absorption. It is best to avoid oral rehydration therapy with soda, sports drinks, or fruit juice as many contain too little sodium along with high concentrations of carbohydrates which may lead to or worsen electrolyte imbalance and diarrheal symptoms. Circling back to your ABCDE approach, does this patient have a compromised airway, difficulty breathing, or disability that would impair their ability to tolerate liquids by mouth? If not, oral hydration is a mainstay when treating dehydration. While no current literature endorses its use in school

Table 27.1 Signs of pediatric dehydration based on severity [6, 7]

	No dehydration	Some dehydration	Severe dehydration
Mental status	Alert	Normal, confused, foggy	Confused, altered
Activity level	Normal, active	Tired/irritable	Lethargic
Eyes	Normal	Sunken	Sunken, no tear production
Thirst	Drinks normally, thirsty	Thirsty, eager to drink	Drinks poorly or unable
Mouth	Normal, wet	Tacky	Dry
Skin pinch/turgor	Skin returns quickly	Skin returns slowly	Delayed tenting of skin (>2 s before return)
Heart rate	Normal for age	Normal/tachycardic	Tachycardia for age
Peripheral pulses	Normal, easily palpable	Weak	Faint, thready
Urine output	Normal	Normal/decreased	Decreased/oliguria
Capillary refill	<2 s	2–3 s	>3 s

settings at this time, ondansetron (Zofran) is an effective and commonly used anti-nausea medication prescribed by doctors in the clinic, urgent care, and hospital settings. As more research is done, this may become another tool for the school nurse to utilize.

27.2 Etiology of Vomiting and Diarrhea in Children and Adolescents [8, 9]

Vomiting and diarrhea are exceedingly common presenting symptoms of many pediatric conditions ranging from benign to life threatening, most commonly these symptoms are due to communicable disease, often viral in origin. Many infectious causes will present with a combination of fever, diarrhea, and vomiting. Despite common things being common, it is critically important to remain vigilant about other possible etiologies beyond infectious causes. Tables 27.2 and 27.3 demonstrate common causes of vomiting and diarrhea, respectively.

If a child presents with vomiting and/or diarrhea, contact the child's guardian. This child should be evaluated by a pediatric healthcare provider in an urgent care center or primary care provider's office prior to return to school, academic, or athletic activities. Children with red flags associated with vomiting or diarrhea should be evaluated in an emergency department (Table 27.4). Of note, bilious emesis is dark green in color and may indicate gastrointestinal obstruction.

Table 27.2 Common causes of vomiting by system in children

Neurologic
Seizure, migraine headache, abdominal migraine, meningitis
Infectious
Viral/bacterial gastroenteritis, parasitic infection
Respiratory
Pneumonia, sinusitis, pharyngitis
Endocrine
Diabetic ketoacidosis, adrenal insufficiency
Renal
Urinary tract infection, kidney stone
Gastrointestinal
Reflux, foreign body, constipation, appendicitis, inflammatory bowel disease, cholecystitis, gastroparesis
Miscellaneous
Anaphylaxis, allergy, toxic ingestion, pain, anxiety, medication side effect, trauma, eating disorder, pregnancy

Table 27.3 Common causes of diarrhea in children

Infectious causes	Non-infectious causes
Viral gastroenteritis—Most common	Dietary: Lactose intolerance, food allergy, excessive juice intake
Bacterial gastroenteritis	Anatomic abnormality: Intussusception, malrotation, Hirschsprung disease
Parasitic infections	Systemic disease: Inflammatory bowel disease
	Medication side effect
	Toxic ingestion
	Eating disorder
	Constipation

Table 27.4 Red flag symptoms with vomiting and dehydration

Vomiting	Diarrhea
Recent head trauma	Bloody diarrhea
Abdominal distension	Marked irritability
High fever	High fever
Bilious emesis (dark green emesis)	Refusal to eat or drink
Severe abdominal pain	Severe abdominal pain
Lethargy	Lethargy
Altered mental status	
Nuchal rigidity or photophobia	

27.3 Stop the Spread

If available, disposable gloves should be worn during the evaluation of patients with vomiting or diarrhea to limit contact with potentially infectious bodily discharge. Remember to wash hands before and after examining the patient. Hand hygiene should be performed with soap and water, be sure to follow proper technique and timing to ensure the safety of yourself, staff, and students.

27.4 Disposition and Return to School

Your school/institution may have established, documented criteria for which students cannot remain in the educational setting and what criteria the student must meet before returning (Table 27.5). Please use this resource as a guide and refer to your specific institutional guidelines for final determination of eligibility.

Table 27.5 Criteria to exclude a student from school and criteria for a student to return to school

	Criteria to exclude a student from school	Criteria to return to school
Vomiting [10, 11]	– Illness preventing participation in school activities – Staff concern for health and safety of other children in class – Vomiting and fever – Vomit that is green or bloody in appearance – Signs of dehydration – Meets other exclusion criteria as set by your institution	– If child is without fever or other symptoms and improvement is seen with short period of rest in an area that allows for privacy – With resolution of vomiting related acute illness – When child is again able to meaningfully participate in education activities – Vomiting is due to a known condition and has a care plan when it occurs
Diarrhea [12, 13]	– Loose/watery stool output more frequent than child's normal – Causing "accidents" in toilet trained children – Blood or mucus in an ill child's stool – Clinical signs of dehydration – Meets other exclusion criteria as set by your institution	– Resolution of blood or mucus if present in stool and cleared by qualified health professional – Frequency of bowel movements in no more than 2 stools above normal for that child – Following diarrhea outbreak: Seek guidance from local health department authorities – If illness due to bacterial infection, check state laws/regulations and institutional guidelines to determine need for negative stool cultures

27.5 Cases Conclusions

1. Deb presents with symptoms of mild dehydration that occurred in the setting of physical exertion but responded well to oral rehydration and rest, when she arrives to you, she is well appearing with a reassuring physical exam. She is tolerating oral hydration and symptom free. Her parents are updated, and she remains at school.
2. Sean presents with symptoms seen in infectious gastroenteritis. It would be most appropriate to exclude this child from the school setting as he has fever, diarrhea, vomiting, signs of dehydration, and his level of discomfort. He is taken home and returns after symptoms and fever subside.
3. Jasper presents to you and is the most acutely ill of the patients in this chapter. You evaluate Jasper after an episode of emesis and note fever, signs of dehydration, inability to tolerate oral hydration, and significant abdominal pain. You recognize red flag symptoms in a sick appearing patient and correctly determine exclusion from the school setting and urgent medical attention are required. He is treated for appendicitis during an inpatient hospital admission and returns to school after medical clearance.

Extra Credit Points

1. Be familiar with age-appropriate vitals and red flag symptoms signaling the need for further evaluation by their pediatrician, urgent care, or emergency department.
2. Limit infection spread by wearing gloves and practicing good hand hygiene.
3. Contact appropriate health authorities if a suspected outbreak/multiple patients presenting with similar symptoms.
4. Oral rehydration should be initiated in patients with suspected fluid status deficit who are at neurologic baseline, with intact airway.
5. Identify disposition and return to school criteria.

References

1. Cunningham RM, Walton MA, Carter PM. The major causes of death in children and adolescents in the United States. N Engl J Med. 2018;379(25):2468–75. https://doi.org/10.1056/NEJMsr1804754.
2. Diarrhoeal disease. World Health Organization. 7 Mar 2024. https://www.who.int/news-room/fact-sheets/detail/diarrhoeal-disease. Accessed 22 Mar 2024.
3. King CK, Glass R, Bresee JS, Duggan C. Managing acute gastroenteritis among children: oral rehydration, maintenance, and nutritional therapy. Centers for Disease Control and Prevention. 21 Nov 2003. https://www.cdc.gov/mmwr/preview/mmwrhtml/rr5216a1.htm. Accessed 3 Mar 2024.
4. Kenney EL, Long MW, Cradock AL, Gortmaker SL. Prevalence of inadequate hydration among US children and disparities by gender and race/ethnicity: National Health and Nutrition Examination Survey, 2009-2012. Am J Public Health. 2015;105(8):e113–8. https://doi.org/10.2105/AJPH.2015.302572.
5. Popkin BM, D'Anci KE, Rosenberg IH. Water, hydration, and health. Nutr Rev. 2010;68(8).439–58. https://doi.org/10.1111/j.1753-4887.2010.00304.x.
6. World Health Organization. The treatment of diarrhoea: a manual for physicians and other senior health workers, 4th rev. World Health Organization; 2005. https://iris.who.int/handle/10665/43209.
7. Vega RM, Avva U. Pediatric dehydration. [Updated 2023 Aug 13]. In: StatPearls [Internet]. Treasure Island (FL): StatPearls Publishing; 2024. https://www.ncbi.nlm.nih.gov/books/NBK436022/.
8. Kotloff KL, Kliegman RM, St. Geme JW III. Chapter 366. Acute gastroenteritis in children. In: Nelson textbook of pediatrics, vol. 2. 21st ed. Elsevier; 2019.
9. Cossey MG, Gambill LK. Pediatric hospital medicine: a case-based educational guide. American Academy of Pediatrics; 2022.
10. Shope T. Vomiting. Managing infectious disease in child care and schools. 6th ed. American Academy of Pediatrics; 2023. https://www-r2library-com.proxy1.library.jhu.edu/Resource/Title/1610026594/ch0006s0652.
11. Vomiting—child care and schools. Pediatric Patient Education 2023. https://doi.org/10.1542/ppe_document08.
12. Shope T. Diarrhea. Managing infectious disease in child care and schools. 6th ed. American Academy of Pediatrics; 2023. https://www-r2library-com.proxy1.library.jhu.edu/Resource/Title/1610026594/ch0006s0232.
13. Diarrhea—child care and schools. Pediatric Patient Education 2023. https://doi.org/10.1542/ppe_document047.

Chapter 28
Syncope

Alana Hughes Boone

Case 1 **You have been called to the choir room because Jamie, a 10-year-old student, has passed out. When you walk into the room she is sitting by the bleachers surrounded by her classmates. She is awake and alert, and is in no distress. After standing on a crowded bleacher for 45 min, she moved to walk off stage, she felt warm and then everything went black. She admitted to having a sense that she was going to pass out right before she lost consciousness. She denies any chest pain, shortness of breath, or palpitations prior to the event. Those around her noticed brief twitching of her arms and legs for a few seconds, and reported that she starting waking up approximately 1 min after passing out. Jamie is alert, her vital signs are within normal limits, and her physical examination is normal. Your glucometer shows a glucose of 108. On review of her medical chart, she has no significant past medical history. What should you do next?**

Case 2 **Timothy, a 6-year-old student has just passed out during a group lesson. His teacher recalls it as a precipitous fall to the ground, as he waited his turn to help read out loud. He hit his head on the soft carpet, but has no obvious injuries. His teacher does think he had a brief loss of consciousness without witnessed seizure activity. He woke up shortly after hitting his head, cried but was consolable.**

He has a history of an Atrial Septal Defect (ASD) that required surgical closure 3 years prior. He is not on any medications. His exam is unremarkable and he is back to baseline. Vital signs are significant for a heart rate of 102 beats per minute with regular rhythm, he is afebrile and his blood pressure is normal for age. You are considering your next steps with respect to evaluation.

A. H. Boone (✉)
Children's National Hospital, Richmond, VA, USA
e-mail: ahboone@childrensnational.org

R. P. Olympia, J. Brady-Olympia (eds.), *Clinical Considerations in School-based Health*, https://doi.org/10.1007/978-3-031-85765-2_28

Case 3 **Tiffany, an 11-year-old student, has just fainted in her classroom. It is at the end of the day and the students were preparing to be dismissed. She quickly stood up from her desk and immediately fell to the ground. She does not remember falling. Her classmates report no head injury. She appears well, face flushed, without fever and normal heart rate with regular rhythm. She is well enough to walk to the school nurse's office where she discloses that she has not had much to drink during the school day because she was worried about an examination that afternoon. She cannot recall the last time she voided since leaving home this morning. Her orthostatic vitals show a 22 mmHg drop in systolic blood pressure when moving from a lying to standing position. Her orthostatic heart rate response is normal. Tiffany is back to her baseline after drinking some water and wants to know if she can go home with her mother.**

Case 4 **You are walking by the cafeteria, and you spot a student that looks a little unsteady. Susie is a 16-year-old new student, and you have not had a chance to meet her yet. She was standing in line with a food tray, waiting her turn and fainted, falling onto the student behind her who caught her before she injured herself. You rush over and help her to the floor, continuing your assessment. She appears pale and anxious. She eventually is well enough to get up and ambulate to the school clinic. While there you review her health records and notice that she has a diagnosis of Postural Orthostatic Tachycardia (POTS). She explains that this is not the first time she has passed out, and has a history of symptoms that include palpitations and chronic weakness. She feels more tired than her baseline and you notice she does have a tremor in both her hands. Her blood pressure is normal, and her heart rate is 80 beats per minute with regular rhythm. She informs you that she has not had much to eat since the night prior. You obtain a point of care glucose, and her serum glucose is 50.**

Syncope (also known as "passing out" or "fainting") occurs across all ages. The incidence of syncope in children aged 2–18 years is approximately 20% [1]. Syncope is a symptom that presents with an abrupt, transient, complete loss of consciousness, associated with inability to maintain postural tone, with rapid and spontaneous recovery [2]. The chances of encountering this in a school setting is likely, and understanding how to quickly access and make plans for further care can vary depending on what caused the child to have a syncopal episode. The most identified type of syncope is vasovagal (21.2%), cardiac (9.5%) is second followed by orthostatic (9.4%); 36.6% fall into the category of unknown cause [3]. Unknown categories include metabolic, toxins and environmental causes. For both vasovagal and orthostatic syncope, reassurance and lifestyle changes are suggested such as improving hydration, getting adequate sleep, exercising regularly, and eating a well-balanced diet. This contrasts with cardiac causes of syncope which almost always needs follow up, and sometimes urgently. Distinguishing between the two is critical. Prior to evaluating a student presenting with syncope, a review of key terms and definitions helps when building a differential diagnosis (Table 28.1).

Table 28.1 Syncope terms and definitions

Term	Definition
Syncope	A symptom that presents with an abrupt, transient, complete loss of consciousness, associated with inability to maintain postural tone, with rapid and spontaneous recovery
Pre- syncope (near syncope)	The symptoms before syncope. These symptoms could include extreme lightheadedness; visual sensations, such as "tunnel vision" or "graying out"; and variable degrees of altered consciousness without complete loss of consciousness. Presyncope could progress to syncope, or it could abort without syncope
Vaso-vagal syncope (VVS)	The most common form of reflex syncope mediated by the vasovagal reflex. VVS (1) may occur with upright posture (standing or seated or with exposure to emotional stress, pain, or medical settings; (2) typically is characterized by diaphoresis, warmth, nausea, and pallor; (3) is associated with vasodepressor hypotension and or inappropriate bradycardia; and (4) is often followed by fatigue
Loss of consciousness	A cognitive state in which on lacks awareness of oneself and one's situation, with an inability to respond to stimuli
Transient loss of consciousness	Can be divided into syncope and non-syncope conditions. Nonsyncope conditions include but are not limited to seizures, hypoglycemia, metabolic conditions, drug or alcohol intoxication, and concussion due to head trauma. The underlying mechanism of syncope is presumed to be cerebral hypoperfusion, whereas nonsyncope conditions are attributed to different mechanisms
Orthostatic intolerance	A syndrome consisting of a constellation of symptoms that include frequent, recurrent, or persistent lightheadedness, palpitations, tremulousness, generalized weakness, blurred vision, exercise intolerance, and fatigue upon standing
Orthostatic hypotension (OH)	A drop in systolic BP of ≥20 mmHg or a diastolic BP of ≥10 mmHg with assumption of an upright position [2]
Postural orthostatic tachycardia syndrome (POTS)	A clinical syndrome usually characterized by the following (1) frequent symptoms that occur with standing (e.g., lightheadedness, palpitations, tremulousness, generalized weakness, blurred vision, exercise intolerance, and fatigue); and (2) an increase in heart rate of >/−30b beats per minute during positional change from supine to standing (or >/− 40 beats per minute in those 12–19 years of age); and (3) the absence of OH (>20 mmHg reduction in systolic blood pressure). Symptoms associated with POTS include those that occur with standing (i.e., lightheadedness, palpitations); those not associated with postures (e.g., bloating, nausea, diarrhea, abdominal pain); and those that re systemic (e.g., fatigue, sleep disturbance, migraine headaches [4]. The standing heart rate is often >120 beats per minute [3]
Psychogenic Pseudosyncope	A syndrome of apparent but not true loss of consciousness that may occur in the absence of identifiable cardiac, reflex, neurological, or metabolic causes

(continued)

Table 28.1 (continued)

Term	Definition
Hypoglycemia	Defined by a plasma glucose concentration below 70 mg/dL; however, signs and symptoms may not occur until plasma glucose concentrations drop below 55 mg/dL [5]

VVS Vasovagal syncope, *BP* blood pressure, *OH* orthostatic hypotension
[a] The definitions in this table were adopted from the 2017 American College of Cardiology/ American Heart Association/ Heart Rhythm Society guidelines for the evaluation and management of patients with Syncope [2]

28.1 Initial Evaluation and Disposition of a Student Presenting with Syncope

The initial assessment of the student with syncope should start with application of the Pediatric Assessment Triangle (appearance, work of breathing, and circulation to the skin), the interpretation of vital signs, the utilization of the ABCDE approach (airway, breathing, circulation, disability, and exposure), the implementation of the SAMPLE mnemonic, and determination of disposition (Chap. 23). Additional considerations should be given with respect to measuring orthostatic blood pressure which includes having the patient lie down for 5 min then measure the blood pressure and heart rate, followed by having the student stand, repeating the blood pressure and heart rate measurements after standing for 1 and 3 min. Orthostatic hypotension is classically defined as a systolic blood pressure decrease greater than or equal to 20 mmHg or a diastolic BP decrease greater than or equal to 10 mmHg and/or experiencing lightheadedness or dizziness while collecting orthostatic vitals. Lastly, measuring a point of care serum glucose may be helpful to evaluate for hypoglycemia as a cause of syncope if a glucometer is available.

Determine the events surrounding the syncopal event and who was there to witness it. Were there any symptoms prior to the event (chest pain, shortness of breath, palpitations, fever, vomiting or diarrhea, dizziness or lightheadedness, headache, etc.)? Was there a loss of consciousness or seizure activity? How long was the event? Was there apnea or cyanosis associated with the event? Were there any traumatic injuries sustained? Any significant past medical history? Information regarding the syncopal event can be obtained from the student (if back to baseline) or witnesses of the event.

In terms of disposition after a syncopal event, many students can follow up with a primary care physician or at an urgent care center, with exceptions noted in Table 28.2 ("SYNCOPE RED FLAGS" mnemonic) and Table 28.3 (Red Flags based on suspected etiology) that may require immediate transfer to an emergency department for evaluation and stabilization.

Table 28.2 "Syncope red flags" mnemonic

S	Seizure >5 min
Y	Why did this happen (unknown etiology)
N	Neurologic status depressed (prolonged)
C	Central cyanosis
O	Overdose/intoxication
P	Pain (headache/chest pain/abdominal pain—Severe)
E	Exertional
R	Repeated episodes with increasing frequency
E	Environmental (heat related illness)
D	Dehydration (moderate to severe)
F	Family history of sudden cardiac death
L	Loss of pulses (requiring CPR)
A	Anemia or significant blood loss
G	Glucose (hypoglycemia or hyperglycemia)
S	Shortness of breath or apnea

Table 28.3 Syncope red flags [6]

Neurology	Cardiology	Other
Prolonged unresponsiveness following event	Any child that has a history of needing cardiopulmonary resuscitation	Heat related illness
Seizures greater than 5 min	Exertional syncope	Severe anemia or blood loss
Seizure associated with significant respiratory compromise and evidence of central cyanosis	Chest pain, palpitations, shortness of breath, apnea, cyanosis, diaphoresis	Severe dehydration
	Multiple episodes of syncope with increase in frequency	Concern for intoxication
	Family history of sudden death	Possible ingestion

28.2 Case Resolutions

Case 1 This is an example of reflex (neural mediated) syncope. Reflex syncope is passing out due to something that causes a symptomatic hypotension, bradycardia, vasodilation, or combination of these responses. The most common type of reflex syncope is vasovagal syncope (VVS). An episode of VVS is typically associated with a prodrome of diaphoresis, warmth, and pallor, with fatigue after the event [2]. The student in this scenario had been standing for a prolonged amount of time, and once movement was initiated there was a prodrome of warmth and a feeling that they were going to lose their balance. These are the details that suggest a reflexive mechanism. Jamie's symptoms slowly improved following rest and hydration in the nurse's office.

This student also had some associated twitching noticed by classmates which is not an uncommon association with VVS. A retrospective study has shown that while performing head-up tilt test (HUT) induced syncope in those with VVS about 66% had observed seizure like activity [7]. Seizures can present similarly to syncope but there are a few helpful clinical clues to take into consideration when evaluating the mechanism of seizure like activity. When an individual has a seizure, they are typically less likely to have a spontaneous neurological recovery and more likely to experience a postictal state where their consciousness is still altered for a period of time before they reach their baseline. Additionally, students who experience a seizure may have involuntary voiding or stooling, or sustain mouth injuries (from biting oral mucosa or tongue).

Other types of reflex syncope include situational syncope. This occurs when there is a syncopal event following a cough, laugh, swallowing, defecation, micturition, or anxiety provoking event (such as a blood draw). It is typical for children with reflex syncope to have recurrent events, as well as normal cardiac anatomy and unremarkable physical examinations.

Case 2 This is an example of cardiac syncope. Timothy has a history of congenital heart disease with subsequent surgical repair. In cardiac mediated syncope there is little to no prodrome and can appear as a precipitous collapse, syncope with exertion, or fainting while in the supine position. These children can have histories of structural heart disease, arrhythmias, and/or prior surgical interventions that can place them at increased risk. Cardiac syncope carries a significantly worse prognosis than does reflex and orthostatic syncope, although students who experience cardiac syncope often have less recurrent events than students who experience reflex and orthostatic syncope [8].

Although recovering quickly and remaining hemodynamically stable during the event, Timothy should be evaluated and have an electrocardiogram performed in an urgent care center or in an emergency department to rule out an underlying arrhythmia as a cause for his syncopal event. In the emergency department, Timothy was noted to have a heart rate of 213 beats per minute, requiring an intravenous does of Adenosine to convert to normal sinus rhythm. Although his heart rate was normal for his age on initial evaluation, it was suspected that Timothy was going in and out of supraventricular tachycardia (SVT). Timothy will need further work up and a more in-depth evaluation by a pediatric cardiologist. Having a cardiac emergency response plan and automated external defibrillator readily available at your school is of utmost importance, especially when dealing with a student who experiences cardiac related syncope and is hemodynamically unstable (Chap. 4).

Case 3 This is an example of Orthostatic Hypotension (OH). Tiffany experienced a syncopal event after a quick change in body position (going from a seated to standing position) as well as associated dehydration from decreased oral liquid intake. Tiffany's symptoms significantly improved after drinking some water and was able to return home with her mother.

OH is an autonomic nervous system dysfunction. There are three different forms of orthostatic intolerance [7–9], which stresses the need to obtain accurate orthostatic measurements using appropriately sized cuffs and measuring at the appropriate body position and time intervals:

1. Transient hypotension is as a variant of OH, defined as a decrease in systolic blood pressure ≥40 mmHg or diastolic BP ≥20 mmHg within 15 s of standing up, and usually resolving within a minute.
2. Classical OH is defined by a decrease of systolic BP of ≥20 mmHg or diastolic BP of ≥10 mmHg within 3 min of assuming and upright position.
3. Delayed OH is defined as a symptomatic hypotension beyond 3 min of standing up.

Orthostatic hypotension and reflex syncope can be difficult to distinguish. Table 28.4 highlights some of the similarities and differences between the two etiologies. The treatment for orthostatic and reflex syncope is initially conservative, such as increasing hydration and salt content, ensuring an adequate, well-balanced diet, as well as being mindful of changes in position to reduce your chances of falling. Regular exercise and adequate rest are typically encouraged as well.

Case 4 This is an example of a patient who has a known diagnosis of POTS, presenting with a syncopal event and who was found to be hypoglycemic. Symptoms related to POTS and hypoglycemia are similar, including generalized weakness, orthostatic intolerance, and tremors. Syncope may occur in approximately 30% of children with POTS [11]. Studies have shown a correlation between carbohydrate consumption and insulin regulation in patients with POTS, with a large carbohydrate intake leading to worsening tachycardia when upright and a decrease in stroke volume [12]. It is not uncommon for patients with POTS to avoid large meals for

Table 28.4 Reflex vs orthostatic syncope [10]

Reflex syncope	Orthostatic syncope
Long history of recurrent syncope, in particular occurring before the age of 40 years	While or after standing
After unpleasant sight, sound, smell or pain	Prolonged standing
Prolonged standing	Standing after exertion
During meal	Post-prandial hypotension
Being in crowded and or hot places	Temporal relationship with start or changes of doses of vasodepressive drugs or diuretics leading to hypotension
Autonomic activation before syncope; pallor, sweating, and/or nausea/vomiting	Presence of autonomic neuropathy or parkinsonism
With head rotation or pressure on carotid sinus (as in tumors, shaving, tight collars)	
Absence of heart disease	

fear of worsening symptoms. Therefore, eating small, more frequent meals throughout the day is recommended to avoid hypoglycemia [12]. Susie's hypoglycemia was treated with oral administration of a readily absorbable carbohydrate in the form of juice. Her symptoms improved and repeated glucose measurement was normal.

Postural Orthostatic Tachycardia Syndrome (POTS) is a type of dysautonomia, affecting multiple somatic systems in children and adults that can cause significant disability [13]. The autonomic system controls non voluntary bodily functions such as digestion or increasing and decreasing heart rate and blood pressure. Other types of dysautonomia include orthostatic intolerance, inappropriate sinus tachycardia and vasovagal syncope to name a few. Patients with POTS experience chronic symptoms of orthostatic intolerance, in the absence of hypotension. They can present with a wide variety of symptoms such as dizziness, headache, fatigue, gastrointestinal complaints, visual disturbances, chest pain, palpitations, brain fog, insomnia, exercise intolerance, venous pooling, joint hypermobility, and muscle pain. The symptoms can fluctuate and can often increase with certain triggers such as stress, overeating, under eating, menstrual cycle, change in season, or concussion. The diagnosis of POTS may have overlapping diagnoses including migraine, functional GI disorders, joint hypermobility and Elhers Danlos syndrome. The exact pathophysiology is not well understood and there are no biomarkers that exist to indicate its presence [11]. Achieving complete resolution of symptoms can be challenging. Lifestyle changes including increasing hydration and regular exercise is the foundation of treatment. The diagnostic criterion for POTS includes symptoms of chronic orthostatic intolerance for greater than or equal to 3 months, persistent symptomatic increase in heart rate by greater than or equal to 40 beats per minute in the first 10 min of upright position after supine position without orthostatic hypotension, and the absence of other potential etiologies. Treatment of POTS is multimodal, and often requires referrals to pediatric cardiology, rheumatology, neurology, and gastroenterology.

Extra Credit Points

1. The contextual clues of what was happening prior to the syncopal event, during and immediately following can help narrow down the etiology of syncope.
2. Obtaining vital signs, particularly orthostatic measurements, can be helpful when distinguishing orthostatic hypotension from reflex syncope.
3. In cardiac mediated syncope there is little to no prodrome and can appear as a precipitous collapse, syncope with exertion, or fainting while in the supine position. Consider referral for an electrocardiogram in these scenarios, or if the student has a significant cardiac history.
4. Although syncope may present with seizure like activity, consider referral to a pediatric neurologist if the student has a prolong post-ictal course, urinary or bowel incontinence, or significant traumatic injuries (head or mouth injuries, etc.)
5. The mnemonic "SYNCOPE RED FLAGS" can be helpful when determining whether a student who experiences a syncopal event requires transfer to a higher level of care.

References

1. Hu E, Liu X, Chen Q, Wang C. Investigation on the incidence of syncope in children and adolescents aged 2-18 years in Changsha. Front Pediatr. 2021;9:638394. Epub 2021 Mar 22.
2. Shen W, Sheldon RS, Benditt DG, et al. Guideline for the evaluation and management of patients with syncope. AHA/ASA J. 2017;136:e60–e122.
3. Soteriades ES, Evans JC, Larson MG, et al. Incidence and prognosis of syncope. N Engl J Med. 2002;341:878–85.
4. Thieben MJ, Sandroni P, Sletten DM. Postural orthostatic tachycardia syndrome: the Mayo Clinic experience. May Clin Proc. 2007;82(3):308–13.
5. Mathew P, Thoppil D. Hypoglycemia. [Updated 2022 Dec 26]. In: StatPearls [Internet]. Treasure Island (FL): StatPearls Publishing; 2024. https://www.ncbi.nlm.nih.gov/books/NBK534841/.
6. Hackett G, Brady J, Olympia RP. School nurses on the front lines of medicine the approach to a student after a syncopal event: don't PASS OUT. NASN Sch Nurse. 2018;33:222–7.
7. Probst MA, Kanzaria HK, Gbedemah M, et al. National trends in resource utilization associated with ED visits for syncope. Am J Emerg Med. 2015;33:998–1001.
8. Freeman R, Wieling W, Axelrod FB, et al. Consensus statement on the definition of orthostatic hypotension, neurally mediated syncope and the postural tachycardia syndrome. Clin Auton Res. 2011;21(2):69–72.
9. Yeom JS, Woo H. Pediatric syncope: pearls and pitfalls in history taking. Clin Exp Pediatr. 2023;66:88–97.
10. Brignole M, Moya A, de Lange FJ. 2018 ESC Guidelines for the diagnosis and management of syncope. Eur Heart J. 2018;39:1883–948.
11. Boris JR, Bernadzikowski T. Demographics of a large paediatric postural orthostatic tachycardia syndrome program. Cardiol Young. 2018;28(5):668–74.
12. Breier NC, Paranjape S, Scudder S. Worsening postural tachycardia syndrome is associated with increased glucose-dependent insulinotropic polypeptide secretion. Hypertension. 2022;79(5):e89–99.
13. Shaw BH, Stiles LE, Bourne K, et al. The face of postural tachycardia syndrome—insights from a large cross sectional online community-based survey. J Intern Med. 2019;286:438–48.

Chapter 29
Fever

Paige Reese and Angela Ropka

Fever is often the first sign of a presenting illness. It is important that you are comfortable with conducting a thorough history and screening physical examination, developing a comprehensive differential diagnosis for fever, and recognizing signs and symptoms associated with fever that requires immediate transport to either an urgent care center or emergency department (ED). We often say that "Fever is your friend" as it is evidence of the body fighting an infection, but yet we as a health profession often respond negatively when a child or adolescent has a fever, promoting "Fever Phobia". Sometimes we focus on the presence of a fever or the height of the fever or duration of a fever, instead of focusing on how the child is acting or interacting with you, how they are breathing, if they are exhibiting signs of significant dehydration, or if they are complaining of a lot of pain.

Let's test your basic knowledge of fever with the following True or False questions (Table 29.1):

Case 1 Samantha, a 10-year-old female, was playing at recess when she came up to her teacher and told them she had a headache. The teacher gave Samantha some water, but 30 min later she was still complaining of headache and started to complain of neck pain. In your office her vital signs include a heart rate of 124 beats per minute, respiratory rate of 22 breaths per minute, an oxygen saturation of 99%, blood pressure of 110/76, and a temperature of 101.3 °F by forehead thermometer. She is able to have a conversation with you, is able to follow commands, and does not have neck stiffness. She does complain of a sore throat. What do you do next?

Fever is an elevation of body temperature that exceeds the normal daily variation and occurs in conjunction with an increase in the set point [1]. When the body

P. Reese (✉) · A. Ropka
Penn State Hershey Medical Center, Hershey, PA, USA
e-mail: preese3@pennstatehealth.psu.edu; aropka@pennstatehealth.psu.edu

R. P. Olympia, J. Brady-Olympia (eds.), *Clinical Considerations in School-based Health*, https://doi.org/10.1007/978-3-031-85765-2_29

Table 29.1 True or false questions regarding fever

1. Fever is the body's natural response to an invasion of the immune system
2. High fevers can lead to brain damage
3. High fevers can cause seizures
4. A high fever means that the student has a serious infection
5. Every fever needs to be treated with a dose of Acetaminophen or Ibuprofen
6. A lack of reduction of a fever after being given antipyretics means that the child has more serious bacterial infection
7. A high fever can result in a student "not acting right"
8. A high fever does not change a student's heart rate and respiratory rate
9. It is important to know the exact temperature associated with every fever
10. A fever lasting more than 5 days means that the student has a more serious infection

attempts to fight off a bacterial or viral illness, the body responds by setting forth a cascade of events leading to a fever. Fever is any temperature above 38 °C or 100.4 °F. Some of the symptoms associated with having a fever include feeling tired, sweating, or shivering, or complaining of headache, abdominal pain, muscle aches, or feeling hot or cold. Cold and clammy hands and feet is often due to the shunting of blood internally and away from the periphery. At the same time, this can also produce shivering, which produces heat from the muscles.

When a student presents to your office with a potential elevation of temperature, confirm the temperature with either a digital thermometer (oral or axillary), a tympanic (ear) thermometer, or a temporal artery (temperature taken across the forehead area) [2]. Axillary, tympanic, and temporal temperatures are approximately 1 °F lower than oral temperatures, which are 1° lower than rectal temperatures [3].

The initial assessment of the student with fever should start with application of the Pediatric Assessment Triangle (appearance, work of breathing, and circulation to the skin), the interpretation of vital signs, the utilization of the ABCDE approach (airway, breathing, circulation, disability, and exposure), the implementation of the SAMPLE mnemonic, and determination of disposition (Chap. 23). Of note, students may have multiple vital sign abnormalities when they have a fever, including both tachycardia and tachypnea.

Treatment of a student with fever includes either acetaminophen (15 mg/kg) or ibuprofen (10 mg/kg). Remember that treatment of a fever in a student is not always necessary, and should be used to make the child or adolescent more comfortable if they do not feel well. Avoid salicylates as this may lead to Reye's syndrome (acute onset encephalopathy, liver dysfunction, and fatty infiltration of the liver) [4]. Other treatment approaches to fever include cool compresses applied to the forehead, back of the neck, axilla, and extremities (loss of heat by evaporation) and starting oral hydration. Be careful to not use very cold water as this may lead to shivering and increasing the core body temperature.

The most common infectious causes of fever are due to viral infections (Chaps. 100, 101, and 103), so determining evidence of a bacterial infection is of utmost importance for diagnosis and disposition (Table 29.2).

Table 29.2 Common bacterial causes for fever

Infection	Presenting signs and symptoms in addition to fever	Associated chapter
Septic shock	– Depressed mental status – Cool mottled or pale extremities, thready pulses, prolonged capillary refill – Petechiae or purpura	88
Meningitis	– Depressed or altered mental status – Stiff neck – Seizures	89
Pneumonia	– Evidence of respiratory distress – Significant cough – Cyanosis	90
Appendicitis	– Significant abdominal pain – Unable to ambulate or jump up and down – Poor appetite – Vomiting	91
Urinary tract infections	– Lower abdominal or flank pain – Painful urination – Urinary frequency – Blood in urine	92
Septic arthritis or osteomyelitis	– Painful extremities or back – Decreased range of motion of the extremity – Joint pain or swelling – Unable to ambulate	93
Cellulitis	– Painful, red, warm skin – Red streaks	96
Gastroenteritis	– Severe abdominal pain – Persistent vomiting – Bloody diarrhea – Dehydration	95
Infections of the head or neck	– Thick nasal discharge and congestion – Ear pain – Sore throat – Neck swelling and pain	94

Case 2 A 7-year-old female, Hailey, is sent to your office by her teacher due to "not acting right". Hailey has been out of school for the last 5 days due to illness, including fever, vomiting, and muscle aches. In your office she is pale, her extremities are cold, and she does not respond to voice but has minimal response to sternal rub. Her vital signs include a heart rate of 150 beats per minute, respiratory rate of 40 breaths per minute, an oxygen saturation of 90%, blood pressure of 82/50, and a temperature of 102.3 °F by forehead thermometer. What should you do next?

When evaluating a child with a fever, it is important to differentiate between a child that looks well and a child that is toxic appearing. A child that has a toxic appearance is one that is unwilling to interact at their normal level, such as preferring to lie down or avoiding making eye contact. They may only respond to noxious stimuli and have a decreased level of alertness [3]. Sometimes it may be difficult to distinguish between a student who doesn't feel well with a fever and a student who is truly "lethargic" due to an underlying bacterial infection, so if you are unsure, transfer the student to a higher level of care. It appears that Hailey has evidence of septic shock and hypoperfusion (Chap. 88), and should be immediately transported to your nearest ED. Table 29.3 lists "red flags" in a student with fever that would require immediate transfer by Emergency Medical Services to your nearest ED [5].

Although daily fever for greater than 5 days is most likely due to a viral infection, differential diagnosis should include latent bacterial infections (such as pneumonia or urinary tract infections or sinusitis), malignancy, and rheumatologic/connective tissue conditions, including Kawasaki's disease or Multisystem Inflammatory Syndrome in Children (MIS-C) [6]. Kawasaki's disease is a condition where the child has high fevers for at least 5 days, plus any 4 of the following 5 findings: bilateral, non-purulent, limbus sparing conjunctivitis; mucous membrane changes (red, dry, cracked lips, strawberry tongue); cervical lymphadenopathy (unilateral, >1.5 cm); generalized polymorphous rash; swelling of the hands/feet. Diagnosis is clinical, but laboratory findings (including elevated inflammatory markers) may support the diagnosis. Treatment with intravenous immunoglobulins and high dose aspirin within 10 days of the beginning of the fever help to decrease the risk of coronary artery aneurysms. MIS-C has many signs and symptoms that overlap with Kawasaki's disease, but usually presents 4–6 weeks after a COVID infection, gastrointestinal symptoms and renal/hepatic dysfunction are more

Table 29.3 Red flag signs and symptoms prompting ED referral in a student with fever

Severe tachycardia
Severe tachypnea
Respiratory Distress with retractions, accessory muscle use
Hypotension
Altered mental status
Lethargy
Lightheadedness or dizziness
Severe headache
Trouble swallowing
Stiff neck
Severe chest pain or abdominal pain
Moderate to severe dehydration shown as decreased skin turgor
Petechiae or purpura
Sloughing of the skin or mucous membrane changes
Unable to ambulate
Severe extremity pain
Pale or cool extremities, mottling of the skin
Joint swelling or decreased range of motion of the joints
Immunocompromised
Unvaccinated
Indwelling devices (tracheostomy, central venous devices, foley catheters)
Recent surgery
Heat related illnesses (heat stroke)
Clinical suspicion for an overdose

common in MIS-C than Kawasaki's disease, 50–80% of children with MIS-C present with shock, 60% of children with MIS-C present with myocardial dysfunction (with abnormal electrocardiogram, elevated NT-proBNP and troponin levels), and often children with MIS-C are older than Kawasaki's disease (average 10 years of age) and are African-American or Hispanic.

Students may present with fever and seizures, with the concern that the seizure may be associated with infection, such as meningitis or encephalitis, or that an infection has decreased the threshold for a seizure in a student with epilepsy. Initial assessment and management is similar to that described in Chap. 23. A "simple" febrile seizure occurs in a child aged 5 months to 6 years without an anatomical reason for seizures (such as a ventriculo-peritoneal shunt), is generalized tonic-clonic in nature, lasts less than 15 min, is limited to one episode in a 24 h period of time, and the child recovers spontaneously and shortly after the seizure without the use of rescue anti-epileptic medication. Febrile seizures that are not defined by "simple" criteria would be considered "complex", and likely requires evaluation in an ED. For seizures associated with fever, the seizure is often associated with a rapid rise in temperature and not due to the temperature reaching a specific, high number. Febrile seizures do not cause brain damage in and of itself (unless the student's airway and breathing is compromised by hypoxia), so concentrating on the ABC's of resuscitation and appropriate transport to an ED is key to management. In cases of prolonged febrile seizure lasting longer than 5 min, rectal diazepam or intranasal versed can be administered as prescribed by the student's primary care provider.

Case 3 You respond to an urgent call from a homeroom teacher reporting that she found one of her students collapsed in the bathroom. You respond to the scene and find Sheila, a 14 year old female who is groggy and not responding appropriately to questions. Her mouth is dry and her skin is red, dry, and very warm to the touch. Her vital signs include a heart rate of 160 beats per minute, respiratory rate of 36 breaths per minute, an oxygen saturation of 96%, blood pressure of 136/86, and she feels warm to the touch. You find out that Sheila has been depressed since the death of her best friend 1 month ago. What should you do next?

The concern with this presentation is for anti-cholinergic toxicity [7]. This is due to an overdose of anticholinergic medications (such as diphenhydramine). The anti-cholinergic toxidrome can be remembered by the saying "Hot as a hare (fever), mad as a hatter (altered mental status, confused), red as a beet (red flushed skin), dry as a bone (dry mouth, dry skin), blind as a bat (mydriasis), and the heart runs along (tachycardia). Management and treatment of this toxidrome should occur in an ED (Chap. 25). Non-infectious causes of fever are listed in Table 29.4. Keep an open mind when evaluating a student with fever … not all fevers are infectious! (Fig. 29.1).

Table 29.4 Non-infectious causes of fever

Medications
Chemotherapy
Neuroleptic malignant syndrome
Malignant hyperthermia
Serotonin Syndrome toxidrome
Anticholinergic toxicity
Drug use: amphetamine, cocaine, PCP, ecstasy
Inflammatory, like: Juvenile Rheumatoid Arthritis, Vasculitis
Autoimmune disorders, like: Systemic Lupus
Malignancies, like: Leukemia, Lymphoma, Solid organ tumors
Intracranial, like: Increased ICP, intracranial hemorrhage, neoplasm
Thromboembolic, like: Renal infarct, Pulmonary Embolism(PE), Deep Vein Thrombosis (DVT)
Metabolic Disorders, like: Thyroid storm, Thyroiditis, Acute Adrenal crisis
Heat related illnesses, like heat exhaustion or heat stroke

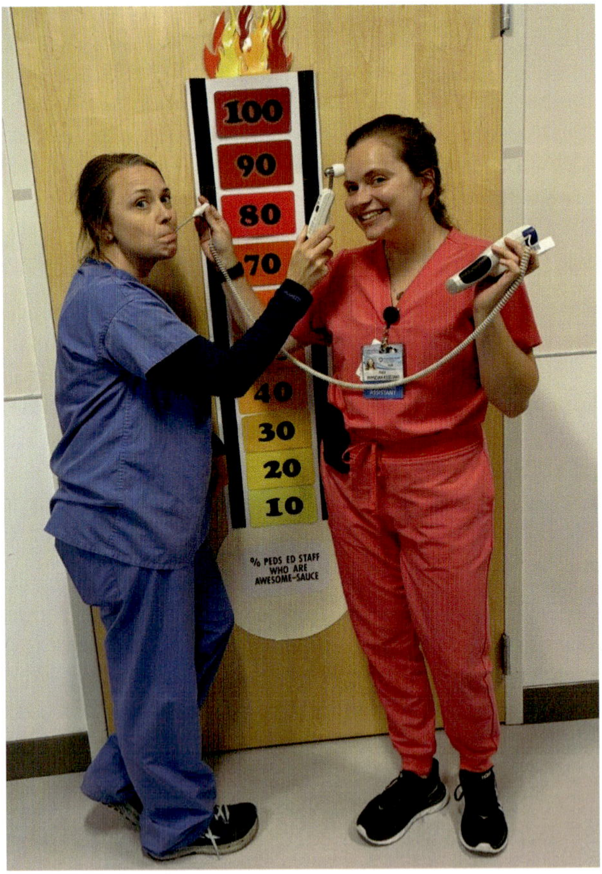

Fig. 29.1 Combining our love for others creates a boundless force that knows no measure

Extra Credit Points

1. Fever is the body's natural response to an invasion of the immune system. **TRUE**: Fever due to an infection is a response to foreign pathogens and is a sign that the immune system is working.
2. High fevers can lead to brain damage. **FALSE**: Fever is a change in set point in relation to foreign pathogens and does not cause brain damage. The exception is environmental causes of fever (such as heat stroke) or if the fever is caused by an infection that potentially damages the brain (such as meningitis).
3. High fevers can cause seizures. **TRUE**: Young children (up to the age of 5 years) or students with epilepsy can present with a seizure due to a fever, but this is often due to the rapid rise of temperature and not because the temperature reaches a certain number.
4. A high fever means that the student has a serious infection. **FALSE**: Often high temperatures are associated with viral infections and not serious bacterial infections. A fever over 102 °F does not automatically mean EMS transport to an ED (as most protocols dictate), but should depend on how the student is acting or interacting with you, how they are breathing, if they are exhibiting signs of significant dehydration, or if they are complaining of a lot of pain.
5. Every fever needs to be treated with a dose of Acetaminophen or Ibuprofen. **FALSE:** As long as the child is acting appropriately and keeping themselves hydrated, no need to administer antipyretic medication for every fever.
6. A lack of reduction of fever after being given antipyretics means a more serious bacterial infection. **FALSE**: A fever may, and often, persist after administering antipyretic medications. This does not mean that the child has a more serious infection or that the child needs transport to a higher level of care.
7. A high fever can result in a student "not acting right". **TRUE**: A fever may cause a child to appear "lethargic" or "sleepy" or "disinterested". If a student continues to have an altered mental status despite antipyretics and fever reduction, or if there is concern for sepsis or meningitis or severe dehydration, the student needs immediate transport to a higher level of care.
8. A fever does not change a student's heart rate and respiratory rate. **FALSE**: Tachycardia and tachypnea is often present when a child has a fever.
9. It is important to know the exact temperature associated with every fever. **FALSE**: Although many school protocols are based on the exact number associated with a fever, when dealing with infectious causes of fever, an exact number is of critical importance in a student who is considered immunocompromised, has had recent surgery or invasive procedure, or is technology dependent (ventriculo-peritoneal shunt, central venous catheter devices, gastric tubes, other indwelling catheters, etc.)
10. A fever lasting more than 5 days means that the student has a more serious infection. **FALSE**: Many viral causes of fever can last more than 5 days, although consider other etiologies such as malignancy, rheumatologic or connective tissue disorders, etc.

References

1. Nadler PL, Gonzales R. Fever & hyperthermia. In: Papadakis MA, McPhee SJ, Rabow MW, McQuaid KR, Gandhi M, editors. Current medical diagnosis & treatment 2024. McGraw-Hill Education; 2024. https://accessmedicine-mhmedical-com.ezaccess.libraries.psu.edu/content.aspx?bookid=3343&sectionid=279900721. Accessed 27 Mar 2024.
2. The Johns Hopkins University, The John Hopkins Hospital, and John Hopkins Health System. Fever. Published 2024. https://www.hopkinsmedicine.org/health/conditions-and-diseases/fever.
3. Rodriguez DM, Nesiama JO, Wang VJ. Fever and serious bacterial illness in infants and children. In: Tintinalli JE, Ma O, Yealy DM, Meckler GD, Stapczynski J, Cline DM, Thomas SH, editors. Tintinalli's emergency medicine: a comprehensive study guide. 9th ed. McGraw-Hill Education; 2020. https://accessmedicine-mhmedical-com.ezaccess.libraries.psu.edu/content.aspx?bookid=2353&sectionid=219644573. Accessed 28 Mar 2024.
4. Grosser T, Ricciotti E, FitzGerald GA. Pharmacotherapy of inflammation, fever, pain, and gout. In: Brunton LL, Knollmann BC, editors. [publicationyear2] Goodman & Gilman's: the pharmacological basis of therapeutics. 14th ed. McGraw-Hill Education. https://accessmedicine-mhmedical-com.ezaccess.libraries.psu.edu/content.aspx?bookid=3191&sectionid=267338476.
5. Tess AV. Chapter 8. Fever. In: Henderson MC, Tierney LM Jr, Smetana GW, editors. The patient history: an evidence-based approach to differential diagnosis. The McGraw-Hill Companies; 2012. https://accessmedicine-mhmedical-com.ezaccess.libraries.psu.edu/content.aspx?bookid=500&sectionid=41026551. Accessed 28 Mar 2024.
6. Rivas MN, Arditi M. Kawasaki disease and multisystem inflammatory syndrome in children: common inflammatory pathways of two distinct diseases. Rheum Dis Clin North Am. 2023;49(3):647–59.
7. LoVecchio F. Anticholinergics. In: Tintinalli JE, Ma O, Yealy DM, Meckler GD, Stapczynski J, Cline DM, Thomas SH, editors. Tintinalli's emergency medicine: a comprehensive study guide, 9e. McGraw-Hill Education; 2020. https://accessmedicine-mhmedical-com.ezaccess.libraries.psu.edu/content.aspx?bookid=2353&sectionid=220746000. Accessed 31 Jul 2024.

Chapter 30
Headache

Kara K. Seaton

Case 1 A 12-year-old student presents to the office complaining of headache. She reports the headache started earlier today. She has no history of frequent headaches. The headache started after taking a test in math class. She says her whole head hurts, but she does not have nausea, has not vomited, and she is acting normally. She is otherwise generally healthy.

Headache is a common complaint in children and adolescents. As many as a third of children will experience headaches during childhood, with the incidence reaching as high as 80% during adolescence [1]. Headaches are rarely caused by a serious underlying disorder or cause for significant concern. However, it is important to identify which children might be at higher risk of serious underlying pathology. Once identified, these children should be referred for further evaluation and management. Children with mild symptoms may be referred to their pediatricians for further evaluation, but any child with concerning or severe symptoms should be sent to the Emergency Department for evaluation. Further discussion of these types of symptoms occurs later in the chapter.

Generally, headaches are classified as primary or secondary. Primary headaches include migraines with or without aura, tension type headaches, and cluster headaches (although these are relatively rare in children, especially younger children). Secondary headache disorders occur when the headache is caused by a secondary process. Table 30.1 provides examples of secondary processes that may cause headaches.

K. K. Seaton (✉)
Children's Minnesota, Minneapolis, MN, USA
e-mail: kara.seaton@childrensmn.org

R. P. Olympia, J. Brady-Olympia (eds.), *Clinical Considerations in School-based Health*, https://doi.org/10.1007/978-3-031-85765-2_30

Table 30.1 Secondary causes of headache

Acute febrile illnesses—Upper respiratory infections, influenza, strep pharyngitis, sinusitis, etc.
Dehydration
Post-traumatic headache
Medication—side effects of medications, medication overuse, drug use/abuse
Hypertension
Intracranial infection—meningitis, encephalitis
Space occupying lesion—mass, tumor, abscess
Increased intracranial pressure—hydrocephalus, idiopathic intracranial hypertension
Intracranial hemorrhage—subdural, subarachnoid, epidural, intraventricular
Stroke—ischemic or hemorrhagic
Visual acuity disturbances
Stressful situations
Sleep disturbances

When initially approached with a child complaining of headache, it is important to ask questions related to headache history and characteristics to determine if it is more likely a primary or secondary disorder. Questions should focus on onset and duration of symptoms, location of pain, associated symptoms, and determining underlying medical risks. Associated symptoms might include those related to a minor acute illness, such as fever, sore throat, rhinorrhea, cough, nausea, or vomiting. More concerning associated symptoms include visual changes, stiff neck, or confusion. Red flag symptoms that should prompt emergency evaluation are discussed later in this chapter. Knowing a student's medical history is important, as it can help delineate students where a lower threshold for emergent evaluation is needed. Table 30.2 outlines examples of medical conditions that may predispose children to more serious causes of headaches.

It is also imperative in the case of headache to obtain a thorough physical exam, as this will help guide diagnosis and management. This includes obtaining a set of vital signs, including blood pressure. While blood pressure is often not obtained in children, omitting this step could prevent the diagnosis of hypertension as a cause of headache. While this is far less common in children compared to adults, it does rapidly identify a potentially serious underlying cause of headache [2]. Other important exam elements include assessment of mental status using the AVPU scale (alert, voice, pain, unresponsive) and determining if children are oriented to person, place, and time. Pupils can be assessed for responsiveness. Checking gait helps assess for ataxia, but also assesses strength in the lower extremities. Having children reach for an object or complete finger-to-nose exercises rapidly assesses coordination.

Categorizing headaches by onset and temporal pattern can be helpful in terms of differential diagnosis. Headaches generally fall into classifications of acute, episodic or recurrent, chronic progressive, and chronic non-progressive [3]. Acute

Table 30.2 Select medical disorders that may increase the risk of serious underlying cause of headache

Hematologic	• Coagulopathy (examples: factor V Leiden, anti-phospholipid syndrome) • Sickle cell disease • Bleeding disorders (examples: hemophilia, von Willenbrand's disease)
Oncologic	• Active malignancy • History of malignancy
Immunologic/ Rheumatologic	• Immunodeficiency • HIV • Lupus
Neurologic	• Hydrocephalus • Implanted Ventriculo peritoneal (VP) shunt
Genetic	• Neurofibromatosis type 1 • Tuberous sclerosis
Cardiac	• Unrepaired congenital heart disease • Implanted cardiovascular shunt
Vascular	• Aneurysm • Arteriovenous malformation • Moya Moya • History of stroke • Hypertension

headaches are most common in children. These may be primary, such as tension type headaches, or secondary due to an acute illness. Many acute illnesses are associated with headache in children, including influenza, strep pharyngitis, sinusitis, COVID, and acute otitis media. Acute headaches are not commonly associated with concerning features, do not have focal neurologic symptoms, and often do not require extensive evaluation. Treatment with acetaminophen or NSAIDs is generally effective and safe, with additional treatments directed at the underlying cause for secondary headaches. These children may benefit from a visit to the pediatrician's office or a nearby urgent care, who may be able to provide additional diagnostics and prescription medications if needed.

Episodic or recurrent headaches include migraines with and without aura, as well as migraine variants. Cluster headaches are also usually episodic, but are rare in children, especially prior to adolescence. Treatments for these types of headaches, especially when chronic in nature, is more challenging. While use of medications such as acetaminophen or NSAIDs is often helpful, medication overuse can lead to rebound headaches [4]. Children with chronic headaches should be managed with direction from a pediatrician or pediatric neurologist. More detailed descriptions of the common primary headaches in pediatrics can be found in Table 30.3.

Children with acute or episodic headaches without other concerning findings generally do not require extensive work ups. The American Academy of Neurology recommends that children with a normal neurologic exam and headache or recurrent headache should not undergo routine neuroimaging, such as CT scan or MRI of the brain [5]. Further work up such as bloodwork, lumbar puncture to assess for

Table 30.3 Classification of episodic headache syndromes

Primary headache type	Severity	Characteristics
Tension type headache	Mild to moderate	• May be infrequent, frequent, or chronic • Duration: 30 min to several days • Often bilateral, band-like or tightening • Not associated with nausea or vomiting; rarely associated with photophobia or phonophobia • Not worsened by activity/cause avoidance of activity
Migraine without aura	Moderate to severe	• Intermittent, recurrent episodes • Duration: 30 min to 48 h • Unilateral more common, often pulsating • Often associated with nausea and/or vomiting, photophobia, phonophobia • More common in adolescents, females
Migraine with aura	Moderate to severe	• Involve one or more reversible neurologic symptoms: visual, sensory, motor, speech/language • Aura may be present prior to onset of headache or without headache
Abdominal migraine	Moderate to severe	• Abdominal pain that is poorly localized • Duration: 2–72 h • May be associated with nausea/vomiting • Family history of migraines is common; may be a precursor to migraine in younger children
Cyclic vomiting syndrome	Severe, recurrent attacks	• Recurrent attacks of intense nausea and vomiting • Duration: 1 h to several days • Attacks are often predictable and present similarly each time • Average age at onset: 5 years
Benign positional vertigo of childhood		• Abrupt onset of vertigo without warning and with spontaneous resolution • Associated with vomiting, nystagmus, ataxia • Average age at onset: 2–5 years • Family history of migraine is common
Cluster headache	Severe	• May be episodic or chronic • Duration: 15 min to 3 h • Unilateral orbital or frontal pain • Associated with ipsilateral autonomic symptoms: conjunctival injection, lacrimation, rhinorrhea, eyelid edema, ptosis • Average age at onset: adolescence • More common in males

meningitis, or EEG to assess for seizure is rarely needed in these cases, as these are not helpful in establishing a diagnosis.

Case 2 A 9 year old student presents to the office shortly after the school day starts complaining of headache. He reports that he has frequently been waking up in the morning with headaches, and they have been worsening. He has had a few episodes of vomiting in the morning as well. He does not have a fever or neck pain, but reports double vision currently.

Table 30.4 Concerning characteristics of pediatric headache

History	Characteristics	Exam findings
Age less than 3 years	"Thunderclap" onset	GCS < 15
Significant change in personality, behavior, or school work	Headache awakens child from sleep or occurs at waking on a consistent basis	Abnormal neurologic exam or focal neurologic deficits
Concerning medical history or conditions with increased risk of intracranial pathology	Worsened with recumbent position, straining, or with physical activity	Neck stiffness/nuchal rigidity
Recent onset (< 6 months) with progressive worsening	Change in pattern of headaches	Reported trauma or signs of trauma
	Lack of response to common medical therapies	Seizure
	Occipital location of pain	

This child's headache would fall under the classification of chronic progressive headache. While most underlying causes of headache are benign, chronic progressive headaches are more concerning. When obtaining a history and physical exam, one should be careful to assess for "red flag" symptoms that may point to a more serious underlying pathology. Examples of worrisome characteristics of headaches are outlined in Table 30.4.

It should be noted that any child with red flag symptoms or an abnormal neurologic exam should have emergent evaluation and imaging (CT and/or MRI). Any child with thunderclap onset, altered mental status, abnormal neurologic findings, or seizure must be referred to the Emergency Department. Children without abnormal neurologic exam but with recurrent but non-progressive headaches should be referred for further evaluation. In these cases, assessment by the child's pediatrician may be an appropriate first step, and may help guide further evaluation and treatment. A pediatrician may recommend referral to a pediatric neurologist for help with management.

Case 3 A 16 year old student has been coming to your office multiple times a week complaining of headache. She says the headaches are pulsating, worsen with gym class or physical activity and she requests to rest in the office or leave school early. She often experiences nausea and photophobia with the headache. Although the headaches are severe when she experiences them, she recovers completely between episodes, and there has not been an increase in frequency recently. She has been missing an increasing amount of school recently, which is starting to affect her grades.

This teenager is experiencing recurrent headache with additional features of nausea and photophobia. Her symptoms point to recurrent or chronic migraine as the likely cause. Children with poorly managed chronic headaches may experience stress and anxiety related to headaches, poor school attendance and/or performance, and avoid activities they once enjoyed. These children may also be mistakenly thought of as having psychogenic symptoms. While emergent evaluation or imaging is not necessarily needed, working with a physician who is comfortable managing chronic headaches is of utmost importance. This might be a pediatrician or pediatric neurologist. Physicians should work with patients and families to focus on improving general health and healthy habits regarding sleeping, exercise, and stress, encourage school attendance, early treatment of migraine exacerbations and mitigating side effects [6]. Some patients will require chronic medication to decrease the severity and frequency of attacks. Commonly used medications for prevention of migraine in children and adolescents include topiramate, propranolol, and amitriptyline. There is good evidence that topiramate decreases the frequency of headaches compared to placebo, and propranolol has been shown to lead to at least a 50% reduction in headache attacks compared to placebo [7]. When combined with cognitive behavioral therapy, amitriptyline does show improved frequency of headaches, but families should be aware of side effects, including a black box warning regarding suicidal thoughts and behaviors [7]. School nurses should work with pediatricians and neurologists on a feasible management plan and employ strategies to keep students positively engaged with school.

30.1 Case Conclusions

Case 1 The student described here has a tension headache, possibly brought on by stress related to the math test. She does not have any concerning historical findings, neurologic deficits, or relevant medical history. With permission from her parents, the patient was given a dose of acetaminophen and returned to class to finish the school day.

Case 2 This student has red flag symptoms, including morning headaches with vomiting and new double vision. These symptoms are concerning for increased intracranial pressure. The patient was transported to the emergency department where he had imaging that revealed hydrocephalus and an intracranial mass. He was admitted to the hospital for management.

Case 3 In this case, we see an example of an adolescent with chronic migraines. She has recurrent headaches that worsen with activity and are associated with nausea and photophobia. Given the frequency of headaches, she was referred to a pediatric neurologist for evaluation. The neurologist started daily medication and worked with the family and school to plan for when her headaches occur. After this, the student had a significant decrease in the frequency of her headaches, and her school performance improved.

Extra Credit Points

1. Headache is a common complaint in school aged children, and most underlying causes of headache are benign.
2. A student reporting headache should be evaluated with a full set of vital signs, including blood pressure, and a complete exam to assess for neurologic abnormalities.

ID: 10722272 S: 0005 PS1000-1 TS: 155x235 Pg: 268/1144 BS: 220x251 H: 2 T: 13 PB

3. Children with headache that have concerning medical histories, "red flag" symptoms, or an abnormal neurologic exam require urgent medical evaluation.
4. Chronic or recurrent headache syndromes may appear during children and have a variety of presentations. These children should be managed with help of a physician who is comfortable caring for patients with such conditions.

References

1. Jacobs H, Gladstein J. Pediatric headache: a clinical review. Headache J Head Face Pain. 2012;52(2):333–9. https://doi.org/10.1111/j.1526-4610.2011.02086.x.
2. Meckler G, Sheridan D. Headache. In: Hoffman RJ, Wang VJ, Scarfone RJ, Godambe SA, Nagler J, editors. Fleisher and Ludwig's 5-minute pediatric emergency medicine consult. 2nd ed. LWW; 2019. p. 394–5.
3. Kelly M, Strelzik J, Langdon R, DiSabella M. Pediatric headache: overview. Curr Opin Pediatr. 2018;30(6):748–54. https://doi.org/10.1097/MOP.0000000000000688.
4. Pauze D, Malabanan C. Pain: headache. In: Shaw KN, Bachur RG, Chamberlain J, Lavelle J, Nagler J, Shook JE, editors. Fleisher & Ludwig's textbook of pediatric emergency medicine. 8th ed. LWW; 2020. p. 394–401.
5. Klein J, Koch T. Headache in children. Pediatr Rev. 2020;41(4):159–71. https://doi.org/10.1542/pir.2017-0012.
6. Lewis DW, Ashwal S, Dahl G, et al. Practice parameter: evaluation of children and adolescents with recurrent headaches: report of the Quality Standards Subcommittee of the American Academy of Neurology and the Practice Committee of the Child Neurology Society. Neurology. 2002;59(4):490–8. https://doi.org/10.1212/wnl.59.4.490.
7. Oskoui M, Pringsheim T, Billinghurst L, et al. Practice guideline update summary: pharmacologic treatment for pediatric migraine prevention: Report of the Guideline Development, Dissemination, and Implementation Subcommittee of the American Academy of Neurology and the American Headache Society [published correction appears in Neurology. 2020 Jan 7;94(1):50. doi: 10.1212/WNL.0000000000008750]. Neurology. 2019;93(11):500–9. https://doi.org/10.1212/WNL.0000000000008105.

Chapter 31
Eye and Ear Complaints

Kari N. Schweiger

Case 1 Milo is a 7-year-old boy with a history of type 1 diabetes who presents to the school nurse office complaining of left ear pain. It started a couple of days ago, at the time was seen by his pediatrician and was given "watch and wait" Augmentin for a possible brewing otitis media. He is crying, holding his ear in pain and not acting like himself. Temperature of 101 °F. What should you do?

Ear infections are very common in school-aged children. There are a range of infectious disease processes associated with the ear from otitis externa to otitis media and even more serious complications like mastoiditis. Initial assessment should be centered on obtaining vitals and examination. If there are significant vital sign derangements like tachycardia, hypotension, and fever or a combination thereof this is more indicative of an urgent etiology. Simple otitis externa and otitis media should not cause vital sign derangements. Ominous clinical signs to look out for are facial nerve palsy, facial paralysis, or confusion in a child with complaints of ear pain.

The examination of the ear should comprise an external inspection, palpation of the pinna and other external structures as well as visualization of the external auditory canal and tympanic membrane, however, these last two can be optional depending on available resources. Additional physical exam findings to look for include proptosis of the ear, swelling or erythema or tenderness of the mastoid area just posterior to the ear. Other signs of mastoiditis or more systemic infection are development of alterations in mentation, lethargy, or cranial nerve 7 palsy (facial weakness). Identifiable risk factors for mastoiditis include recurrent acute otitis media, immunocompromised individuals and patients less than 2 years [1].

K. N. Schweiger (✉)
Penn State Hershey Medical Center, Hershey, PA, USA
e-mail: kschweiger@pennstatehealth.psu.edu

R. P. Olympia, J. Brady-Olympia (eds.), *Clinical Considerations in School-based Health*, https://doi.org/10.1007/978-3-031-85765-2_31

It is important to recognize that there is a large differential for infectious and noninfectious ear complaints and disposition should be based on your assessment and differential (Table 31.1).

Appropriate evaluation and disposition of infectious diseases of the ear is paramount as serious complications can arise such as facial nerve paralysis, meningitis, encephalitis, brain abscess, venous sinus thrombosis, or sepsis.

Case 2 Harper is a 15-year-old female with no significant past medical history who presents to the school nursing office with a painful and red right eye that started earlier at school after gym class. What should you do?

The "red eye" has numerous etiologies but in this case we will discuss some of the more common causes of the traumatic and nontraumatic red eye in children (Table 31.2). Examination of the eye consists of visual inspection, pupil reactivity, extraocular muscles and visual acuity. These comprise part of the vital signs of the eye that can be quickly and easily assessed.

Initial evaluation of eye complaints should start with the vital signs of the eye as mentioned above [2]. External inspection of the eye can be done rapidly as part of your assessment. It is important to understand basic eye anatomy to assist in honing the differential diagnosis further. Next step is checking the patient's extraocular motility which assesses the function of cranial nerves III, IV and VI [3]. Have the child follow your finger in an "H-pattern" while keeping their head still. They should be able to do this without difficulty or pain. Then assess the child's pupils: looking for symmetry between the pupils' size and appropriate constriction to both direct and indirect light. Lastly assess visual acuity with a Snellen eye chart.

Additional testing commonly performed for complaints of eye pain include fluorescein staining and examination under a Wood's lamp. Using fluorescein dye to stain the patient's cornea and then examine under blue light. This examination helps identify corneal defects like those in abrasions/lacerations, foreign objects and for full-thickness defects to the cornea/sclera. The Seidel sign is identified with fluorescein testing and is positive when there is flow of aqueous humor/dilution of the dye due to a full-thickness corneal defect. This sign is indicative of a globe rupture.

Conjunctivitis is the most common atraumatic cause of the acutely red eye in children [4]. Typically presents as conjunctival injection with limbal sparing. Eye pain is not typical but presents with more of an irritated feeling or discomfort. There are many etiologies of conjunctivitis and some of the more common causes are viral, allergic and bacterial conjunctivitis (see Table 31.3 for additional distinguishing features). Typical treatments for conjunctivitis should target common bacterial causes such as *S. aureus*, *S. pneumoniae*, *H. influenzae*, and additional Pseudomonal coverage is required in patients who wear contact lens.

Infectious conjunctivitis is most commonly a viral etiology followed by bacterial. The majority of viral conjunctivitis is due to adenovirus. Greater than 60% of cases of bacterial conjunctivitis will resolve spontaneously in 1–2 weeks and serious complications are rare [5]. When a patient presents with symptoms of a "red eye" while it is often presumed to be conjunctivitis it is imperative to rule out serious ocular conditions that can present similarly. Initial steps to help differentiate

Table 31.1 Differential diagnosis of ear pain

Diagnosis	Risk factors	Initial presentation	Disposition/treatment
Otitis externa	Swimming Instrumentation (q-tip use)	Rapid onset of symptoms (<48 h) Otalgia Hearing loss Tenderness of pinna/ tragus Edema and erythema of the ear canal Otorrhea	Refer to pediatrician or urgent care Anti-inflammatories Avoidance of q-tip/ foreign bodies and keep canal dry Otic drops (ofloxacin or ciprofloxacin)
Malignant otitis externa	Diabetes Immunosuppression	Rapid onset Fever, toxic appearing Otalgia Edema of EAC Facial nerve involvement (facial weakness)	Refer to ED for evaluation Advanced imaging (CT) Antipseudomonal antibiotics
Otitis media	Age—predominantly affects younger kids due to anatomical differences	Otalgia Fever Nontoxic appearing ME effusion, bulging TM, erythema of TM	Refer to pediatrician or urgent care Antipyretics Anti-inflammatories Antibiotics or observation period (watch and wait)
Mastoiditis	Secondary to or concurrent with otitis media	Abnormal TM findings Erythema, edema, tenderness of mastoid Proptosis of the auricle Cranial nerve VI and VII palsies	Referral to ED Advanced imaging (CT)
Foreign body	Young children; Button batteries are very corrosive and need prompt removal	Reported by child, ear pain, visible FB, drainage from the area	Referral to pediatrician, urgent care or ED Requires removal of FB
Cellulitis/ perichondritis	Trauma, burns, chondral ear piercings and immunosuppression	Dull ear pain progressing to severe otalgia, erythema and tenderness of the auricle without involvement of the ear lobe	Refer to pediatrician or urgent care Antipseudomonal antibiotics and possible drainage by specialist
Auricular hematoma	Caused by blunt trauma to the ear RF: wrestling, boxing	Gross deformity of the pinna, loss of normal ear anatomy, blood commonly collects in the scaphoid fossa and concha of the ear	Refer to ED Requires drainage within 7 days to prevent neocartilage formation

Abbreviations: *TM* tympanic membrane, *CT* computed tomography, *EAC* external auditory canal, *ME* middle ear, *EMS* emergency medical services

Table 31.2 Differential Diagnosis of atraumatic and traumatic eye pain

Diagnosis	Initial presentation	Disposition/treatment
Ocular foreign body	Symptoms: eye pain, foreign body sensation, blurred vision, tearing Possible high impact History is important for diagnosis Hammering during metal workshop or use of power tools Non-high impact (dirt, dust, wood, etc.)	Referral to urgent care or ED Slit lamp exam w/ fluorescein IOP Extensive exam with lid eversion High impact or concern for intraocular FB CT imaging Removal of FB Ophthalmic antibiotic drops +/– tetanus booster If concern for globe injury or intraocular FB recommend EMS activation to ED
Corneal abrasion	FB sensation Photophobia +/– decreased visual acuity Eye pain	Referral to urgent care or ED Must rule out intraocular FB Extensive exam with lid eversion Fluorescein exam w/ woods lamp or slit lamp Ophthalmic antibiotic drops Systemic NSAIDs Cycloplegics or ophthalmic NSAIDs
Caustic keratoconjunctivitis	Chemical burn to eye Alkali (basic pH) are more severe Symptoms: severe ocular pain, reduced visual acuity, altered ocular pH (normal 7.0–7.2) Conjunctival injection or blanching, corneal loss or edema or perilimbal ischemia Alkali examples: Drain cleaners, grease remover (Sodium hydroxide and potassium hydroxide) Oven cleaners, swimming pool chlorinator, bleach (sodium hypochlorite and ammonia) Acidic examples: hydrochloric acid, hydrofluoric acid, sulfuric acid, phosphoric acid, acetic acid Found in auto batteries, drain cleaners, toilet bowl cleaners, rust remover, nail remover	Refer to ED for evaluation Immediate irrigation is most important and should be started prior to comprehensive evaluation *Tap water is acceptable in prehospital setting Goal restore normal ocular pH (7.0–7.2) Do not attempt to neutralize pH by adding base to acidic burn or vice versa Topical anesthetics, antibiotics and steroids are additional treatment modalities

(continued)

Table 31.2 (continued)

Diagnosis	Initial presentation	Disposition/treatment
Retrobulbar hemorrhage/hematoma	RF: blunt orbital trauma Eye pain Proptosis Decreased visual acuity Elevated IOP *Can cause vision loss rapidly secondary to orbital compartment syndrome	Refer to ED CT orbits Consider lateral canthotomy Additional medical management modalities are available in conjunction with cantholysis
Globe rupture	RF: blunt eye trauma or penetrating eye trauma Suspect in any puncture/laceration of eyelid or periorbital area Symptoms: eye pain +/− decreased visual acuity Tear drop shaped pupil Extrusion of ocular contents 360° subconjunctival hemorrhage	EMS activation to ED Do not put pressure on eye Place eye cover such as paper cup but be careful to make sure it does not touch globe Detailed inspection of lids, lashes, cornea, sclera and pupils, visual acuity testing Do not do IOP testing Fluorescein testing can be done (contraindicated in obvious globe rupture) CT orbits to evaluate for intraocular FB +Seidel's sign is indicative (leakage of aqueous humor) +/− tetanus booster if indicated IV antibiotics Surgical repair
Subconjunctival hemorrhage	Etiology: spontaneous (forceful coughing/vomiting) or secondary to trauma Symptoms: painless No effect on visual acuity Area is not significantly raised Masks conjunctival vessels	Referral to pediatrician or urgent care Must maintain suspicion for globe rupture Consider fluorescein staining to evaluate for corneal injury Resolve spontaneously
Corneal ulcer	Eye pain, FB sensation +/− decreased visual acuity Photophobia Gray/white corneal lesion Delayed pain 2-3 days after inciting event RF: contact lens use or incomplete eyelid closure	Referral to urgent care or ED Extensive exam with lid eversion Fluorescein exam w/ woods lamp or slit lamp Commonly circular and visible w/ white light (unlike corneal abrasion) Ophthalmic antibiotic drops +/− cycloplegic

Abbreviations: *IOP* intraocular pressure, *FB* foreign body, *CT* computed tomography, *EMS* emergency medical services, *ED* emergency department, *RF* risk factors

Table 31.3 Conjunctivitis subtypes

	Bacterial	Viral	Allergic
Distribution	Unilateral or bilateral	Unilateral or bilateral	Typically bilateral
Discharge	Mucopurulent	Watery/clear	None, cobblestoning of conjunctiva
Pruritus	Rarely	Rarely	Yes
Associated findings/ treatment	Tx: topical antibiotics	Viral prodrome Tx: good hygiene	Congestion, sneezing, cough, allergic shiner Tx: antihistamine eye drops
Disposition	Refer to pediatrician, urgent care or ED	Refer to pediatrician, but only requires symptomatic treatment	Can refer to pediatrician but not always required

between different etiologies include obtaining a detailed history, ophthalmologic evaluation and recognizing when a higher level of care is needed.

Case 3 Ariadne is a 6 year old girl who presents to the nursing office with frequent headaches and blurred vision. What should you do?

There are many causes for blurred vision in children from simple refractive errors to more concerning problems such as elevated intracranial pressure (Table 31.4). Children require certain vision skills in order to read and learn appropriately such as eye-hand coordination, visual perception, eye tracking, ability to focus and visual acuity. Oftentimes children can present with signs and symptoms of eye and visual problems but it can be subtle. Some common signs/symptoms of visual problems in children are frequent eye rubbing/blinking, short attention span, headaches, avoiding reading, covering one eye, head tilting, seeing double or blurred vision, etc. [6]. It is important to catch these issues early and intervene.

It is paramount to keep a broad differential as oftentimes the etiologies that can cause blurry vision can also overlap with those that cause a red or painful eye.

31.1 Case Conclusion

Case 1 Milo likely has mastoiditis based on his complaints and examination findings (swelling, tenderness, erythema and bogginess of the mastoid process). He would require referral to the ED for advanced imaging, specialty consultation for possible surgical intervention and IV antibiotic.

Case 2 Harper likely has developed a corneal abrasion during gym class causing a painful and red eye. She will require evaluation at either an urgent care or ED as well as antibiotic eye drops and follow up with ophthalmology.

Table 31.4 Differential diagnosis for blurred vision

Diagnosis	Risk factors	Initial presentation	Disposition/treatment
Refractive errors	Family history and younger age	Often subtle but frequent blinking, eye rubbing, headaches, trouble reading/ focusing	Refer to pediatrician or optometrist Tx: refractive lenses
Migraine headaches	Family history, female, certain triggers	Unilateral headache, nausea/vomiting, photophobia, phonophobia, avoidance of physical activity, can have aura symptoms	Refer to pediatrician or ED for treatment and possible prophylaxis Tx: NSAIDs, tylenol, compazine, benadryl, steroids, etc.
Trauma	Recent head trauma	Headache, confusion, blurred vision, amnesia	Refer to ED Tx: depends on clinical presentation and severity and underlying injuries
Concussion	Blunt force injury or acceleration-deceleration injury	Trouble with memory, executive functioning, attention, headaches, dizziness, insomnia, blurred vision, behavioral changes	Refer to urgent care or ED Tx: limitations in activities to avoid repeat head injury, f/u with pediatrician if simple; if complex may need referral to sports medicine
Hyper/ hypoglycemia	Diabetes, certain genetic syndromes, decreased oral intake	Hyper: blurred vision, increased thirst, increased urination Hypo: blurred vision, anxiousness, tremors, unresponsiveness, seizures	Refer to ED Tx: dependent on underlying cause for derangement
Idiopathic intracranial hypertension	Obesity, female, certain medications (OCP, vitamin A, cyclosporine)	Headache worse at night or in the AM, nausea/ vomiting, blurred vision	Refer to ED Tx: testing including imaging, ruling out other causes of increased ICP, lumbar puncture Often treated with medications or repeat LP
Preseptal vs orbital cellulitis	Prespetal: due to contiguous infection of face/eye structures Orbital: sinusitis, trauma, infection within the teeth or middle ear	Preseptal: swelling/ erythema of the eyelids Orbital: proptosis, pain or limitation with EOM, chemosis, double vision or vision loss	Refer to ED if concern for orbital cellulitis Tx preseptal: oral or IV antibiotics Tx orbital: IV antibiotics, admission and ophthalmology

(continued)

Table 31.4 (continued)

Diagnosis	Risk factors	Initial presentation	Disposition/treatment
Hordeolum vs chalazion	Hordeolum: blockage of various glands (internal vs external) Chalazion: chronic inflammation from a blocked gland often from a healing hordeolum	Hordeolum: painful pustule with associated erythema and edema Chalazion: painless rubbery/nodular lesion more commonly on upper eyelid	Refer to pediatrician Hordeolum tx: warm compresses, avoid makeup and antibiotics if surrounding periorbital cellulitis Chalazion tx: warm compresses, antibiotics not indicated

Case 3 Ariadne is suffering from a refractive error and could benefit from evaluation by optometrist and refractive lenses. However, it is important to consider other more dangerous etiologies of blurred vision and be able to rule them out.

Extra Credit Points

1. Children who present with simple cases of AOM and OE should not have significant vital sign derangements or other concerning features (altered mentation, facial nerve palsies, etc.). If present, be wary of more serious etiologies/complications.
2. Chemical eye burns—begin irrigation immediately and in the prehospital setting tap water is acceptable
3. Obtaining eye "vital signs" can help guide appropriate triage and disposition of various conditions
4. The VISION & HEARING mnemonic (Table 31.5) can be helpful to identify causes that would require immediate ED referral

Table 31.5 VISION & HEARING mnemonic—reasons for ED referral

V—vision loss (complete)
I—injury (significant trauma to the eye/ear)
S—swelling over the mastoid process
I—intraocular pressure (headaches, blurry vision, eye redness, pain)
O—orbital cellulitis (proptosis of the eye)
N—Noxious chemical conjunctivitis
H—hearing loss (complete)
E—extraocular movement pain or limitation
A—auditory canal foreign body (button battery)
R—red eye in contact lens wearer
I—immunocompromised (malignant otitis externa, orbital cellulitis, mastoiditis)
N—nerve involvement (facial nerve palsy or facial paralysis)
G—globe rupture (abnormally shaped pupil)

References

1. Cassano P, Ciprandi G, Passali D. Acute mastoiditis in children. Acta Biomed. 2020;91(1-S):54–9. Published 2020 Feb 17. https://doi.org/10.23750/abm.v91i1-S.9259.
2. Noble J, Lloyd JC. The red eye. CMAJ. 2011;183(1):81. https://doi.org/10.1503/cmaj.090379.
3. McNickle L, Olympia RP. School nurses on the front lines of healthcare: Infectious diseases popularized in the news. NASN Sch Nurse. 2020;35(4):212–6. https://doi.org/10.1177/1942602X20921426.
4. Varu DM, Rhee MK, Akpek EK, et al. Conjunctivitis preferred practice pattern®. Ophthalmology. 2019;126(1):P94–P169. https://doi.org/10.1016/j.ophtha.2018.10.020.
5. Azari AA, Arabi A. Conjunctivitis: a systematic review. J Ophthalmic Vis Res. 2020;15(3):372–95. Published 2020 Aug 6. https://doi.org/10.18502/jovr.v15i3.7456.
6. American Optometric Association. School-Aged Vision: 6–18 years of age. www.aoa.org. https://www.aoa.org/healthy-eyes/eye-health-for-life/school-aged-vision?sso=y

Chapter 32
Chest Pain

MaryAnn Mansour

Case 1 9 year old Chelsea presents to the office with pain in the middle of her chest. Her pain is worse when she takes a deep breath. She appears well, speaks in full sentences and does not have work of breathing. Vital signs are Heart Rate (HR) 90 beats per minute, Respiratory Rate (RR) 16 breaths per minute, Blood Pressure (BP) 110/70, Temperature (T) 98F Oxygen Saturation (O2) is 99% on Room Air (RA). Her lung sounds are clear and she has no murmurs. The chest wall is normal on appearance with midsternal tenderness on palpation.

Case 2 Ryan is a 17 year old male with no significant past medical history. He comes to you with a sudden onset of chest pain and shortness of breath. On exam, he is tall and thin. He appears uncomfortable but is speaking full sentences and there is no work of breathing. He is well perfused and there are no signs of cyanosis. His vital signs are T 98.6F HR 100 beats per minute RR 18 breaths per minute O2 sat 95% on RA and BP 126/78. His chest wall is normal in appearance and there is no reproducible chest wall tenderness or crepitus. He has decreased breath sounds on the left side of chest.

Case 3 Jason is an 8 year old male who presents to the office with chest pain and fatigue. He has been having cold symptoms for the past few days. On exam, he appears tired. His vital signs are T 100.4F, HR160 beats per minute, RR18 breaths per minute, BP 120/70, 02 saturation is 99% on room air. His lungs are clear to auscultation and there are no murmurs on cardiac exam. His extremities are warm and well perfused. Capillary refill is 2 s.

Chest pain is a common complaint prompting children and adolescents to seek medical attention [1, 2]. It causes great anxiety due to the belief that chest pain is

M. Mansour (✉)
NYU Grossman School of Medicine, New York, NY, USA
e-mail: maryann.mansour@nyulangone.org

R. P. Olympia, J. Brady-Olympia (eds.), *Clinical Considerations in School-based Health*, https://doi.org/10.1007/978-3-031-85765-2_32

usually related to cardiac causes in adults. Fortunately, most cases of pediatric chest pain are benign in nature and cardiac chest pain is rare [1]. The differential is broad and can be divided into cardiac and non-cardiac causes. Common causes of chest pain by etiology are musculoskeletal and/or idiopathic (38.7–86.3%), respiratory (1.8–12.8%), psychogenic (5.1–83.6%), gastrointestinal (0.3–9.3%), and cardiac (0.3–8.0%) [3]. Younger children are more likely to have a cardiorespiratory cause of chest pain while adolescents are more likely to have a psychogenic cause [3, 4]. A thorough history and physical exam is key to differentiate the benign from serious cases and determine which patients will need referral to an ED or activation of [Emergency Medical Services (EMS). Table 32.1 lists differentials and dispositions of chest pain using the *"CHEST PAIN"* mnemonic.

The child's general appearance, assessment of ABC's and vital signs will provide the initial information on whether or not your patient will need to be referred to the emergency department. Refer to Chap. 23 on the Pediatric Assessment Triangle for more information on initial assessment of ill children and assessing ABC's.

Once ABC's have been addressed, the patient's vital signs will help stratify the severity of the chest pain. Tachycardia, tachypnea, hypertension or oxygen desaturations are concerning for more serious causes of chest pain. However, be aware that psychogenic causes of chest pain may also cause hyperventilation, mild tachycardia [5]. EMS should be activated immediately if there are any ABC or serious vital sign abnormalities.

A thorough history will often help reveal the etiology of chest pain [4, 5]. The *"OPQRSTU"* Mnemonic used in Table 32.2 can be used to gather details about and characterize the patient's pain [6].

Chest pain that is described as crushing, radiating to jaw, shoulder or left arm is concerning for myocardial infarction and EMS should be activated immediately. Pain associated with running or exercise is more likely due to cardiac disease or exercise induced asthma [3, 7]. Chest pain after eating is more likely due to gastrointestinal disease [3].

A good review of systems will also provide important information to narrow the differential. Symptoms such as fever, fatigue, shortness of breath, syncope will alert you to patients that need more urgent care. Finally, a review of the patient's past medical history and family history will also alert you to patients that are more at risk for serious causes of chest pain. Patients with an oncology history, acquired or congenital heart disease, sickle cell disease, family history of sudden cardiac death before 40 should prompt you to consider more serious causes of chest pain. Please refer to Table 32.3 for life threatening signs and symptoms of chest pain that require EMS activation.

The chest should be visualized and inspected for bruising, swelling or asymmetry that would point to a traumatic cause of pain. Reproducible chest pain is more likely to be due to musculoskeletal pain such as costochondritis. Pneumomediastinum may present with palpable crepitus. Finally, auscultating the heart and lungs for wheezes, crackles, murmurs or frictions rubs. Children with wheezing may have relief of their chest pain once given an albuterol treatment. Inspection and palpation of the abdomen is important as abdominal pain may be radiating to the chest

Table 32.1 Differential diagnosis and disposition for student's presenting with chest pain using the "CHEST PAIN" mnemonic

	Etiology	Presenting signs and symptoms	Disposition and treatment
Chest Wall	Costochondritis Muscle strain	Pain worse with inspiration Reproducible wall tenderness No shortness of breath, URI symptoms or fevers	Reassurance Anti-inflammatory Refer to PCP
	Precordial Catch	sharp, localized stabbing pain	Refer to PCP
Heart	Coronary Ischemia	Classic left sided crushing chest pain, radiating to jaw	Activate EMS to ED
	Arrhythmias	Palpitations, Shortness of breath, Syncope, weak pulses	Activate EMS to ED
	Pericarditis	Pain worsened with laying down Pericardial rub on auscultation	Activate EMS to ED
	Hypertrophic cardiomyopathy	Syncope with exertion Murmur louder with valsalva maneuver	Activate EMS to ED
Esophageal	Esophagitis	Burning pain, pain after eating, difficulty swallowing	Refer to PCP
	Esophageal foreign body	Younger children, drooling, stridor, cough	Activate EMS to ED
"Syche"	Anxiety, Depression, hyperventilation	Palpitations, numbness and tingling of extremities	Refer to PCP or therapist If actively suicidal, homicidal or psychotic then refer to ED
Trauma	Blunt Chest Trauma	Pain for chest wall Contusions, pulmonary contusions may present with shortness of breath, tachypnea, hypoxia Cardiac contusion may present with evidence of shock	Pain control Activate EMS to ED
Pulmonary	Asthma/Reactive Airway	wheezing, retractions, difficulty speaking	Start albuterol nebulizer treatments Activate EMS to ED for respiratory distress PCP or urgent care if patient is not in respiratory distress
	Sickle Cell Acute Chest	Chest pain, fevers, shortness of breath	Pain control and Activate EMS to ED
	Pulmonary Embolism	Pleuritic chest pain, Shortness of breath, leg swelling, diaphoresis, fevers, tachycardia, tachypnea	Activate EMS to ED

(continued)

Table 32.1 (continued)

	Etiology	Presenting signs and symptoms	Disposition and treatment
	Pneumothorax	Pleuritic chest pain, tachypnea, shortness of breath	Activate EMS to ED
Abdominal	Gastritis	Sharp burning pain radiating from epigastric area to chest	Refer to PCP
Infectious	Pneumonia	Fevers, tachypnea, hypoxia, tachycardia crackles and rales	Fever and pain control Refer to urgent care or ED depending on severity
	Myocarditis	fevers, shortness of breath, chest pain, syncope, ill appearing, poorly perfused	Activate EMS to ED
	Endocarditis	Chest pain, fevers, ill appearing, poor perfusion	Activate EMS to ED
Neck	Pharyngitis, peritonsillar abscess, retropharyngeal abscess	Referred pain from neck, sore throat, fevers, drooling, neck stiffness	Fever and pain control Refer to ED or Activate EMS if patient is toxic or in respiratory distress

Abbreviations: *ED* emergency department, *EMS* emergency medical services, *PCP* primary care provider

Table 32.2 Assessment of pain using the "OPQRSTU" Mnemonic

Onset	When did the pain start?
Provocation	What makes pain better or worse?
Quality	Description of pain such as crushing, stabbing, burning?
Region and Radiation	Where is the pain? Does it travel anywhere?
Severity	How severe is the pain on a scale of 1–10? Younger children can use Wong Baker Faces scale for pain
Timing	When did the pain start? Is it worsening or improving? Have medications helped
Understanding	What do you believe is causing the pain?

causing referred pain. Epigastric pain is more likely to be a gastrointestinal cause of chest pain [4].

If the pain is deemed benign or musculoskeletal the patient may be treated with over the counter pain medicine and reassurance. Patients with concerning findings as described in Table 32.3 should be referred to an emergency department.

Table 32.3 Life threatening presentations of chest pain requiring immediate EMS transport

Patients who received CPR
Significant Vital Sign abnormalities
Signs of respiratory distress: retractions, grunting, nasal flaring, inability to speak full sentences, decreased breath sounds
Significant trauma to chest
Drug use such as Cocaine or amphetamines
Syncope with exertion
Chest pain with exertion
Severe pleuritic chest pain
History of heart disease, cardiac surgery or arrhythmias
Family history of early sudden death or early cardiac death <35 years of age
History of sickle cell disease, hypercoagulable state or hypercholesterolemia
Severe abdominal pain
Altered mental status

32.1 Case Resolutions

Case 1 Chelsea is experiencing costochondritis, a musculoskeletal cause of chest pain. It is a benign and often temporary inflammation of the cartilage that joins the ribs to the sternum. Chest pain due to musculoskeletal causes is usually sharp, brief and worsened by deep inspiration. It is often reproducible upon palpation of the chest wall. Please refer to Table 32.1 lists common causes of musculoskeletal chest pain.

She is given a dose of weight-based ibuprofen and observed in your office. She feels better after observation and is able to go back to class. You let her parents know so they can follow up with her pediatrician.

Case 2 You activate EMS who transport Ryan to the emergency department. A Chest X-ray shows a small, left sided pneumothorax. He is observed overnight for progression of symptoms. Since his pneumothorax remains stable, he does not have dyspnea or oxygen requirement. He is discharged to home the next day. Pneumothorax is gas in the pleural space. This air in the pleural space causes equalization of atmospheric and pleural space that leads to collapse of the lung. Spontaneous pneumothorax usually presents suddenly at rest but may occur with exertion. It typically affects individuals with tall, thin body habitus. The level of dyspnea and work of breathing will depend on the size of the pneumothorax. Most pneumothoraces are treated with conservative measures. However, larger pneumothoraces may need chest tube placement.

Case 3 You give Jason a dose of acetaminophen for his fever and call his father who takes him to an urgent care. Urgent care finds he is persistently tachycardic despite fever control. A chest x-ray shows mild cardiomegaly and EKG showed tachycardia with ST segment changes. He was promptly transferred to an emergency room where a diagnosis of myocarditis was made after he was found to have elevated troponins and decreased cardiac function on echocardiogram. Myocarditis can present very subtly and usually due to viral illness in children. There should be a higher index of suspicion if tachycardia persists despite fever and pain control. He was admitted to pediatric ICU for continuous cardiorespiratory monitoring. He is managed with oral diuretics and ACE inhibitors. He eventually makes a full recovery and is discharged home after 1 week.

Extra Credit Points

1. Pediatric chest pain is usually due to musculoskeletal or idiopathic causes. Cardiac chest pain is rare in children
2. Younger children are more likely to have a cardiorespiratory cause of chest pain
3. Adolescents are more likely to have psychogenic chest pain
4. A through history and physical will often help make the diagnosis of chest pain

References

1. Aygun E, Aygun ST, Uysal T, Aygun F, Dursun H, Irdem A. Aetiological evaluation of chest pain in childhood and adolescence. Cardiol Young. 2020;30(5):617–23. https://doi.org/10.1017/S1047951120000621.
2. Chen L, Duan H, Li X, et al. The causes of chest pain in children and the criteria for targeted myocardial enzyme testing in identifying the causes of chest pain in children. Front Cardiovasc Med. 2021;8:582129. https://doi.org/10.3389/fcvm.2021.582129.
3. Huang SW, Liu YK. Pediatric chest pain: a review of diagnostic tools in the pediatric emergency department. Diagnostics. 2024;14(5):526. https://doi.org/10.3390/diagnostics14050526.
4. Barbut G, Needleman JP. Pediatric chest pain. Pediatr Rev. 2020;41(9):469–80. https://doi.org/10.1542/pir.2019-0058.
5. Sumski CA, Goot BH. Evaluating chest pain and heart murmurs in pediatric and adolescent patients. Pediatr Clin N Am. 2020;67(5):783–99. https://doi.org/10.1016/j.pcl.2020.05.003.
6. Gay T, Olympia RP. Distress in my chest: the approach to a student presenting with "chest pain". NASN Sch Nurse. 2018;33(6):366–71. https://doi.org/10.1177/1942602X18789257.
7. Statuta SM, Barnes ES, MacKnight JM. Non-cardiac conditions that mimic cardiac symptoms in athletes. Clin Sports Med. 2022;41(3):389–404. https://doi.org/10.1016/j.csm.2022.02.003.

Chapter 33
Abdominal Pain

William Bruno

You are the school nurse on a busy Monday morning, and 6 students present to your office with the following presentations (Table 33.1).

Abdominal pain can affect children of all ages, with between 10–20% of children experiencing recurrent pain. Abdominal pain can significantly impact academic performance, attendance, and overall well-being, making it critically important for school-aged patients [1].

The historical roots of understanding abdominal pain can be traced back to ancient Greece, where prominent figures like Aristotle and Hippocrates made significant contributions to medical knowledge. Aristotle's anatomical observations laid the groundwork for understanding human physiology, while Hippocrates, often regarded as the "Father of Medicine," emphasized the importance of clinical observation and detailed case histories in diagnosing and treating abdominal disorders. These foundational principles continue to influence modern medical practices and are particularly relevant in the school setting, where careful assessment and timely intervention are crucial [2].

For descriptive purposes, the abdomen is generally divided into either four quadrants (left upper, right upper, left lower, and right lower), or into nine regions for greater specificity. Below are the nine regions with associated etiologies of pain (Table 33.2) as well as a photo illustrating the regions (Fig. 33.1).

Screening, Recognition, and Diagnosis

- Obtain a detailed medical history, including onset, duration, frequency, and nature of the pain, utilizing the SOCRATES method (Table 33.3). Inquire about associated symptoms such as nausea, vomiting, diarrhea, constipation, and fever [1]. Explore any recent dietary changes, stressors, or family history of

W. Bruno (✉)
Penn State Health Hershey Medical Center, Hershey, PA, USA
e-mail: william.bruno17@houghton.edu

R. P. Olympia, J. Brady-Olympia (eds.), *Clinical Considerations in School-based Health*, https://doi.org/10.1007/978-3-031-85765-2_33

Table 33.1 Abdominal pain cases

Case 1	• Presentation: A 12-year-old boy reports acute right lower quadrant pain, fever, and nausea. • General Appearance: The patient appears pale and in distress. • Vital Signs: Temperature: 38.5 °C (101.3 °F), Heart rate: 110 bpm, Blood pressure: 100/60 mmHg. • Movement: The patient has a hard time moving around the room and is reluctant to jump up and down. • Rebound/Guarding: Positive rebound tenderness and guarding noted on examination. • Assessment: Physical examination reveals significant tenderness in the lower right abdomen
Case 2	• Presentation: A 13-year-old girl presents with sudden, severe lower abdominal pain, mainly on the right side. • General Appearance: The patient is in significant pain and has a distressed appearance. • Vital Signs: Temperature: 37.5 °C (99.5 °F), Heart rate: 120 bpm, Blood pressure: 105/65 mmHg. • Movement: The patient is having a hard time moving around the room and avoids jumping. • Rebound/Guarding: Guarding is present, and there is significant rebound tenderness. • Assessment: Palpation of the abdomen shows marked tenderness in the right lower quadrant.
Case 3	• Presentation: A 14-year-old boy presents with acute lower abdominal pain and scrotal swelling. • General Appearance: The patient appears anxious and is holding his abdomen. • Vital Signs: Temperature: 37.2 °C (99 °F), Heart rate: 115 bpm, Blood pressure: 100/60 mmHg. • Movement: The patient is unable to move around comfortably and refuses to jump. • Rebound/Guarding: Guarding is noted, but rebound tenderness is less prominent. • Assessment: Examination reveals swollen, tender testicle with high-riding appearance.
Case 4	• Presentation: A 4-year-old boy presents with intermittent, severe abdominal pain, and recent history of sore throat. • General Appearance: The patient is pale and lethargic between pain episodes. • Vital Signs: Temperature: 38 °C (100.4 °F), Heart rate: 130 bpm, Blood pressure: 90/50 mmHg. • Movement: The child has difficulty moving around and cries when asked to jump. • Rebound/Guarding: Rebound tenderness is present, and guarding is observed. • Assessment: Palpation reveals a sausage-shaped mass in the right upper quadrant.
Case 5	• Presentation: A 10-year-old girl presents with lower abdominal pain, dysuria, and fever. • General Appearance: The patient appears uncomfortable and febrile. • Vital Signs: Temperature: 38.8 °C (101.8 °F), Heart rate: 105 bpm, Blood pressure: 95/55 mmHg. • Movement: The patient is reluctant to move around and experiences pain with jumping. • Rebound/Guarding: Guarding is present, but there is no significant rebound tenderness. • Assessment: Abdominal examination shows tenderness in the lower abdomen and costovertebral angle.

(continued)

Table 33.1 (continued)

Case 6	• Presentation: A 7-year-old girl complains of lower abdominal pain and infrequent bowel movements. • General Appearance: The patient appears uncomfortable but not in acute distress. • Vital Signs: Temperature: 37.2 °C (99 °F), Heart rate: 90 bpm, Blood pressure: 105/65 mmHg. • Movement: The patient is able to move around but complains of discomfort when jumping. • Rebound/Guarding: Mild guarding is present, but no rebound tenderness. • Assessment: Examination reveals a distended abdomen with some tenderness.

Table 33.2 Nine regions of the abdomen with associated etiologies of pain

Abdominal region	Etiology of pain
Right Hypochondrium	Gallbladder disease (cholecystitis, gallstones), liver diseases (hepatitis, liver abscess), pleuritis or pneumonia of the lower right lung
Epigastrium	Peptic ulcer disease, gastritis, pancreatitis, myocardial infarction, esophagitis or GERD (gastroesophageal reflux disease)
Left Hypochondrium	Spleen conditions (splenomegaly, splenic infarct), pleuritis or pneumonia of the lower left lung, gastric ulcers
Right Lumbar (or Right Lateral)	Kidney stones or infection (pyelonephritis), ureteric colic, lumbar hernia
Umbilical	Small intestine issues (obstruction, Crohn's disease), early appendicitis, aortic aneurysm, pancreatitis
Left Lumbar (or Left Lateral)	Kidney stones or infection (pyelonephritis), ureteric colic, lumbar hernia
Right Iliac (or Right Inguinal)	Appendicitis, cecal diverticulitis, ovarian cysts or torsion, ectopic pregnancy
Hypogastrium	Urinary bladder issues (cystitis), uterine conditions (fibroids, pregnancy), prostatitis, inflammatory bowel disease
Left Iliac (or Left Inguinal)	Sigmoid diverticulitis, ovarian cysts or torsion, ectopic pregnancy, hernia

gastrointestinal disorders. Review general past medical history (PMH), previous surgeries, current medications, and allergies.

- Conduct a thorough physical examination, starting off with general appearance, vital signs, and positioning of the student (writhing in pain, wanting to stay as still as possible, unable to walk). Remember that cardiac and respiratory problems, as well as dehydration, can present with abdominal pain, so focus on these examination elements. Lastly, perform an abdominal examination (Table 33.4), focusing on the nine regions of the abdomen.
- Based on your initial assessment, formulate a differential diagnosis, utilizing the mnemonic "ABDOMINAL PAINS HURT" (Table 33.5).
- Red flags for a student presenting with abdominal pain that requires immediate transport to an Emergency Department include:
  - Debilitating or escalating pain with inability to walk or jump
  - Abdominal pain localized to the right lower quadrant

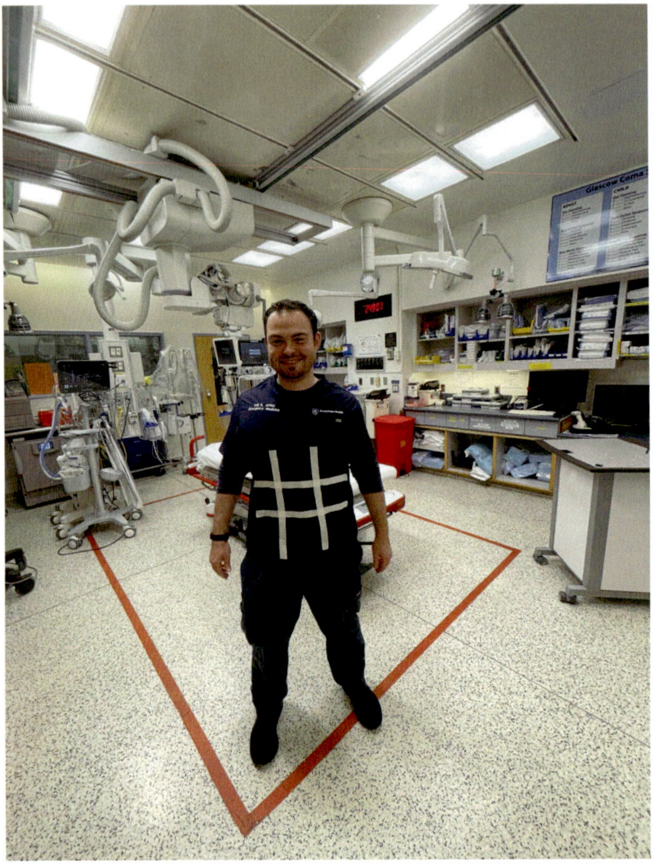

Fig. 33.1 William Bruno demonstrating the nine regions of the abdomen

- Persistent vomiting.
- Hematemesis (vomiting blood).
- Hematochezia (blood in stool).
- Signs of significant dehydration (skin tenting, dry mucus membranes).
- Abdominal distension with tenderness.
- Concern for testicular or ovarian process
- Pregnancy related abdominal pain

For non-emergent cases of abdominal pain, initial management includes reassurance, hydration, dietary modifications, and over-the-counter pain relief if appropriate. School nurses should provide education and counseling to both the child and caregivers about potential abdominal pain triggers and necessary lifestyle modifications. Encouraging regular bowel habits, a balanced fiber-rich diet, and adequate hydration is essential. It is important to monitor symptoms closely and provide follow-up care as needed. Students and caregivers should be advised to keep detailed

Table 33.3 Medical History: SOCRATES mnemonic

	Questions to ask
Site	■ Where did the pain start? ■ Where is the pain now? ■ Where does it hurt the most? □ "Point with one finger"
Onset	■ When did the pain start? ■ Was it sudden or gradual?
Character	■ What is the pain like? ■ Sharp or stabbing? □ Obstruction or infarction ■ Dull or pressure?
Radiation	■ Does the pain go anywhere? □ Kehr's sign □ Epigastric □ Flank to groin
Association	■ Fever ■ Headache ■ Sore throat ■ Cough or SOB or Chest pain ■ Change in appetite ■ Nausea/vomiting (bilious?) ■ Diarrhea/constipation/bloody stool ■ Urinary or vaginal symptoms ■ Weight loss ■ Rashes ■ Joint pain or swelling
Time Course	■ Does the pain follow any pattern? ■ Constant ■ Intermittent—"colicky" ■ Does the pain ever completely go away?
Exacerbating/ relieving factors	■ Does anything change the pain? ■ Make the pain better? ■ Make the pain worse? ■ Medications? ■ Associated with meals? ■ Associated with BMs? ■ Associated with menstrual cycles?
Severity	■ Age-appropriate pain scale such as identifying which face they feel fits their current condition, or, if old enough, rating pain on a 1–10 scale.

records of pain episodes, interventions, and outcomes. Ensuring the student has a pediatric primary care provider for follow-up is also crucial. Collaboration with pediatricians, urologists, gastroenterologists, and mental health professionals can ensure comprehensive care. Timely referrals for persistent or severe cases should be made to appropriate specialists, as necessary, to prevent complications and ensure proper management [3].

Innovations such as telehealth can increase access to specialist consultations via telehealth platforms, improving the speed and accuracy of diagnosis and treatment.

Table 33.4 Key elements of the physical examination in a student presenting with abdominal pain

Abdomen examination	Signs
Inspection • Distension • Skin exam (hives, petechiae/purpura) • Ecchymosis • Abrasions • Lacerations	Murphy's Murphy's sign is a clinical test for cholecystitis, where pain and interruption of deep inspiration upon palpation of the RUQ suggest inflammation of the gallbladder.
Palpation • Tenderness • Guarding • Rebound • Soft vs. Rigid • Hepatosplenomegaly	Rovsing's Rovsing's sign is a diagnostic indication of appendicitis, where pain in the RLQ is elicited by applying and then releasing pressure in the LLQ, suggesting referred pain from an inflamed appendix.
Percussion Dullness, tympany, or resonance	Obturator's Obturator's sign is a clinical indication of appendicitis, where pain is elicited by internal rotation of the right hip, pointing to inflammation involving the obturator internus muscle.
	Psoas' The patient lies on their left side, and the right thigh is extended backward. Pain elicited in the right lower quadrant (RLQ) during this maneuver suggests irritation of the psoas muscle due to an inflamed appendix, indicating appendicitis.
	Modified J-Up Test Ability to perform 10 jumping jacks can help rule out appendicitis

Wearable technology can be used to monitor hydration and physiological parameters, providing real-time data that can help in the management of abdominal pain. Enhanced training for school nurses in pediatric gastroenterology through educational programs will equip them with the necessary skills to manage these cases effectively. Ongoing research includes studies on the effectiveness of school-based interventions for managing functional abdominal pain and the impact of stress reduction programs on psychosomatic abdominal pain [4, 5].

Table 33.5 Common causes of abdominal pain: ABDOMINAL PAINS HURT mnemonic

	Condition	Key symptoms
A	Appendicitis	Right lower quadrant pain, fever, nausea
B	Blockage (Constipation)	Lower abdominal pain, infrequent bowel movements
D	Dehydration	Abdominal discomfort, dry mouth, decreased urine
O	Ovarian Cyst/Torsion	Acute lower abdominal pain, often unilateral
M	Migraine (Atypical/Abdominal)	Severe abdominal pain, no clear GI cause
I	Injury (Musculoskeletal, Intra-Abdominal)	Pain depending on injury location
N	Nausea/Vomiting/Diarrhea (Gastroenteritis)	Acute pain, diarrhea, vomiting
A	Allergies/Anaphylaxis	Abdominal pain with systemic symptoms
L	Lipase (Pancreatitis)	Upper abdominal pain radiating to the back
P	Pregnancy	Consider in female adolescents of reproductive age with abdominal pain
A	Anxiety/Stress	Abdominal pain related to psychological factors
I	Inflammation (GERD, Gastritis, IBD)	Chronic or recurrent pain
N	Neoplasms	Rare in children, but tumors can cause abdominal pain
S	Stones (Gallbladder, Renal)	Severe, acute abdominal pain
H	Hepatosplenomegaly	Pain from enlarged liver or spleen
U	Urinary or Genital Tract Infections	Pain with urinary symptoms
R	Referred Pain	Pain from other conditions like pharyngitis
T	Testicular Torsion and Others	Acute scrotal pain, sometimes referred

Case resolutions utilizing the SOCRATES method.

SOCRATES Element	Case #1	Case #2	Case #3
Site	Right lower quadrant	Right lower quadrant	Lower abdomen and scrotum
Onset	Acute	Sudden	Acute
Character	Sharp, constant	Sharp, severe	Sharp, severe
Radiation	None	None	Radiates to groin
Association	Nausea, fever	None	Scrotal swelling
Time Course	Progressive	Sudden onset, persistent	Sudden onset, persistent
Exacerbating/Relieving Factors	Movement exacerbates	Movement exacerbates	Movement exacerbates
Severity	Severe	Severe	Severe
Case Resolution: diagnosis and disposition	Appendicitis, emergency surgery	Ovarian torsion, gynecological evaluation	Testicular torsion, urological evaluation and surgery

(continued)

SOCRATES Element	Case #4	Case #5	Case #6
Site	Generalized, right upper quadrant	Lower abdomen	Lower abdomen
Onset	Intermittent	Gradual	Gradual
Character	Cramping	Dull, aching	Dull, cramping
Radiation	None	None	None
Association	Recent sore throat	Dysuria, fever	Infrequent bowel movements
Time Course	Intermittent, worsening	Persistent, worsening	Persistent
Exacerbating/ Relieving Factors	Movement exacerbates	Urination exacerbates	None
Severity	Severe	Moderate	Moderate
Case Resolution: diagnosis and disposition	Intussusception, emergency radiological evaluation	Pyelonephritis, antibiotic therapy	Constipation, dietary and hydration management

Extra-Credit Points

1. Always consider appendicitis in cases of acute right lower quadrant pain.
2. Educate students and caregivers on hydration and regular bowel habits.
3. Be vigilant for red flags that necessitate immediate medical referral.
4. Collaboration with healthcare providers is crucial for comprehensive care.
5. Utilize telehealth resources to enhance access to specialist care.

References

1. Bandyopadhyay A, Kanti Mondal P. Recurrent abdominal pain in children and adolescents: a hospital-based study. Int J Contemp Pediatr. 2017;4(3):726–8.
2. Sánchez I, Swain S. Chapter 4 Greek physicians to whom hippocrates transmitted the art of medicine. A literary history of medicine. Leiden: Brill; 2019. p. 63–188.
3. Santucci N, Chogle A, Leiby A, et al. Non-pharmacologic approach to pediatric constipation. Complement Ther Med. 2021:59.
4. Goddard A, Sullivan E, Fields P, et al. The future of telehealth in school-based health centers: lessons from COVID-19. J Pediatr Health Care. 2021;35:304–9.
5. Cozzi G, Lucarelli A, Borrometi F, et al. How to recognize and manage psychosomatic pain in the pediatric emergency department. Ital J Pediatr. 2021;47:74.

Chapter 34
Limp

Nicholas A. Roberts and Joseph A. Gehrz

Case 1 A 7-year-old student, Jessica, presents to the nurse with a limp and significant pain in her right knee. She started feeling generally unwell yesterday but was able to walk onto the bus this morning. Now, after sitting down in class all morning with worsening pain in her right knee, she cannot put weight on the right leg to walk to lunch. She has a temperature of 102.4 °F and on examination, there is marked swelling, erythema, and warmth over the right knee joint. Jessica is unable to bear weight on the affected leg and cries when attempting to move the knee.

Limp is defined as an abnormal gait caused by pain, weakness, or deformity [1]. A common complaint encountered by school nurses, limping can result from musculoskeletal, neurologic, infectious, inflammatory, or referred conditions [2]. Any child with joint pain requires a Look-Feel-Move exam (Table 34.1) [1–5]. Visual inspection can identify infection or inflammation, rashes or petechiae indicating systemic infection, or evidence of trauma. Palpation of the affected extremity and referred pain sites can reveal focal tenderness and identify neurovascular issues. Lastly, range the joint through its full motion arc both passively by moving the extremity and actively by having the patient move it; pain on active and not passive motion suggests soft tissue involvement while pain on both suggests joint space involvement. Also, keep in mind that hip pathology can manifest as pain in the anterior thigh, knee, or medial upper leg.

Case 1 Conclusion Jessica should be transferred emergently to a healthcare facility for further evaluation, joint aspiration, and initiation of intravenous antibiotics due to a concern for septic arthritis (Chap. 93). Septic arthritis is an acute bacterial infection of a joint which most commonly affects large joints such as the knees and hips. The classic clinical features include fever, severe joint pain, swell-

N. A. Roberts · J. A. Gehrz (✉)
Naval Medical Center San Diego, San Diego, CA, USA
e-mail: nicholas.a.roberts40.mil@health.mil; joseph.a.gehrz.mil@health.mil

R. P. Olympia, J. Brady-Olympia (eds.), *Clinical Considerations in School-based Health*, https://doi.org/10.1007/978-3-031-85765-2_34

Table 34.1 The Look-Feel-Move exam

<table>
<tr><td rowspan="3">Look</td><td colspan="4">Examine the child and the affected extremity for signs of:</td><td>Red Flags</td></tr>
<tr><td>Systemic Infection*</td><td colspan="2">Focal Infection*</td><td>Trauma</td><td rowspan="8">Acute onset
Fever
Limp >7 days
Nocturnal pain
Weight loss
Diffuse Rash
Refusal to bear weight
Presence of any of the above requires Emergency Department evaluation</td></tr>
<tr><td>– Diaphoretic, Fever
– Diffuse Rash
– Petechiae</td><td colspan="2">– Red swollen skin or joints
– Spreading redness
– Blisters or pustules</td><td>– Bruising, Swelling
– Deformities
– Skin injuries</td></tr>
<tr><td rowspan="4">Feel</td><td colspan="4">• Assess all extremities for sensation, motor, and pulses.
• Palpate referred pain sites: Back, Abdomen, Groin (see Table 34.7)</td></tr>
<tr><td colspan="4">Palpate extremities for focal areas of pain indicating:</td></tr>
<tr><td>Joints</td><td colspan="2">Long Bones</td><td>Soft Tissue</td></tr>
<tr><td>• Joint infection
• Intra-articular fracture
• Ligament/ tendon injury
• Cartilage injury</td><td colspan="2">• Fracture
• Bone infection
• Periostitis "bone bruise"</td><td>• Cellulitis
• Abscess
• Soft tissue injury
• Hematomas</td></tr>
<tr><td rowspan="3">Move</td><td colspan="4">Fully range all joints through both active and passive range of motion:</td></tr>
<tr><td>Shoulders + Hips
• Flex, Extend
• Adduct, Abduct
• Rotate: In/ external</td><td>Elbows
• Flex, Extend
• Pronate
• Supinate</td><td>Knees
• Flex, Extend
• Stress laterally and medially</td><td>Wrists + Ankles
• Flex, Extend
• Rotate: Internal and external</td></tr>
<tr><td colspan="4">See Table 34.6 for provocative tests of specific joints</td><td></td></tr>
</table>

ing, erythema, warmth, and limited range of motion. Prompt recognition and intervention are essential to prevent complications such as joint destruction and systemic spread of infection [3]. Septic arthritis can be confused with transient synovitis, and the Kocher criteria have been developed to help make this distinction (Table 34.2). Transient synovitis is a common, non-infectious, inflammatory process involving the hip joint synovium in young (3–10 years old) children. Though its etiology is poorly understood, it is frequently seen following a recent upper respiratory infection [6]. As it can present similarly to septic arthritis with fever and joint pain, the diagnosis of transient synovitis should only be made after X-ray, ultrasound, and laboratory studies including CBC with differential, ESR, and CRP have adequately decreased concern for septic arthritis (Fig. 34.1). These patients may have low-grade fevers and joint pain but less commonly have swelling, redness, and severe pain on passive range of motion seen in septic arthritis. Another disease process on the differential diagnosis of a student with joint pain, swelling and warmth is osteomyelitis (Chap. 93), a serious infection of long bones with fevers, redness, and bony tenderness that requires emergent evaluation and treatment in the hospital setting [7].

Table 34.2 Kocher criteria for prediction of pediatric septic arthritis

Kocher criteria	Probability of septic arthritis
Fever >38.5	4/4 = 99%
Unable to Bear Weight	3/4 = 93%
WBC > 12	2/4 = 40%
ESR > 40	1/4 = 3%

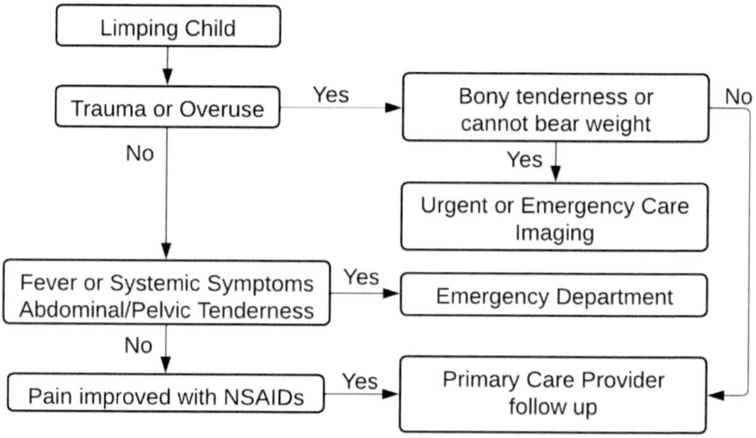

Fig. 34.1 Disposition of the limping child

Case 2 Emma, a 10-year-old student, presents to the school nurse limping with abrasions to her hands and left knee after falling at recess. She reports she was running down the sidewalk and tripped off the curb, falling onto the pavement. Cleaning the left knee, she only has mild tenderness on her abrasions. Palpating the rest of the extremity, she has exquisite point tenderness overlying her fifth metatarsal head on her lateral foot. She can bear weight but flinches while trying to ambulate.

In children presenting after traumatic injury, examine the entire extremity, using the Look-Feel-Move exam to identify injuries. Limping patients who can walk, have no systemic symptoms, and whose pain is non-focal and improves with oral analgesia can follow up with a primary care provider (Fig. 34.1) [5]. If a fracture is suspected based on examination, ensure the extremity is neurovascularly intact by checking pulses, capillary refill, and sensation throughout the entire extremity and especially distally. Compartment syndrome (any combination of the 6 P's: pain, paresthesias, poikilothermia, pallor, paralysis, and pulselessness) should prompt immediate transport to an emergency department. Management of suspected fractures in the school-based setting should focus on splinting unstable bones or joints, analgesia, and arranging for the child to be evaluated urgently with imaging in an urgent care setting or emergency department.

Table 34.3 Traumatic extremity orthopedic injuries [8]

Definition	Findings	Management
Sprain Ligament tear	Tenderness or laxity of a joint. Laxity correlates with severity. Swelling and bruising common.	Ice, compression, and NSAIDs, then early mobility as tolerated. Severe sprain may require surgery.
Strain Muscle tear	Pain on movement with contraction of muscle. Severe strains will have bruising and tenderness.	Ice and NSAIDs with return to mobility as tolerated.
Dislocation[a] Displacement of a bone from a joint.	Obvious deformity to a joint with restriction and pain on passive or active joint range of motion.	Rapid reduction if possible, hospital management if not. Imaging post-reduction to evaluate for concurrent fracture.
Fracture[a] Disruption of the bone cortex.	Tenderness on palpation of fracture site. Swelling and bruising. Displaced fractures have obvious deformity. Open fractures have overlying skin injury.	Pain control. Imaging at Urgent Care or Emergency Care. Displaced or open fractures require emergency evaluation.

[a]Fractures and dislocations require a neurovascular exam. Any deficits require emergent management

Assessment of a child with traumatic extremity injuries should prompt consideration of sprains, strains, dislocations, and fractures in the differential diagnosis (Tables 34.3 and 34.4). A thorough extremity exam and application of the Ottawa Rules (Table 34.5) can identify injuries requiring imaging. Individual joints can be further assessed with provocative tests (Table 34.6).

Case 2 Conclusion Emma has a fifth metatarsal head fracture from stepping awkwardly off a curb. Her fall produced skin injuries which can distract from underlying fractures, so make sure you utilize the Look-Feel-Move examination to identify injuries that may be subtle.

Case 3 A 7-year-old boy, Javier, limps into the exam room complaining of pain in his right hip while walking. He also “doesn’t feel well” and did not eat his lunch. On his exam he is afebrile and complains of hip pain worse when extending his right hip on passive and active range of motion. Pressing around the hip, he has pain on palpation of the abdominal soft tissues superior to the inguinal ligament.

Case 3 Conclusion Javier presents with psoas muscle pain due to a retrocecal appendix, and his exam is concerning for appendicitis (Chap. 91). Appendicitis and testicular or ovarian torsion are two surgical emergencies which can mimic joint pain, though torsions are often exquisitely more painful. His systemic symptoms would suggest this is more than a musculoskeletal cause of hip pain, and a thorough Look-Feel-Move exam will uncover the location of his tenderness. Similar referred pain syndromes that may present as limp are covered in Table 34.7. Comparing pain on active and passive range of motion can uncover the actual source of pain and localize the exam.

Table 34.4 Common pediatric long bone fracture patterns

Fracture		Management[a]
Salter Harris Fractures (Fractures of the Physeal Plate)	Type 1: fracture through the physis	Immobilization. Orthopedic evaluation within 5 days
	Type 2: metaphysis and physis fracture	Immobilization. Orthopedic evaluation within 5 days
	Type 3: epiphysis and physis fracture	Immobilization. ED for Orthopedic evaluation.
	Type 4: fracture of the metaphysis, physis, and epiphysis	Immobilization. ED for Orthopedic evaluation.
	Type 5: physis compression fracture	Frequently missed. Immobilization. ED for Orthopedic evaluation.
Torus "Buckle"	Compression of the bony cortex	Immobilization. Orthopedic evaluation within 5 days
Greenstick	Partial thickness fracture involving only one side of the bony cortex	Immobilization. Orthopedic evaluation within 5 days
Transverse "Complete"	Fracture of the complete bony cortex. Angulation: distal fragment tilted off the axis of proximal bone Displacement: fracture resulting in loss of axial alignment	Reduce and immobilize. Requires orthopedic evaluation. Management dependent on alignment and displacement.
Comminuted	Multiple bone fragments	Immobilization. ED for Orthopedic evaluation.

a. All obviously deformed fractures should be evaluated in the Emergency Department (ED)

Table 34.5 Ottawa rules for identifying injuries requiring imaging

Ottawa Knee Rules	• Isolated patellar tenderness • Inability to flex knee to 90° • Inability to bear weight
Ottawa Ankle Rules	• Bony tenderness in the distal 6 cm of the lateral or medial malleolus • Inability to bear weight
Ottawa Foot Rules	• Point tenderness at the fifth metatarsal base • Point tenderness of the navicular • Inability to bear weight

Table 34.6 Provocative testing of the lower extremity [8]

	Test	Brief description	Disposition
Back	Straight Leg Raise	Assess for sciatic nerve root impingement. Lift the supine patient's leg while keeping the knee straight. Pain radiating down the leg is positive.	Primary Care NSAIDs
Hip	FABER	Assess for sacroiliac or hip joint pathology. Supine patient, flex and abduct and externally rotate the hip, crossing the ankle over the opposite knee.	Orthopedic evaluation NSAIDs
	Trendelenburg	Assess for hip abductor and gluteus weakness. The patient stands on one leg while the examiner observes for pelvic drop on the opposite side.	Primary Care
	Passive Range of Motion	Assess for septic arthritis or slipped capital femoral epiphysis. Passively move the hip joint through its full ROM. Pain or restriction suggests hip joint pathology.	Orthopedic evaluation
Knee	Varus + Valgus Stress	Assess for LCL/MCL injury. Knee held in slight flexion with varus/valgus stress placed on the knee joint. Laxity compared to uninjured side indicates injury.	Emergency department for orthopedic evaluation
	Anterior/ Posterior Drawer	Assess for ACL (anterior) and PCL (posterior) injury. Stabilize femur, flex knee to 90°, and apply anterior/posterior traction to tibia. Increased translation indicates injury.	Emergency department for orthopedic evaluation
	McMurray and Apley	Assess for meniscal tears. Flex knee and rotate while extending; or prone patient, flex knee to 90° and axially load and rotate the tibia. Pain indicates injury.	Orthopedic evaluation
Lower Leg	Squeeze	Assess for ankle syndesmosis sprain. At the midcalf, compress the tibia and fibula. Pain at the anterior ankle indicates ankle syndesmosis sprain.	Primary Care or Urgent Care NSAIDs
	Axial Torsion	Assess for tibia fracture in toddlers. Stabilize the knee, grasp the ankle, and internally and externally rotate the lower leg. Tibia pain indicates fracture.	Orthopedic evaluation
	Thompson	Assess for Achilles tendon rupture. Prone patient with feet off a table, squeeze the calf. Lack of plantarflexion of foot is positive.	Orthopedic evaluation
Ankle	Anterior and Posterior Drawer	Assess for ankle ligament instability. Stabilize the lower leg and pull foot anteriorly. Increased laxity indicates ligamentous injury.	Primary Care or Urgent Care
	Medial and Lateral Glide	Assess for medial and lateral ligament injury. Apply medial or lateral force to the forefoot. Increased translation indicates injury.	Primary Care or Urgent Care

ROM range of motion, *LCL* lateral collateral ligament, *MCL* medial collateral ligament, *ACL* anterior collateral ligament, *PCL* posterior collateral ligament, *Ant* anterior, *Post* posterior

Table 34.7 Referred Pain Syndromes Causing Limp [1, 4, 5, 9]

		Presentation	Treatment
Back Pain	Spinal Nerve Compression	Electric pain radiating into the buttock causing pain on walking.	Primary Care NSAIDs
	Spinal Cord Compression	Spinal pain + leg weakness or pain	Emergency
	Discitis	Spinal point tenderness, refusal to move back	Emergency
	Epidural Abscess	Spinal point tenderness, fever.	Emergency
	Muscular Pain	Muscle syndromes resulting in compression of nerves to the leg i.e. Piriformis Syndrome	Primary Care and NSAIDs
	Psoas Abscess	Pain on hip extension, tenderness, +/− fever	Emergency
Abdominal Pain	Appendicitis	Abdominal tenderness, anorexia	Emergency
	Inguinal Hernia	Pain in testicle or inguinal canal worsened with exertion or lower extremity movement.	Primary care
	Torso Muscle Strain	Torso muscle tenderness on movement.	NSAIDs
Pelvic or Groin Pain	Testicular Torsion	Abdominal or testicular tenderness/ swelling with pain worsened by movement.	Emergency
	Ovarian Torsion or Cyst	Pelvic tenderness with pain or lower extremity movement.	Emergency
	Pelvic Inflammatory Disease	Gradually worsening pelvic pain and tenderness exacerbated with leg movement.	Emergency
Thigh or Knee Pain	Hip and Pelvis Injury	Complaints of thigh/knee pain but with tenderness only over the hip joint.	Emergency

Extra-Credit Points

1. Limping children should be evaluated for systemic symptoms and then assessed with a "look, feel, move" exam on the entire affected extremity. Any child who is refusing to bear weight on an extremity should be referred for further evaluation and testing.
2. Always evaluate for systemic symptoms. Fever and acute joint pain should prompt close examination of the entire affected extremity and rapid referral to a higher level of care.
3. Trauma is the most common cause of joint pain and limps. Always assess for neurovascular status. Use provocative testing to identify injuries and their severity.
4. Always consider referred pain in limping children and perform a thorough physical examination.
5. "AMBULATION – DYSFUNCTION" is a mnemonic you can use to determine etiologies of pediatric limp (Table 34.8)

Table 34.8 Mnemonic for etiologies of pediatric limp [1, 4, 5, 9]

A	Arthritis	Fever + joint pain (Chap. 93)
M	Myositis	Fever + muscle pain
B	Bone infection	Fever + bony tenderness (Chap. 93)
U	Urinary	Dysuria, hematuria, and/or flank pain (Chap. 92)
L	Laceration	Dermatologic trauma (Chap. 36)
A	Appendicitis	Abdominal tenderness and anorexia (Chap. 91)
T	Toxic synovitis	(see Case #1)
I	Inguinal	Hernia or inguinal lymphadenopathy
O	Obstruction	Constipation (Chap. 44)
N	Neoplasm	Weight loss or unexplained fracture. Common malignancies: Ewings Sarcoma, osteosarcoma, leukemia (Chap. 41)
D	Dislocation	Joint dislocation or subluxation
Y	EpiphYsis (SCFE)	Slipped capital femoral epiphysis (SCFE). Adolescents.
S	Soft tissue	Sprains or strain
F	Foreign body	Examine for splinters, etc.
U	Urologic	Testicular (male) or Pelvic (female) tenderness
N	Necrotizing fasciitis	Exquisite tenderness overlying skin infection
C	Cellulitis/ Abscess	Tenderness and erythema of the skin (Chap. 96)
T	Traumatic fractures	Bony tenderness
I	Inflammation	Fevers or joint pains, rheumatologic history. Vasculitis (Chap. 54)
O	Overuse injuries	Common etiologies: Osgood Schlatter, Osteochondritis dissecans, stress fracture, jumper's knee, chondromalacia patella (Chap. 118)
N	Necrosis	Avascular necrosis of the femoral head

References

1. Herman MJ, Martinek M. The limping child. Pediatr Rev. 2015;36:184–95. quiz 196–187
2. Duey-Holtz AD, Collins SL, Hunt LB, Husske AM, Lange AM. Acute and non-acute lower extremity pain in the pediatric population: part I. J Pediatr Health Care. 2012;26:62–8.
3. Brown DW, Sheffer BW. Pediatric septic arthritis: an update. Orthop Clin North Am. 2019;50:461–70.
4. Khan SA, Raja H, Waheed A. The limping child – when to worry and when to refer: a GP's guide. Br J Gen Pract. 2020;70:467.
5. Melbourne TRCsH. Clinical practice guideline: the limping or non-weight bearing child. Vol 20242020. https://www.rch.org.au/clinicalguide/guideline_index/Child_with_limp/.
6. Kastrissianakis K, Beattie TF. Transient synovitis of the hip: more evidence for a viral aetiology. Eur J Emerg Med. 2010;17:270–3.

7. Tse SM, Laxer RM. Approach to acute limb pain in childhood. Pediatr Rev. 2006;27:170–9. quiz 180
8. Sarwark JF, LaBella CR, American Academy of Pediatrics. Pediatric orthopaedics and sports injuries : a quick reference guide. 3rd ed. Elk Grove Village, IL: American Academy of Pediatrics; 2021.
9. Sawyer JR, Kapoor M. The limping child: a systematic approach to diagnosis. Am Fam Physician. 2009;79:215–24.

Chapter 35
Rashes

Joshua Belfer and Ashlyn Katz

When children present with rashes in a school-based health setting, the rash itself may not be their primary complaint or the initial reason for the visit. Often, rashes accompany systemic symptoms such as fever, fatigue, or respiratory issues. It is crucial for clinicians to determine whether the rash and associated symptoms indicate a condition that requires urgent or emergent medical attention. Prompt identification of potentially serious conditions can significantly impact the child's health outcome, making a systematic approach to identifying rashes crucial in a school-based health setting.

A brief but thorough history can greatly assist clinicians in triaging a child presenting with a rash. The RASHES approach (Table 35.1) to history-taking encompasses many of the important elements to identifying the etiology for rashes.

A standardized approach to examining and describing a rash can prove crucial in allowing you to identify the rash. As a single rash can have multiple morphologies, examining a rash systematically can make assessment less overwhelming and less confusing. The SCRIPTS approach (Table 35.2), created by Dr. Robert Olympia, has been utilized as an organized way to assess a rash [1].

Case 1 A 6-year-old male presents to the school nurse's office with a high fever, malaise, headache, and vomiting. The nurse initially notes an erythematous maculopapular rash and cool extremities. Vital signs: T-103.4, HR-136, BP-86/52, RR-20, SaO2–92% on room air.

Using the RASHES approach: Recent Exposures: Recently visited his 18-year-old brother in college last week. Allergies: None. Symptoms: High fever, neck

J. Belfer (✉)
Perelman School of Medicine, University of Pennsylvania, Philadelphia, PA, USA
e-mail: belferj1@chop.edu

A. Katz
The Brooklyn Hospital Center, Brooklyn, NY, USA

R. P. Olympia, J. Brady-Olympia (eds.), *Clinical Considerations in School-based Health*, https://doi.org/10.1007/978-3-031-85765-2_35

Table 35.1 RASHES approach to history-taking

R	Recent Exposures	Exposures to new soaps, lotions, or detergents. Also consider: Plant or animal exposures.
A	Allergies	Known allergies to foods, medications, or environmental allergens.
S	Symptoms	Associated symptoms, including itching, pain, burning, or fever (addressed in more depth below).
H	History	Patient history of past skin conditions, family history of skin disorders.
E	Evolution	How the rash started and has changed (addressed in more depth below).
S	Site	Location and spread of the rash.

Table 35.2 The SCRIPTS approach to assessing a rash

S	Shape (including size and morphology, see Fig. 35.1)
C	Color
R	Region (where did the rash start, where had it progressed to, does it come and go)
I	Itchy?
P	Painful?
T	Trauma-related?
S	Systemic symptoms (Fever, headache, mucous membrane changes, joint swelling or pain, abdominal pain, swelling of the extremities, myalgias, generalized weakness, etc.)

stiffness, malaise, headache, vomiting. History: Eczema. Evolution: Initially started as an erythematous maculopapular rash but has quickly become more petechial with areas of purpura; non-blanching. Site: Trunk and extremities, worse on the legs.

Likely one of the most alarming rashes that a clinician can see, meningococcemia is due to the gram-negative *Neisseria meningitidis* bacteria. Some fast facts:

- 422 cases were reported in 2023—the highest annual amount since 2014 [2].
- Meningococcal disease risk is reduced by meningococcal vaccines, recommended for all 11–12-year-olds (MenACWY vaccine), with a booster at 16 years old, and a MenB vaccine available for 16–23-year-olds [2].
- Most cases are sporadic, but outbreaks do occur; you may recall that there have been several meningococcal serogroup B infection outbreaks at college campuses since 2009, making vigilance of school-based clinicians, especially those at boarding schools, of utmost importance.

The clinical presentation of meningococcal infection can be variable, presenting after an incubation period that can be as short as one day but sometimes as long as ten days. While disease is often considered for children with signs of sepsis and meningitis, the rash in meningococcal disease presents early in the illness (within hours) and can rapidly progress. Beginning as maculopapular or urticarial in nature, the quickly evolving rash can become petechial. Early meningococcal disease may present with fever and nonspecific viral-like symptoms, including vomiting, diarrhea, poor feeding, and dehydration. It is important for clinicians to keep in mind that sepsis, caused by meningococcal disease or by another organism, can lead to disseminated intravascular coagulation (DIC), which can present with similar rash

Term	Description	Term	Description	Term	Description
Macule 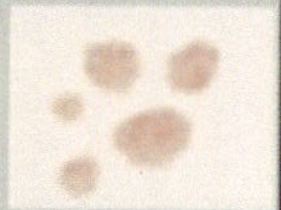	Flat, non-palpable, change in skin color, <1cm.	Patch 	Flat, non-palpable, change in skin color, > 1cm.	Plaque 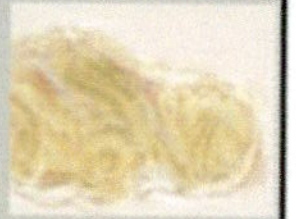	Raised but flat, solid, > 1 cm, often confluent.
Vesicle 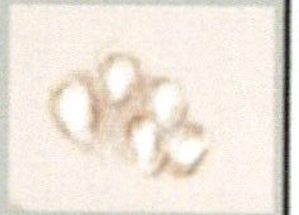	Elevated, Fluid-filled, < 1 cm.	Bullae 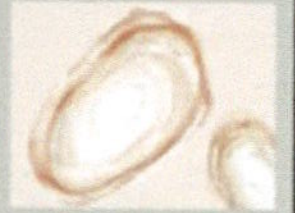	Elevated, Fluid-filled, >1cm.	Pustule 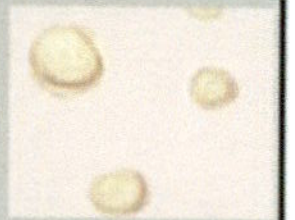	Elevated, contains pus, < 1 cm.
Papule 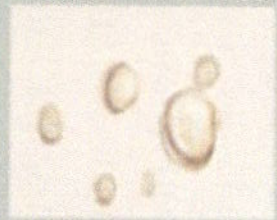	Elevated, solid, palpable, typically inflamed, no pus < 1cm.	Nodule 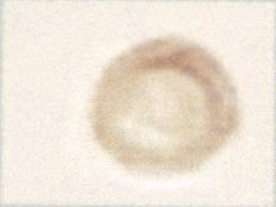	Elevated, solid, palpable, typically inflamed, no pus, > 1cm.	Wheal 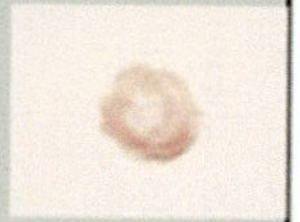	Raised, pruritic area, usually resolves in 24 hours- often associated with allergies.
Petechiae 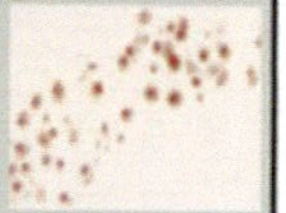	Flat or raised, red or purple, non-blanching, < 3 mm.	Purpura 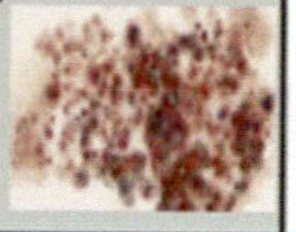	Flat or raised, red or purple, non-blanching, > 3 mm.	Urticaria 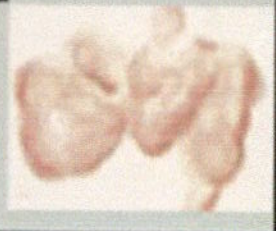	Coalescence of wheals with inflammation to deeper dermis.

Fig. 35.1 Rash Morphologies

characteristics to meningococcal infection. Similarly, viral rashes—specifically enterovirus, Epstein-Barr virus, cytomegalovirus, and measles—can mimic meningococcal rashes.

Early recognition of meningococcal disease can be lifesaving, leading to improved outcomes. Individuals with suspected meningococcal infection should be immediately isolated while emergency transport is arranged. If there is the ability to give antibiotics while arranging or awaiting transport, a third-generation cephalosporin, such as ceftriaxone, would be the antimicrobial of choice. Studies have shown improved mortality with early administration of antibiotics. With the assistance of public health authorities, chemoprophylaxis should be initiated for those who have been in close contact to a patient with meningococcal disease.

Want a comprehensive review on meningococcal disease? Check out Pediatrics in Review: Meningococcal Disease [3].

Case 1 Conclusion Due to the ill-appearance of the child, along with the concerning vital signs and petechial, quickly evolving rash, the school nurse is immediately concerned for meningococcal disease. She isolates the child, calls 911 and he is immediately taken to the Emergency Department. The nurse works with the local Department of Health to ensure that close contacts receive antibiotic prophylaxis.

Case 2 A 12-year-old girl presents to the school nurse's office with targetoid lesions on her hands and forearms. She has no recent illnesses but reports being on an antibiotic for a urinary tract infection. Vital signs: T-98.6/HR-75, BP-116/75, RR-16, SaO2–98% on room air.

Using the RASHES approach: Recent Exposures: Recently started on an antibiotic for a UTI. Allergies: None. Symptoms: Feels wells, no associated symptoms. History: None. Evolution: Rash started a day ago, continues to spread. Site: Worst on arms and legs, with several small lesions in the mouth.

Erythema multiforme (EM) is an immune-mediated skin condition. While infections are frequent triggers (with herpes simplex virus being the most common), medications (NSAIDs, anticonvulsants, antibiotics), malignancy, vaccines, radiation, allergic contact dermatitis, and even menstruation have also been cited as precipitating triggers.

EM skin lesions can exhibit many different characteristics (hence the name "multiforme"). The typical lesions are small (<3 cm), have a targetoid appearance, with a classical acral distribution (hands, feet, limbs). The target lesions have a dusky center. Mucosal involvement can and does commonly occur, most frequently in the oral mucosa. Of note, erythema multiforme can be divided into "minor" and "major" categories based on the extent of the skin involvement; both can have mucosal involvement, with the "major" subset having severe involvement with associated severe symptoms, including fever and arthralgias.

Evolving over several days, EM lesions typically resolve after several weeks. The presence and severity of mucosal involvement and associated symptoms help direct clinicians to the necessity and urgency of management. Most mild cases of EM, those without significant mucosal involvement and/or severe symptoms, can be managed in an outpatient setting. If there is a known medication trigger, that should be removed, while supportive care should be given with a close eye to alleviating discomfort from skin lesions and ensuring hydration in the setting of oral mucosa involvement. Corticosteroids can play a role in treating EM, with topical forms used for skin discomfort, and systemic steroids used for more extensive mucosal involvement.

There are several clinical mimics to erythema multiforme, many of which deserve urgent or emergent evaluation in the emergency department (Table 35.3). Additionally, rashes involving the palms and soles can also be associated with Hand, Foot, and Mouth Disease; secondary syphilis; Rocky Mountain spotted fever; and meningococcemia.

> Want more on Erythema multiforme vs Urticaria multiforme vs Serum sickness-like reaction? Check out Pediatrics in Review: Visual Diagnosis [4].

Case 2 Conclusion Recognizing the potential medication trigger to the patient's illness, the school nurse identifies that there is a broad differential to this patient's presentation. While mild at the time of assessment, the nurse recommends urgent pediatrician follow up due to concern that the rash may worsen over the subsequent 24–48 h and may require emergency management in the hospital.

Case 3 A 4-year-old boy is brought to the school nurse's office with a cough and runny nose. The nurse notes the boy to have an erythematous macular rash on his entire body that does not seem to be bothersome. He says that he feels fine and that his sister stayed home from school since she was sick. Vital signs: T-100, HR-114, BP-100/74, RR-20, SaO2–99% on room air.

Using the RASHES approach: Recent Exposures: Sister is a sick contact. Allergies: None. Symptoms: Cough, nasal congestion, and rhinorrhea for the past 3 days. Low grade fever 2 days ago, no fever in the last 24 h. History: None. Evolution: Appeared gradually. Site: Started on chest and back, no palm or sole involvement.

The word exanthem, coming from the Greek "*exanthema*" meaning "break out," typically refers to a rash that accompanies a viral infection. The rash associated with a virus is thought to be secondary to a hypersensitivity reaction triggered by the virus. Some viruses may present with pathognomonic or characteristic features, but one of the frustrating aspects of viral exanthems is that they are, as some have described, "a great imitator." They can present at any time of the illness (first symptom of a virus or later on in the course) and can take on different morphologies. Even more confusing: they can look different at different times!

Table 35.3 Clinical Mimics of Erythema Multiforme

Stevens-Johnson Syndrome (SJS): Historically, had been referred to as "erythema multiforme major," but this terminology has fallen out of favor as evidence has suggested they are two separate entities. *History*: Typically triggered by medications, with anticonvulsants (Lamotrigine, Carbamazepine) and sulfonamide antibiotics (Bactrim) being among the most common. Preceded by fever, myalgias, and malaise. *Appearance*: Rapid and widespread evolution of painful bullae that involve the trunk, extremities, and mucous membranes. Toxic epidermal necrolysis (TEN) is when >30% of the body surface area is involved. *Treatment*: Requires immediate evaluation in the emergency department. Supportive care with fluid resuscitation, electrolyte management, pain control, and wound care. Typically managed by a multidisciplinary team and carries significant mortality risk.	Mycoplasma-induced Rash and Mucositis (MIRM) AKA Reactive Infectious Mucocutaneous Eruption (RIME) *History*: Prodromal symptoms of atypical Mycoplasma pneumoniae pneumonia, including fever, cough, and congestion. Typically not triggered by medication, which can help differentiate from other diagnoses. *Appearance*: Like its name, significant mucositis, often with more than one mucous membrane involved. Can have limited skin involvement, but when present, skin lesions appear vesicular, bullous, and/or targetoid. *Treatment*: Requires immediate evaluation in the emergency department. Supportive care similar to SJS/TEN, patients may benefit from antibiotic treatment for atypical pneumonia. Location and extent of mucosal involvement may warrant a multidisciplinary care team.
Serum Sickness-Like Reaction: *History*: Hypersensitivity reaction triggered by medications, including antibiotics. Presents 1–3 weeks after initiation of the medication, and is associated with fever, rash, and arthralgias, sometimes with joint swelling. *Appearance*: Urticarial, maculopapular, or purpuric lesions, sometimes referred to as morbilliform ("measles-like"). No mucous membrane involvement. Sometimes also described as "purple urticaria" due to its violaceous hue. *Treatment*: Removal of triggering agent, supportive care with antihistamines and antipyretics. Consider systemic corticosteroids for severe symptoms.	Urticaria multiforme: *History*: Thought to be a histamine-mediated hypersensitivity reaction. May have precipitating infections or medication use (most commonly antibiotics and antipyretics). May have concomitant fever or upper respiratory symptoms. *Appearance*: Large, annular, polycyclic wheals. May have a dusky center or central clearing. *Treatment*: Self-resolving, usually within 24 h. Discontinue any medication triggers.

Despite the varied characteristics of viral exanthems, there are several more typical presentations that can suggest viruses as the etiology for a rash. Gianotti-Crosti syndrome, named after the Italian dermatologists who originally described the skin disorder, was originally found to be associated with Hepatitis B but is now known to be precipitated by many other viral illnesses, including but not limited to Epstein-Barr virus, cytomegalovirus, coxsackievirus, and parvovirus B19. Also known as papular acrodermatitis, the rash is self-limiting and typically presents as a symmetric, monomorphic papular or papulovesicular eruption. Classic locations for this rash include the face, buttocks, extensor aspects of the forearms and legs, and feet. Clinical mimics include Henoch-Schonlein purpura, acute hemorrhagic edema, insect bites, and lichen planus. Lesions from Gianotti-Crosti are self-limited, but can last longer than typical viral exanthem, usually resolving in three to four weeks but may last for several months.

Papular-purpuric gloves and socks syndrome (PPGSS) is a symmetrical, painful or pruritic rash that is most commonly associated with parvovirus B19. The syndrome is usually seen in the spring and summer seasons, and can start as a bright red exanthem with edema of the hands and feet (an acute acral exanthem) progressing to purpuric papules and petechiae. The "gloves and socks" nomenclature refers to the well demarcated lesions on the wrists and ankles, although the presence of lesions on other parts of the body does not exclude this diagnosis. Clinical mimics include Rocky Mountain Spotted Fever, Henoch-Schonlein purpura, Kawasaki disease, and meningococcemia. As with other viral-related rashes, PPGSS spontaneously resolves in one to two weeks. Table 35.4 demonstrates a few other characteristic or pathognomonic viral exanthems.

> Want more on Viral, Bacterial, Fungal, and Allergic Rashes – with pictures? Check out Rashes in School: Can They Stay, or Should They Go? [5].

Case 3 Conclusion Considering the boy's sister as a sick contact, in addition to the patient being well appearing with associated cough and congestion, the school nurse believes the rash to be secondary to a viral upper respiratory illness. She advises the boy's mom to monitor his respiratory status and make sure he is drinking plenty of fluids, and recommends following up with his pediatrician if needed. No specific treatment is indicated for the rash.

In summary, rashes can be CHALLENGING! They can be worrisome, they can be benign, they can look one way and then change, and a lot of rashes look the same! Hopefully, we have provided you with the tools to assess and diagnose a rash. And remember, you don't always have to know exactly what the rash is—sometimes it is enough to just know whether your patient needs to be seen urgently or emergently in the emergency department. So next time you have a patient present with a rash: Use the RASHES approach to take a detailed history, the SCRIPTS

Table 35.4 Viral exanthems

Coxsackievirus (Hand, Foot, and Mouth Disease) Typically presents with an erythematous macular, maculopapular, or vesicular rash and fever. Younger children can often present with poor oral intake, due to painful oropharyngeal lesions.
Roseola Presents with several days of fever (sometimes >104 °F) that suddenly stops, with the subsequent appearance of an erythematous macular or maculopapular rash that lasts for one to two days.
Varicella A vesicular, pruritic rash that appears in different stages on different parts of the body. See Chap. 103 for more on Varicella.

approach to assess and describe the rash, and keep an eye out for worrisome aspects of the history or physical exam that should prompt you to send your patient for immediate care in the emergency department.

Extra Credit Points

1. Recognize if the rash is serious: Signs of severe rashes include petechiae and purpura (indicative of conditions like meningococcemia or thrombocytopenia); widespread blistering (staphylococcal scalded skin syndrome); and desquamation (toxic shock syndrome).
2. Be vigilant for red flag symptoms that accompany a rash: Including high fever, lethargy, severe pain, difficulty breathing, and neurological changes.
3. Is the rash secondary to an allergy or hypersensitivity: A thorough history can identify potential triggers for the rash.
4. Communication and Care Coordination: Use standard terminology and the SCRIPTS approach to ensure proper handoff when referring to the emergency department.

References

1. Olympia RP. School nurses on the front lines of medicine: connecting the dots: SCRIPTS for success in the evaluation of pediatric rashes. NASN Sch Nurse. 2017;32(3):172–7.
2. Cases of Meningococcal Disease Are Increasing in the United States. April 16, 2024. Accessed May 29, 2024. https://www.cdc.gov/ncird/whats-new/meningococcal-disease-cases-increasing-us.html#:~:text=CDC%20issued%20a%20health%20advisory%20notice,highest%20annual%20figure%20since%202014.
3. Vaz LE. Meningococcal disease [published correction appears in Pediatr Rev. 2017 Jun;38(6):279]. Pediatr Rev. 2017;38(4):158–69.
4. Boehm BA, Kolodziejski K, Roy A, Kumar G. Targetoid rash in an infant-hit the target! Pediatr Rev. 2023;44(8):477–80.
5. Jakubowski TL, Perron TJ, Teixeira E. Rashes in school: can they stay, or should they go? [published correction appears in NASN Sch Nurse. 2016 Jan;31(1):61–2]. NASN Sch Nurse. 2015;30(5):274–82.

Chapter 36
Traumatic Skin Emergencies

Masrur Khan and Ee Tein Tay

When evaluating a student with an acute traumatic injury, use the DERM mnemonic (Table 36.1) to initially assess the injury and determine the need for a higher level of care.

Case 1 During recess, 6-year-old girl Tiffany was attempting to go down the slide but didn't realize that her classmate was at the bottom of the slide when she started her descent. In an attempt to stop herself from colliding with her classmate, she grabbed onto the slide and fell over the edge. She was brought into the nurse's office for a traumatic injury to her left forearm that was initially bloody. She is crying but can move her elbow and wrist without any pain. The bleeding stops with direct pressure and there is an underlying superficial abrasion and no active bleeding. A review of her chart demonstrates that she is up to date on all her vaccinations. What should you do?

Abrasions are caused by superficial wounds to the skin and usually involve only the epidermis. These injuries typically heal well with thorough cleaning and otherwise minimal intervention. *Avulsion injury* involving the dermis or hypodermis can increase the risk of scarring or excessive bleeding.

There are three main types of abrasions: linear, grazed or brush, and patterned abrasions. A linear abrasion is caused by an external factor stripping away a layer of epidermis, such as an aggressive nail scratching. A grazed or brush abrasion might be caused by friction forces that cause the separation of skin layers, such as a road rash. A patterned abrasion is caused by excessive pressure on the skin that leaves behind a mark, such as excessive compression from wearing tight socks.

For the majority of abrasions, there might be an initial period of bleeding that stops with direct pressure, followed secondarily by a period of redness, swelling, pain, or bruising around the affected area. The treatment includes thorough

M. Khan (✉) · E. T. Tay
NYU Langone Health, New York, NY, USA

R. P. Olympia, J. Brady-Olympia (eds.), *Clinical Considerations in School-based Health*, https://doi.org/10.1007/978-3-031-85765-2_36

Table 36.1 DERM mnemonic describing the initial evaluation of a student with a traumatic skin injury

D	Depth (Layers of the skin)	Determine the depth of the injury: Epidermis—the outermost layer, consisting of mostly keratin, and provides barrier protection from external elements, such as water, sun, bacteria, and other environmental toxins. Dermis—the layer that provides structural integrity to the skin and is the thickest of the layers of skin. It consists of collagen and elastin to allow for strength and flexibility of the skin. Oil glands here keep the skin smooth and maintain water balance while the sweat glands regulate temperature. This layer also consists of terminal nerve branches to help sense temperature, pain, and pressure. Hypodermis—the layer of fat that cushions the body, protects the underlying muscles, and helps with temperature regulation. The nerves and blood vessels that connect the skin to the rest of the body exist in this layer.
E	Extent	Perform a neurovascular assessment distal to the trauma—check for pulse, sensation, motor strength, capillary refill, temperature, and color.
R	Region	Determine the location of the trauma, noting proximity to major blood vessels, joints/tendons/ligaments, etc.
M	Management	Stabilize airway/breathing/circulation; apply pressure dressing or tourniquet for significant bleeding; cover traumatic lesions with saline soaked gauze; determine disposition to emergency department (ED), urgent care center or primary care physician's office

cleansing with soap and water, application of topical antibiotic ointment, and bandage to help prevent infections. Avoid additional frictional injury from excessive rubbing, but gentle scrubbing with a soft sponge and copious irrigation using sterile water or sterile saline may be necessary to remove foreign bodies. The majority of abrasions can be managed in the school's health office. However, if bleeding persists despite direct pressure for more than 15 minutes, or if there is concern for abrasions involving deeper skin layers, further evaluation may be warranted in an acute care setting. Urgent care should be sufficient for the initial evaluation of most abrasions.

Lacerations are deeper skin openings that, depending on the depth and severity, may involve the dermis, hypodermis, or deeper structures. The likelihood of scarring increases if a laceration extends beyond the epidermis. Superficial and linear lacerations may be closed with bandages or surgical strips. The majority of lacerations will involve more layers than the epidermis, may have prolonged bleeding, may be greater than 0.5 cm in length, and require additional evaluation for possible closure with sutures or skin glue. Students should be referred to the closest ED for lacerations with neurovascular compromise (distal lack of pulses, weakness or lack of motor function, or distal paresthesia); concern for joint space injury or underlying fracture; concern for embedded foreign bodies; or significant blood loss or signs of shock. If there is concern for significant blood loss, tourniquets can and should be used to minimize blood loss (see Chap. 5). The patient's vaccination status for tetanus should be obtained and updated if the vaccination status has lapsed or if the wound has a high likelihood of infectious contamination. For any children unvaccinated or incompletely vaccinated against tetanus, prophylaxis should be administered. Wounds should be irrigated and cleaned to prevent infection. It is recommended that for each 1 cm of laceration, 50 mL of sterile water or sterile saline should be used for irrigation.

Case 2 During his high school AP chemistry class, 16-year-old non-binary adolescent Samuel had a spill on their skin. While handling a flask with corrosive contents, they were not wearing protective equipment (gown, gloves) as instructed, and they accidentally dropped the flask. The contents spilled off the table onto their right forearm and on their abdomen. They report to the school nurse's office immediately with a partial thickness burn on their arm that is exquisitely tender to touch. What should you do?

There are four categories of burns as classified by source. *Thermal burns* are caused by hot sources that can cause cell death due to elevated temperature, such as a spill from boiling water. *Radiation burns* are caused by prolonged exposure to radiation sources, such as sunburn. *Chemical burns* are caused by substances that cause changes in the composition of the skin layer and cause damage, such as exposure to strong acids or alkalis. *Electrical burns* are caused by electricity moving from an external source through the skin layer, such as exposure to electric current from an outlet to a metallic object.

Of these, chemical and electrical burns require immediate medical attention and should be referred to the nearest ED. Thermal and radiation burns may be less emergent, and acuity will be dependent on the degree of burns sustained. There are four degrees of burns as classified by depth (Table 36.2).

Table 36.2 Description of burns

Degree of burn	Depth/skin layer involvement	Signs and symptoms	Disposition	Treatment
First (superficial)	Epidermis only	Redness, pain (i.e. sunburn)	Urgent care center	Cool water, saline-soaked gauze bandages, topical antibiotics, pain control
Second (partial thickness)	Epidermis and dermis	Redness, pain, blistering of skin	ED	Topical antibiotics, topical silver sulfadiazine, elevation of affected areas
Third (full thickness)	Epidermis, dermis, and hypodermis	Charring, painless	ED (Burn Center)	Surgical evaluation, debridement, skin grafting
Fourth	Epidermis, dermis, hypodermis, and underlying tissue (muscles, bone)	Charring, painless, neurovascular concerns, systemic symptoms possible (ex: arrhythmia, shock, organ failure)	ED (Burn Center)	Surgical evaluation, debridement, skin grafting

It is also important to note the pattern distribution or the locations of burns. Any burns to the *face, hands, feet, groin, genitals, or any circumferential burns involving the limb or neck* will require immediate evaluation at an ED or burn center. Further medical evaluation may be warranted if there is an unclear or inconsistent medical history not correlating with exam findings for suspected abuse or non-accidental trauma.

It is important to have the appropriate burns evaluated promptly, as early intervention is important for cosmetic purposes as well as evaluation of additional possible medical sequelae. For initial burn management, one may rinse the area with cool water for 10 min. Be sure to remove any tight items from the area (such as rings, bracelets, etc.) in anticipation of swelling. If the skin has denuded at all, you may apply topical antibiotic ointment. Consider pain control as necessary with acetaminophen or ibuprofen. Apply a sterile bandage to the area (can consider saline-soaked gauze) while they are en route to their nearest ED for further evaluation.

Case 3 While out on the playground during recess, 8-year-old boy Abid yells in pain and runs over to you crying. He is brought to the school nurse after a suspected insect bite. The stinger is intact and it appears the bite was committed by a honey bee. Aside from pain and itchiness at the site of the bite, Abid begins to develop a rash all over his body and is now complaining of a scratchy sensation in his throat. After 5 min, he has one episode of non-bloody, non-bilious emesis. What should you do?

A *bite* describes when an animal uses its mouth to penetrate the skin, whereas a *sting* is when an animal uses a different body part, such as a stinger, to penetrate the skin for defense purposes. Animal bites are uncommon in a school setting and include (but are not limited to) classroom pets such as rodents or reptiles. Human bites may require serum studies and communicable disease prophylaxis and should be referred to an acute care facility. For minor wounds, evaluation at urgent care centers is sufficient. Larger wounds that require skin closure should also be referred for further medical attention at an ED All bites breaking the skin will require antibiotics prophylaxis. Affected skin should be irrigated thoroughly with sterile water or sterile saline and patients should be assessed for tetanus status.

Common stings on school grounds include those from bees, wasps, and mosquitoes. Stings may cause local reactions such as pain, swelling, or pruritus. Allergic reactions leading to anaphylaxis (involvement of the cardiovascular, respiratory, gastrointestinal, and/or skin/mucous membranes organ systems) may occur in patients who sustained stings. If available, intramuscular epinephrine injection should be administered for patients with respiratory distress or swelling involving the face or airway after a sting, and seek immediate medical attention in the ED. Patients with superficial bites and minor stings can be managed supportively in the school health office. Cold compresses to minimize swelling, pruritus, and pain relief may provide comfort to the patient. Avoidance of additional trauma to bite or sting sites such as scratching affected skin may reduce the risk of secondary infection.

Case 4 Two weeks after presenting to her primary pediatrician for mosquito bites, a 5-year-old girl Fatoumata presents to the school nurse with tenderness to her right leg. She reportedly has been scratching her itchy mosquito bites constantly over the last week. However, today she reports that her entire leg has become red, itchy, and very painful. She is afebrile and her vitals are within normal limits. However, she has a confluent, indurated, linear erythematous lesion on her right leg. It is warm to the touch, and there is some yellow crusting around the area. What should you do?

While many traumatic skin injuries can be supportively managed or referred for urgent care/ED evaluation per the guidelines above, it is important to note that there could be secondary superinfection and local sequelae of any traumatic skin injuries (Table 36.3).

Extra Credit Points

1. When evaluating a student with an acute traumatic injury, use the DERM mnemonic (Table 36.1) to initially assess the injury and determine the need for a higher level of care.
2. The majority of traumatic skin emergencies can be assessed and managed in an urgent care setting or primary care physician's office. Red flags for traumatic skin emergencies that require immediate ED referral utilizes the mnemonic "EPIDERMIS":

E—Exsanguination/shock	Significant blood loss (hypovolemic shock) or infection (sepsis) can lead to signs of hypoperfusion (altered mental status, cool pale skin, tachycardia)
P—Pulselessness	Neurovascular compromise from deep laceration or burns
I—Infection	Warm, tender to touch, severe pain or swelling, fever
D—Deep laceration or burns of bites	Into the hypodermis, and underlying tissue (muscles, bone)
E—Epinephrine use for severe allergic reactions	Stings leading to severe allergic reactions involving cardiovascular, respiratory, gastrointestinal and/or skin/mucous membrane organ systems
R—Region of the burn	Burns to the face, hands, feet, groin, genitals, or any circumferential burns involving the limb or neck
M—Motor weakness	Neurovascular compromise from deep laceration or burns
I—Insensitivity to pain	Neurovascular compromise from deep laceration or burns
S—Substances	Embedded foreign bodies, teeth from animal bites, etc.

Table 36.3 Possible complications of traumatic skin injuries and associated signs/symptoms, dispositions, and treatment plans

Complication	Signs and symptoms	Disposition	Treatment
Cellulitis	Tender, indurated, erythematous wound; +/− fever	Urgent care or home	Oral antibiotics (cephalexin)
Impetigo	Honey-crusted discharge from wound	Urgent care or home	Topical antibiotics (mupirocin); consider oral antibiotics (ex: amoxicillin, clindamycin) if several lesions
Abscess	Tender wound with fluctuance	Urgent care or ED	Oral antibiotics with MRSA coverage (Bactrim) and incision + drainage
Necrotizing fasciitis	Exquisitely tender, erythematous or gangrenous wound	ED, admission to hospital	Intravenous antibiotics and surgical debridement
Lymphadenopathy	Enlarged lymph nodes, especially regional nodes close to original wound(s)	Home	Reassurance
Lymphadenitis	Tender, erythematous lymph nodes +/− fever	Urgent care or ED	Pain control and oral antibiotics (cephalexin)
Tenosynovitis	Significant swelling and tenderness of joints or fingers/extremities with limitation of range of motion, fever	ED, possible surgical intervention	Pain control, intravenous antibiotics, and surgical debridement
Osteomyelitis or septic joint	Exquisite tenderness at affected joints, reduced range of motion of joint, fevers	ED	Intravenous antibiotics, orthopedic surgery consultation, imaging, synovial tap
Keloids	Discoloration, extraneous and firm tissue near site of wound	Home	Supportive management, consultation with dermatology/plastic surgery for cosmesis
Scar tissue	Discoloration at site of wound	Home	Supportive management, consultation with dermatology/plastic surgery for cosmesis
Sepsis	Fever, tachycardia, tachypnea, signs of end organ damage (decreased urine output, altered mental status)	Emergency department, admission to the hospital	Intravenous antibiotics and volume resuscitation

Part IV
Managing a Student with Chronic Medical Conditions

Chapter 37
Individualized Health Care Plans

Ashley Kane and Kimberly Matthews

Children with special health care needs are a broad population of student learners who may experience challenges within the educational environment [1]. The term "special health care needs" is used to describe "those who have or are at risk for a chronic physical, developmental, behavior, or emotional condition and who also require health and related services of a type or amount beyond that required by children generally" [2]. Some of these students may have chronic medical conditions which persist for one year or more, require on-going medical intervention, and impair functioning or limit activities of daily living [3]. It is believed that between 10-30% of student learners have a chronic medical condition [3]. These conditions can also be associated with psycho-social consequences across the lifespan, as well as other negative sequalae such as chronic pain, discrimination, social difficulties, missed school days, and academic impairment [3]. As students with chronic medical conditions may require more frequent treatment in the outpatient setting or through inpatient hospitalization, these students may experience an increased rate of school absences [1, 3].

Attending school during scheduled hours allows for the development of peer relationships, socialization opportunities, and increased academic success as students who attend school on a regular basis are more likely to perform well in school [4]. As it is important to keep students engaged and motivated, the inclusion of students who have chronic or complex health care needs into educational settings has been prioritized and enhanced through clarification of federal special education law, changes in federal health insurance rules, federal health care initiatives, and

A. Kane (✉)
Penn State Health Milton S. Hershey Medical Center, Hershey, PA, USA
e-mail: akane@pennstatehealth.psu.edu

K. Matthews
Penn State Health Children's Hospital, Hershey, PA, USA
e-mail: kmatthews2@pennstatehealth.psu.edu

R. P. Olympia, J. Brady-Olympia (eds.), *Clinical Considerations in School-based Health*, https://doi.org/10.1007/978-3-031-85765-2_37

changes in the roles and responsibilities of school-based teachers and nurses [2]. Not all children with special health care needs will require special education services; some may simply require specialized technology and/or health-related support during the school day.

Given the possibility for extra support and the potential for frequent absences and impacts on student learning, children with chronic medical conditions may require a 504 Plan, outlined by Sect. 504 of the Rehabilitation Act of 1973, which permits for academic accommodations at school. While most clinicians are familiar with Individualized Education Plans (IEPs), few may be aware of, or have experience with, 504 plans for medical conditions [3]. IEPs can be considered an educational road map for children with disabilities as required by the federal Individuals with Disabilities Education Act (IDEA). These plans are regularly updated and include specific goals and milestones customized to each student's needs. A 504 Plan focuses on equitable access to a learning environment for students with a broader range of disabilities and needs compared to IEPs. Unlike IEPs, 504 Plans can continue into post-secondary education settings.

Some children will not require a 504 Plan or an IEP, and an Individualized Health Plan (IHP) may be of benefit to the child with a chronic health condition, the child's family, and the school system [4]. In 1987, The Surgeon General's Campaign on Children with Special Health Care Needs funded a project at Boston Children's Hospital, Project School Care, which provided guidance to assist school systems in responding to the challenge of integrating children assisted by medical technology into educational settings. From this project, the authors developed a model for designing Individualized Health Care Plans for students with special health care needs who received their care in school settings, which have served as a critical resource guide for school nurses and others [2].

Individualized health plans are clear and efficient documented plans which are determined to be appropriate generally by the school nurse and are developed by the school nurse in collaboration with a multidisciplinary team [4]. The multidisciplinary team can include school personnel such as nurses, teachers, social workers, school administrators and/or psychologists, and should utilize information from the parent(s) and/or guardian(s) of the student as the primary source of information. When an IHP is implemented, communication between school personnel, health care providers, and the child's parent(s) and/or guardian(s) is of utmost importance to convey the health-related concerns of the student. Health care agency consent forms must be completed to release medical information about the child to school personnel, in compliance with Health Insurance Portability and Accountability Act (HIPAA) regulations [4]. Table 37.1 includes an IHP template that can be utilized as a reference point.

The benefits of IHPs include addressing concerns and easing the transition from the hospital or health care clinic back into school by providing information specific to the child's condition, helping to facilitate the child's ability to attend school on a regular basis by decreasing the obstacles that hinder the child from returning to school, and increasing the teacher's knowledge of chronic conditions in children

Table 37.1 Individualized Healthcare Plan (IHP) example

Student Information	
Primary Language:	
Name:	Date of Birth:
Address:	School Name:
City, State, Zip:	Grade:
Parent/Guardian Information	
Mother/Guardian	Father/Guardian
Name:	Name:
Address:	Address:
City, State, Zip:	City, State, Zip:
Phone Number(s):	Phone Number(s):
Additional Emergency Contact Information	
Preferred Hospital:	
Primary Care Physician:	Specialty Care Physician:
Name:	Name:
Phone Number:	Phone Number:
Insurance Information	
Primary Insurance	Secondary Insurance
Name:	Name:
Policy Number:	Policy Number:
Health Information	
Primary Diagnosis: (Please add any additional diagnoses)	
Food and Medication Allergies:	

Medication				
Medication Name	Dosage	Frequency	Method of Administration	Given at Home or School
–	–	–	–	–
–	–	–	–	–

Medical Equipment		
Type of Equipment	Describe How to Use	Trained Staff
–	–	–
–	–	–

Potential Medical Issues and Treatment Plan *Please list any possible interventions or treatments that may occur during the school day*			
Problems and Triggers	Signs of the Problems	Interventions	Treatments
–	–	–	–

(continued)

Table 37.1 (continued)

Potential Medical Issues and Treatment Plan *Please list any possible interventions or treatments that may occur during the school day*			
Problems and Triggers	Signs of the Problems	Interventions	Treatments
–	–	–	–

Crisis Plan	
In a situation, if the following behaviors or conditions occur…	Please apply these action steps
In an Emergency, please do the following:	
1. Call 911 2. Designate an adult to stay with the student – clear area of any potential hazards 3. Call the school nurse, principal or other designated personnel to assist 4. If the event occurs in an area where other students are present, have a designated adult lead other students to another room 5. Contact parent/guardian	
Please add any additional emergency steps needed for optimum care	

and facilitating his or her confidence in dealing with issues that may arise in the school setting [4, 5].

Consider the case study examples in Table 37.2: a 10-year-old male in elementary school and a 17-year-old female high school student. What actions might you take to ensure that these students have the necessary academic support in place to optimize learning in the classroom environment and beyond? Would Case Study 1 benefit from a 504 Plan? How might an IHP for Case Study 2 provide support and would this student also benefit from a 504 Plan?

Table 37.2 Case studies

	Case Study 1—Elementary	Case Study 2—Late High School-College Transition
Gender	Male (he, him)	Female (she, her)
Age	10	17
Grade	4- *Regular Education*	11—Special *Education—Other Health Impairment (OHI) IHP embedded in IEP*
Diagnosis	Irritable Bowel Disease (IBD)—Diagnosed at age 10	Sickle Cell Disease—Diagnosed at birth through newborn sickle cell screening
Symptoms	Bloody diarrhea Weight loss Fatigue Malnutrition Chronic abdominal pain	Pain crises with temperature changes Fatigue Silent Strokes Prone to Acute chest syndrome

(continued)

Table 37.2 (continued)

	Case Study 1—Elementary	Case Study 2—Late High School-College Transition
Case Study Background	During a holiday break, 10-year-old Benjamin began to have consistent diarrhea and was extremely fatigued. As he began to feel worse, he noticed that he had blood in his stool and had severe stomach pain. His parents took him to the closest children's hospital, where he was admitted for a work-up of IBD for Crohn's Disease vs. Ulcerative Colitis. After several diagnostic tests, Benjamin was diagnosed with Ulcerative Colitis and was prescribed a biologic medication for the management of his symptoms. As holiday break was coming to an end, the topic of school was discussed and the accommodations that may be needed in the academic and educational environment for Benjamin. What would you do to support Benjamin in the education/academic environment?	Carmen is a 17-year-old female who was diagnosed with sickle cell anemia as a result of the Unites States mandated newborn screening for Hb SS-Disease. During her elementary and middle school years, Carmen had at least 3 hospitalizations a year due to pain crises and occasional instances of acute chest syndrome. It was also found during that time that Carmen was experiencing silent strokes that impacted her executive functioning abilities. The main areas of concern, which were identified during the evaluation stage of the IEP process, were memory, concentration, and organization. Carmen's disability category for the IEP is Other Health Impairment, as her diagnosis has greatly impacted her academic success. She receives specially designed instruction and support to assist in her academics for executive functioning deficits. In her IEP, Carmen has an Individual Health Plan (IHP) that includes any needs that must be met during the school day, such as having the ability to carry water and the ability to move her seat in class due to the forceful air of the heater or air conditioner that could exacerbate a pain crisis. Carmen, who is going into her senior year of high school has plans of going to a 4-year university to study nursing. Her IEP expires at the end of her 12th grade year and will not carry over to the college level. What would you do to assist Carmen in having the correct tools to assist her academics that would transfer to the college level?

(continued)

Table 37.2 (continued)

	Case Study 1—Elementary	Case Study 2—Late High School-College Transition
Solution for the School and Academic Environment	Students that have been diagnosed with a chronic health condition can experience many absences from school. These absences have an impact on a child's overall performance in the academic setting [4]. Addressing the impact of school absences can positively impact a student's academic needs, social needs, and their medical needs. Since the student in the case study does not have a chronic health condition that would necessitate a modified curriculum, a 504 Plan would be in their best interest.	Students that have an IEP in place during their years in grade school, may not realize that their document does not follow them to the collegiate level. Many students, along with their families, have to figure out a solution to having the same supports in college that aided in their overall academic success in grade school. In this scenario, empowering the student to self-advocate is in everyone's best interest [6]. Also, meeting with the school's disability office and campus medical staff can positively impact their experience. In meeting with school personnel, the student can share their IHP and develop a 504 Plan to distribute to their professors to meet their medical and academic needs.

Extra Credit Points

1. Students with chronic conditions or health care needs are commonly educated in general education classrooms. These students may need health and related services of a type or amount greater than their peers.
2. Individualized health care plans (IHPs) can be an option for students with special health care needs or chronic medical conditions to ensure a plan is in place to foster academic success and support optimal attendance.
3. IHPs are created by school nurses with input from healthcare professionals caring for the student, parents and caregivers, and other education professionals.
4. Individualized Education Plans (IEPs), 504 Plans, and Individualized Health Care Plans (IHPs) are implemented to serve different purposes, as seen in the following table:

Individualized Education Plan (IEP)	504 Plan	Individualized Health Care Plan (IHP)
• Governed by a federal special education law: Individuals with Disabilities Education Act (IDEA) • Utilized for students with one or more of 13 disabilities as defined by IDEA • Contains formal, written learning goals that are measured and updated frequently.	• Governed by a federal civil rights law: Section 504 of the Rehabilitation Act of 1973. • Broader requirements for students with any type of disability, or medical condition, that interferes with the ability to learn in a general or special education classroom. • No formal template but would generally include specific accommodations, services, or supports for the student, the names of those individuals who provide each service, and the individual responsible for ensuring the plan is implemented. • Can be used in conjunction with an IEP to focus on accommodations that provide a student with non-discriminatory inclusion.	• Not governed by any federal or state law. • Follows professional nursing standards of care. • Addresses medical concerns or needs that might arise during the school day but do not directly impact the student's learning. • Can be used alone, or in conjunction with a 504 Plan and/or IEP, which are governed by federal law.

References

1. Wikel K, Markelz AM. Chronic health conditions, school attendance, and socioeconomic factors: a literature review. J Special Educ Apprenticeship. 2023;12(2) https://scholarworks.lib.csusb.edu/josea/vol12/iss2/9
2. Lehr DH. Placement of students with severe disabilities who have complex health care needs in general education classes. Res Practice Persons Severe Disab. 2019;45(1):39–44. https://doi.org/10.1177/1540796919895971.
3. Russo K. Assessment and treatment of adolescents with chronic medical conditions. J Health Serv Psychol. 2022;48(2):69–78. https://doi.org/10.1007/s42843-022-00059-4.
4. Hopkins AF, Hughes M. Individualized health care plans: supporting children with chronic conditions in the classroom. Young Exceptional Children. 2016;19(2):33–43. https://doi.org/10.1177/1096250614566538.
5. Cabat TL, Shafer K. Resources for facilitating back to school programs. Cancer Pract. 2002;10(2):105–8. https://doi.org/10.1046/j.1523-5394.2002.102009.x.
6. Ju S, Zeng W, Landmark LJ. Self-determination and academic success of students with disabilities in postsecondary education: a review. J Disab Policy Stud. 2017;28(3):180–9. https://doi.org/10.1177/1044207317739402.

Chapter 38
Anaphylaxis and Food Allergies

John Park and Joseph Schwob

Case 1 Sarah, a 10-year-old transfer student, arrives at Elementary School with a history of food allergies. She has been diagnosed with multiple food allergies, including peanuts and tree nuts, and is currently receiving treatment with Omalizumab (Xolair) under the care of a pediatric allergist.

Food allergies are a major public health concern in the United States, impacting up to 8% of children in this country [1]. Research has shown that up to 20% of allergic reactions in children occur at school or daycare [2]. Although it is possible for a child to develop an allergic reaction to any food item, there are 8 foods which have been shown to cause the most serious allergic reactions in the United States: milk, eggs, fish, crustacean shellfish, wheat, soy, peanuts and treenuts [3]. It's vital for school staff to safeguard children with food allergies, especially since about 25% of peanut allergy reactions happen in a school setting [4]. The diagnosis of food allergies involves a thorough medical history, skin prick tests, and occasionally blood tests to identify specific allergens. Some known risk factors that can predispose a child to allergic reactions include genetic predisposition, asthma, the route and timing of exposure to food allergens, skin barrier defects, vitamin D deficiency, dietary fat, and exposure to infection [5]. Food allergies can present in a variety of ways, and it is crucial for staff members in school and daycare to protect and care for children with food allergies when they are not in the care of their parents. Sometimes, children may have difficulty expressing or identifying how they're feeling when experiencing an allergic reaction to a food, and one should be aware of some of the more common ways that children may communicate a reaction. Children may say that their mouth or tongue is burning, itching, or feels "funny", or that their lips or their throat feel tight [6].

J. Park (✉) · J. Schwob
Maria Fareri Children's Hospital at Westchester Medical Center, Valhalla, NY, USA

R. P. Olympia, J. Brady-Olympia (eds.), *Clinical Considerations in School-based Health*, https://doi.org/10.1007/978-3-031-85765-2_38

Widespread hives are the most common manifestation of food allergies in children. If a child presents with any life threatening symptoms, such as low blood pressure, difficulty breathing, or symptoms that involve more than one body system (such as vomiting and a rash), Intramuscular Epinephrine (Epipen) should be immediately administered and Emergency Medical Services contacted. If a child is hemodynamically stable and the only manifestation of the allergic reaction is the rash, correctly dosed antihistamine can be given for patients that are not allergic to that class of medications. However, not all schools stock Benadryl for use in students without a history of allergies. The availability of Benadryl and other medications in schools varies by district and state regulations. While some schools may have Benadryl on hand as part of their emergency medication supplies, it is not universally required or provided. The use of Benadryl in schools generally depends on local policies and the specific needs of the student population. For students with known allergies, schools often focus on maintaining emergency epinephrine for anaphylaxis, as it is the critical treatment for severe allergic reactions. If a patient has a history of an anaphylactic reaction to a particular food in the past, and now is only presenting with a rash or hives, Epinephrine should still be considered and ready for administration, as prior anaphylaxis is a risk factor for subsequent anaphylaxis episodes.

It is imperative that schools implement comprehensive safety measures for students with food allergies, including having a comprehensive emergency plan with immediate access to epinephrine. Schools should also consider nut-free areas and collaborate with parents and healthcare professionals to ensure effective management and staff training.

Recent advancements in food allergy treatments include Omalizumab, which reduces allergic reactions by inhibiting IgE, though it can cause headaches, dizziness, and injection site reactions. Other FDA-approved treatments include epicutaneous immunotherapy, which involves a patch to desensitize the immune system but may cause skin reactions, and oral immunotherapy, which gradually increases allergen exposure and may lead to gastrointestinal symptoms.

Referring a student to a pediatric allergist is essential when they experience severe or persistent symptoms unresponsive to standard treatments, have unclear diagnosis, or suffer from frequent severe reactions like anaphylaxis. Additionally, a specialist should be consulted for students with significant family histories of allergies or whose symptoms notably impact their school performance. Specialists can also help to identify patients with complex symptoms and uncover other diseases associated with food allergies (Table 38.1).

Case 2 During lunch hour one day at school, 11 year old Emily started vomiting, her face turned red, and she also started to complain that she felt like her throat was closing. Emily was immediately taken to the nurse's office where vitals were taken, and she was found to have an increased respiratory rate, increased work of breathing, and low blood pressure. What is the immediate next step that should be taken?

Table 38.1 Diseases associated with food allergies

Disease	Clinical symptoms	Diagnosis	Treatment
FPIES (Food Protein-Induced Enterocolitis Syndrome)	Severe vomiting, diarrhea, lethargy	Clinical history, elimination diet	Intravenous fluids, supportive care
Eosinophilic Esophagitis	Difficulty swallowing, abdominal pain, reflux	Endoscopy with biopsy, elimination diet	Steroids, proton pump inhibitors
Celiac Disease	Abdominal pain, diarrhea, weight loss	Blood tests (anti-tTG, EMA), biopsy	Gluten-free diet

Table 38.2 Common signs and symptoms of anaphylaxis in children

Body system	Symptom presentation
Skin	Erythema, urticaria, flushing, angioedema
Eyes	Edema/chemosis, pruritus, tearing, conjunctival injection
Respiratory	Cough, rhinorrhea, sneeze, stridor, laryngeal edema, shortness of breath, wheezing, hypoxemia
Cardiovascular	Palpitations, syncope, dizziness, chest pain, cyanosis, pallor, tachycardia, hypotension
Abdominal	Throat tightness, difficulty swallowing, vomiting, diarrhea, abdominal cramps
Neurological	Headache, blurry vision, dizziness, mood changes, agitation, depressed mental status

Most anaphylactic reactions occur outside a hospital setting [7], and it is very important for school health departments to be aware of how this severe reaction can present. Usually, anaphylaxis that is caused by a food allergen occurs within minutes to several hours after the food was ingested [8]. Anaphylaxis, according to the Brighton Collaboration Working Group in 2022, presents acutely and leads to a marked change in an individual's previous stable condition and is characterized by the following: rapid progression of symptoms and signs which typically affects multiple body systems (skin/mucosa/respiratory/cardiovascular/gastrointestinal) at the same time or sequentially but occurring in a short period of time (within 1 hour of onset of the first symptoms or signs). It has the potential to quickly turn into a life threatening emergency. Anaphylaxis should be considered when children exhibit severe symptoms or any symptoms that involve more than one body system (Table 38.2). Although most reactions to food allergens are mild and closely resemble a standard reaction, the symptoms of anaphylaxis can also often initially appear mild, and therefore, any child that has a known or suspected food allergy needs to be closely monitored. Children who have a history of having an anaphylactic reaction in the past, or those who have a known food allergy, and those with poorly controlled asthma are at an increased risk of having severe reactions to food items. Other significant risk factors to be aware of include a delay in the administration of epinephrine or in situations where health care providers rely on antihistamine medications in situations when epinephrine needs to be given.

It is incredibly important to stress that intramuscular epinephrine is the **only** first line treatment for anaphylaxis. It should be administered immediately in any situation of an obvious or suspected anaphylactic reaction. Other medications like antihistamines or bronchodilators should never be given prior to or in place of epinephrine. The American Academy of Pediatrics (AAP) recommends that the epinephrine be given in the anterolateral thigh intramuscularly to ensure safety and adequate absorption. The recommended dose (according to the AAP) of the epinephrine is 0.01 mg/kg/dose of the 1 mg/mL concentration with maximum dose of 0.3 mg in the prepubertal child and 0.5 mg in the adolescent given intramuscularly, and should be repeated every 5 to 15 min as needed. Lastly, as of August 2024, the US Food and Drug Administration approved the use of an epinephrine nasal spray for the emergency treatment of life threatening anaphylaxis in adult and pediatric patients who weigh at least 30 kilograms (66 pounds).

The AAP also strongly recommends that all pediatric patients who are at risk for anaphylaxis should have an Allergy and Anaphylaxis Emergency Plan at school. The form should identify what the child's allergies and risk factors are, it should be easily accessible and comprehensible to those caring for the child in the school setting. The Emergency Plan stresses the importance of intramuscular epinephrine, and clearly instructs caretakers to immediately call 911 after administering epinephrine. Additionally, it is very important that schools be well stocked with epinephrine so that it is readily available in times of need. Having non-student-specific epinephrine available in schools enables school nurses and staff to address anaphylaxis on-site while waiting for Emergency Medical Services to arrive. However, it's important to note that not all states require K-12 schools to keep epinephrine on hand. In states where stocking epinephrine is permitted but not mandated, schools have the option to choose not to stock it [9].

38.1 Case Conclusions

Case 1 This case study illustrates the importance of proactive management of food allergies in schools to ensure the safety and well-being of students like Sarah. By understanding the complexities of food allergies and implementing appropriate accommodations and emergency plans, schools can create a supportive environment conducive to learning and growth for all students.

Case 2 Emily was given the correct dose of epinephrine, and 911 was called, with a special request to send an ambulance stocked with epinephrine. Her vomiting persisted while waiting for the ambulance to arrive, and she was kept on her side to avoid aspiration. While en route to the hospital, Emily required another dose of the epinephrine about 15 minutes after the first one was given. She required two more doses of epinephrine while in the Emergency Department and was admitted for observation and discharged home the following day. As a side note, in an emergency department, treatments for anaphylaxis, in addition to epinephrine, may include antihistamines like diphenhydramine for symptom relief, bronchodilators like albuterol for respiratory issues, and supplemental oxygen if needed. Intravenous fluids and, in severe cases, vasopressors such as norepinephrine are used to manage hypotension and support circulation. Corticosteroids are not used as the main treatment for anaphylaxis but may be given as an additional measure to help reduce the risk of a secondary or prolonged reaction. However, it is important to note that the evidence supporting this use is quite weak.

Extra Credit Points

1. Intramuscular epinephrine administration in the anterolateral thigh is the first line treatment for anaphylaxis.
2. In a severe or suspicious allergic reaction, do not rely on antihistamines, steroids, bronchodilators or other medications; intramuscular epinephrine should always be given right away without hesitation.
3. All patients at risk for an anaphylactic reaction should have an emergency action plan given to school health care providers in order to provide them with clear instructions on how to manage potential emergency scenarios.

References

1. Gupta RS, Warren CM, Smith BM, Blumenstock JA, Jiang J, Davis MM, Nadeau KC. The public health impact of parent-reported childhood food allergies in the United States. Pediatrics. 2018;142(6):e20181235. https://doi.org/10.1542/peds.2018-1235. Epub 2018 Nov 19. Erratum in: Pediatrics. 2019 Mar;143(3): PMID: 30455345; PMCID: PMC6317772
2. Waserman S, Cruickshank H, Hildebrand KJ, Mack D, Bantock L, Bingemann T, Chu DK, Cuello-Garcia C, Ebisawa M, Fahmy D, Fleischer DM, Galloway L, Gartrell G, Greenhawt M, Hamilton N, Hourihane J, Langlois M, Loh R, Muraro A, Rosenfield L, Schoessler S, Tang MLK, Weitzner B, Wang J, Brozek JL. Prevention and management of allergic reactions to food in child care centers and schools: practice guidelines. J Allergy Clin Immunol. 2021;147(5):1561–78. https://doi.org/10.1016/j.jaci.2021.01.034.
3. Boyce JA, Assa'ad A, Burks AW, et al. NIAID-sponsored expert panel. Guidelines for the diagnosis and management of food allergy in the United States: report of the NIAID-sponsored expert panel. J Allergy Clin Immunol. 2010;126(suppl 6):S1–S58.
4. Sicherer SH, Furlong TJ, DeSimone J, Sampson HA. The US peanut and tree nut allergy registry: characteristics of reactions in schools and day care. J Pediatr. 2001;138:560–5.
5. Lack G. Update on risk factors for food allergy. J Allergy Clin Immunol. 2012;129(5):1187–97. https://doi.org/10.1016/j.jaci.2012.02.036. Epub 2012 Mar 30
6. The Food Allergy & Anaphylaxis Network. Food Allergy News. 2003;13:2.
7. Wood RA, Camargo CA, Lieberman P, et al. Anaphylaxis in America: the prevalence and characteristics of anaphylaxis in the United States. J Allergy Clin Immunol. 2014;133(2):461–7.
8. Joyce JA, Assa'ad A, Burks AW, et al. NIAID-sponsored expert panel. Guidelines for the diagnosis and management of food allergy in the United States: report of the NIAID-sponsored expert panel. J Allergy Clin Immunol. 2010;126(Suppl 6):S1–S58.
9. Russell AF, Bingemann TA, Cooke AT, Ponda P, Pistiner M, Jean T, Nanda A, Jobrack J, Hoyt AEW, Young MC. The need for required stock epinephrine in all schools: a work group report of the AAAAI adverse reactions to foods committee. J Allergy Clin Immunol Pract. 2023;11(4):1068–1082.e1.

Chapter 39
Asthma

Timothy P. Roach and Amy A. Dooley

Case 1 8 year old Ben, who has intermittent asthma, comes to your office in the middle of gym class complaining of difficulty breathing while playing basketball. This is the third time this month that he has come to your office during gym class asking to use his albuterol. He has a dry cough with mild supraclavicular retractions and prolonged expiratory phase on auscultation. His respiratory rate is 30 breaths per minute, pulse oximetry is 97% on room air, and heart rate is 116 beats per minute.

Asthma is a chronic inflammatory state which exists in both persistent and intermittent forms. Within each subset of asthma, a child can have either controlled or uncontrolled asthma. In addition, it is common for children to have comorbidities than can be allergic (rhinitis, eczema, food allergies) or non-allergic (obesity, sleep disordered breathing, prematurity) in nature. The National Heart Lung and Blood Institute (NHLBI) Guidelines for the Diagnosis and Management of Asthma defined asthma as "a chronic inflammatory disorder of the airways in which many cells and cellular elements play a role... In susceptible individuals, this inflammation causes recurrent episodes of wheezing, breathlessness, chest tightness, and coughing, particularly at night or in the early morning. These episodes are usually associated with widespread but variable airflow obstruction that is often reversible either spontaneously or with treatment. The inflammation also causes an associated increase in the existing bronchial hyperresponsiveness to a variety of stimuli." [1] These stimuli are

T. P. Roach
Penn State Milton S. Hershey Medical Center, Hershey, PA, USA
e-mail: troach@pennstatehealth.psu.edu

A. A. Dooley (✉)
Penn State Children's Hospital, Hershey, PA, USA
e-mail: adooley@pennstatehealth.psu.edu

R. P. Olympia, J. Brady-Olympia (eds.), *Clinical Considerations in School-based Health*, https://doi.org/10.1007/978-3-031-85765-2_39

Table 39.1 Common asthma triggers can be allergic, environmental, illness, or other exposures

Allergic: dust, cockroaches, pet dander, mold, pollen
Environmental: wood fires, smoke, air pollution, chemicals, fragrances, weather
Respiratory illness
Other exposures: exercise, stress, strong emotions,

often more commonly known as "triggers" (Table 39.1). There is no one trigger that is universal among all asthmatics, so knowing which ones impact your patients is important.

Recognizing triggers may take some time and be difficult to identify, especially in younger children who are inconsistent historians. In observing times when they start to have symptoms of asthma, trying to find a correlating exposure can help with prevention. If a known trigger can be avoided or mitigated, the asthma symptoms can be avoided. Unfortunately, often triggers cannot be avoided and "pre-treatment" can be a way to allow patients to continue engaging in activities they enjoy. Given the rapid onset of action of albuterol, it can be given prior to a planned activity to prevent the development of symptoms or need for rescue medication. Other medications may be used as "rescue" medications instead of albuterol, so it is always important to review a child's Asthma Action Plan (AAP) prior to giving medication.

In addition to providing the appropriate medication and dose of rescue medication, it is also important to consider the modality. The two most common ways of providing bronchodilator is through a nebulizer or metered dose inhaler (MDI) with valved holding chamber—often called a spacer for simplicity. Evidence has shown that inhalers with spacers are non-inferior to nebulizers when providing medication with decreased side effect and shortened duration of treatment [2]. Spacers continue to be recommended for all children using metered dose inhalers regardless of age. There are two common ways to give an inhaler with spacer device as detailed in Table 39.2.

There are many commercially available inhaler devices on the market today, so be sure to check to see if the inhaler you're supposed to be giving is a metered dose inhaler (MDI/HFA), breath actuated inhaler (respiclick), soft mist inhaler (Respimat), or dry powder inhaler (DPI) as they will all have slightly different modes of delivery. In addition to bronchodilators, other common asthma medications available to prevent and treat asthma are described in Table 39.3.

Case 1 Conclusion *You give Ben 2 puffs of albuterol with his spacer and, after about 15 min, his cough has resolved to the point where he feels ready to go back to gym. You call his parents and discuss the idea of pre-treating him with albuterol for gym class. The family sends in an updated asthma action plan and you start giving him 2 puffs of albuterol with his spacer prior to starting gym. He stops coming to you during activity for the remainder of the school year.*

Table 39.2 Two common spacer methods to deliver inhaled medications to children

MDI with spacer and mask	MDI with spacer and mouthpiece
• Allows for coordination of breath in a younger child or one with delays • Steps: ○ Shake inhaler and insert into spacer ○ Create a seal around the nose and mouth with mask ○ Puff inhaler into chamber ○ Count 10 breaths ▪ Watch the valve on the spacer or feel/watch for chest movement ○ Remove mask from face ○ Repeat as indicated in 30–60 s	• Works best for children who can create a mouth seal • Steps: ○ Shake inhaler and insert into spacer ○ Take a deep breath in and blow it all out ○ Place spacer in mouth ○ Puff inhaler into chamber ○ Take a slow deep breath in ▪ Don't let the spacer whistle! ○ Count to 10 ○ Slowly exhale out ○ Repeat as indicated in 30–60 s

Case 2 11 year old Zoe is a student with asthma who you know well as she often comes to your office to use her inhaler before going outside for recess. She has just come back to school after being out for a few days due to a viral induced asthma exacerbation. Before lunchtime, she comes to your office because she's starting to cough and feel like her chest is "tight" more than it was this morning. She also thinks she remembers something about her mom saying she needed to take her emergency inhaler when she's at school, but she's not sure when. Her respiratory rate is 18 breaths per minute, heart rate is 96 beats per minute, and pulse oximetry is 98% on room air. She is speaking comfortably in sentences with intermittent, harsh cough and a faint end-expiratory wheeze.

Children with asthma will often miss a significant amount of school when dealing with an exacerbation. Often, they will feel well enough to return to school prior to their symptoms being completely gone. During this time, the use of their Asthma Action Plan (AAP) is vital in continuing their recovery back to baseline. Their AAP, provided by their primary or specialty care provider, will detail medications which should be given both at baseline and at times of exacerbation. Many areas will have their own specific AAPs, though they often follow the standard GREEN-YELLOW-RED arrangement [3]. (Fig. 39.1).

The GREEN zone is when children are at their well baseline. For many, it may include their daily controller medications, as needed allergy medications, and possibly pre-treatment medications. Many children will spend much of their time within the GREEN zone. Some will require their controller medications to be taken during school hours, but this is not common.

The YELLOW zone is a warning zone, letting patients and families know that symptoms are starting and how best to avoid an exacerbation. This zone will include instructions for their "as needed" medications to help them manage their symptoms better. For many children, this medication will be albuterol. However, in recent years, studies have found that other medications may be as beneficial as albuterol

Table 39.3 Common medications used for the prevention and treatment of asthma

	Medication	Formulation	Indication	Side effects
Preventive	Corticosteroids			
	• Fluticasone • Mometasone • Budesonide	• MDI • MDI/DPI • Nebulizer/ DPI	Frequent symptoms and need for bronchodilators in setting of triggers	Oral thrush
	Combination inhalers			
	• Budesonide/ formoterol • Mometasone/ formoterol • fluticasone/salmeterol	• MDI/DPI • MDI • MDI/DPI	Frequent albuterol use while on controllers, used as step-up therapy	Oral thrush Jitteriness
	Leukotriene receptor antagonist			
	• Montelukast	• Pill/ granules	Exercise induced asthma, possible allergic triggers	Headaches nightmares behavior change
	Antihistamines			
	• Loratadine • Cetirizine • Fexofenadine	• Pill/liquid • Pill/liquid • Pill/liquid	Allergic triggers of asthma symptoms, upper airways cough	Dry eyes/mouth Sleepiness Hyperactivity
	Long-acting muscarinic antagonist			
	• Tiotropium	• Respimat	Need for further step-up therapy	Pupillary changes
Acute	Bronchodilators			
	• Albuterol/ Levalbuterol • Ipratropium bromide	• MDI/ nebulizer • MDI/ nebulizer	Increased cough, shortness of breath, chest tightness, or wheezing	Tachycardia Jitteriness Anxiety QT prolongation
	Systemic Steroids			
	• Prednisone • Methylprednisone • Dexamethasone	• Liquid/pill • Pill/IV • Liquid/Pill/ IV/IM	Persistent symptoms in the setting of a trigger, need for frequent bronchodilators	Hyperglycemia Agitation Fluid retention
Emergency	• Epinephrine (catecholamine)	• IM	Status asthmaticus with impending respiratory failure	Tachycardia Anxiety
	• Magnesium sulfate (smooth muscle relaxant)	• IV	Poor air entry with hypoxemia and difficulties oxygenating	Hypotension Syncope
	• Terbutaline (systemic beta agonist)	• IM/IV	Poor air entry with hypoxemia and difficulties oxygenating	Tachycardia Jitteriness Anxiety

Abbreviations: *DPI* dry powdered inhaler, *IV* intravenous, *IM* intramuscular, *MDI* meter dose inhaler

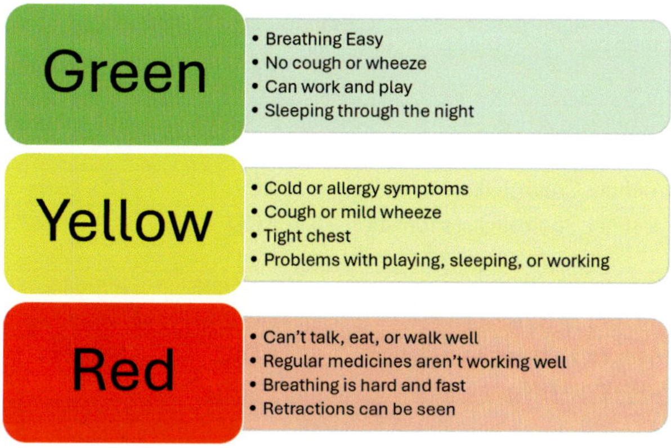

Fig. 39.1 Asthma Action Plan guidelines in the common GREEN-YELLOW-RED set up

when used at times of exacerbation. One of these approaches is called **SMART** therapy where there is a **S**ingle **M**aintenance **A**nd **R**eliever **T**herapy for the patient which has them using one inhaler as both their controller and their rescue. The recommended inhaler in this instance is budesonide-formoterol as the long-acting beta agonist component has a fast onset, similar to albuterol [4].

The RED zone is often a time for alarm that a child's asthma is not well controlled and they are at risk of having a severe exacerbation. This zone will often include instruction for the use of repeated treatments of the child's rescue medication—typically, three treatments spaced 15 min apart are recommended. This may be the same medication and dose used in the child's YELLOW zone or may be different. At this time, it is also typically recommended that the child seek medical attention at an urgent care or emergency department as they may need more aggressive treatments and monitoring.

Many AAPs may include areas for a child's peak flow as it had been standard in adult asthma care for decades. Literature has shown that peak flow in children is a very variable measure based on effort and may not correlate well with clinical symptoms or progress. Unless specifically requested, documentation of peak flows is not typically recommended for children with asthma nor is it followed during times of exacerbation. But, as always, each child is an individual and care may vary widely [5].

Another aspect of the AAP is the determination as to whether children can administer their own inhaled medications and if they are able to "self-carry" their inhalers. There is no standard age recommendation for when a child is ready to start carrying their inhaler with them for self-treatment. These decisions are often made in partnership with the patient, their caregivers, and the school the patient attends.

Case 2 Conclusion *You review Zoe's asthma action plan, which indicates that she should get 2 puffs of albuterol with spacer every 4–6 h while in the "yellow zone". You provide her treatment and she returns to class. She visits you around the same time the next two days for treatments, but by the end of the week she reports that she is feeling much better and doesn't need her "midday puffs" anymore.*

Table 39.4 Validated control measures for children with asthma that can be followed serially to gauge control over seasons or the school year

Test	Abbreviation	Age	Design
Childhood Asthma Control Test	C-ACT	4–11 years	7 items: 4 for the child, 3 for the caregiver
Asthma Control Test	ACT	12+ years	5 items
Asthma Control Questionnaire	ACQ	12+ years	6 questions and FEV1 measurement
Test for Respiratory and Asthma Control in Kids	TRACK	< 5 years	5 items
Asthma Therapy Assessment Questionnaire	ATAQ	5+ years	20 items, 4 in the control domain

Case 3 Destiny is a 10 year old female who has missed multiple days of school for her asthma and was hospitalized once this winter. She comes to get her albuterol inhaler infrequently outside of colds and does not use it routinely prior to gym class. During Spring Field Day, she is out running on the lawn when she starts to cough and complains that she can't breathe. She arrives at your office speaking in 1–2 word sentences, breathing 34 times per minute, with a heart rate of 114 beats per minute. Her pulse oximetry is 91% on room air and she has diffuse inspiratory and expiratory wheezes.

Asthma, despite having known triggers and patterns, can be a very unpredictable and sudden onset emergency. Over time, triggers for an individual can even evolve and ones that were not problematic for them before could be life threatening. Assessing asthma control can be helpful to determine a baseline for patients with frequent exacerbations. There are several standardized measures for asthma control presented in Table 39.4 [6]:

These measures can clarify aspects of a child's life that are impacted by their asthma and how limiting it may be for them. While they cannot be used to predict a severe exacerbation, they provide a better sense of the level of control an asthmatic has over their disease. Identifying poorly controlled asthma can also be remembered by using the Rule of Twos: using their rescue inhaler more than TWO times a week, waking up with asthma symptoms more than TWO times a month, and refilling their albuterol more than TWO times a year. If a patient is having these baseline symptoms or more, they may be at higher risk of having an exacerbation [7].

Knowing which patients have poorly controlled asthma at baseline can help with being prepared for when emergencies happen. During known triggering seasons (viral, allergen, poor air quality), make sure students have enough of their rescue medications available and that all appropriate paperwork is on file. While preventing attacks can be a large task and sometimes impossible, preparation can help get through exacerbations. Regardless of control status, an asthmatic should always have easy access to their inhaler both while in school and off grounds for school sponsored activities.

Case 3 Conclusion *After three treatments of 4 puffs of albuterol given 15 min apart, Destiny continues to have increased work of breathing, borderline oxygen saturation, and persistent wheeze. Her mother is on the way into the school and EMS has just arrived to provide additional treatments.*

Extra Credit Points

1. Asthma is the most common chronic illness of childhood and is very variable from child to child. Individualizing care and providing the treatment that is appropriate for that patient utilizing their GREEN-YELLOW-RED Asthma Action Plan is of utmost importance.
2. An exacerbation can occur at any time and often without warning, always make sure to have rescue medications available for all asthmatic patients you care for.
3. Asthma care is changing rapidly with the advent of injectable medications for asthma (biologics) that can be used to downregulate the body's response to triggers which can reduce both exacerbations and controller need.

References

1. Expert Panel Report 3: Guidelines for the Diagnosis and Management of Asthma. National Institute of Health: National Heart, Lung, and Blood Institute (2007).
2. Castro-Rodriguez JA, Rodrigo GJ. beta-agonists through metered-dose inhaler with valved holding chamber versus nebulizer for acute exacerbation of wheezing or asthma in children under 5 years of age: a systematic review with meta-analysis. J Pediatr. 2004;145(2):172–7.
3. Simon AE, Akinbami LJ. Asthma action plan receipt among children with asthma 2–17 years of age, United States, 2002–2013. J Pediatr. 2016;171:283–9.e1.
4. Beasley R, Harrison T, Peterson S, et al. Evaluation of budesonide-formoterol for maintenance and reliever therapy among patients with poorly controlled asthma: a systematic review and meta-analysis. JAMA Netw Open. 2022;5(3):e220615.
5. Sly PD. Peak expiratory flow monitoring in pediatric asthma: is there a role? J Asthma. 1996;33(5):277–87.
6. Dinakar C, Chipps BE, et al. Clinical tools to assess asthma control in children. Pediatrics. 2017;139(1)
7. Millard M, Hart M, Barnes S. Validation of rules of Two™ as a paradigm for assessing asthma control. Baylor Univ Med Cent Proc. 2014;27(2):79–82.

Chapter 40
Bleeding Disorders and Anemia

Marlliny Sullivan, Carla Reale, and Ellen M. Benitah Bulbarelli

Case 1 Emma, a 12-year-old female, presents to the school clinic with a 3-month history of progressive fatigue and exercise intolerance. Emma has been more tired than usual, often requiring naps after school. Emma used to participate in soccer but has stopped attending practices after passing out during a practice. Emma's mother has also noticed that she has been craving and eating ice, which she finds unusual. Menarche occurred at age 11 years old, and she reports regular menstrual cycles, duration 5–6 days with heavy flow on the first two days. There is no history of recent illness, weight loss, fever, or night sweats. Physical Examination: normal vital signs. Pale-appearing, alert. Conjunctivae are pale. Mild angular cheilitis noted. Normal respiratory and cardiovascular exam. Abdomen: soft and no hepatosplenomegaly. You obtain the following diagnostic tests: Complete Blood Count (CBC): Hemoglobin (Hgb): 9.2 g/dL (Low), hematocrit (Hct): 28% (Low), Mean Corpuscular Volume (MCV): 70 fL (Low), Red Blood Cell Count (RBC): 4.0 million/μL (Low), Red Cell Distribution Width (RDW): 17% (High), normal white blood cell count and platelets. Serum Iron: 20 μg/dL (Low), Ferritin: 8 ng/mL (Low), Total Iron-Binding Capacity (TIBC): 420 μg/dL (High), Transferrin Saturation: 5% (Low), Peripheral Blood Smear: Microcytic, hypochromic RBCs with mild anisocytosis. What is Emma's diagnosis?

M. Sullivan
SUNY Upstate Medical University, Syracuse, NY, USA

C. Reale · E. M. Benitah Bulbarelli (✉)
Jefferson Einstein Philadelphia Hospital, Philadelphia, PA, USA

R. P. Olympia, J. Brady-Olympia (eds.), *Clinical Considerations in School-based Health*, https://doi.org/10.1007/978-3-031-85765-2_40

Emma has iron deficiency anemia based on history, physical examination, and confirmed by laboratory studies. Anemia is a common hematological condition characterized by a decrease in the number of red blood cells (RBCs) or the hemoglobin concentration in the blood, leading to a diminished capacity to carry oxygen to tissues. Anemia is defined as a reduction of hemoglobin concentration or red blood cell mass. The reference range for hemoglobin in children from 6 to 12 years old is approximately 11.2 to 14.5 g/dL. The range for hematocrit in children ages 6 to 12 years old is 35 to 44% [1–3]. Chronic and severe anemia in the pediatric population can lead to neurodevelopmental and cognitive deficits in early childhood, impaired growth, and increased susceptibility to infections. Significant acute anemia leads to shortness of breath, chest pain, tachycardia, dizziness, and syncope. Worldwide, the most common nutritional disorder is iron deficiency anemia. Table 40.1 shows the most common causes of anemia in children.

The diagnostic approach to a child with symptoms of anemia includes performing a complete history and physical examination, and confirmed with laboratory testing (Table 40.2) [4–8] Children with significant symptoms (generalized weakness, exercise intolerance, inability to ambulate without dizziness or lightheadedness, tachycardia or hypotension) should be referred to an emergency department for stabilization, possible blood transfusion, and consultation with hematology/oncology.

Case 2 David is a 14-year-old male with a history of Hemophilia A who presents to the school nurse's office with pain and swelling in his right knee after a fall during a soccer game. David reports that he fell while playing soccer about 2 h ago. He initially experienced minor discomfort, but the pain in his right knee has been progressively getting worse. He describes the pain as throbbing and severe, with associated swelling and difficulty to move the knee. On physical examination, David appears in moderate distress due to pain. He is afebrile, heart rate is 80 beats per minute, blood pressure 110/70 mmHg, and respiratory rate 17 breaths per minute. Physical examination of his right lower extremity demonstrates right knee swelling, tender to touch, with limited range of motion due to pain. No open wounds, bruising, or deformities on inspection. No other joint involvement noted. Cardiovascular, respiratory, and neurological exams are unremarkable. What should you do?

Bleeding disorders are a group of medical conditions that affect the body's blood clotting ability, potentially leading to excessive bleeding (Table 40.3). In school-age children, bleeding disorders can present in different ways and often affect daily activities and participation in sports or other physical activities [9, 10].

If a child exhibits signs of a bleeding disorder, it's essential to inform the parents and consult a pediatric hematologist/oncologist for proper diagnosis and treatment. Children should be referred to the emergency department for the following: severe bleeding episodes (e.g. bleeding does not stop after applying pressure for 10 minutes or if there is bleeding from a cut that requires more than basic first aid);

Table 40.1 Types of anemia in children

Etiology	Description	Signs/symptoms	Diagnosis	Treatment
– Iron Deficiency Anemia (IDA)	Most prevalent Typically, due to inadequate dietary iron intake [7], increased growth demands, or chronic blood loss.	Fatigue, pallor, irritability, dizziness, dyspnea on exertion, and developmental delays, pica—an appetite for non-food substances (e.g., ice, clay, cloth, dirt, paper, or metal)	History of present illness Physical examination CBC and iron studies	Dietary changes encouraging the consumption of iron-rich foods, such as lean meats, beans, and fortified cereals. Iron supplements
– Vitamin B12 Deficiency	Often occurs in children with dietary restrictions or malabsorption issues.	Fatigue, neurological changes (e.g., weakness, ataxia, paresthesia), macrocytic anemia	History of present illness Physical examination CBC and iron studies Vitamin B12 levels	Treatment of B12 deficiency cause Vitamin B12 supplements
– Folate Deficiency	Inadequate folate intake, often found in children with poor dietary habits or malabsorption syndromes.	Similar symptoms to B12 deficiency, macrocytic anemia	History of present illness Physical examination CBC and iron studies Folate levels	Treatment of folate deficiency cause Folate supplements

(continued)

Table 40.1 (continued)

Etiology	Description	Signs/symptoms	Diagnosis	Treatment
Hemolytic Anemia	Occurs when RBCs are destroyed faster than they are produced. Genetic disorders (e.g., sickle cell disease, hereditary spherocytosis), autoimmune conditions (e.g., autoimmune hemolytic anemia)	Fatigue, jaundice, dark urine, weakness	CBC and peripheral blood smear Reticulocyte count Haptoglobin Lactate dehydrogenase Indirect bilirubin	Treatment may involve corticosteroids, immunosuppressive agents, or even splenectomy in certain cases, depending on the underlying cause.
Anemia of Chronic Disease	Common in chronic conditions such as infections (e.g., chronic sinusitis, H. pylori), inflammatory diseases (e.g., IBD, cystic fibrosis), or malignancies.	Fatigue, pale skin, inflammation-related symptoms	History of present illness Physical examination CBC and iron studies Characterized by normal or high ferritin with low serum iron.	Effective management of the underlying cause.
Genetic Factors	Exposure to lead or other toxins can interfere with hemoglobin synthesis, leading to anemia through hemolysis.	Fatigue, irritability, developmental delays	CBC Lead levels Other toxins levels	Effective management of the underlying cause.

Table 40.2 Laboratory testing for anemia

Complete blood count	Essential for evaluating hemoglobin levels and red blood cell indices. Low hemoglobin and hematocrit levels indicate anemia. MCV (mean cell or corpuscular volume) measures average size of red blood cells. MCV helps classifying type of anemia based on rather cells are smaller, normal or larger in size
Peripheral Blood Smear	Assesses red blood cell morphology, helping differentiate between microcytic, macrocytic, and normocytic anemias
Iron Studies	Essential for diagnosing iron deficiency anemia, including serum iron, ferritin, TIBC, and transferrin saturation
Reticulocyte Count	Evaluates bone marrow response to anemia. High reticulocyte counts indicate increased red blood cell production
Additional Tests	Depending on clinical suspicion, tests for vitamin B12, folate, and hemolytic anemia markers (like haptoglobin and lactic dehydrogenase-LDH) may be performed

Table 40.3 Bleeding disorders in children

Bleeding disorder	Description	Common symptoms
Hemophilia A, B or C	A genetic disorder caused by a coagulation defect. A: deficiency of Factor VIII B: deficiency of Factor IX C: deficiency of Factor XI	• Easy bruising, • Prolonged bleeding, • Joint bleeding • Joint pain or swelling after injury
Von Willebrand Disease	The most common inherited bleeding disorder. Deficiency in von Willebrand factor causing defect in platelet plug formation.	• Easy bruising • Heavy menstrual bleeding in girls • Frequent nosebleeds
Thrombocytopenia	Low platelet count. Caused by autoimmune disorders, viral illness, malignancy, or drug reactions.	• Easy bruising, • Petechiae (tiny red or purple spots), • Prolonged bleeding from cuts.
Vitamin K Deficiency	Lack of vitamin K. Often due to insufficient dietary intake or absorption issues.	• Easy bruising, • Bleeding gums
Acquired Coagulation Disorders	Conditions caused by other medical issues, such as liver disease or certain medications use.	• Variable presentation • Easy bruising • Prolonged bleeding
Disseminated Intravascular Coagulation (DIC)	Uncontrollable bleeding. Triggered by severe medical conditions including infections, trauma, snake bites, malignancy.	• Bleeding from multiple sites, such as the nose, gums, mouth, or wounds • Bruising • Chest pain, shortness of breath • Confusion, memory loss, or behavioral changes • Fever

significant joint bleeding (hemarthrosis); internal bleeding signs such as blood in urine, stools or severe abdominal pain, head Injuries with altered mental status or neurologic signs/symptoms; or any evidence of shock [11, 12] Children who are referred to the emergency department require stabilization, possible diagnostic testing or imaging (complete blood counts, X-rays of extremities, CT scan of the brain), and possible treatment (factor replacement, platelet transfusion, antibiotics). Tranexamic acid (TXA) is a newer medication that can be used to prevent or treat excessive bleeding. It is commonly used to treat heavy menstrual bleeding, prevent bleeding during surgeries, and manage bleeding disorders such as hemophilia. Oral doses of TXA may be prescribed for those with bleeding disorders, and may be administered intravenously or nebulized in the event of acute hemorrhages associated with trauma or following surgery (such as dental procedures or oral/pharyngeal surgeries [13, 14].

Case 3 Sara, a 10-year-old girl, was referred to the school nurse after her teacher noticed unusual bruising on her legs and arms during a routine classroom activity. The bruises seemed to appear without any known injury. The school nurse noted multiple small purple spots (petechiae) and bruises on Sara's arms and legs, was concerned about either a bleeding disorder or non-accidental injury, and was referred to the local emergency department. A complete blood count (CBC) revealed a significantly low platelet count of 20,000/μL (normal range: 150,000 to 450,000/μL). The rest of her blood work was within normal limits. Based on her clinical presentation and laboratory results, the consulting pediatric hematologist diagnosed her with Immune Thrombocytopenic Purpura (Table 40.4) [15, 16]**.**

Sara was started on a short course of corticosteroids to help boost her platelet production. She was advised to avoid contact sports and other physical activities that could put her at risk of injury. Sara's school staff was informed about the diagnosis, and in coordination with her healthcare team and parents, a safety plan and proper accommodations were established. Her platelet count gradually improved with treatment and Sara was able to return to her normal activities.

Table 40.4 Immune thrombocytopenia purpura (ITP)

Etiology	– Autoimmune Response: The immune system produces antibodies that target and destroy platelets. – Infections: Commonly triggered by viral infections (e.g., EBV, CMV, varicella). – Idiopathic: Unknown cause.
Clinical Presentation	– Bruising: Unexplained or excessive bruising (ecchymosis). – Petechiae: Small red spots under the skin. – Mucosal Bleeding: Nosebleeds, gum bleeding, blood in urine/stools. – Fatigue: Feeling tired.
Most common treatments	– Watchful Waiting: Observation in mild cases. – Corticosteroids: Prednisone or dexamethasone to increase platelet count. – IVIG: For rapid increase in platelets.
Less common treatments	– Anti-D Immunoglobulin (Rh-positive). – Rituximab: For chronic or severe cases. – TPO-RAs: Eltrombopag, romiplostim to stimulate platelet production. – Splenectomy: Considered in chronic refractory cases.
Supportive Care	– Avoid NSAIDs (e.g., ibuprofen). – Restrict contact sports and high-risk physical activities.
When to Refer to Emergency Department	– Severe Bleeding: Intracranial hemorrhage (severe headache, confusion, seizures), severe fatigue or dizziness, uncontrollable nosebleeds, or blood in vomit/stools/urine. – Platelet Count <10,000/μL with any bleeding. – Head Trauma: Immediate.

Coordination of care for children with bleeding disorders or anemia at the school setting

1. Communication with the school personnel: Set up meetings with the child's teachers, school nurse, and administrator. Foster open communication with the child's family.
2. Education and training: Provide training for school staff about hematologic disorders, signs of bleeding and appropriate responses. Foster an environment of understanding and support among child's classmates.
3. Care plan: Develop an individualized health plan. Identify the child's specific needs and risks related to their hematologic disorder. Identify steps to take in case of a bleeding episode, including contact information for healthcare providers and emergency medical services. Have the child's physician or specialist provide written care plans.

Extra Credit Points

1. Having a high index of suspicion for students with anemia based on signs and symptoms can lead to prompt diagnosis and treatment, preventing neurodevelopmental and cognitive deficits in early childhood, impaired growth, and increased susceptibility to infections.
2. Regular communication and education with school staff are vital to promoting a positive school experience for students with anemia and bleeding disorders.
3. Students should be referred in an emergency department for signs of severe anemia (generalized weakness, exercise intolerance, inability to ambulate without dizziness or lightheadedness, tachycardia or hypotension) or significant bleeding disorder signs/symptoms (uncontrollable bleeding, significant joint bleeding, blood in urine, stools or severe abdominal pain, head Injuries with altered mental status or neurologic signs/symptoms, or any evidence of shock).

References

1. World Health Organization (WHO). (2021). Global Health Observatory (GHO) data: prevalence of anemia among children under five years.
2. Staffa SJ, Joerger JD, Henry E, Christensen RD, Brugnara C, Zurakowski D. Pediatric hematology normal ranges derived from pediatric primary care patients. Am J Hematol. 2020;95(10):E255–7. https://doi.org/10.1002/ajh.25904. Epub 2020 Aug 12
3. Higgins V, Tahmasebi H, Bohn MK, Hall A, Adeli K. CALIPER Hematology Reference Standards (II). Am J Clin Pathol. 2020;154(3):342–52. https://doi.org/10.1093/ajcp/aqaa057. PMID: 32525543; PMCID: PMC7403758
4. Iron Deficiency Anemia: A Clinical Practice Guideline. (2020). American Society of Hematology.
5. Johnson-Wimbley TD, Graham DY. Diagnosis and management of iron deficiency anemia in the 21st century. Ther Adv Gastroenterol. 2011;4(3):177–84. https://doi.org/10.1177/1756283X11398736. PMID: 21694802; PMCID: PMC3105608
6. Recommendations to prevent and control iron deficiency in the United States. Centers for Disease Control and Prevention. MMWR Recomm Rep. 1998;47(RR-3):1–29.

7. Leung AKC, Lam JM, Wong AHC, Hon KL, Li X. Iron deficiency anemia: an updated review. Curr Pediatr Rev. 2024;20(3):339–56. https://doi.org/10.2174/1573396320666230727102042.
8. Short MW, Domagalski JE. Iron deficiency anemia: evaluation and management. Am Fam Physician. 2013;87(2):98–104.
9. American Society of Hematology: Educational resources and guidelines on the management of bleeding disorders. 2024. Accessed on September 27, 2024. https://www.hematology.org/education/patients/bleeding-disorders
10. Centers for Disease Control and Prevention (CDC): Information on hemophilia and other bleeding disorders. May 15, 2024. Accessed on September 28, 2024. https://www.cdc.gov/hemophilia/about/?CDC_AAref_Val=https://www.cdc.gov/ncbddd/hemophilia/facts.html.
11. The hemophilia society. Bleeding Disorders and School 2023. Accessed September 28, 2024. https://haemophilia.org.uk/wp-content/uploads/2021/01/THS_A5_Booklet_school_JC_FINAL_V1_Interactive19.pdf
12. Omole O, Reed J, Dunn AL, Gleason CN. Mild hemophilia in a competitive high school soccer player: a case report. J Athl Train. 2023;58(7–8):669–72. Published online 2023 Oct 9. https://doi.org/10.4085/1062-6050-0402.22.
13. ACOG committee opinion no. 557: Management of acute abnormal uterine bleeding in non-pregnant reproductive-aged women. Obstet Gynecol 2013;121(4):891–896. doi: https://doi.org/10.1097/01.AOG.0000428646.67925.9a.
14. Nomura S. Current status and challenges in delivering comprehensive care for patients with hemophilia. J Blood Med. 2023;14:629–37. Published online 2023 Dec 15. https://doi.org/10.2147/JBM.S446204.
15. Pietras NM, Gupta N, Vaillant A, Pearson-Shaver A. Immune thrombocytopenia. Treasure Island (FL): StatPearls Publishing; 2024. https://www.ncbi.nlm.nih.gov/books/NBK562282/
16. Schifferli A, Moulis G, Godeau B, Leblanc T, Aladjidi N, Michel M, Leverger G, Elalfy M, Grainger J, Chitlur M, Heiri A, Holzhauer S, Le Gavrian G, Imbach P, Kühne T. Adolescents and young adults with newly diagnosed primary immune thrombocytopenia. Haematologica. 2023;108(10):2783–93. [PMC free article] [PubMed]

Chapter 41
Cancers

Christy Lucas

Attending school is a normalizing childhood experience. It is widely accepted that return to school after a cancer diagnosis promotes a positive adjustment for children and adolescents [1]. There are perceived risks, including infection, but the benefits of school, including maintaining peer relationships and continuing education, most often outweigh the risks [2]. Children with cancer may have physical changes, including hair loss, decreased energy, increased risk of bleeding/bruising, weight gain or loss, facial fullness, muscle weakness, or motor control difficulties [2]. The stress of having cancer, along with medication side effects, can lead to mood swings [2]. Cancer can also lead to a new vocabulary for both the child, family, and school (Tables 41.1 and 41.2) [3]. It is important to note that no two children with cancer are the same, even if they carry the same diagnosis.

It is vital for a school nurse to be aware of general side effects of chemotherapy, particularly those that they may need to "**TAME**" (Table 41.3) in the school environment. School nurses must also recognize that fatigue is a common side effect of cancer treatment and can make children feel tried, weak, and/or sad; children with cancer may need special accommodations, including a nap during the school day, half-day attendance, or limited participation in physical activity, which a school nurse is primed to help advocate for, along with the primary oncology team [2, 4]. Teachers and school nurses can help prepare the physical and emotional environment of school by taking a proactive approach in the child's care plan and educating colleagues and peers to reduce the potential for uninformed comments or actions [4, 5]. It may be challenging to know where to begin, but many organizations, including the Coalition Against Childhood Cancer and the Leukemia and Lymphoma

C. Lucas (✉)
Dana-Farber Cancer Institute/Boston Children's Cancer and Blood Disorders Center, Boston, MA, USA
e-mail: christym_lucas@dfci.harvard.edu

R. P. Olympia, J. Brady-Olympia (eds.), *Clinical Considerations in School-based Health*, https://doi.org/10.1007/978-3-031-85765-2_41

Table 41.1 Descriptions of commonly encountered pediatric cancers in school-aged children [3]

Brain Tumors	Brain tumors are the second most common childhood cancer after leukemia. There are many different types of brain tumors, but generally treatment consists of surgery with potential for chemotherapy and radiation depending on the type of tumor, location of the tumor, patient age, and success of the surgery. Children with brain tumors can be at risk for seizures and may also commonly present with severe or persistent headache, nausea/vomiting, and vision changes. The location of the brain tumor and size determine the symptoms that a child might experience.
Hepatoblastoma	Hepatoblastoma is a cancer of the liver, and it mostly affects babies and toddlers. It is the most common childhood liver cancer. It is most often treated with chemotherapy and surgery with the potential for a liver transplant.
Leukemia	Leukemia is the most common childhood cancer and is a white blood cell cancer. In leukemia, the bone marrow (aka the blood cell factory) accidentally makes immature, malignant white blood cells called "blasts." The blasts rapidly grow and divide and outcompete "normal" white blood cells, red blood cells, and platelets for "room" in the bone marrow like weeds in a garden, resulting in risk of infection, anemia, and thrombocytopenia. In addition, blasts can accumulate in the blood stream and other organs, including the eyes, lungs, and brain. Leukemia requires chemotherapy, and some high-risk types require a stem cell transplant.
Lymphoma	Lymphoma is also considered to be a blood cancer but affects the lymphatic system, which includes the bone marrow, lymph nodes, spleen, and an immune organ called the thymus. Lymphoma can present as a persistently enlarged lymph node, or more insidiously with a mediastinal chest mass that makes it hard to breathe. Examples of lymphoma include Hodgkin's lymphoma and non-Hodgkin's lymphoma, which can both be broken down into further subgroups based on pathology testing. Most children with lymphoma will be treated with chemotherapy. Some may be treated with radiation.
Neuroblastoma	Neuroblastoma is a cancer of nerve tissue, called the sympathetic nervous system (i.e., "fight or flight"). It is not a brain tumor. It is the most common solid tumor in children after brain tumors. Neuroblastoma can present anywhere along the sympathetic nerve tracts, but it frequently occurs in the adrenal gland on top of the kidney and in the chest or pelvis. It is treated with chemotherapy. Surgery and/or radiation may also play a role in treatment.
Sarcoma	Sarcoma is the general name for a cancer arising from the bone or connective tissues of the body. Commonly encountered sarcomas may include osteosarcoma, which is a bone cancer frequently occurring in the large bones of the arm or leg, Ewing's sarcoma, which is a bone cancer more likely to occur in the axial skeleton like the ribs, spine, or pelvis, and rhabdomyosarcoma, which arises from the soft tissue, most commonly in the head, neck, abdomen, or pelvis. Chemotherapy and local control of the tumor with surgery and/or radiation is part of treatment.
Wilm's Tumor	Wilm's tumors are a kidney cancer, most frequently occurring in toddlers. Wilm's tumors are at risk for rupture. Surgery to remove the mass (and kidney) and chemotherapy are part of the treatment. Some children may require radiation. Children with one kidney after Wilm's tumor removal should be encouraged to maintain good hydration and may be told to avoid medicines that may be toxic to the remaining kidney, such as NSAIDs.

Table 41.2 Common cancer terminology explained

Absolute Neutrophil Count (ANC)	Neutrophils are a type of white blood cell that is important for fighting bacteria. Chemotherapy causes decreased blood counts, including neutrophils. Neutropenia (low neutrophils) can cause fatigue, mouth sores, and gastrointestinal upset. Severe neutropenia is an ANC of less than 500. Fever with an ANC of less than 500 is a medical emergency and requires antibiotics within one hour.
Central line	Many chemotherapies are not safe to be given in a peripheral vein, and children with cancer require frequent lab monitoring. Central lines, such as implanted ports, tunneled catheters, and peripherally inserted central catheters (PICCs), help provide stable vascular access. The line is threaded through a vein, and the tip of the catheter should sit at the top of the right atrium of the heart.
Chemotherapy	Chemotherapy is the general term for oral, intravenous, or intrathecal (i.e., given into the spinal fluid) medications that kill rapidly dividing cells in the body, including cancer cells.
Fever	Fever is an emergency in oncology patients given the presence of a central line and potential for neutropenia, both increasing risk of a blood stream infection. Different institutions define fever differently, and even multiple low-grade fevers of temperatures as "low" as 100.4F may necessitate emergency care for a blood culture, blood counts, and antibiotics within an hour of fever. Children with cancer should not be given fever-reducing medications, and if a medicine such as acetaminophen is given for pain, a temperature should be checked beforehand to ensure one is not masking a fever. Fever in a child with cancer should prompt a call to the parent/guardian and potentially a referral to the emergency department.
Radiation	Radiation uses strong beams of energy, usually x-rays, to kill cancer cells and shrink tumors. Children may have radiation "tattoos" to make sure the radiation field can be consistent with each radiation session. Side effects of radiation depend on what location is being irradiated.

Society offer informal and formal coursework to learn how to best care for children with cancer in the school environment [6, 7].

Case 1 A 14-year-old girl named Jenny with metastatic osteosarcoma has returned to school for the first time after starting treatment for her cancer. Her treatment has resulted in changes to her appearance, including the loss of her hair, and requiring a wheelchair to help her with ambulation. She was feeling well this week after starting her last cycle of chemotherapy ten days ago and came to school, eager for a sense of normalcy and to see her classmates. She takes medication as needed for nausea and pain. You notice in the lunch room that she is sitting off by herself and appears distressed trying to eat, so you go to check-on her. She shares that she underestimated the discomfort of her mouth ulcers and does not feel as well as she had hoped. You ask additional symptomatic questions, and she endorses fatigue, lightheadedness, and some nausea. She has not had any nose bleeds or other bleeding symptoms. You take her back to the school nurse's office to check her vitals. She does not have a fever. Her heart rate is mildly elevated for age at 100 beats per minute (bpm). Her respiratory rate is normal. Her blood pressure is normal at 112/60. Jenny expresses that she is overwhelmed and does not feel well today. What do you do next?

Table 41.3 How to recognize and "**TAME**" common chemotherapy side effects

Side effect	Definition	Management
Thrombocytopenia	Thrombocytopenia refers to low platelets. This can present as prolonged bleeding or oozing with cuts, trauma, or nose bleeds, excessive menstrual bleeding, and easy bruising	Symptoms of bleeding can be treated, for example, (1) Afrin® and nasal pressure for a nose bleed or (2) holding pressure on a wound. The definitive treatment for thrombocytopenia with or without bleeding is a platelet transfusion at a hospital. Call the child's parent to inform them of your concern. Bleeding >10 min in spite of attempts at intervention should prompt emergency care. Abnormal vital signs or altered mental status with bleeding symptoms should also prompt emergency care.
Anemia	Anemia refers to low hemoglobin, the molecule in the blood needed to give oxygen to the tissues. Symptoms of anemia can include fatigue, headache, lightheadedness, pallor, decreased exercise tolerance, and/or tachycardia.	Children feeling lightheaded or fatigued should be directed to lie down in the nurse's office and provided with oral fluids to decrease symptoms of orthostasis. After a child is triaged, their parent should be notified of the concern for anemia. Call the child's parent to inform them of your concern. The definitive treatment of anemia with or without symptoms is a blood transfusion at a hospital. Syncope, shortness of breath, severe headache, and persistent tachycardia should prompt emergency care.

(continued)

Table 41.3 (continued)

Side effect	Definition	Management
Mucositis	Mucositis is inflammation of the mucus membrane surfaces in the body, most commonly the mouth, throat, gastrointestinal tract, and genitourinary tract. The most common presentation of mucositis on physical exam is oral ulcers, which may make eating, drinking, and speaking painful. Mucositis occurs when the white blood cells are very low, particularly the neutrophils (i.e., neutropenia). Children with mucositis are at risk for dehydration.	With parental permission, children can be given acetaminophen for pain. They should never be given non-steroidal anti-inflammatories (NSAIDs) like ibuprofen, naproxen, or aspirin for pain due to the anti-platelet effect that increases bleeding risk. Cold and/or hot foods can sometimes provide relief. Children should be monitored for signs and symptoms of dehydration. Call the child's parent to inform them of your concern. Significant dehydration, significant pain, drooling, and/or difficulty opening the mouth or swallowing should prompt emergency care.

(continued)

Table 41.3 (continued)

Side effect	Definition	Management
Extremity Pain	Children with cancer are at risk for numerous musculoskeletal (MSK) symptoms. For example, certain cancers, particularly hematologic malignancies, require high doses of steroids as part of chemotherapy that can cause painful bone changes called avascular necrosis (AVN), aka osteonecrosis. Steroids also increase risk of bone fracture and can cause muscle weakness. In addition to bone and muscle pain, certain chemotherapies that are used for blood cancers, solid tumors, and central nervous system tumors, can cause nerve changes. Nerve changes, known as neuropathy, can include electrical shocks or tingling in the hands or feet and changes in walking or running, including frequent tripping or a foot slapping. Lastly, with extremity pain, blood vessels must be considered since cancer and having a central venous catheter, like many children with cancer have for chemotherapy, are a risk for blood clots. Symptoms of a blood clot in an extremity can include redness, swelling, pain, and/or warmth, but all symptoms may not be present. A swollen extremity without a history of trauma should be particularly concerning.	With parental permission, children can be given acetaminophen for pain. They should never be given non-steroidal anti-inflammatories (NSAIDs) such as ibuprofen, naproxen, or aspirin for pain due to the anti-platelet effect that increases bleeding risk. Call the child's parent to inform them of your concern. *Bone* Bone pain should prompt a medical evaluation for a physical exam and consideration of imaging. Inability to bear weight, deformity, swelling, numbness/tingling, and/or color changes should prompt emergency care for bone pain. *Muscle* Physical therapy exercises to promote strength can sometimes be helpful. *Nerve* Unfortunately, many over the counter pain medicines are not helpful for nerve pain. Physical therapy exercises can sometimes be helpful, but symptom management would require input from an Oncologist and possibly a physician with expertise in pain management. *Blood Vessels* If there is concern for symptoms of a blood clot, a child should be referred to emergency care.

Jenny is experiencing symptoms of her cancer treatment, specifically mucositis, and her elevated heart rate and fatigue are concerning for symptoms of anemia. Many children with cancer will come to know the timing in a chemotherapy cycle when they will feel most symptomatic and experience their lowest blood counts. The mnemonic "**TAME**" (Table 41.3) can help a school nurse become familiar with chemotherapy side effects, their management, and when emergency care is warranted. Jenny is not only experiencing physical side effects of cancer and treatment, but also psychosocial distress. It is vital to holistically understand and prepare for school reentry of children with cancer. Cancer is a new experience for the child, their classmates, and school staff. Taking a proactive approach with education and communication can ease the transition from hospital or clinic to school. Most hospitals have an oncology psychosocial provider or nurse available to coordinate communication between the family, school, and medical team, in addition to informing school staff about the impact of cancer and treatment on the school experience [1]. School reentry support should include should open communication between the oncology team and school, an individualized learning plan for the student, a plan with the child's parents/guardians for acute medical issues or emergencies, and developmentally appropriate education for peers and school staff [1]. You call Jenny's parent who gives permission to offer her acetaminophen, which you check a temperature prior to administering. Her parent also arranges for a lab check at the Oncology clinic given her symptoms concerning for anemia. You reach out to Jenny's Oncology social worker to discuss strategies to collaborate with her healthcare team and teachers to support Jenny's reentry into school, and look into resources through the Leukemia and Lymphoma Society to develop a presentation to talk to her classmates [7].

Case 2 Micah, a 17-year-old year old boy undergoing treatment for leukemia for the last 18-months, comes to your office noting right ankle pain that limited his participation in gym class. You ask a series of questions about how long the pain has been occurring, in addition to the onset, duration, and intensity of the pain. You inquire about factors that exacerbated the pain versus made it better, in addition to the quality and location of the pain. He shares that the pain has been smoldering over the last week but has progressively worsened. He denies any trauma or injury. The pain is present at rest and with activity and has caused him to limp with limitations in the range of motion. He notes subtle swelling along his ankle. He does not have any numbness or tingling, and his posterior tibial and dorsalis pedis pulses are present and equal. What do you do next?

Cancer-directed therapy can affect the musculoskeletal system in numerous ways, impacting bones, muscles, nerves, and blood vessels, summarized in Table 41.3. Micah is undergoing treatment for leukemia, and steroids are an important part of the chemotherapy backbone for leukemia. However, steroids can cause changes in the integrity of the bone and cause muscle weakness. Adolescents in particular are at risk for a steroid-related complication called avascular necrosis (AVN), where the blood supply to the bone is altered and bone starts to die. This can be incredibly painful and may not be on the top of the differential for joint pain in a child unless one is familiar with the diagnosis. In triaging the chief complaint, it is important to ensure that the child is neurovascularly intact (e.g., palpable and equal pulses, normal sensation, no report of numbness/tingling), as compromises to the nerves or blood flow should always prompt emergency treatment. You call Micah's parent, and they notify his oncologist, who arranges for imaging of his ankle to prepare for an orthopedic evaluation given the progressive, joint-threatening nature of AVN.

Case 3 A 7-year-old girl named Max is sent to your office by her teacher. Max is typically an active and outgoing child. Over the last few weeks, she has been falling sleep in the classroom and has also come to your office for pain in her legs with a normal exam and sporadic nose bleeds. She has not been able to fully participate in gym class and asked to sit out today. She appears pale, with loss of the rosy appearance to her lips and cheeks. Max tells you that she feels tired and does not feel hungry to eat lunch. You take Max's vitals and she has a fever to 100.8F with tachycardia to 140 bpm. Her blood pressure is normal. You notice many bruises on her body and see a fine pinpoint polka-dot-like rash on her extremities. You assess that Max is sick. What do you do next?

Max is demonstrating several red flag symptoms for malignancy, including changes in energy, weight, and appetite in addition to bone pain and signs of abnormal blood counts (e.g., pallor, easy bruising, increased bleeding, and tachycardia out of proportion to fever). You call her parent and recommend that she is either urgently seen by her primary care doctor for blood work or at the emergency department. School nurses are on the frontlines and may be able to pick up subtle symptoms of cancer, such as fatigue, pallor, easy bleeding/bruising, weight changes, abdominal distension, persistent headaches, persistent nausea or vomiting, changes in behavior, or abnormal gait.

Extra Credit Points

1. School is a normalizing experience for children with cancer, and they may require special accommodations to be able to engage with school, for example: permission to wear a hat or scarf in school, half-day attendance, a time and space for a nap, a 504 plan, the ability to leave school for doctors' appointments or labs, and an emergency contact plan.
2. Cancer diagnosis and treatment leads to a new vocabulary for both families and the school to become familiar with; no two children with cancer (even the same cancer) are the same.
3. A school nurse may encounter side effects of chemotherapy in the school environment that they can help "**TAME**," triaging to a higher level of care if needed, particularly if concern for abnormal vital signs, disruptions in motor or sensory function, persistent bleeding, altered mental status, fatigue, syncope, fracture, blood clot, or fever.
4. Children may present with insidious signs or symptoms of cancer at school, and a school nurse has the potential to recognize red flag symptoms for malignancy and advocate for a referral to care.
5. It is vital for a school nurse to form a relationship not only with the child, but also with the family, medical care team, and psychosocial providers of a child with cancer, who know the child best and can help troubleshoot concerns that arise at school through both preventative and reactive measures. The education in this chapter should not be seen as professional medical advice or replace any relationship with a physician or healthcare provider who knows the child.

References

1. Thompson AL, Christiansen HL, Elam M, et al. Academic continuity and school reentry support as a standard of care in pediatric oncology. Pediatr Blood Cancer. 2015;62(Suppl 5):S805–17. https://doi.org/10.1002/pbc.25760.
2. School Support. Children's Oncology Group (COG). 2023. Accessed April 6, 2024. https://childrensoncologygroup.org/school-support
3. Glossary. The Morgan Adams Foundation. 204. Accessed April 16, 2024. https://www.morgan-adamsfoundation.org/about-pediatric-cancer/brain-tumor-glossary/.
4. Managing School During and After Cancer. American Society of Clinical Oncology. June 2019. Accessed April 6, 2024. https://www.cancer.net/navigating-cancer-care/young-adults-and-teenagers/school-and-work-during-cancer/managing-school-during-and-after-cancer
5. Accommodating Children with Cancer in Child Care or School. HealthChildren.org, from the American Academy of Pediatrics. Updated March 16, 2020. Accessed April 6, 2024. https://www.healthychildren.org/English/health-issues/conditions/cancer/Pages/Children-with-Cancer-in-Child-Care-or-School.aspx#:~:text=Children%20may%20come%20to%20school,attend%20child%20care%20or%20school.
6. CAC2 Survivorship Toolkit: Educational Guidance and Planning. Coalition Against Childhood Cancer. 2020. Accessed April 6, 2024. https://cac2.org/impact-areas/survivorship/survivorship-toolkit/educational-guidance-and-planning/
7. Staying Connected®: Facilitating the Learning Experience During & After Cancer Treatment. Leukemia and Lymphoma Society. Accessed April 6, 2024. https://www.lls.org/professional-education-webcasts/staying-connectedr-facilitating-learning-experience-during-after

Chapter 42
Celiac Disease

Patrick Lin and Janice Joseph

Case 1 You receive a letter from the pediatrician of Michelle, an 11-year-old student, stating that she was recently diagnosed with celiac disease. The letter recommends that she follow a gluten-free diet. What types of precautions should you take?

Celiac disease is an autoimmune disorder in which exposure to gluten, a protein found in wheat, barley, or rye, leads to inflammation and damage to the lining of the small intestine [1]. Individuals with celiac disease are born with a genetic predisposition to the disease and exposure to gluten triggers the cascade of events that leads to chronic inflammation. Celiac disease can be highly variable in its presentation. The more classic gastrointestinal symptoms include abdominal pain, bloating, diarrhea, constipation, or poor weight gain (Table 42.1). There can also be extraintestinal symptoms such as chronic fatigue, headaches, dental erosions, or typically painful, blistering, and itchy rash called dermatitis herpetiformis (Table 42.2).

Celiac disease is diagnosed via blood tests, such as tissue transglutaminase IGA antibody (tTG-IGA) that is a highly sensitive screening test. Other blood tests, including tissue transglutaminase IGG antibody (tTG-IGG), deaminated gliadin antibody, or endomysial antibody, can lend support for a diagnosis of celiac disease in certain situations. Ultimately, individuals with positive blood tests as above or with otherwise continued concern for the disease, should be referred to a Pediatric Gastroenterologist for further evaluation and workup. The gold standard for diagnosis of celiac disease remains tissue biopsies taken from the small intestine during an upper endoscopy that demonstrate histologic findings for specific markers of chronic inflammation, such as villous blunting [1]. The treatment is strict gluten avoidance for life. This will allow for healing of the affected areas of the small intestine and

P. Lin (✉) · J. Joseph
Lehigh Valley Reilly Children's Hospital, Allentown, PA, USA
e-mail: Patrick.Lin@lvhn.org; Janice.joseph@lvhn.org

R. P. Olympia, J. Brady-Olympia (eds.), *Clinical Considerations in School-based Health*, https://doi.org/10.1007/978-3-031-85765-2_42

Table 42.1 Gastrointestinal manifestations of celiac disease

Abdominal distention	Diarrhea
Abdominal pain	Poor weight gain
Anorexia	Vomiting
Constipation	Weight loss

Table 42.2 Non-Gastrointestinal manifestations of celiac disease

Alopecia	Chronic fatigue	Hypotonia
Amenorrhea	Dental enamel defects	Infertility
Anemia or iron deficiency	Depression	Neuropathy
Aphthous stomatitis	Dermatitis herpetiformis	Osteopenia/osteoporosis
Arthritis/joint pain	Epilepsy with intracranial calcifications	Pubertal delay
Ataxia	Foggy mind	Short stature
Behavioral problems	Headaches	Transaminitis

resolution of the above symptoms, although this healing process can take up to a year on average. Generally, improvement is monitored clinically and with follow-up blood tests. Follow up endoscopy is reserved for children who do not demonstrate clinical improvement or continued to have abnormal blood tests despite adherence to the gluten-free diet [2].

All children with celiac disease should have a 504 Plan in place to allow them to have a gluten-free learning environment. School caretakers should be aware of most gluten-containing and gluten-free foods (Table 42.3) as well as some common non-food items that contain gluten (Table 42.4). A more comprehensive list of gluten-free foods can be found in the Gluten-Free Ingredients Glossary in the *Voluntary Recommendations for MANAGING CELIAC DISEASE IN LEARNING ENVIRONMENTS* [3]. Appropriate accommodations should be discussed for children with celiac disease, but with emphasis on not singling out the child for requiring something different than the other children. To that end, care should be taken to consistently provide gluten-free options for school lunches, activities, field trips, or classroom parties/events.

Case Takeaway For Michelle, or any other child with celiac disease, adhering to a strict gluten-free diet is paramount. Good care should be undertaken to ensure that their school learning environment is safe for her by enabling a gluten-free environment as well as establishing school accommodations for her to avoid any gluten exposures.

Table 42.3 Unsafe (gluten-containing) foods and safe (gluten-free) foods

Common Gluten-Containing Foods	• Grains (wheat, barley, rye) • Breading, bread crumbs, and coating mixes • Brewer's yeast • Communion wafers/hosts • Challah • Croutons • Licorice • Malt, malt flavoring, malt extract derived from barley, and malt vinegar, • Matzah and matzah meal • Soy sauce
Foods that MAY contain Gluten	• Broth, bouillon, and soup stock • Brown rice syrup • Cake frosting • Candy • Drink mixes • Energy bars • Flavored teas and coffees • Imitation seafood • Oats (unless labeled "gluten free") • Processed meats • Packaged rice pilaf, other rice mixes
Common Gluten–Free Foods	• Fresh fruits/vegetables • Dairy - milk, cheese, yogurt • Eggs • Unprocessed meats, poultry, fish • Beans • Nuts • Gluten-free grains and starches – Rice – Corn – Potato – Amaranth – Buckwheat – Quinoa – Teff – Millet

Table 42.4 Unsafe non-food items

Non-food Items that may contain gluten	• Play-Doh • Paper mâché • Glue • Vitamin/gummy vitamins • Cosmetics/Makeup

Case 2 Steven, 7-year-old boy with a history of celiac disease, is sent to the nurse's office after lunch. He is complaining of abdominal pain and is crying due to the pain. Shortly thereafter, he starts to have vomiting and is complaining of worsening pain. When asked, he admits that during lunch, he ate half of his friend's sandwich that was made with regular bread.

Accidental exposures to gluten-containing items (whether food or not) can be hazardous to patients with celiac disease. While some patients may not have any symptoms with ingestion of gluten, others may develop symptoms such as abdominal pain, vomiting, or diarrhea, within a few minutes to hours after exposure. In these cases, it is important to have the child assessed quickly, remove the offending food/item from the child's possession, and allow them unrestricted access to a bathroom. As symptoms can differ amongst individuals, the child's 504 plan should document their typical symptoms with gluten exposure. The child's parents/caretakers should be informed about the exposure as soon as possible. The child will need to be closely monitored, may need to be sent home, or, if the child is having severe symptoms such as continuous vomiting, severe/worsening abdominal pain, or dehydration, then they will need to be evaluated in a medical facility for treatments such as Intravenous (IV) fluids for rehydration, electrolyte boluses for electrolyte abnormalities, and pain medications and anti-emetics for symptom relief [3].

Good cleaning and sanitation practices are vitally important to minimize risk of accidental exposures. For example, if students are eating lunch at their desks or at a shared common desk, wiping down the tables with soap/water or all-purpose cleaner after lunch would help prevent any cross contamination. It is important to note the alcohol-based hand sanitizers are not sufficient in removing gluten [3]. Cross-contamination of gluten into gluten-free foods or spaces can pose additional challenges. While a few breadcrumbs may not be a major issue to some children, there are others who would develop symptoms from even such small exposures. Similarly, there should be care in selecting gluten-free products for school art supplies and activities, such as gluten-free pastas for crafts, Play-Doh, glues, or paper mâché. While it is unlikely that topical exposure to gluten will lead to issues, there is concern for accidental ingestion of these products or from aerosolization of gluten particles that could cause symptoms [3].

Case Takeaway Given Steven's symptoms, further medical evaluation was recommended. His parents were contacted and he was brought to the closest Emergency Room for evaluation and treatment that included intravenous (IV) fluids, anti-emetic medications such as Ondansetron, and Ketorolac for pain control. After a period of time, his symptoms improved and he was able to be discharged to home. In Steven's 504 Plan, an Action Plan should be written out that lists his symptoms after exposure to gluten and steps for management.

Extra Credit Points

1. Celiac disease is an autoimmune disease that can cause a variety of symptoms triggered by exposure to gluten. Treatment is a strict gluten-free diet.
2. Have lists of gluten-containing and gluten-free foods and non-food items available in order to help prevent any exposures/cross-contamination.

3. Develop Action/Care Plans for students with celiac disease and incorporate 504 Plans that list out necessary accommodations to keep individual students gluten-free, as well as the child's known symptoms with exposure to gluten and contingency plan for accidental exposure to gluten.

Additional Resources

- Celiac Disease Foundation: www.celiac.org
- Gluten-free Passport: www.glutenfreepassport.com
- National Celiac Association: www.nationalceliac.org

References

1. Hill ID, Fasano A, Guandalini S, et al. NASPGHAN Clinical report on the diagnosis and treatment of gluten-related disorders. J Pediatr Gastroenterol Nutr. 2016;63(1):156–65.
2. Rubio-Tapia A, Hill ID, Semrad C, et al. American college of gastroenterology guidelines update: diagnosis and management of celiac disease. Am J Gastroenterol. 2023;118(1):59–76.
3. Celiac Disease Foundation and Children's National Hospital. Voluntary Recommendations for Managing Celiac Disease in Learning Environments 2020. https://celiac.org/main/wp-content/uploads/2020/05/Celiac-Disease-School-Management-Plan.pdf

Chapter 43
Cerebral Palsy

Rebecca Wilding and Laura Owens

Case 1 **Chelsea is a 7-year-old female diagnosed with spastic left-sided hemiplegic CP as the result of a pre-natal stroke. She is currently a second grader in a regular education classroom and does not use any mobility aids at school but does wear an ankle-foot orthosis (AFO) on her left leg. She communicates verbally and wears prescription glasses due to her low vision. Chelsea presents to the school clinic after recess on an especially hot day complaining of pain and redness on her left ankle.**

Case 2 **Andrew is a 6-year-old male with spastic quadriplegic CP secondary to an anoxic brain injury at birth. He is currently a kindergartener in a regular education classroom with paraprofessional support. He uses a power wheelchair to navigate the school which he is able to independently control with the joystick control. He communicates very efficiently with his alternative communication program on his iPad and a few words and signs. He presents to the school clinic on his first day back at school from having a device implanted to help with his tone. His paraprofessional reports that he has been using his communication device and saying he was seeing cats on the ceiling, but they thought he was just being silly. They became concerned when he became very sweaty and itchy.**

Case 3 **Mallory is a 15-year-old female diagnosed with spastic quadriplegic CP due to a traumatic brain injury at age 18 months. She is currently in her first year of the life skills program, and she will remain in the school system until age 21. She is dependent for mobility in her manual wheelchair and requires a chest harness to maintain her seated positioning. Mallory communi-**

R. Wilding · L. Owens (✉)
Nemours Children's Health, Wilmington, DE, USA
e-mail: rebecca.wilding@nemours.org; laura.owens@nemours.org

R. P. Olympia, J. Brady-Olympia (eds.), *Clinical Considerations in School-based Health*, https://doi.org/10.1007/978-3-031-85765-2_43

cates using a manual picture board and requires G tube feeds for nutrition. Mallory presents to the school clinic with her paraprofessional who is concerned that Mallory's muscles seem tighter, and she has been grimacing throughout the day. She has otherwise been acting like herself.

Cerebral palsy (CP) describes a group of disorders of movement and posture causing activity limitations as the result of non-progressive disturbances to the brain during infancy or early childhood [1]. Cerebral palsy is the most common motor disorder of childhood, affecting 1.5 to 4/1000 live births or 1 out of every 345 children in the United States [2]. Children with CP may have a variety of presentations, including which areas of the body are affected (Table 43.1), mobility limitations, and other associated comorbidities. Spastic CP comprises up to 80% of cases and is the most common type encountered [3]. Spasticity refers to an increase in muscle tone, with sustained or intermittent involuntary activation of muscles (Table 43.2). Children may also have dystonia, which appears as more repetitive or posturing increases in tone, or other abnormal muscle/movement patterns such as choreoathetosis, hypotonia, or impairment in coordination, such as ataxia [1, 2].

Cerebral palsy describes only the motor disorder these children have; however, most children with CP also have additional diagnoses that can add complexity to their medical care. Children with CP are at higher risk for common childhood conditions such as reflux, constipation, epilepsy, vision or hearing deficits, as well as learning challenges, including attention disorders and learning disabilities [4]. Cognitive and language abilities can vary widely, from normal to significantly impaired, and special attention must be taken to help optimize a student's ability to self-advocate and communicate. In this chapter, we will focus on the musculoskeletal factors in CP; however, many of these other conditions are featured in other areas of this book and are important to review.

43.1 Mobility

With the wide variation in motor ability that exists for children with CP, it is important to recognize that over 50% of children with CP can walk independently or with handheld mobility devices [3]. Although many children with CP can walk, deficits in coordination, endurance, and higher-level activities are still present. Students may have an identified Gross Motor Function Classification Scale (GMFCS) level (Table 43.3). This tool helps to describe the mobility and gross motor function of people with CP and can be helpful to understand a child's mobility needs [5].

Table 43.1 Cerebral palsy spasticity patterns

Hemiplegic	One side of the body is affected
Diplegic	Lower body significantly affected, variable upper body involvement, at least some trunk control
Quadriplegic	All four limbs and trunk are significantly affected

Table 43.2 Abnormal movement patterns

Spasticity	Increased muscle tone resulting in stiffness and movement difficulty
Dystonia	Intermittent contractions or increased tone causing repetitive motions or abnormal postures
Choreoathetosis	Continuous or frequent involuntary movements, may be writing, twisting or irregular and involve the face, trunk, and/or extremities

In addition to mobility devices such as walkers or wheelchairs, many children with CP will use various types of bracing or orthotics to help give additional support or assist with positioning. Children may wear orthotics on their lower extremities to support ankle or knee joints, braces that support the spine, or arm/hand bracing. Typically, a sock or thin layer of clothing is worn beneath the orthotic to prevent irritation and rubbing. If the fabric becomes wet or sweaty, this can increase the risk of skin breakdown and thus may need to be changed throughout the day.

43.2 Neuromusculoskeletal Issues

Increased muscle tone and spasticity (passive movement related tone) is a common issue for children with cerebral palsy. While CP is non-progressive, spasticity and tone can be dynamic and change based on factors such as pain, illness, growth, or even mood [4]. Children with CP may also have contractures, or a fixed shortening of the muscles limiting motion, which can affect positioning and comfort in different assistive equipment. Children with CP, especially those with limited mobility, are at higher risk for complications such as skin breakdown or pressure wounds, fractures, and hip dislocations which all can cause increases in tone due to pain [5]; however, it is important to remember common childhood and adolescent sources of discomfort, such as menstrual cramps, constipation pain, or headache, can also lead to increases in tone. This is especially important to keep in mind if the child is unable to communicate if they are in pain or to localize the discomfort.

Many children with increased spasticity and tone may be on medication to help decrease tightness, manage pain or spasms, and maintain range of motion. Most enteral tone medications, including baclofen and diazepam, may cause sedation, and use should be monitored, especially in combination with other sedating medications (antiepileptics, pain medication etc.) [5]. Baclofen is the most common medication used, most often oral or via enteral tube but some children may be managed with an implanted intrathecal baclofen pump. Withdrawal from oral tone management medications is uncommon but may occur when an issue arises with the intrathecal baclofen system. Symptoms of baclofen withdrawal may include sudden increase in tone/spasticity, hallucination, hyperthermia (fever, sweating), pruritis, or seizure [6]. Overdose with baclofen or similarly sedating agents may lead to drastically low tone and hyporeflexia, decreased alertness, hypotension, and respiratory

Table 43.3 Gross motor function classification scale (age > 6) with special considerations

GMFCS Levels	Level I	Level II	Level III	Level IV	Level V
Description	• Independently walk and climb stairs • Performs skills such as running, jumping but balance, coordination limited	• Walks in most settings, may need rail for stairs or handheld mobility devices for longer distances • Minimal running, jumping	• Walks with handheld mobility device (like a walker) in most settings, uses wheeled mobility for longer distances • Can self-propel a manual wheelchair	• Walking is limited even with assistive devices • Uses a wheelchair as their main form of mobility, may drive a power wheelchair	• Dependently transported in a manual wheelchair • Limited head, truncal control
Special Considerations	• At risk for falls during recess and in unfamiliar environments like on field trips	• May have difficulty walking long distances, on uneven terrain, or crowded areas. • High risk for falls during recess and in unfamiliar environments like on field trips • May benefit from use of elevator in school in place of stairs to decrease risk of falls	• May need additional help with propelling manual wheelchair for longer distances or uneven surfaces • Benefits from use of elevator	• Ill-fitting equipment can increase the risk of skin breakdown and injury, children may or may not be able to localize and communicate where discomfort is coming from • Adequate room is required to navigate the school setting in a power wheelchair	• Ill-fitting equipment can increase the risk of skin breakdown and injury, children may or may not be able to localize and communicate where discomfort is coming from. • Require 1:1 support for mobility, self-care

failure [6]. If you suspect a child is experiencing baclofen withdrawal or toxicity, please immediately seek emergency care!

43.3 Case Conclusions

Case 1 Chelsea had an area of erythema over her left lateral malleolus where her orthotic was rubbing. She was able to take a break from her AFO to allow time for her socks to dry from the sweat before continuing with her day. You can consider sending a note asking the family to provide additional socks for her to change into if needed and may monitor for need to adjust her orthotic.

Case 2 In further discussion with Andrew's mother via phone, she tells you that he had an intrathecal baclofen pump implanted in the last week and stopped all his oral baclofen he had previously been on. You recognize that his symptoms are consistent with baclofen withdrawal (hallucinations, sweating, pruritis) and know this is a medical emergency. You immediately call 911, and Andrew was transported to the closest ED for appropriate care.

Case 3 On review of systems, you and her paraprofessional noted no concerns for injury or illness, but her paraprofessional did remember that Mallory is currently on her menstrual period. Using her picture board, Mallory was able to indicate "yes" when asked if she was in pain and point to the stomach region on the body picture when asked where the pain was. Mallory's mom had previously sent ibuprofen and appropriate documentation to the school clinic allowing it to be given for Mallory's menstrual cramps. Following ibuprofen administration, Mallory was able to return to class and completed her day with improvements in her tone and relief of her discomfort.

Extra Credit Points

1. Children with CP can have a wide variety of presentations and use a variety of different mobility and assistive devices/technology. Being familiar with common injuries and complications associated can be helpful to help prevent accidents and injuries while at school.
2. Remember, kids with complex medical needs still experience "typical" childhood ailments like their peers, but they may not be able to communicate what they are feeling in the same way as their peers.
3. Baclofen withdrawal and overdose are medical emergencies! If you have concern for withdrawal or overdose, children should be sent for emergent evaluation.

References

1. Rosenbaum PL, Paneth NS, Leviton A, Goldstein M, Bax MC, Damiano DL, Dan B, Jacobsson B. A report: the definition and classification of cerebral palsy April 2006. Dev Med Child Neurol. 2007;49.
2. Noritz G, Davidson L, Steingass K, Council on children with disabilities, and the American academy for cerebral palsy and developmental medicine. Executive summary: providing a primary care medical home for children and youth with cerebral palsy. Pediatrics. 2022;150(6):e2022060056. https://doi.org/10.1542/peds.2022-060056.
3. Vitrikas K, Dalton H, Breish D. Cerebral palsy: an overview. Am Fam Physician. 2020;101(4):213–20.
4. Ogoke CC. Clinical classification of cerebral palsy. Cerebral Palsy – Clinical and Therapeutic Aspects. 2018.
5. Palisano RJ, Rosenbaum P, Walter S, Russell DJ, Wood EP, Galuppi BE. Development and reliability of a system to classify gross motor function in children with cerebral palsy. Dev Med Child Neurol. 1997;39.
6. Romito JW, Turner ER, Rosener JA, Coldiron L, Udipi A, Nohrn L, Tausiani J, Romito BT (2021) Baclofen therapeutics, toxicity, and withdrawal: a narrative review. SAGE Open Medicine. 9.

Chapter 44
Constipation

Brianna Koehnke and Adam Michael Sunday

Case 1 8-year-old Lily presents to your school-based clinic due to abdominal pain. She has not had a bowel movement in a couple days, and complains of lower abdominal and rectal pain, as well as burning on urination. Her appetite has been decreased for the past week and she admits to having intermittent nausea without vomiting. She denies fever, sore throat, or cough. You call her mother who says that Lily has a history of constipation, but is not on any medications. What do you think is going on?

Constipation is a relatively common problem in the pediatric population. Approximately 30% of children are affected by constipation at some point in their lives [1]. Constipation is defined as a condition in which the bowel movements occur less frequently than usual or stools tend to be hard, painful, and difficult to pass, and depends upon the usual pattern and consistency of the child's stool [2]. The widely accepted adage is that the patient will eventually get better on their own. While this is true occasionally, there are times when intervention is necessary. A constipated child or adolescent can develop complications such as poor feeding and dehydration, nausea and vomiting, urinary tract infections, anal fissures, and fecal incontinence. On the other hand, a child or adolescent may have a large fecal burden, and have minimal symptoms, including normal and frequent bowel movements without straining to stool or hard stools (consider constipation in a child with chronic abdominal pain). A low index of suspicion is necessary in order to diagnosis constipation, to treat the child appropriately, and to prevent associated complications. Treatment of constipation involves educating the caregivers, implementing dietary changes, providing appropriate toileting behaviors, and starting pharmacotherapy [3].

B. Koehnke (✉) · A. M. Sunday
The Milton S. Hershey Medical Center, Hershey, PA, USA
e-mail: bkoehnke@pennstatehealth.psu.edu; asunday@pennstatehealth.psu.edu

R. P. Olympia, J. Brady-Olympia (eds.), *Clinical Considerations in School-based Health*, https://doi.org/10.1007/978-3-031-85765-2_44

Pediatric constipation is usually functional meaning that there is no anatomical or physiological causes that could explain the child's symptoms [4]. In students, constipation may be associated with stool withholding; when this occurs, colonic stasis occurs allowing the colon to reabsorb additional fluid creating harder and larger stools. As the stools grow, abdominal distention occurs, and the patient becomes uncomfortable and develops abdominal pain. Pediatric constipation can also be multifactorial, often associated with diet or recent infection (post infectious gastroparesis) [2–4]. Furthermore, conditions that may be associated with constipation include Hirschprung's disease, thyroid dysfunction, celiac disease, lead poisoning, cystic fibrosis, spinal cord injury, calcium issues, chronic narcotic use/abuse, or history of abdominal surgery. Performing a thorough history includes eliciting the following information: nature and character of the stool, frequency of bowel movements, bowel movement patterns at school and at home, pain or straining with bowel movements, abdominal or rectal pain, urinary symptoms, bowel or urinary incontinence, nausea or vomiting, weight loss, appetite and fluid intake, recent or current illness, medical history and medication prescribed, and life stressors. The Bristol stool scale, which characterizes stool into 7 categories, may help children describe their stool better and assist health care providers formulate a differential diagnosis based on the character of the child's bowel movements (Fig. 44.1).

Physical examination should include a review of the patient's growth parameters and thorough abdominal examination to rule out acute and surgical causes of abdominal pain. Often an internal rectal examination is deferred due the discomfort associated with this procedure, but consider an external rectal examination to evaluate for anal fissures or hemorrhoids associated with constipation. Functional constipation is classically associated with a rectal vault filled with stool, while obstructive causes of constipation may be associated with an empty rectal vault. While the diagnosis of constipation is clinical, X-rays of the abdomen may assist in evaluating fecal load and guide treatment [5].

Management of constipation involves both non-pharmacologic and pharmacologic interventions. The non-pharmacological route should be pursued first, as these interventions are often less invasive. This approach should focus on optimizing the patient's diet to include fruits and vegetables that are high in fiber; encouraging sufficient water intake; and promoting physical activity. When this approach fails to alleviate constipation, then pharmacological measures should be implemented. Relief of constipation can be accomplished with oral, nasogastric, rectal medications or a combination. Oral medications are recommended as they are less invasive. In a randomized trial, an oral laxative (polyethylene glycol 3350) was as effective as enemas in treating impaction, and relieved constipation in 95% of children with chronic constipation [1]. This laxative is generally palatable and well tolerated by children. The dose of polyethylene glycol 3350 for disimpaction is 1 to 1.5 g/kg/day by mouth for up to six days. It is dissolved in approximately 10 mL/kg body weight of water. If constipation is not relieved after six days of oral treatment or if there are signs of obstruction, then the child may potentially need hospitalization for aggressive nasogastric treatments (with or without enemas) or manual disimpaction, with

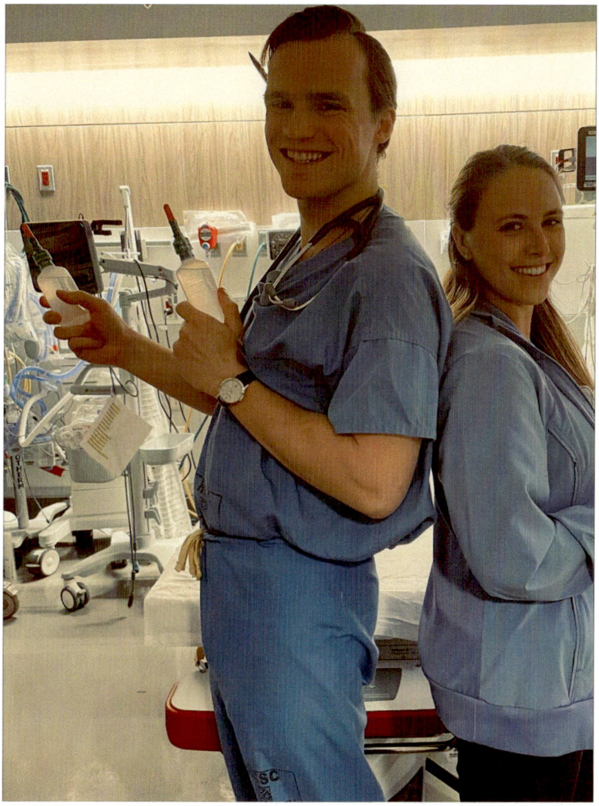

Fig. 44.1 Our authors demonstrating a pharmacologic intervention effective in the treatment of pediatric constipation

attention to electrolyte abnormalities and hydration status. Enemas may consist of sodium phosphate, saline, soap suds, fleet, pink lady and mineral oil.

Once the patient is successfully disimpacted, it is imperative that the patient be started on maintenance therapy to prevent constipation and promote healthy bowel health. Pharmacologic options for the treatment of acute and chronic constipation can be seen in Table 44.1.

Case Resolution Lily is referred to your local urgent care center where she is diagnosed with constipation and a urinary tract infection, often associated with constipation [6]. She is started on Miralax for one week and a 7 day course of Omnicef, with complete resolution of her symptoms within a few weeks. She is started on a maintenance bowel regimen, and encouraged to increase her water intake.

Case 2 Grayson is a 7-year-old male with a past medical history of cystic fibrosis. He is presenting to your school-based clinic due to fevers, lethargy, and severe abdominal pain. He has a history of constipation and has not had a bowel movement in at least 8 days. He has been vomiting for 3 days and has not been able to tolerate any oral intake over the past 24 h. Grayson had an antegrade continence enemas (ACE) procedure last year to treat his chronic consti-

Table 44.1 Types of laxatives for acute or chronic constipation in children

Type of laxative	Mechanism of action	Uses	Examples	Time to take effect	Side effects
Stool Softeners	Allows the surface of the stool to soften so it passes easier	To prevent straining, fissures or hemorrhoids, frequently used in combo with other laxatives	Docusate sodium. Liquid paraffin	24–72 h	– Abdominal cramps – Diarrhea/ nausea – Lipid pneumonia – Rash
Bulking Agents	Increases stool size, stimulates peristalsis, and improves stool form	Chronic/Not acute constipation	Psyllium, Sterculia	48–72 h	– Bowel obstruction if not appropriately hydrated – Flatulence – Abdominal pain, bloating, distension
Osmotic Laxatives (PEG & Magnesium Sulfate	Ions are used to keep fluid in the stool because are the ions are poorly absorbable. Stimulates peristalsis. Must be taken with water	Fecal impaction, severe and acute constipation	PEG, Magnesium Phosphate	0.5–48 h	– Electrolyte imbalance – Dehydration – Nausea, vomiting, diarrhea, – Bloating or distension – Flatulence
Osmotic Laxatives (Lactulose/ Sorbitol)	Poorly or nonabsorbable sugar which will pull fluid into stool. Works to stimulate peristalsis	Constipation management	Sorbitol, Lactulose	24–72 h	– Abdominal pain – Abdominal distension – Electrolyte imbalance – Diarrhea – Flatulence
Stimulant Laxatives	Colon wall is stimulated which will increase stool movement in the colon	Severe constipation, spinal cord injury, intermittent constipation, neuromuscular conditions	Senna, Sodium Picosulfate, Bisacodyl	6–12 h, often given at night	– Fecal incontinence – Diarrhea – Electrolyte imbalance – Dehydration – Abdominal pain – Nausea

Chart created by Brianna Koehnke, PA-C

pation. In your office, Grayson appears dehydrated and lethargic, his vitals are a temperature of 38.2 °C, heart rate of 142 beats per minute, blood pressure of 80/46, and his neurologic examination is "alert to painful stimuli" on the AVPU scale. What do you do?

ACE, which stands for antegrade continence enemas, is a surgical procedure in which a catheter is placed through the right lower quadrant of the abdomen, usually into the cecum (cecostomy tube) or appendix (appendicostomy tube). The goal of this procedure is to evacuate colonic stool by giving fluids through the catheter at the proximal colon causing the irrigation of stool and improvement of fecal load [7]. More than 90% of children have improvement after this procedure. Saline flushes can be done at home and as needed.

There are different reasons why the ACE procedure may be indicated. Typically, the procedure is indicated for children who have chronic constipation that does not improve with routine pharmacologic and non-pharmacologic treatment, or those who have bowel incontinence, often secondary to significant constipation. Alternative methods are usually attempted over many months before moving to an ACE procedure, as this requires a full surgical procedure. Other indications for an ACE procedure include congenital abnormalities that affect the anus or rectum, spinal abnormalities, or congenital abnormalities such as spina bifida or cystic fibrosis [8].

As with any procedure, there are associated risks. Complications at the time of the procedure include bleeding, bowel perforation and necrosis of the tissue that is used to form the ACE channel [8]. Late complications following the procedure include bleeding at the site, wound infections, leaking of feces around the catheter, blockage of the catheter, accidental catheter removal, displacement of the catheter into the bowel, stenosis of the tract, creation of a false passage, and adhesions leading to obstruction.

Severely constipated children are 6.8 times more likely to develop urinary tract infections and obstruction/hydronephrosis than non-constipated children. Significant stool in the abdomen can lead to urinary retention or only partial emptying of the bladder increasing the risk for urinary tract infections and obstruction.

Case Resolution You recognize septic shock, likely associated with a urinary tract infection. Greyson is transported to your local emergency department where he receives fluid resuscitation, intravenous antibiotics, and vasopressors, and is admitted to the intensive care unit. Specialists believe that significant stool burden was the trigger for Greyson's urosepsis, and his bowel regimen was modified after his discharge from the hospital.

Extra Credit Points

1. Constipation is a very common diagnosis in the pediatric population and is found to be the culprit in many children with acute and chronic abdominal pain.
2. Constipation is a clinical diagnosis but abdominal x-rays are often utilized to evaluate fecal load and guide treatment.

3. If mildly constipated, dietary changes are the first choice of treatment as it is the least invasive, however, laxatives are an appropriate choice as well.
4. In certain instances, severe constipation can cause additional problems that can be life threatening and result in hospitalization, such as significant dehydration or urosepsis.
5. ACE is used for chronic constipation but even with this procedure, you cannot always guarantee resolution of the problem.

References

1. Good MS. Chronic functional constipation and fecal incontinence in infants, children, and adolescents: treatment. UpToDate. 2023. Accessed May 30, 2024. https://www.uptodate.com/contents/chronic-functional-constipation-and-fecal-incontinence-in-infants-children-and-adolescents-treatment?search=management+of+pediatric+constipation&source=search_result&selectedTitle=1~150&usage_type=default&display_rank=1#H3.
2. Nurko S, Zimmerman LA. Evaluation and treatment of constipation in children and adolescents. Am Family Physician. July 15, 2014. Accessed May 30, 2024. https://www.aafp.org/pubs/afp/issues/2014/0715/p82.html#afp20140715p82-b2.
3. de Geus A, Koppen IJN, Flint RB, Benninga MA, Tabbers MM. An update of pharmacological management in children with functional constipation. Paediatric Drugs. May 2023. Accessed May 30, 2024. https://www.ncbi.nlm.nih.gov/pmc/articles/PMC10097737/.
4. Tabbers MM, DiLorenzo C, Berger MY, et al. Evaluation and treatment of functional constipation in infants and children. J Pediatr Gastroenterol Nutr. 2014;58(2):258–74. https://doi.org/10.1097/mpg.0000000000000266.
5. Moylan S, Armstrong J, Diaz-Saldano D, Saker M, Yerkes EB, Lindgren BW. Are abdominal x-rays a reliable way to assess for constipation? J Urol. August 21, 2010. Accessed May 31, 2024. https://pubmed.ncbi.nlm.nih.gov/20728159/.
6. Sampaio C, Sousa AS, Fraga LGA, Veiga ML, Bastos Netto JM, Barroso U. Constipation and lower urinary tract dysfunction in children and adolescents: a population-based study. Front Pediatrics. October 3, 2016. Accessed August 2, 2024. https://www.ncbi.nlm.nih.gov/pmc/articles/PMC5046079/.
7. Larowe E. Antegrade continence enema bowel management … med.umich.edu. Accessed August 2, 2024. https://www.med.umich.edu/1libr/PedSurgery/ColorectalProgram/ACE.pdf.
8. Antegrade continence enema (ACE): surgical formation and continuing care in children. NHS choices. July 24, 2023. Accessed August 2, 2024. https://www.cuh.nhs.uk/patient-information/antegrade-continence-enema-ace-surgical-formation-and-continuing-care-in-children/.

Chapter 45
Cystic Fibrosis

Kelly M. Lynch and Pritish Mondal

Case 1 Chase is a second-grader with a known history of cystic fibrosis (CF). His teacher sent him to your office for a breathing treatment for persistent coughing fits. His teacher reports that he has been having increased cough and fatigue and seems to be struggling more with normal activities during school hours. His parents separated last year, and Chase reports that he has not been getting his vest and cough assist device when he is at his mother's house. You are concerned about adherence to medical therapies affecting his symptom control and disease progression.

The incidence of CF in the United States is approximately one in 4000 children. However, it is more common among Caucasians, including in the Amish community. Reported incidence in South America and East Asia is low, though lack of CF registries and availability of newborn screening may contribute to underestimation [1]. In the United States, newborn screening helps to identify over half of the CF cases. If a screening test is positive, the diagnosis is confirmed by sweat chloride testing as the standard of care. Genetic testing helps identify the specific mutated cystic fibrosis transmembrane conductance regulator (CFTR) gene and can help direct treatment options. Genetic testing can also be performed before and during pregnancy [1]. Children with CF may present with symptoms like wet cough, wheezing, and constipation [2]. Depending on the specific gene mutation and organs affected, they may also present with:

- Sinusitis and pulmonary infections
- Chronic diarrhea
- Poor weight gain, short stature
- Chronic hypoxia leading to breathlessness and clubbing of fingers and toes

K. M. Lynch (✉) · P. Mondal
Penn State Hershey Medical Center, Hershey, PA, USA
e-mail: klynch@pennstatehealth.psu.edu; pmondal@pennstatehealth.psu.edu

R. P. Olympia, J. Brady-Olympia (eds.), *Clinical Considerations in School-based Health*, https://doi.org/10.1007/978-3-031-85765-2_45

- Delayed puberty
- Infertility in males
- Pancreatitis

When students with CF present with acute disease exacerbation, school nurses and providers are often the first point of contact. Children who are followed at CF centers typically have a care plan consisting of airway clearance, nutritional supplements, and a sick plan to supplement their routine CF care. However, the family and school system need to collaborate to integrate the child's healthcare plan into their weekday routine or individualized education plan (IEP) to ensure that all care providers at home and in school understand the child's disease condition and care goals. The school-based healthcare provider is pivotal in implementing the CF care plan and maintaining the continuity of care. Parents of CF children often experience burnout due to medical care demands, financial burdens, and emotional strain. Parents often report insufficient support for their mental health and financial needs, along with inadequate community services, healthcare services, and suboptimal school support systems [3]. Care providers should educate families about available resources and facilitate interventions that support parents' well-being and confidence in caring for their children [4]. When a school-based healthcare provider, such as a school nurse, identifies a child with CF who may not be receiving adequate care at home, they can offer an additional layer of vigilance. In such cases, the school-based healthcare provider may intervene, offer additional medical care, and collaborate with the parents and medical providers to enhance adherence to treatment (Table 45.1). For instance, implementing airway clearance therapies (ACT) during school hours with the support of a school-based provider would be advisable in these situations. ACT, which typically takes about 30–45 minutes twice daily when the child is well, should be integrated into the child's learning plan. ACT often includes:

- albuterol/bronchodilator (to relax and open up the airways),
- mucolytic agents and inhaled antibiotics (if indicated) to be administered via a nebulizer machine (to thin and break up mucus),
- chest physiotherapy or vest therapy (to mobilize the mucus)
- cough assist or huff cough (to expel the mucus)
- administration of nutritional supplementation
- oral medications, including CFTR modulators

While supplementing CF care at school requires a significant time commitment, studies have shown that school-based ACT improves adherence and health outcomes [5]. Without ACT, students with CF experience frequent pulmonary exacerbations which aggravate disease progression, leading to a permanent decline in lung function, poor quality of life, and diminished life expectancy [6]. In conclusion, the school-based healthcare provider can alleviate some family burdens, educate and support the child, prevent exacerbations, and promote a healthier life for children with CF.

Table 45.1 Common CF Medications/Supplements

Medication	Indication	Mechanism of action	Side effects/potential complications
Bronchodilators	Reduce obstruction, supplement airway clearance, and improve the effectiveness of other medications, such as inhaled mucolytics and antibiotics	Relaxes muscles in the airways to improve airflow and ensure optimal deposition and absorption of subsequent inhaled therapies	• Rapid heart rate, palpitations • Nervous, jittery, hyper feelings • Tremors • Nausea
Hypertonic saline/inhaled mucolytics	Thins mucus and decreases obstructions, making it easier to clear mucus from the airways, and helps to reduce lung infections	Increase concentration of sodium in the airways, which attracts water to secretions to reduce the viscosity of the mucus; may also inhibit biofilm formation and improve management of bacterial infections	• Increased cough • Sore throat • Chest tightness
Inhaled antibiotics	Maintenance therapy to prevent/treat lung infections, reduce bacterial burden, decrease frequency of exacerbations, allow delivery of high concentration antibiotic directly to the lung tissue, and slow disease progression	Inhibit protein synthesis or bacterial cell wall synthesis and/or disrupt bacterial cell wall membrane	• Cough • Oropharyngeal pain • Abnormal taste • Tinnitus • Alteration of the voice • Transient increases in creatinine
Inhaled corticosteroids	Reduce lung damage from airway inflammation; prevent and treat wheezing	Reduce formation of mucus and edema; inhibit chemotaxis, adhesion, and activation of leukocytes; inhibit nuclear factor activation; interfere with inflammatory mediators	• Thrush • Slowed growth (typically only with high doses, but generally, the final height is unaffected) • Hoarse voice (rare)

(continued)

Table 45.1 (continued)

Medication	Indication	Mechanism of action	Side effects/potential complications
Oral antibiotics	Treat bacterial infections, limit inflammation, preserve lung function	Inhibit or interfere with protein synthesis, attack cell wall, prevent replication, interfere with folic acid synthesis	• Nausea/Vomiting • Diarrhea • Skin rash • Changes in taste or smell • Headaches • Photosensitivity • Allergic reactions • Hard-to-treat bacterial infections, like *C. diff* • Antibiotic resistance
CFTR modulators	Helps the CFTR protein perform better by augmenting the malfunctioning protein and/or the chloride channel to reduce the symptoms of CF	Current modulators are effective only for specific mutations; correctors help the CFTR protein form the right shape, traffic to the cell surface, stay at the surface longer; potentiators open the chloride channel and hold the gate open, allowing chloride to flow to optimize flow of water and chloride in and out of cells lining the lungs and other organs	• Headaches • Upset stomach • Nasal congestion/ rhinorrhea • Chest tightness • Mood changes
Enzymes	pancreatic enzyme replacement therapy (PERT) to prevent malnutrition	break down fat, protein, and starches in the small intestine to improve absorption of nutrients and fat-soluble vitamins	• Constipation • Diarrhea • Upset stomach • Gas • Bloating • Headache
Vitamins	Prevent vitamin deficiencies secondary to poor absorption, malnutrition, or liver disease	Support many physiologic functions, such as cellular proliferation, antioxidant benefits, anti-inflammatory activity, bone health, and immunity	• Toxicity • GI upset

Case 2 Jake is a seventh grader with CF. He is diligent with his medical regimen and tries to stay active with the middle school track team. He is shorter than other students on the team and works hard to keep up. He is well-liked and generally seems to have a positive outlook. When anyone on the team is sick, Jake will wear a mask, and he has to maintain separation from that teammate. His family will arrange his transportation to track meets so that he can avoid the crowded bus. When Jake gets sick, he will miss several days. This all creates significant social distancing between him and his teammates.

Parents of CF children often experience difficulties keeping up with daily health maintenance therapies and educational needs. ACT adherence frequently falls below 50%, which can lead to poor disease outcomes [5]. CF care routine tends to be organized around educational and school activities, and ACT treatments may be compromised when completing both is not feasible. At times, families report that treatments are a barrier to educational progress. Additionally, time-consuming treatment routines can significantly impact socialization and friendships. Thus, CF healthcare teams should consider incorporating treatments into the family's routines and other priorities when planning to manage CF [7]. In addition to health and education, families are also concerned about their child's social experience and exposure. While parents recognize their primary role in facilitating social experiences, they seek greater support from schools, social networks, and peers to create opportunities for social development [8]. Families often express concern that peers may lack understanding and empathy, leading to bullying and peer pressure. This presents an opportunity for school-based healthcare providers to promote education and awareness through social skills groups.

The school-based healthcare provider plays a crucial role in supporting adolescents with CF by collaborating with their care team to ensure school-based assistance that promotes disease management, safety, academic progress, and peer relationships. They can help the care team plan accommodations during extended health-related absences, such as virtual learning and peer engagement through the safe use of social media, to address missed educational experiences and reduce social isolation [11].

Contraindications for Exercise/Sports with CF.

Children with CF should have a high-salt diet to prevent dehydration, especially during exercise and summer months. CF children lose more salt in their sweat and can develop hyponatremia if adequate supplementations are not provided. While regular exercise and participation in sports are encouraged and may help improve health conditioning and enhance airway clearance, participation in exercise should sometimes be considered with caution or even be contraindicated. For example, outdoor games in the afternoon during summer months should be discouraged, as running outside in heat can lead to acute hyponatremia. Usually, hyponatremia can be managed and prevented by supplementing salt in the diet and drinks [9]. Activities such as scuba diving, skydiving, bungee jumping, or high-intensity activities (running, hiking, mountain climbing) at high altitudes are contraindicated in CF children due to diminished lung function and poor oxygen exchange at their baseline [10]. CF children with liver or spleen enlargement should avoid contact sports like football, basketball, wrestling, or soccer [10].

CF care providers should be aware of following warning signs of hyponatremia:

- Headache
- Stomach pain
- Muscle cramping
- Nausea or vomiting
- Confusion or fatigue
- Low blood pressure
- Weakness or loss of energy

In summary, the school-based healthcare provider should take the responsibility to implement accommodations for medication administration at school, infection control procedures, changes to the student's schedule to integrate ACT, and/or modifications to the academic plan, and optimizing social interaction and sports participation in alignment with the disease severity [12].

Case 3 Hazel is a tenth grader with CF who has been doing reasonably well from a respiratory standpoint. However, she has been in your office a few times in the past month, complaining of stomach cramps, and has asked to lie down. You also note abdominal bloating and gas. She is typically quiet and polite but does not make good eye contact.

Teenagers naturally seek to fit in with their peers. However, adolescents with CF may struggle to connect with their fellow students. Coping with their chronic illness can be emotionally challenging for teens, often resulting in anger and resentment, which can lead to neglecting self-care [13]. A student with CF may have to take up to 40 pills per day, including antibiotics, CFTR modulators, enzymes, and vitamins. They often feel stigmatized having to take pills or perform therapies in front of peers. Families and care providers must recognize compliance concerns and intervene to provide care while encouraging autonomy [13]. School-based healthcare providers should work with the student and family to determine the appropriate level of independence and desired level of privacy, such as performing ACT at the nurse's office, and then develop a plan to have in place at school [14].

In children with CF, the gastrointestinal (GI) system is second to the respiratory system in terms of the number of complications. Constipation is common in children with CF, and distal intestinal obstruction syndrome (DIOS) is a serious complication that school-based healthcare providers should be aware of. DIOS can occur if children with CF do not adhere to dietary recommendations, get dehydrated, or miss daily pancreatic enzyme replacement therapy (PERT). PERT is recommended to be taken at school before every meal or snack to aid digestion. Older students should be authorized to carry and administer their enzymes to avoid frequent trips to the nurse's office [15]. It is important to monitor whether the student follows specific medication instructions. For instance, enzyme capsules must not be crushed or chewed. If swallowing the pill is difficult, capsules should be opened, sprinkled on a small amount of acidic food, such as applesauce, and consumed immediately [16].

Constipation is common with CF and likely occurs due to an underlying salt transport defect that affects water reabsorption in the colon, along with bowel dysmotility and fat malabsorption. In addition, sticky mucus, underlying bowel inflammation, and abnormal gut microbiota increase the risk for constipation. Typically, constipation presents with abdominal discomfort, bloating or distention, decreased stool frequency, and increased stool consistency. Constipation can typically be improved with an oral laxative in combination with hydration, adequate physical activity, nutrition, and diligence with PERT [13].

Poor adherence to their GI regimen can lead to intestinal obstruction in CF [17], and school nurses should be aware of the symptoms of DIOS, which often require a high index of suspicion and urgent referral [8]. DIOS occurs less frequently than constipation but is not uncommon. The annual prevalence of DIOS is 5–12 episodes per 1000 CF patients [8]. DIOS often clinically presents with features of incomplete obstruction, such as abdominal pain and non-resolving constipation. If not treated in a timely manner, it can progress to complete obstruction, which may become life-threatening. Abdominal tenderness and bilious vomiting, along with worsening constipation, should raise suspicion, especially in children with a recent history of diet changes, dehydration, or concerns for poor adherence to PERT [8, 13]. Urgent referral of the child to the emergency department or CF center is crucial for ensuring prompt evaluation and treatment, as DIOS with complete obstruction would likely require hospitalization with bowel rest, nasogastric lavage and aspiration, IV rehydration, and pain medications [8].

Extra Credit Points

1. A typical day for a child with CF includes medications, supplements, and respiratory treatments every morning and evening. Even at baseline, mid-day treatments may be necessary at school.
2. When a CF child is sick, an individualized care plan should incorporate wearing a mask and isolation, increased frequency of treatments, special transportation, and accommodating missed days by providing additional support such as virtual learning.
3. If the school-based healthcare provider notices concerns such as inadequate care, mental health concerns, poor compliance, or medical decline, they should immediately communicate these concerns to the CF healthcare team.
4. Table 45.2 shows common concerning presentations of students with CF.

Table 45.2 Common concerning presentations of students with CF

Common concerns	Signs and symptoms children may present with at school	Acute management at school	Disposition (PCP, urgent care and/or emergency department)	Treatment
Upper respiratory infection	increased cough, nasal congestion, sinus pressure, poor appetite	Increased fluids, nasal saline spray, saline nebs, increased airway clearance therapies. Allow student to keep water, tissues, trash can, and hand sanitizer at or near desk.	For patients needing more frequent treatments, reach out to PCP. If associated with increased work of breathing or oxygen desaturations not improving with treatments, refer to ED.	• Increased airway clearance therapies • Inhaled antibiotics • Saline nebs • Oral steroids • Oral antibiotics
Cough (can be normal for CF patients, even without URI)	Increased mucus, coughing to clear mucus	Do not draw attention to coughing, allow student to leave room to cough (f needed), encourage student not to hold the cough in, some students may need to Huff Cough if the mucus is not able to be expelled with coughing	Consider reaching out to PCP for students who may need instructions for Huff Cough or need to increase mucolytics or airway clearance before/ after school	• Increased airway clearance therapies • May not always require additional treatment • Do not draw attention to cough • Allow student to take a break or go to nurse
Constipation	Pain, cramping, gas, bloating	Increase water intake, encourage high fiber diet, ensure adherence with enzymes, promote exercise	Contact PCP for recommendations for improved management for mild symptoms. For abdominal bloating with severe GI pain, blood in stool, inability to stool, or vomiting, refer to ED	• Fluids • Laxatives and/or stool softeners • Nasogastric tube • Surgery may be required in severe cases

(continued)

Table 45.2 (continued)

Common concerns	Signs and symptoms children may present with at school	Acute management at school	Disposition (PCP, urgent care and/or emergency department)	Treatment
Hyponatremia	Headache, stomach pain, muscle cramping, nausea or vomiting, confusion or fatigue, low blood pressure, weakness or loss of energy, seizures	High salt foods, add salt to fluids, monitor for increased symptoms on hot days or after exercise	PCP may consider increasing salt supplements, adding medication, checking blood levels, or evaluating for underlying causes (infection, CF complications). For students whose symptoms are severe, or who are not improving with acute management, refer to ED.	• Sodium replacement with close monitoring • Fluid restriction • Hypertonic saline via intravenous infusion may be needed for critically low sodium levels • Medications
Gastroesophageal Reflux	Heartburn, acid taste in mouth, sore throat, emesis, throat clearing, trouble swallowing, stomach pain; more frequent respiratory illnesses, increased cough, or more severe lung disease	Smaller, more frequent meals, avoiding spicy foods and carbonated drinks.	PCP may consider increasing or adding medication, or ordering further evaluations/testing	• Lifestyle modifications • Proton pump inhibitors • H2 blockers • Nissen
Malabsorption	malodorous oily stools that can be difficult to flush, chronic diarrhea, failure to thrive, weight loss, bloating, and dyspepsia	Ensure adherence with enzymes and provide adequate opportunities for high-calorie snacks and lunch.	For patients who are not adherent, reach out to PCP. For concerns for access to high-calorie foods, reach out to PCP, nutritionist, or social worker.	• High calorie diet • Pancreatic enzymes • Frequent meals

Abbreviations: *ED* emergency department, *PCP* primary care provider

References

1. Scotet V, L'Hostis C, Férec C. The changing epidemiology of cystic fibrosis: incidence, survival and impact of the CFTR gene discovery. Genes. 2020;11(6):589. https://doi.org/10.3390/genes11060589.
2. NIH. Cystic Fibrosis – Symptoms | NHLBI, NIH. www.nhlbi.nih.gov. Published March 24, 2022. https://www.nhlbi.nih.gov/health/cystic-fibrosis/symptoms
3. Robertson EG, Kelada L, Ilin R, et al. Psychological well-being among parents of a child living with a serious chronic illness: a cross-sectional survey study. J Child Health Care. Published online March 29, 2024. https://doi.org/10.1177/13674935241238485.
4. Spurr S, Bally J, Burles M, et al. A investigation into hope, self-efficacy, distress and uncertainty in parents who have a child with a life-threatening or life-limiting illness. J Pediatr Nurs. 2022;66:e9–e15. https://doi.org/10.1016/j.pedn.2022.07.002.
5. Byrwa DJ, Perez GF, Roach CM, et al. Airway clearance therapy in the school environment: retrospective analysis of a cohort of pediatric patients with cystic fibrosis. J Cyst Fibros. 2023;22(5):811–5. https://doi.org/10.1016/j.jcf.2023.01.006.
6. Burgel P-R, Southern KW, Addy C, et al. Standards for the care of people with cystic fibrosis (CF); recognising and addressing CF Health issues. J Cyst Fibros. 2024;23(2):187–202. https://doi.org/10.1016/j.jcf.2024.01.005.
7. Gathercole K. Managing cystic fibrosis alongside children's schooling: family, nurse and teacher perspectives. J Child Health Care. 2019;23(3):425–36. https://doi.org/10.1177/1367493518814930.
8. Janin MM, Ellis SJ, Lum A, et al. Parents' perspectives on their child's social experience in the context of childhood chronic illness: a qualitative study. J Pediatr Nurs. 2018;42:e10–8. https://doi.org/10.1016/j.pedn.2018.06.010.
9. Minerals | Cystic Fibrosis Foundation. www.cff.org. https://www.cff.org/managing-cf/minerals
10. Cystic Fibrosis and Exercise. www.cincinnatichildrens.org. https://www.cincinnatichildrens.org/health/c/cystic-fibrosis-exercise
11. Grieve AJ, Tluczek A, Racine-Gilles CN, et al. Associations between academic achievement and psychosocial variables in adolescents with cystic fibrosis. J Sch Health. 2011;81(11):713–20. https://doi.org/10.1111/j.1746-1561.2011.00648.x.
12. Hjelm M, Hente E, Schuler CL, et al. Education-related needs for children with cystic fibrosis: perspectives of US pediatric care teams. Pediatr Pulmonol. 2023;59(1):95–100. https://doi.org/10.1002/ppul.26716.
13. Rego TD, de Moraes JR, Cabral IE, et al. Self-care deficits reported by school children with cystic fibrosis. J Pediatric Nursing. Published online May 2024. https://doi.org/10.1016/j.pedn.2024.04.049.
14. Segal TY. Adolescence: what the cystic fibrosis team needs to know. J R Soc Med. 2008;101(1_suppl):15–27. https://doi.org/10.1258/jrsm.2008.s18005.
15. Coughing and huffing. Cystic Fibrosis Foundation. Accessed May 1, 2024. https://www.cff.org/managing-cf/coughing-and-huffing.
16. Mennitt D. What is the current FDA-approved therapy to treat pancreatic insufficiency for children with cystic fibrosis? NASN Sch Nurse. 2012;27(2):67–8. https://doi.org/10.1177/1942602x11425930.
17. Cystic Fibrosis Canada. Accessed May 1, 2024. https://www.cysticfibrosis.ca/distal-intestinal-obstruction-syndrome-dios.

Chapter 46
Diabetes Mellitus

Lina Huerta-Saenz

Case 1 **Alexander is a 6-year-old boy diagnosed with T1D one month ago, who will be starting first grade soon. Parents feel nervous about the transitioning of T1D care from the home setting to the school setting. He is a very smart, talkative, and previously healthy boy who was attending kindergarten 3 days per week before the diagnosis of T1D. After his recent diagnosis, his parents decided to keep him at home, and since then his mother has been the main caretaker. There are no language barriers at home, and he is also the only child at home. He loves school but is concerned about attending a new school for first grade. Parents are feeling overwhelmed about the transition to school. The elementary school where Alexander will be starting classes soon has 2 school nurses, but parents are uncertain about the level of experience of the school nursing staff related to T1D care. What needs to be done to help Alexander's diabetes care transitioning process to school be successful?**

Diabetes mellitus (DM) is one of the most common chronic conditions in children and it can impact their lifestyle significantly [1]. In the USA, 352,000 children and adolescents younger than age 20 years or 35 per 10,000 U.S. youths have been diagnosed with diabetes mellitus, and a total of 304,000 children and adolescents have diagnosis type 1 diabetes (T1D). DM is diagnosed based on the American Diabetes Association criteria including: a) Plasma fasting glucose above 126 mg/dL, and/or random plasma glucose above 200 mg/dL, and/or hemoglobin A1C $\geq$ 6.5% and/or in an individual with classic symptoms of hyperglycemia (polydipsia, polyuria and/or polyphagia) or hyperglycemic crisis, a random plasma glucose $\geq$200 mg/dL [2].

L. Huerta-Saenz (✉)
Division of Pediatric Endocrinology and Diabetes, Penn State Health Children's Hospital, Penn State College of Medicine, Hershey, PA, USA
e-mail: lhuertasaenz@pennstatehealth.psu.edu

R. P. Olympia, J. Brady-Olympia (eds.), *Clinical Considerations in School-based Health*, https://doi.org/10.1007/978-3-031-85765-2_46

There are many types of DM, but the most common ones are T1D and type 2 diabetes (T2D). Both types of DM can be diagnosed in children and adolescents, and family history can also be present in both types, however the crucial difference is that T1D is an autoimmune disease, and T2D is not. Additionally, patients with T1D are insulin dependent due to progressive destruction of the pancreatic cells (insulitis) and have evidence of autoimmunity at diagnosis (at least one positive T1D antibody). There are some other features to distinguish T1D from T2D, but are weaker discriminators. There are five T1D antibodies available for testing: Glutamic acid decarboxylase (GAD), islet cell antibody (ICA), Zinc transporter 8 antibody (ZnT8), insulin antibody and islet-2 antigen (I2) (Table 46.1).

Routine care of children with T1D includes frequent monitoring of glucose levels, adherence to carbohydrate counting, daily administration of insulin, frequent visits to the diabetes clinic, and regular communication with the diabetes care team for insulin therapy adjustments [3]. Diabetes technology is daily used for monitoring of glucose levels. Glucose monitoring can be completed through frequent finger pricks during the day, and this technique is called blood glucose monitoring (BGM) and is based on the use of glucometers. The other methodology is the 24-hour continuous glucose monitoring (CGM). For those children on BGM, the clinical guidelines recommend monitoring pre-prandial glucose levels before the three main meals of the days, 2-hours after meals and bedtime [4]. After initial diagnosis of DM and in those children initiating treatment with basal insulin therapy (24-hour long-acting insulin), it is also recommended to check glucose levels at 2–3am for the first few days after initial diagnosis. Therefore, during school days, it is recommended to check glucose levels either with a glucometer or with a 24-hour CGM before breakfast, lunch and whenever the child with DM is showing or reporting symptoms concerning for hypoglycemia (palpitations, tremors, anxiety, sweating, pallor, hunger, paresthesias, lethargy, irritability, hypothermia, confusion, coma, seizures) or hyperglycemia (polydipsia, polyphagia, frequent urination, headache, blurred vision, fatigue, weight loss, nausea/vomiting, dehydration, abdominal pain, fruity-smelling breath, deep labored breathing or hyperventilation, rapid heartbeat, confusion and disorientation, loss of consciousness) [5].

Table 46.1 Typical Characteristics to distinguish T1D from T2D

Type 1 Diabetes	Type 2 Diabetes
• *Autoimmunity present (Positive T1D antibodies)* • Younger age at diagnosis (after 1 year of life) • Ketosis with acidosis (Diabetic ketoacidosis) • Family history of T1D • History of unintentional weight loss at diagnosis • History of suboptimal linear growth (6–12 months before clinical diagnosis)	• *Absent autoimmunity* • Any age at onset but older than 1 year, but incidence increases near to puberty age • Ketosis without acidosis • Family history of T2D • History of long-time weight gain prior diagnosis of insulin resistance, and/or prediabetes • History of being born SGA, LGA and early puberty onset

Insulin therapy is the main cornerstone of T1D treatment, as endogenous insulin production in these patients is absent or near-absent. Insulin treatment can be provided as insulin injections (Multiple dose injections = MDI) or as subcutaneous insulin infusion (also called continuous subcutaneous insulin infusion= CSII or insulin pump). Intensive insulin therapy may be associated with a higher rate of hypoglycemia, however patients with better glucose control have fewer macrovascular and microvascular complications [6].

Insulin replacement therapy consists of basal insulin, mealtime insulin, and correction insulin [7]. Basal insulin includes NPH insulin, long-acting insulin analogs, and continuous delivery of rapid-acting insulin via an insulin pump. Most insulin pumps work through automated insulin delivery (AID) and require connection to CGMs using algorithms to determine the amount of short acting insulin to be delivered. AID systems are preferred and should be considered for children with T1D who are capable of using the device safely (either by themselves or with a caregiver) to improve time in range and reduce A1C and hypoglycemia [8, 4]. When choosing among insulin delivery systems, individual preferences, cost, insulin type, dosing plan, and self-management capabilities should be considered.

During the last 20 years, the more frequent use of CGMs have modernized DM care. These devices are able to measured interstitial glucose levels every 5 minutes avoiding the need to perform multiple finger pricks in children with DM. Even though, these devices are incredibly helpful, as any technology device, CGMs can also fail, and it the reported glucose level does not match the physical exam or symptoms of the child with DM, the recommended next step is to measure glucose level with a traditional glucometer.

When children with DM start school, diabetes care professionals need to create a diabetes school management plan (DSMP) to ensure this plan is followed and implemented successfully at school. Coordination of care is crucial to support school personnel, so they can receive adequate education and training for better care of children with DM [3]. The level of diabetes care supervision at school can vary based on the age of the child and the ability to self-care. Regardless of the age of the child with DM, supervision by the school personnel and strict adherence to the diabetes school plan are still required [9].

46.1 National and International Policies Ruling the Need for Structural Support for Children with T1D

In the United States of America, the standard-of-care clinical guidelines by the American Diabetes Association released annually provide the theoretical framework for recommended guidelines for children with diabetes, [3] while at the international level, the International Society of Pediatric and Adolescent Diabetes (ISPAD) guidelines fulfill that role [10, 11].

46.1.1 Diabetes School Management Plans (DSMP)

A typical template for diabetes school orders includes detailed information about the recommended diabetes treatment regimen during school hours. For those children receiving either a multiple dose injection (MDI) regimen or on an insulin pump, these instructions need to describe the carbohydrate counting ratio for the meals eaten at school, the fasting target glucose level and the insulin sensitivity factor (ISF). Glucose levels requiring monitoring of urine or plasma ketones also need to be specified, in addition to instructions for the treatment of hypoglycemia. Further details related to the instructions for glucose monitoring frequency, permission to wear continuous glucose monitors at school, and sick day management are also needed. Glucagon dosing (needed for hypoglycemia treatment) also needs to be described.

46.1.2 The 504 Plan

The 504 plan is a personalized plan for the medical care of a child with a chronic illness at school. Diabetes care in the school setting can be challenging as children with T1D require frequent use of the restroom, the potential need to monitor blood or urine ketones, frequent glucose monitoring, use of CGMs, treatment of acute hyperglycemia and/or hypoglycemia, permission for bathroom breaks, etc. A 504 Plan sets out the actions the school personnel will take to make sure the student with DM is medically safe, has the same access to education as other children, and is treated fairly.

Each 504 plan needs to be individualized to the specific needs, and abilities of the student. The submission of this plan supports the implementation of the requested facilities. Organizations such as the Juvenile Diabetes Research Foundation (https://www.breakthrought1d.org/t1d-resources/school/) and the American Diabetes Association have online templates for free download (http://main.diabetes.org/dorg/PDFs/Advocacy/Discrimination/504-plan.pdf) [12, 13].

46.1.3 Individual Educational Plan (IEP)

The IEP is another plan to implement at school for students who qualify for services under the Individuals with Disabilities in Education Act (IDEA) [14], All children with DM should have an Individualized Education Program (IEP) instead of a 504 plan at school. The IEP is the document that sets out what the school is going to do to meet the individual educational needs of the child with DM. As the IEPs are very detailed and have specific requirements, school districts often use their form. Although students with diabetes who qualify for services under IDEA are also covered by Section 504, there is no need to write two separate plans as both 504 Plan and the IEP aim to support the best coordination of care of children with DM.

It is important to re-evaluate the 504 or the IEP plans at least once a year, and during transitioning phases of development (E.g. childhood to adolescence, elementary to middle school) as there could be challenges in the school-based diabetes care due to internal or external factors [15].

46.2 Coordination of Diabetes Care with the School Personnel

There are multiple steps to follow when coordinating the diabetes care of children with DM with the school personnel. First, *a) parents/caregivers need to request the primary diabetes care team for the preparation of a detailed diabetes school management plan, and b) parents/caregivers need to notify the school staff members about the need to execute the diabetes care plan.* The ultimate goal of the school personnel role is to provide support, encouragement, and supervision of the children with DM.

Families of children with DM and the school personnel need to develop planning strategies to support these children. We will discuss the important role of active coordination between the diabetes care professionals, the child's caregivers, and the school personnel for optimal diabetes care outcomes. School liaisons may be needed. Table 46.2 summarizes the process of care coordination with the school staff in more detail.

46.3 Training and Knowledge of School Staff Members

Pediatric diabetes care teams also play a role in the coordination of education of the school nursing staff. While self-management tasks in pediatric diabetes are highly encouraged, this is not always possible when the child is very young or has a recent diagnosis of diabetes mellitus. Therefore, for those children with diabetes mellitus who are not independent yet with their diabetes care, it is vital to ensure they receive adequate support from school staff members with appropriate training. The school plan of care can only be effective if implementation is successful at the school setting.

Table 46.2 Initial Steps in the Coordination of Care of Children with Diabetes Mellitus at the School Setting

1. Communication with the Diabetes Care Team
a. Notify the diabetes care team about the initiation of school classes
b. Learn more about the diabetes school orders and provide the school contact information to the diabetes care professionals
c. Obtain information about how to prepare a 504 plan for the school
2. Communication with the School Personnel
a. Contact the school nurse and request a meeting
b. Obtain information about the school staff's expertise with children with T1D
c. Share the Diabetes School Management Plan (DSMP) with the school personnel
d. Request a 504 Plan meeting in writing
e. Request the implementation of an Individual Educational Plan (IEP) if needed
f. Explore the availability of peer support at school
3. The 504 Plan
a. The 504 Plan should include important details such as:
i. Easy access to food, water, and restrooms
ii. Permission to use cell phones (T1D-related technology such as CGMs and insulin pumps require 24-hour use of cell phones for close monitoring of sugar levels)
iii. Training needed for school personnel including bus drivers
iv. Who will be responsible for monitoring student for hypoglycemic control and hyperglycemic events
v. When and where insulin will be administered
vi. Who will be administering insulin
b. Complete a 504 Plan formal meeting to discuss the implementation of the plan at school
4. The Individual Educational Plan(IEP)
a. To be completed if the student qualifies for services due to disabilities in education

46.3.1 Specific Instructions Related to the Performance of Physical Activity and Sports At School

Intensive physical activity impacts glucose levels. School personnel including the sports coaches and gym teachers must be aware of the risks of severe hypoglycemia in children receiving insulin therapy who are undergoing physical exertion. Glucose disturbances after exercise are hard to predict, but school personnel need to be ready to treat hypoglycemic events to prevent life-threatening consequences (Table 46.3) [16, 17].

Case 2 Camille is a 14-year-old girl diagnosed with T1D at age 9 years old. Her parents used to be the main diabetes caregivers until she started middle school. Her glucose control used to be within range (HbA1C ≤7%) until recently. She no longer seems to be interested in her diabetes care. Her most recent HbA1C was 10%, and she has been missing many days at school due to hyperglycemia and ketonuria. Parents and school personnel are very concerned, and a meeting including the school counselor has been scheduled for further discussion of her recent suboptimal diabetes control.

Table 46.3 Recommendations for the Physical Education Teachers or Sports Coaches at School

• Encourage participation in exercise and physical activities/sports
• Make sure that glucose monitoring equipment and devices are available at school
• Confirm the availability of a hypoglycemia emergency kit (Nasal or glucagon injections) availability
• Verify that the student always measures glucose levels before exercise and that glucose level before starting sports practice is within the recommended range
• Be aware of the signs and symptoms of hypoglycemia and hyperglycemia and follow the diabetes school management plan (DSMP)
• Maintain close communication with the school nurse and/or trained diabetes personnel and parents regarding any concerns about the student.

46.3.2 The Role of Mental and Behavioral Health in the Diabetes Care of School-Aged Children

Children with diabetes mellitus are at high risk of developing anxiety, depression, adjustment disorder, and other associated conditions [18]. When compared with children and adolescents without diabetes, those with diabetes had almost 2-fold higher prevalence of mental, behavioral, and developmental disorders. [19] The reported prevalence of depression and anxiety in children with DM are 22.2% and 17.7% respectively. Mental and behavioral health evaluation and support are needed, especially when children transition into the adolescent development phase. Coping techniques are also needed for them and their caregivers [20].

Disturbances of mental and/or behavioral health are often very subtle and frequently, anxiety and depression symptoms are not easily identified. Some circumstances suggesting the need to screen the child or adolescent with DM for underlying mental/behavioral conditions are unexplained deterioration of the HbA1C, frequent visits to the emergency department, ketonuria, hypoglycemic seizures, frequent diabetic ketoacidosis admissions, and decreased performance at school. The co-existence of psychiatric disorders and T1D is linked to underachievement in school [21]. Routine screenings for depression and anxiety are frequently completed as part of the annual surveillance evaluation at pediatric diabetes clinics, and one of the most common screening tools for depression and suicidal ideation is the Patient Health Questionnaire 9 (PHQ-9) [22]. It is important to watch for symptoms of depression and anxiety in the school setting. The school counselors can play an important role in this process, as very frequently, they are the initial behavioral support at school. Case 2 illustrates clearly the importance of screening adolescents with T1D for mental/behavioral health disease.

46.4 Potential Challenges in the Communication Process

Family involvement in the diabetes care of a child with diabetes mellitus is a crucial component of optimal diabetes management. However, once the child starts school, other factors and challenges play a role in this process. Some potential barriers to a

Table 46.4 Diabetes Care and School Personnel Involved in the Regular Care of Children with Diabetes Mellitus

School Care Team	Diabetes Care Team
– Teacher – Teacher aids – School nurse – Administrator – Office Staff – Coaches – Counselors – Transportation staff	– Physicians – Physician assistants – Nurse practitioners – Diabetes educators – Dietitians – Social workers – Nurses – Administrative staff (e.g. schedulers, assistants, etc.)

good communication process are fear of hypoglycemia, (b) DM technology literacy, (c) language barriers, and (d) cultural barriers. It is also important to clearly describe the roles of each person involved in the diabetes care of these children. Table 46.4 describes some of the designated contact/support team members involved.

Extra Credit Points

1. Close communication and coordination between the diabetes care professionals and the school personnel is vital for successful outcomes of diabetes care in the school setting
2. Preparation and implementation of the 504 Plan and/or an IEP are legal documents to support to accommodate the individual needs of school-aged children with diabetes on their learning environment
3. Monitoring and surveillance of symptoms suggesting mental or behavioral health problems in school-aged children with diabetes is highly recommended. Parents should partner with the school counselor and the diabetes care professionals for a holistic evaluation of these children

References

1. Miller GF, Coffield E, Leroy Z, Wallin R. Prevalence and costs of five chronic conditions in children. J Sch Nurs. 2016;32(5):357–64.
2. American Diabetes Association Professional Practice Committee. Section 2. Diagnosis and Classification of Diabetes: *Standards of Care in Diabetes—2024*. Diabetes Care. 2024;47:S20–42.
3. Elsayed NA, Aleppo G, Bannuru RR, Bruemmer D, Collins BS, Ekhlaspour L, et al. 14. Children and adolescents: standards of care in diabetes—2024. Diabetes Care. 2024;47(Supplement_1):S258–S81.
4. American Diabetes Association Professional Practice Committee. Section 7. Diabetes Technology: *Standards of Care in Diabetes—2024*. Diabetes Care. 2024;47:S126–S44.
5. Jackson CC, Albanese-O'Neill A, Butler KL, Chiang JL, Deeb LC, Hathaway K, et al. Diabetes care in the school setting: a position statement of the American Diabetes Association. Diabetes Care. 2015;38(10):1958–63.
6. Lachin JM, Nathan DM, Group DER. Understanding metabolic memory: the prolonged influence of Glycemia during the diabetes control and complications trial (DCCT) on future risks

of complications during the study of the epidemiology of diabetes interventions and complications (EDIC). Diabetes Care. 2021;44(10):2216–24.

7. American Diabetes Association Professional Practice Committee. Section 9. Pharmacologic Approaches to Glycemic Treatment: *Standards of Care in Diabetes—2024*. Diabetes Care. 2024;47:S158–S78.
8. Phillip M, Nimri R, Bergenstal RM, Barnard-Kelly K, Danne T, Hovorka R, et al. Consensus recommendations for the use of automated insulin delivery technologies in clinical practice. Endocr Rev. 2023;44(2):254–80.
9. McCollum DC, O'Grady MJ. Diminished school-based support for the management of type 1 diabetes in adolescents compared to younger children. Diabet Med. 2020;37(5):779–84.
10. Codner E, Acerini CL, Craig ME, Hofer SE, Maahs DM. ISPAD clinical practice consensus guidelines 2018: what is new in diabetes care? Pediatr Diabetes. 2018;19(Suppl 27):5–6.
11. Lawrence SE, Albanese-O'Neill A, Besançon S, Black T, Bratina N, Chaney D, et al. ISPAD clinical practice consensus guidelines 2022: management and support of children and adolescents with diabetes in school. Pediatr Diabetes. 2022;23(8):1478–95.
12. Juvenile Diabetes Research Foundation (JDRF). 504 Plans & Legal Resources for Parents of Children with T1D.
13. American Diabetes Association Professional Practice Committee. Safe at School: Section 504 Plan. 2016.
14. American Diabetes Association Professional Practice Committee. Safe at School: Individualized Educational Program (IEP). 2024.
15. March CA, Siminerio LM, Kazmerski TM, Albanese-O'Neill A, Miller E, Libman I. School-based diabetes care: a national survey of U.S. pediatric diabetes providers. Pediatr Diabetes. 2023;1–10.
16. Riddell MC, Gal RL, Bergford S, Patton SR, Clements MA, Calhoun P, et al. The acute effects of real-world physical activity on glycemia in adolescents with Type 1 diabetes: the Type 1 diabetes exercise initiative pediatric (T1DEXIP) study. Diabetes Care. 2024;47(1):132–9.
17. Sherr JL, Bergford S, Gal RL, Clements MA, Patton SR, Calhoun P, et al. Exploring factors that influence postexercise glycemia in youth with type 1 diabetes in the real world: the type 1 diabetes exercise initiative pediatric (T1DEXIP) study. Diabetes Care. 2024;47(5):849–57.
18. Khemakhem R, Dridi Y, Hamza M, Ben Hamouda A, Khlayfia Z, Ouerda H, et al. Living with type 1 diabetes mellitus: How does the condition affect children's and adolescents' quality of life? Arch Pediatr. 2020;27(1):24–8.
19. Barrett CE, Zhou X, Mendez I, Park J, Koyama AK, Claussen AH, et al. Prevalence of mental, behavioral, and developmental disorders among children and adolescents with diabetes, United States (2016–2019). J Pediatr. 2023;253:25–32.
20. Khemakhem R, Dridi Y, Hamza M, Ben Hamouda A, Khlayfia Z, Ouerda H, et al. How do parents of children with type 1 diabetes mellitus cope and how does this condition affect caregivers' mental health? Arch Pediatr. 2020;27(5):265–9.
21. Liu S, Ludvigsson JF, Lichtenstein P, Gudbjörnsdottir S, Taylor MJ, Larsson H, et al. Educational outcomes in children and adolescents with type 1 diabetes and psychiatric disorders. JAMA Netw Open. 2023;6(4):e238135.
22. Moss AC, Roberts AJ, Yi-Frazier JP, Read KL, Taplin CE, Weaver KW, et al. Identifying suicide risk in adolescents and young adults with type 1 diabetes: are depression screeners sufficient? Diabetes Care. 2022;45(5):1288–91.

Chapter 47
Down Syndrome and Other Common Genetic Disorders

Timothy Lequang and Ermal Aliu

Case 1 Sarah is a delightful 10-year-old girl with Down Syndrome who lives with her parents and two older siblings in a supportive family environment. Sarah is enrolled in an elementary school where efforts are made to provide inclusive education. What medical challenges could Sarah expect to face in her school environment and what are some recommendations to address them?

Trisomy 21, due to an extra chromosome 21, results in a group of clinical recognizable features that are collectively known as Down Syndrome (DS) (Table 47.1). Common manifestations of DS include intellectual disability, autism, hearing loss, cataracts, congenital heart defects, neurologic dysfunction, atlantoaxial instability, gastrointestinal atresia, hip abnormalities and dislocations, and thyroid disease [1–3]. The American Academy of Pediatrics recommends annual counseling by a clinical geneticist or genetic counselor throughout childhood to assess: "personal support available to family; participation in a family-centered medical home; age-specific Down syndrome-related medical and developmental conditions; financial and medical support programs and long-term financial planning for which the child and family may be eligible; injury and abuse prevention, with special consideration of developmental skills and intellectual ability; and nutrition and activity to maintain appropriate weight [4]".

Focusing on school-aged children, in early childhood, from ages 1–5 years, the American Academy of Pediatrics recommends following the *Bright Futures/ American Academy of Pediatrics schedule*, including monitoring weight and height, changes in feeding, and signs of anemia [4]. Because of the increased risk for

T. Lequang
Penn State College of Medicine, Hershey, PA, USA
e-mail: tlequang@pennstatehealth.psu.edu

E. Aliu (✉)
Penn State Children's Hospital, Hershey, PA, USA
e-mail: ealiu@pennstatehealth.psu.edu

R. P. Olympia, J. Brady-Olympia (eds.), *Clinical Considerations in School-based Health*, https://doi.org/10.1007/978-3-031-85765-2_47

Table 47.1 Common Manifestations of Down Syndrome

Organ System	Disease, Syndrome, Symptoms
Head and Neck	– Otitis media with effusions – Nasolacrimal duct occlusion – Hypodontia – Delayed dental eruption
Ophthalmic	– Refractive errors – Strabismus – Nystagmus – Cataracts – Glaucoma – Keratoconus
Cardiovascular	– Atrioventricular septal defect, – Persistent ductus arteriosus – Tetralogy of Fallot
Respiratory	– Obstructive sleep apnea – Upper and lower respiratory tract infections
Gastrointestinal	– Gastrointestinal atresia – Celiac disease – Hirschsprung Disease
Endocrine	– Hashimoto thyroiditis – Graves' Disease – Hyperthyroidism – Type 1 Diabetes
Dermatologic	– Seborrheic dermatitis – Atopic dermatitis – Xerosis – Alopecia
Neurologic/Psychiatric/Developmental	– Autism – Alzheimer disease – Seizure – Moyamoya disease
Hematologic	– Iron deficiency anemia – Transient abnormal myelopoiesis – Leukemia
Musculoskeletal/Rheumatologic	– Atlantoaxial instability – Juvenile idiopathic arthritis

auditory and visual disorders associated with DS, children with DS should be screened at the appropriate developmental milestones and suspicion for these conditions should be considered in children with DS who exhibit changes in behavioral patterns in the classroom. Behavioral changes in these children may also indicate possible obstructive sleep apnea, and referral to a pediatric sleep laboratory should be made [5]. Additional common causes of sleep related disturbances include low ferritin [6]. Atlantoaxial instability is a feature of DS due to hypotonia, ligamentous laxity, and bony changes, and cervical spine precautions should be discussed with parents [7]. At school, recognition of myelopathic presentations including abnormal cervical tenderness, head positioning, gait disturbances, weakness, and/or bowel or bladder incontinence should prompt emergent evaluation. In children with DS, autism spectrum disorder (ASD) may be difficult to identify due to the complex interplay between the two conditions. It is important to recognize that symptoms of ASD may overlap with or modify developmental delays that are typically associated with DS. Therefore, the American Academy of Pediatrics recommend expert screening for all children with DS between ages 18 and 24 months [4].

In late childhood, ages 5–12 years, the American Academy of Pediatrics similarly recommends following the *Bright Futures/American Academy of Pediatrics schedule*. Appropriate screening and preventive measures are recommended during this age group, such as weight, height, head circumference, diet, lifestyle, and vision and hearing screening. In this age group, atlantoaxial instability should continue to be monitored, and special attention to developmentally appropriate skills and responsibilities at home and in school should be given. Continued management of chronic or evaluation for acute behavioral changes, including medical causes, is recommended to allow for proper and timely intervention [8]. Patients with DS may enter puberty during this period and may require additional counseling to help them navigate these changes.

From adolescence to early adulthood, ages 12 to 21 years, recommended screenings and preventive measures can be found in the *Bright Futures /American Academy of Pediatrics schedule*. In this age range, particular emphasis should be placed on cardiac evaluation due to the high prevalence of congenital heart defects, typically mitral or aortic valvular diseases, in the DS population [9]. Patients with progressive fatigue, shortness of breath, exertional dyspnea, new murmurs, or gallops should be evaluated. In addition, there should be continued attention to behavioral changes, myelopathic signs due to atlantoaxial instability, and sexual development.

There is no cure or treatments currently approved for Down Syndrome. Rather, goals of care involve: (1) prevention and management of known DS symptoms, (2) early recognition and intervention of complications, and 3) measures that improve quality of life and burden for the patient and their families.

Case 2 Emma is a vivacious 7-year old girl diagnosed with achondroplasia, the most common form of short stature. She lives with her parents and two siblings in a supportive family environment. Emma attends an elementary school where efforts are made to provide inclusive education. What are common medical and psychiatric complications that may be seen while at school?

Achondroplasia is an autosomal dominant disorder that affects the fibroblast growth factor receptor type 3 (*FGFR3*) gene, which primarily leads to disproportionately short stature [10]. Clinical features include shortened upper and lower extremities, normal trunk length, and relative macrocephaly. Quality of life for those with achondroplasia is an important consideration, particularly in adolescence. Early recognition of common complications may expedite intervention and significantly improve quality of life and prevent potential future complications.

Physical complications of achondroplasia include motor developmental delay, spinal stenosis and/or compression, pain, and weight management. In young children with achondroplasia, motor development may be delayed, and the American Academy of Pediatrics recommends using a specialized achondroplasia milestone chart. Spinal stenosis can cause motor, sensory, and coordination dysfunction, as well as bowel and bladder incontinence. Children who exhibit these symptoms should be promptly evaluated by a provider. Chronic pain is a common complication of achondroplasia and may affect a child's quality of life, as well as performance in school [11]. Careful attention should be given for those who exhibit symptoms of pain, such as preferring to use one limb compared to the other gait abnormalities, and general poor physical function. Children exhibiting these symptoms should be referred to their pediatrician for evaluation and management. For children with achondroplasia, maintaining a healthy weight and an active lifestyle during adolescence is particularly important for mitigating potential future complications of achondroplasia [12].

Patients with achondroplasia may experience mental health burdens due to their functional limitations, but also from the social impact of their condition. It is important to rule out medical causes that may mimic psychiatric disorders such as depression. Children with achondroplasia who present with progressive behavioral changes, such as irritability, should be evaluated for sleep apnea, which is a common complication of the disease. School-based healthcare providers can advocate for accessibility assist devices or accommodations that lessen the functional burden of the disorder, such as specialized seating and equipment placement. Peer education and awareness may help to foster a culture of acceptance and inclusivity among students by promoting understanding and empathy towards individual differences.

Although the natural history of achondroplasia has been well elucidated, research into improving quality of life is still in its nascency. Patients and families are highly recommended to follow a multidisciplinary team that has experience in managing achondroplasia.

Extra Credit Points

1. The phenotypic expressions of genetic disorders are varied and complex, but the challenges of these phenotypic expressions at an individual level are unique and require a personalized and interdisciplinary management approach. Table 47.2 lists several genetic disorders that you may encounter with several of your students.
2. Management of genetic disorders and syndromes in school-based health should be anticipatory and preventative to optimize quality of life and goal attainment.
3. Along with following the guidelines and recommendations set by the American Academy of Pediatrics, school-based health should be focused on emphasizing and maximizing the abilities of children with genetic conditions instead focusing on their limitations and disabilities.

Table 47.2 Pediatric genetic disorders

Genetic disorder	Features
Ataxia Telangiectasia	• Onset typically before age 4 years • Progressive cerebellar ataxia (starts after initiation of walking) • Oculocutaneous telangiectasias (+ 3 years) • Various T- and B-cell abnormalities • Chronic sinopulmonary disease
Axenfeld-Rieger Syndrome	• Eye manifestations: Photophobia, visual acuity loss, strabismus, glaucoma • Systemic manifestations: Congenital heart defect, dysmorphic features, microdontia/hypodontia
CHARGE Association	• Colobomas • Heart defects (TOF, PDA) • Atresia of choanal • Retarded growth / mental capacity • Genital hypoplasia (males) • Ear anomalies or deafness
DiGeorge Syndrome	• Cardiac: Interrupted aortic arch, truncus arteriosus • Hypoparathyroidism: Hypocalcemic seizures • Immunologic: Thymic hypoplasia, T-cell defects • Facies: Micrognathia, hypertelorism, low-set ears
Ehlers-Danlos Syndrome	• Hyperextensibility of joints and skin • Poor wound healing with thin (atrophic) scars • Easy bruising • Soft skin • MVP or aortic root dilatation
Fragile X Syndrome	• Autism spectrum disorder • Characteristic facial features (elongated face, broad forehead, large and protruding ears, prominent lower jaw) • Hypotonia • Increased joint mobility • Macro-orchidism
Klinefelter Syndrome	• Musculoskeletal: Tall stature, gynecomastia • Urologic: Small testes, infertile • CNS: Mild intellectual impairment • Behavior problems
Leber's Hereditary Optic Neuropathy	• Mitochondrial inheritance • Age of onset between 15-35 years with decreased penetrance, M>F affected • Visual acuity loss (blurry vision, fogging, color loss) • Visual field defects (typically central vision) • Optic nerve atrophy

(continued)

Table 47.2 (continued)

Genetic disorder	Features
Marfan Syndrome	• Cardiac: Aortic or mitral regurgitation, MVP, dilation of ascending aorta • Sudden death / Aortic dissection • Pulmonary: Apical blebs, spontaneous pneumothorax • Musculoskeletal: Tall stature with long slim limbs, pectus excavatum, scoliosis, hyperextensible joints, arachnodactyly • Ophthalmologic: Lens subluxation
Neurofibromatosis Type 1	• Café au lait macules (6 +, greater than 5 mm before puberty and greater than15 mm after puberty) • Neurofibromas • Axillary or inguinal freckling • Optic gliomas • Lisch nodules • Osseous lesions (scoliosis, pectus excavatum) • Seizures, learning disability, behavioral difficulties • Increased risk for malignancies (sarcoma, schwannoma, Wilms', pheochromocytoma, leukemia)
Noonan Syndrome	• "Male Turner Syndrome" • Intellectual impairment • Short stature • Webbed neck • Pectus excavatum • Pulmonic stenosis
Oculocutaneous Albinism	• Eyes: vision loss, nystagmus, macular hypoplasia, strabismus, decreased iris pigmentation • Skin color changes
Osteogenesis imperfecta	• Fragile bones / blue sclera / early deafness • Type I (mild): Joint laxity, fracture decrease post puberty, dentin hypoplasia • Type II (lethal): Numerous intrauterine fractures, stillborn or death in newborn period • Type III (progressive deforming): Severest non-lethal form, wormian bones (undermineralized calvarium) • Type IV (moderately severe): Bowing of lower long bones but attain ambulation
Sturge-Weber Syndrome	• Seizures (90%) • Port-wine stain in first and second branches of trigeminal nerves • Cognitive deterioration • Glaucoma • Venous leptomeningeal angiomatomas
Turner Syndrome	• Musculoskeletal: Prenatal nuchal pad thickening, lymphedema of hands/feet during infancy, webbed neck, wide-spaced nipples, short stature, low posterior hairline • Cardiac: Coarctation of the aorta, bicuspid aortic valve, aortic stenosis • Renal: Horseshoe kidney, duplicated collecting system • Gynecologic: gonadal dysgenesis

(continued)

Table 47.2 (continued)

Genetic disorder	Features
Tuberous Sclerosis	• Triad: Intellectual impairment, seizures, adenoma sebaceum (+ 5 years) • Shagreen patches • Hypopigmented macules (ash leaf macules) • Cortical tubers • Ungal fibromas • Cardiac rhabdomyomas • Retinal hamartomas
VACTERL association	• Vertebral defects • Anal atresia • Cardiac malformations • Tracheoesophageal fistula • Renal anomalies • Limb anomalies
Wiskott-Aldrich syndrome	• Triad: Eczema, thrombocytopenia, increased risk of infections • Cellular and humoral immunity defects • Susceptible to capsular bacterial organisms

References

1. Stoll C, Dott B, Alembik Y, Roth MP. Associated congenital anomalies among cases with Down syndrome. Eur J Med Genet. 2015;58(12):674–80.
2. Shaw EDBR, Beals RK. The hip joint in Down syndrome. A study of its structure and associated disease. Clin Orthop Relat Res. 1992;278:101–7.
3. Kent L, Evans J, Paul M, Sharp M. Comorbidity of autistic spectrum disorders in children with Down syndrome. Dev Med Child Neurol. 1999;41(3):153–8.
4. Bull MJ, Trotter T, Santoro SL, Christensen C, Grout RW. The council on genetics; health supervision for children and adolescents with down syndrome. Pediatrics. 2022;149(5):e2022057010. https://doi.org/10.1542/peds.2022-057010.
5. Shott SR, Amin R, Chini B, Heubi C, Hotze S, Akers R. Obstructive sleep apnea: should all children with Down syndrome be tested? Arch Otolaryngol Head Neck Surg. 2006;132(4):432–6.
6. Dosman C, Witmans M, Zwaigenbaum L. Iron's role in paediatric restless legs syndrome – a review. Paediatr Child Health. 2012;17(4):193–7.
7. Brockmeyer D. Down syndrome and craniovertebral instability. Topic review and treatment recommendations. Pediatr Neurosurg. 1999;31(2):71–7.
8. Worley G, Crissman BG, Cadogan E, Milleson C, Adkins DW, Kishnani PS. Down syndrome disintegrative disorder: new-onset autistic regression, dementia, and insomnia in older children and adolescents with Down syndrome. J Child Neurol. 2015;30(9):1147–52.
9. Dimopoulos K, Constantine A, Clift P, Condliffe R, Moledina S, Jansen K, Inuzuka R, Veldtman GR, Cua CL, Tay ELW, Opotowsky AR, Giannakoulas G, Alonso-Gonzalez R, Cordina R, Capone G, Namuyonga J, Scott CH, D'Alto M, Gamero FJ, Chicoine B, Gu H, Limsuwan A, Majekodunmi T, Budts W, Coghlan G, Broberg CS; for Down Syndrome International (DSi). Cardiovascular complications of down syndrome: scoping review and expert consensus. Circulation. 2023;147(5):425–41. https://doi.org/10.1161/CIRCULATIONAHA.122.059706. Epub 2023 Jan 30. PMID: 36716257; PMCID: PMC9977420.

10. Shiang R, Thompson LM, Zhu YZ, et al. Mutations in the transmembrane domain of FGFR3 cause the most common genetic form of dwarfism, achondroplasia. Cell. 1994;78(2):335–42.
11. Cormier-Daire V, AlSayed M, Ben-Omran T, de Sousa SB, Boero S, Fredwall SO, Guillen-Navarro E, Irving M, Lampe C, Maghnie M, Mortier G, Peijin Z, Mohnike K. The first European consensus on principles of management for achondroplasia. Orphanet J Rare Dis. 2021;16(1):333. https://doi.org/10.1186/s13023-021-01971-6. PMID: 34332609; PMCID: PMC8325831
12. Hoover-Fong J, Scott CI, Jones ME. AAP Committee on Genetics Health supervision for people with achondroplasia. Pediatrics. 2020;145:e20201010. https://doi.org/10.1542/peds.2020-1010.

Chapter 48
Epilepsy

Gayatra Mainali and Sita Paudel

Case 1 While in math class, 7-year-old Rick has a generalized tonic-clonic seizure with left eye deviation lasting approximately 5 min. Following his seizure, he appears unresponsive but is not cyanotic. Records show that he has a diagnosis of epilepsy and is taking daily anti-seizure medications. What should you do?

A seizure is a sudden surge of abnormal electrical activity in the brain. Clinical manifestations may include episodic changes in motor, sensory or cognitive function. Seizures can be categorized as generalized (abnormal electrical activity affects the entire brain) or focal (abnormal electrical activity starts in one part of the brain) [1]. They are further divided into several subtypes (Table 48.1).

Epilepsy is a chronic medical condition characterized by recurrent unprovoked seizures [2, 3]. The etiology of epilepsy can be unknown or be caused by a genetic disorder, structural brain abnormality, metabolic abnormality, infectious (meningitis/encephalitis), or a combination of these (Table 48.2). Children with autism have higher risk of developing epilepsy by around 30% compared to developmentally normal children. In school, having a student with epilepsy requires knowledge of their emergency action plan, including the recognition of their specific seizure type and indications for the administration of rescue medications.

Most students with seizures will have had brain magnetic resonance imaging (MRI) to evaluate the cause of their seizures and an electroencephalogram (EEG) to know the type of seizures. Sometimes students may need to undergo extended EEG monitoring which may lead to significant absenteeism from school.

Students with known epilepsy will likely be prescribed daily antiseizure medications and seizure rescue medications (Table 48.3). If a student exhibits possible side effects, it may be worthwhile asking family if there has been recent change in doses

G. Mainali (✉) · S. Paudel
Penn State Children's Hospital, Hershey, PA, USA
e-mail: gmainali@pennstatehealth.psu.edu; spaudel@pennstatehealth.psu.edu

R. P. Olympia, J. Brady-Olympia (eds.), *Clinical Considerations in School-based Health*, https://doi.org/10.1007/978-3-031-85765-2_48

Table 48.1 Common subtypes of pediatric seizures

Seizure types	Description of the seizure	Common Ages	Common medications used	Important facts
Tonic-clonic seizure	Stiffening and rhythmic body jerking, with foaming at the mouth, urinary or stool incontinence, loss of consciousness	Any ages	Levetiracetam, Lamotrigine, Topiramate, Zonisamide, Valproate	Associated with Juvenile Myoclonic Epilepsy (JME), Lennox Gastaut Syndrome (LGS), Idiopathic generalized epilepsy
Tonic seizure	Stiffening of body and abnormal posture sustained for several seconds	Any age	Levetiracetam, Lamotrigine, Topiramate, Zonisamide, Valproate, Clobazam, Rufinamide	Commonly seen with Lennox Gastaut Syndrome Usually requires a combination of antiseizure medications
Absence seizure	Staring with arrest of motor activity and rhythmic/rapid eyes blinking, lip smacking lasting 5–15 s	Typical onset 4 to 10 years	Ethosuximide, Valproate, Lamotrigine	Associated with Absence epilepsy Often misdiagnosed as "day dreamer" or ADHD
Focal onset seizure	Sustained head and eyes turn to one side, one sided body jerking	Any age	Carbamazepine, Oxcarbazepine, Lacosamide, Phenytoin	Temporal lobe seizures are type of focal seizures where there is altered consciousness and automatic behavior like lips smacking, hand fumbling, repeating words
Myoclonic seizure	Shock like jerk of limbs particularly if affecting both sides	Any age If part of JME, can be seen in adolescence	Levetiracetam, Valproate, Clonazepam	Can be confused with tics, clumsiness. Many also have absence seizure and tonic clonic seizures
Atonic seizure	Muscle relaxes/ losses muscle tone, falls over	Infants, toddlers and school age	Levetiracetam, Lamotrigine, Topiramate, Zonisamide, Valproate, Clobazam, Rufinamide	Can be associated with sudden fall and risk of head injury, developmental delay can be seen after seizure onset Can be seen with epilepsy syndromes like Lennox Gastaut, Doose Syndrome

or regimen. Most daily antiseizure medications are given twice a day (at home), however some regimens may require an addition dose to be given while at school. Some students with refractory epilepsy may have a device called a Vagus Nerve

Table 48.2 Common etiologies of pediatric epilepsy

Causes of Epilepsy	Common abnormalities	Important facts
Genetic	1. Single gene disorders like SCN1A mutation 2. Rett Syndrome: MECP2 gene 3. Sometimes single gene not identified, as in Lennox Gastaut syndrome, absence epilepsy	SCN1A mutation causes refractory seizures triggered by a fever Some medications like phenytoin or carbamazepine can make seizures worse. Rett syndrome only seen in girls with severe speech regression, loss of purposeful hand function and frequent seizures
Structural	Brain MRI shows acquired lesions like stroke, tumors, bleeds, and infections Genetic related lesions like tubers in Tuberous Sclerosis Complex (TSC)	Brain MRI is test of choice and has better diagnostic capabilities than head CT scan. CT scan may be helpful urgently to evaluate bleed or large tumors
Metabolic	Usually present as seizures in neonates, can be identified in new born screening. Usually associated with developmental delay and seizures later in childhood	Vitamin responsive conditions such as Pyridoxine responsive seizures, Hyperglycinemia. Temporary biochemical abnormalities such as hypoglycemia or hyponatremia can cause acute seizures but not epilepsy

Table 48.3 Commonly prescribed antiseizure medications

Drugs	Common side effects	Indications
Levetiracetam	Behavioral changes, irritability	Focal, myoclonic, generalized
Lamotrigine	Rash, nausea	Focal, generalized
Valproic acid	Elevation of liver transaminase (ALT, AST), weight gain, hair loss, easy bruising	Focal, myoclonic, generalized
Ethosuximide	Nausea, vomiting	Absence
Topiramate	Weight loss, paresthesia, fatigue	Focal, absence, generalized
Zonisamide	Nausea, decrease appetite	Focal, absence, generalized
Clobazam	Increase salivation, nausea, vomiting, fatigue	Atonic, tonic, generalized, focal
Oxcarbazepine	Nausea, rash, hyponatremia	Focal
Cannabidiol	Fatigue, elevation of liver transaminase (ALT, AST), diarrhea	Focal, generalized

Stimulator (VNS) [4]. This device has a magnet which can be swiped over the device implanted usually in their left upper chest in the event of a seizure. Online training videos are available via the Epilepsy foundation (https://www.epilepsy.com/treatment/devices/vagus-nerve-stimulation-therapy)

The evaluation of a student who presents with seizure-like activity begins with a thorough history and physical examination, focusing on airway, breathing, and circulation. A student should be transported to an emergency department if there is compromise of ABCs, first time seizure, prolonged seizures (>5 min), depressed mental status or abnormal neurologic examination, seizures associated with a concerning history (trauma, meningitis, overdose, hypoglycemia, significant dehydration, history of brain tumor or ventriculoperitoneal shunt, etc.), or if the student is administered a rescue seizure medication and does not return to baseline. Commonly prescribed rescue medications include rectal diazepam (Diastat), nasal spray diazepam (Valtoco), nasal spray midazolam (Nayzilam), buccal clonazepam tablets, and buccal midazolam [5]. Indication for the administration of a rescue medication include if the seizure lasts longer than 3 min or if there are seizure clusters i.e. 2 or more seizures in a 2-hour timeframe. Rectal diazepam is commonly used in children less than 6 years, while nasal spray medications such as Valtoco or Nayzilam are prescribed in older children. School nurses and school staff should become familiar with the administration of rectal (https://www.epilepsy.com/treatment/seizure-rescue-therapies/rectal-rescue-medicines) and nasal (https://www.epilepsy.com/treatment/seizure-rescue-therapies/nasal-rescue-medicines?gad_source=1&gclid=Cj0KCQjw6PGxBhCVARIsAIumnWZDmpSLtj7wd-ZTL9QTyfsTk6OwX9FYHqiXijPyBFF4XK5rzxy7YLcaAp-8EALw_wcB) rescue medications.

Case 2 You are called to see 16-year-old Luna who collapsed during gym class. She is having violent abnormal body movements, back arching, pelvis thrusting, and side to side head movements. Her eyes are closed and she is moaning in pain. Vitals appears normal. She is able to follow commands.

It is important to differentiate epileptic seizures from seizure mimics. Seizure like episodes can be physiological (such as syncope or migraine phenomena) or psychogenic. Psychogenic Nonepileptic Events/Seizures (PNEE or PNES) are very common particularly in adolescent students who have significant daily stressors. Differentiating them from epileptic seizures can be challenging. Some movements are very atypical for epileptic seizures and can point toward psychogenic non-epileptic episode which include:

- Reciprocating movements (back and forth, to and fro movements including side to side head movements, alternating kicking movements of arms or legs).
- Eye closure (particularly forceful eye closure) during the episode
- Pelvic thrusting
- Talking or crying during the episode
- Each episode looks different than previous episode
- Waxing and waning (Stop-go stop). Episode stops for a while but starts again
- Episode occurring in presence of others
- Event duration can be helpful as well. Seizures usually are brief seconds to minutes. Episodes lasting more than 30 min without significant changes in vitals are unlikely to be an epileptic seizure [6].

In a student without a diagnosis of PNES/PNEE that presents with seizure-like activity, initial management is similar to that discussed in Case 1. However, in a student with a diagnosis of PNES/PNEE, ensure the following [7]:

- Choose one person in the school to be the "PNES response" person. No one else should respond or attend to the student while he/she is exhibiting an event.
- We recommend that you do not send the student home if they have an event. Teachers may wish to notify the school nurse after a class period if they have an event during their class. The student's parents can be contacted to record that an event has occurred.
- When an event occurs, the student should be left in the same place where the event began while ensuring physical safety. Removal of unsafe objects while they have symptoms is recommended.
- Teachers and students should continue what they have been doing in the classroom.
- When the event stops, the student should return to what they were doing prior to the event.
- If the student misses work because of the event, they should make up the work.

48.1 Case Conclusions

Case 1 Rick is given his seizure rescue medication (nasal spray diazepam), which promptly stops the seizure and he returns to baseline. His family is informed who takes him home.

Case 2 Luna is transported to her local emergency department. Her labs (basic metabolic panel, liver function tests, complete blood counts, urine toxicology screen, and urine pregnancy test) and head CT scan were normal. She is hospitalized and undergoes extended video EEG monitoring for 24 h. Her EEG is normal. She has several jerking and thrashing episodes while on EEG without any changes in EEG background which suggests these episodes are psychogenic non-epileptic events (PNEE/PNES). She is seen by a psychiatrist and a referral is made to an outpatient counselling service.

Extra Credit Points

1. Having a student with epilepsy requires knowledge of their emergency action plan, including the recognition of their specific seizure type and the use of rescue medications.
2. A student should be transported to an emergency department if there is compromise of ABCs, first time seizure, prolonged seizures (>5 min), depressed mental status or abnormal neurologic examination, seizures associated with a concerning history (trauma, meningitis, overdose, hypoglycemia, significant dehydration, history of brain tumor or ventriculoperitoneal shunt, etc.), or if the student is administered a rescue seizure medication and does not return to baseline.
3. Brain MRI and EEG are the tests of choice to evaluate seizures but can be done in an outpatient setting. Head CT scan and routine labs including toxicology panel are usually done in an ED while evaluating new onset seizure activity.

4. Behavior Plan for PNES: Ensure physical safety, minimize attention, remain at school, return to typical activity immediately after symptoms stop, inform parent.

References

1. Fisher RS. The new classification of seizures by the international league against Epilepsy 2017. Curr Neurol Neurosci Rep. 2017;17(6):48. https://doi.org/10.1007/s11910-017-0758-6. PMID: 28425015
2. Gogou M. Seizures and epilepsy in childhood. Continuum. 2022;28(2):428–56. https://doi.org/10.1212/CON.0000000000001087.
3. Wirrell E. Evaluation of first seizure and newly diagnosed epilepsy. Continuum. 2022;28(2):230–60. https://doi.org/10.1212/CON.0000000000001074.
4. Jain P, Arya R. Vagus nerve stimulation and seizure outcomes in pediatric refractory epilepsy: systematic review and meta-analysis. Neurology. 2021;96(22):1041–51.
5. Romanowski EMF, McNamara NA, Neil EE, Gottlieb-Smith R, Dang LT. Seizure rescue medications for out-of-hospital use in children. J Pediatr. 2021;229:19–25.
6. Devinsky O, Gazzola D, LaFrance WC Jr. Differentiating between nonepileptic and epileptic seizures. Nat Rev Neurol. 2011;7(4):210–20. https://doi.org/10.1038/nrneurol.2011.24. Epub 2011 Mar 8. PMID: 21386814
7. Hopp J. Nonepileptic episodic events. Continuum. 2019;25(2):492–507. https://doi.org/10.1212/CON.0000000000000711.

Chapter 49
Heart Conditions

Christopher Collin Hayes and Robert D. Tunks

Case 1 Jillian is a 6-year-old girl who developed shortness of breath after running during recess. A heart murmur was heard by a physician in a school-based clinic. After rest, she is no longer short of breath and appears well.

Detection of a heart murmur is the most common reason for referral to most pediatric cardiology practices [1]. Murmurs are characterized as either pathologic or innocent depending on the presence or absence of structural heart disease. Murmurs are graded on their intensity and are described as being systolic, diastolic, holosystolic, or continuous. Systolic murmurs louder than a grade 3/6, holosystolic murmurs, and all diastolic murmurs are considered pathologic and warrant referral to a pediatric cardiologist for evaluation [2]. Innocent murmurs result from blood coursing through a structurally normal heart and as such, children are asymptomatic. Innocent murmurs tend to be louder when the patient assumes a supine position, frequently have a vibratory quality, and can be accentuated during times of increased cardiac output (i.e. increased activity level, fever, anemia, etc.). Tables 49.1 and 49.2 describe features of common innocent and pathologic murmurs in children. In cases of uncertainty about the auscultatory findings, concern for potential pathology, or should the child have cardiovascular symptoms, referral to a pediatric cardiologist for further evaluation is warranted [2].

Chest pain, syncope, palpitations, and family history of arrhythmia or sudden death are other common reasons for referral to a pediatric cardiologist. Symptoms during times of physical activity are concerning and warrant additional evaluation. Table 49.3 lists other suggested reasons for referral for subspecialty evaluation.

Case 2 Sarah is a 16-year-old girl who experiences sudden onset palpitations and dizziness while sitting in class. She feels uncomfortable and goes to the

C. C. Hayes · R. D. Tunks (✉)
Penn State Children's Hospital, Hershey, PA, USA
e-mail: chayes3@pennstatehealth.psu.edu; rtunks@pennstatehealth.psu.edu

R. P. Olympia, J. Brady-Olympia (eds.), *Clinical Considerations in School-based Health*, https://doi.org/10.1007/978-3-031-85765-2_49

Table 49.1 Examples of Innocent Heart Murmurs

Murmur Type	Description
Pulmonary flow murmur	Grade 1–3 SEM best at LUSB; no click or thrill; normal S2
Venous hum	Continuous murmur best at left or right upper chest; softens or becomes inaudible when supine, with head rotation, or compression of jugular vein
Still's murmur	Low frequency SEM with vibratory/musical quality, louder in supine position

LUSB left upper sternal border, *SEM* systolic ejection murmur

Table 49.2 Examples of Pathologic Heart Murmurs

Murmur Etiology	Description
ASD	Widely fixed split S2 with systolic ejection murmur along LUSB +/− diastolic rumble
VSD	Harsh holosystolic murmur, best at LMSB and LLSB +/− diastolic rumble
Aortic stenosis	Harsh SEM along left sternal border with radiation to RUSB, +/− ejection click
Mitral or tricuspid regurgitation	Blowing holosystolic murmur along LLSB (tricuspid) or apex (mitral)
Coarctation of the aorta	Grade 2–3 systolic ejection murmur, harsh, often radiates to the mid-scapular region of the back; decreased lower extremity pulses

ASD atrial septal defect, *VSD* ventricular septal defect, *LUSB* left upper sternal border, *LMSB* left middle sternal border, *LLSB* left lower sternal border, *RUSB* right upper sternal border, *SEM* systolic ejection murmur [For further reading and audio examples of innocent and pathologic heart murmurs in children, please refer to the following source: Geggel, R. L., & Lorin, M. I. (2021). Approach to the infant or child with a cardiac murmur. *UpToDate*]

Table 49.3 Other Potential Reasons for Referral to a Pediatric Cardiologist

Patient Symptoms	Family History
Chest pain with exertion	Congenital heart disease, particularly in a first degree relative
Syncope and presyncope, dizziness especially during exertion	Sudden unexplained death
Palpitations or heart racing, especially with sudden onset and/or termination	Arrhythmia syndrome (Long QT, Brugada) or symptoms suggestive of possible arrhythmia issue (drowning, or congenital deafness)
Cyanosis	Cardiomyopathy (hypertrophic, dilated, restrictive, arrhythmogenic)
Pathologic heart murmur; provider concern	Myocardial infarction or stroke before age of 55

nurse where her heart rate is 220 beats/minute. Her blood pressure is normal. She drinks a glass of cold water and her heart rate abruptly falls below 100 beats/minute. What are the next steps?

Supraventricular tachycardia (SVT) is the most common arrythmia in childhood, affecting as many as 1 in 250 otherwise healthy children [3]. SVT, can affect infants, older children, and adolescents [3]. SVT is a term that describes tachycardias which originate above the ventricle. SVT is almost always a narrow complex rhythm. Some examples include ectopic atrial tachycardia (EAT), atrial flutter, and atrioventricular reciprocating tachycardia (AVRT). Many SVT rhythms affecting children involve an accessory pathway and AV nodal mediated reentry. In some cases, conduction across an accessory pathway leads to pre-excitation in the form of delta waves seen on an ECG, confirming the diagnosis of Wolff-Parkinson-White Syndrome (WPW).

Symptoms suggestive of SVT include a sudden onset and offset of palpitations with associated dizziness, presyncope, shortness of breath, chest pain, and fatigue. Young children can have vague complaints including poor appetite, decreased activity level, or pallor. While only rarely life-threatening [4], SVT can lead to development of tachycardia induced cardiomyopathy if the rhythm remains unrecognized or untreated. Rhythm assessment via 24 or 48-hour monitoring can be utilized to characterize the rhythm and its correlation to symptoms. Often, rhythm monitors may be extended for as long as 30 days if clinical suspicion persists. Table 49.4 lists common symptoms of SVT and its mimickers in the school-aged child:

Clinically, SVT in the school-aged child has a number of important considerations. If a child is in SVT for 15 minutes or longer despite vagal maneuvers, the authors recommend evaluation in the Emergency Department for further assessment and potential conversion to normal sinus rhythm. Management of SVT can include medication therapy, with beta blockers being a commonly used and well tolerated choice. Some SVT rhythms can be difficult to control and require multiple antiarrhythmic medications. In older children, catheter ablation can be performed to disrupt the electrical pathway responsible for SVT and thus offers a potentially curative treatment option.

Case 3 John is a 14-year-old male who had flu-like symptoms 3 days ago. He now has complaints of persistent chest pain and shortness of breath when lying flat. His heart rate is 115 beats/minute and his blood pressure is 95/50 mmHg. What do you do?

Myocarditis has been cited as one of the leading causes of sudden cardiac death in children and young athletes, representing 7% of deaths in a large US registry

Table 49.4 Symptoms of SVT versus Common Mimickers

Signs and symptoms of SVT	Potential Mimickers of SVT
Sudden onset and offset of tachycardia	Anxiety
Persistently elevated heart rate (220 beats/minute for infants; 180–220 beats/minute for adolescents)	Exercise mediated tachycardia
Dizziness	Dehydration
Presyncope/syncope	Fever/illness
Shortness of breath	Autonomic dysfunction/postural orthostatic tachycardia syndrome
Chest discomfort	Caffeine or other drug/medication induced tachycardia

cohort of over 886 youth athletes [5]. Myocarditis involves inflammation of the myocardium and is most commonly caused by a preceding viral infection. Coxsackie B, Adenovirus, Human Herpes Virus-6, and Parvovirus B19 are relatively common etiologies. Cases of Covid-19 myocarditis, bacterial, and non-infectious cases have also been described [6]. Myocarditis can affect people of all ages.

Patients with myocarditis can have complaints of fever, chest pain, dyspnea, palpitations, and gastrointestinal symptoms in some cases. Any patient with suspected myocarditis should be promptly evaluated by a pediatric cardiologist, and potentially in the Emergency Department depending on the severity of presentation and level of testing available in the outpatient setting. Electrocardiographic changes and elevated serum troponin levels suggest evidence of myocardial damage and, if present, warrant additional evaluation and imaging. An echocardiogram is a commonly used modality to quickly evaluate myocardial performance and to evaluate for presence of a pericardial effusion [6] (Fig. 49.1).

Cardiac MRI, with its unique ability to quantify ventricular function and delineate areas of myocardial edema and fibrosis, is now regularly used as the confirmatory diagnostic tool of choice in lieu of an endomyocardial biopsy [7]. A patient's initial management ultimately depends on the degree of symptoms, ranging from patients who are relatively asymptomatic to severely affected individuals with overt heart failure and shock. Following the acute phase of myocarditis, it is generally recommended that children avoid vigorous exercise and sports participation until cleared by a pediatric cardiologist [8].

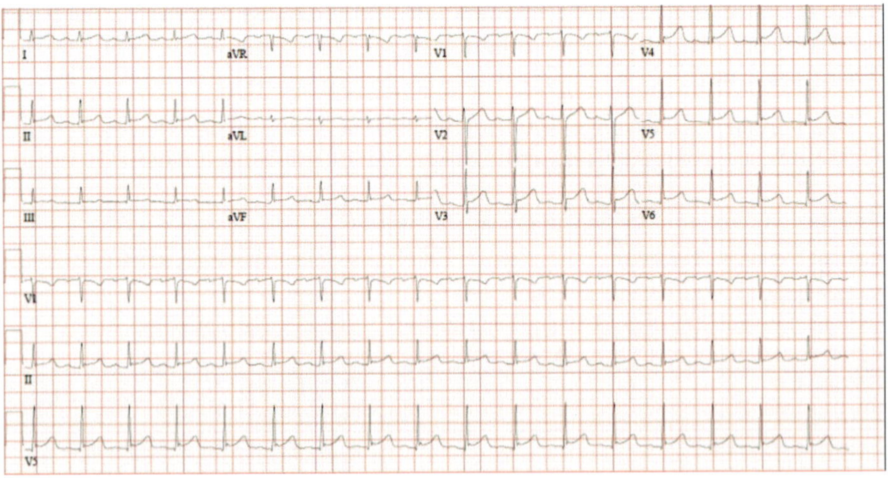

Fig. 49.1 ECG demonstrating sinus tachycardia with inferolateral PR depression and ST segment elevation suggestive of myocarditis

49.1 Case Conclusions

Case 1
Jillian was referred to a pediatric cardiologist who described that she had a grade 2/6, vibratory quality systolic ejection murmur that was heard loudest when she was in a supine position. This was consistent with a functional Still's Murmur. Given that she was diagnosed with an innocent murmur, no additional testing (ECG, echocardiogram) was required. She was discharged with no activity restrictions.

Case 2
Sarah experienced intermittent episodes of palpitations over the next several days and went to her pediatrician where she was referred to a pediatric cardiologist. She had an ECG in the office that showed ventricular pre-excitation (i.e. Wolff-Parkinson-White Syndrome). A 30-day event monitor documented episodes of supraventricular tachycardia. She subsequently underwent a successful ablation procedure after which she has remained asymptomatic. After her procedure, she did not require treatment with anti-arrhythmic medications.

Case 3
John was brought to the Emergency Department where he had persistent chest pain. A chest X-ray showed borderline cardiomegaly and his serum troponin level was elevated. An ECG showed T-wave inversions in the lateral precordial leads. An echocardiogram revealed depressed left ventricular systolic function. He was admitted to the intensive care unit and was supported with inotropic medications. Cardiac MRI later confirmed evidence of myocardial edema and fibrotic changes. His cardiac function eventually recovered. He continues to follow up with a pediatric cardiologist.

Extra Credit Points
1. Innocent murmurs are due to blood flow in a structurally normal heart and are not associated with cardiac symptoms. Innocent heart murmurs have certain features on physical exam and do not require additional cardiac testing. Refer to a pediatric cardiologist if concerned for any pathologic murmur.
2. SVT is usually a narrow complex tachycardia that frequently presents with palpitations, dizziness, and chest discomfort. SVT can lead to tachycardia-induced cardiomyopathy if unrecognized. SVT can be managed with anti-arrhythmic medications or definitively treated through a catheter ablation procedure.
3. Patients with myocarditis can have preserved ventricular function or can have severe dysfunction and clinical evidence of shock. A high index of suspicion should exist for a child who presents with cardiovascular-related symptoms following a recent viral illness. Management ultimately depends on a child's degree of heart failure. Cardiac MRI is a powerful tool that can confirm the diagnosis of myocarditis.
4. Consider the following mnemonic (CARDS RECS) for reasons to refer to a pediatric cardiologist:
   C—Chest pain.

A—Auscultated pathologic murmurs.
R—Racing heart (palpitations).
D—Dizziness.
S—Syncope.
R—Respiratory complaints (shortness of breath).
E—ECG Abnormalities.
C—Cyanosis.
S—Sudden death (family history).

References

1. Sumski CA, Goot BH. Evaluating chest pain and heart murmurs in pediatric and adolescent patients. Pediatr Clin N Am. 2020;67(5):783–99.
2. Ford B, Lara S, Park J. Heart murmurs in children: evaluation and management. Am Fam Physician. 2022;105(3):250–61.
3. Salerno J, Seslar S. Supraventricular Tachycardia. Archiv Pediatr Adolescent Med. 2009;163(3):268–74.
4. Etheridge S, Escudero C, Blaufox A, et al. Life-threatening event risk in children with Wolff-Parkinson-white syndrome: a Multicenter international study. J Am Coll Cardiol: Clin Electrophysiol. 2018;4(4):433–44.
5. Maron B, Haas T, Ahluwalia A. Demographics and epidemiology of sudden deaths in young competitive athletes: from the United States National Registry. Am J Med. 2016;129(11):1170–7.
6. Williams J, Jacobs H, Lee S. Pediatric myocarditis. Cardiol Therapy. 2023;12:243–60.
7. Law Y, Lal A, Chen S, et al. Diagnosis and management of myocarditis in children a scientific statement from the American Heart Association. Circulation. 2021;144(6):e123–35.
8. Maron B, Zipes D, Kovacs R. Eligibility and disqualification recommendations for competitive athletes with cardiovascular abnormalities: preamble, principles, and general considerations a scientific statement from the American Heart Association and American College of Cardiology. Circulation. 2015;152:e256–61.

Chapter 50
Immunocompromised Disorders

Lorie-Mae Nicolas and Kristen Lutzkanin

Case #1 Lisa is an 8-year-old female diagnosed IgA deficiency who is brought to the school nurse's office due to coughing episodes, congestion and reports of chills. Currently, there is an outbreak of Rhino/Entero Virus at the school. She is febrile, with temperature of 102.3F, her heart rate was 120 bpm, respiratory rate of 14 with normal pressure. She appears in no acute distress. What is the next step?

Inborn errors of immunity are rare disorders of the immune system in children that are due to genetic abnormalities, involving the adaptive or innate immunity. Signs and symptoms include frequent or repeat infections e.g. otitis media, pneumonia, sinusitis, bronchitis, skin infections and chronic diarrhea with increase susceptibility to autoimmune diseases and malignancy [1–3]. Infections often are severe and last longer than the usual course. Table 50.1 demonstrate examples of inborn errors of immunity.

Management of a Child with Inborn Errors of Immunity in a School Setting

- Assess Child's Clinical Status
  - Obtain vitals: Temperature, Heart Rate, Respiratory Rate, Blood Pressure, Oxygen Saturations
  - Identify red flags (Table 50.2 and Fig. 50.1)

If a clear source of infection is identified, such as a viral upper respiratory infection (URI), otitis media, or strep pharyngitis, referral to the Emergency Department (ED) may not be necessary unless the child is exhibiting red flags (Table 50.2). The primary immunologist should be notified as antibiotics may be required. Urgent Care evaluation is essential for assessment.

L.-M. Nicolas · K. Lutzkanin (✉)
Penn State Children's Hospital, Hershey, PA, USA
e-mail: lnicolas@pennstatehealth.psu.edu; klutzkanin@pennstatehealth.psu.edu

R. P. Olympia, J. Brady-Olympia (eds.), *Clinical Considerations in School-based Health*, https://doi.org/10.1007/978-3-031-85765-2_50

Table 50.1 Examples of Inborn Errors of Immunity [3, 4]

Inborn Errors of Immunity	Examples	Clinical Features
Primary B Cell Immunodeficiency	● *Common Variable Immunodeficiency (CVID)* ● *X-Linked Agammaglobulinemia (XLA) (aka Bruton agammaglobulinemia)* ● *Hyper-IgM Syndrome* ● *Selective IgA Deficiency*	● Recurrent sinopulmonary infections including encapsulated bacteria, gastrointestinal infections ● Sepsis ● Chronic diarrhea
Primary T Cell Immunodeficiency	● *DiGeorge Syndrome (22q11.2 Deletion Syndrome)*	● Absent thymus ● Chronic diarrhea ● Severe or chronic viral infections e.g. Epstein-Barr Virus (EBV), Cytomegalovirus (CMV) ● Congenital heart disease ● Opportunistic infections e.g. Candidiasis, CMV and Pneumocystis Jirovecii Pneumonia (PJP)
Combined B- and T-Cell Immunodeficiency	● *Severe Combined Immunodeficiency (SCID)* ● *Wiskott-Aldrich Syndrome* ● *Ataxia-Telangiectasia*	● Combination of the infections mentioned above
Phagocyte Disorders	● *Chronic Granulomatous Disease (CGD)* ● *Leukocyte Adhesion Deficiency (LAD)* ● *Chediak-Higashi Syndrome* ● *Neutropenia*	● Skin and organ abscesses with additionally delayed wound healing, eczema and stomatitis ● Bacterial and Fungal infections ● Poor growth ● Inflammatory bowel disease
Complement Disorders	● *Early Complement Deficiency (C1-C4)* ● *Terminal Complement Deficiency (C5-C9 aka MAC complex)*	● Severe pyogenic infections (*Step Pneumonia*) ● Meningitis or sepsis due to encapsulated bacteria *(Neisseria meningitidis, H. Influenzae Type B)* ● Sepsis

Table 50.2 Red Flags for Students with Inborn Errors of Immunity

High Fevers (>= 102.4°F)	Confusion	Difficulty breathing or shortness of breath
Severe headache	Rapid Heart Rate (>120 bpm)	Persistent vomiting or diarrhea
Seizures	Dizziness	Low blood pressure (<90/60)

Classroom Outbreaks Viral respiratory tract infections are common in children and may present a more serious clinical picture in those who are immunocompromised [5]. All classroom outbreaks including viral infections, upper respiratory tract

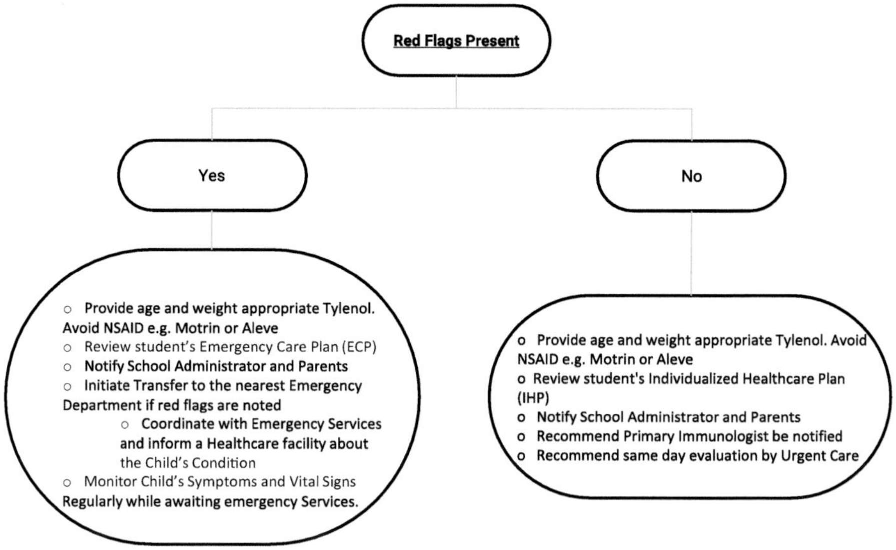

Fig. 50.1 Recommended workup by clinicians based on the presence of red flags

infections, diarrhea, chickenpox, measles, should be reported to parents. Good hygiene, including washing hands with soap and water before meals, after using the restroom should be routine. In the event where a classmate is experiencing a viral respiratory tract infection, students with inborn errors of immunity can still comfortably attend the classroom. However, for precautionary measure, they should be seated separately from the affected classmate and offered a mask to minimize the protentional risk of acquiring infections and ensuring a safe and inclusive learning environment for all. Additionally, some students may have Individualized Healthcare Plan (IHP) and/or Emergency Care Plan (ECP) which should be referred to for further information.

Absenteeism Children with immunocompromised disorder often miss more school than their classmates due to illnesses, side effect from medication (Table 50.3), scheduled treatments and appointments. Some students may have Individualized Education program (IEP) and/or Section 504 Plan which should be referred to further assess additional services which the student would quality for.

Immunization Children with congenital immunodeficiency, receiving immunosuppressive therapy or undergoing stem cell treatment are NOT vaccinated against live viruses. Live vaccines include MMR, Varicella, Rotavirus, Oral Poliovirus and Intranasal influenza. These vaccinations pose a life-threatening risk for severe infections and are NOT recommended. Additionally, parents should be notified of any vaccination program within the school due to risk of contracting infections from another individual who recently received live virus. Vaccination should NOT be administered without parental permission.

Table 50.3 Common Medical Therapies in Immunocompromised Children [6, 7]

Medical therapies	Purpose	Common side effects
Immunoglobulin (IVIG)	Provides antibodies to boost immunity (Primary B-Cell Immunodeficiency)	Headache, chills, fatigue, allergic reaction, thrombosis
Antibiotics (e.g. amoxicillin, Bactrim, Ciprofloxacin, Azithromycin)	Prevents and treat bacterial infections	Nausea, vomiting, diarrhea
Antifungals (e.g. Fluconazole, Voriconazole, Amphotericin B)	Treats fungal infections (CGD, SCID, AIDS, DiGeorge)	Liver toxicity, renal injury, rash, nausea, vomiting, diarrhea
Antivirals (e.g. Acyclovir, Valacyclovir, ganciclovir, Oseltamivir)	Treats Viral infections (e.g. SCID, DiGeorge, HIV/AIDS)	Nausea, vomiting, headache fatigue
Bone Marrow or Hematopoietic Stem Cell Transplant	Replaces defective or damaged immune cells with healthy ones (SCID, Wiskott-Aldrich Syndrome)	Graft-versus-host disease (GVHD), infection, organ damage, mucositis
Hematopoietic Growth Factors	Stimulates white blood cell production (e.g. chemotherapy-induced neutropenia, Bone marrow patients with severe neutropenia)	Fever, bone pain, injection site reaction
Interferon Gamma	Improves bacterial killing by phagocytes in individuals with CGD	Flu-like symptoms, fever, fatigue, muscle pain, injection site reactions, liver enzyme elevation

Case #1 Resolution

Parents should be notified immediately. She should be given antipyretic e.g. Tylenol and her vitals should be monitored. She should be picked up from school and seen at an Urgent Care center. Recommend to family to contact her Immunologist as she may benefit from antibiotics regardless of viral etiology. Parents should be advised that if she is exhibiting red flags (Table 50.2), she should be taken to the Emergency Department.

Case #2 Tommy is a 3rd grade student diagnosed with Acute Lymphoblastic Leukemia currently undergoing chemotherapy. She told her teacher that she is not feeling well, so she was sent to the school nurse for evaluation. In the office, she has a fever of 101.3F with normal blood pressure, respiratory rate and oxygen saturations. What is the next step?

Case # 3 Sarah is a 7th grade student with known HIV currently on antiretroviral therapy. While on the playground during recess, she fell and scraped her elbow and is currently bleeding. She was sent to the school nurse for wound evaluation. Her vitals are normal. The school nurse irrigates the wound and applies bandage over it though it continues to slowly ooze. Sarah asks if she is able to go back to the playground to play with her friends. What is the next step?

Secondary immunodeficiency results from infections, immunosuppressive medications, malnutrition and neoplastic diseases with the most common being Acquired Immunodeficiency Syndrome (AIDS) [8].

Chemotherapy Induced Neutropenia Chemotherapy drugs decrease cell counts including neutrophils which are one of the first immune cells to respond in an infection [9, 10]. They travel to the site and destroy the microorganism. It is a life-threatening, treatment-related toxicity which can lead to shock and death [9, 10]. It is traditionally treated in the inpatient setting. Febrile Neutropenia is defined as a single oral temperature of at least 100.9°F or a temperature of at least 100.4°F for 1 hour with absolute neutrophil count of 500 cells/μL or less [11].

Management of Febrile Child Undergoing Chemotherapy or Stem Cell Transplant

- Obtain vital signs including Temperature, Blood Pressure, Respiratory Rate, Oxygen Saturations
- Administer Antipyretics as Necessary (avoid NSAIDs)
  - Notify School Administration for Support
  - Contact Parent/Guardian Immediately and Recommend Immediate Medical Attention
  - Emergency Department (ED) evaluation is Required:

    Coordinate with Emergency Services and Inform Healthcare Facility About Child's Condition
    Provide Necessary Medical Information to Healthcare Facility

  - Monitor Child's Symptoms and Vital Signs Regularly while waiting for Emergency Services
- ED workup and management
  - Diagnostic Tests: CBC with differential, complete metabolic panel, Urinalysis, Inflammatory markers, blood culture, urine culture. If having respiratory symptoms, will obtain CXR, Respiratory Viral Panel and Sputum Culture
  - Antibiotics is started empirically. Plan, continuation of antibiotics and disposition depends on Absolute Neutrophil Count (ANC) obtained from the CBC with differential and Oncologist Recommendation

    ANC < 500 → Admit to the Hospital and continue Cefepime
    ANC > 500 → can be discharge if stable, without serious infections identified, reliable follow up and discussion with Oncologist

Human Immunodeficiency Virus (HIV) affects the immune system and can lead to Acquired Immunodeficiency Syndrome (AIDS) if left untreated [8]. It is spread via contact with the mucous membrane or openings in the skin with infected blood and body fluids [8]. Children can also be infected via mother to infant breastfeeding, contaminated needles or sharp instruments or sexual contact [12]. It is NOT spread by non-bloody saliva, tears, stools or urine [13]. Indications for exclusion a child

Table 50.4 HIV Transmission Information

Body Fluids that Transmit HIV	Ways HIV is NOT Transmitted
Blood	Sharing dishes
Vaginal Fluids	Saliva
Breast milk	Tears
Rectal fluids	Sweat
Semen	Through Air
Pre-seminal fluid	Hugging/Kissing
	Insect Bites

with HIV from group settings include active bleeding or open weeping skin lesions. Table 50.4 gives some HIV transmission information.

Case #2 and #3 Resolution

Case #2: The school nurse should call Tommy's parents to inform them of his fever and recommend that he be taken to the ED due to concerns for neutropenic fever.

Case #3: Sarah should be kept in the nurse's office until the bleeding has stopped. Her wound should be fully irrigated and covered. Her parents should additionally be notified.

Extra Credit Points

1. Children with known Inborn Errors of Immunity exhibiting red flags (Table 50.2) should be immediately seen by healthcare professional at a hospital due to risk of life-threatening infections. See Fig. 50.1 for recommended workup in school setting.
2. If a clear source of infection is identified, such as a viral upper respiratory infection (URI), otitis media, or strep pharyngitis, referral to the Emergency Department (ED) may not be necessary unless the child is exhibiting red flags (Table 50.2).
3. For children undergoing stem cell transplant and chemotherapy, it is ALWAYS recommended to seek emergency department care if febrile.
4. Be aware that live vaccination is NOT recommended for children with congenital immunodeficiency, receiving immunosuppressive therapy or undergoing stem cell treatment.
5. Children with HIV with active bleeding or seeping wound should be excluded from group settings.

References

1. Amrol D. Immunodeficiency. American Academy of PediatricsItasca, IL eBooks. Published online January 1, 2018. https://doi.org/10.1542/9781610021159-63
2. McCusker C, et al. Primary immunodeficiency. Allergy Asthma Clin Immunol. 2018;14(S2) https://doi.org/10.1186/s13223-018-0290-5.
3. Justiz Vaillant AA, Qurie A. Immunodeficiency. PubMed. Published 2020. https://www.ncbi.nlm.nih.gov/books/NBK500027/

4. "Primary Immunodeficiency (PI) | CDC." Www.cdc.gov, 1 July 2020, www.cdc.gov/genomics/disease/primary_immunodeficiency.htm.
5. Barr RS, Drysdale SB. Viral respiratory tract infections in the immunocompromised child. J. Pediatr. Infect. Dis. 2023. Publish Ahead of Print; https://doi.org/10.1097/inf.0000000000003855.
6. Paris K, Wall LA. The treatment of primary immune deficiencies: lessons learned and future opportunities. Clin Rev Allergy Immunol. 2023;65(1):19–30. https://doi.org/10.1007/s12016-022-08950-0.
7. Peddi NC, Vuppalapati S, Sreenivasulu H, Muppalla SK, Reddy PA. Guardians of immunity: advances in primary immunodeficiency disorders and management. Cureus. 2023;15(9):e44865. Published 2023 Sep 7. https://doi.org/10.7759/cureus.44865.
8. Chinen J, Shearer WT. Secondary immunodeficiencies, including HIV infection. J Allergy Clin Immunol. 2010;125(2):S195–203. https://doi.org/10.1016/j.jaci.2009.08.040.
9. Punnapuzha S, Edemobi PK, Elmoheen A. Febrile Neutropenia. PubMed. Published 2024. Accessed July 8, 2024. http://www.ncbi.nlm.nih.gov/books/NBK541102/
10. Davis K, Wilson S. Febrile neutropenia in paediatric oncology. Paediatr Child Health (Oxford). 2020;30(3):93–7. https://doi.org/10.1016/j.paed.2019.12.002.
11. Sung L, Johnston DL. Approach to febrile neutropenia in the general paediatric setting. Paediatr Child Health. 2007;12(1):19–21. https://doi.org/10.1093/pch/12.1.19.
12. Centers for Disease Control and Prevention. "Body Fluids That Transmit HIV | HIV Transmission | HIV Basics | HIV/AIDS | CDC." Www.cdc.gov, 28 Oct. 2020, www.cdc.gov/hiv/basics/hiv-transmission/body-fluids.html.
13. "Ways HIV Is Not Transmitted | HIV Transmission | HIV Basics | HIV/AIDS | CDC." www.cdc.gov, 28 Oct. 2020, www.cdc.gov/hiv/basics/hiv-transmission/not-transmitted.html.

Chapter 51
Inflammatory Bowel Disease

Marc E. Schaefer

Case 1 For the first two months of Billy's 5th grade school year, his teacher and school nurse have noticed a pattern of multiple visits to the nurse's office for complaints of abdominal pain after lunch. He also has to use the bathroom multiple times daily for an extended duration, especially after lunch. When the school nurse recently checked his weight, she noticed he had lost five pounds since the first nurse visit at the beginning of the school year. What should the school nurse do?

It is estimated that 25% of all Inflammatory bowel disease (IBD) cases are diagnosed before the age of 20, with the peak incidence in adolescence [1]. Ulcerative colitis (UC) and Crohn's disease (CD) result in inflammation of the gastrointestinal tract, and some of the most common symptoms are abdominal pain, diarrhea, blood in the stool, vomiting, poor appetite, and weight loss.

This patient demonstrates characteristic signs of IBD, and therefore, it is imperative to begin the appropriate evaluation (Table 51.1) and expedite a referral to a pediatric gastroenterologist. It is also necessary to rule out other conditions that can mimic IBD, such as infections and other inflammatory conditions (Table 51.2). The lab evaluation and imaging help rule out other conditions and assess the severity/ complications of IBD. Still, the gold standard for diagnosing IBD is an upper endoscopy and colonoscopy. In addition, pediatric IBD has a variety of severe presentations that often necessitate referral to the emergency room (Table 51.3).

M. E. Schaefer (✉)
Penn State Health Children's Hospital, Hershey, PA, USA
e-mail: mschaefer@pennstatehealth.psu.edu

R. P. Olympia, J. Brady-Olympia (eds.), *Clinical Considerations in School-based Health*, https://doi.org/10.1007/978-3-031-85765-2_51

Table 51.1 Evaluation for IBD

History and Physical Exam	Labs	Imaging	Definitive Diagnosis
Abdominal pain Diarrhea with or without blood or tenesmus Decreased appetite/early satiety Weight loss/Poor weight gain (Review weight curve) Growth delay (Review growth curve) Family history of IBD Oral ulcers Unexplained fevers Arthralgias or arthritis Erythema nodosum Pyoderma gangrenosum	Complete blood counts (CBC) with differential C-reactive protein (CRP) Erythrocyte Sedimentation Rate (ESR) Liver functional tests (with albumin and GGT) Iron deficiency panel Stool pathogen testing Fecal calprotectin or lactoferrin	Magnetic resonance enterography (MRE) Magnetic resonance imaging of the pelvis (Concern for perianal fistula/abscess) CT enterography (CTE) (emergent presentations) Bone age	Ileocolonoscopy with biopsies Upper endoscopy with biopsies

Adapted from [2] Picoraro JA, Moore H, LeLeiko NS. Inflammatory Bowel Disease: An Update. Pediatr Rev. 2023 Mar 1;44 (3): 139–152

Case 2 Julie is a 12-year-old girl attending middle school. At her annual school health assessment, the school-based physician notices her weight has decreased from the 50th percentile to the 5th percentile, and her height has decreased from the 25th percentile to <5th percentile over the past three years (Fig. 51.1). On history and physical exam, the only significant finding is the patient reporting vague chronic abdominal pain. What are the next steps for evaluating this presentation?

This patient should have a lab evaluation (Table 51.1) ordered and be referred to a pediatric gastroenterologist. Given the lack of significant gastrointestinal symptom history, a bone age and pediatric endocrinology referral would also be appropriate.

Poor weight gain and poor growth can be a unique presentation of pediatric IBD (more often with Crohn's disease) that sometimes does present with minimal to no gastrointestinal symptoms. Chronic weight and growth concerns can be challenging to pick up on routine annual health assessments, especially if weights and heights over the previous years are unavailable. The chronicity of this subtle presentation places the patient at risk for vitamin deficiencies [4–6] (Table 51.4) and other nutritional complications such as delayed puberty, low bone mineral density, and decreased final adult height.

Table 51.2 Differential Diagnosis of IBD

Infectious	C. difficile Salmonella Shigella Campylobacter Yersinia Giardia Cryptosporidium Enteroviruses Other bacterial, viral, or parasitic infections
Inflammatory	Appendicitis Celiac disease Microscopic colitis
Malabsorptive	Lactose intolerance Small intestinal bacterial overgrowth Pancreatic insufficiency (cystic fibrosis)
Allergy/Immunology	Eosinophilic GI diseases Food protein-induced enterocolitis (FPIES) Immunodeficiencies Autoimmune enteropathy
Rheumatology	Henoch-Schõnlein purpura Bechet syndrome Systemic lupus erythematosus
Oncologic	Lymphoma Other malignancies
Other	Irritable bowel syndrome Eating disorders Endocrinopathies (Hypothyroidism) Laxative abuse Radiation enteritis Ischemia

Adapted from [3] Conrad MA, Rosh JR. Pediatric Inflammatory Bowel Disease. Pediatr Clin North Am. 2017 Jun;64(3):577–591

Table 51.3 Reasons to Consider Referral to the Emergency Department in Pediatric IBD

Clinical
Concern for fulminant colitis (e.g. toxic megacolon)
Profuse bloody diarrhea, fever, chills, nausea/vomiting, abdominal distention, and abdominal tenderness (All or many of these symptoms) [2]
Concern for intestinal obstruction (often presents as abdominal pain with nausea/vomiting and inability to tolerate oral liquids)
Dehydration
Symptomatic anemia (dyspnea, impaired consciousness, orthostatic changes, and/or hemodynamic changes)
Severe abdominal pain
Perianal abscess
Severe malnutrition
Right lower quadrant pain with mass palpated (possible intra-abdominal abscess)
Laboratory Concerns
Asymptomatic with significant anemia
Electrolyte imbalance

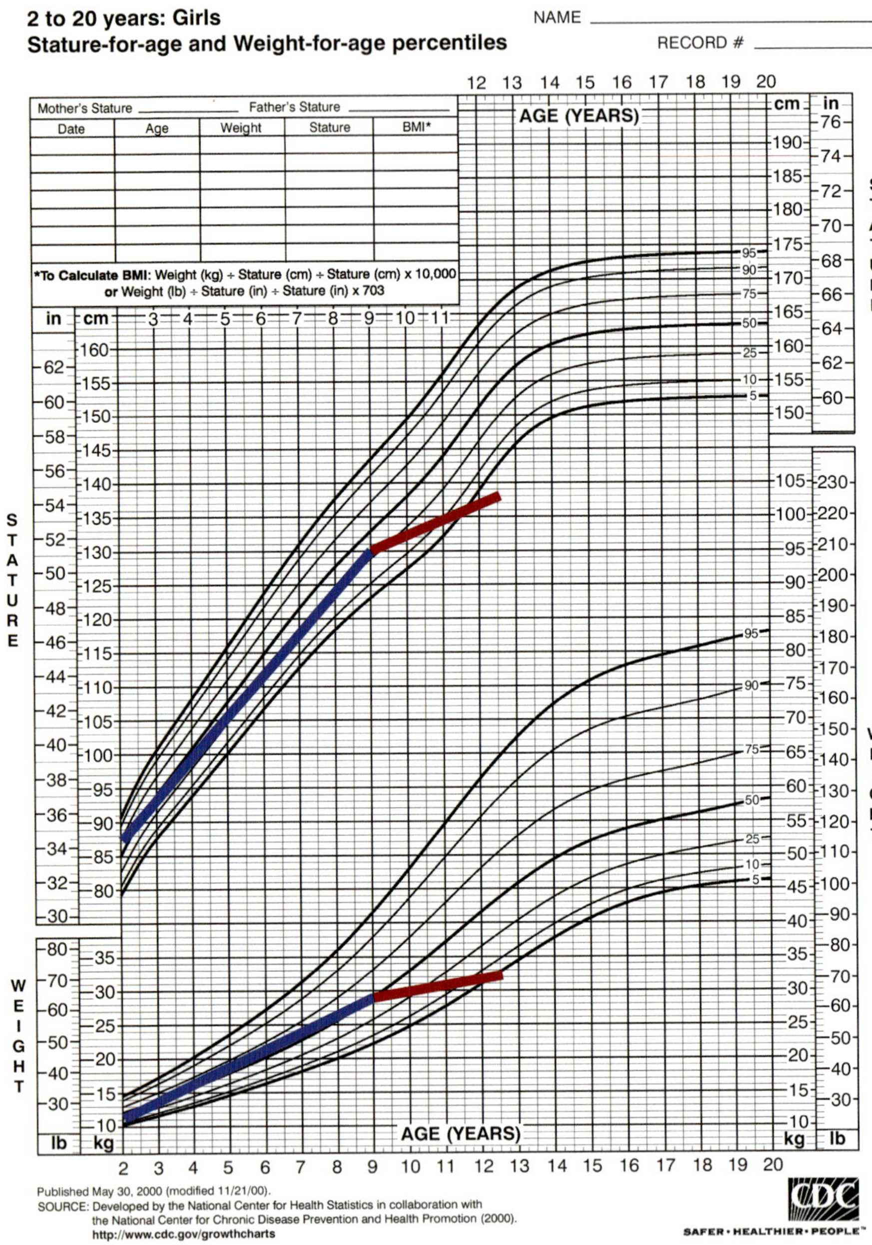

Fig. 51.1 Weight and stature charts for Case 2

Table 51.4 Common Vitamin/Mineral Deficiencies in IBD Patients

Vitamin/Mineral	Deficiency Manifestations
Iron	Fatigue, lethargy, dizziness, microcytic anemia, behavioral abnormalities
Vitamin D	Osteopenia, Increased risk for fractures, Rickets (genu varum or valgum)
Vitamin B12	Megaloblastic anemia, loss of deep tendon reflexes (neuropathy), developmental regression, hypotonia, paresthesia, glossitis, neuropsychiatric changes (e.g., depression)
Folate	Megaloblastic anemia, stomatitis, paresthesia, glossitis
Zinc	Perioral and perianal rashes, poor wound healing, growth failure, alopecia

Table 51.5 Recommended Vaccinations for IBD Patients

Inactivated Vaccines
Diphtheria, pertussis, and acellular tetanus
Haemophilus influenza
Inactivated Polio
Influenza (flu shot)
Pneumococcus
Hepatitis A
Hepatitis B
HPV
Meningococcal disease
Live Vaccines (if not on immunosuppression)
MMR
Varicella
Influenza (The Nasal Spray Flu Vaccine/FluMist) [10]

Case 3 Tim is a 16-year-old who was diagnosed with ulcerative colitis (UC) six months ago. He did initially require hospitalization for severe anemia associated with chronic rectal bleeding. Tim was placed on Infliximab (anti-TNF immunosuppressive treatment) for treatment of his UC, which continues every eight weeks by infusion at a local infusion clinic. He is clinically doing well. There is a chicken pox outbreak at his school. What precautions should be taken by the school?

Up-to-date immunizations are crucial to the health of patients with chronic diseases or immunocompromised conditions because the hosts are more susceptible to infection [7]. It is recommended that pediatric and adolescent IBD patients receive all inactivated vaccines (Table 51.5) that have been recommended by the American Academy of Pediatrics [4].

Regarding live vaccines (Varicella and MMR), ideally, these vaccines should be given and brought up to date in IBD patients before they start immunosuppressive treatment. Live vaccines have been contraindicated in immunosuppressed patients due to the risk and fears of disseminated vaccine-induced disease [8, 9]. Immunosuppression is defined as ≥ prednisone 2 mg/kg/day or equivalent, or prednisone 20 mg/day or equivalent, for ≥14 days, cyclosporine, tacrolimus, thiopurines, methotrexate, or advanced therapies (biologics and synthetic small molecules). No immunosuppressive therapy should be received three months before and six weeks after administering live virus vaccines. If there is no documentation of varicella and measles vaccinations, then titers can be checked. [4] However, data have shown that patients with chronic diseases or on immunosuppressive treatment tend to be under-immunized or have inadequate seroprotection levels after immunization [7].

The risk of infection secondary to immunosuppression is just one of several complications that can develop in pediatric patients with IBD. Table 51.6 categorizes these complications into intestinal (Table 51.6A), extraintestinal (Table 51.6B), and treatment (Table 51.6C) related. Many of these complications have a range of severity. Identifying the specific complication or the severity of the complication can help one determine the disposition, such as contacting the primary care provider (PCP), the pediatric gastroenterologist (Pediatric GI), or sending immediately to the emergency department (ED).

Table 51.6 Complications in IBD patients

Complication	Signs/symptoms	Disposition
A. Intestinal complications in IBD patients		
Disease relapse (Flare)	Typically, an exacerbation of patient's initial symptoms at diagnosis (symptoms vary)	Pediatric GI (ER in severe cases)
Clostridium difficile infection	Acute onset, watery, profuse diarrhea [11] (can mimic an IBD flare)	Pediatric GI
Stricture	Post-prandial abdominal pain, nausea/vomiting, early satiety	Acute severe abdominal pain/ dehydration- ER Chronic and not dehydrated- Contact pediatric GI/Surgery referral
Perianal fistula	Perianal pain, mucus and/or blood drainage	Pediatric GI
Perianal abscess	Perianal pain, pain with sitting and/ or walking	ER
Intraabdominal abscess	Abdominal mass palpated, abdominal pain, unexplained fevers	ER
Bowel perforation	Abdominal pain, abdominal distention, toxic appearance	ER
Severe bleeding (Hematochezia)	Tachycardia, dyspnea/tachypnea, pallor, impaired consciousness, orthostatic changes	ER
Toxic megacolon	Abdominal pain (often with peritoneal signs), abdominal distention, sepsis, marked colonic dilation on AXR [12]	ER
B. Extraintestinal complications in IBD patients		
Erythema nodosum	Tender, subcutaneous, erythematous nodules typically on the lower legs [13]	PCP or pediatric GI

(continued)

Table 51.6 (continued)

Complication	Signs/symptoms	Disposition
Pyoderma gangrenosum	Painful ulcerating skin lesion [13]	PCP or pediatric GI
Arthritis	Ranges in severity and can vary from axial to peripheral joint pain [13]	Mild chronic- PCP/pediatric GI Severe- ER
Uveitis	Acute/subacute eye pain, headache, photophobia, and blurred vision; to asymptomatic [13]	ER or Emergency Eye clinic
Episcleritis	Eye redness and burning, no vision impairment [13]	PCP or Eye clinic
Primary sclerosing cholangitis (PSC)	Often nonspecific, but can include fatigue, anorexia, jaundice, pruritus, & hepatomegaly [13]	Pediatric GI
Autoimmune hepatitis	Often nonspecific and asymptomatic, but can include fatigue, anorexia, nausea, abdominal pain, & pruritus [14]	Pediatric GI
Nephrolithiasis	Acute abdominal/flank pain, dysuria, urgency, and hematuria [15]	PCP or ER (depending on severity)
Venous thromboembolism	Asymptomatic to swelling/ discoloration of the affected limb [16]	ER
Mental Health (Anxiety and/or Depression)	Changes in mood, appetite, and/or concerns about level of social, athletic, or academic functioning [17]	PCP (ER for suicidal concerns)
C. Treatment complications in IBD patients		
Opportunistic Infections [18, 19]	Pneumonia Cellulitis TB Reactivation Abscess Parasites/Fungi/Viruses	PCP or ER (Depends on severity)
Delayed Infusion Reaction (serum sickness)	Arthralgias, back pain, myalgias, fever, skin rash, and leukocytosis (4–9 days after an infusion) [19]	PCP or pediatric GI
Drug induced lupus	Fever, arthralgias/arthritis, myalgias, and rash [20]	PCP or pediatric GI
Skin [21]	Injection site reactions (localized) Psoriasis/psoriasiform like rash Eczematiform lesions Stevens-Johnson syndrome	Pediatric GI PCP and/or Dermatologist PCP and/or Dermatologist ER
Lymphoma	Enlarging, non-tender lymphadenopathy. Possible abdominal mass. Additional symptoms vary [22]	PCP or Pediatric GI

51.1 Case Conclusions

Case 1 The school nurse contacts the patient's primary care provider (PCP). The PCP orders the appropriate labs and places an urgent referral to the local pediatric gastroenterology practice. The labs show mild iron deficiency anemia, elevated CRP, ESR, fecal calprotectin, and negative stool studies for enteric pathogens. The pediatric gastroenterology group performs an upper endoscopy and colonoscopy within a few weeks, consistent with Crohn's disease. The patient is started on medical therapy.

Case 2 This 12-year-old girl is referred to a pediatric gastroenterologist and is found to have Crohn's disease involving the terminal ileum. Subsequent lab evaluations include findings of mild iron deficiency anemia, vitamin D deficiency, and B12 deficiency. In addition to being started on treatment to decrease her small bowel inflammation, she receives supplemental Iron, Vitamin D, and B12. She responds well to her Crohn's disease treatment, and her weight and height trend back towards the 25th percentile over the next few years.

Case 3 The medical director/school nurse checks the patient's immunization record and that the patient only received the initial Varicella vaccine at one year old. Some studies show that one dose of the Varicella vaccine provides some immune protection [8]. It is recommended that the patient have their Varicella titer checked. If the patient had direct contact with one of the Varicella cases, one could consider a dose of VZIG as prophylaxis. The decision to give VZIG prophylaxis should be discussed with the patient's pediatric gastroenterologist or an infectious disease specialist. The general recommendation is to isolate those individuals with positive Varicella until their lesions are crusted over. The patient's Varicella titer does come back positive. The patient does not develop any signs of active Varicella. A booster Varicella vaccine is not given due to the patient's immunosuppressed state.

Extra-Credit Points

(1) There is a broad spectrum of clinical presentations in pediatric IBD that can include subtle presentations in poor weight gain and/or growth and extra-intestinal manifestations.
(2) IBD is often associated with vitamin and mineral deficiencies that can cause significant symptoms and complications in pediatric patients.
(3) IBD patients who are immunosuppressed are often under-immunized. It is ideal to immunize IBD patients with the live vaccines (MMR and Varicella) before starting immunosuppression.
(4) Intestinal, extraintestinal, and treatment complications can develop in pediatric IBD patients at any time in their disease course. Recognizing the complication and determining the severity help with referring the patient to the most appropriate medical provider.

References

1. Rosen MJ, Dhawan A, Saeed SA. Inflammatory bowel disease in children and adolescents. JAMA Pediatr. 2015;169(11):1053–60.
2. Picoraro JA, Moore H, LeLeiko NS. Inflammatory bowel disease: an update. Pediatr Rev. 2023;44(3):139–52.
3. Conrad MA, Rosh JR. Pediatric inflammatory bowel disease. Pediatr Clin North Am. 2017;64(3):577–91.
4. Steinberg JM, Charabaty A. The management approach to the adolescent IBD patient: health maintenance and medical considerations. Curr Gastroenterol Rep. 2020;22(1):5.
5. DeFilippis EM, Sockolow R, Barfield E. Healthcare maintenance for the pediatric patient with inflammatory bowel disease. Pediatrics. 2016;138(3) Published online Aug. 3, 2016
6. Kleinman RE. Iron deficiency, trace elements, and vitamins. pediatric nutrition handbook, vol. 299–300, 313–314. 5th ed. Itasca: AAP; 2003. p. 340–57.
7. Lu Y, Jacobson D, Bousvaros A. Immunizations in patients with inflammatory bowel disease. Inflamm Bowel Dis. 2009;15(9):1417–23.
8. Weinberg A, Horslen SP, Kaufman SS, et al. Safety and immunogenicity of varicella-zoster vaccine in pediatric liver and intestine transplant recipients. Am J Transplant. 2006;6(3):565–8.
9. Nguyen HT, Minar P, Jackson K, et al. Vaccinations in immunosuppressive-dependent pediatric inflammatory bowel disease. World J Gastroenterol. 2017;23(42):7644–52.
10. Live Attenuated Influenza Vaccine [LAIV] (The Nasal Spray Flu Vaccine). Centers for Disease Control and Prevention, National Center for Immunization and Respiratory Diseases (NCIRD). Updated August 25, 2022. Accessed May 30, 2024. https://www.cdc.gov/flu/prevent/nasalspray.htm
11. Crews J, Nicholson MR. *Clostridioides difficile* infection in children: Clinical features and diagnosis. UpToDate. Updated July 9, 2024. Accessed July 13, 2024. Clostridioides difficile infection in children: Clinical features and diagnosis - UpToDate
12. Mattei P, Rombeau JL, Surgical Treatment of Ulcerative Colitis, Mamula P, Markowitz JE, Baldassano RN. Pediatric inflammatory bowel disease. 1st ed. New York: Springer; 2008. p. 470.
13. Rabizadeh S, Oliva-Hemker M. Extraintestinal manifestations of pediatric inflammatory bowel disease. In: Mamula P, Markowitz JE, Baldassano RN, editors. Pediatric inflammatory bowel disease. 1st ed. New York: Springer; 2008. p. 94–7.
14. Heneghan MA. Overview of Autoimmune hepatitis. UpToDate. Updated September 19, 2023. Accessed July 13.2024. Overview of autoimmune hepatitis - UpToDate
15. Smith J, Stapleton FB. Kidney Stones in children: Clinical features and diagnosis. UpToDate. Updated February 1, 2024. Accessed July 14, 2024. Kidney stones in children: Clinical features and diagnosis - UpToDate
16. Albisetti M, Chan AK. Venous thrombosis and thromboembolism (VTE) in children: Risk factors, clinical manifestations, and diagnosis. UpToDate. Updated January 22, 2024. Accessed July 14, 2024. Venous thrombosis and thromboembolism (VTE) in children: Risk factors, clinical manifestations, and diagnosis - UpToDate
17. Rufo PA, Denson LA, Sylvester FA, et al. Health supervision in the management of children and adolescents with IBD: NASPGHAN recommendations. J Pediatr Gastroenterol Nutr. 2012;55(1):93–108.
18. Veereman-Wauters G, de Ridder L, Veres G, et al. Risk of infection and prevention in pediatric patients with IBD: ESPGHAN IBD Porto Group commentary. J Pediatr Gastroenterol Nutr. 2012;54(6):830–7.
19. Vermeire S, Van Assche G, Rutgeerts P, Infliximab Therapy. In: Mamula P, Markowitz JE, Baldassano RN, editors. Pediatric inflammatory bowel disease. 1st ed. New York: Springer; 2008. p. 393–6.

20. Merola JF. Drug-Induced Lupus. UpToDate. Updated May 24, 2024. Accessed July 21, 2024. Drug-induced lupus - UpToDate
21. Freling E, Baumann C, Cuny JF, et al. Cumulative incidence of risk factors for, and outcome of dermatological complications of anti-TNF therapy in inflammatory bowel disease: a 14-year experience. Am J Gastroenterol. 2015;110(8):1186–96.
22. Termuhlen AM, Gross TG. Overview of non-Hodgkin lymphoma in children and adolescents. UpToDate. Updated December 6, 202. Accessed July 13, 2024. Overview of non-Hodgkin lymphoma in children and adolescents – UpToDate

Chapter 52
Kidney Disorders

Pankhuri Mohan and Deborah Kees-Folts

Case 1 14-year old Micah presents to your office after his blood pressure was found to be elevated during a health fair. You check a set of vital signs including heart rate, blood pressure and temperature. You find that his blood pressure is elevated to 138/90. You check it again manually and continue to get similar values. He tells you he feels completely fine and denies headaches, lightheadedness, chest pain, shortness of breath or pain elsewhere in his body. What should you do?

High blood pressure (hypertension) in children is defined by blood pressure *percentiles* which are based on the child's age, sex and height, determining normal and abnormal ranges of blood pressure. Hypertension is defined as sustained blood pressure on separate occasions that is >95th percentile for age, sex and height (Table 52.1). Pediatric blood pressure percentiles are available in table form in a number of publications or can be calculated using on-line apps [1, 2]. Childhood hypertension can be classified as primary or secondary, based on whether an underlying etiology can be established. Primary hypertension is the most common form of hypertension, defined by the absence of an obvious underlying cause. Secondary hypertension refers to high blood pressure occurring as a symptom of an underlying condition, which can include kidney disorders (such as glomerular diseases, parenchymal scarring from reflux, or chronic kidney disease of any cause), or endocrine causes (such as hyper-/hypothyroidism and Cushing's syndrome) and cardiac causes (such as coarctation of the aorta). Certain drugs can cause hypertension such as oral contraceptive drugs. Caffeine, other energy drinks, pain and anxiety can raise blood pressure as well. Regardless of the etiology, it is important to identify a child with high blood pressure because untreated hypertension poses significant risk of long-term cardiovascular complications. High blood pressure can contribute to hardened

P. Mohan (✉) · D. Kees-Folts
Penn State Hershey Medical School, Hershey, PA, USA
e-mail: pmohan1@pennstatehealth.psu.edu; dkeesfolts@pennstatehealth.psu.edu

R. P. Olympia, J. Brady-Olympia (eds.), *Clinical Considerations in School-based Health*, https://doi.org/10.1007/978-3-031-85765-2_52

Table 52.1 Hypertension values in children of average size (1, 2)

Age	>95th Percentile BP
5–6 years	114/73
7–8 years	116/75
9–10 years	119/77
11–12 years	122/79
>13	130/80

vessels and plaque build-up, causing the arteries to narrow and ultimately potentially affecting blood flow to the heart.

When an elevated blood pressure is identified, it is important to distinguish when immediate stabilization and treatment is required. First and foremost, ensure that the blood pressure is being taken correctly. Proper blood pressure technique requires an appropriately sized cuff, defined as width measuring about 40% of the child's upper arm length and 80-100% of the mid-arm circumference. Note that smaller cuffs frequently artificially elevate the blood pressure [3, 4]. Figure 52.1 demonstrates the appropriate way to take blood pressures.

Any child with symptoms associated with hypertension including severe headaches, seizures, changes in mental status, vomiting, visual disturbances, chest pain, palpitations or shortness of breath should be immediately evaluated in an emergency department. It is important in these cases for a medical provider to determine if high blood pressure has caused any *end organ damage* and to prevent further damage by carefully lowering the child's blood pressure in a controlled environment [1]. In the case above, since Micah is asymptomatic, it is appropriate to advise Micah's parents that he should have an appointment with his pediatrician for a recheck of his blood pressure and further evaluation.

Pediatric hypertension is a common problem for which a child may be evaluated and followed by their primary care provider, a pediatric nephrologist or pediatric cardiologist. Most children with hypertension require daily medication to maintain blood pressure in an appropriate range. Although medication is usually necessary, lifestyle modifications are equally important; there is clear data supporting the association of obesity and inactivity with hypertension [1]. School programs focused on an active and healthy lifestyle can therefore contribute to both prevention and management of pediatric hypertension.

Case 2 Peggy is a 6 year old girl who is brought in to the school nurse by her teacher, who is concerned that she might be having an allergic reaction after noticing that her eyes are very swollen. On closer look, she does have significant periorbital edema, her ankles also appear somewhat swollen and her abdomen is rather full. She does not have any rash or itching, and she does not have any appearance of respiratory distress. In speaking with her mother, you discover that the family has noticed over the past couple of weeks that her clothes are fitting much more tightly than usual, and have been concerned that she might need to go on a diet due to excess weight gain. You ask Peggy to give

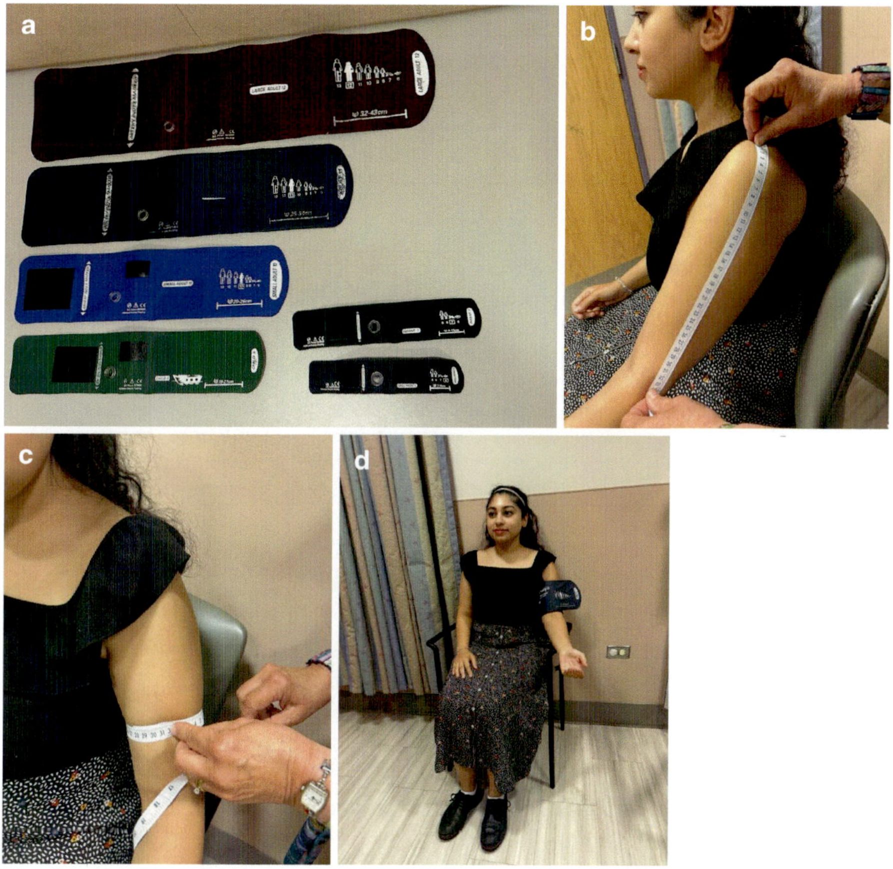

Fig. 52.1 Appropriate blood pressure measurement technique. (**a**) A variety of sizes of blood pressure cuffs are available for use in pediatric patients. Choice of an appropriately sized cuff and adherence to established blood pressure monitoring technique is imperative in obtaining an accurate blood pressure. Blood pressure cuff choice should be based on arm size, and not on age or weight. (**b** and **c**) Blood pressure cuff size should be determined based on measurement of the circumference of the upper arm (**c**) at the mid-point between the acromion (shoulder) and olecranon (elbow.) Cuff bladder length should be at least 80–100% of mid-arm circumference and cuff width should be at least 40% of arm circumference. When there is overlap between cuff size choices, the larger cuff is usually the best choice. (**d**) Blood pressures are most accurate when a correctly sized cuff is used and the patient is seated with the back supported, legs uncrossed and feet on the floor. Pediatric blood pressure norms are based on auscultated ("manual") blood pressures obtained following all of these guidelines

you a urine specimen, and are concerned that it appears to be grossly bloody. You saw Peggy about 2 weeks ago when she had a strep throat infection which has since resolved. What should you do?

The evaluation of a child with obvious edema, in the absence of obvious signs/symptoms of cardiac disease or severe liver disease, should focus on renal causes of

Table 52.2 Nephritis vs. Nephrosis

Signs/Symptoms	Glomerulopathies	
	Nephritis	Nephrosis
Edema	Yes	Yes
Blood pressure	Elevated	Normal
Urinalysis	Prominent hematuria, often gross hematuria Moderate proteinuria	Heavy proteinuria Variable microhematuria
Kidney function	Elevated creatinine	Normal creatinine
Serum albumin	Normal or slightly low	Very low
Common pediatric diagnoses	Acute post-streptococcal glomerulonephritis IgA nephropathy IgA vasculitis (Henoch Schonlein Purpura) Familial nephritis	Minimal change nephrotic syndrome Focal segmental glomerulosclerosis
Less common pediatric diagnoses	Membranoproliferative glomerulonephritis Systemic vasculitis with associated kidney disease Systemic lupus erythematosus ANCA positive vasculitis	Congenital nephrotic syndrome Membranoproliferative glomerulonephritis

edema, with the most likely diagnoses being either a nephrotic syndrome or a nephritic syndrome. Both nephrotic syndrome ("nephrosis") and nephritic syndrome ("nephritis") are terms that describe a group of signs and symptoms which can be due to several more specific diagnoses. Nephrotic syndromes and nephritic syndromes both fall into an overarching category of glomerular disease. Features that differentiate nephrotic syndromes from nephritic syndromes are listed in Table 52.2. Frequently, initial physical exam, including assessment of blood pressure, and office urinalysis provide enough data to distinguish between nephrosis and nephritis in an edematous child.

Although both nephritic syndromes and nephrotic syndromes are both due to glomerular disease, and both include edema as a primary manifestation, the pathophysiology of edema in these two disease sets is different. In a pure nephrotic syndrome, increased glomerular permeability to protein leads to heavy urinary protein loss (often defined as daily urine protein loss of >3.5 gm, or a urine protein/creatinine ratio >2–4; in children, daily urine protein loss >40 mg/m^2/hour is also sometimes used) [5]. The resultant hypoalbuminemia leads to low capillary oncotic pressure, and secondarily, increased flow of fluid from capillaries to the interstitial space. The causes low intravascular volume, with subsequent upregulation of both anti-diuretic hormone, and the renin-angiotensin system, leading to enhanced renal reabsorption of both water and salt, which contributes to edema formation. Individuals with pure nephrotic syndrome are said to have vascular "underfill;" they are subsequently normotensive and even with edema, may easily develop symptomatology of volume depletion. Nephritic syndromes, on the other hand, are vascular overfill conditions, due to decreased glomerular filtration of sodium, causing both sodium and water retention. Although fluid still ultimately leaks into the interstitium, the leak occurs due to increased capillary hydrostatic pressure. With vascular overfill, elevated blood pressure is common, and pulmonary edema may also occur.

It's important to recognize that some chronic glomerular diseases may demonstrate components of both nephrosis and nephritis.

Most children with nephrotic syndrome come to medical attention due to marked edema. With a first episode of nephrotic syndrome, it isn't unusual for edema to initially be attributed to allergies or excess true body weight gain. In the pediatric population, the majority of children with nephrotic syndrome are ultimately found to have minimal change disease. In children 2–6 years of age, minimal change disease is especially common—90–95% of children with nephrotic syndrome in that age range have minimal change nephrotic syndrome. Minimal change nephrotic syndrome uniformly responds to steroid treatment with resolution of proteinuria and subsequent resolution of edema; average response time is 7–14 days, but the range can be up to 6 weeks. The necessary course of prednisone treatment is lengthy; a common regimen for the initial episode of nephrotic syndrome is 6 weeks of daily high-dose prednisone followed by a 6-week alternate day wean. Even with a prednisone response, relapses are common. Although minimal change nephrotic syndrome usually ultimately entirely resolves. Frequent relapses may necessitate treatment with alternate maintenance immunosuppression. Absence of prednisone response is highly suggestive of another form of nephrotic syndrome, with the most common diagnosis in steroid-non-responsive patients being focal segmental glomerulosclerosis. Other less common causes of nephrotic syndrome include congenital (genetic) nephrotic syndromes and chronic glomerulopathies. Membranoproliferative glomerulonephritis (MPGN) may present with manifestations of both nephrosis and nephritis; MPGN may be either idiopathic or secondary to chronic infections such a hepatitis B or C. Minimal change disease is uniformly responsive to prednisone, treatment response is used as the primary criteria for diagnosis of minimal change disease. In children <10 years of age, often the only necessary work-up is confirmation of typical findings of nephrotic syndrome (heavy proteinuria, hypoalbuminemia, normal kidney function) and assessment of steroid response. More extensive work-up, including serologic testing and kidney biopsy is generally only necessary in steroid-non-responsive disease, or in older children/teenagers who present with nephrotic syndrome. Even in older children and adolescents, many practitioners opt to evaluate for steroid-responsive disease before embarking on a broad-based work-up for glomerular disease.

A sizeable minority of children with minimal change nephrotic syndrome show microhematuria on urinalysis, but gross hematuria is quite unusual. Therefore, although Peggy presented with edema, the presence of gross hematuria makes it much less likely that her edema is due to nephrotic syndrome.

The differential diagnosis of gross hematuria is broad, and on initial evaluation can include discoloration of urine with substances other than blood. Urine can often look pink or red due to consumption of certain foods such as beets, blackberries or rhubarb. Drugs such as phenazopyridine can also cause urine to look "bloody" as well. This can be easily differentiated with a urine dipstick testing the urine for blood. Microscopic hematuria (blood in the urine) is a common finding in children that is often benign. Gross (visible) hematuria occurs much less frequently and is almost always associated with some kind of pathology affecting the genitourinary tract, though not necessarily serious. Common causes of gross hematuria (Table 52.3) are outlined below; the most common associated diagnosis is urinary tract infection.

During the assessment of gross hematuria, it is often helpful to determine if associated signs and symptoms point toward a lower urinary tract origin or upper tract (glomerular) disease. (Table 52.2.) Signs suggesting lower urinary tract origin of gross hematuria include voiding symptoms (dysuria, urgency, and frequency), the presence of clots or sandy material in the urine, lower abdominal pain or recent trauma or very vigorous exercise [7]. The presence of hypertension, edema, associated proteinuria and symptoms of systemic vasculitis (fever, rash, joint pain) suggest some form of glomerulonephritis. Bright red urine is more suggestive of lower tract hematuria, while tea or cola-colored urine suggests glomerular disease, though this is not an absolute [6]. Microscopic urinalysis or urine dipstick is helpful and should be one of the first diagnostic tests obtained. Positive leukocyte esterase and/or nitrites and elevated white blood cells in the urine can point towards a urinary

Table 52.3 Common causes of Gross Hematuria [6, 7]

Anatomical location	Diagnosis	History & Exam Clues	Pathology
Lower Genitourinary Tract	Urinary Tract Infection	Fevers, flank pain, abdominal pain, dysuria, urinary frequency	Ascending bacterial infection of the uroepithelial cells
	Local trauma	Irritation to the perineum	Perineal sloughing of skin cells with local irritation and bleeding
	Trauma or vigorous exercise induced hematuria	Contact sports, bruising, extreme exercise	Direct trauma to kidneys or bladder or potential kidney ischemia during non-traumatic vigorous exercise
	Kidney stones	Unilateral flank pain, radiation to groin; poor fluid intake; nausea, vomiting	Formation of stone in kidney, bladder or urethra, most commonly calcium oxalate and calcium phosphate stones
Upper Genitourinary Tract	Post-infectious acute glomerulonephritis	Antecedent illness (pharyngitis or impetigo or upper respiratory infection), periorbital edema	Immune complex formation inducing glomerular inflammation and injury
	Henoch-Schonlein Nephritis	Abdominal pain, bloody stools, purpuric rash, arthralgia	IgA immune deposition in glomerulus, skin and GI tract
	IgA Nephropathy	Hematuria with acute illness (GI illness or upper respiratory illness) or strenuous exercise; adolescent predisposition	Formation of IgA immune complexes causing glomerular injury and inflammation

tract infection. If urinary tract infection is suspected, referral to a provider is warranted as the child will need antibiotics.

Trauma may also cause gross hematuria in children. This includes local trauma to the perineum or urethral meatus. Physical exam of the genital area is key to identifying this diagnosis. Trauma to the kidneys or bladder due to contact sports can also lead to gross hematuria, which generally requires emergency department evaluation. "Exercise-induced" hematuria most commonly occurs after very vigorous exercise such as marathons or triathlons, or forced military marches [7].

Returning to our case, however, Peggy's' presentation with a combination of edema and gross hematuria points strongly to some form of glomerulonephritis. It is also important to note that she developed gross hematuria after a strep throat infection 2 weeks previously. Post-infectious glomerulonephritis (which encompasses post-streptococcal glomerulonephritis) is the most common cause of glomerulonephritis in children worldwide. The term "glomerulonephritis" refers to kidney glomerular inflammation, resulting in abnormal filtration of red blood cells. Red blood cell casts may form as filtered blood collects in the renal tubules and may be visible on microscopic urinalysis. In Peggy's case, it is likely that immune complexes formed due to the strep infection deposited in the kidneys, inciting glomerular inflammation. This ultimately results in a fall in glomerular filtration, fluid and sodium retention and increasing serum creatinine signaling acute kidney injury.

Another common form of glomerulonephritis is IgA nephropathy, in which IgA immune complexes are deposited in the glomeruli, which can result in gross hematuria concurrently with (rather than after) a viral infection, usually an upper respiratory infection or a gastrointestinal illness. Sometimes, the associated infections in these conditions aren't obvious. Henoch-Schonlein purpura (HSP) is another systemic vasculitis associated with IgA immune complex formation that can affect the kidneys, GI tract, skin and joints, causing a variety of symptoms including gross hematuria, abdominal pain and bloody stools, rash and arthralgias [7].

Children with symptoms suggesting glomerulonephritis can be referred to their primary care provider. If the child with suspected glomerulonephritis has vital sign instability such as severe hypertension or respiratory distress associated with fluid gain, evaluation in the ED and/or hospital admission may be warranted.

Case 3 Katie, an 8-year-old 3rd grader, has been into your office 3 times in the last two weeks after having wet her pants. She tells you that she has to urinate very suddenly and doesn't have time to get permission to get to the bathroom. She denies any pain with urination, but she does complain of frequent stomach aches. You obtain a dipstick urinalysis which shows a specific gravity of 1.030, and is negative for glucose, blood, protein, nitrites and leukocyte esterase. You call her mother to suggest bringing in a couple of changes of clothes and she explains that she is very frustrated that Katie has also started wetting the bed frequently after having been dry both daytime and nighttime for a number of years. What advice do you give?

Although most children are dry by age 4–5, both daytime and nighttime enuresis are still common in older children. Some degree of daytime wetting occurs in upwards of 15% of 6–8 year-olds [8], and 25% of both day and night enuresis is secondary (occurring after primary dryness is achieved) [9]. Enuresis is very rarely due to kidney disease or systemic disease, and often, the only necessary work-up is a urinalysis to demonstrate urinary concentrating ability and rule out glucosuria. A large majority of children with daytime wetting have uninhibited bladder contractions associated with constipation; constipation is also very commonly associated with recurrent urinary tract infections [10]. A good stooling history is a key part of the work-up, and often the only necessary work-up other than urinalysis. Although bladder anti-spasmodics such as oxybutanin are sometimes used, most daytime enuresis, and associated nighttime wetting ultimately responds to constipation treatment.

Case Conclusions

Case 1: Micah's parents were contacted and Micah had follow up with his primary care physician where his blood pressure was confirmed to be elevated. He underwent evaluation for an etiology of his hypertension including complete blood count, comprehensive metabolic panel, lipid profile, urinalysis, and renal ultrasound, which all came back normal. He was diagnosed with primary (essential) hypertension and treated with Lisinopril with improvement in his blood pressure in the subsequent checks.

Case 2: Peggy's parents were contacted and she was taken to her primary care physician. She had mild hypertension and edema on evaluation. Lab studies showed slightly elevated serum creatinine and a low C3 complement. She was diagnosed with post-infectious acute glomerulonephritis and was followed closely as an outpatient. She was treated for several days with an oral diuretic due to hypertension and edema. Gross hematuria resolved within 3 days, and blood pressure and kidney function returned to normal within one week.

Case 3: Katie was seen by her primary care physician and a clear history of constipation was obtained. After an appropriate initial "clean-out" regimen and ongoing treatment for constipation with both medication and diet change, both daytime and nighttime enuresis resolved.

Extra Credit Points

(1) Pediatric hypertension is identified utilizing blood pressure percentiles based on the child's sex, age, and height and is defined as blood pressure that is >95th %ile.
(2) Pediatric hypertension associated with signs and symptoms of headaches, seizures, mental status changes, shortness of breath and chest pain is a medical emergency which should lead to immediate medical care.
(3) Children with significant edema usually have some form of glomerular disease. Nephrotic syndrome usually shows heavy proteinuria, minimal hematuria, normal blood pressure and normal kidney function, while nephritis syndromes more commonly result in significant hematuria, mild proteinuria, elevated blood pressure and decreased kidney function.
(4) UTIs are the most common cause of gross hematuria in children; hematuria due to UTI should be associated with typical lower urinary tract symptomatology.

(5) Gross hematuria can be caused by a variety of forms glomerulonephritis, most commonly post-infectious, and requires evaluation by a provider to assess the extent of kidney involvement.
(6) The majority of daytime wetting in school-aged children, as well as recurrent urinary tract infections, are associated with constipation and respond to treatment for constipation.

References

1. Flynn JT, Kaelber DC, Baker-Smith CM, et al. Clinical practice guideline for screening and management of high blood pressure in children and adolescents. Pediatrics. 2017;140(3):e20171904. https://doi.org/10.1542/peds.2017-1904.
2. MDCalc - Medical calculators, equations, scores, and guidelines. MDCalc. http://mdcalc.com
3. Brady TM. Hypertension. Pediatr Rev. 2012;33(12):541–52. https://doi.org/10.1542/pir.33-12-541.
4. Normal Blood Pressure for Child 5-12 Years. www.brightfuturesny.com. Published February 9, 2024. Accessed May 29, 2024. https://www.brightfuturesny.com/post/normal-blood-pressure-for-child
5. Rodriguez-Ballestas E, Reid-Adam J. Nephrotic Syndrome. Pediatr Rev. 2022;43(2):87–99. https://doi.org/10.1542/pir.2020-001230.
6. Keskinyan VS, Lattanza B, Reid-Adam J. Glomerulonephritis. Pediatr Rev. 2023;44(9):498–512. https://doi.org/10.1542/pir.2021-005259.
7. Sureshkumar P, Jones M, Cumming R, Craig J. A population based study of 2,856 school-age children with urinary incontinence. J Urol. 2009;181(2):808–16. https://doi.org/10.1016/j.juro.2008.10.044.
8. Viteri B, Reid-Adam J. Hematuria and proteinuria in children. Pediatr Rev. 2018;39(12):573–87. https://doi.org/10.1542/pir.2017-0300.
9. Marjo-Riitta Järvelin L, Vikeväinen-Tervonen MI, Huttunen NP. Enuresis in seven-year-old children. Acta Paediatr Scand. 1988;77(1):148–53. https://doi.org/10.1111/j.1651-2227.1988.tb10614.x.
10. Loening-Baucke V. Urinary incontinence and urinary tract infection and their resolution with treatment of chronic constipation of childhood. Pediatrics. 1997;100(2):228–32. https://doi.org/10.1542/peds.100.2.228.

Chapter 53
Muscular Dystrophy and Other Muscle Disorders

Sarah Ghattas and Eileen Shieh

Case 1 Matthew is a 5-year-old boy who presents to your office due to toe walking. His mother says that he has always been a toe walker. He has also been delayed with his gross motor development: he started walking a few months late, has trouble with stairs, and falls more frequently than his sisters. You notice that when he stands up from sitting on the floor, he uses his hands to push on his thighs to get upright. Matthew's maternal uncle also had similar weakness. He used a wheelchair starting in middle school and died in his early 20s. He was diagnosed with Duchenne Muscular Dystrophy through a genetic work up. What are some challenges and comorbidities that may impact Matthew's school experience?

Duchenne Muscular Dystrophy (DMD) is the most common hereditary neuromuscular disease with increased severity when compared to other muscle disorders. The disease is caused by the lack of an anchoring protein, dystrophin, which leads to progressive muscle breakdown. DMD typically presents in males at approximately years 4-5 with proximal muscle weakness that manifests as toe walking, difficulty climbing stairs, as well as frequent tripping and falling [1]. The phases of disease progression can be classified in Table 53.1.

The mainstay of treatment is corticosteroids (prednisone, deflazacort), but there are promising new treatment options currently in development that are intended to repair the genetic defects resulting in the lack of the dystrophin protein. In addition to the musculoskeletal system, other systems are also compromised (either as a primary process of the disease or as a secondary effect of its treatment) and must be monitored. Health imperatives for the treatment of DMD can be remembered by the

S. Ghattas (✉) · E. Shieh
Nemours Children's Health, Jacksonville, FL, USA
e-mail: sarah.ghattas@nemours.org; eshieh@nemours.org

R. P. Olympia, J. Brady-Olympia (eds.), *Clinical Considerations in School-based Health*, https://doi.org/10.1007/978-3-031-85765-2_53

ID: 10722273 S: 0005 PS1000-1 TS: 155x235 Pg: 447/1144 BS: 220x251 H: 3 T: 13 PB

Table 53.1 DMD phases of disease[a]

Presymptomatic (1–3 years old)	Early Ambulatory (4–9 years old)	Late Ambulatory (10–13 years old)	Early Non-Ambulatory (14–18 years old)	Late Non-Ambulatory (18+ years old)
Diagnosis by family history or ↑Creatnine Kinase	Gower's sign: patients use their hands to "walk" up their legs due to proximal hip weakness	More labored gait	Can self propel for some time	Limited upper limb function
± Delayed milestones	Waddling gait	Difficulty climbing stairs	Able to maintain posture	Very difficult to maintain posture
No gait disturbance	± Toe walking	Difficulty rising from floor	± Scoliosis	
	Can climb stairs			

[a]Age ranges are based on the natural history of disease and treatment with steroids. The time course may differ with newer treatment options (Patterson et al. 2023).

acronym **DUCHENNE MD** (Table 53.2), which was developed by the Parent Project Muscular Dystrophy [2]. The table below gives important treatment considerations for the medical team and reminds us of the different comorbidities that these children often face.

Case 2 Jonathan is a 12-year-old boy with Duchenne Muscular Dystrophy. His teachers notice that he is struggling to keep up academically and has trouble with concentration. He has also started to have more trouble walking and is falling more frequently. Jonathan struggles with interacting with his classmates and has had a difficult time making friends. He is often made fun of for being different.

A large portion of boys with DMD will have neurocognitive and neurobehavioral disorders. In fact, about 30% of those with DMD have cognitive impairment as evidenced by a non-progressive lower IQ [3]. Other associated disorders include autism, attention deficit hyperactivity disorder, anxiety, depression, and obsessive-compulsive disorder [4]. It is important for school-based health professionals to be aware of these disorders as many symptoms of these disorders can often arise or be most prominent in the academic setting as students are expected to achieve academic success and maintain societal norms. These expectations can lead to significant social isolation with further elevation of pre-existing anxiety and depression. Neuropsychological testing can be beneficial for this population during the school aged years as the results can be used for diagnostic purposes as well as aide in specific recommendations for an individualized education plan (IEP). This testing can be repeated throughout the different grades and can be used as an objective tool to help with changes in neurocognitive status. Furthermore, screening assessments

Table 53.2 DMD Health Imperatives

D DIAGNOSIS	The mainstay of diagnosis is genetic testing for the dystrophin gene. A muscle biopsy can help with prognostication of the disease course.
U UNDERSTAND BREATHING PROBLEMS	Many patients will suffer from hypoventilation overnight as the disease progresses that can manifest as fatigue or morning headaches. **All DMD patients should have a sick plan for respiratory illnesses and any cold symptoms should be promptly identified and treated!** Immunizations should also be up to date.
C CORTICOSTEROIDS	Steroids remain the mainstay of treatment. Monitor for common side effects (see extra credit points) such as osteoporosis, mood changes, weight gain, cataract formation, an immunocompromised state, adrenal insufficiency, and hypertension.
H HEART	Dilated cardiomyopathy can progress to heart failure and arrhythmias that can ultimately lead to death. Patients should be seen by a cardiologist annually.
E ENDOCRINE	Poor bone health and osteoporosis can occur from chronic steroid use and impaired ambulation. Fractures should be ruled out in any child with DMD who has fallen and has localized pain. Be aware of possible compression fractures as well, which typically present as chronic back pain and midline spinal tenderness.
N NEVER FORGET PHYSICAL & OCCUPATIONAL THERAPY	It is important that these students receive the appropriate therapies to maintain range of motion and strength. **Therapy should focus on *maintaining* skills rather than *gaining* strength/endurance (as overuse of muscles can cause pain and hasten muscle breakdown)**.
N NUTRITION & GASTROINTESTINAL	Early in the disease course, steroids may cause children with DMD to be overweight or obese. Progressive muscle weakness will impair older students' ability to self-feed and swallow safely. Thus, their weight should be monitored closely as well as their nutritional status.
E EMERGENCY	Patients should always carry a list of their medications with them and should be educated on their disease course so that they can be treated appropriately in case of emergency.
M MENTAL HEALTH	There is a high morbidity of anxiety and depression in this population due to its prognosis and associated behavioral challenges and emotional disorders. The patients' teachers and medical team should have ongoing honest conversations and provide screening and support as needed.
D DON'T DO IT ALONE	This population should be treated from a multidisciplinary approach and every part of the team is important to their care.

Table 53.3 SMA Subtypes

SMA Subtypes			
	Disease Onset	Life Expectancy	Expected Functional Status
Type 0	Prenatally to birth	< 6 months	Severely impaired
Type 1	0–6 months	< 2 years	Inability to sit independently
Type 2	6–18 months	Adulthood	Needs assistance for ambulation
Type 3	18 months—teenage years	Unaffected	Independent ambulator
Type 4	Adulthood	Unaffected	Independent ambulator

such as a PHQ-9 can be regularly distributed to help assess this population's mood and what level of treatment should be pursued. Both pharmacologic and nonpharmacologic treatment methods should be utilized for most neurocognitive and mental health disorders. Medications including stimulants, antidepressants, and antipsychotics can be used to help with underlying neurocognitive disorders. Some medications may need to be administered at school, and the student should be monitored for unwanted side effects as with any medication. These patients may benefit from psychology services to provide regular counseling and coping strategies for underlying diagnoses.

Case 3 Shelby is a 4-year-old girl who was diagnosed with Spinal Muscular Atrophy type 2 on her newborn screen. She has never been able to walk and uses her wheelchair as her primary means of mobility. She also has leg braces and a stander to help promote independence and avoid secondary complications of her disease. Her parents are requesting guidelines to help guide her school team to use her equipment safely and appropriately.

Spinal Muscular Atrophy (SMA) is a group of genetic disorders that affect the anterior horn cells within the spinal cord. This leads to progressive proximal more than distal weakness and muscle atrophy. In some states, the newborn screen looks for abnormalities at the survival motor neuron 1 gene (SMN1); the gene affected in SMA. However, to confirm the diagnosis, genetic testing should be performed. There are 4 subtypes of spinal muscular atrophy (Table 53.3).

This student has SMA type 2 and thus will need bracing to help assist her with standing. This will promote bone health through active weight bearing and can help with contracture prevention. There are many types of orthoses that can be used depending on a child's underlying strength, tone, and functional goals. One common type of brace that may be used to help with stability in a stander is an ankle foot orthosis (AFO). It is important to ensure proper fit of the brace (Fig. 53.1).

When a child first starts wearing braces, they may be instructed to gradually ramp up time in their new brace. Frequent skin monitoring should be performed throughout this process and their prescribing medical provider and/or orthotist should be notified of any wounds or non-blanching redness of the skin that lasts for 15 min or more, as these findings would indicate the need for brace modifications. In addition to bracing, many patients with SMA will use wheelchairs to promote independent mobility and interaction with their environments. Depending on a child's functional level, they may be prescribed a manual or power wheelchair. It is important to realize that students who use wheelchairs may have the capability to

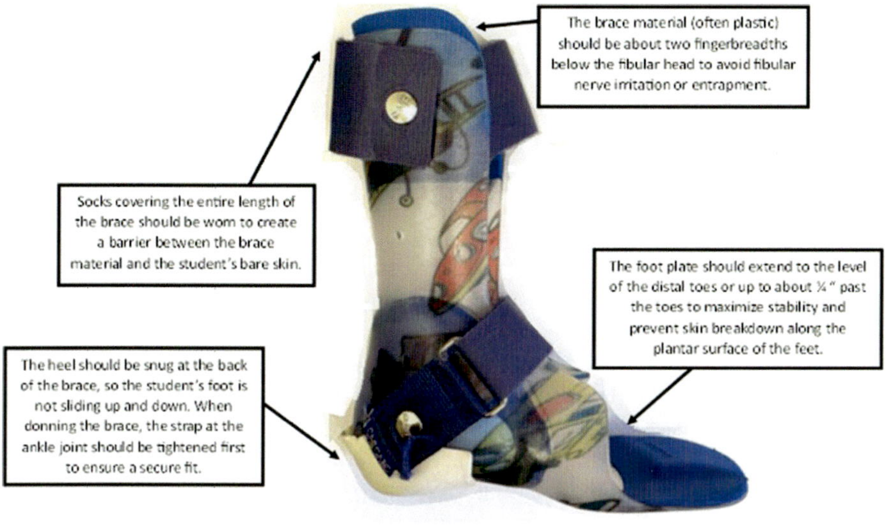

Fig. 53.1 Ankle foot orthosis

transfer and walk short distances with assistance. While they technically can perform these functions without a wheelchair, these children may be quite fatigued or have pain after completion of these tasks. Thus, it is often wiser to use a wheelchair to preserve a student's energy level to ensure their best function in school—academically and socially, just like any other child. Power mobility requires that the user have intact executive functioning and safety awareness [5], which is not typically an issue in students with SMA. All wheelchairs should be assessed for appropriate fit to prevent wounds, contractures, and pain. The "Rule of 90's" can be applied to assess for appropriate wheelchair fit: a child should be able to sit in their wheelchair with their hips, knees and ankles at 90 degrees.

Case Conclusions

Case 1: Matthew was started on oral steroids shortly after being diagnosed with Duchenne muscular dystrophy. He receives treatment at a certified Duchenne center where he can follow with all his medical specialists. He is starting first grade in the fall and is enjoying age-appropriate activities with his peers.

Case 2: Jonathan's teachers reached out to his parents expressing their concerns of inattention and difficulty with socializing. This was further discussed with his medical team. He underwent neuropsychology testing and was given diagnoses of autism and ADHD. The neuropsychologist provided recommendations for strategies to support him in classroom learning. He was also started on Ritalin to help with his concentration; he continues to be monitored for medication side effects including appetite suppression, abdominal pain, insomnia, and headaches.

Case 3: Shelby's parents were able to meet with upcoming teacher, the school nurse, and the school administration to create specific accommodations placed in her IEP to ensure that Shelby would receive the appropriate assistive equipment and therapy services to help her best succeed at school.

Extra Credit Points

(1) DMD or SMA are neuromuscular diseases that cause progressive weakness. This population should be referred to rehab medicine as early as possible in their disease course as students with these diseases should be monitored closely through each phase of disease. Equipment needs, therapies, level of assistance, and school accommodations differ in each functional period. It is important that the medical team anticipate the needs for the following stage to maintain function and prevent unnecessary complications.

(2) There are many comorbidities in DMD that can be attributed to steroid treatment including osteoporosis, mood changes, weight gain, cataract formation, an immunocompromised state, adrenal insufficiency, and hypertension. If a child with DMD is ill at school, further medical attention should be promptly sought since their status can decline quickly, especially respiratory compromise or adrenal crisis. Symptoms of adrenal crisis include findings of dehydration (vital sign changes—hypotension, tachycardia), new weakness, and change in mental status. These patients should be sent to the emergency room if there has been a significant fall, their breathing is labored, if they are having persistent fevers, or findings of adrenal crisis as aforementioned.

(3) School and health providers should regularly assess patients with disabilities for mental health concerns. Physical disabilities place children at increased risk for anxiety, depression, and bullying, and these concerns can be compounded by pre-existing risk for neurocognitive and neurobehavioral differences such as in DMD. It is especially important to offer teenagers independent time (away from their caregivers) to discuss their concerns.

(4) Many new medications including Eteplirsen, Ataluren, Vyondys, and Viltepso are being researched or have been approved to help modify the disease courses of Duchenne Muscular Dystrophy and Spinal Muscular Atrophy. These interventions are promising in changing the rate of disease progression and level of disability of these patients.

References

1. Muscular Dystrophy Association. Duchenne Muscular Dystrophy (DMD). Muscular Dystrophy Association. Published 2018. https://www.mda.org/disease/duchenne-muscular-dystrophy
2. Diagnosis & Early Phase. Parent Project Muscular Dystrophy. https://www.parentprojectmd.org/care/care-guidelines/by-stage/early-ambulatory/
3. Hellebrekers DMJ, van Abeelen SAM, Catsman CE, et al. Cognitive and behavioral functioning in two neurogenetic disorders; how different are these aspects in Duchenne muscular dystrophy and Neurofibromatosis type 1?. PLoS One. 2022;17(10):e0275803. Published 2022 Oct 10. https://doi.org/10.1371/journal.pone.0275803
4. Banihani R, Smile S, Yoon G, et al. Cognitive and neurobehavioral profile in boys with duchenne muscular dystrophy. J Child Neurol. 2015;30(11):1472–82. https://doi.org/10.1177/0883073815570154W.
5. Murphy KP, McMahon MA, Houtrow AJ. Pediatric rehabilitation principles and practice. Springer Publishing Company; 2021.

Further Reading

Patterson G, Conner H, Groneman M, et al. Duchenne muscular dystrophy: Current treatment and emerging exon skipping and gene therapy approach. Eur J Pharmacol. 2023;947:175675. https://doi.org/10.1016/j.ejphar.2023.175675.

Chapter 54
Rheumatologic and Connective Tissue Disorders

Andrew Kung and Timothy Hahn

Rheumatologic diseases encompass a spectrum of conditions that can present with diverse clinical manifestations. While more common conditions such as juvenile arthritis can present with non-traumatic joint swelling and morning stiffness, other more systemic diseases can present with recurrent fevers, extreme fatigue, muscle weakness, and photosensitive rashes. These symptoms should raise concern for rheumatic diseases should you encompass them in clinical practice.

Case 1 James is a 6-year-old male who presents to the nurses' office with a swollen left knee. His teachers have noted that he has been limping for the last 2–3 weeks when he arrives to school but by 2nd period he denies any pain or stiffness. At recess he has been able to run and play with only occasional trouble squatting. He denies any recent trauma or recent illnesses. On exam, his left knee appears larger than the right knee. Otherwise his vital signs are normal and he appears well.

Idiopathic Arthritis (JIA) is the most common pediatric rheumatologic disease in children. JIA is an autoimmune disease resulting in persistent joint inflammation for at least 6 weeks, with onset prior to 16 years of age [1]. The most important clinical feature of JIA is **arthritis**, which is defined as either joint swelling or the presence of two or more of the following: limitation in range of motion, pain on motion, or increased heat. This is in contrast to isolated joint pain, or **arthralgia**, which is nonspecific and can be seen in a variety of different conditions such as hypermobility, overuse, trauma, or infection.

On examination, children with juvenile arthritis may not complain of pain at rest but movement of the joint elicits pain, which can be expressed by guarding and resistance to bending or straightening the joint. This can also result in subtle

A. Kung · T. Hahn (✉)
Penn State Hershey Medical Center, Hershey, PA, USA
e-mail: akung@pennstatehealth.psu.edu; thahn@pennstatehealth.psu.edu

R. P. Olympia, J. Brady-Olympia (eds.), *Clinical Considerations in School-based Health*, https://doi.org/10.1007/978-3-031-85765-2_54

findings such as persistent limping, gait alteration, decreased interest or activity in physical activity, or dysfunction with hand writing or typing. Importantly, the above findings may occur in the absence of reported pain and so astute observation is required to identify the abnormality. Another hallmark symptom for JIA is stiffness which is usually most prominent in the morning or after prolonged periods of rest and frequently resolves throughout the day.

The diagnosis is clinical but can involve laboratory studies such as complete blood count, inflammatory markers, Lyme titers, and synovial fluid analysis to rule out other causes of joint swelling such as Lyme disease, post-streptococcus reactive arthritis, or septic arthritis (if the child appears ill or is febrile). Imaging such as X-rays can evaluate for trauma or malignant processes. Other imaging modalities such as MRI or ultrasound can be used if the diagnosis is in question [2].

The treatment for JIA is tailored to the patient based on factors including subtype of JIA, age, symptoms, and other comorbidities. Common treatment plans include intra-articular joint injections, oral non-steroidal anti-inflammatory drugs (NSAIDs) or disease-modifying antirheumatic drugs (DMARDs) such as methotrexate or adalimumab (Table 54.1). The majority of these treatments are administered in the home or clinic setting. Some medications are given via IV infusion which could cause school absenteeism but this should be predictable and scheduled ahead of time. Physical and occupational therapy are helpful to maintain joint mobility and function.

In the initial evaluation of a child presenting with joint swelling, with or without known JIA, careful consideration should be made to other causes such as trauma or infection. The child can be asked about recent trauma and observation of ecchymosis or soft tissue swelling around the area would not be consistent with JIA. Infectious arthritis can present with rapid onset of swelling, overlying erythema, significant pain, and fever which should be evaluated immediately in an emergency department

Table 54.1 Common Rheumatic Medications and Side Effects

Common medications used in rheumatic disease	Common side effects
Non-steroidal anti-inflammatory (ibuprofen, naproxen, etc.)	Abdominal discomfort, reflux, peptic ulcers, pseudo porphyria, hepatitis, headaches, renal insufficiency
Methotrexate (conventional DMARD)	Abdominal discomfort, nausea, hepatitis, immunosuppression, hematological toxicity, teratogenicity
Adalimumab, Infliximab	Immunosuppression, hematological toxicity, injection site reactions
Hydroxychloroquine	Retinal toxicity, hyperpigmentation of the skin, GI intolerance, CNS side effects
Corticosteroids	Weight gain, insomnia, mood changes, growth suppression, osteoporosis or avascular necrosis, immunosuppression, psychosis, cataracts or glaucoma, Cushing Syndrome, adrenal crisis if abruptly discontinued
Mycophenolate Mofetil	GI toxicity, hematological toxicity (cytopenia), and immunosuppression, teratogenicity

setting (refer to Chapter 93). Other infection related conditions such as Lyme disease, post-streptococcal arthritis, or reactive arthritis from a recent viral or bacterial infection present weeks after the infection and often require careful history and laboratory evaluation in a clinic, urgent care, or emergency department setting. In the setting of known JIA, without history of trauma or infection, patients with new onset swelling should be evaluated on a routine basis by their provider.

In the school setting, proper accommodations should be given in order to keep children at the least restrictive environment possible for learning and development. Examples of accommodations are found in Table 54.2 [1]. In regard to school absences, the majority should be planned, including frequent medical appointments, and there should be an option to make up schoolwork or participate in extracurricular activities despite frequent absences. Some children may require biologic medications given via infusion which would also cause absenteeism. Even with proper treatment, a small percentage of children will develop destructive joint changes may result in permanent functional limitations, which is important to clarify with the family when determining accommodations.

Case 2 Lucia is a 14-year-old Hispanic female with history of Lupus who presents to the office after a fall while walking upstairs resulting in a prolonged nosebleed. She also admits to fatigue, nausea, lightheadedness, joint pain, and

Table 54.2 Accommodation Examples for Rheumatologic Diseases Based on Manifestations

Lower Extremity Arthritis, Myositis, or generalized weakness	• Classroom activities involving movement to prevent stiffness such as collecting papers (arthritis only) • Seated in back or side of classroom to allow movement without classroom disruption (arthritis only) • Extra time between classes • Use of an elevator or wheelchair as needed • Providing multiple sets of books • Determine cafeteria assistance plan with help carrying trays • Encouragement of gym class and recess with modification as tolerated by the student
Upper Extremity Arthritis	• No grades for hand writing or typing • Extra time for tests or writing assignments or use of oral tests • Note taking services • Use of pencil grips or other modifiers
Uveitis	• Sunglasses as needed during flares • Preferential seating at the front of the class
Dermatologic manifestations in Lupus or JDM	• Frequent application of sunscreen SPF 30 or higher • Application of UV light shades on classroom windows or fluorescent lights
Neurocognitive effects	• Consideration for neuropsychiatric testing or IEP evaluation
Vascular Changes (Raynaud's phenomenon)	• Allow gloves or hand warmers • Preferential participation in indoor activities during winter months

a worsening of her facial rash over the past few weeks. She has been out of her daily medications for the last 3 weeks including her prednisone and hydroxychloroquine. Her vitals are reassuring in your office and her nosebleed stops after 15 min of pressure.

Systemic lupus erythematosus (SLE or Lupus) is a chronic autoimmune disease that can affect multiple body systems including skin, joints, kidneys, heart, lungs, blood vessels, and brain resulting in immune-complex depositions into these tissues. Lupus is rare prior to 5 years of age and increases in prevalence every decade afterwards. The cause of Lupus remains unknown but is suspected from a combination of genetic, immunological, and environmental factors.

The clinical manifestations of Lupus are numerous and include persistent fever, weight loss, **malar rash** (erythema on the malar eminence and nose which tends to spare the nasolabial folds), white color change of the fingers, oral or nasal ulcers (painful or painless), chest pain from pericarditis or pleuritis, shortness of breath, fatigue, alopecia, arthralgia, arthritis, delirium, cognitive dysfunction, depression, anxiety, headache, seizures, or strokes [1]. Due to these broad manifestations, children with lupus have significantly lower quality of life compared with healthy controls. The laboratory evaluation includes CBC for cytopenia, inflammatory markers such as ESR and CRP, complements, and autoantibodies including ANA. If the ANA is positive, further tests including anti-dsDNA, anti-Smith, anti-RNP, anti-SSA, and anti-SSB are ordered and are more specific to Lupus. Importantly, low-titer ANAs can be elevated in infections, malignancies, drug exposures, other autoimmune conditions such as thyroid or liver diseases, and can even be present in the healthy adolescent [3]. Therefore, a positive ANA without other signs or symptoms of rheumatic disease would not be worrisome.

The major goals of treatment are to suppress the patient's improper immune response to contain disease activity and prevent organ specific damage. Treatment options are based upon symptoms at diagnosis but typically includes hydroxychloroquine to improve musculoskeletal symptoms, alopecia, and skin rashes. Systemic corticosteroids are frequently used at diagnosis and can be used thereafter based on the relapsing nature of the disease. Corticosteroids have significant side effects and need to be tapered appropriately in order to prevent adrenal crisis symptoms including nausea, abdominal pain, weight loss, confusion, and hypoglycemia, such as in Case 2. Additional treatment of lupus is dependent on which organs are involved. For example, a patient with malar rash, mild arthritis, and cytopenia could be treated with medications such as hydroxychloroquine, azathioprine, and/or methotrexate. Patients with more severe manifestations or organ may need more aggressive immunosuppression. Application of broad-spectrum sunscreen (SPF 30 or higher), applied at least 30 min prior to sun exposure is critical as UV light is a known trigger of disease. Other pivotal treatment modalities for Lupus include behavioral counseling, physical or occupational therapy, and age appropriate vaccines to prevent infections.

Given the broad range of symptoms, triage of a patient with Lupus can be quite challenging. Their symptoms should be taken seriously and careful consideration should be given to updating their Rheumatologist, unless emergent symptoms which would require evaluation in the emergency department. Special consideration should be given to a proper medication reconciliation for adherence and the potential for withdrawal symptoms. Unfortunately, a frequent trigger for flares in Lupus includes discontinuation of medications, whether intentionally due to frustration with side effects or unintentionally due to missed appointments, loss of insurance, transportation issues to the pharmacy, or cost of medications. Please reference Table 54.1 for common medication side effects.

In regard to accommodations, special attention should be given to the dermatologic, neurocognitive, and vascular changes that can be seen with Lupus (see Table 54.2). In addition to planned absences for medical appointments, infusion medications, and therapies, children with Lupus may have prolonged, unplanned absences secondary to a disease flare which could result in hospitalization. Even with excellent medication compliance, Lupus is a chronic disease that can flare with unknown triggers and results in significant impact on quality of life.

Case 3 Lily is a 7-year-old female presenting to the nurses' office after a recent fall on the playground while jumping rope. She denies any head trauma during the injury. She endorses frequent falls over the last few weeks as well as trouble climbing stairs and standing up from chairs. Her gym teacher reports that Lily has suddenly become uninterested in gym and cried during a recent game of duck-duck-goose as she was unable to stand up quickly and run around the room. On examination she is well appearing but you notice extensive use of her arms to push up from a seated position. She has a normal gait without ataxia. You also notice a red rash on her upper eyelids and red bumps across her knuckles.

Juvenile Dermatomyositis (JDM) is a systemic autoimmune disease with particular involvement of the muscles and skin. The cause of JDM remains unknown but is suspected from a combination of genetic, immunological, and environmental factors. Symptoms of JDM can include fatigue and anorexia but the hallmark is muscle inflammation (**myositis**) with weakness and dermatologic manifestations including a rash on the eyelids (heliotrope rash—Fig. 54.1) and raised papules on the knuckles, knees, or elbows (Gottron papules). Muscle weakness is typically symmetric and involves the limb-girdle muscles including the shoulders, upper arms, neck, pelvis, and thighs. Children typically have difficulty climbing stairs, raising their arms above their head to brush their hair, and standing up without using their arms. In severe disease, pharyngeal and respiratory muscle weakness can occur resulting in trouble swallowing, aspiration, shortness of breath, or respiratory failure [4].

The diagnosis of JDM is clinical and involves evaluation for aforementioned signs and symptoms. Testing of muscle enzyme breakdown with creatine kinase, aldolase, lactate dehydrogenase, or aspartate aminotransferase can be helpful but elevation is not always present, even in active disease [4]. MRI is typically used to assess for muscle inflammation and the use if Muscle biopsy or electromyography is less common in the pediatric population. The differential can include other

Fig. 54.1 Heliotrope rash of JDM

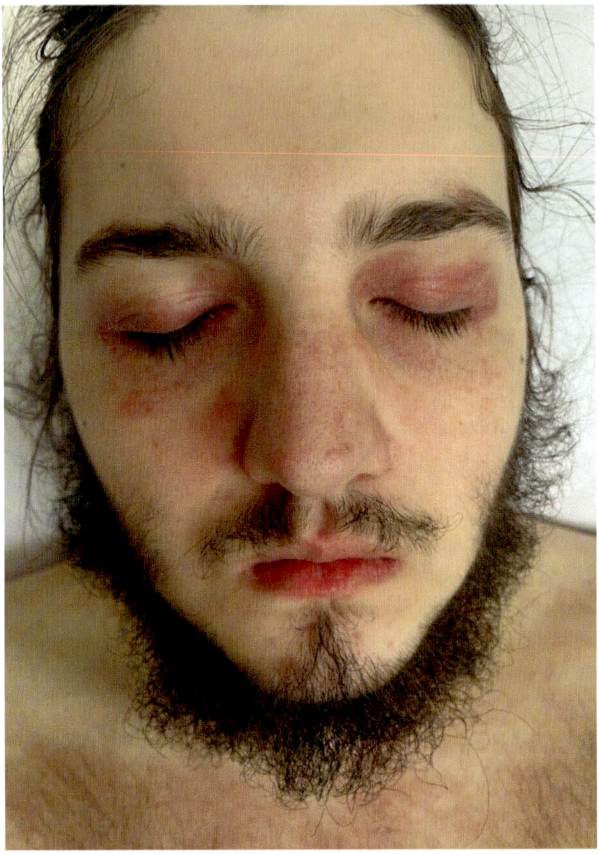

autoimmune conditions, postinfectious rhabdomyolysis, or noninflammatory myopathies. For postinfectious myopathies, a current or recent viral or bacterial trigger can often be identified, including influenza, parvovirus, coxsackievirus, staphylococcus or streptococcus. Post-infectious myopathies typically resolve with appropriate treatment of the illness, supportive care, and IV fluids. Noninflammatory myopathies include multiple genetic conditions such as muscular dystrophies, metabolic myopathies, drugs, or endocrinological disorders such as thyroid or parathyroid disorders.

The hallmark of pharmacologic treatment includes systemic corticosteroids at diagnosis with tapering as feasible over months based on the patient's response [4]. Other medications can include methotrexate, intravenous immunoglobulin, cyclosporine, cyclophosphamide, tacrolimus, or biologic agents such as rituximab. Nonpharmacological treatment is also pivotal for this chronic condition and could include physical or occupational therapy and behavioral counseling. Similarly to Lupus, exacerbation can be caused by UV light and frequent, liberal use of broad-spectrum SPF 30 or higher sunscreen should be allowed.

In an established patient with JDM, common triage concerns may include worsening fatigue, weakness, and rash. Weakness may present with frequent falls or decreased participation in physical fitness. Traumatic falls or injuries should be triaged as normal. Other common symptoms may include medication reactions such as nausea, vomiting, abdominal discomfort, and fatigue secondary to methotrexate or acute corticosteroid effects as discussed previously.

Accommodations for JDM are similar in nature to both JIA and Lupus and can be found in Table 54.2. Even with proper treatment, JDM manifestations can slowly worsen but should rarely result in a significant flare. With adequate disease control, school absenteeism should be similar to JIA with frequent but scheduled and expected absences.

Extra-Credit Points

(1) The hallmark of juvenile idiopathic arthritis includes joint swelling, limited range of motion, and morning stiffness. Flares can occur and should be evaluated by their Rheumatologist, unless there are other concerning symptoms such as fever or severe pain at which point referral to an Emergency Department would be appropriate.
(2) Lupus is a complex autoimmune condition which can affect nearly any organ system. Special consideration for joints, skin, and cognitive manifestations should be given in the school setting.
(3) Juvenile Dermatomyositis primarily affects the skin and muscles resulting in significant weakness.
(4) Referral to a Pediatric Rheumatologist should be considered with symptoms including joint swelling, joint stiffness, recurrent fevers, muscle weakness, or photosensitive rashes on the face or hands.

References

1. Petty RE, Laxer RM, Lindsley CB, Wedderburn LR, Mellins E, Fuhlbrigge R. Textbook of pediatric rheumatology. 8th ed. Elsevier, Inc; 2020.
2. Malattia C, Tzaribachev N, van den Berg JM, Magni-Manzoni S. Juvenile idiopathic arthritis - the role of imaging from a rheumatologist's perspective. Pediatr Radiol. 2018;48(6):785–91. https://doi.org/10.1007/s00247-017-4014-7.
3. Ostrov BE. Reliability and reproducibility of antinuclear antibody testing in pediatric rheumatology practice. Front Med (Lausanne). 2022;9:1071115. https://doi.org/10.3389/fmed.2022.1071115.
4. Leung AKC, Lam JM, Alobaida S, Leong KF, Wong AHC. Juvenile dermatomyositis: advances in pathogenesis, assessment, and management. Curr Pediatr Rev. 2021;17(4):273–87. https://doi.org/10.2174/15733963176662104261050454.

Chapter 55
Sickle Cell Disease

Gayle M. Smink

Case 1 Jeremy is a 7-year-old child with a history of sickle cell SS disease. He comes to the school nurse complaining of "not feeling well." You notice that he is warm to touch and has mild increased work of breathing. His vital signs are: Temperature 102.7° Fahrenheit, Heart Rate (HR) 105 beats per minute, Respiratory Rate (RR) 22 breaths per minute, Blood Pressure (BP) 117/85. You do not have access to a pulse oximeter.

Case 2 Shelly is a 16-year-old female with sickle cell SC disease who presents to your office with complaints of right leg pain. She states that she developed leg pain yesterday, but it has progressively gotten worse. Her leg is painful in the right mid-thigh, and she rates her pain as a 7 out of 10. She states that this feels similar to her previous sickle cell vaso-occlusive painful events. Her vital signs are: Temperature 97.2, Heart Rate (HR) 85 beats per minute, Respiratory rate (RR) 16 breaths per minute, Blood Pressure (BP) 130/88.

Sickle cell disease is a rare inherited, lifelong blood disorder affecting an estimated 100,000 individuals in the United States [1]. Sickle cell disease (SCD) is a genetic disorder of red blood cells that is more commonly seen in individuals of African, Hispanic, Southern European, Middle Eastern, or Asian descent [2]. SCD occurs in about 1 in every 365 African American births, and 1 in every 36,000 Hispanic-American births [1]. Sickle cell disease has multiple genotypes the most common being sickle cell SS and SC. Since school nurses often care for patients with chronic medical conditions, they may care for patients with SCD. These children may have sickle cell related complications at school necessitating the school nurse to triage and care for these complications.

G. M. Smink (✉)
Penn State Hershey Medical Center, Hershey, PA, USA
e-mail: gsmink@pennstatehealth.psu.edu

R. P. Olympia, J. Brady-Olympia (eds.), *Clinical Considerations in School-based Health*, https://doi.org/10.1007/978-3-031-85765-2_55

SCD results from a single nucleotide change in the beta globin gene, which is the substitution of a valine for glutamic acid [3]. This mutation, when inherited with another beta globin abnormality, can lead to sickle cell disease. This genetic alteration impacts the hemoglobin molecule, leading to a change in the shape of the red blood cell. The cell changes from a disc shape to the shape of a sickle or crescent moon. The sickled red blood cell also becomes rigid due to the polymerization of hemoglobin within the cell. This results in the potential to become "stuck" in blood vessels leading to vaso-occlusion and reduced downstream blood flow. The reduced blood flow results in tissue damage, vasculopathy, and reperfusion injury. The change in the shape of the red blood cell also results in a reduced lifespan and hemolysis resulting in anemia. Complications of sickle cell disease requires prompt evaluation, recognition, and treatment (Table 55.1).

Table 55.1 Common complications in sickle cell disease

Complication	Common symptoms	Disposition
Vaso-oclussive Crisis (VOC)	- Pain - Swelling - Warmth of the skin	- Primary care physician for mild-moderate pain - ED for moderate-severe pain
Infection	- Fever (101.3°F/38.5°C or higher) - Increased work of breathing	- ED
Anemia	- Pallor - Jaundice - Fatigue - Difficulty breathing - Headache - Dark Urine	- Primary care physician for mild symptoms - ED for moderate-severe symptoms
Stroke	- Paralysis - Facial droop - Sudden weakness - Trouble speaking or slurred speech - Blurred or double vision - Altered mental status - Sudden and severe headache	- ED
Acute chest syndrome	- Fever - Cough - Difficulty breathing - Chest pain	- ED
Splenic sequestration	- Pallor - Fatigue - Abdominal pain - Headache - Shortness of breath	- ED
Aplastic anemia	- Pallor - Fatigue - Shortness of breath - Exercise intolerance	- ED

Abbreviations: Emergency Department (ED)

Vaso-Occlusive Crisis (VOC) The most common complication of sickle cell disease is painful events called vaso-occlusive crisis events. VOCs typically present with sudden onset of pain, although some individuals can have a gradual onset of pain. VOCs are unpredictable and may not have a precipitating cause. Extremity, chest, and back are the most common locations for VOCs in children, but pain can occur anywhere in the body. There are no laboratory or imaging tests to diagnose a VOC. Obtaining a history, as well as evaluating for other potential causes of pain (injury, infection, etc.), should be the initial step in the assessment of a student with sickle cell disease and pain. Treatment is guided by the severity of the pain as well as the presence of any accompanying symptoms (fever, swelling, erythema, etc.). Assessment should include vital signs (including pulse oximetry if available), evaluation of the area of pain, and evaluation for any other symptoms (fever, shortness of breath, swelling, etc.). Students experiencing mild to moderate pain which improves with NSAIDS can continue this treatment in the absence of contraindications [4]. Pain medications should start as soon as the pain begins, if possible. Other non-pharmacologic interventions can also be utilized including applying heat to the painful area and increasing fluid intake. It is recommended to avoid the use of ice in the setting of a VOC. Routine medications for VOC events, such as ibuprofen and acetaminophen, should be available at school. Individuals experiencing moderate to severe pain may require referral to medical provider or the Emergency Department to initiate treatment with opioids and intravenous fluids. Students experiencing severe pain or pain not improving within an hour of initial treatment should have their parents contacted for further care. The school nurse should work in partnership with parents to determine the best treatment plan for individuals experiencing sickle cell pain at school.

Infection Individuals with sickle cell disease have an increased risk of infection, including bacteremia, sepsis, and osteomyelitis, due to poor splenic function. People with sickle cell disease are at risk for invasive bacterial infections, most commonly encapsulated organisms such as pneumococcal and meningococcal infections. Individuals with SCD and fever have a 1.1% chance of bacteremia, and those with a history of bacteremia, central line-associated bloodstream infections, and apheresis had a higher risk of bacteremia [7]. Initiation of penicillin prophylaxis, as well as improvement in vaccinations against these bacterial infections, has resulted in lower incidence of invasive infections. The National Heart, Lung, and Blood Institute (NHLBI) guidelines recommend that all individuals with SCD be vaccinated according to the CDC guidelines including vaccinations against Streptococcus pneumonia, and meningococcus [4]. Fever in the setting of SCD is considered a medical emergency and requires prompt evaluation. Digital thermometers should be available in schools to assess for fever in students with SCD. Fever-reducing medications should be withheld until a temperature has been obtained. Individuals with SCD should seek medical care whenever they develop fever of 101.3°F or 38.5°C or higher, due to the risk of severe infection [4]. In the Emergency Department patients should have laboratory testing including a complete blood count and a blood culture drawn. Prompt treatment with intravenous antibiotics (Ceftriaxone) should be initiated to reduce risk of morbidity. Individuals with history of bacteremia, central venous lines, symptoms of acute chest syndrome, or high fevers should be considered for hospitalization.

Anemia Individuals with SCD have chronic anemia due to the shortened red blood cell lifespan associated with the disease process. Baseline hemoglobin values can vary between individuals with SCD. Acute anemia can occur in patients with SCD and is defined as a decline in hemoglobin by 2 g/dL or more below baseline. Causes of acute anemia in SCD can include aplastic crisis, splenic sequestration, and increased hemolysis [4]. Aplastic crisis results when the production of red blood cells suddenly stops which results in severe anemia. Splenic sequestration occurs when blood becomes trapped in the spleen, and the spleen becomes enlarged. Increased hemolysis occurs when the red blood cell lifespan declines, and red blood cells are hemolyzing at an increased rate. All of these entities result in acute anemia in the setting of SCD. Individuals exhibiting signs of acute anemia, including fatigue, lethargy, increased jaundice, should seek emergent evaluation. Emergency Department management should include intravenous fluids, and possible blood transfusion. The school nurse can work in partnership with the parents to determine the best treatment plan in the setting of signs or symptoms of worsening anemia.

Stroke Stroke is a devastating complication of SCD and is most commonly due to stenosis or occlusion of the internal carotid or middle cerebral artery. Approximately 10% of children with sickle cell anemia (HbSS) will have an overt (symptomatic) stroke without primary prevention. National guidelines recommend individuals with SCD have emergent evaluation if they develop changes in level of consciousness, changes in speech patterns, paralysis, or seizures as these could be signs of an overt stroke. A student who develops signs or symptoms concerning for stroke should be evaluated immediately in the Emergency Department. Individuals who have an overt stroke have a high rate of having a recurrent stroke without appropriate treatment [4, 5]. Individuals with SCD that have had an overt stroke can have cognitive and motor deficits following a stroke that may impact school performance. Also, up to 35% of children with sickle cell SS disease will have silent cerebral infarcts (no overt signs or symptoms of stroke) which can present with school difficulties and cognitive decline [6]. In individuals with SCD exhibiting declining school performance, silent strokes should be considered. Both ischemic and hemorrhagic strokes can occur in individuals with sickle cell anemia. Stroke is a medical emergency and individuals with signs or symptoms of stroke should be emergently evaluated in the Emergency Department. Emergency Department management should include head computerized tomography (CT) followed by magnetic resonance imaging (MRI) and magnetic resonance angiography (MRA) if these tests are available. Red blood cell exchange transfusion should be initiated in patients with sickle cell disease and acute stroke [4].

Acute Chest Syndrome Acute chest syndrome is clinically similar to pneumonia and typically presents with fever, respiratory symptoms (cough, wheezing, increased work of breathing, retractions), hypoxia, and chest pain [4]. Acute chest syndrome is a common cause for morbidity and mortality in SCD. Acute chest syndrome is seen with increased frequency in individuals who have other pulmonary diseases, including chronic lung disease and asthma. Acute chest syndrome commonly presents with fever, increased work of breathing, chest pain, and hypoxia. Children with sickle cell disease who exhibit these symptoms should be evaluated emergently. If a student with SCD were to develops these symptoms, close collaboration with the parents to determine the best treatment plan is warranted. The child's guardian should be contacted immediately to determine if referral to the Emergency Department is needed. Emergency Department management should include laboratory testing, including blood culture, chest x-ray, and initiation of broad-spectrum antibiotics including intravenous cephalosporin and an oral macrolide. Supplemental oxygen should be administered to maintain oxygen saturations greater than 95% and incentive spirometry should be encouraged [4]. Individuals with a worsening anemia associated with acute chest syndrome can be treated with a blood transfusion to improve oxygen carrying capacity.

Caring for children living with sickle cell disease includes a collaborative approach between school nurses, caregivers, and medical providers. Many children with SCD will need a unique healthcare action plan at school to help facilitate understanding of their disease and recommendations for medical care (Table 55.2). Healthcare action plans can be useful to provide instructions on how to care for sickle cell emergencies as well as other sickle cell disease complications that may occur while under the care of a school nurse. In addition to healthcare action plans, students with SCD may require accommodations including transportation, 504 Plans, and Individualized Education Plans (IEPs) to help foster their success. Lastly, school healthcare providers should be familiar with common medications that students with SCD may be prescribed and the side effects associated with these medications (Table 55.3).

Sickle cell disease is a genetic disorder of the red blood cell that can lead to complications including, but not limited to, pain, anemia, infection, pneumonia/acute chest syndrome, and stroke. Children with sickle cell disease can lead normal lives and attend school. It is important for school nurses to be aware of the potential complications of sickle cell disease should they arise. Understanding of the pathophysiology of the disease, as well as recognition of complications, is key to caring for these children.

55.1 Case Resolution

Case 1 Jeremy has a fever along with respiratory symptoms. Due to his risk for invasive infections, including encapsulated organisms, fever 101.3°F or higher requires prompt evaluation. Due to his respiratory symptoms, he is also at risk for acute chest syndrome, which can be a severe complication of sickle cell disease.

Table 55.2 Interventions to Reduce the Risk of Sickle Cell Complications

Things to do:	- Access to fluids, especially water, throughout the day - Accommodations during extremes of temperature - Wear warm clothes during cool and cold weather - Resting during physical activity - Prompt evaluation in the setting of feeling unwell or developing pain - Access to educational services - Institute a healthcare action plan in the event of a SCD complication occurring during school
Things to avoid:	- Being near a heating or cooling vent - Restricted access to water - Utilization of ice in the setting of injury - Excessive physical activity (individuals with SCD should be able to rest at their discretion) - High altitude
Potential Accommodations:	- Environmental accommodations (avoiding heating or cooling vents, assistance with transportation, access to water and the bathroom) - Excused absences for scheduled medical appointments, hospitalizations, or medically documented illnesses - Instructional provisions for increased rest during physical educations - Instructional provisions for testing and homework (increased time, deadline extensions, makeup homework, etc.) - Caregiver involvement in healthcare action planning and regular communication about student needs - A 504 at school can help to delineate necessary accommodations at school including unlimited nurse visits, water breaks, rest during physical activity, and modified physical education and/or recess - Children with cognitive deficits secondary to SCD may qualify for individualized learning program (IEP) and other educational services

Prompt discussion with the family to determine the best course of action is warranted. The patient should be evaluated by a healthcare provider which could occur in a hematology clinic or emergency department. If a parent or caregiver is unavailable this patient should be evaluated in the Emergency Department for further care.

Case 2 Shelly is experiencing a vaso-occlusive crisis event due to her sickle cell disease. Prompt evaluation for other potential causes should be done. Without other concerns, and in the setting of mild to moderate pain, a trial of NSAIDs would be a reasonable treatment strategy if she has written medication administration consent. Other interventions could include increased hydration and heat to the area of pain. In the setting of severe pain evaluation in the Emergency Department for further therapy, including intravenous opioids, may be necessary.

Extra Credit Points

(1) Sickle cell disease is a rare genetic red blood cell disorder seen in the United States and worldwide.
(2) Sickle cell disease results in a change in the shape of the red blood cell from a disc to a crescent moon. The cell also becomes more rigid and fragile.

Table 55.3 Common Medications Utilized in Sickle Cell Disease

Medication	Use	Side effects
Hydroxyurea	- Increases fetal hemoglobin production - Increases hemoglobin - Reduces number of painful events	- Skin rash - Neutropenia, thrombocytopenia, anemia - Headache
Glutamine	- Reduces vaso-occlusive events	- Chest pain - Abdominal pain - Constipation - Nausea - Headache - Cough
Crizanlizumab	- Reduces vaso-occlusive events	- Abdominal pain - Diarrhea - Nausea - Fatigue - Headache - Arthralgias - Fever

(3) Vaso-occlusion, tissue damage, and vasculopathy lead to the common complications of sickle cell disease.
(4) There are varying genotypes that can lead to sickle cell disease and phenotype varies between individuals.
(5) Individuals with sickle cell disease are at increased risk for invasive bacterial infections due to functional asplenia.
(6) Painful events (vaso-occlusive events) are the most common complication of SCD.

References

1. Centers for Disease Control and Prevention. Sickle Cell Disease (SCD). [n.d.] https://www.cdc.gov/ncbddd/sicklecell/index.html
2. What Is Sickle Cell Disease? [n.d.] NHLBI. https://www.nhlbi.nih.gov/health/sickle-cell-disease
3. Sundd P, Gladwin MT, Novelli EM. Pathophysiology of sickle cell disease. Ann Rev Pathol. 2019; https://doi.org/10.1146/annurev-pathmechdis-012418-012838.
4. Evidence-Based Management of Sickle Cell Disease, Expert Panel Report, 2014. National Heart, Llung, and Blood Institute. https://www.nhlbi.nih.gov/sites/default/files/media/docs/sickle-cell-disease-report%20020816_0.pdf
5. Ware RE, Zimmerman SA, Schultz WH. Hydroxyurea as an alternative to blood transfusions for the prevention of recurrent stroke in children with sickle cell disease. Blood. 1999;94(9):3022–6.
6. Miller ST, Macklin EA, Pegelow CH, Kinney TR, Sleeper LA, Bello JA, et al. Silent infarction as a risk factor for overt stroke in children with sickle cell anemia: a report from the Cooperative Study of Sickle Cell Disease. J Pediatr. 2001;139(3):385–90.
7. Rineer S, Walsh PS, Smart LR, Harun N, Schnadower D, Lipshaw MJ. Risk of bacteremia in febrile children and young adults with sickle cell disease in a multicenter emergency department cohort. JAMA Netw Open. 2023;6(6):e2318904.

Chapter 56
Spina Bifida

Maya Sevrin and Rochelle Haas

Case 1 Anna is a 7-year-old with a history of myelomeningocele (sacral level) who presents to the nurse's office after running around in recess. For the second time in the day, her teacher notifies her that her clothing is wet and sends her to you. Anna typically comes to the office 2–3 times a day to perform her clean intermittent catheterization routine but being wet like this is not usual for her. What should you do?

Spina bifida is the second most common occurring complex congenital birth defect [1, 2]. When we refer to spina bifida we are most commonly referring to the open neural tube defect, myelomeningocele. Myelomeningocele occurs when there is an opening of the neural tube with leakage of spinal fluid and exposed neural tissue in a sac. This can be repaired prenatally or postnatally. Myelomeningocele is often associated with lower extremity weakness, sensory deficits, bowel and bladder difficulties, Chiari II malformations, hydrocephalus and learning differences [3]. Infants born with Myelomeningocele have complex medical needs that extend into childhood and adulthood.

The majority of individuals with myelomeningocele have some degree of neurogenic bladder or neurogenic bowel, regardless of the "level" of spinal cord involvement [3]. Both higher spinal levels and the presence of shunted hydrocephalus increases the likelihood of incontinence [4]. Because of the high rates of incontinence, bladder and bowel management are a common focus of care for individuals with myelomeningocele across their lifespan. Frequent visits to the nurse's office throughout their school age years is likely – sometimes for routine bowel and

M. Sevrin
Moorestown Friends School, Moorestown, NJ, USA
e-mail: sevrinm@mfriends.org

R. Haas (✉)
Nemours Children's Health, Delaware Campus, Wilmington, DE, USA
e-mail: rhaas@nemours.org

R. P. Olympia, J. Brady-Olympia (eds.), *Clinical Considerations in School-based Health*, https://doi.org/10.1007/978-3-031-85765-2_56

bladder program needs and sometimes for "accidents". Without students participating in a regular bladder program and bowel program, continence is difficult to achieve. Individuals with open neural tube defects work closely with Urology and their Rehabilitation Medicine team to achieve continence.

Common neurogenic bladder programs include timed voiding, clean intermittent catheterization (CIC) through the urethra or a surgically created stoma (Mitrofanoff), or less commonly, surgical creation of a suprapubic stoma which can be accessed with a catheter or drain passively. Often individuals use anticholinergic medications (such as oxybutynin, tolterodine, or mirabegron) to encourage the bladder to hold onto the urine and improve bladder health and continence.

A bowel program typically consists of 3 types of medications—a stool softener, a laxative and a suppository or enema. Higher volume enemas may help improve continence. Surgical options include a Malone or MACE procedure or a cecostomy placement to allow for an antegrade continence enema (ACE). More recently trans-anal irrigation systems, such as Peristeen, have allowed individuals to achieve improved continence without surgical procedures [5]. Typical signs of constipation include abdominal pain, changes in appetite, hard stool, loose stool, bowel leakage, and bowel incontinence [6].

Lower levels of the spinal cord, at the S2–S4 segments, are responsible for the contraction of the bladder and relaxation of the internal sphincter allowing for bladder emptying. The higher levels of the spinal cord, at the T11-L2 segments, are responsible for facilitating relaxation of the bladder wall and contraction of the internal sphincter allowing the bladder to hold on to the urine [7]. Depending on the level of the spinal lesion and function of the spinal nerves, this pattern of holding onto urine and subsequently emptying the bladder can be affected in multiple ways. Students can have a paralyzed pelvic floor, an overactive pelvic floor or an overactive detrusor muscle. Sometimes the signal from the spinal nerve levels to the bladder send mixed signals and can result in detrusor sphincter dyssynergy. When this occurs, the bladder contracts despite there being a tight internal sphincter. This increase in bladder pressure increases the likelihood of kidney damage [8]. The differential diagnosis of new or worsening urinary incontinence is quite broad.

Neurogenic bladder increases the risk of urinary tract infections. The two most common organisms that cause a urinary tract infection in youth with spina bifida are Escherichia coli and Klebsiella species [9]. Both incomplete bladder emptying, and urinary stasis increase this risk. In the setting of dyssynergy and higher pressure, this can result in kidney damage. Routine use of antimicrobial prophylaxis is no longer routinely recommended as they have not been shown to reduce the rate of urinary tract infections [10]. By school age more than three quarters of individuals with spina bifida have experienced a urinary tract infection [8].

When a student with spina bifida presents to the Nurses office with new or worsening incontinence they need to be referred for evaluation to their primary care doctor or local urgent care if they are well appearing or the emergency department if they are ill appearing. Concern for a urinary tract infection should be high. Common signs or symptoms of a urinary tract infection which can range from mild to severe and can be focal or directly bladder related or more generalized with fever and malaise (Table 56.1).

Individuals with suprapubic catheters are particularly vulnerable to infection and other complications including bleeding, bladder spasms, catheter-related trauma, and urinary leakage. In the absence of an infection, there can be many causes of new or worsening incontinence (bowel or bladder) for individuals with spina bifida, ranging from non-urgent to urgent triggers that require immediate attention (Table 56.2).

Bladder incontinence and "accidents" can be very difficult for children to cope with. It is very common for children and adolescents with spina bifida to never discuss their bladder (or bowel) differences with their peers. Individuals with frequent incontinent episodes may not feel the wetness due to sensory differences and can habituate to the smells associated with the incontinence. They may be completely unaware of their "accidents". School nurses, teachers, and others should not blame the child for their incontinence or lack of awareness of incontinence, rather they should normalize the importance of addressing incontinence and the teamwork needed to help make it easier for the student.

Case 2 Jamal is a 12yo with L4 level myelomeningocele with associated neurogenic bowel, neurogenic bladder, and shunted hydrocephalus. He wears leg braces (AFOs) and uses forearm crutches for ambulation. He does not use a wheelchair at school. Although you have seen Jamal many times and he uses the bathroom in the office for his bladder care while at school, he almost never complains of pain or looks uncomfortable. You have noticed that he has gained some weight and height over the course of the school year. He presents to the nurse's office complaining of back pain and asking for some ibuprofen. You remember overhearing his teachers commenting earlier in the day that Jamal is arriving late to class because he seems to be moving slower in the hallways. Jamal denies any changes in his bowel or bladder continence. He does feel like his walking has changed and he is tripping more. What should you do?

Motor and sensory deficits are commonly associated with myelomeningocele. Typically, the lower the level of the spinal lesion the fewer the mobility deficits. For

Table 56.1 Signs and Symptoms of UTI [11, 12]

Sign/Symptom	Description
Fever	Temperature of 100.4°F (38 °C) or higher
Changes in Urinary Patterns	Increased frequency, urgency, difficulty urinating, incontinence
Painful Urination	Discomfort or pain during urination
Cloudy or Foul-Smelling Urine	Urine that appears unusually cloudy or has a strong, unpleasant odor
Blood in the Urine	Presence of blood in the urine (hematuria)
Abdominal Pain or Discomfort	Pain or discomfort in the lower abdomen or back
General Malaise or Lethargy	A general sense of feeling unwell or unusually tired

Table 56.2 Causes of Bladder Incontinence in Spina Bifida [11, 12]

Cause	Description
Tethered Cord Syndrome	Abnormal attachment of the spinal cord to surrounding tissues leads to increased tension and damage, exacerbating neurogenic bladder symptoms.
Bladder Compliance Issues	Changes in the bladder's ability to stretch and store urine can lead to high-pressure storage and increased risk of leakage.
Detrusor Sphincter Dyssynergia (DSD)	Lack of coordination between the bladder muscle and sphincter can worsen, causing inefficient bladder emptying and overflow incontinence.
Changes in Neurogenic Bladder Function	Growth, additional nerve damage, or other factors can lead to deterioration in bladder control.
Bladder Outlet Obstruction	Structural abnormalities or changes can cause or worsen obstruction, making bladder emptying difficult and leading to worsening incontinence.
Medication Side Effects	Some medications including diuretics, some antidepressants, antihistamines, and decongestants can have side effects that worsen incontinence.
Dietary and Fluid Intake Changes	Changes in diet or fluid intake, including consuming bladder irritants like caffeine, can exacerbate incontinence.

individuals with myelomeningocele the tip of the spinal cord, known as the conus medullaris, remains attached to surrounding tissues, interfering with the normal migration of the conus to the L1-2 position [13]. That means that on imaging studies like an MRI they have evidence of a "tethered cord". The attachment increases the risk of spinal related nerve dysfunction during periods of growth, usually throughout childhood. This can result in back pain, leg pain, scoliosis, changes in walking, changes in bowel or bladder function, and changes in the neurologic exam—including the presence of new upper motor neuron signs such as increased reflexes or clonus. This is called a tethered cord syndrome. As many as 30% of individuals with myelomeningocele experience a tethered cord syndrome [13]. A tethered cord syndrome requires surgery to relieve the tethering and ideally, prevent further neurologic damage [14].

In the absence of a tethered cord syndrome, back pain, weakness and/or sensory deficits, changes in posture, changes in bowel/bladder may signal a different neurosurgical/neurological issue. Myelomeningocele can also be associated with development of a syrinx, brainstem dysfunction or symptomatic hydrocephalus from a shunt malfunction or a failed treatment alternative. New weakness involving the upper extremities should be cause for concern. Changes in grip/arm strength, manual dexterity and handwriting should be assessed for. If there is a new concern interfering with function, referral to a neurosurgeon is warranted. The differential diagnosis of new pain and weakness in a student with spina bifida is broad (Table 56.3).

As individuals with spina bifida go through puberty, they typically get taller, heavier and their center of gravity changes. These biomechanical changes can be associated with back pain and changes in gait/ambulation/mobility. Approximately

Table 56.3 Neurosurgical Concerns in Spina Bifida [15]

	Signs and Symptoms
Acute Shunt Failure	- Headache - Vomiting - Lethargy/Sleepiness
Chronic Shunt Failure	- Low-grade recurring headache - Neck pain - Loss of developmental milestones
Signs of Brainstem Dysfunction (in this age range)	- Poor control of oral secretions - Swallowing dysfunction - Stridor - Impaired language acquisition
Signs of Tethered Spinal Cord (TSC) and Urologic Dysfunction	- Back pain - Declining lower extremity sensorimotor function - Urologic dysfunction
Signs of Syringomyelia	- Back pain - Sensory changes in hands, worsening scoliosis

45% of individuals with spina bifida that are community ambulators at age 9 are no longer walking by age 50 [16]. Once more urgent neurosurgical causes for back pain and changes in gait have been ruled out by the medical team, biomechanically related triggers jump to the top of the differential diagnosis. These individuals will frequently be referred to physical therapy to address the changes; however, children with myelomeningocele should also be encouraged to participate in recreational and physical activities.

Children and adolescents with spina bifida have multidisciplinary health care needs and frequently present to their school health care team for management. Multidisciplinary team members often include: neurosurgeons, orthopedists, physical medicine and rehabilitation specialists, urologists, physical therapists, occupational therapists, neuropsychologists and social workers. Although two common scenarios were presented, the needs and issues that may arise are quite broad. In order to optimize care for this vulnerable population, there are published guidelines with recommendations to serve as a resource for care providers. They can be founded at: http://www.spinabifidaassociation.org/guidelines/

Case Conclusions

Case 1: Anna's parent/guardian was notified of the incontinence episodes. Anna should be referred to her medical team for evaluation for a urinary tract infection or other cause for her new/worsening incontinence. A urinalysis was performed, and a urine culture was sent. Anna's laboratory evaluation was concerning for a lower urinary tract infection- she did not have systemic symptoms, including fever, malaise or pain and she was started on cephalexin to treat E Coli based on culture results and sensitivities. Anna's bladder continence returned to her baseline.

Case 2: Jamal's pain improved after he was given ibuprofen. His parent was notified and feedback from his visit with you and his teaching team was shared with his parent. The concern that he may have a neurologic based trigger for his pain and change in function was conveyed to his parent and evaluation with his spina bifida specialty care team was recommended. Jamal was evaluated by the team and tethered cord syndrome was diagnosed. Jamal underwent a surgical release of his tethered cord without any further progression of his symptoms. His gait improved some, but did not quite return to his pre-tethered baseline.

Extra Credit Points

1. Spina bifida is a neural tube defect that commonly results in differences in motor/sensory function, bladder function, bowel function and cognitive function.
2. Neurogenic bladder and Neurogenic bowel are frequent consequences of an open NTD which can result in incontinence and interfere with kidney/bladder health. Bladder and bowel management are often a challenge across the lifespan and students aren't always aware of their incontinent episodes.
3. New pain, weakness and/or a change in function can signal a neurosurgical concern and referral for medical evaluation is warranted.

References

1. Kancherla V, et al. Scorecard for spina bifida research, prevention, and policy: score analysis by human development index and WHO region. Prev Med. 2019;123:1–7.
2. Hopson B, et al. The development of a lifetime care model in comprehensive spina bifida care. J Pediatr Rehabil Med. 2018;11(4):323–34.
3. McComb JG. A practical clinical classification of spinal neural tube defects. Childs Nerv Syst. 2015;31(10):1641–57.
4. Wiener JS, Suson KD, Castillo J, et al. Bladder management and continence outcomes in adults with spina bifida: results from the National Spina Bifida Patient Registry, 2009 to 2015. J Urol. 2018;200(1):187–94. https://doi.org/10.1016/j.juro.2018.02.3101.
5. Choi E, Shin S, Im Y, et al. The effects of transanal irrigation as a stepwise bowel management program on the quality of life of children with spina bifida and their caregivers. Spinal Cord. 2013;51:384–8. https://doi.org/10.1038/sc.2013.8.
6. Schletker J, Edmonds T, Jacobson R, Ketzer J, Hall J, Trecartin A, Peña A, Bischoff A. Bowel management program in patients with spina bifida. Pediatr Surg Int. 2019;35(2):243–5. https://doi.org/10.1007/s00383-018-4403-5. Epub 2018 Nov 7. PMID: 30402681
7. Neurogenic bladder. Medscape. https://reference.medscape.com/drugs/neurogenic-bladder.
8. de Jong TP, Chrzan R, Klijn AJ, Dik P. Treatment of the neurogenic bladder in spina bifida. Pediatr Nephrol. 2008;23(6):889–96. https://doi.org/10.1007/s00467-008-0780-7. PMID: 18350321; PMCID: PMC2335291
9. Ortiz TK, Velazquez N, Ding L, Routh JC, Wiener JS, Seed PC, Ross SS. Predominant bacteria and patterns of antibiotic susceptibility in urinary tract infection in children with spina bifida. J Pediatr Urol. 2018;14(5):444.e1–8. https://doi.org/10.1016/j.jpurol.2018.03.017. Epub 2018 Apr 20. PMID: 29709445.
10. Zegers B, Uiterwaal C, Kimpen J, van Gool J, de Jong T, Winkler-Seinstra P, Houterman S, Verpoorten C, de Jong-de Vos van Steenwijk C. Antibiotic prophylaxis for urinary tract infections in children with spina bifida on intermittent catheterization. J Urol. 2011;186(6):2365–70. https://doi.org/10.1016/j.juro.2011.07.108. Epub 2011 Oct 22. PMID: 22019031.
11. Forster CS, Kowalewski NN, Atienza M, Reines K, Ross S. Defining urinary tract infections in children with Spina Bifida: a systematic review. Hosp Pediatr. 2021;11(11):1280–7. https://doi.org/10.1542/hpeds.2021-005934.
12. Spina Bifida Association. Urology Guideline. Available at: https://www.spinabifidaassociation.org.
13. Agarwalla PK, Dunn IF, Scott RM, Smith ER. Tethered cord syndrome. Neurosurg Clin N Am. 2007;18(3):531–47. https://doi.org/10.1016/j.nec.2007.04.001. PMID: 17678753.
14. Ferreira Furtado LM, Da Costa Val Filho JA, Dantas F, Moura de Sousa C. Tethered cord syndrome after myelomeningocele repair: a literature update. Cureus. 2020;12(10):e10949. https://doi.org/10.7759/cureus.10949. PMID: 33072445; PMCID: PMC7560491.

15. Spina Bifida Association. Neurosurgery Guideline. Available at: https://www.spinabifidaassociation.org.
16. Oakeshott P, Poulton A, Hunt GM, Reid F. Walking and living independently with spina bifida: a 50-year prospective cohort study. Dev Med Child Neurol. 2019;61(10):1202–7. https://doi.org/10.1111/dmcn.14168.

Chapter 57
Students with Medical Devices: Ventricular Shunts

Kyle Tuohy

Hydrocephalus is an abnormal accumulation of CSF within the ventricles of the brain, which can lead to increased intracranial pressure if left untreated [1]. Most cases are congenital (one cause being myelomeningocele, which is discussed in Chapter 56), but can be acquired from infections (meningitis), perinatal hemorrhage, or tumors. Shunts divert CSF from the ventricle to another body cavity where it can be absorbed more readily. The most common location is the abdomen (peritoneum), but other distal locations are possible (e.g. atrium of the heart, pleural space, or gallbladder) as shown in Fig. 57.1.

Malfunction or infection of a shunt system is a medical emergency and requires prompt recognition and referral. If suspected, the child should be referred immediately to the emergency department (ED), ideally one with access to neurosurgical services. The most common findings in older children with shunt malfunction are a result of increased intracranial pressure: headache, lethargy, nausea, vomiting, gait instability, eye findings (upgaze or abduction palsy), or papilledema [3]. Shunt infections often present with non-specific findings, such as fever, lethargy, and anorexia, but may also have erythema and/or tenderness along the shunt tubing, meningitis, or peritonitis (if a distal infection of a VP shunt) [3]. They may also present as shunt malfunction, with the associated findings of such.

However, signs and symptoms can be highly individualized for each child. Therefore, it is essential that all children with shunted hydrocephalus have an Individualized Healthcare Plan (IHP) on file with the school nurse, created with the assistance of the child's parents and primary physician [4, 5]. In addition, referral should ideally be made to the facility in which the child receives their hydrocephalus care if feasible, as they will be most familiar with the child's previous shunt history. Table 57.1 lists the minimum components of the child's shunt history that

K. Tuohy (✉)
Department of Neurosurgery, Penn State Hershey Medical Center, Hershey, PA, USA
e-mail: ktuohy@pennstatehealth.psu.edu

R. P. Olympia, J. Brady-Olympia (eds.), *Clinical Considerations in School-based Health*, https://doi.org/10.1007/978-3-031-85765-2_57

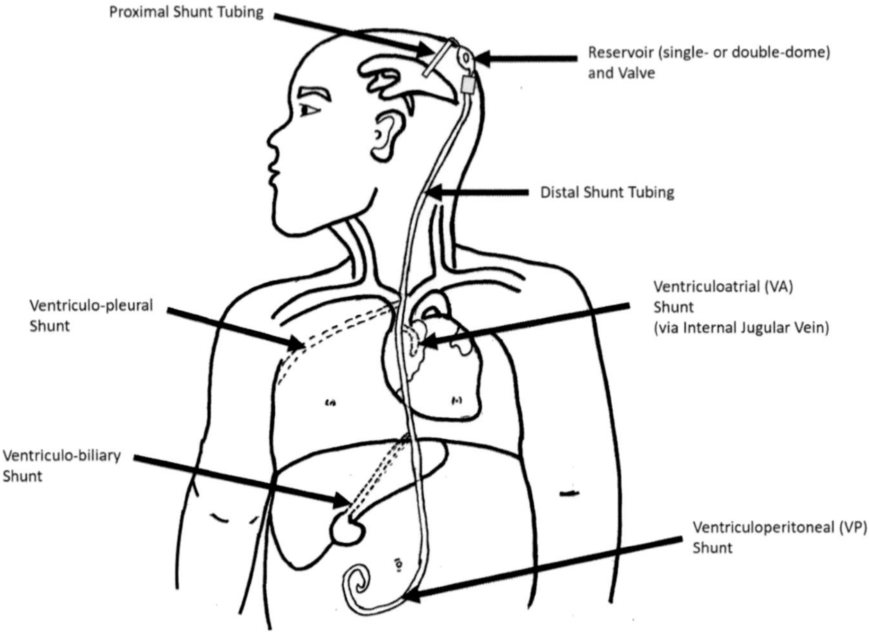

Fig. 57.1 Anatomy of various shunt systems (adapted from Farou et al. [2]). A shunt has three main components: the ventricular catheter that enters the CSF cavities of the brain, a valve that regulates flow (which may also contain a reservoir that can be palpated as a small bubble under the skin, and can be used to aspirate CSF by a physician), and the distal catheter that goes to a distal drainage site (this image depicts multiple distal catheters to demonstrate the possible variations, but most children have only one distal catheter)

Table 57.1 Essential items to be included in the Individualized Healthcare Plan for children with a shunt

Type of shunt (ventriculoperitoneal, ventriculo-atrial, ventriculo-pleural, ventriculo-biliary)
Initial placement: reason (myelomeningocele, post-infectious, etc.) and patient age
Last surgical revision and why
Type of valve and setting (e.g. Certas at 3, Codman at 150, etc.)
Restriction/accommodations: physical activity, position, magnets, need for straight catheterization, history of seizures, etc.
Failure symptoms (typical signs and symptoms of a shunt malfunction)
Primary neurosurgeon and preferred hospital

should be included in their IHP. This information should also be provided to the ED staff when referring a patient with suspected shunt malfunction. An excellent example is provided by Obst and Roesler 2017 [6].

Case James, an 11-year-old boy, comes to your office because of neck pain. He also notes difficulty taking notes with his right hand today in class. After reviewing his IHP, you remember that he has a history of myelomeningocele

and shunted hydrocephalus, with a Strata valve set at 1.5. His last revision was one year ago for a proximal catheter obstruction, at which time his failure symptoms were neck pain with new-onset right hand weakness and loss of fine motor control. What is the next step in management for this child?

Although we previously discussed common signs and symptoms of shunt malfunction, it is again important to highlight that each individual child may have unique symptoms that do not follow conventional patterns. The atypical presentation listed here can also be a sign of failure in shunted myelomeningocele patients. Thankfully, you had a documented IHP for this child which helped to clue you in to a more serious problem. This child's parents should be notified, and he should be referred to the emergency department for evaluation of his shunt.

In the ED, after a thorough history (expedited thanks to a copy of his IHP you provided) and physical exam, the next step in evaluation is an X-ray of the entire length of the shunt system to evaluate for disconnection or kinking, and intracranial imaging to evaluate ventricle size and proximal catheter placement. This imaging should ideally be fast-sequence magnetic resonance imaging (MRI) to minimize the lifetime risk of fatal cancer due to ionizing radiation from frequent use of computed tomography (CT) scan [7, 8]. Low-dose non-contrast CT can be used if no MRI is available, or if the child has a contraindication to MRI. Often the ventricles will be enlarged compared to imaging obtained while the shunt was functioning appropriately. However, a small number of children will not demonstrate an increase in ventricle size (slit ventricle syndrome), due to chronic shunting and reduced compliance of the ventricular system [9].

On fast-sequence MRI, James was found to have an increase in his ventricle size, consistent with imaging obtained prior to his last malfunction. He subsequently went to the operating room emergently for shunt exploration, where an obstruction was noted in the proximal catheter which needed to be replaced. James spent the rest of that day under observation in the hospital and was discharged the following day, which is customary for most uncomplicated shunt revisions.

Upon return to school, most children are prescribed only light activity for the first 3-4 weeks and may need accommodations for physical education during that time. After their first post-operative visit, there are generally no restrictions on activity or sports, but ask the child's physician regarding contact sports as occasionally they are avoided to prevent damage from a direct blow to the shunt system. Aside from over-the-counter pain medication right after surgery, there are no medication or dietary changes necessary. Of note, many children with myelomeningocele develop a latex allergy. Although most healthcare facilities now avoid latex for all patients, it is especially important to consider in this patient population.

James will likely have incisions on the top of his head (which requires a generous shaving of hair over that area, leaving a bald spot) and possibly behind his ear or belly depending on the site of malfunction. He may prefer to wear a cap or scarf to cover these areas if sensitive about them; these preferences should be observed and may require special permission depending on dress code. The setting of an adjustable valve (such as the one James has) may inadvertently be changed upon exposure to strong magnetic fields, such as MRI. Children with these valves should have their setting checked by a healthcare professional experienced in doing so after any MRI. Children are advised to keep magnet-containing products at least 2 inches from the valve and use the ear opposite of the shunt, when possible, but the Food and Drug Administration does not advise against the use of any specific electronics currently [10]. Lastly, the highest risk for shunt infection is in the months following a revision, and therefore should be closely monitored for, as we will now see:

About a month after returning to school, James comes to your office again after an episode of emesis in the bathroom. He also has headache and continues to be nauseous. His temperature is 100.5°F, he is tachycardic, and his proximal shunt tubing is erythematous and tender to palpate. What is the next step in management for this child?

In someone without shunted hydrocephalus, it may be reasonable to send a child home with plans for evaluation by his primary pediatrician or urgent care later that day or tomorrow. However, in a child with a shunt, especially one that was recently revised, he is at high risk for healthcare-associated ventriculitis and meningitis. He again needs referral to the ED for further evaluation. The reservoir beneath his scalp can be accessed by the neurosurgery team to obtain a CSF sample for testing. There will often be abnormalities in CSF cell count, glucose, and protein, but these values by themselves are not reliable indicators of infection [11]. The best diagnostic evaluation is CSF culture to identify a causative organism, which will also allow for a tailored antibiotic regimen specific to that organism.

Shunt infections are extremely serious and require removal of the shunt system, followed by placement of a temporary external ventricular drain to divert CSF while the child is treated with antibiotics [11]. The shunt can be replaced after 3-10 days of antibiotics, depending on the causative bacteria. However, children often require 1–3 weeks of intravenous (IV) antibiotics after replacement and may be sent home with a central venous access device to complete their course (see Chapter 60 for more information on managing these devices).

Although this situation may sound unlikely, it is unfortunately quite common for children with shunts. The rate of failure in the first year is between 11–25%, with a roughly 10% risk of obstruction per year thereafter [3]. The rate of infection is 5–7%, with 50% occurring in the first 2 weeks after surgery and 70% within 2 months [3]. The "Rule of 2's" can be used to help in the evaluation of a child with suspected shunt issues [1]. In the first 2 days after surgery, complications include hemorrhage, stroke, or mispositioned hardware, which are often identified prior to the child leaving the hospital but not always. In the first 2 months, the risk for infection is highest as previously discussed. Lastly, the first 2 years represents the highest risk for malfunction, mostly commonly obstruction of the proximal catheter.

Each child should have an individual education plan (IEP), 504 plan, or Individual service plan (ISP) created in collaboration with the child's teachers and parents. This should include accommodations and modification as necessary, especially regarding extended and frequent medical absences such as in this case. Children with hydrocephalus may have other medical conditions as well, and some deal with seizures, headaches (outside of those associated with malfunction), vision problems, and issues with fine motor skills and coordination. Each child is different, but it is important to identify these associated symptoms early so that appropriate accommodations can be made.

A brief mention should be made about endoscopic third ventriculostomy (ETV). Some cases of hydrocephalus can be treated by surgically creating a new pathway for CSF to travel outside of the normal ventricular system [1]. Although there is a higher upfront risk associated with the surgery itself, this procedure eliminates the need for implanted hardware and therefore removes the risk of infection associated with a shunt. There is still a possibility of "failure" if the new pathway shuts down, which is dependent on several patient-specific factors, but the rate is generally lower than the rate of shunt malfunction [3]. If failure should occur, a child will likely present similarly to a child with shunt malfunction.

Extra Credit Points

1. There should be a high index of suspicion for shunt malfunction/infection in children with a known VP shunt presenting with typical "failure symptoms" or infectious signs and symptoms (see Table 57.2).
2. If malfunction/infection is suspected, the patient should promptly be referred to the emergency department, ideally one with neurosurgical services available and ideally to the facility in which the patient receives their hydrocephalus care if this will not overly delay referral.
3. All children with a VP shunt should have an IHP, created in collaboration with the child's parents and primary physician managing their hydrocephalus.
4. Children with VP shunts often require accommodations in school, and should have an IEP, 504 plan, or ISP on file, which should be reviewed at least annually and updated as needed.

Table 57.2 Characteristics and differentiating factors between shunt malfunction and infection

Characteristic	Malfunction	Infection
Timing	Highest risk in the first 2 years Failure rates anywhere between 11–25% in the 1st year after placement	50% of staph infections occur within 2 weeks of placement/revision 70% occur within 2 months
Signs and symptoms	Headache (may be affected by posture, position, or activity), nausea, vomiting, diplopia, lethargy, ataxia, seizures (new, or if pre-existing, an increase in frequency)	Can present with shunt malfunction, but also fever, irritability, chills, pain/stiffness/erythema around shunt tubing, rarely fulminant meningitis, or peritonitis (distal infection)
Diagnosis	Intracranial imaging, ideally with fast MRI to evaluate ventricle size, and "X-ray shunt series" to visualize entire length of shunt tubing and inspect for disconnection/kinking	CSF analysis, gold standard is fluid culture for causative organism, but may also see abnormalities in cell count, glucose, and protein
Treatment	Shunt exploration and revision. All parts may be tested, but often only the non-functioning portions are replaced	Removal or partial externalization of shunt hardware, followed by prolonged course of IV antibiotics before replacement

5. Use the "Rule of 2's" to aid in the evaluation of a child with shunt complications.

Additional Resources for Clinicians and Families

Hydrocephalus Association (https://www.hydroassoc.org): Good resources for anyone, but especially parents and teachers.

International Society for Pediatric Neurosurgery (https://ispn.guide): Clinician-oriented site with general hydrocephalus information and very detailed overview of different valve types.

National Association of School Nurses (NASN) School Nurse journal: articles on shunts [2, 6] and position statements [4, 5], requires membership to NASN to access.

References

1. Wright Z, Larrew TW, Eskandari R. Pediatric hydrocephalus: current state of diagnosis and treatment. Pediatr Rev. 2016;37(11):478–90. https://doi.org/10.1542/pir.2015-0134.
2. Farou N, Lucas C, Olympia RP. School nurses on the front lines of healthcare: children with medical devices—shunt system malfunctions and infections. NASN School Nurse. 2021;36(2):86–91. https://doi.org/10.1177/1942602X20940036.
3. Greenberg M. Greenberg's handbook of neurosurgery. 10th ed. Thieme; 2023.
4. National Association of School Nurses. Wearable medical technology in schools: The role of the school nurse (Position brief). Published online 2018.
5. National Association of School Nurses. Use of individualized healthcare plans to support school health services (Position statement). Published online 2020.
6. Obst B, Roesler M. Hidden devices in the school setting: what the nurse needs to know about shunts. NASN School Nurse. 2017;32(3):154–8. https://doi.org/10.1177/1942602X17697026.
7. O'Neill BR, Pruthi S, Bains H, et al. Rapid sequence magnetic resonance imaging in the assessment of children with hydrocephalus. World Neurosurg. 2013;80(6):e307–12. https://doi.org/10.1016/j.wneu.2012.10.066.
8. Choosing Wisely Recommendations: Don't routinely order a head computed tomography to assess for shunt failure in children with hydrocephalus. https://www.aafp.org/pubs/afp/collections/choosing-wisely/534.html.
9. Rekate HL. Classification of slit-ventricle syndromes using intracranial pressure monitoring. Pediatr Neurosurg. 1993;19(1):15–20. https://doi.org/10.1159/000120694.
10. Food and Drug Administration. Magnetic field interference with programmable CSF shunts. Published online 2019.
11. Tunkel AR, Hasbun R, Bhimraj A, et al. 2017 Infectious Diseases Society of America's clinical practice guidelines for healthcare-associated ventriculitis and meningitis*. Clin Infect Dis. 2017;64(6):e34–65. https://doi.org/10.1093/cid/ciw861.

Chapter 58
Students with Medical Devices: Tracheostomies

Robin Kingston

Case Aleena is a 5-year-old female with a medical diagnosis of ACTA1 Nemaline Myopathy Type 3. She has profound neuromuscular weakness that necessitates her being ventilator dependent 24 hours per day via tracheostomy tube. Aleena will be starting Kindergarten in the Fall.

The reasons for tracheostomies in children are varied but can include upper airway obstruction caused by craniofacial abnormalities like Pierre-Robin sequence or trauma, for secretion management, vocal cord paralysis, or to provide a means for long-term mechanical ventilation such as needed for children with neuromuscular diseases. Whatever the reason for tracheostomy, increasing numbers of children with tracheostomies are in school settings and the care needed for these children is complex and needs to be carefully planned for.

It is the right of every child to have free public education provided to them, even those with complex health care needs. With the passing of the Education Act (1981, 1996) and the Special Education Needs Code of Practice (2021) there has been a push to include children with special educational needs in mainstream schools [2]. The means for providing care for these children in mainstream schools can be somewhat of a challenge. Children with tracheostomies require trained caregivers to manage their tracheostomy tube and specialized equipment. Planning for these children to be in the school setting needs to start early.

Students with tracheostomies can be supported in school with various supports and plans. Each school district can assist families to determine the most appropriate level of support for their child. The "care plan" can be included in an Individualized Education Plan (IEP) or 504 Plan which allows parents to request classroom adaptations for their child's learning needs and a medical care plan that outlines the specific medical needs of the student. Assembling a team of individuals to be involved

R. Kingston (✉)
Penn State Children's Hospital, Hershey, PA, USA
e-mail: rkingston@pennstatehealth.psu.edu

R. P. Olympia, J. Brady-Olympia (eds.), *Clinical Considerations in School-based Health*, https://doi.org/10.1007/978-3-031-85765-2_58

to assist with the creation of these plans is vital and should include the family caregivers, special education coordinator, principal, teacher, school nurse and potentially the child's health care providers and home nursing agency [3].

58.1 Equipment

One of the first things to consider is the equipment that will be necessary to care for the child in school. (Table 58.1) A "Go Bag" with emergency tracheostomy equipment is essential for any child with a tracheostomy tube. This bag includes a tracheostomy tube of the same size and one that is a size smaller or the "downsize tube", extra trach tube holders, lubricant, saline, syringe, and tracheal stoma dressings. This "Go Bag" should stay with the child at all times.

It is recommended that there be oxygen available in the school for emergencies. Some children may require oxygen at all times or when ill. If a child needs oxygen in the school they need to have a portable oxygen source. This could be in the way of a portable oxygen concentrator or portable oxygen tanks. The child's Durable Medical Equipment (DME) Company usually provides the portable oxygen. The parents may be able to transport the oxygen daily with the child or there may need to be extra oxygen stored at the school. Oxygen needs to be safely stored and secured in a well-ventilated area away from a furnace or open flame [3].

Other equipment may also need to be stored at the school including nebulizers or cough assist devices. The student's care plan will need to include where this equipment will be stored and where the child will utilize the equipment or receive "treatments". Any equipment stored at the school will need to have ongoing maintenance and safety checks. If the equipment is being supplied by the DME Company, they can assist with this.

Table 58.1 Equipment that might be needed for child with tracheostomy tube

"Go Bag"
• Same size tracheostomy tube
• Downsize tracheotomy tube
• Trach tube holders
• Lubricant
• Saline for suctioning
• Syringe if cuffed trach tube
• Tracheal stoma dressing supplies
• Suction machine and suction catheter
Pulse-oximeter
Oxygen
Ambu® Bag
Ventilator
Cough Assist Machine
Nebulizer equipment
Inhalers

58.2 Transportation

Transporting the child to and from school also needs to be considered and planned for. Will the parent transport the child or will the school district transport the child? There are many things to consider if the school district will be providing the transportation. Does the child need any type of specialized seating or wheelchair accessibility? What equipment needs to be with the child in the vehicle? Does there need to be a nurse with the child? What is the plan in the event of an emergency?

58.3 Caregivers

Also to be considered for a child with a tracheostomy to attend school, is who will be providing care for the child at school. Per the American Thoracic Society, there should be a trained caregiver with these children at all times [4]. In the United States, this care is usually provided by a nurse or in some cases a respiratory therapist as well as the parent who is trained in the child's care. It is often not feasible for the school nurse to be providing the one on one care that these children require. It needs to be clearly identified in the child's IEP or 504 Plan who is to be providing this care. While federal law stipulates that the school district must provide for whatever accommodations are outlined in the IEP or 504 Plan, providing for one on one nursing can be a great financial strain for a school district. Often the child's health care insurance will include a nurse caring for the child in the school setting as part of the home skilled nursing authorization. With current nursing shortages, however, it may be difficult to provide a nurse to be with a student on a daily basis. The IEP or 504 Plan should include what services will be provided for a child who cannot attend school due to lack of nursing services.

Some states have utilized trained lay caregivers to care for these students due to the extreme nursing shortages. If it is determined that a school nurse or lay caregiver will be providing the care for the child while in school, that nurse or caregiver will need to be trained regarding the care for that child including tracheostomy tube changes, tracheal suctioning, the administration of inhaled medications, and what is to be done in the event of an emergency.

58.4 Restrictions

The child's health care provider along with the parent will need to determine if there are any restrictions for the child while in school including when or if a child should not participate in gym class or outdoor recess. The health care provider can provide for a particular range of temperatures for when the child should stay inside.

58.5 Emergency Planning

Part of planning for a child with a tracheostomy to be in school is to devise an emergency plan.

Caregivers need to be well-versed as to how to provide care for tracheostomy emergencies (Table 58.2). All necessary equipment including the student's "Go Bag", suction equipment, Ambu® bag and oxygen should be available all times. There should be written guidelines for care for the child in the event of emergency, including phone numbers for who needs to be called. All important numbers including the health care provider's numbers should be included in the plan.

Table 58.2 Tracheostomy Emergencies

Problem	Presenting signs/ symptoms	Acute management	Disposition
Respiratory distress	• Increased work of breathing – Tachypnea – Retractions – Desaturation – Adventitious breath sounds – Generally looking uncomfortable	• Suction trach tube • Other airway clearance device – Cough assist • **Change trach tube** • Oxygen • Consider albuterol	• Back to classroom if initial steps resolve the problem. • Call EMS if symptoms persist
Obstructed trach tube	• Signs/symptoms of respiratory distress • Unable to pass suction catheter.	**Change the trach tube**	• Back to classroom if no additional problems after changing the tube
Dislodged trach tube	• Signs/symptoms of respiratory distress • Trach tube not in stoma	**Replace the trach tube**	• Back to classroom if no additional problems after replacing the tube • Call EMS if unable to replace tube
Infection—tracheitis	• Increased tracheal secretions • Discolored tracheal secretions – Yellow – Tan – Blood-tinged • Fever • Oxygen requirement	• Increased airway clearance – Albuterol – Chest PT – Suctioning – Other airway clearance devices	• Contact PCP or pulmonary specialist

58.6 Challenges

There are many challenges with children with tracheostomy tubes who likely have other complex medical issues to attend school. In addition to nursing shortages as already mentioned, parents may not want to transport the multiple pieces of equipment needed to care for the child back and forth to school every day. The DME Company may be able to provide additional equipment to be kept at school, however, it can be difficult to obtain insurance authorization for this extra equipment.

Parents are often concerned about their children becoming ill or having more frequent illnesses due to being in school around other children who are sick. Parents may request that the child be home-schooled during "cold and flu" season in an attempt to reduce illnesses for their child. It can also be challenging to determine when a child should be in school or kept at home with minor illnesses or when they should return to school after an illness or hospitalization.

Ongoing and good communication are crucial for all of the potential issues for caring for a child in school with a tracheostomy tube. The IEP or 504 plan may need to be updated more frequently than just yearly. Providing for a safe school environment while also providing for the child's education and socialization can be challenging but totally achievable with early planning and teamwork.

58.7 Case Study

Planning for Aleena to attend school was initiated approximately a year prior to her starting school. Aleena is receiving services through the Intermediate Unit (IU) in her county including therapies such as physical, occupational, and speech therapies and preschool education from a teacher. The IU has initiated the plans for transition from IU services to the public-school district. The parents were contacted to set up an initial meeting to initiate planning. This meeting included school district representatives including the Special Education Department, a representative from the State Department of Education, coordinator from the IU, speech language pathologist and the parent. The child was not required to attend the meeting. The parents were informed of Aleena's rights as a student of the district and the state's responsibilities to her in that district. The various elementary schools that might be able to accommodate AD were reviewed as well as an explanation of the testing to be completed. Aleena currently has an IEP through the IU. The team along with the parent discussed the current IEP and changes that might need to be addressed.

Accommodations were made for Aleena to complete her pre-Kindergarten cognitive and social testing at a different time from the other students. She was evaluated by an occupational therapist, physical therapist, speech language pathologist, psychologist, IT specialist and social worker. They not only completed cognitive testing but assessed her physical limitations and needs. The IU also completed a school transition evaluation. The school physical and occupational therapists visited

Aleena's home to better understand what specialized equipment she uses in order to plan for what will be needed for her at school.

A second meeting with the parents occurred in February prior to Aleena starting Kindergarten that included updating her current IEP. Included in Aleena's IEP:

- Nurse will accompany her to school to attend to medical needs
- An aide will be provided for any school related activities
- School district will provide transportation and nurse will accompany
  - She will be transported in her wheelchair
- Medical equipment will travel with Aleena to and from school
- School will provide equipment such as a stander or activity seat
- Diapering will take place in nurse's office
- Gastrostomy tube feeds will be done during school lunch time

The school has offered storage for any supplies that could be kept in school such as spare change of clothing, adaptive equipment or devices that she may need to use, etc. Kindergarten in Aleena's school district is only half day. As she also needs to have her therapies including physical, occupational, and speech therapies during school hours, the district is considering having her attend full day with classroom work occurring with the students and her therapies the other half of the day. As Aleena has no cognitive limitations, her parents are advocating for her to be mainstreamed rather than in a specialized classroom. At this time the school that Aleena will attend has not been determined. The school will need to be able to accommodate her physical needs including wheelchair accommodations to be able to reach all areas of the school.

Aleena's educational journey is just beginning. The consideration for her needs is extensive and will require multiple updates to her IEP. It is a working relationship with the school district, school, and her parents that requires extensive planning and ongoing communication (Fig. 58.1).

Extra Credit point

1. Respiratory emergencies with tracheostomy tubes are often related to mucous obstruction. With any change in child's respiratory status always consider trach tube change if initial steps like suctioning do not fix the problem. When in doubt change it out!!

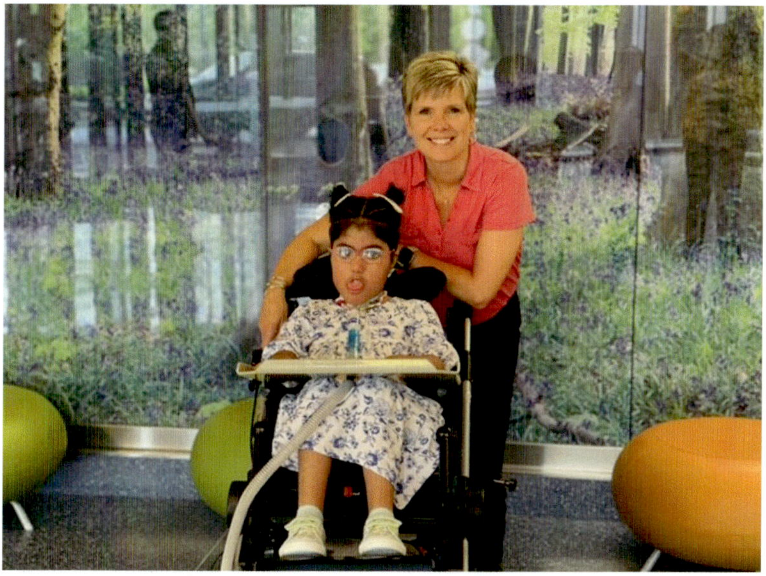

Fig. 58.1 Aleena and Robin Kingston at a recent clinic visit

References

1. Singh A, Zubair A. Pediatric tracheostomy. StatPearls [Internet]. August 17, 2023. Accessed April 21, 2024. https://www.ncbi.nlm.nih.gov/books/NBK560622/.
2. Smith J, Williams J, Gibbin K. Children with a tracheostomy: experience of their careers in school. Child Care Health Dev. 2003;29(4):291–6. https://doi.org/10.1046/j.1365-2214.2003.00344.x.
3. Hornick I. A clinician's how-to guide for sending a child on ventilation to school. Healio. June 6, 2023. Accessed 21 April 2024. https://www.healio.com/news/pulmonology/20230606/a--clinicians-howto-guide-for-sending-a-child-on-ventilation-to-school
4. Care of the child with a chronic tracheostomy. Am J Respir Crit Care Med. 2000;161(1):297–308. https://doi.org/10.1164/ajrccm.161.1.ats1-00.

Chapter 59
Students with Medical Devices: Gastrostomy Tubes

Raul E. Sanchez

Children have frequently required use of gastrostomy tubes, frequently known as "G tubes," for a variety of reasons including providing supplemental nutrition, hydration, medications, or even venting of gas from the stomach. These G tubes have provided easy access to the gastrointestinal (GI) tract for pediatric patients often used in the school setting for various conditions. Some of these conditions include developmental delays, poor weight gain, aspiration, craniofacial abnormalities, vomiting syndromes, and other upper tract abnormalities. [1] Per ESPEN guidelines on artificial enteral nutrition, gastrostomy tube feeding should be considered when nasogastric tube feeding is required for more than 6 weeks. [2] G tubes are seen in as many as 83.7 per 100,000 children. [3] This means that there is a chance of encountering a student with a gastrostomy in your local classroom.

It is important to know that G tubes can be placed surgically or endoscopically in children. [4] There are typically two surgical approaches, open or laparoscopic. An open approach includes a midline incision, while the laparoscopic approach includes two small laparoscopic incisions and one of which is via the umbilicus. One advantage in the past of a surgical approach has been the immediate placement of a "low profile" gastrostomy which will be discussed later with the types of tubes utilized. G tubes can also be placed endoscopically, with one technique is a pull through percutaneous endoscopic gastrostomy (PEG) placement. The advantage of an endoscopic procedure is it being a quick procedure with one small incision made at the insertion site. The disadvantage has been that there has been a long piece of the tube extending out of the patient until the first tube change. Now there can be low profile G tubes placed endoscopically via a push one-step placement. This involves a trochar inserted into the stomach lumen and allows for a dilator to create a stoma wide

R. E. Sanchez (✉)
Division of Gastroenterology, Hepatology, and Nutrition, Nationwide Children's Hospital, Columbus, OH, USA
e-mail: Raul.sanchez@nationwidechildrens.org

R. P. Olympia, J. Brady-Olympia (eds.), *Clinical Considerations in School-based Health*, https://doi.org/10.1007/978-3-031-85765-2_59

enough for a new low profile G tube to be placed. There are 3 fasteners that help anchor the stomach to the anterior abdominal wall. [5] Due to lower complication rate, it can be recommended for endoscopic placement rather than surgical placement. [2, 5]

As mentioned earlier there are a few types of G tubes. The more common type is a low-profile G tube which can have an internal balloon bumper or internal rubber bolster to hold it in place. These tubes are frequently referred to as "buttons" or also known as the brand "Mic-key." The difference between the two is the balloon low profile G tubes are changed every 3–6 months while the internal rubber bolsters are meant to stay in for longer periods of time. There are G tubes with longer external extensions from the patient as well. The standard PEG typically has a plastic internal disk with about 10 cm of tube outside of the patient with an external bumper and angle piece to have the tube typically take a right-angle turn. A "standard" G tube can have a longer external extension and have an internal balloon bumper to anchor the tube internal to the patient and an external disk that can slide along the external extension to allow a snug fit on the abdominal wall, known as "MIC" or "Cor-pak" tubes but these are the brand names/manufacturer. Importantly, balloon bumpers should be filled with water, sterile or tap but not saline, as saline can gradually weaken the balloon and can crystallize leading to difficulty instilling into the port. [4] There are other types of G tubes, but they would infrequently be seen out of the neonatal period and in the school setting. Additionally, some children need feeds or medicines to be given into the small intestine, jejunum, rather than the stomach. These are called GJ (gastrojejunal) tubes. These GJ tubes generally have the same low profile or longer external extension with sliding external disk on the outside of the patient. But the differences of GJ tubes is that there are typically two infusion ports on the outside of the body and a longer extension tube extending into the small intestine on the inside of the child.

G tubes can have a variety of uses for students with them; including providing nutrition, hydration, medications, or venting of gas. Typically, the child should have a feeding plan from their medical team such as the type of feed (formula or blenderized diet), how it is mixed (if needed), the rate the feed should be infused, and the duration of the feed is to be given over. The same type of instructions should be followed if any fluids, water or Pedialyte, are given regarding rate and for how long that is infused into the G tube. Many medications given via a G tube are liquid, but sometimes tablets can be crushed, mixed with water, and given via the tube. Sometimes there are developmentally delayed patients who swallow significant amounts of air, aerophagia, which can lead to abdominal distention, pain, nausea, or vomiting. [6] These patients can have gas vented from their G tube, with an extension tube attached to the G tube, which is connected to an empty syringe. These ventings can be done before a feed or at specified times during the day for the student to improve abdominal distention.

Case 1 You have a 7-year-old male student with a history of cerebral palsy, mild developmental delays, and history of poor weight gain due to picky eating currently with a gastrostomy tube placed about 4 months prior. He typically receives bolus feeds over 1 hour via an enteral pump via his G tube four times

a day with two of those feeds given during the school hours. He receives a blenderized diet, which contains whole foods such as fruits, vegetables, meats, and liquids that have been pureed. [7] As the second feed of the day is being given, their feeding pump continues to alarm due to high pressure and is not infusing. What are some important aspects of this case to note? And what would you do to solve the problem?

59.1 Complications Associated with Gastrostomy Tubes That May Present in the School Setting

There are a few complications of a G tube a clinician in the school setting should be familiar with such as site infection, dislodgement, leakage, bleeding, and clogging. [1, 4, 8, 9] Infection is more frequently encountered in the perioperative setting but can occur at any time and is typically minor. Rates of infection can range from 2%-30%. [1, 5] Findings of infection or peristomal site cellulitis typically include erythema, induration, significant pain at the site, purulent drainage around the site, and rarely fevers. Typically, a course or topical or enteral antibiotics are sufficient for treatment which can be managed in the primary care office or in the urgent care setting. [8, 9] But anytime concern for infection exists, there could be risk for developing sepsis, which is a life-threatening complication of an infection. Anytime there is serious signs such as fatigue, fast heart rate, low blood pressure, fever, hypothermia, chills, rigors, confusion or significant agitation there should be concern for the development of sepsis which would be best initially managed in the emergency department.

Dislodgement can frequently happen in pediatric patients due to how active children are, as well as the rate of G tubes who are placed in neurodevelopmentally delayed children who may pull at the tube without realizing. [10] The tract needs to mature after initial placement so early dislodgement, within 4–6 weeks of primary placement, requires immediate medical attention as there could be injury to the peritoneal cavity with blind placement. [1, 4, 8] This ideally is managed in the emergency department. If after 2–3 months from primary placement, the tube can be replaced immediately if no additional concerns (bleeding at the site or significant pain). [1] If the tube is malfunctioning for some reason, balloon does not inflate and no replacement is available, the tube or a Foley catheter can be placed into the site to hold the stoma site open until medical care is reached urgently. [1, 8] This is done so the opening or stoma of the tract does not close quickly, as some tracts may close within 24 h.

Leakage around the tube is another common issue that is encountered which can lead to skin irritation/breakdown. [9] It can occur due to decreased internal balloon volume, excessive tension or pulling in many different directions, poor fit of the tube, loose bumpers, or granulation tissue. [1, 4, 8, 9] First steps would be evaluating the volume in the balloon if it is still an adequate amount. Next, trying to eliminate the traction forces leading to tension, such as disconnecting the feeding extension from the G tube when student is not receiving feeds. [4] Sometimes layering dressings around the G tube which is thought to help dry the area provides vertical traction, can create pressure injuries to the skin and internal stomach tissue which can make leaks worse. [4] If the external bumper is loose, this can make the tube more mobile leading to leakage, so making sure external bumper is snug but not tight is a good step. [8] If excessive granulation tissue, which is normal part of the healing process with pink or red, irregular, friable and moist tissue, is present it can lead to the G tube not sitting flush in its proper position at the skin level which can lead to leakage. [1, 4] Typically a health care clinician can provide cauterization with silver nitrate to remove the granulation tissue as frequently as every 2–5 days. [1, 8, 9]

Bleeding from the site can be a significant complication. It can be in the perioperative setting or in the delayed setting from ulcerated superficial skin or ulceration of the stomach tissue. [8] Bleeds are quite rare, only occurring in 1% of cases. [11] It is important to know if there is bleeding through the tube or around the tube. Blood seen through the tube indicates the blood is coming from within the gastrointestinal tract, which small amounts are usually tolerated and often require proton pump inhibitor therapy or even sucralfate. [4] Bleeding around the tube is generally from hyper-granulation tissue or mucosal prolapse of stomach tissue. Hyper-granulation tissue appears as a bumpy or cauliflower-like texture versus a more velvet-like texture of mucosal prolapse. [4] The hyper-granulation tissue can be treated with silver nitrate cautery or topical corticosteroid cream, while prolapse is often treated with surgical revision or placing tube at a new site. [4]

Clogging of the G tube is also a common issue. This is especially an issue with the use of blenderized diets due to the increased viscosity of these feeds, thought to be up to 40–200 times the viscosity of typical formulas. [7] Typical prevention includes flushing with water before and after medication or feeding administration. [1, 12] There are reports of carbonated beverages, juices, pancreatic enzymes, and commercial enzymatic agents used but these options seem unreliable and can even make clogging worse in situations. Water is the best de-clogging solution which can be instilled for 20 min before flushing or using a back and forth motion with a syringe plunger to break the clog. [12] If unsuccessful at de-clogging, the G tube may end up needing replaced which can be done at home or at school if replacement G tube is available. [1]

59.2 Returning to the Case

It would be important to note the timing of G tube placement—being 4 months ago, the tract should be matured. But we would also want to know if there has been the first G tube change by the clinician who placed it as that is usually done around 3 months post operatively. The school-based clinician could flush via the infusion port with water and a little pressure to see if that opens the infusion port, could also consider a back and forth motion with a syringe plunger. If still unsuccessful, one could consider replacing the G tube if a replacement is available. Generally, if the tube has been changed before, there does not have to be a dye contrast study to confirm it is located within the stomach. There is data to show that commercial blenderized formulas vary in viscosity and leads to variable amounts being delivered via standard enteral pumps. [13] This variability of amount can lead to more formula left in the line of the tube that can pre-dispose to clogging.

59.3 The Future of Gastrostomy Tubes

While much has advanced in the area of G tubes, there is still room for improvement. The current data on antimicrobial agents and duration for peristomal infections remains variable. There are also further complicated patients who have chronic illness, frequently in the healthcare setting, and more susceptible to multi drug resistant organisms. This is always an area that is ever evolving and improving.

Much is changing with the type of feeds or nutrition that patients receive. There are new formulas on the market such a pea protein based nutrition supplements compared to the typical cow's milk based formulas. The commercialization of blenderized diet has led to many different viscosities that the medical team and subsequently all care takers need to be aware of. [7] There needs to be continued attention to detail of these viscosities to help prevent tube clogging and assuring proper mixture with water to achieve this.

There is also an ever-improving culture of education of parents, guardians, and care takers relating to the medical equipment that they are expected to have some care skills while at home. Current research and development is going on right now leveraging the use of virtual reality to help educate parents and care takers on medical devices such as G tubes, tracheostomy tubes, PICC lines, and other central venous catheters. [14] The hope would be to set the parent in the virtual setting with hands on experience to build the confidence to care for their child with the particular medical device after leaving the support of the inpatient hospital setting.

Extra-Credit Points

1. There are many different types of G tubes with different lengths of time they may remain in
2. G tubes, can have a variety of uses for students with them; including providing nutrition, hydration, medications, or venting of gas
3. Complications of G tubes can include infection, dislodgement, leakage, bleeding, and clogging of the tube (Table 59.1)
4. Care around G tubes for parents, guardians, and care takers is constantly evolving.

Table 59.1 Complications of Gastrostomy tubes

Complication	Signs and symptoms of complication	Disposition from school	Treatment
Infection	Erythema, induration, significant pain at the site, purulent drainage around the site, and rarely fevers	PCP or Urgent care If concern for sepsis with VS changes, would plan for ED evaluation	Enteral or IV antibiotics
Dislodgement	Visualization of the tube out of the tract at abdominal wall	If > 6 weeks—replace the tube and refer to their PCP or the clinician who placed the tube If <6 weeks—replace tube and immediately seek ED care	After replacement of appropriate tube, may need contrast study to evaluate location of tube, especially if the tube has not been changed before
Leakage	Drainage of fluid around G tube, erythematous tissue around tube	PCP	Check water volume in balloon Replace tube Find ways to decease tension on the tube
Bleeding	Blood seen from around tube or coming out of the tube	PCP if stable ED if large amounts of blood seen or if not stable	Proton pump inhibitor Sucralfate Endoscopy
Clogging	Inability to infuse feeds, fluids, or medications into the tube	ED	Flush with water – back and forth motion Next, replace G tube

Abbreviations: *ED* emergency department, *IV* intravenous, *PCP* primary care physician

References

1. Novak I, Velazco NK. Gastrostomy tubes: indications, types, and care. Pediatr Rev. 2024;45:175–87.
2. Bischoff SC, Austin P, Boeykens K, et al. ESPEN practical guideline: home enteral nutrition. Clin Nutr. 2022;41:468–88.
3. Pardy C, Kharma N, Lau R, et al. Point prevalence of gastrostomy in a paediatric population. J Pediatr Gastroenterol Nutr. 2021;72:528–31.
4. Blinman T, Hiller D. Troubleshooting the pediatric gastrostomy. Nutr Clin Pract. 2023;38:240–56.
5. Bitar R, Azaz A, Rawat D, et al. Advances and challenges of gastrostomy insertion in children. World J Gastrointest Surg. 2023;15:1871–8.
6. de Jesus LE, Cestari AB, Filho OC, et al. Aerofagia patológica: uma causa rara de distensão abdominal crônica [Pathologic aerophagia: a rare cause of chronic abdominal distension]. Rev Paul Pediatr. 2015;33:372–6.
7. Chandrasekar N, Dehlsen K, Leach ST, et al. Exploring clinical outcomes and feasibility of blended tube feeds in children. JPEN J Parenter Enteral Nutr. 2021;45:685–98.
8. Abdelfattah T, Kaspar M. Gastroenterologist's guide to gastrostomies. Dig Dis Sci. 2022;67:3488–96.

9. Rahnemai-Azar AA, Rahnemaiazar AA, Naghshizadian R, et al. Percutaneous endoscopic gastrostomy: indications, technique, complications and management. World J Gastroenterol. 2014;20:7739–51.
10. Backman E, Sjögreen L. Gastrostomy tube insertion in children with developmental or acquired disorders: a register-based study. Dev Med Child Neurol. 2020;62:1191–7.
11. Rajan A, Wangrattanapranee P, Kessler J, et al. Gastrostomy tubes: Fundamentals, periprocedural considerations, and best practices. World J Gastrointest Surg. 2022;14:286–303.
12. Boullata JI, Carrera AL, Harvey L, et al. ASPEN safe practices for enteral nutrition therapy. JPEN J Parenter Enteral Nutr. 2017;41:15–103.
13. Murayi JA, Evenson E, Verkin-Siebert D, et al. Thickness of commercial blenderized formulas adversely affects successful delivery via enteral feeding pumps. Nutr Clin Pract. 2023;38:1354–9.
14. CHOC partners buzzing about new virtual reality app that will teach parents about their child's surgical devices. Choc.org. https://care.choc.org/choc-partners-buzzing-about-new-virtual-reality-app-that-will-teach-parents-about-their-childs-surgical-devices/. May 18, 2021. Accessed: May 5, 2024.

Chapter 60
Students with Central Venous Access Devices (CVADs)

Catherine Considine and Christy Lucas

Central venous access devices (CVADs) are intravenous (IV) lines that are inserted into large veins. These devices are essential for the treatment of children with chronic health conditions, including cancer, short-gut syndrome, and blood disorders. They are often utilized to administer IV nutrition, fluids, or medications. When a CVAD is indicated, a multi disciplinary conversation will occur to determine which line is best for the patient (Table 60.1 and Fig. 60.1). Factors to consider when discussing the type of line can include: diagnosis, length of treatment, weight, and developmental age. A central venous catheter (CVC) or line (CVL), as well as a peripheral inserted catheter (PICC), may be considered more frequently for patients who require multiple access points, as these devices can be extended from a single lumen up to a triple lumen. As the number of entry portals increases, however, the risk of complications and infections also increases [1]. Pediatric patients will almost always have CVADs placed under general anesthesia or heavy sedation. When treatment is complete, the line is no longer needed, or complications of the line put the patient in great danger, the line will be removed in a similar fashion to how it was placed. PICC lines are the one exception, as they can often be removed by bedside nurses at most institutions.

C. Considine
Dana-Farber Cancer Institute, Boston, MA, USA
e-mail: catherine_considine@dfci.harvard.edu

C. Lucas (✉)
Dana-Farber Cancer Institute/Boston Children's Cancer and Blood Disorders Center, Boston, MA, USA
e-mail: christym_lucas@dfci.harvard.edu

R. P. Olympia, J. Brady-Olympia (eds.), *Clinical Considerations in School-based Health*, https://doi.org/10.1007/978-3-031-85765-2_60

Table 60.1 Descriptions and Diagrams of Common Central Venous Access Devices (CVADs)

Line Type	Description	Other Common Names
Central Venous Catheter (CVC) or Central Venous Line (CVL)	Inserted into the internal jugular or subclavian vein; can be tunneled or non-tunneled, extending into the superior vena cava (SVC) at the confluence of the right atrium. They can have one, two, or three lumens.	Broviac® or Hickman®
Peripherally Inserted Catheter (PICC)	Inserted into the basilic, brachial, or cephalic vein in the arm, extending into the superior vena cava (SVC) at the confluence of the right atrium. They can have one, two, or three lumens.	
Implanted Port	Inserted under the skin with a catheter extending into the superior vena cava (SVC) at the confluence of the right atrium.	Mediport, Port-a-Cath, Powerport

Case 1 Grace is an 11-year-old girl undergoing treatment for leukemia, who comes to your office today for a fever. She has a central line, specifically a right chest implanted port. You check her temperature, which is 102.3°F orally. She has mild tachycardia to 110 beats per minute (bpm) with a normal blood pressure for age of 98/60 mmHg. Her peripheral perfusion is normal with a capillary refill of <2 s. Her mental status is normal; she is alert and talkative, denying pain. What do you do next?

Though fevers are often a sign of infection in all children, a fever in an oncology patient is a medical emergency. Fevers may be the only sign of infection, and for those undergoing chemotherapy, it can be life-threatening. It is important to know fever criteria and to follow the specific algorithm laid out by the patient's care team. Generally speaking, one temperature above 100.4°F (38 °C) is significant enough to seek additional support. For children with CVADs (in this case, an implanted port), it is crucial to suspect an infection until proven otherwise. Patients with a new fever must present to the emergency department (ED) where they will obtain a blood culture and receive antibiotics within 60 min of the first fever [2]. Each hospital has specific guidelines when triaging a pediatric oncology patient with fever, however blood cultures are often obtained from *all* points of access. Broad-spectrum antibiotics (e.g., cefepime) with coverage of key, life-threatening bacteria, are then given through the CVAD and have been shown to be the best therapeutic and preventive approach to bacterial infections for those ill-appearing or presenting with fever [3]. While the antibiotic is infusing through the CVAD, the ED will obtain labs closely to monitor the white blood cell count (WBC), the absolute neutrophil count (ANC), procalcitonin, and c-reactive protein (CRP), all of which help diagnose and risk stratify sepsis [4]. Though it is standard to give acetaminophen (Tylenol) to most pediatric patients, oncology patients should not receive antipyretics until a comprehensive fever work-up is completed. Oncology patients should also never receive non-steroidal anti-inflammatories (NSAIDs) such as ibuprofen (Motrin, Advil) or naproxen (Aleeve) given anti-platelet effects that increase risk for bleeding.

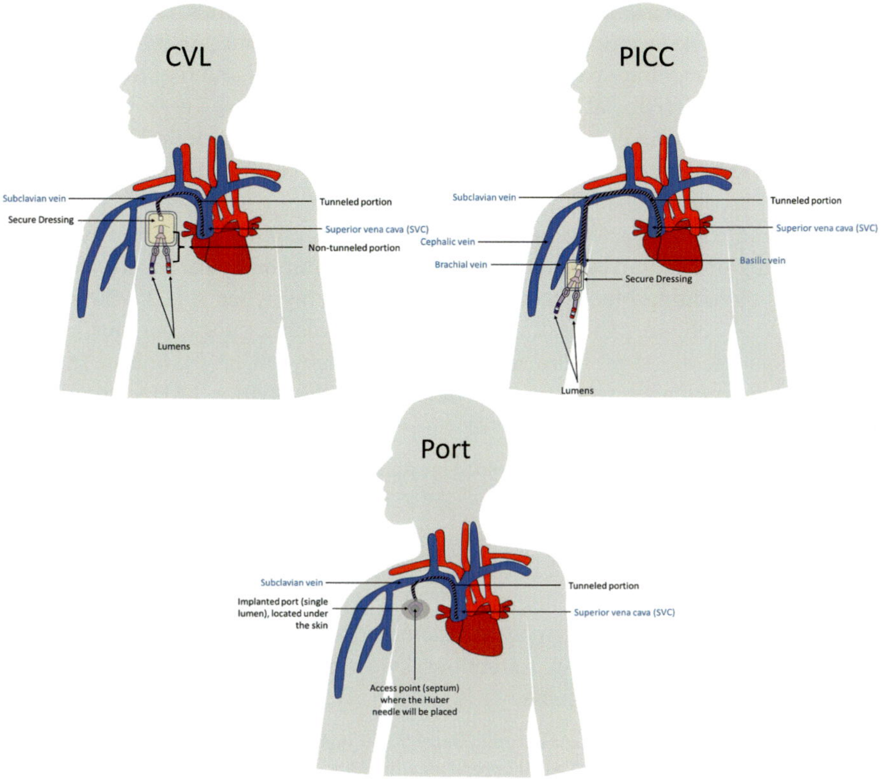

Fig. 60.1 Examples of common CVADs and anatomical positions (internal and external). *Graphics created by Christy Lucas, MD*

In Your Office Grace is presenting with a high-grade fever. Contact her parent/caregiver to ensure that she can be seen in the ED for further evaluation. While awaiting pick-up, continue to monitor for any change in vital signs or signs of distress. Do not administer Tylenol or any additional antipyretics. Due to the fact that Grace only has a single lumen port, she will have one blood culture drawn and antibiotics must be administered within 60 minutes.

Case 2 Ace is a 15-year-old boy undergoing treatment for leukemia, who comes to your office today for chills. He has a central line, specifically a right chest implanted port. You check his temperature, which is 101.8°F orally. He looks pale. He is tachycardic to 160bpm, tachypneic to 30 breaths per minute, with an oxygen saturation of 93% on room air. The highest blood pressure you can obtain is 80/50 mmHg. His peripheral perfusion is not normal with a prolonged nail bed capillary refill of 5 s. He responds to voice but seems to be falling asleep in your office. What do you do next?

Even if you are in a small nurse's office with minimal supplies, rely on the basic yet key indicators of an emergency: vital signs and presentation. As previously mentioned, fevers in oncology patients are a medical emergency and require immediate intervention. Though facial coloring can often be subjective, it is important to remember that coloring can be indicative of anemia: a laboratory finding reflecting a decrease in the number of red blood cells. Frequently, children with cancer may be anemic after receiving chemotherapy as their bone marrow is suppressed post treatment. Anemia requires prompt medical attention and often a blood transfusion. A child's hemoglobin is lowest on average 7–10 days after he or she receives chemotherapy. As circulating blood volume decreases, notably when it is 25–30% of the effective blood volume, patients can enter into hypovolemic shock, demonstrated by a drop in systolic blood pressure accompanied by tachycardia [5]. Follow standard blood pressure guidance from the American Heart Association (AHA) to evaluate and monitor for hypotension.

Hypotension is defined by the *systolic* blood pressure less than the 5th percentile of normal for age: <70 mm Hg + (2× age in years) in children 1–10 years of age and <90 mm Hg in children ≥10 years of age [6].

The lack of oxygen-rich blood circulating throughout the body may also lead to respiratory distress, displayed in a number of ways including but not limited to: an increased breathing rate (tachypnea), increased heart rate (tachycardia), color changes, grunting, nasal flaring, retractions, sweating, wheezing, stridor, accessory muscle use, or change in alertness.

To assess tachycardia, follow AHA guidelines: >140 beats per minute (bpm) for school aged children (2–10 years) and >100 bpm in an adult [6].

Though a capillary refill time alone is not a foolproof indicator of circulatory volume, assessing such is a quick and easy way to monitor dehydration and oxygen perfusion.

A capillary refill time >2 s is notable for further action according to the AHA [6].

In Your Office Immediately upon seeing Ace, your gut instinct is correct: he needs help. Remain calm, and obtain baseline vital signs. Use the algorithm outlined by the AHA to determine that not only is he febrile, but he is also hypotensive and tachycardic. In this case, you have a pulse oximeter and determine his oxygen saturation is 93% on room air. However, if you did not have this device, the initial presentation consisting of an increased respiratory rate and extended capillary refill time alone is indicative that Ace is not getting enough oxygen. Knowing Ace's vital signs, coupled with his inability to maintain a conversation and the presence of a CVAD (an implanted port in this case), you must call 911 immediately, followed by a call to his parent/caregiver; you are worried that Ace is septic. If possible, administer oxygen via nasal cannula to assist with his work of breathing as you wait for further instruction from the paramedics. Upon arriving to the hospital, the medical team will access his implanted port, obtain blood cultures, collect lab work, administer antibiotics within 60 minutes of initial fever, and provide supportive care consisting of: oxygen, antipyretics, and fluid resuscitation. As lab work begins to result, the team will note that Ace has a low hemoglobin, which you expected based on his facial coloring and timing of his last chemotherapy treatment. He will receive a red blood cell transfusion and be admitted to the hospital for further monitoring.

Case 3 Holly is an 18-year-old young woman undergoing treatment for Hodgkin lymphoma. She has a PICC line in her left arm. She is an avid basketball player and comes to your office today for concerns of swelling in her left arm. She has not had any recent trauma, and she denies numbness or tingling. She notes a feeling of "tightness." Holly overall has preserved range of motion, but her left bicep, forearm, and hand are noticeably swollen in comparison to her right. There is not overlying redness. Her PICC dressing site appears clean. Her arm feels warm to the touch. Holly asks you if she can have some acetaminophen so that she can return to practice and promises to tell her mother later. What do you do next?

Many patients undergoing treatment for Hodgkin lymphoma will often have a peripherally inserted catheter (PICC) as the primary access for therapy. Though PICCs are more "external" than an implanted port, they come with similar risk factors. PICCs specifically can cause blood clots to form inside the vein. For that reason, there are often detailed notes from the care team with instructions of how to flush the line with either saline or heparin. Clots can be divided into two categories: superficial vein thrombosis (SVT) and deep vein thrombosis (DVT). SVTs appear in the smaller surface veins (superficial) of the upper arm, forearm, and hand. DVTs appear in the larger deeper veins, frequently in the veins above the elbow that extend in the internal jugular vein in the neck. Though there can be general irritation or inflammation from initial insertion of a PICC, any change in appearance should be noted and taken seriously. If patients experience discomfort, redness, tenderness, and/or swelling over the affected vein, a clot workup should be completed in the ED [7]. After diagnosing a thrombus by a duplex ultrasound and evaluating coagulation factors, including a D-dimer [8], pediatric patients are often started on anticoagulation therapy (i.e., a blood thinner). Current recommendations indicate low-molecular weight heparin such as enoxaparin (Lovenox) for three to six months, the timeline often dictated by location of the clot, cause of the clot, and symptomatic improvement vs. progression. For those who fail to respond to anticoagulation, additional thrombolytic therapy may be pursued. CVAD removal may be indicated if the patient fails to respond to treatment and/or symptoms progress.

All patients with a thrombus are at a higher risk of developing a pulmonary embolism, which is the result of a clot that detaches and travels through the venous blood stream into the pulmonary artery tree. Though patients may remain asymptomatic, they often present with shortness of breath, chest pain, and/or bloody cough [9]. Due to this risk, patients are watched very closely in a hospital setting to confirm continued free exchange of oxygen and carbon dioxide.

In Your Office Though Holly is an independent 18-year-old, who is responsible for the saline and heparin locking of her PICC, her presence already in your office

Table 60.2 Touch, Look, Compare Method

TLC METHOD	
TOUCH	Is the area warm, soft, dry, pain-free?
LOOK	Is the dressing dry and intact? Is the coloring normal?
COMPARE	Compare one extremity to the other to ensure similar size and no swelling.

should trigger you to think twice about why she is requesting Tylenol. Though she is adamant to return to basketball practice, perform a thorough assessment using the "**TLC: Touch, Look, Compare**" method. (Table 60.2) Despite the fact that her range of motion is consistent in both arms, you take special note of the swelling, tightness, and warmth. You inform her that she will need to skip practice today, call her healthcare team, and go to the hospital for a further work-up, likely consisting of an ultrasound to evaluate for a venous blood clot. You take a set of vital signs to confirm no fever, and administer Tylenol to aid with the discomfort. You also encourage elevation and warm compresses to aid in symptom relief.

Holly is sent to the ED, and after completing the ultrasound, her team confirms a DVT requiring anticoagulation therapy. She is admitted to the floor for initiation of low-molecular weight heparin and monitoring. In Holly's case, she is started on the subcutaneous injection, enoxaparin (Lovenox), which she will continue for the next several weeks. She will continue the injections at home and will be instructed to closely monitor for additional signs of thrombocytopenia (low platelet levels).

Case 4 Pete, a 6-year-old boy in kindergarten undergoing treatment for relapsed neuroblastoma, was enjoying recess with his friends. He fell from the swings, and part of his central line, a double lumen tunneled line in his left chest, cracked off. What do you do next?

Many patients being treated for neuroblastoma will have two points of access, i.e., either a double port or a double lumen tunneled Broviac. This allows many different medications to be given simultaneously, which is vital in treatment. Though Broviacs are helpful in a medical setting, they are challenging for families to manage at home, especially for school age children. Despite it being an "internally" placed catheter, the majority of the device is external. Parents and caregivers need to be mindful of what activities their child can safely participate in and also minimize any activities that would cause the dressing to become wet or soiled. Like most CVADs, Broviacs are made up of a catheter, a clamp (to open and close access), an access cap, an insertion site, and a dressing to cover and protect the tube. Given the many different components, it is crucial to be aware of how to troubleshoot complications. The school nurse should be equipped and familiar with an emergency kit specific to the child's line which would include items such as: gloves, mask, extra dressing, tape, sterile gauze, alcohol wipes, and a clamp [10]. As always, hand

Table 60.3 Troubleshooting CVAD Complications [5]

Complication	Action
Line is pulled out	The child will likely be bleeding. Remain calm and apply pressure with gauze to the line insertion site and apply pressure directly above the site on the side of the neck. Hold pressure for a minimum of 10 min to stop the bleeding. Contact the child's parents/caregivers.
Dressing is loose or lifting	If the edges are lifting, reinforce with additional Tegaderm or tape. If the dressing comes off completely, change the dressing using sterile technique if educated properly and comfortable. Inform the child's parents/caregivers of actions.
The cap falls off the line	Ensure the clamp is closed. Scrub the end of the line for 15 s, being careful not to push any debris into the line. Place a new cap back onto the line. Contact the child's parents/caregivers.
CVAD line breaks, is cut, or cracks	The child will be likely be bleeding. Remain calm. Take out the clamps (that mimic scissors) and secure the line above the break (closer to the child's body). Clean the broken area with an alcohol swap, wrap the end of the line with sterile gauze and secure with tape. Contact the child's parents/ caregivers.

hygiene should be performed prior to any interventions with CVAD's and the patient should seek further medical care immediately. Refer to Table 60.3 for case-by-case situations.

In Your Office

Knowing that Pete will likely be very scared, remain calm and obtain the CVAD emergency kit. Perform proper hand-hygiene. Depending on the area of breakage, he may be bleeding. If he is bleeding, clamp the line above the breakage point, clean the broken area with an alcohol swab, wrap the end of the line with sterile gauze, and secure with tape. Contact the child's parents/caregivers and inform them that Pete will need to be immediately in the ED for his line break.

Extra Credit Points

- Fevers may be a sign of a serious infection for those undergoing chemotherapy or other cancer treatment and are a medical emergency.
- Though vital signs are a simple act that you can complete in the office, they often give great meaning to a patient's presentation. Pediatric oncology patients have a tendency to need transfusions (i.e., blood and platelets) throughout their treatment, but they can also be hypovolemic due to shock. Act quickly on any altered vital signs you notice on exam.
- PICCs are known to cause small clots that can sometimes escalate to SVT's and DVT's. Use the **TLC method** to monitor the site and act quickly with any change or concern.
- Though CVADs are well secured, children are accident-prone and complications can arise. Be sure to familiarize yourself with the emergency kit supplied by the family and review proper steps specific to the child, his/her line, and institutional guidelines.

References

1. Huang H, Chang Q, Zhou Y, Liao L. Risk factors of central catheter bloodstream infections in intensive care units: A systematic review and meta-analysis. PLoS One. 2024;19(4):e0296723. Published 2024 Apr 23. https://doi.org/10.1371/journal.pone.0296723.
2. Lehrnbecher T, Robinson P, Fisher B, et al. Guideline for the management of fever and neutropenia in children with cancer and hematopoietic stem-cell transplantation recipients: 2017 update. J Clin Oncol. 2017;35(18):2082–94. https://doi.org/10.1200/JCO.2016.71.7017.
3. Boeriu E, Borda A, Vulcanescu DD, et al. Diagnosis and management of febrile neutropenia in pediatric oncology patients-A systematic review. Diagnostics (Basel). 2022;12(8):1800. Published 2022 July 25. https://doi.org/10.3390/diagnostics12081800
4. Pierrakos C, Velissaris D, Bisdorff M, Marshall JC, Vincent JL. Biomarkers of sepsis: time for a reappraisal. Crit Care. 2020;24(1) https://doi.org/10.1186/s13054-020-02993-5.
5. Levy MM, Fink MP, Marshall JC, et al. 2001 SCCM/ESICM/ACCP/ATS/SIS international sepsis definitions conference. Crit Care Med. 2003;31(4):1250–6. https://doi.org/10.1097/01.CCM.0000050454.01978.3B.
6. Part 12: Pediatric Advanced Life Support. Circulation. 2005;112(24_suppl):IV-167IV-187. https://doi.org/10.1161/circulationaha.105.166573
7. Evans NS, Ratchford EV. Catheter-related venous thrombosis. Vasc Med. 2018;23(4):411–3. https://doi.org/10.1177/1358863x18779695.
8. Audu CO, Wakefield TW, Coleman DM. Pediatric deep venous thrombosis. J Vasc Surg Venous Lymphatic Disord. 2019;7(3):452–62. https://doi.org/10.1016/j.jvsv.2018.12.012.
9. Wenger N, Sebastian T, Engelberger RP, Kucher N, Spirk D. Pulmonary embolism and deep vein thrombosis: similar but different. Thrombosis Res. 2021;206:88–98. https://doi.org/10.1016/j.thromres.2021.08.015.
10. Corrigan ML, Huang S, Weaver A, et al. Resources for the provision of nutrition support to children in educational environments. Nutr Clin Pract. 2017;32(6):834–43. https://doi.org/10.1177/0884533617718471.

Chapter 61
Tics and Tourette Syndrome

Jaclyn Tencer and Debra Byler

Case 1 A 9-year-old boy presents to your office for abnormal movements. He has a history of Attention- deficit/hyperactivity disorder (ADHD) for which he has an Individualized Education Plan (IEP) in school. For the last month, his family and teachers have noted that he is frequently blinking his eyes and clearing his throat. It does not seem to bother him significantly however classmates and teachers have been asking him about this. What should you do?

Tics are unintentional, repetitive, stereotyped, movements or sounds that people make. The exact cause of tic disorders is unknown. Tics can be classified as motor tics (such as blinking, sniffing, moving their face or head, shoulder shrugs, etc.) or as vocal tics (grunting, whistling, expressing words). Sniffing or throat clearing can be a type of tic and may be mistaken for allergies. Tics can also be classified as simple or complex depending on the quality of the movements or vocalizations. Of note, one form of vocal tic known as coprolalia which consists of patients shouting out swear words is often what people associate with tics and Tourette syndrome (TS), however this tends to be quite rare. Tics may be referred to as "semi-voluntary" as some patients may be able to briefly suppress the movements, however many patients are unable to do so and there is often significant discomfort associated with the temporary suppression. There are various tic disorders which vary based on the type of tics and the duration of symptoms (Table 61.1) [1].

The true incidence of tic disorders in the population is very challenging to measure as a substantial percentage of patients with tics go undiagnosed. Some studies have suggested that 1 in 50 children aged 5–14 years old may be affected by persistent tic disorders (including TS) [2] and others have noted transient tic disorder affecting about 3% of children [3]. Tics often begin around 5–10 years of age. The

J. Tencer (✉) · D. Byler
Penn State Children's Hospital, Hershey, PA, USA
e-mail: jtencer@pennstatehealth.psu.edu; dbyler@pennstatehealth.psu.edu

R. P. Olympia, J. Brady-Olympia (eds.), *Clinical Considerations in School-based Health*, https://doi.org/10.1007/978-3-031-85765-2_61

Table 61.1 Spectrum of Tic Disorders

Provisional/Transient Tic Disorder	Persistent (Chronic) Motor or Vocal Tic Disorder	Tourette Syndrome
• Have motor and/or vocal tics • Symptoms have been present for <1 year • Tics started <18 years old	• Have motor OR vocal tics- but not both • Symptoms have been present >1 year • Tics started <18 years old	• Have at least 2 motor tics AND at least 1 vocal tics (don't have to be at the same time just over the course of the patient's life) • Symptoms have been present >1 year • Tics started <18 years old

types and characteristics of the tics may change over time and often have a waxing and waning quality with periods of increased symptoms intermixed with periods of relative quiescence. In most cases, tics improve during adolescence and often fully resolve by adulthood however some patients may have ongoing symptoms [4].

Comorbidities: It has become very clear over time that for many patients, tics are merely one symptom of a broader neurodevelopmental disorder. Comorbid ADHD and Obsessive compulsive disorder (OCD) is quite common for patients with tics and in patients with Tourette Syndrome, higher rates of anxiety, oppositional defiant disorder (ODD) and mood disorders have been found [5]. It is crucial to evaluate for and treat these conditions as this may also have secondary benefit on tic severity. In addition, the morbidity from the associated conditions may be much greater than that from tics and treatment may need to be focused on the psychiatric symptoms.

Evaluation: Most of the time laboratory testing, brain imaging and EEG testing are not needed for the diagnosis. A video of the movements in question or seeing the movements during a visit are often the most helpful tools for the medical professional evaluating the child. If there is a typical time course and pattern, further testing is not typically done. A medical evaluation is indicated to confirm the diagnosis, assess the severity of symptoms and screen for comorbidities. Management of tics can be done by a primary care physician, neurologist or psychiatrist depending on the severity and comorbidities and on the provider's comfort and scope. In neurology clinic, some patients are referred immediately at the onset of a tic diagnosis while others are referred following unsuccessful treatment trials carried out by the primary provider. It often depends on the comfort and expertise of the PCP and both options can be appropriate. A psychiatric or neuropsychological evaluation for comorbid conditions is often appropriate.

Treatment: Treatment for tic disorders is not required and should be initiated specifically for patients whose tics are causing functional, physical or significant social challenges. When it comes to medications there is no clear evidence that earlier treatment has a better long-term outcome so treatment decisions should be symptom based. Many patients do not treat their tics. When it comes to treatment there are three main categories which include Cognitive Behavioral Therapy, specifically Cognitive Behavioral Intervention for Tics (CBIT), medications, and procedural/surgical options in refractory cases.

- Cognitive Behavioral Intervention for Tics (CBIT)
  - CBIT is a specific therapeutic program consisting of habit reversal training (HRT), relaxation and cognitive training. For patients who are able to trial this and can find a trained provider, this can be a very positive treatment with benefits over medications which come with inherent potential for side effects. The American Academy of Neurology (ANN) published a practice guideline for treatment of tics and stated that "For people with tics who have access to CBIT, clinicians should offer CBIT as an initial treatment option relative to medication" [6].
- Medications
  - The goal of treatment is to improve quality of life as elimination of all tics may not be possible. While the FDA approved treatments for Tourette Syndrome are in the antipsychotic group, the usual approach is to try medications with fewer potential side effects first such as alpha 2 agonists or topiramate. (Table 61.2).
- Procedural/Surgical Treatment Options
  - Botulinum Toxin Injections may be appropriate for patients with localized and problematic motor tics and possibly aggressive vocal tics [6].
  - Deep Brain Stimulation (DBS) may be considered in patients with severe tics who have been refractory to other treatment trials.

Differential Diagnosis: While most often classic tics do not require further workup as described above, there are rare alternatives to consider should the tics have unusual features or the patient have other clinical findings. Here are red flags that might prompt additional referral or testing (Table 61.3).

Another topic that comes up in regards to tics is PANS (Pediatric Acute-onset Neuropsychiatric Syndrome or PANDAS (Pediatric Acute-onset Neuropsychiatric Disorders Associated with Streptococcus) These terms are used to describe a constellation of sudden onset symptoms typically involving behavioral and psychiatric changes, at times with associated movement disorder, thought to occur following a Streptococcus infection. There is significant controversy about the mechanism of this symptom complex, and the treatment is typically symptom based. Immunologic therapies have been proposed, but are yet to be proven as the standard of care for treatment [7].

Table 61.2 Medication Options for Tics

Category	Typical Medication Choices	Notable Side Effects
Alpha-2 Agonists	Clonidine or Guanfacine	Sedation, hypotension, bradycardia, QTc prolongation
Anti-Seizure medications	Topiramate	Cognitive challenges, weight loss, increased risk of renal stones
Antipsychotic medications	Risperidone, Ariprazole, Pimozide among others	Weight gain, extrapyramidal signs, QT prolongation, hormonal effects

Table 61.3 Red flags for students presenting with tics that require referral or testing

Symptom	Possible Alternative Diagnosis
Additional movement disorders other than tics (tremor, dystonia, etc.)	Alternative pediatric movement disorder
Temporal relationship with medications	Tics as a medication side effect
Other systemic symptoms such as liver, kidney, ocular disease	Rare genetic conditions (Wilson's disease, metabolic disease, etc.)
Associated asymmetric weakness	Structural cause (i.e. remote stroke)
Tics are specifically eye flutter seen with eye closure or quick body jerks	Epilepsy with eyelid Myoclonia or myoclonic epilepsy
Movements are provoked by change in position or action	Paroxysmal kinesigenic dyskinesia (PKD)

Case 2 A 14-year-old girl presents to your office for abnormal movements. They seemed to start acutely yesterday with near constant arm flailing, clicking, vocalizations and difficulty walking due to frequent sudden jerking movements. When distracted by being on her phone when the provider leaves the room the movements seem to stop and restart when the provider re-enters the room. In gathering history you learn that she has seen other kids on social media who have similar symptoms to her. What should you do?

An important condition to keep in the differential diagnosis for patients who present with abnormal movements is Functional Tic-Like Disorder, a form of Functional Neurologic Disorder (FND). FND also known as conversion disorder, or psychogenic symptoms, describes a group of conditions that manifest with varying neurologic symptoms that lack a clear underlying physical basis and often have a close tie to psychologic processes and mental health. Functional movement disorders are one of the most common causes of movement disorders in children and adolescents [8].

Notably, since the COVID-19 pandemic, providers in several countries concomitantly have seen a significant rise in the frequency of adolescents presenting with acute functional tic-like behaviors. Many of these patients had been exposed to social media content of others manifesting functional tics as well [8]. While the movements are not thought to be under voluntary control, there is often significant psychological comorbidity.

Differentiating tics from functional tic-like disorder can be a significant challenge (Table 61.4). One especially nebulous feature is that some patients may have both tics and functional movement disorder. While every patient is unique and these patterns do not apply to all presentations, there are some factors which may help the provider assess these diagnoses when seeing a patient [8–10].

When a patient presents with functional movement disorder, psychologic intervention is the appropriate treatment.

Table 61.4 Tics vs Functional Movement Disorders

	Tic Movement Disorder	Functional Movement Disorder
Onset	– Gradual onset	– Abrupt and explosive onset.
Pattern	– Typically present with simple motor or vocal tics – Typically begin around 5–10 years old	– Often present with complex tics- often flailing, significant vocal tics, sometimes with self-injurious behavior or large functional limitations, sometimes leading to patients presenting to the ER – Age of onset is often older than that for tics
Variability	Even though stress or different environments may act as a trigger, tics often wax and wane	Symptoms may cease when the patient is distracted or is not being knowingly observed
Suppressibility	Often with great focus, movements can be temporarily suppressed	Patients often will not be able to suppress the movements when asked

61.1 Case Conclusions

Case 1: This boy is diagnosed with Transient Tic Disorder. Given that the symptoms do not seem to bother him, his provider makes a plan to keep clinically monitoring without targeted treatment at this time. The provider suggests that his family talk to his teachers to make sure they are all on the same page and that the teachers can monitor symptoms but that tics will not be given unnecessary attention and if any classmates seem to be bullying the patient, this can be addressed. The provider discussed with the family that if tics become more prominent or bothersome, a trial of CBIT could be tried and if there is no improvement and tics are causing significant issues, then guanfacine or clonidine can be trialed. Support and treatment for ADHD should continue.

Case 2: This patient and her family are counseled that functional tic-like disorder appears most likely at this time. The provider talks to the patient and her family, screening for underlying anxiety, depression or other psychiatric symptoms. The provider stresses the importance of establishing care with a psychologist and supports them as they begin therapy.

Extra Credit Points

1. Tics are very common in the pediatric population
2. Tourette Syndrome criteria are
   (a) The person has had at least 2 motor tics and 1 vocal tic at some point
   (b) Symptoms have been present for >1 year
   (c) Symptoms started <18 years of age
3. Tics only need to be treated if they are causing functional, physical or significant social challenges and if treated, it is important to consider CBIT as a first line followed by alpha-2 agonists or Topiramate

4. Patients with Tics and Tourette Syndrome are at high risk of other comorbidities such as ADHD, OCD and anxiety for which screening and treatment is crucial and may help tics
5. Functional tic-like disorder is a common diagnosis to consider in patients presenting with abnormal movements.

References

1. Tourette Syndrome. Updated May 31, 2023. Accessed April 8, 2024. https://www.cdc.gov/ncbddd/tourette/diagnosis.html.
2. Tinker SC, Bitsko RH, Danielson ML, Newsome K, Kaminski JW. Estimating the number of people with Tourette syndrome and persistent tic disorder in the United States. Psychiatry Res. 2022;314:114684.
3. Knight T, Steeves T, Day L, Lowerison M, Jette N, Pringsheim T. Prevalence of tic disorders: a systematic review and meta-analysis. Pediatr Neurol. 2012;47(2):77–90.
4. Groth C, Mol Debes N, Rask CU, Lange T, Skov L. Course of Tourette syndrome and comorbidities in a large prospective clinical study. J Am Acad Child Adolesc Psychiatry. 2017;56(4):304–12.
5. Hirschtritt ME, Lee PC, Pauls DL, et al. Lifetime prevalence, age of risk, and genetic relationships of comorbid psychiatric disorders in Tourette syndrome. JAMA Psychiatry. 2015;72(4):325–33.
6. Pringsheim T, Okun MS, Müller-Vahl K, et al. Practice guideline recommendations summary: treatment of tics in people with Tourette syndrome and chronic tic disorders. Neurology. 2019;92(19):896–906.
7. Gilbert DL. Inflammation in tic disorders and obsessive-compulsive disorder: are PANS and PANDAS a path forward? J Child Neurol. 2019;34(10):598–611.
8. Amorelli G, Martino D, Pringsheim T. Rapid onset functional tic-like disorder outbreak: a challenging differential diagnosis in the COVID-19 pandemic. J Can Acad Child Adolesc Psychiatry. 2022;31(3):144–51.
9. Chouksey A, Pandey S. Functional movement disorders in children. Front Neurol. 2020;11:570151.
10. Garone G, Graziola F, Grasso M, Capuano A. Acute movement disorders in childhood. J Clin Med. 2021;10(12):2671.

Chapter 62
Weight Management and Nutrition

Corey McBrayer

While 'you are what you eat' is not entirely true, nutrition is a key player in childhood and adolescent development. Healthy nutrition and physical activity during the school-age years set the trajectory for the rest of a child's life. Around 20% of 5–19-year-olds are affected by obesity in the United States. Obesity and its sequelae disproportionately affect Black and Hispanic children (up to 25%) [1]. Adolescents with obesity become adults with obesity in over 80% of cases [2]. Obesity is a multi-factorial disease, and it is important that it is treated within a chronic disease framework [1].

62.1 The Growth Chart

Body mass index (BMI) can be calculated with the following formula: $BMI = \frac{Weight(kg)}{Height(m)^2}$. Although adult BMI does not always accurately reflect body composition (for example, Arnold Schwarzenegger had a BMI of 30 at his peak fitness, placing him within the obese range [3]), for the pediatric population the CDC has developed accurate height, weight, and BMI charts allowing practitioners to compare children across the US population (Figs. 62.1 and 62.2).

C. McBrayer (✉)
Penn State Health Medical Center, Hershey, PA, USA
e-mail: cmcbrayer@pennstatehealth.psu.edu

R. P. Olympia, J. Brady-Olympia (eds.), *Clinical Considerations in School-based Health*, https://doi.org/10.1007/978-3-031-85765-2_62

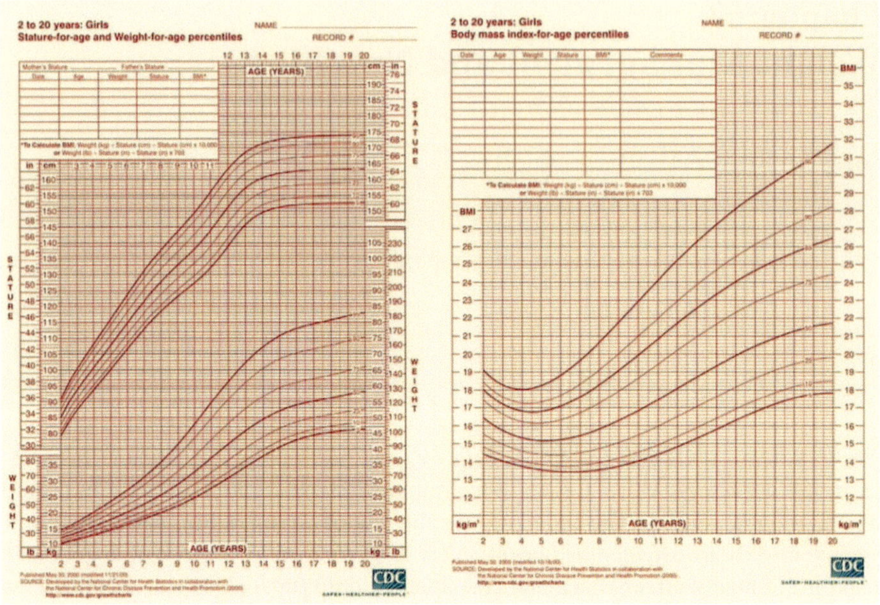

Fig. 62.1 Height, weight, and BMI percentiles for girls [4]. (Adapted from: Centers for Disease Control and Prevention, National Center for Health Statistics. CDC growth charts: United States. http://www.cdc.gov/growthcharts/. May 30, 2000)

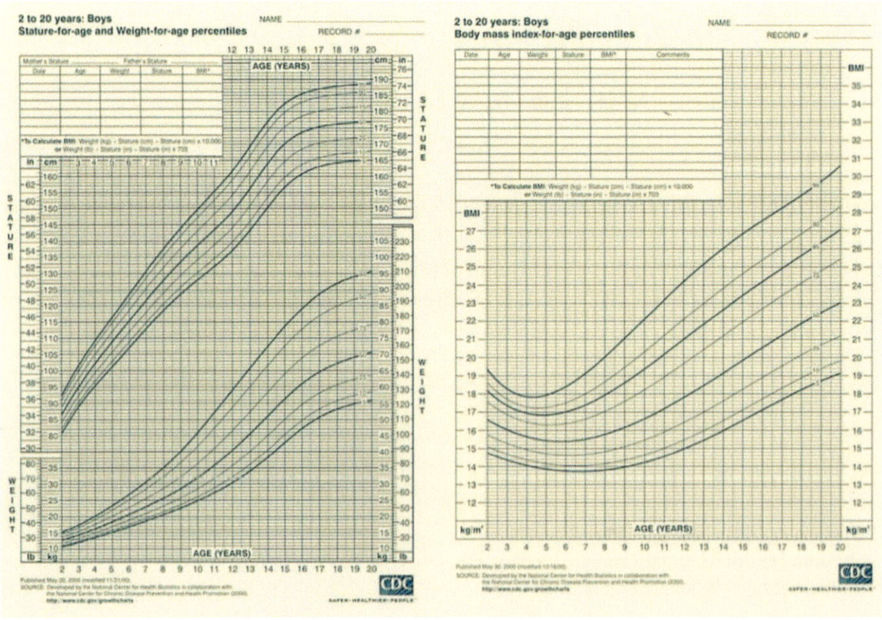

Fig. 62.2 Height, weight, and BMI percentiles for boys [4]. (Adapted from: Centers for Disease Control and Prevention, National Center for Health Statistics. CDC growth charts: United States. http://www.cdc.gov/growthcharts/. May 30, 2000)

Table 62.1 Weight definitions [5]

Underweight	<5th percentile for BMI
Normal weight	5th–85th percentile for BMI
Overweight	85th–<95th percentile for BMI
Obese	≥95th percentile for BMI
Severe obesity	**Class 2**: ≥120% to <140% of the 95th percentile BMI or ≥35 to <40 BMI, whichever is lower **Class 3:** ≥140% of the 95th percentile BMI or ≥40 BMI, whichever is lower

Table 62.2 Fluid and macronutrient requirements [7, 8]

Nutrient	Amount	Examples
Calories	- 5-year-old: 70 kcal/kg/day - 6–8-year-old: 60–65 kcal/kg/day - 9+ year-old: 35–45 kcal/kg/day - Add 200–400 kcal+ for active patients	All macronutrients
Carbohydrates	- 50–55% of caloric intake (1 g = 4 kcal) - Simple sugars limited to 5–10% of caloric intake - Fiber: age+5 g (example: a 9-year-old should consume 9 + 5 = 14 g of fiber daily)	Beans, bread, fruit, rice
Protein	20% of caloric intake (1 g = 4 kcal)	Meat, fish, legumes, dairy
Fat	- 25–30% of caloric intake (1 g = 9 kcal) - <10% of fat should be saturated	Oil, butter, lard
Water	20 kg+: 1500 mL for first 20 kg plus 20 mL/kg for each kg above 20 kg per day (those with larger fluid losses, such as athletes will need more)	All fluids

These charts exist for specific populations as well, such as those with Down syndrome. Table 62.1 defines weight based on the CDC growth chart [5, 6].

Case 1 Allie is a 9-year-old girl presenting for a wellness visit. She recently became vegetarian after visiting a farm, and her mom is supportive but concerned that Allie won't be able to eat enough protein. How would you counsel Allie and her mom about nutritional requirements at this stage of development?

62.2 Components of Nutrition

Components of nutrition are macronutrients (Table 62.2: carbohydrates, protein, and fat), micronutrients (Table 62.3: minerals, vitamins), and water [7]. Balance between food groups provides adequate energy requirements via macronutrients, while variety within food groups (e.g. eating many types of vegetables or protein sources) optimizes micronutrient consumption. The NIH has both consumer and professional fact sheets available on various nutritional supplements (https://ods.od.nih.gov/factsheets/list-all/).

Table 62.3 Select micronutrient requirements [5, 9]

Nutrient	Amount	Examples
Calcium	- 5–8-year-olds: 800 mg/day - 9–18-year-olds: 1,300 mg/day	Dairy, fortified non-dairy 'milks'
Vitamin D	600 IU/day	Fortified cereals, milk
Iron	- 5–8-year-olds: 10 mg/day - 9–13-year-olds: 8 mg/day - Female 14–18-year-olds: 15 mg/day - Male 14–18-year-olds: 11 mg/day	Red meat, legumes, spinach
Folate	Adolescents capable of becoming pregnant: 400 μg/day	Fortified cereals, bread, leafy greens
Sodium	Should be limited to <6 g/day	Most highly processed foods, frozen foods

62.3 Physical Activity Requirements

The American Academy of Pediatrics (AAP) dedicates a chapter of Bright Futures to physical activity, highlighting its importance (Table 62.4). Habits developed in childhood and adolescence can lead to a healthier adulthood. Parental attitudes towards physical activity greatly influences young child and early adolescent engagement [5], however school policy and practice around daily activity also affects activity levels. It is important that children and adolescents are allowed daily, fun, developmentally appropriate physical activity. The CDC has a guide for healthy activity before, during, and after school (https://www.cdc.gov/healthyschools/physicalactivity/index.htm).

Case 1 Resolution You spend some time during the visit discussing the importance of eating a variety of foods, including protein-rich foods such as nuts and legumes, dairy products, and eggs. You provide handouts from the CDC and AAP regarding healthy nutrition at her stage of development and let the mom know that a dietitian consult can be placed if there are weight or nutritional concerns in the future. You discuss with mom a follow-up date that is comfortable for her given her daughter's new dietary requirements.

Case 2 Ethan is a 16-year-old male who presents with right knee pain. You note that he is 101 kg, well over the 99th percentile for weight and BMI. After you ask permission to discuss his weight and overall health, his dad becomes concerned and asks what health issues Ethan is at risk for 'at such a young age.'

62.4 Obesity Comorbidities

Children and adolescents with overweight or obesity are at risk of a multitude of diseases that were once thought to affect only adults (Table 62.5). For example, type 2 diabetes is on the rise in adolescents and can no longer be considered

Table 62.4 Physical activity [1, 5]

Age	Time	Appropriate activities
5–6	- ≥60 min daily, most of which is moderate or intense (sweating, limited ability to converse) - 3x+/week aerobic exercise - 3x/week muscle-strengthening - 3x/week bone-strengthening	Fun, motor skill development, repetitive
7–9		Simple, fun, motor skill development
10–11		Fun, teamwork, can introduce competition
12–18		Weight-bearing, competition

Table 62.5 Overweight and obesity sequelae [6, 8]

Disease	Potential symptoms	Screening/imaging
Prediabetes/insulin resistance	Generally none, +/− family history	Fasting blood glucose
Obstructive sleep apnea	Snoring, daytime sleepiness, morning headache, apnea, decreased concentration	Ask about symptoms; polysomnography
Polycystic ovarian syndrome (PCOS)	Oligomenorrhea, acne, hirsutism	Ask about symptoms; labs including free and total testosterone
Hypertension	Generally none	Office blood pressure reading with correct sized cuff
Non-alcoholic fatty liver disease	Generally none	Liver function testing
Idiopathic intracranial hypertension	Headaches (generally persistent, throbbing), vision changes	Papilledema on eye exam→MRI→lumbar puncture
Dyslipidemia	Generally none, +/− family history	Fasting lipid panel
Slipped capital femoral epiphysis (SCFE)	Knee and/or hip and groin pain, limp, no history of trauma	AP and lateral hip x-ray
Mood disorder	Anxiety, depression, body image issues	Various mental health screening tools available

'late-onset diabetes' [6]. The AAP recently published their first clinical practice guideline for the treatment of overweight and obesity, using a chronic disease framework. Within a chronic disease framework, obesity is treated as a health issue which requires life-long prevention and/or treatment, with screening for the sequelae associated. By treating obesity similar to asthma, type 1 diabetes, or any other pediatric chronic illness, blame is shifted from the patient so that medical decision-making is directed towards prevention of long-term consequences of obesity. With a recommendation for immediate, intensive treatment including pharmacotherapy or surgery for many adolescents with obesity, the hope is to avoid much of the sequelae into adulthood [6].

62.5 Treatment of Overweight and Obesity

The AAP recommends that all patients with overweight and obesity have a medical home where they can be screened for the above-mentioned disorders and treated in a chronic disease model. The language surrounding weight management is evolving, and the most respectful language should be used when both referring to and documenting about patients with weight concerns. For example, instead of documenting 'obese patient,' it is best to say 'patient with obesity.' When discussing weight with a patient and their family, ask permission prior to the discussion and keep tabs on emotions that evolve over the course of the visit. The risk for development of disordered eating is low while following evidence-based treatment. Community messaging and self-directed dieting increase risk of disordered eating, lending even more importance to compassionate medical involvement [6].

There is limited evidence around school-based programs that monitor student BMI. Ideally schools will provide evidence-based nutrition and nutritional counseling along with age-appropriate daily activity. Students who are part of a weight management clinic can be supported in their journey and assisted with medications if they require administration around meals or during the day, such as orlistat (Table 62.6). Language surrounding weight should be strength-based and focused on current and future health and functionality as opposed to size or a specific number [1].

Goals of treatment for those with overweight revolve around slowing or halting the weight gain trajectory [5]. Depending on the age and height of the patient, their BMI may trend to normal with this approach. For those aged 6–11 years and obese, the goal shifts to slow weight loss of no more than 1 pound per month. In this age range with severe obesity this can increase to a loss of up to 2 pounds per week, particularly if there are comorbidities [5]. For 12–18-year-olds who are overweight, the goal is similarly to stop weight gain and monitor. If comorbid conditions exist then slow weight loss can be considered, but for most patients maintenance will be the goal as they continue to grow. For those in the obese and severe obesity categories, weight loss of no more than 2 pounds weekly can occur [5].

Non-pharmacologic treatment depends on the age of the child. For those 5–11 years old, parents are highly involved as they make most food and activity choices for their child. Motivational interviewing at this age focuses on parental motivation to change within the family structure. Providing parents with general health information and nutrition and activity guidance is part of the process. Ideally, motivational interviewing will occur frequently over the course of 3–12 months and may include groups, nutrition, and individual counseling. Rarely, a patient in the 8–11-year-old age group may require medication management (see Table 62.6), but lifestyle intervention and motivational interviewing are first-line at this age [6].

For those ages 12–18 years, the recommendation shifts to motivational interviewing focusing on goals of the adolescent along with parental support. Medication management and/or bariatric surgery involvement, as indicated, are much more common. Anyone over the 95th percentile for BMI should be offered the chance to

Table 62.6 Medications used to treat obesity [6]

Medication	Mechanism	Side effects	Notes
Metformin	Reduces insulin resistance, used in PCOS to induce ovulation	Diarrhea and nausea most common; rare lactic acidosis	Not FDA approved for weight loss or PCOS; performs poorly for weight loss in studies
Topiramate	Appetite suppression	Cognitive slowing; is a teratogen so birth control should be discussed in those who could become pregnant	Used off-label for weight management; FDA approved for binge eating disorder in 18+; can be used in conjunction with phentermine
Phentermine	Appetite suppression	Elevated blood pressure, headache, abdominal pain, tremor	FDA approved for ages 16+ for 12 weeks; schedule 4 narcotic
Lisdexamfetamine	Appetite suppression	Abdominal pain, headache, elevated blood pressure, anxiety, tics; misuse potential	FDA approved for binge eating disorder in 18+; used off-label for weight management; schedule 2 narcotic
Orlistat	Blocks fat absorption	Steatorrhea, diarrhea most common	FDA approved for weight loss in ages 12+; must be taken with each meal to be most effective
GLP-1 agonists	Slows gastric emptying, assists with satiety and fullness cues	Nausea most common, diarrhea; rare pancreatitis or gastroparesis; contraindicated in those with a family or personal history of medullary thyroid cancer (though human studies have not found an increase with use)	Liraglutide and semaglutide are FDA approved for weight loss in ages 12+; injections
MC4R agonists	Appetite regulation for those with genetic defects related to interaction with the MC4 receptor	Nausea	Setmelanotide is FDA approved for ages 6+ with proven genetic defect

start medication. Those above 140% of the 95th percentile for BMI (or a BMI ≥40, whichever is less), or those with comorbid condition(s) who are 120% of the 95th percentile for BMI (or a BMI ≥35, whichever is less), should be offered a consultation with bariatric surgery if there are no contraindications such as pregnancy, current substance use disorder, or reversable causes of obesity (such as hypothyroidism) [6].

Case 2 Resolution Your discussion with Ethan and his dad revolves not around his weight number but instead known risk factors of obesity in children and adolescents. While most of the health issues associated with obesity have traditionally been thought of as adult health problems, you explain to dad that this is no longer the case. You provide a handout explaining short- and long-term effects of obesity in adolescents. Due to his hip pain, you recommend immediate right hip X-Ray to rule out SCFE, and if there are exam findings concerning for instability of the hip, he will leave the office on crutches.

Extra-Credit Points

1. Obesity is a chronic disease and should be treated within that framework
2. Healthy nutrition and activity choices should be encouraged from a young age
3. All children and adolescents with a BMI ≥95th percentile should be offered intensive services including motivational interviewing
4. All adolescents ages 12+ with a BMI ≥95th percentile should be offered medication management as part of their care
5. All children and adolescents with overweight or obese should be screened for comorbid conditions

References

1. Obesity. Division of Population Health, National Center for Chronic Disease Prevention and Health Promotion. https://www.cdc.gov/healthyschools/obesity/index.htm#print
2. Simmonds M, Llewellyn A, Owen CG, Woolacott N. Predicting adult obesity from childhood obesity: a systematic review and meta-analysis. Obes Rev. 2016;17(2):95–107. https://doi.org/10.1111/obr.12334.
3. Staley L. Big fat beat up. IPA Review. 2008:24–28.
4. Centers for Disease Control and Prevention, National Center for Health Statistics. CDC growth charts: United States. May 30, 2000. http://www.cdc.gov/growthcharts/.
5. Bright futures: guidelines for health supervision of infants, children, and adolescents. 4th ed. American Academy of Pediatrics; 2017.
6. Hampl SE, Hassink SG, Skinner AC, et al. Clinical practice guideline for the evaluation and treatment of children and adolescents with obesity. Pediatrics. 2023;151(2). https://doi.org/10.1542/peds.2022-060640
7. Faizan U, Rouster A. Nutrition and hydration requirements in children and adults. StatPearls: StatPearls Publishing; 2023.
8. Neinstein LS, Katzman DK, Callahan ST, Gordon CM, Joffe A, Rickert VI. Neinstein's adolescent and young adult health care a practical guide. 6th ed. Wolters Kluwer; 2016.
9. Iron Fact Sheet for Professionals (NIH) (2023).

Part V
Managing a Student with Mental and Behavioral Health Disorders

Chapter 63
Providing School-Based Comprehensive Mental and Behavioral Health Services

Theodore Miller, Jessica Santucci, and Fiana Klein

There is no official data on how many schools in the US have programs that would qualify under CBMHS, yet according to the National Center for Education Statistics report on mental health services in schools in 2022, only 3% of public schools did not provide any mental health services to students and 56% of public schools reported they moderately or strongly agree that their school is able to effectively provide mental health services to all students in need. Close to 70% of public schools reported increasing the mental health services they provide since the start of the pandemic [1].

These increases in services are welcome and necessary given the rates of mental health needs of children and adolescents. The ramifications of the mental health crisis are vast with schools being on the front lines and in a unique position to intervene with preventative as well as therapeutic measures. Regardless of this potential, there are still limitations to the impact that schools can make. Emergency departments across the nation have been challenged with increasing rates of children and adolescents presenting for psychiatric evaluations. Approximately 30–40% of total emergency department evaluations for behavioral health concerns are referred from schools, and most of these referrals are avoidable. While the reasons for school-initiated referrals are complex and include school district policies and litigation concerns, there is evidence that the rates of inappropriate referrals dropped by 52% when a screening was performed by school-based health staff (with most screenings being performed by nurses and counselors). Over 80% of US schools have school nurses, so even without the additional supports offered by CSBMHS, screening by school nurses can decrease the burden on emergency departments [2].

T. Miller (✉) · J. Santucci
Penn State College of Medicine, Hershey, PA, USA
e-mail: tmiller51@pennstatehealth.psu.edu; jsantucci@pennstatehealth.psu.edu

F. Klein
North Shore Child and Family Guidance Center, Plainview, NY, USA

R. P. Olympia, J. Brady-Olympia (eds.), *Clinical Considerations in School-based Health*, https://doi.org/10.1007/978-3-031-85765-2_63

The drive for mental health care in schools has been supported by both state and federal legislation initiatives, including the "Every Student Succeeds Act" (ESSA) which was signed into law in 2015. Aimed at prioritizing the need for general tiered school supports, an estimated 74% of US schools and districts now take advantage of these hierarchical support modalities and incorporate frameworks like the Multi-Tiered Systems of Support (MTSS) model into their curriculum [3]. MTSS is a three-tiered framework for supporting the various academic and emotional needs of students [4]. (Fig. 63.1)

Our focus will be on how the MTSS framework addresses children's mental health needs in educational settings and through the lens of common presentations of different age groups. Prevention is the thread that runs through all three tiers. Tier 1 is a universal approach that focuses on promoting mental wellbeing and preventing the occurrence of problems. Tier 2's aim is preventing risk factors or addressing problems in their early stage to prevent them from progressing. Tier 3 focuses on individual student needs and interventions that address more serious concerns and prevents the worsening of symptoms that can impact daily functioning [5].

Using the MTSS framework allows for the tiers to build on one another, with increasing levels of support based on the needs of the student. Movement between tiers does not need to be exclusive to one tier or another, as interventions can be in place at multiple tiers at once. Another important element of MTSS and school based mental health services is the personnel who deliver the services. Teachers, school counselors, school social workers, and school psychologists can all provide services to students. In school based mental health centers, school mental health personnel develop collaborations with outside mental health treatment teams, incorporating the expertise of social workers, psychologists, nurses, and psychiatrists.

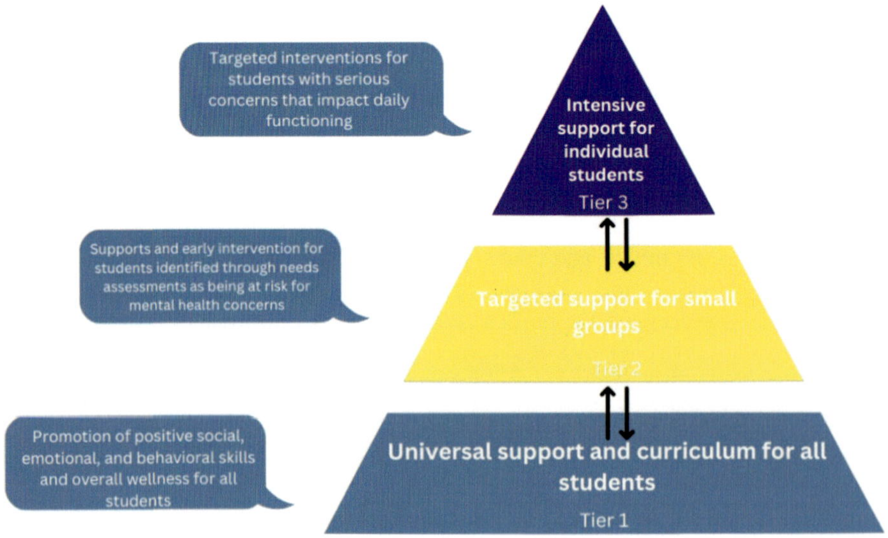

Fig. 63.1 MTSS framework

These outside treatment teams provide support in the school building or in community-based clinics. Other mental health professionals and school staff—teachers, administrators, and support faculty—have additional expertise in typical child behavior and development that holds significant utility in optimizing school supports. This knowledge of typical behaviors allows for detection of children who may have mental health concerns that would have initially gone unnoticed. Once a school professional notices a difference in behavior, the potential for early identification leads to improved prognosis as interventions can be implemented in a timely fashion. Teachers can identify the existence of behavioral problems and rate their severity [6].

Standardized screening tools and the involvement of professionals from various disciplines can then help to better characterize emotional problems and more nuanced presentations of mental health disorders. School districts choose the screening tools they use based on several factors including their ease of use and the cost of the tools. The School Health Assessment and Performance Evaluation System (SHAPE) is a resource from the National Center for School Mental Health that helps schools and districts improve their schools' mental health systems and have various resources including many screenings tools.

Our first case discusses behavioral concerns stemming from Attention-deficit/hyperactivity disorder (ADHD) and Oppositional Defiant disorder (ODD), as these are often what brings an elementary school student's mental health to the attention of schools. In our second case, we explore depressive disorders, anxiety disorders, suicidality, and the impact of bullying in the middle and high school populations. According to the Youth Risk Behavior Survey, "nearly all indicators of poor mental health and suicidal thoughts and behaviors increased from 2011 to 2021" [7]. These concerning trends have highlighted the importance of increased support for children and adolescents in the school setting and beyond.

Case 1 Mrs. Breslow is a 1st grade teacher. Her district has adopted the MTSS Framework. The district decided to use the DESSA-mini, an 8- item assessment tool that teachers use to screen for social and emotional competencies in students in grades K–8. In conducting the screening on her students, one child, Stanley, screened positive. Mrs. Breslow has noticed that Stanley often requires reminders of the classroom and school-wide rules and has had a difficult time getting along with peers alongside episodes of aggressive behaviors toward staff.

Universal interventions should go beyond screening measures. At the school level, Positive Behavior Intervention and Support (PBIS) is a proactive framework which falls under the MTSS umbrella. PBIS promotes positive behavior among students by establishing clear expectations, teaching desired behaviors, and implementing consistent rewards and consequences to create a supportive and inclusive environment for all student [8]. When using the PBIS framework, rather than establishing specifically what NOT to do, schools define and teach expectations and skills they want to see. An example of rewards that students can receive for positive behaviors are having breakfast or lunch with the principal or offering positive tickets that teachers hand out to students who are demonstrating their school's core

PBIS values. Classroom management strategies implemented by teachers are another universal intervention. Classroom management is the process teachers use to limit disruptive behaviors from students and therefore ensure that classroom lessons run smoothly. Classroom management techniques have shown to improve classroom behavior, build relationships for a better classroom community, and foster a positive classroom environment where student learning is the number one collective goal [9].

Appropriate teacher responses to challenging behaviors exhibited by students are associated with significantly lower rates of retained behaviors throughout the child's lifetime [10]. Elementary school students with behavioral concerns often have academic and social difficulties as well. For common disorders presenting in the elementary school age population like ADHD, evidence supports the positive impact classroom interventions have on reducing future challenging behaviors exhibited by children. Interventions like those aimed at replacing a socially undesirable behavior with a socially appropriate equivalent and targeted interventions, such as organizational skills training and self-regulation strategies, have considerable utility in managing disruptive classroom actions and improving future prognoses of problematic behaviors [11].

Mrs. Breslow reviewed class wide expectations and posted classroom rules in a visible location. She began to publicly praise Stanley when he was able to adhere to classroom rules and ignored minor disruptive behaviors. Stanley began to meet with the school social worker to learn to manage his emotions and self-monitor his behaviors. As his behaviors would often escalate in the classroom when he was frustrated, his teacher sectioned off a small area of the classroom to be a "calm down corner." The "calm down corner" was made available for all the students, and Stanley received support on when and how to use the area during his sessions with the school social worker.

Case 2 Mr. Lott is a school social worker at the local school. Last week, he met with a student, Melissa, after she overheard two peers in her class talking about her and making fun of her appearance. Mr. Lott reassured Melissa, and she returned to class following that incident. Today, Mr. Lott receives an email from Melissa's mother stating that Melissa has been out of school for the last few days because she had been refusing to go to school after there was a cyberbullying incident over the weekend. Melissa also made a post on social media indicating that she did not want to live. The school district recently expanded its services to include a school based mental health center, and Mr. Lott asks the team for support.

For Melissa, as is often the case for victims of bullying, the impacts of bullying intersect with other symptoms and contribute to dysfunction. First, there needs to be a risk assessment due to the suicidal statement she made. Suicide is the second leading cause of death among children ages 10 through 17 years nationwide [12], and prevention measures require an understanding of risk factors as well as protective factors. Treatment and supportive measures can mitigate modifiable risk factors such as current substance abuse, lack of mental health treatment, and limited relationships. Non-modifiable risk factors, like a personal or family history of suicide, early life adversity, and genetic predisposition, are not changeable. To determine the risk of suicide in an individual at any given time, there needs to be an assessment of risk factors, protective factors, and warning signs [13]. (Fig. 63.2)

The school based mental health center's psychiatrist reaches out to Melissa's mother and arranges for Melissa's assessment at the community-based site. It is determined that although Melissa made a statement about suicidal thoughts, a prominent warning sign of suicide, and has risk factors of being a victim of bullying and symptoms of generalized anxiety disorder, she has protective factors of no prior history of suicide attempts or inpatient hospitalizations. Further, she has no family history of suicidality, no history of substances abuse, and reinforced family support. The psychiatrist works with Melissa to create a suicide safety plan using an app (Table 63.1) that Melissa downloads on her phone, and Melissa shares the plan with her mother. Counseling is provided to Melissa's mother about means restriction measures to limit her access to potentially lethal means of suicide.

By addressing the other modifiable risk factors of Melissa's symptoms of anxiety, including her lack of treatment, her disengagement from school, and her bullying experiences, her risk of suicide can further be reduced. The psychiatrist arranges

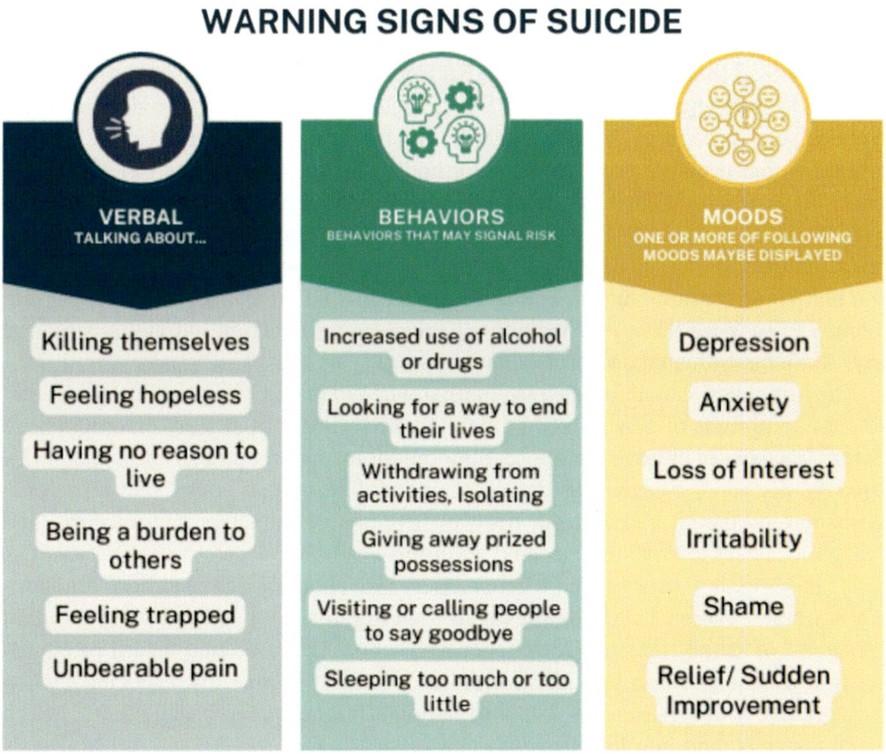

Fig. 63.2 Warning signs of suicide [9]

Table 63.1 Suicide safety planning apps

App	IOS	Android
Suicide safety plan	Yes	Yes
Stanley-Brown safety plan	Yes	Yes
Suicide Safe by SAMHSA	Yes	Yes
Safety plan	Yes	Yes
Suicide safe	Yes	Yes

for a team meeting with the school psychologist and helps to link Melissa with ongoing treatment at the school based mental health clinic.

An important exacerbating factor in Melissa's presentation is the presence of bullying by peers. Bullying is defined as "unwanted, aggressive behavior among school aged children that involves a real or perceived power imbalance. The behavior is repeated, or has the potential to be repeated, over time" [14]. As children reach the middle and high school years, there are changes in social dynamics and increasing complexity of relationships which are further complicated through social media and other online forums. These factors often create opportunities for bullying to occur both in school and online [15]. Bullying's negative outcomes of depression and anxiety are pervasive to multiple parties, involving not only the victim but the bully and bystanders as well. Evidence shows that both victims and perpetrators of bullying have increased risk of suicidal behavior. The highest risk group is made of those who report both bullying others and being victims of bullying [16].

It is critical that schools play an active role in bullying prevention due to bullying's wide spanning impact. The MTSS framework lends itself to providing a comprehensive approach to addressing bullying in schools. Universal tools include programs that promote positive behavior and foster a culture of respect and inclusion. These programs establish clear expectations for behavior and provide students with the skills needed to navigate social interactions effectively. Following the identification of bullying, students who are bullies or victims of bullying receive tier 2 and tier 3 interventions such as counseling, peer mediation, and skill-building group therapy [17]. With these interventions, further assessments on individual's mental health can be evaluated and properly addressed.

The initial assessment by the psychiatrist who evaluated Melissa determined that she has symptoms of generalized anxiety disorder. Rates of anxiety disorders have been increasing in child and adolescent populations over the last several years [18]. Anxiety disorders can disrupt the acquisition of important social and emotional skills that lay the groundwork for healthy development, positive relationships, and academic success in adolescence and adulthood.

As in Melissa's case, an area where anxiety most notably affects school functioning is when it causes a child to be fearful of going to school and results in avoidant behaviors of school refusal. Comprehensive school based mental health programs are in a unique position to address children's anxiety symptoms, especially when they present with school refusal. Coordination with the school-based mental health team, teachers, and families are important pillars to successfully support Melissa's academic, social, and emotional needs. Evidence has shown that interventions for anxiety-related school refusal should be those using a Cognitive Behavioral Therapy framework in which gradual desensitization and exposure techniques can help Melissa first gain comfort on school property without the presence of peers. She can then slowly work towards attending all classes with peers, given the newly developed support she has at multiple levels of the school system [19]. Once Melissa is back in the classroom, the SBMH clinic will provide ongoing treatment of her anxiety and assessment for suicidal thinking. It is through this plan that Melissa and her care team will develop interventions to improve her resilience and self-efficacy while also reducing incidences of bullying.

Extra Credit Points

1. In the era of a mental health crisis among young people, comprehensive school-based mental health services are an important and effective strategy in addressing the social, emotional, and mental health needs of children and adolescents.
2. The integration of mental health support in educational settings fosters emotional well-being, academic success, and needed interventions for all students. CSBMHS can prevent, recognize, and treat mental illness in youths.
3. Among US school districts, the most used framework for implementation of CSBMHS is the Multi-Tiered Systems of Support (MTSS) framework. MTSS encompasses three tiers and emphasizes prevention, early intervention, and individualized support based on students' needs.
4. Services under the CSBMHS umbrella are typically delivered by school-employed personnel like teachers, school nurses, school counselors, and school psychologists. CSBMHS-related services are enhanced through collaborations with community based mental health providers.
5. Community mental health providers complement the efforts of school-employed professionals, expanding the scope of mental health support available to students.

References

1. National Center for Education Statistics. Mental health and well-being of students and staff during the pandemic. 2022. https://ies.ed.gov/schoolsurvey/spp/SPP_April_Infographic_Mental_Health_and_Well_Being.pdf
2. Grudnikoff E, Taneli T, Correll CU. Characteristics and disposition of youth referred from schools for emergency psychiatric evaluation. Eur Child Adolesc Psychiatry. 2014;24(7):731–43. https://doi.org/10.1007/s00787-014-0618-8.
3. Pendharkar E. What we know about Multi-Tiered Systems of Supports (MTSS), in charts. Education Week. November 9, 2023. https://www.edweek.org/teaching-learning/what-we-know-about-multi-tiered-system-of-supports-mtss-in-charts/2023/11. Accessed 27 May 2024.
4. Crocker J, Franks R, Sosnowski D, et al. Mental health and schools: best practices to support our students. 2023. https://www.bakercenter.org/resources/library/mental-health-and-schools-best-practices-to-support-our-students. Accessed 27 May 2024
5. Hoover S, Lever N, Sachdev N, et al., Advancing comprehensive school mental health: guidance from the field. 2019. https://www.schoolmentalhealth.org/media/som/microsites/ncsmh/documents/bainum/Advancing-CSMHS_September-2019.pdf. Accessed 27 May 2024.

6. Loades ME, Mastroyannopoulou K. Teachers' recognition of children's mental health problems. Child Adolesc Ment Health. 2010;15(3):150–6. https://doi.org/10.1111/j.1475-3588.2009.00551.x.
7. Centers for Disease Control and Prevention. Youth risk behavior survey data summary & trends report 2011–2021. April 27, 2023. https://www.cdc.gov/healthyyouth/data/yrbs/pdf/YRBS_Data-Summary Trends_Report2023_508.pdf. Accessed 27 May 2024
8. Simonsen B, Sugai G. School-wide positive behavioral interventions and supports: A systems-level application of behavioral principles. Behavioral interventions in schools: evidence-based positive strategies. 2nd ed. American Psychological Association; 2019. p. 35–60. https://doi.org/10.1037/0000126-003.
9. Simon DJ. Foundations of mental health services in school. In School-centered interventions: evidence-based strategies for social, emotional, and academic success. Washington (DC): American Psychological Association; 2016. https://doi.org/10.1037/14779-001.
10. Owens JS, Holdaway AS, Smith J, et al. Rates of common classroom behavior management strategies and their associations with challenging student behavior in elementary school. J Emot Behav Disord 2018;26(3):156–169. https://doi.org/10.1177/1063426617712501.
11. DuPaul GJ, Gormley MJ, Daffner-Deming M. School-based interventions for elementary school students with attention-deficit/hyperactivity disorder. Child Adolesc Psychiatr Clin N Am. 2022;31(1):149–66. https://doi.org/10.1016/j.chc.2021.08.003.
12. Hughes JL, Horowitz LM, Ackerman JP, Adrian MC, Campo JV, Bridge JA. Suicide in young people: screening, risk assessment, and intervention. BMJ. Apr 24, 2023;381:e070630. https://doi.org/10.1136/bmj-2022-070630
13. American Foundation for Suicide Prevention. Risk factors, protective factors, and warning signs. December 18, 2023. https://afsp.org/risk-factors-protective-factors-and-warning-signs. Accessed 27 May 2024
14. U.S. Department of Health and Human Services. Facts about bullying. StopBullying.gov. September 9, 2021. https://www.stopbullying.gov/resources/facts. Accessed 27 May 2024
15. Pellegrini AD, Long JD. A longitudinal study of bullying, dominance, and victimization during the transition from primary school through secondary school. Br J Dev Psychol. 2002;20(2):259–80. https://doi.org/10.1348/026151002166442.
16. Wolke D, Lereya ST. Long-term effects of bullying. Arch Dis Child. 2015;100(9):879–85. https://doi.org/10.1136/archdischild-2014-306667.
17. Rivara F, Le Menestrel S. Committee on the Biological and Psychosocial Effects of Peer Victimization: Lessons for Bullying Prevention; Board on Children, Youth, and Families; Committee on Law and Justice; Preventing bullying through science, policy, and practice. Washington (DC): National Academies Press (US); September 14, 2016. https://doi.org/10.17226/23482.
18. Goger P, Rozenman M, Gonzalez A, et al. Early indicators of response to transdiagnostic treatment of pediatric anxiety and depression. J Child Psychol Psychiatry. 2023;64(12):1689–98. https://doi.org/10.1111/jcpp.13881.
19. Johnsen DB, Lomholt JJ, Heyne D, et al. The effectiveness of modular transdiagnostic cognitive behavioral therapy versus treatment as usual for youths displaying school attendance problems: a randomized controlled trial. Res Child Adolesc Psychopathol. May 13, 2024. https://doi.org/10.1007/s10802-024-01196-8

Chapter 64
Emotional Regulation in the School Setting

Andrew Yeich and Meenal Pathak

Case 1 **A 12-year-old girl named Sarah is brought to your office at the end of the school day. A teacher who was supervising bus pick-up reports that Sarah was sitting by the door to the school inconsolably crying. It is hard to make out what Sarah is saying, but as you review her file you find reports by several of her teachers of inattention and "daydreaming" during classes. You also read a message from her parents last year describing Sarah's hospitalization after a serious but non-lethal car accident. Through her sobbing, which has continued for almost ten minutes now, you hear her repeatedly say that she doesn't want to go back to the parking lot. What underlying condition may be associated with the extended negative emotions Sarah is struggling with?**

Case 2 **A 16-year-old boy named Thomas is brought to your office after being removed from his classroom. His teacher reports that Thomas seemed fine at the start of class but began to act out after a group of boys began taunting on him for requiring extra assistance with an assignment. The teacher's attempts at consolation turned into a high-volume argument. Thomas became more and more combative, eventually throwing his desk chair across the room. Presently, Thomas sits in the chair of your office looking down at his feet. His initially rapid breathing has slowed to a more natural pace, and his hands are no longer clenched, but he appears withdrawn and still does not respond to conversation. What interventions may have prevented Thomas' outburst from occurring, and when would they have been most effective?**

A. Yeich (✉)
Penn State College of Medicine, Hershey, PA, USA
e-mail: ayeich@pennstatehealth.psu.edu

M. Pathak
Penn State Health, Hershey, PA, USA
e-mail: mpathak@pennstatehealth.psu.edu

R. P. Olympia, J. Brady-Olympia (eds.), *Clinical Considerations in School-based Health*, https://doi.org/10.1007/978-3-031-85765-2_64

Case 3 Several months after his initial outburst, Thomas and his parents arrive 30 minutes late to a meeting with school staff to address his behaviors. Through the discussion, you learn that all his teachers have had difficulty managing Thomas' tendency to lash out after encountering small difficulties in academic assignments. A particular group of peers that share several classes with Thomas have taken to bullying him in these moments. Individually, the teaching staff have tried several different strategies in their respective classes and encounter resistance from Thomas who often refutes attempts to moderate his behavior by citing the policies of another classroom. What types of interventions can address Thomas' behavior in the future?

Emotional regulation (ER) is broadly defined as an individual's ability to manage emotions in a non-destructive and socially acceptable manner. It is a crucial skill for social function across all ages, but particularly so for school age children, as ER correlates significantly with both academic and social performance in the school setting [1]. Development of ER begins as early as birth. Babies learn to differentiate primary emotion states (neutral, pleasurable, and non-pleasurable) and their intensity through interactions with caregivers. By the age of 7, children develop primary regulation strategies to modify their emotional states, including seeking, avoiding, redirecting attention, suppressing impulses, and problem solving. ER development is affected by a complex set of internal and external factors, including genetic predisposition, temperament, and the caregiving environment that the child is exposed to are particularly important influences [2].

Emotional dysregulation (ED) refers to a deficit in ER skills. Multiple aspects of social communication and internal regulation can be affected. For example, a common problem is an underdeveloped ability to withstand negative emotions while in a social setting. Children may also lack appropriate recognition towards the types of emotional responses that others display to their words and actions, leading to poor social functioning. Even when properly identified, some children have difficulty accepting responses that run counter to their own social desires. Some children struggle with expressing their own emotions clearly, particularly in nuanced scenarios [3]. ED can present as either an isolated deficit or as a symptom of a developmental pathology or psychiatric condition. For many of the disorders with which ED is associated, the presence of ED as a comorbidity worsens prognosis. Fortunately, adequate treatment of the underlying disorder often has the potential to improve the child's ER abilities in addition to other symptoms. Table 64.1 lists the developmental and psychiatric disorders commonly associated with ED in school aged children.

Table 64.1 Disorders associated with emotional dysregulation

Comorbid condition	Association of disorder with ED
Attention deficit hyperactivity disorder (ADHD)	Children with ADHD have a high prevalence of ED that often persists into adulthood, and ED may be a more specific marker of ADHD than many other symptoms [4].
Autism spectrum disorder	The social deficits inherent to autism spectrum disorder can complicate emotional expression and interpretation, and ED can manifest as aggression, tantrums, mood lability, and self-injurious behavior [5].
Major depressive disorder	Children experiencing depressive symptoms commonly use rumination instead of more effective ER strategies, leading to worsening symptoms [6].
Bipolar disorder	Children with bipolar disorder are less able to accurately differentiate subtle emotional expressions on the faces of others [7].
Post-traumatic stress disorder	Intrusion symptoms of PTSD are linked to emotional under-regulation, while emotional over-regulation leads to numbness, avoidance, and dissociation symptoms [8].
Conduct disorder	Emotional dysregulation may manifest as aggression to people or animals, destruction of property, theft, or violation of major age-appropriate social norms such as running away from home or truancy [9].
Disruptive mood dysregulation disorder (DMDD)	Children with DMDD experience frequent dysregulation of mood, increased impulsivity often out of proportion to triggers [10].

64.1 Recommendations for a Student in Acute Emotional Distress

Episodes of acute emotional distress can be relatively common amongst school-aged children yet challenging to manage in the school setting. As detailed in Sect. 64.1, there are many different pathways through which negative emotions can grow beyond a child's ability to cope. However, regardless of cause, most instances of behavioral disturbances escalate and de-escalate along a predictable pattern [11]. Recognizing the stage at which a particular child is struggling during an acute episode allows for targeted interventions to prevent further escalation. Table 64.2 displays Colvin and Scott's model of these behaviors, along with suggested interventions for each stage.

Table 64.2 Stages of acute emotional distress [11]

Stage	Characteristics	Interventions
Calm	Although the student may already have deficient ER skills or prior exacerbating experiences, their current behavior is indistinguishable from baseline	Continue providing supportive supervision as afforded to other students Implement previously established behavioral plan/IEP Pre-correct known or anticipated triggers
Triggers	An event or situation places emotional distress on a student, including conflicts, changes in routine, peer provocations, academic pressures or mistakes, disciplinary actions, or circumstances outside of school	Identify the inciting events or contexts that may have acted as the trigger Clarify which behaviors are acceptable coping strategies vs. unacceptable responses If possible, modify the environment to avoid triggers with a systematic plan that minimizes and normalizes changes to routine

(continued)

Table 64.2 (continued)

Stage	Characteristics	Interventions
Agitation	Following a triggering event that overwhelms the student's ER capacity, their behavior changes to either hyperactivity (attention target fluctuation, physical restlessness, rapid entering and exiting of social/work groups, lability of tasks) or hypoactivity (zoning out, avoidance of eye contact, non-conversational language, social withdrawal)	Demonstrate that the student's concerns, feelings, and perspectives are being heard, even if full agreement is impossible Consider implementing small, short-term accommodations to prevent further escalations such as additional space, time, instructor attention, or preferred activities Provide clear choices for possible remedies Garner momentum for cooperation by getting the student to agree to multiple simple and easy requests
Acceleration	A previously agitated student begins to test limits, seeks out confrontation with authority figures, or engages with peers antagonistically	Avoid escalating reactions to the student's behavior, including power struggles, violations of personal space, defensive body language Project composure and a calm respect for the student by using corrective language directed at the behaviors rather than the individual Present consequences (preferably those that were pre-established) as clear choices and follow through with them
Peak	The student's behaviors have escalated to a level that completely disrupts a learning environment or jeopardizes the safety of the student or others, hyperventilation is often present	Immediately implement the school district's crisis plan with a primary focus on safety of students and staff Referral to home or the emergency department may be warranted if safety concerns persist

(continued)

Table 64.2 (continued)

Stage	Characteristics	Interventions
De-escalation	The student has discontinued the most intensive outbursts of emotional distress and begins to either reintegrate to the social environment or disengage, cooperation and focus are still impaired	Isolate the student, provide adequate supervision, and allow time to cool off Engage in achievable independent work with clear criteria, preferably a standardized behavior form that can be used in debriefing Determine consequences (can include restoring the environment if it was disrupted by the outburst) and resume the regular schedule
Recovery	The student returns to the non-agitated state that allows for some level of classroom participation	Maintain a strong focus on routines, supportive communication, reinforcement of positive behaviors, and a heightened vigilance for new triggers Consider a debriefing session to revisit the incident to foster the student's insight into their behaviors Carry out any consequences as they were determined, and avoid minimizing them in response to initial cooperation

64.2 Recommendations for Long-Term Emotional Regulation Interventions

The most effective interventions for facilitating ER in the school setting are done before an acute episode of emotional distress occurs. As shown in Table 64.2, the early stages of the acting out cycle can often be addressed through pre-correcting known triggers. For students with frequent outbursts that are not amenable to simple vigilance, a formal assessment of behavioral patterns allowing for systematic interventions may be necessary. A Functional Behavioral Assessment (FBA) seeks to identify the precipitants surrounding episodes of an acute emotional distress for the purposes of revealing possible secondary gains that may be motivating an individual student to repeat their behaviors [12]. The information gained through an FBA allows for a Behavioral Intervention Plan (BIP) to be designed for the student. BIPs can involve prevention strategies that target environmental factors exacerbating a child's distress, teaching strategies that address possible underlying ER skill deficits, and response strategies that equip instructors with a standardized protocol for managing future incidents [13].

For some children, FBA will reveal the primary cause driving repeated behaviors is an underdeveloped set of ER skills. Although all children experience intense emotions at different points in their life, it is important to remember that that emotional disturbance is a formal category of disability under the Individuals with Disabilities Education Act. Students with a suspected disability should undergo a special education evaluation to determine eligibility for special education services. This is performed by a multidisciplinary team of school-based professionals, and the assessment of a consulting psychiatrist or behavioral health specialist may be included in the evaluation. If a child is found to have a disability, the school-based team may develop either an Individualized Education Plan (IEP) or a 504. Students who receive these special education services for ED should also be provided evaluation for undiagnosed or untreated psychopathology that may act as a contributing factor [14].

There are several other forms of intervention that have demonstrated efficacy in helping students develop ER skills. Selective Prevention Programs and Indicated Prevention Programs are broad categories of initiatives that seek to deliver resources to students in need. They can be implemented to facilitate evaluation and treatment for underlying psychopathology and subsequent referral to counseling or advisory groups as appropriate. A Selective Prevention Program targets students likely to meet criteria for underlying psychiatric conditions, while an Indicated Prevention Program has less strict admission requirements and can include high-risk students not meeting full criteria for an identifiable disorder [15]. Universal Prevention Programs are initiatives through which psychiatrists and other mental health professionals visit to provide the school community with education on relevant topics such as interpersonal problem solving, social interaction, and management techniques. Instruction can take many forms including school-wide assemblies, classroom talks, or seminars at parent-teacher organizations. School systems without existing prevention programs may benefit from partnerships with local healthcare systems to develop these resources for their students. Psychiatrists and other mental health professionals can collaborate with school personnel to conduct a needs assessment to bolster existing mental health resources [16].

Case Resolutions

Case 1: Given her recent accident, Sarah is possibly displaying signs of PTSD. Her current emotional distress is likely grounded in avoiding parking lots and vehicles. The acute change in her concentration reported by her teachers may represent dissociative symptoms commonly experienced by children after traumatic events. In this case, evaluation and subsequent psychiatric treatment of the underlying disorder is crucial.

Case 2: Several points of intervention could have de-escalated Thomas' outburst. Behavioral plans based on prior incidents may have adjusted the classroom environment in a way that mitigated the stressors he faced. Vigilant pre-correction of known triggers, such as the group of peers that began taunting Thomas, would be useful in addressing new problems as they arise. Attempts at consolation should prioritize avoiding power struggles and project a calm tone respect for the student once agitated. Presentation of clear choices and consequences, including voluntarily leaving the classroom for an alternative activity, may have given Thomas an off-ramp before he chose his explosive behavior of throwing the chair. In the subsequent de-escalation phase that Thomas presents to the office in, engagement in achievable independent work like a standardized behavior sheet may stimulate insight and facilitate return to classroom learning.

Case 3: Subsequent behavioral incidents have made clear the need for systematic intervention. A functional behavioral assessment should be conducted to identify triggers, and a behavioral intervention plan would provide a platform upon which Thomas' teachers can address future problems in a fair but consistent manner. Some themes have already been identified through this meeting. Thomas seems to have difficulty coping with academic failures and should be evaluated for learning deficits in case an individualized education plan is needed. Bullying clearly contributes to his stressors as well; separating him from the peers involved and implementing disciplinary action according to school policy may help him further. As with any student, possible stressors outside of school should also be considered.

Extra Credit Points

1. ER is a complex skill that contains multiple different domains, and an individual student may need assistance in particular domains but not others.
2. Many students with ER deficits have undiagnosed or untreated psychopathology. Triggers outside of the school setting can also play a significant contributing role.
3. Planned behavioral interventions depend on consistent implementation. School personnel must follow through on previously determined responses as a united front.
4. Widespread unmet needs exist in for mental health services within schools. Students and families may not be aware of resources that are available to them.
5. In some counties, educational advocates may be available to help families navigate the process of accessing resources.

References

1. Adynski H, Propper C, Beeber L, et al. The role of emotional regulation on early child school adjustment outcomes. Arch Psychiatr Nurs. 2024;51:201–11.
2. Paulus FW, Ohmann S, Mohler E, et al. Emotional dysregulation in children and adolescents with psychiatric disorders. A narrative review. Front Psychiatry. 2021;12:628252.
3. Gratz KL, Roemer L. Multidimensional assessment of emotion regulation and dysregulation: development, factor structure, and initial validation of the difficulties in emotion regulation scale. J Psychopathol Behav Assess. 2004;26:41–54.
4. Faranone SV, Rostain AL, Blader J, et al. Practitioner review: emotional dysregulation in attention-deficit/hyperactivity disorder—implications for clinical recognition and intervention. J Child Psychol Psychiatry. 2019;60:133–50.

5. Pablo GS, Jorda CP, Vaquerizo-Serrano J, et al. Systematic review and meta-analysis: efficacy of pharmacological interventions for irritability and emotional dysregulation in autism spectrum disorder and predictors of response. J Am Acad Child Adolesc Psychiatry. 2023;62:151–68.
6. Stegge H, Meerum TM. Awareness and regulation of emotion in typical and atypical development. In: Gross JJ, editor. Handbook of emotion regulation. New York: Guilford Press; 2007. p. 269–86.
7. Schenkel LS, Pavuluri MN, Herbener ES, et al. Facial processing in acutely ill and euthymic patients with pediatric bipolar disorder. J Am Acad Child Adolesc Psychiatry. 2007;46:1070–9.
8. Lanius RA, Vermettten E, Loewenstein RJ, et al. Emotion modulation in PTSD: Clinical and neurobiological evidence for a dissociative subtype. Am J Psychiatry. 2010;167:640–7.
9. Moehler E, Brunner R, Sharp C. Editorial: Emotional dysregulation in children and adolescents. Front Psychiatry. 2022;7:883753.
10. Frick PJ. Developmental pathways to conduct disorder: Implications for serving youth who show severe aggressive and antisocial behavior. Psychol Sch. 2004;41:823–34.
11. Colvin G, Scott TM. Managing the cycle of acting-out behavior in the classroom. 2nd ed. Thousand Oaks: Corwin Press; 2014.
12. https://cdn.prod.website-files.com/5d3725188825e071f1670246/61fda7bcc5646e5e20ea845f_Tier%203%20Comprehensive%20Functional%20Behavior%20Assessment%20(FBA)%20Guide.pdf
13. Bostic JQ, Mattison R, Cunningham D. Explosive outbursts at school. Child Adolesc Psychiatr Clin N Am. 2000;3:223–41.
14. Walker HJ, Berkovitz IH. Practice parameter for psychiatric consultation to schools. J Am Acad Child Adolesc Psychiatry. 2005;44:1068–83.
15. Mattison RE. School consultation: a review of research on issues unique to the school environment. J Am Acad Child Adolesc Psychiatry. 2000;39:402–13.
16. Grunbaum JA, Gingiss P, Orpinas P, et al. A comprehensive approach to school health program needs assessments. J Sch Health. 1995;65:54–9.

Chapter 65
Pharmacology of Mental and Behavioral Health Disorders

Ramnarine Boodoo and Thejasvi N. Lingamchetty

Case 1 **12 year old Jasmine comes to your office with her mother, for complaints of refusal to prepare for the school day, vomiting and headaches especially on Monday mornings, quitting softball, and not wanting to hang out with friends. This has resulted in missing 25% of school days in the past 2 months. Jasmine first saw you a month ago, psychotherapy was recommended, but despite 4 sessions her symptoms are worsening. The school is now moving forward with charges of truancy against student and parent.**

Case 2 **17 year old James sees you at your school-based practice. He complains of a two year history of difficulty concentrating, despite having exemplary grades, along with extra-curricular activities. He states he does so well because he spends twice as much time as colleagues on schoolwork. James graduates in one year, and is hoping to be accepted to a pre-medicine college program. He believes he has attention-deficit hyperactivity disorder (ADHD) and wishes to start a medication for this. Today he is diagnosed with ADHD, predominantly inattentive presentation and is given a prescription for extended-release mixed amphetamine salts (Adderall XR).**

School-based prescribers are often tasked with having to start, adjust or discontinue psychiatric medications. Being able to do so competently and safely requires an understanding of the range of psychiatric medication options available, their indications, contraindications, and adverse effects. Also necessary is an understanding of general psychiatric prescribing principles in the pediatric population.

R. Boodoo (✉) · T. N. Lingamchetty
Penn State Hershey Medical Center, Hershey, PA, USA
e-mail: rboodoo@pennstatehealth.psu.edu; tlingamchetty@pennstatehealth.psu.edu

R. P. Olympia, J. Brady-Olympia (eds.), *Clinical Considerations in School-based Health*, https://doi.org/10.1007/978-3-031-85765-2_65

65.1 General Principles for Prescribing Psychiatric Medication in Youth

1. **Treat syndromes, not symptoms: [1]** Although we may sometimes use medications to target discrete symptoms such as insomnia, or bouts of anxiety, we should try as much as possible to diagnose and treat the psychiatric conditions which may be causing these.
2. **Psychotherapy is first-line treatment:** Due to the much higher risk of adverse effects from medications when compared to psychotherapy, a trial of psychotherapy (also referred to as counseling or just "therapy") should be considered prior to prescribing a medication. However, a medication may be prescribed even without a patient having had psychotherapy under the following circumstances—

   a. The patient's presentation is so severe that psychotherapy alone is unlikely to be effective, or take effect quickly enough, to prevent deterioration
   b. Psychotherapy services are unavailable or available only after an extended period
   c. Clear and definitive history of ADHD in youth 6 years of age and above, without psychiatric co-morbidities and psychosocial stressors

It should be noted that medication prescribed before initiation of psychotherapy may be tapered off after psychotherapy is started and clinical stability achieved.

3. **Understand that psychiatric prescribing in youth is often off-label [1]**: Due to the dearth of research studies on psychiatric medication use in youth when compared to adults, many psychiatric medications that are commonly used in youth are not FDA-approved. Nevertheless, these medications are used safely and effectively in the pediatric population.
4. **Ensure there are no medical or psychiatric contraindications to medication being considered:** Patients being prescribed any psychiatric medications must be screened for conditions which may be exacerbated by these medications. Examples include cardiac disease being a relative contraindication to stimulant and escitalopram use, and a seizure disorder or eating disorder being a contraindication to bupropion use.
5. **Obtain informed consent from necessary parties [1]:** Obtaining informed consent before prescribing any medication for psychiatric purposes is always necessary. In fact, based on the age of the child, consent may need to be obtained before a clinical evaluation is conducted. At a minimum, informed consent for medication consists of a discussion of medication risks, benefits and alternatives, and giving an opportunity to ask questions about these. For young children, a parent or guardian will have to provide informed consent. In such cases, obtaining the assent of the child is also desirable. Depending on state law, the age at which an adolescent may consent on their own for psychiatric medication will vary. It is therefore imperative to be aware of the laws governing informed consent in the state in which prescribing is undertaken.

6. **Consider using a controlled substance agreement [2]:** When prescribing controlled substances such as stimulants, consider having the patient or guardian sign a contract (commonly referred to as a controlled substance agreement) outlining the circumstances under which the medication will no longer be prescribed. Such situations include lost or stolen medication, sharing or selling medication, obtaining prescriptions from a different provider or multiple pharmacies, and concurrent illicit drug use. If the patient or parent refuses to sign the agreement, no controlled substance should be prescribed.
7. **Start low, go slow:** When starting medication in the pediatric population, starting doses are often lower than those for adults. Additionally, intervals between dose increases are often longer. This prevents the occurrence of adverse effects, but such doses may also be sub-therapeutic. Intervals between dose increases may be shortened to facilitate reaching a therapeutic dose, but close monitoring for adverse effects must be undertaken.
8. **Medications take 2 weeks to start working:** Most psychiatric medications, when taken at therapeutic doses, take at least 2 weeks before effects are noticed. Therefore, patients must be advised to wait at least this long before suspecting that their medication is ineffective. Once active, the effects are continuous. Exceptions to this occur with stimulants, and medications that are given on an as needed basis, such as immediate-release alpha-2 agonists and hydroxyzine. The effects of these medications typically begin within an hour, and the effects last several hours at most.
9. **Refer to a specialist psychiatric prescriber if necessary**: If not a specialist psychiatric prescriber yourself, consider referring to one in cases of significant medical or psychiatric co-morbidity, failure of two or more adequate medication trials, use of more than two medications for clinical stability, and increased possibility of danger to self or to others. Of course, any suspicion of imminent danger to self or to others should trigger referral to a higher level of care such as a hospital emergency department.

Psychiatric medications may be broadly divided into antidepressants, anxiolytics, mood stabilizers, antipsychotics, and others (including those used for the treatment of ADHD). Medications used for ADHD may then be divided into stimulants and non-stimulants. Although a thorough review of all types of psychiatric medication is beyond the scope of this chapter, Table 65.1 describes commonly used psychiatric medications.

65.2 Points to Keep in Mind

1. Selective serotonin reuptake inhibitors (SSRIs) are considered first line medications for depressive and anxiety disorders in youth.
2. Benzodiazepines should not be prescribed in youth due to risk of addiction, misuse and disinhibited behavior.

Table 65.1 Selected commonly used psychiatric medications

Medication name and class	Indications	Dosage range (total daily dose)	Important considerations
Fluoxetine (Prozac) Antidepressant, SSRI	**MDD (8+ YO), OCD (7+ YO),** Panic Disorder, Bulimia, PMDD	20–60 mg (initial dose may be 10 mg)	- The only antidepressant approved for treating MDD in younger children. **- Some risk of activation syndrome (emotional lability, irritability, psychomotor restlessness)** - Risk of increased suicidal thinking and behavior in those 24 YO and younger.
Sertraline (Zoloft) Antidepressant, SSRI	**OCD (6+ YO),** MDD, Panic Disorder, PTSD, PMDD, Social Anxiety Disorder	25–200 mg (initial dose may be 12.5–25 mg)	**- Some risk of increased bleeding (prevents platelet aggregation)** - Risk of increased suicidal thinking and behavior in those 24 YO and younger.
Escitalopram (Lexapro) Antidepressant, SSRI	**MDD (12+ YO),** GAD, Social Anxiety Disorder	10–20 mg (initial dose may be 5 mg)	- **Risk of QT prolongation** - Risk of increased suicidal thinking and behavior in those 24 YO and younger.
Duloxetine (Cymbalta) Antidepressant, SNRI	**GAD (7+ YO),** MDD, Diabetic peripheral neuropathy, Fibromyalgia, Chronic pain	30–60 mg (first dose may be 20 mg)	**- Avoid in patients with chronic hepatic disease** - Risk of increased suicidal thinking and behavior in those 24 YO and younger.
Bupropion (Wellbutrin) Antidepressant, DNRI	MDD, Smoking cessation, Seasonal affective disorder SR and XL are commonly used formulations	IR & SR: 150–300 mg (first dose may be 37.5–75 mg) XL: 150–450 mg	- Good option with co-morbid illness such as ADHD or tobacco use disorder. **- Contraindicated in eating disorders and epilepsy due to significant lowering of seizure threshold** **-Monitor for anxiety, agitation, irritability, insomnia, hypertension** - Risk of increased suicidal thinking and behavior in those 24 YO and younger.

(continued)

Table 65.1 (continued)

Medication name and class	Indications	Dosage range (total daily dose)	Important considerations
Buspirone (BuSpar) Anxiolytic, Serotonin modulator	GAD	15–60 mg; may start at 10 mg/day	- Risk of dizziness and headache
Hydroxyzine (Atarax, Vistaril) Anxiolytic, Antihistamine	**Anxiety**	<6 YO: 10–50 mg >6 YO: 10–100 mg	- Typically used on an as needed basis for anxiety or insomnia - May cause grogginess on mornings, or paradoxical excitation
Lamotrigine (Lamictal) Mood stabilizer, anticonvulsant	Bipolar disorder (maintenance); Used off-label for mood stabilization in other disorders	100–200 mg (must start at 25 mg/day for 14 days)	- Risk of headache, nausea, sedation **- Black box warning for potentially life-threatening skin reactions including Stevens-Johnson syndrome/ toxic epidermal necrolysis**
Risperidone (Risperdal) Antipsychotic, atypical	**Schizophrenia (13+ YO), Bipolar mania (10+ YO), Irritability in autism (5+ YO)**	0.25–6 mg	**- Risk of weight gain, hyperglycemia, hyperlipidemia. Must monitor via lab work** **- Risk of tardive dyskinesia. Must complete AIMS exams periodically** **- Risk of gynecomastia**
Aripiprazole (Abilify) Antipsychotic, atypical	**Schizophrenia (13+ YO), Bipolar mania (10+ YO), Irritability in autism (6+ YO), Tourette's disorder (6+ YO)**	2–30 mg	**- Risk of weight gain, hyperglycemia, hyperlipidemia. Must monitor via lab work** **- Risk of tardive dyskinesia. Must complete AIMS exams periodically** - Can counteract antipsychotic induced hyperprolactinemia given partial agonist properties
MPH IR (Ritalin) Stimulant, Controlled Substance	**ADHD, Narcolepsy (6+ YO)**	5–60 mg DOA 4 h	- Tablet may be cut or crushed [3] - Risk of misuse and addiction, appetite suppression leading to weight loss, insomnia, hypertension and tachycardia, tics

(continued)

Table 65.1 (continued)

Medication name and class	Indications	Dosage range (total daily dose)	Important considerations
MPH ER (Concerta) Stimulant, Controlled Substance	**ADHD (6+ YO)**	18–72 mg DOA 12 h	- Capsule must not be cut or crushed [3] - Risk of misuse and addiction, appetite suppression leading to weight loss, insomnia, hypertension and tachycardia, tics
MPH ER (Quillichew ER) Stimulant, Controlled Substance	**ADHD (6+ YO)**	20–60 mg DOA 8 h	- Tablet can be cut or chewed [3] - Risk of misuse and addiction, appetite suppression leading to weight loss, insomnia, hypertension and tachycardia, tics
Dexmethyl-phenidate ER (Focalin XR) Stimulant, Controlled Substance	**ADHD (6+ YO)**	5–30 mg DOA 10–12 h	- Capsule can be opened and sprinkled but not crushed or chewed [3] - Risk of misuse and addiction, appetite suppression leading to weight loss, insomnia, hypertension and tachycardia, tics
AMP IR (Adderall) Stimulant, Controlled Substance	**ADHD (3+ YO), Narcolepsy (6+ YO)**	3–5 YO:2.5–40 mg 6–17 YO: 5–40 mg DOA 4–6 h	- Can be crushed or cut [3] **- Risk of serious cardiovascular adverse events** - Risk of misuse and addiction, appetite suppression leading to weight loss, insomnia, hypertension and tachycardia, tics
AMP ER (Adderall XR) Stimulant, Controlled Substance	**ADHD (6+ YO)**	6–12 YO: 5–30 mg 13–17 YO: 10–40 mg DOA 8–12 h	- Capsule can be opened and sprinkled but not crushed or chewed [3] **- Risk of serious cardiovascular adverse events** - Risk of misuse and addiction, appetite suppression leading to weight loss, insomnia, hypertension and tachycardia, tics

(continued)

Table 65.1 (continued)

Medication name and class	Indications	Dosage range (total daily dose)	Important considerations
AMP ER (Vyvanse) Stimulant, Controlled Substance	**ADHD (6+ YO)**	20–70 mg; DOA 9–12 h	- Liver enzymes must cleave lysine to activate, therefore less risk of misuse - Risk of misuse and addiction, appetite suppression leading to weight loss, insomnia, hypertension and tachycardia, tics - Capsule can be opened and sprinkled [3]
Clonidine (Catapres/ Kapvay) Non-stimulant; A2A	**ADHD (ER formulation only, 6+ YO)**	0.1–0.4 mg	- Risk of sedation, low blood pressure, bradycardia - IR can but cut or crushed, ER must be swallowed whole [3]
Guanfacine (Tenex/Intuniv) Non-stimulant; A2A	**ADHD (ER formulation only, 6+ YO)**	1–7 mg	- Risk of sedation (less than for clonidine), low blood pressure, bradycardia - IR can but cut or crushed, ER must be swallowed whole
Atomoxetine (Strattera) Non-stimulant; NRI	**ADHD (6+ YO)**	0.5–1.4 mg/kg/ day, max 100 mg/ day	- Twice daily dosing has better tolerability - Risk of increased suicidal thinking and behavior in those 24 YO and younger.

Key: FDA approved indications in pediatric population given in **bold.**; A2A—alpha-2 agonist; ADHD –Attention-Deficit and Hyperactivity Disorder; AIMS—abnormal involuntary movement scale; AMP—Amphetamine; ER—extended release; DNRI—dopamine norepinephrine reuptake inhibitor; DOA—duration of action; GAD—Generalized Anxiety Disorder; IR—immediate release; MDD—Major Depressive Disorder; MPH—Methylphenidate; NRI—norepinephrine reuptake inhibitor; OCD –Obsessive Compulsive Disorder; PMDD—Premenstrual Dysphoric Disorder; PTSD—Post-traumatic Stress Disorder; SNRI—serotonin norepinephrine reuptake inhibitor; SSRI—selective serotonin reuptake inhibitor; YO—years old

3. Non-stimulants may be particularly useful for patients with ADHD who have co-morbid anxiety, as they treat both.
4. When discontinuing any psychiatric medication, a gradual taper is always preferred to stopping "cold-turkey." This lowers the risk of withdrawal effects, and recurrence of symptoms. One exception to gradual tapering is when severe or potentially serious adverse effects arise.
5. When prescribing stimulants, it is preferable to start with an extended-release preparation.

Case Resolutions Case 1: Jasmine was diagnosed with social anxiety disorder, and started on escitalopram 5 mg orally once daily. This was increased after a week to 10 mg orally once daily. She initially responded very well, but by day 15 of treatment she began to complain of suicidal ideation. Because there was nothing else to account for such ideation, such as psychosocial stressors or major depressive disorder, escitalopram was discontinued, and sertraline was started at a dose of 12.5 mg orally once daily. This was titrated up to 25 mg orally once daily after a week. She did well at this dose, without adverse effects. School attendance improved and truancy proceedings were halted.

Case 2: After a month James ended up in the emergency department with hypertension, tachycardia and altered mental status. He admitted to overusing his prescribed stimulant in an attempt to perform better on examinations. On returning to clinic, a thorough history from several sources ruled out ADHD as a diagnosis. No other psychiatric conditions were found. James was discharged from the clinic.

Extra Credit Points

1. Know your state's laws regarding the age at which minors may provide consent for their own psychiatric medications.
2. Remember that antidepressants and atomoxetine have a black box warning about increasing the risk of suicidal thinking and behavior in those 24 years of age and younger.
3. Remember that stimulant medications enhance cognitive performance, including sustained attention, in any individual, not just in those with ADHD. As such they may be diverted from those with a prescription to those without. They may also be abused by the patient through taking more than prescribed to achieve a desired effect [4].

References

1. Lee ES, Findling RL. Principles of psychopharmacology. In: Dulcan's textbook of child and adolescent psychiatry. 3rd ed. American Psychiatric Publishing; 2022. p. 677–94.
2. Colaneri N, Keim S, Adesman A. Physician practices to prevent ADHD stimulant diversion and misuse. J Subst Abuse Treat. 2017;74:26–34. https://doi.org/10.1016/j.jsat.2016.12.003.
3. Bostwick JR, Demehri A. Pills to powder: an updated clinician's reference for crushable psychotropics. Current Psychiatry. 2017;16(2):46–50.
4. Bagot KS, Kaminer Y. Efficacy of stimulants for cognitive enhancement in non-attention deficit hyperactivity disorder youth: a systematic review. Addiction. 2014;109(4):547–57. https://doi.org/10.1111/add.12460.

Chapter 66
ADHD

Elizabeth W. Barnhardt and Rohan Patel

Case 1 Emily is a 7-year-old female who was referred to the school-based health clinic by her teacher due to concerns about her inability to focus. Her teacher also has noted that she has trouble following instructions, gets distracted easily, and frequently loses her personal items. Her teacher has noted that she is a very bright child but scores below average on most assignments. What could be your next steps?

Attention-deficit/hyperactivity disorder (ADHD) is one of the most common disorders of childhood, affecting 7.2–15.5% of children in the United States, and can impact cognitive, academic, behavioral, emotional, and social functioning [1]. School-based health clinicians must be able to recognize signs and symptoms of ADHD and are incredibly well-positioned to participate in their ongoing care due to their ability to communicate with both the parent and the child's school team. Most children with ADHD will continue to have symptoms and some degree of impairment into adolescence and beyond. While symptoms of hyperactivity and impulsivity may be predominant in younger children, these symptoms tend to decline into adolescence at which point inattentive symptoms persist [2, 3].

E. W. Barnhardt (✉)
Division of Developmental and Behavioral Pediatrics, Nationwide Children's Hospital/The Ohio State University, Columbus, OH, USA
e-mail: Elizabeth.Barnhardt@nationwidechildrens.org

R. Patel
Division of General Pediatrics and Adolescent Medicine, Unviersity of North Carolina at Chapel Hill, Chapel Hill, NC, USA
e-mail: Rohan.Patel@unc.edu

R. P. Olympia, J. Brady-Olympia (eds.), *Clinical Considerations in School-based Health*, https://doi.org/10.1007/978-3-031-85765-2_66

66.1 How to Diagnose ADHD

When diagnosing ADHD, we must characterize whether the child is presenting with predominantly symptoms of hyperactivity, impulsivity, or a combination of both. The three types of ADHD are ADHD (inattentive subtype), ADHD (hyperactive-impulsive subtype) and ADHD (combined subtype). To make the diagnosis of ADHD, an astute clinician must gather data from multiple sources to verify the presence of symptoms as outlined per the Diagnostic and Statistical Manual of Mental Disorders—5th Edition (DSM-5) (Table 66.1) [4].

It is important to keep in mind that other diagnoses can manifest with symptoms of what appears to be hyperactivity, impulsivity, or inattention (especially in the school environment). Shown in Table 66.2 is a possible list of items which you might consider:

Many of these diagnoses may be differentiated based on an appropriate history and physical examination.

When considering an ADHD diagnosis (such as in Emily's case above), school-based health clinicians should have the parent/caregiver of the child as well as the child's teachers complete behavior rating scales to establish the presence of

Table 66.1 DSM-5 criteria for ADHD

<table>
<tr><td colspan="2">A. For ≥ 6 months, a persistent pattern of inattention and/or hyperactivity-impulsivity exists as described by (1) and/or (2)
• +Symptoms are inconsistent with developmental level and have negatively impacted social, academic, and/or occupational functioning
• The symptoms are not solely a manifestation of oppositional behavior, defiance, hostility, or failure to understand tasks or instructions.</td></tr>
<tr><td colspan="2">B. Several symptoms present before age 12 and occur in 2 or more settings (i.e. home and school)</td></tr>
<tr><td colspan="2">C. Symptoms are not solely a manifestation of another psychiatric disorder, Substance Use Disorder, or medical condition</td></tr>
<tr><td>1. Inattention ≥6 symptoms</td><td>2. Hyperactivity and Impulsivity: ≥6 symptoms</td></tr>
<tr><td>a. Frequently forgets daily activities</td><td>a. Talks excessively</td></tr>
<tr><td>b. Easily distracted by external stimuli</td><td>b. Difficulty waiting turn</td></tr>
<tr><td>c. Unable to listen when spoken to directly</td><td>c. Impulsively blurts out answers</td></tr>
<tr><td>d. Loses items necessary for tasks or activities</td><td>d. Runs or climbs in unacceptable situations</td></tr>
<tr><td>e. Trouble organizing schoolwork and other activities</td><td>e. Inability to remain seated when necessary</td></tr>
<tr><td>f. Difficulty maintaining attention in work or play activities</td><td>f. Fidgets with hands or feet or squirms in seat</td></tr>
<tr><td>g. Unable to follow instructions and falls to finish schoolwork and other tasks</td><td>g. Unable to play or engage in quiet, leisure activities</td></tr>
<tr><td>h. Fails to focus on details or makes careless mistakes in schoolwork or other activities</td><td>h. Often "on the go" or acts as if "drive by a motor"</td></tr>
<tr><td></td><td>i. Interrupts activities or conversations of others or intrudes or takes over for others</td></tr>
</table>

Table 66.2 Differential diagnosis for ADHD in children and adolescents

Developmental abnormalities or variations • Intellectual disability • Giftedness • Normal variation	Psychosocial or environmental problems • Child abuse or neglect • Stressful home environment • Inappropriate educational setting • Frequent school absence Adverse childhood experiences causing prolonged stress response
Developmental disorder • Learning disability • Language or communication disorder • Autism spectrum disorder • Fetal Alcohol Spectrum Disorders • Genetic syndrome (ex: Fragile X syndrome, Klinefelter syndrome) • Metabolic disorders	Medical conditions • Hearing or vision impairment • Sleep disorder • Iron deficiency anemia • Lead poisoning • Endocrine disorders (ex: thyroid disorder, diabetes mellitus) • Cardiac disorders (ex: Heart failure) • Substance abuse • Malnutrition • Medication side effects
Neurologic disorder • Seizure disorder • Sequelae of central nervous system trauma or infection	Emotional/behavioral disorders • Mood disorder/Depression • Anxiety disorder • Oppositional defiant disorder (ODD) • Conduct disorder (CD) • Posttraumatic stress disorder • Adjustment disorder • Obsessive compulsive disorder

symptoms in more than one environment (Table 66.3). Typically, more narrow rating scales such as the Vanderbilt Assessment Scales are able to be used appropriately in the primary care and school-based health clinic setting, however, it is not uncommon for school psychologists to use more broadband rating scales when completing a child's Evaluation Team Report so an astute school-based health clinician may choose to reference previously completed rating scales when considering a diagnosis of ADHD. Unless concerns are identified, the evaluation for ADHD does not require neuroimaging, electroencephalography, blood lead levels, thyroid hormone levels, other bloodwork, or psychological testing unless indicated based on your initial evaluation.

Case 2 Benjamin is an 8-year-old male with a history of Autism Spectrum Disorder who is being seen due to concerns regarding significant impulsivity, difficulty participating in classroom activities, and not turning in homework on time. Academically, he is noted to struggle with reading in particular. Upon further discussion with his caregivers, you discover a longstanding history of sleeping difficulties. On average, he is only sleeping about 5–6 h at night as it takes him up to 2 h to fall asleep. In addition to his autism diagnosis he also has a history of a mixed receptive-expressive language disorder and is receiving school-based speech therapy services.

Table 66.3 Rating scales used to diagnosis ADHD

Rating scale	Behaviors assessed	Age range	Time to complete	Cost
Vanderbilt Assessment Scales (parent/ teacher)	Symptoms of ADHD according to DSM-IV criteria; screen for comorbid conditions (ODD, CD, anxiety, depression)	6–12 years	10–15 min	Free
Conners 3rd edition (parent/ teacher)	Inattention, hyperactivity/impulsivity, learning problems, executive functioning, aggression, peer relations, ODD, CD	6–18 years	15 min	Available for purchase
Conners Early Childhood	Inattention/hyperactivity, defiant/ aggressive behaviors, social functioning/atypical behaviors, anxiety, mood and affect, physical symptoms, developmental milestones (adaptive skills, communication, motor skills, play, and pre-academic/ cognitive)	2–6 years	25 min	Available for purchase
Child Behavior Checklist/ Teacher Report Form (CBCL/ TRF)	Somatic complaints, social/thought/ attention problems, anxiety/ depression, aggressive/delinquent behavior, withdrawal	Version for 1.5–5 years, 6–12 years	10 min	Available for purchase
Behavior Assessment System for Children (BASC) (parent and teacher)	Hyperactivity, aggression, conduct problems, anxiety, depression, somatization, atypicality, withdrawal, attention problems, learning problems, lack of adaptability/social/ leadership/study skills	Versions for 2–5 years, 6–11 years, and 12–21 years	10–20 min	Available for purchase

66.2 Recognizing ADHD and Co-occurring Conditions

ADHD often coexists with mental health, developmental, and medical conditions, which can complicate diagnosis and treatment. When ADHD symptoms are presenting at atypical ages (either <4 years or >12 years), there is diagnostic uncertainty, there are multiple coexisting conditions, or when there is inadequate response to standard treatments, such cases may be categorized as "complex ADHD". In such situations, referring to the Society for Developmental and Behavioral Pediatrics (SDBP) Clinical Practice Guideline for Complex ADHD can provide additional guidance [5]. Although school-based clinicians may not be expected to manage complex ADHD cases independently, being aware of these guidelines ensures that they can help identify and support the need for specialized care.

1. **Emotional and Behavioral Disorders**

Anxiety (30–40%) and depression (15–30%) frequently accompany ADHD, worsening inattention and impulsivity [1]. Children with Oppositional Defiant Disorder

(ODD) or Conduct Disorder (CD) (40–60%) may exhibit defiant or aggressive behaviors, which pose challenges in the classroom [1]. Behavioral interventions are critical for managing these conditions, both at home and in school.

2. **Learning Disabilities and Developmental Disabilities**

Learning disabilities (30–45%), particularly in reading, writing, and mathematics, often co-occur with ADHD. Children may require Individualized Education Programs (IEPs) or 504 Plans to access tailored educational support [6]. Co-existing developmental disabilities like autism spectrum disorder (ASD) require specialized interventions focusing on communication and social skills.

3. **Sleep Disorders and Sensory Impairments**

Sleep problems, such as insomnia or restless sleep, can exacerbate ADHD symptoms. Addressing sleep hygiene and adjusting medication timing can improve school performance. Vision and hearing impairments can mimic ADHD symptoms, so regular screenings are vital to ensure these impairments are properly addressed in school settings. Obstructive sleep apnea notably can manifest with symptoms of inattention and/or hyperactivity during the day so inquiring about snoring during an ADHD evaluation is necessary.

4. **Seizure and Tic Disorders**

Children with ADHD are at higher risk for seizure disorders. Schools should have action plans in place to manage seizures and work closely with healthcare providers regarding medication management. Tic disorders, such as Tourette syndrome, can be managed with environmental accommodations (e.g., stress reduction, providing breaks) in the classroom to reduce triggers [6].

5. **Substance Use, Trauma, and Bipolar Disorder**

Adolescents with ADHD have an increased risk of developing substance use disorders (SUDs), especially if their symptoms of ADHD are inadequately controlled. School-based programs focused on prevention and early intervention are crucial [7]. Children with ADHD who have experienced trauma may develop Post-Traumatic Stress Disorder (PTSD), necessitating trauma-informed care in schools. Bipolar disorder also co-occurs with ADHD and requires environmental modifications and emotional support to manage mood instability [8].

Case 2 Follow-up As seen in Jacob's case, ADHD is a common comorbidity in individuals with autism. Although ADHD is a reasonable diagnosis to explore in his case, it will also be important to first rule out insufficient sleep as being the sole contributing factor to his difficulties with daytime performance. In addition, learning disabilities should also be on the differential. Sometimes difficulties participating in classroom activities or inattention in the school environment can indicate an underlying learning-related difficulty that may warrant additional evaluation and supports. In Jacob's case, the history of having had language delays should increase your suspicion of an underlying language-based learning disability.

66.3 Treatment of ADHD

Treatment for ADHD typically involves behavioral therapy and medication, with an approach tailored to the child's age, developmental needs, and co-morbidities.

1. Treatment by Age Group

For preschool-aged children (ages 3–5 years), behavioral therapy is the first-line treatment. Medications are generally avoided unless behavioral interventions are insufficient, symptoms are severe, and/or there are significant safety concerns [5]. Parent training programs help caregivers manage behaviors at home, while teachers implement similar strategies in the classroom.

For children ages 6–12 years, a combination of behavioral therapy and medication is often the most effective treatment. Medications like stimulants help manage core ADHD symptoms such as attention, focus, and impulse control, while behavioral interventions focus on academic and social skills. Positive reinforcement systems and classroom management techniques are important in promoting engagement and reducing disruptive behaviors [1].

For adolescents (ages 13–18 years), treatment focuses on organizational skills training and study skills, while medication helps manage core symptoms. Adolescents face increasing academic and social pressures, and treatment plans should address these challenges by emphasizing independence, time management, and planning. Ongoing communication with teachers helps ensure that interventions are effective [8].

2. Behavioral Therapy

Behavioral interventions help manage ADHD symptoms by teaching children, parents, and teachers how to improve behavior and daily functioning. School-based strategies include daily report cards, positive reinforcement, and token reward systems, which provide immediate feedback and rewards for achieving behavioral goals [8].

3. Medication Management

For most children, stimulants like methylphenidate and amphetamine-based products are first line medications used to treat ADHD. When medications are used to treat ADHD in children less than 6 years of age, typically short-acting formulations (with a 4–6 h duration of action) are used, whereas for children 6 years and up, extended-release formulations (which typically have a duration of action of 8–12 h) are used. For children who do not tolerate stimulants, there are many nonstimulant options available for use. The ADHD Medication Guide (www.ADHDMedicationGuide.com) is a helpful visual aid which reviews all doses of FDA-approved brand name medications and describes which medications can be chewed, sprinkled on food, dissolved in liquid, or must be taken whole and provides

Table 66.4 Common ADHD medications

Drug	Side effects
Methylphenidate products (Ritalin, Methylin, Metadate CD, Concerta, Ritalin LA)	Insomnia, decreased appetite, weight loss, headache, irritability, stomachache
Dexmethylphenidate (Focalin, Focalin XR)	Insomnia, decreased appetite, weight loss, headache, irritability, stomachache
Mixed amphetamine products (Adderall, Adderall XR)	Insomnia, decreased appetite, weight loss, headache, irritability, stomachache
Atomoxetine	Decreased appetite, GI upset, sedation, lightheadedness
Viloxazine	Increased heart rate and blood pressure, insomnia, somnolence, GI upset, weight loss
Clonidine and Guanfacine	Hypotension, bradycardia, fatigue, lightheadedness

age-specific dosing information. Shown in Table 66.4 are examples of commonly utilized ADHD medications and their side effects.

Teachers, parents, and school-based clinicians can work together to assess efficacy, duration of action, and side effects of medications utilized. Ongoing monitoring tools, such as the Vanderbilt Assessment Scales, help quantify improvements in symptoms and track progress over time. Typically, extended-release formulations last throughout the school day, but occasionally afternoon booster doses (typically of short-acting stimulant doses) might be necessary. Teachers are often the first to notice side effects, such as mood swings, irritability, or appetite suppression. Reporting these observations to healthcare providers helps inform decisions on medication adjustments, ensuring that the benefits outweigh the side effects. For helpful tips on ADHD medication management, clinicians can reference the ADHD Toolkit published by the American Academy of Pediatrics [9].

4. School-Based Treatment and Support

Individualized Education Plans (IEPs) and 504 Plans provide accommodations to support academic success, such as extra time on tests, preferential seating, and structured routines [10]. The AAP ADHD Toolkit [9] also provides excellent guidance on managing ADHD in school settings and helping families navigate requesting formalized supports in the form of IEPs or 504 plans. ADHD is a qualifying disability under Section 504 of the Federal Rehabilitation Act, so at a bare minimum, a child with a diagnosis of ADHD is entitled to classroom accommodations in the form of a 504 plan. A child with ADHD may also qualify for an Individualized Education Plan if they meet criteria for special education services per the criteria set out in the Individuals with Disabilities Education Act (IDEA). Children with ADHD may qualify for an IEP if they have a comorbid diagnosis such as autism, intellectual disability, learning disability, hearing impairment, or speech and language difficulties.

66.4 When to Refer

Primary care providers can manage most ADHD cases, but referral to a specialist and/or directly to the emergency department may be considered in the following situations shown in Table 66.5.

Extra Credit Points

1. To diagnose ADHD, behaviors must be present in at least two different environments
2. The first line treatment for children less than 6 years old diagnosed with ADHD is behavioral therapy unless there are significant safety concerns or the child is exhibiting evidence of significant impairment despite appropriate interventions
3. For children ages 6 years and older, the ideal treatment regimen typically includes a triad of medication (with stimulants being first line), behavioral therapy, and appropriate school-based supports
4. Children with ADHD are eligible for services and an individual accommodation plan (504 plan) but may also qualify for an Individualized Education Plan in the case of a comorbid diagnosis or learning disorder

Table 66.5 When to refer to subspecialists or the emergency department

Developmental-behavioral pediatrics (DBP) or psychiatry	Emergency department
Co-occurring psychiatric disorders: Complex conditions like severe anxiety, bipolar disorder, or depression may require psychiatric intervention.	Suicidal ideation or severe self-harm behaviors.
Non-response to standard treatments: When a child does not respond to first-line stimulant medications or experiences severe side effects.	Severe side effects from ADHD medications, such as fainting or rapid heart rate
Complex developmental disorders: Children with ADHD and significant developmental delays, ASD, or seizure disorders may need specialized care.	Acute psychosis or mania triggered by ADHD medication.
	Uncontrolled aggression or violence that poses a risk to others.

References

1. Wolraich ML, Hagan JF Jr, Allan C, et al. Clinical practice guideline for the diagnosis, evaluation, and treatment of attention-deficit/hyperactivity disorder in children and adolescents. Pediatrics. 2019;144(4):e20192528. https://doi.org/10.1542/peds.2019-2528.
2. Molina BS, Hinshaw SP, Swanson JM, et al. MTA Cooperative Group. The MTA at 8 years: prospective follow-up of children treated for combined-type ADHD in a multisite study. J Am Acad Child Adolesc Psychiatry. 2009;48(5):484–500.
3. Holbrook JR, Cuffe SP, Cai B, et al. Persistence of parent-reported ADHD symptoms from childhood through adolescence in a community sample. J Atten Disord. 2016;20(1):11–20.
4. American Psychiatric Association. Diagnostic and statistical manual of mental disorders. 5th ed. Washington, DC; 2013.
5. Barbaresi WJ, Katusic SK, Voigt RG, et al. SDBP clinical practice guideline for the evaluation and treatment of complex ADHD. J Dev Behav Pediatr. 2020;41(Suppl 1):S35–57. https://doi.org/10.1097/DBP.0000000000000734.
6. Centers for Disease Control and Prevention. ADHD toolkit for clinicians and teachers. CDC ADHD Toolkit. 2019. https://chadd.org.
7. Sibley MH, Pelham WE, Molina BS, et al. The delinquency outcomes of boys with ADHD with and without comorbidity. J Abnorm Child Psychol. 2012;40(4):671–83. https://doi.org/10.1007/s10802-011-9602-9.
8. Pelham WE Jr, Fabiano GA. Evidence-based psychosocial treatments for attention-deficit/hyperactivity disorder. J Clin Child Adolesc Psychol. 2008;37(1):184–214. https://doi.org/10.1080/15374410701818681.
9. Zurhellen W, Lessin HR, Chan E, Allan CC, Wolraich M, Sprecher E, Evans SW. ADHD-Caring for children with ADHD: a practial resource toolkit for clinicians. 3rd ed. American Academy of Pediatrics; 2019. https://publications.aap.org/toolkits/book/337/chapter/5731127/Caring-for-Children-With-ADHD-A-Practical-Resource
10. DuPaul GJ, Chronis-Tuscano A, Danielson ML, Visser SN. Predictors of receipt of school services in a national sample of youth with ADHD. J Atten Disord. 2019;23(11):1303–19. https://doi.org/10.1177/1087054718816169.

Chapter 67
Alcohol and Substance Abuse

Manvita Mareboina and Stephen Sandelich

According to the Diagnostic and Statistical Manual of Mental Disorders Fifth Edition (DSM-5), substance use disorders (SUDs) are characterized by a problematic pattern of use of an intoxicating substance leading to significant impairment or distress. The DSM-5 outlines 11 criteria categorized into impaired control, physical dependence, social issues, and risky use, which can manifest due to substance misuse [1]. Substance use disorders are classified as mild, moderate, or severe based on the number of symptoms a person exhibits. The classification aids in guiding tailored treatment recommendations and interventions [2]. High-risk substance use refers to the consumption of substances by adolescents that dramatically increases the likelihood of serious adverse outcomes, including injury, legal issues, school dropout, or death [3].

To understand the prevalence and impact of alcohol and substance use among adolescents, it is important to consider current statistics and trends. Approximately a quarter of children in America live in households impacted by alcohol abuse and dependence [4]. The use of vaping products and e-cigarettes has also significantly increased among adolescents.[2] Substance use at earlier ages increases a student's risk of developing SUD, further elevating the likelihood of other adverse health and life outcomes, including academic difficulties and less schooling [5, 6]. According to the 2023 Monitoring the Future survey, the percentage of adolescents reporting the use of any illicit substances has continued to hold steady below pre-pandemic levels. Specifically, 10.9% of eighth graders, 19.8% of 10th graders, and 31.2% of 12th graders reported any illicit drug use in the past year. The use of alcohol remained stable for eighth and 10th graders at 15.1% and 30.6% respectively but declined for 12th graders to 45.7% from 51.9% in the previous year. Nicotine vaping remained stable for eighth graders at 11.4% but fell in older grades. Cannabis

M. Mareboina · S. Sandelich (✉)
Penn State Hershey Medical Center, Hershey, PA, USA
e-mail: mmareboina@pennstatehealth.psu.edu; ssandelich@pennstatehealth.psu.edu

R. P. Olympia, J. Brady-Olympia (eds.), *Clinical Considerations in School-based Health*, https://doi.org/10.1007/978-3-031-85765-2_67

use remained stable across all surveyed grades (8.3% amongst eighth graders, 17.8% among 10th graders, and 29% amongst 12th graders) [7, 8].

In light of these challenges, the role of school-based health providers in early recognition and intervention becomes crucial. School-based health centers (SBHCs) can work with schools and community centers to improve substance use services and academic outcomes [9]. Research has shown that SBHCs offer a secure and supportive environment for SUD screening among adolescents [10].

Case 1 A 14-year-old student presents with mood swings, frequent tardiness, and a strong smell of alcohol during a school event. The student's academic performance has recently declined and they have been missing assignments. Teachers have reported noticeable changes in behavior, including increased irritability and withdrawal from previously enjoyed activities. The student's friends have also expressed concern, mentioning that they have seen the student with a different peer group known for risky behaviors. The student has no prior history of behavioral issues or academic struggles.

During a routine school event, a teacher noticed the student smelled strongly of alcohol. When approached, the student was evasive and defensive, refusing to discuss the matter. The student's physical appearance included bloodshot eyes and poor hygiene, which were not typical for this student. What would you do next?

Signs and symptoms of alcohol use and acute intoxication in adolescents can include mood swings, frequent tardiness, a strong smell of alcohol, noticeable changes in behavior such as increased irritability and withdrawal from previously enjoyed activities, and physical signs like bloodshot eyes and poor hygiene. In more severe cases, symptoms may include confusion, agitation, vomiting, seizures, slow breathing, hypothermia, and unresponsiveness. In order to assess adolescent substance use, validated screening tools such as CRAFFT, Problem Oriented Screening Instrument for Teenagers (POSIT), Alcohol Use Disorders Identification Test (AUDIT), and National Institute on Alcohol Abuse and Alcoholism (NIAAA) Screening Guide are recommended (Table 67.1) [2]. The American Academy of Pediatrics (AAP) advises medical providers to familiarize themselves with Screening, Brief Intervention, and Referral to Treatment (SBIRT) initiatives [2]. Screening involves the use of validated tools to quickly assess the severity of substance use and identify the appropriate level of treatment. Brief Intervention focuses on engaging individuals in a conversation while providing advice about substance use, and motivating them to consider making changes. Referral to Treatment involves directing individuals who require more extensive care to specialized treatment services, particularly when alcohol abuse is identified. This approach ensures that patients receive timely, appropriate care, potentially preventing the escalation of substance use issues

Care Plan Engage the student's family, referral to counseling or a substance use program, and monitoring at school. Referral to a specialized substance use program is indicated when the screening tools identify moderate to severe substance use,

Table 67.1 Adolescent substance use assessment tools

Tool	Age group (in years)	Time to administer	Content
AUDIT[11]	13–19	Approximately 2 min	- Questions about alcohol use frequency and quantity—Screening for alcohol-related problems
CRAFFT[12]	14–18	74 s (paper) and 49 s (electronic)	- Six questions covering alcohol and drug use, as well as consequences and treatment history
NIAAA	9–11, 11–14, 14–18	Not specified	- Two questions focused on alcohol use, tailored to each age group
POSIT[13]	12–19	20–30 min	- Comprehensive assessment covering substance use, related problems, and risk factors - Identifies services that may be needed in 10 functional areas

significant behavioral issues, or when the student exhibits high-risk behaviors that pose immediate harm to themselves or others. Screening tools are applicable at any stage of drug use [2, 14]. Additionally, students referred to substance use programs are closely monitored through regular check-ins with school counselors and health-care providers. Progress is tracked through follow-up screenings, behavioral observations, academic performance reviews, and feedback from teachers and family members. Potential complications include academic decline, behavioral issues, use of other illicit substances, and peer influence. Triage/Disposition involves referral to a substance use program, continued school support, and periodic evaluation. Students are evaluated using a combination of self-report questionnaires, clinical interviews, and feedback from family and school staff. Regular assessments help determine the effectiveness of the interventions and whether adjustments are needed.

What Educators/Schools Can Do Utilize the resources Substance Abuse and Mental Health Services Administration (SAMHSA) provides for screening and assessment, including the National Institute on Alcohol Abuse and Alcoholism Screening Guide. Additionally, SAMHSA offers a behavioral health treatment services locator to aid in accessing appropriate support and treatment for adolescents grappling with substance use issues.

Case Resolution The 14-year-old student, identified with mood swings, frequent tardiness, and a strong smell of alcohol, was assessed using tools like the CRAFFT, POSIT, AUDIT, and NIAAA Screening Guide. These assessments confirmed the student's risky alcohol use behaviors. Interventions and outcomes subsequent to the diagnosis include the following:

1. **Family Engagement and Counseling**: The student's family was involved in the intervention process. They participated in counseling sessions to support the student's recovery.
2. **Referral to a Substance Use Program**: The student was referred to a specialized adolescent substance use program, which included therapy sessions to address alcohol use and teach coping mechanisms.
3. **Monitoring and Support at School**: The school implemented a monitoring plan to support the student's recovery, providing additional academic assistance and regular check-ins with the school counselor.
4. **Periodic Evaluation**: The student was regularly evaluated to monitor progress and adherence to the treatment plan.

This case points out several key points:

- Timely recognition by teachers and peers led to a structured and supportive intervention plan.
- Tools like CRAFFT, POSIT, AUDIT, and NIAAA provided a comprehensive assessment of the student's alcohol use.
- The intervention involved the student's family, school, and specialized substance use programs.
- Regular evaluations and continuous support helped the student improve their academic and personal life.

Case 2 A 16-year-old student is found unresponsive on campus during lunch break. Peers reported that the student had been acting strangely, appearing confused and agitated earlier in the day. The student has a known history of experimenting with various substances. Upon initial assessment, the student's airway was patent, but their breathing was shallow with a slow respiratory rate. They had a pulse with a rate of 50 beats per minute and blood pressure, recorded at 80/50 mmHg. The student was unresponsive to verbal stimuli with dilated pupils. No visible signs of trauma were present, but the student appeared flushed and sweating. What would you do next?

Considering the differential diagnosis for mental status depression [15], possible causes included opioid overdose, which would present with pinpoint pupils, respiratory depression, and unresponsiveness. Management would involve administering naloxone, monitoring vitals, and calling 911. Another possibility is gamma-hydroxybutyrate (GHB) overdose, indicated by drowsiness, dizziness, nausea, loss of consciousness, and respiratory depression, managed by monitoring vitals, providing supportive care, and referring to the emergency department. Also, consider alcohol poisoning with signs such as confusion, vomiting, seizures, slow breathing, hypothermia, and unresponsiveness. This will require monitoring of vitals, prevention of aspiration, and referral to the emergency department.

For mania or psychosis, potential causes included methamphetamine intoxication [16], which presents with agitation, increased energy, paranoia, hallucinations, tachycardia, and hyperthermia. Management involved creating a calm environment, monitoring vitals, ensuring hydration, applying cooling measures, and referring to the emergency department. Synthetic cannabinoid intoxication was another consideration, with symptoms of agitation, confusion, hallucinations, tachycardia, vomiting, and seizures managed by monitoring vitals, providing supportive care, and referring to the emergency department. Tables 67.2 and 67.3 describe common designer "street" drugs, stratified by mental status depression and mania/psychosis. Care of a student under the influence of alcohol or drugs includes the assessment and initial stabilization of airway, breathing, and circulation, followed by the activation of Emergency Medical Services.

Prevention and Follow-Up Actions Provide education to students about the dangers of substance use and the importance of seeking help, offer counseling and sup-

Table 67.2 Common designer "street" drugs affecting mania/Psychosis [17]

Drug	Street names	Presenting signs & symptoms	Disposition
Ecstasy (MDMA)	Molly, E, X	Euphoria, increased energy, emotional warmth, distorted perceptions, dehydration, hyperthermia	Hydration, monitor vitals, cooling measures, refer to ED if severe symptoms
Synthetic Cannabinoids	Spice, K2	Agitation, confusion, hallucinations, tachycardia, vomiting, seizures	Monitor vitals, supportive care, refer to ED if severe symptoms
Bath Salts	Flakka, Cloud Nine	Agitation, paranoia, hallucinations, chest pain, increased blood pressure, aggressive behavior	Monitor vitals, supportive care, sedation if necessary, refer to ED
LSD	Acid, Blotter	Hallucinations, dilated pupils, tremors, altered perception of time, paranoia	Calm environment, reassurance, monitor vitals, refer to ED if severe symptoms
GHB	Liquid Ecstasy, G	Drowsiness, dizziness, nausea, loss of consciousness, respiratory depression	Monitor vitals, supportive care, refer to ED if severe symptoms
Methamphetamine	Crystal, Ice, Meth	Increased energy, decreased appetite, rapid heart rate, high blood pressure, hyperthermia, paranoia	Hydration, monitor vitals, cooling measures, refer to ED if severe symptoms
Ketamine	Special K, Kit Kat	Dissociation, hallucinations, confusion, elevated heart rate, nausea	Calm environment, monitor vitals, supportive care, refer to ED if severe symptoms
Psilocybin Mushrooms	Shrooms, Magic Mushrooms	Hallucinations, altered perception, nausea, panic attacks	Calm environment, reassurance, monitor vitals, refer to ED if severe symptoms
Rohypnol	Roofies, Forget-Me-Pill	Drowsiness, confusion, impaired motor skills, memory loss, respiratory depression	Monitor vitals, supportive care, refer to ED if severe symptoms

All exposures and usages should prompt immediate stabilization and ED visit as needed

Table 67.3 Common designer "street" drugs affecting mental status depression [17]

Drug	Street names	Presenting signs & symptoms	Disposition
GHB	Liquid Ecstasy, G	Drowsiness, dizziness, nausea, loss of consciousness, respiratory depression	Monitor vitals, supportive care, refer to ED if severe symptoms
Rohypnol	Roofies, Forget-Me-Pill	Drowsiness, confusion, impaired motor skills, memory loss, respiratory depression	Monitor vitals, supportive care, refer to ED if severe symptoms

port services to students struggling with substance use, and collaborate with local health services and community organizations to create a network of support for students. Implement SBIRT, which screens students for substance use, providing brief interventions for those at risk and facilitating referrals to specialized treatment services when needed (SAMHSA). Referrals are made based on the severity of the situation: immediate medical emergencies require an ED referral, significant behavioral or psychological concerns warrant a child and adolescent psychiatrist, and persistent or severe substance use issues indicate the need for an alcohol and drug treatment facility. By integrating SBIRT into the school nurse's role and collaborating with other school-based health providers, educators, and community resources, early identification of substance use issues can occur, preventing future drug overdoses.

Case Resolution Upon arrival at the emergency department, the student received comprehensive care, including further evaluation, stabilization, and treatment for the identified substance use. The precise substance responsible for the unresponsiveness was confirmed through toxicology screening, allowing for targeted treatment.

67.1 Prevention and Follow-Up Actions

- **Education and Awareness**: The school implemented an educational program to raise awareness about the dangers of substance use and the importance of seeking help.
- **Counseling and Support Services**: The student was referred to counseling and substance use support services to address underlying issues and prevent future incidents.
- **SBIRT Implementation**: The school adopted the Screening, Brief Intervention, and Referral to Treatment (SBIRT) approach to identify and support students at risk of substance use.
- **Collaboration with Community Resources**: Partnerships with local health services and community organizations were established to create a support network for students to reach out to other peers and professionals.

67.2 Future of School-Based Care and Innovations

Looking forward, it is imperative to prioritize the integration of mental health and substance use services within educational settings. This includes expanding school nurses' roles and health centers' roles to provide early intervention, support, and referrals for adolescents facing these challenges. The continual development of innovative approaches in the assessment and intervention of students with alcohol and drug use, such as technology-enabled screening tools and evidence-based interventions tailored to their needs, enhances effective and accessible care. Additionally, integrating telehealth services and digital platforms shows significant promise in broadening access to care for this demographic.

Extra-Credit Points

1. Early Identification: Prompt recognition of signs and symptoms suggestive of substance use or mental health issues in adolescents—such as mood swings, tardiness, or unexplained injuries—allows for timely intervention and support.
2. Utilization of Screening Tools: Incorporating validated screening tools, such as those mentioned in Table 67.1, facilitates early identification of substance use disorders among adolescents.
3. SBIRT Integration: Understanding and implementing Screening, Brief Intervention, and Referral to Treatment (SBIRT) initiatives, as recommended by professional organizations like the American Academy of Pediatrics (AAP), is crucial for early intervention.
4. Collaboration: Effective support for adolescents struggling with substance use or mental health concerns requires collaboration between healthcare providers, educators, and community resources.
5. Prevention and Education: Educating adolescents, families, and school personnel about the risks associated with substance use and mental health disorders, as well as promoting healthy coping mechanisms, plays a vital role in addressing these issues early.

References

1. American Psychiatric Association. Diagnostic and statistical manual of mental disorders. 5th ed. Washington, DC: American Psychiatric Association; 2013.
2. Kulak JA, Griswold KS. Adolescent substance use and misuse: recognition and management. Am Fam Physician. 2019;99:689–96.
3. High risk substance use in youth. Adolescent and school health. CDC. 2023. https://www.cdc.gov/healthyyouth/substance-use/index.htm. Accessed 3 Jun 2024.
4. Grant BF. Estimates of US children exposed to alcohol abuse and dependence in the family. Am J Public Health. 2000;90:112–5.
5. Mrug S, Gaines J, Su W, Windle M. School-level substance use: effects on early adolescents' alcohol, tobacco, and marijuana use. J Stud Alcohol Drugs. 2010;71:488–95.
6. Lee KTH, Vandell DL. Out-of-school time and adolescent substance use. J Adolesc Health Off Publ Soc Adolesc Med. 2015;57:523–9. https://doi.org/10.1016/j.jadohealth.2015.07.003.

7. Miech RA, Johnston LD, Patrick ME, O'Malley PM, Bachman JG. Monitoring the future: national survey results on drug use, 1975–2023: secondary school students. NIDA, University of Michigan Institute for Social Research; n.d.
8. NIDA. Reported drug use among adolescents continued to hold below pre-pandemic levels in 2023. 2023. https://nida.nih.gov/news-events/news-releases/2023/12/reported-drug-use-among-adolescents-continued-to-hold-below-pre-pandemic-levels-in-2023. Accessed 3 June 2024.
9. Kjolhede C, Lee AC, Duncan De Pinto C, O'Leary SC, Baum M, Savio Beers N, et al. School-based health centers and pediatric practice. Pediatrics. 2021;148:e2021053758. https://doi.org/10.1542/peds.2021-053758.
10. Ozechowski TJ, Wilson K. Rates, patterns, and predictors of follow-up care for adolescents at risk for substance use disorder in a school-based health center SBIRT program. J Adolesc Health Off Publ Soc Adolesc Med. 2022;71:S57–64. https://doi.org/10.1016/j.jadohealth.2022.02.024.
11. Alcohol screening and brief intervention for youth: a practitioner's guide. National Institute on Alcohol Abuse and Alcoholism (NIAAA). n.d. https://www.niaaa.nih.gov/alcohols-effects-health/professional-education-materials/alcohol-screening-and-brief-intervention-youth-practitioners-guide/resources. Accessed 3 June 2024.
12. CRAFFT. n.d.. https://crafft.org/. Accessed 3 June 2024.
13. Problem Oriented Screening Instrument for Teenagers (POSIT). Office of justice programs. n.d. https://www.ojp.gov/ncjrs/virtual-library/abstracts/problem-oriented-screening-instrument-teenagers-posit. Accessed 3 June 2024.
14. National Institute of Drug Abuse. Principles of adolescent substance use disorder treatment: A research-based guide. n.d.
15. Change in mental status. StatPearls: NCBI Bookshelf. n.d. https://www.ncbi.nlm.nih.gov/books/NBK441973/. Accessed 3 June 2024.
16. Dailey MW, Saadabadi A. Mania. StatPearls, Treasure Island (FL): StatPearls Publishing; 2024.
17. Street & commercial names. n.d. https://www.nihlibrary.nih.gov/resources/subject-guides/opioids/street-commercial-names. Accessed 3 June 2024.

Chapter 68
Anxiety and PTSD

Stephanie Harvison, Tara Kelly, and Alexis Steefel

It is estimated that nearly 1 in 12 children aged 3–17 years and 1 in 4 adolescents aged 13–18 years are diagnosed with an anxiety related disorder in the United States [1]. Individuals can experience varying levels of impairment and diagnoses range from specific phobias to social anxieties, separation anxiety, panic disorders, and generalized anxiety. In addition, trauma related disorders, including Post-Traumatic Stress Disorder, often result in a heightened degree of common symptoms associated with anxiety.

When considering a child's well-being, their mental health is a large contributing factor to the ways in which they navigate their world and interact with others. Responses to stressors and traumas cause neurological pathways to alter as an individual attempts to cope and survive within their environment. These changes directly impact how a child learns, interacts with others, and manages emotions. Consider the following six students described in Table 68.1.

In 1998, the Adverse Childhood Experiences (ACE) Study concluded that the greater an individual is exposed to stressful experiences in childhood, the more likely they are to develop negative mental health and physical health outcomes as they age [2]. A trauma-informed approach does not necessitate that an individual discloses their trauma. Rather, it assumes that all individuals bring a history of trauma to their relationships with others and the environments that they spend their time in. Healthcare providers in a variety of settings, including educational settings, hold a unique position in that they can implement small changes during each interaction with a patient that are aligned to the beliefs and assumptions of a trauma-informed approach [3]. Universal approaches that can be taken include establishing physical and emotional safety, developing trust, practicing open communication,

S. Harvison (✉) · T. Kelly · A. Steefel
Penn State Hershey Medical Center, Hershey, PA, USA
e-mail: sharvison@pennstatehealth.psu.edu; tkelly3@pennstatehealth.psu.edu; asteefel@pennstatehealth.psu.edu

R. P. Olympia, J. Brady-Olympia (eds.), *Clinical Considerations in School-based Health*, https://doi.org/10.1007/978-3-031-85765-2_68

Table 68.1 Six student presentations: anxiety disorder diagnosis?

Case #1:	Rachel is a 7-year old female demonstrating decreased attendance at school in recent weeks, and, when in attendance, she seems to more frequently check-in with her teacher rather than work independently as she had in the past. Her participation in the classroom is minimal and she requests to visit the school nurse often for complaints of stomachaches. The school nurse spoke to Rachel who revealed she has been spending her nights between the homes of different family members while her parents remain at the hospital with a sibling diagnosed with cancer five weeks ago. She has only seen her parents and sibling for short visits to the hospital on the weekends. She later revealed she has been unable to sleep at night and has developed fears that other members of her family will also develop cancer.
Case #2:	Isabella is a high school senior who has been described by family and friends as a "worry wart". She reports that she has always been a nervous individual since a young age, and worries about things such as her grades, artistic skills, and whether or not she is a good enough soccer player. She has attempted meditation strategies after speaking to her guidance counselor without success because she feels she cannot concentrate and remains restless. Sometimes she asks to stay home from school because she is unable to get a good night's sleep as her mind won't "shut off". Her parents shared that she can often be difficult to be around due to unexplained irritability. Her worrying seems to have worsened this school year as she is preparing to submit college applications.
Case #3:	Johnny is a middle school student. It is known by the school administration that Johnny has witnessed domestic abuse between this biological father and mother. Changes have been noticed within the past 3-months in the school setting. Johnny seems to disengage during specific classes such as gym and music. When this disengagement occurs, he quickly leaves the environment and is found in an entirely different room. There have been noted shifts in participation with previously preferred elective classes, as well as an increase in isolation during recess and lunch. Johnny appears uncomfortable during sudden transitions in the average classroom day as teachers say he reacts "strongly" to student groupings for assignments, and corrections for assignments. These "strongly" seeming reactions have not only challenged the procedures of each day, but also has challenged Johnny's relationships with his peers and his teacher.

(continued)

Table 68.1 (continued)

Case #4:	Ariela is a high school student and is new to the school district with this being her second academic year. Ariela quickly became part of the social activities in the school with sports, academic clubs and participation with the school theatre. Within the past 6-months, Ariela has experienced moments that she describes as feeling "an extreme overwhelm." Peers have escalated their concern to teachers during these episodes as they are worried about Ariela's well-being. When asking Ariela to reflect on these experiences, she shares that she first notices her body sweating and shaking, then her heart pounding with an intense chest pain. Ariela goes on to share that these experiences often repeat with these same symptoms, but they always come with some element of "worry." Oftentimes, the worry comes during the attack with it being about the fear of not surviving those moments. As of the past month, this worry has caused her to drastically change her normal routine by only attending the social events that she can watch and not perform with the fear of the "extreme overwhelm" suddenly happening again.
Case #5:	Marina is an 8-year old third grade student returning to school following a brief hospitalization after her family was a motor vehicle crash two weeks ago. While no one was seriously injured, Marina suffered a broken arm and her mother was diagnosed with a concussion after hitting her head on the window. Since returning to school, Marina has been uncharacteristically irritable and tearful. She appears to be having difficulty focusing on her work and is easily startled by noises in the classroom. Marina has frequently asked her teacher to contact her mother to ensure her safety and wellbeing during the school day. The school counselor followed up with Marina after her teacher expressed concerns. Marina informed the school counselor that she is having difficulty sleeping at night and is having nightmares about her family being hurt. She also reported having difficulty getting in the car, although is able to ride the school bus.
Case #6:	Jackson is a 7th grade student and has been noted to be increasingly withdrawn from his peers since the beginning of the school year. His teachers report that he will often eat lunch alone, sometimes even requesting to go to the nurse or meeting with a teacher during the lunch period. He is also rarely seen engaging with peers during free time. Teachers have not observed any interactions concerning for bullying. Multiple teachers expressed concern to the school counselor. When asked about these concerns, Jackson reports that he does not have any friends and everyone makes fun of him at school. He reports that he avoids the school cafeteria because when he walks in for lunch, he can feel all eyes on him and knows that his peers are scrutinizing him, such as his clothing or something he said. Jackson expressed that he is unable to sleep at night due to worries related to what his peers think of him and replaying the embarrassing events of the school day.

collaborating with other disciplines, and empowering individuals to make choices, which can greatly reduce anxieties and the potential for re-traumatization when implemented during interactions with others [4].

As an individual perceives danger, stress hormones are released that cause physiological changes to prepare the body for response to the threat [5]. Those hormones are often broken down as a threat passes; however, chronic activation can create toxic neurological pathways. Further, if an individual is exposed to a traumatic or life-threatening event, the limbic system may start to respond accordingly with an involuntary fight, flight or freeze reaction [5]. The maturing brain of a child or adolescent typically includes the development of neurological prefrontal-amygdala circuits responsible for emotional regulation of experiences such as fear and anxiety

[6]. Trauma in the developing brain leaves potential for priming the limbic system for frequent alerting, causing the child to respond with involuntary reactions regardless of the level of threat. As threat processes and emotional regulatory systems are impacted by childhood trauma, risk of affective disorders are higher amongst this group [6].

Oftentimes the impact of trauma on a child or adolescent leads to the inability to regulate emotions [7]. Secondary to the neurological impact of trauma, difficulty is often found with identifying, controlling and directing internal feelings. Given the appropriate circumstances to engage in experiences that support an individual in achieving these aims would allow them to appropriately survey an environment and respond to circumstances based on appropriate or improved emotion regulation. Creating opportunity for self-regulation will aim to mitigate the effects of trauma for the benefit of creating neural pathways for alternative mind-body response patterns [7]. Such interventions for mind-body self-regulation, for example: mindfulness, yoga, and focused breathing techniques, allow for establishment of new or improved neurologic pathways. Observable behaviors recognized with this support include increasing calmness, self-control, positive thinking, self-awareness, and other areas significant for functioning within structured learning environments [7]. Since schools are a critical setting to observe changes in a child's disposition and can encourage collaboration between family and community resources to ensure students receive the right support to manage anxiety, recognizing key characteristics of these disorders is vital (Table 68.2) [8].

Individuals may be at higher risk for developing symptoms of anxiety if they have experienced or witnessed a trauma in their life, have pre-existing mental health conditions, are experiencing an increased number of psychosocial stressors, or are they are navigating health concerns or a complex medical diagnosis. In addition, research indicates that there is a genetic pre-disposition to anxiety [9]. Students and their families should connect with their primary care physician to begin the steps of connecting with a licensed mental health provider and/or psychiatrist, if needed, as most treatment for anxiety and PTSD occurs outside of the school environment.

Pediatricians, psychiatrists, and licensed mental health provides will use validated anxiety screening tools and rating scales to assist in the identification and diagnosis of various anxiety and trauma-related disorders, as these standardized tools are more effective than clinical assessment alone. The most commonly used tools in the pediatric population are the Screen for Child Anxiety Related Disorders (SCARED) and the Generalized Anxiety Disorder-7 (GAD-7). The SCARED is an anxiety screening tool validated for children 8 years old and up to assess for a variety of anxiety disorders, including panic disorder, generalized anxiety, specific phobias, separation anxiety, social anxiety, school avoidance, and somatic symptoms. The GAD-7 is a validated rating scale specific to generalized anxiety disorder for children ages 11 to 17 and can be used to track the severity of symptoms over time and treatment [10].

Seeking support early, identifying and practicing coping skills that include components of mindfulness, maintaining a healthy lifestyle with a balanced diet and proper the management of symptoms. Some appropriate intervention treatments

Table 68.2 Defining characteristics of the most commonly diagnosed anxiety and trauma disorders

Separation anxiety disorder	• Developmentally inappropriate and excessive fear or anxiety concerning separation from attachment figure(s) • Recurrent and excessive distress when anticipating or experiencing separation • Persistent and excessive worry about losing attachment figure(s) • Persistent and excessive fear of being alone, including during sleep • Frequent nightmares related to the above • Frequent somatic complaints when separated from attachment figure(s) • Symptoms are persistent for 4 or more weeks in children/adolescents
Specific Phobia	• Marked fear or anxiety about a specific object or situation • Object or situation provokes immediate fear or anxiety • Object or situation is actively avoided • Fear or anxiety is out of proportion to the actual danger posed • Symptoms are persistent for 6 months or more
Social anxiety disorder	• Marked fear or anxiety about one or more social situations in which the individual is exposed to possible scrutiny by others • Fears they will act in a way that will be negatively evaluated • Social situations almost always provoke fear or anxiety • Social situations are actively avoided • Symptoms are persistent for 6 months or more

(continued)

Table 68.2 (continued)

Panic disorder	• Recurrent unexpected panic attacks • Panic attacks are an abrupt surge of intense fear that reaches a peak within minutes and the following symptoms may occur: palpitations, sweating, trembling, shortness of breath, chest pain, nausea, dizziness, numbness or tingling, and fear of losing control or dying • Panic attacks are following by 1 month of persistent concern about additional panic attacks and/or maladaptive change in behavior related to the attacks
Generalized anxiety disorder	• Excessive worry and anxiety occurring more days than not for at least 6 months, about various events or activities • Difficult to control the worry • Worry and anxiety may be associated with the following symptoms: restlessness, fatigue, difficulty concentrating, irritability, muscle tension and sleep disturbance
Posttraumatic stress disorder	• Exposure to actual or threatened death, serious injury, or sexual violence by direct involvement, witnessing event, learning of the event, or extreme exposure to aversive details of the event • Presence of intrusive symptoms, such as: intrusive distressing memories, distressing dreams, and flashbacks • Persistent avoidance of external reminders of the event and/or efforts to avoid distressing memories • Presence of negative alteration in cognition and mood, such as: inability to remember aspects of the event, exaggerated negative beliefs of oneself, inappropriate self-blame, persistent negative emotional state, diminished interest in activities, and/or detachment from others • Alteration in arousal and reactivity, such as: irritability and anger outbursts, reckless behavior, hypervigilance, exaggerated startle response, concentration difficulties, and/or sleep disturbance • Symptoms are persistent for more than 1 month
Acute stress disorder	• Symptoms largely comparable to criteria for Posttraumatic Stress Disorder, outside of duration • Duration of symptoms is 3 days to 1 month

(continued)

Table 68.2 (continued)

Adjustment disorders	• Development of emotional or behavioral symptoms in response to an identifiable stressor(s) occurring within 3 months of onset of symptoms • Symptoms must cause marked distress that is out of proportion to the severity of the stressor and/or cause significant impairment to daily functioning • Specific symptoms can include: depressed mood, anxiety, conduct disturbance, or any combination of the three

may include trauma focuses of cognitive behavior therapy (CBT), and dialectical behavior therapy (DBT). Alternative treatment modalities, such as expressive arts therapies, have also been supportive when processing the physiological sensation, emotions, and cognitions surrounding traumatic or stress related events. Please seek out a mental health provider to receive an appropriate referral for services as all treatment approaches necessitate a trained practitioner. Medications can also be considered with the proper guidance of a healthcare provider, such as SSRI. Without proper, healthy coping strategies to manage anxiety-related disorders, individuals may turn to substance use, disordered eating patterns, or self-harm to ease more severe anxiety symptoms (Table 68.3).

Students may require additional support in the school setting as they navigate appointments, potential side effects of medications, and finding a quiet space in the school setting to use if it is beneficial to their coping plan. Educators in the school setting should encourage students to utilize their coping skills and assist with necessary accommodations to complete assignments in addition to practicing a trauma-informed approach in their interactions with all students. When necessary, a school nurse may encourage caregivers seek an evaluation to the Emergency Department. Indications for Emergency Department evaluation or crisis assessment generally include concerns for the student's safety or the safety of other students. This may look like a student engaging in self-harm requiring medical intervention, a student endorsing thoughts of suicide or significant concerns of a student possibly considering suicide, or a student threatening or engaging in behaviors that put other students in the school in danger.

Extra-Credit Points

1. Response to stress and trauma can directly impact how a child learns, interacts with others, and manages emotions.
2. A good therapeutic relationship, including establishment of physical and emotional safety, trust, and open communication, can have a significant impact on engagement in treatment.
3. Seeking treatment early, utilization of coping skills, having a good support network, and psychotropic medication, if appropriate, can greatly contribute to the management of anxiety-related symptoms.

Table 68.3 Six student presentations: anxiety disorder diagnosis?—case resolutions

Case #1: Rachel, 7 year-old: decreased school attendance, frequent somatic complaints, difficulty with sleep, fears related to safety of family	Likely diagnosis: Separation Anxiety Disorder Differential diagnosis may include: Adjustment Disorder
Case #2: Isabella, high school senior: "worry wart", primarily performance related worries, sleep disturbance and increased irritability	Likely diagnosis: Generalized Anxiety Disorder Differential diagnosis may include: Social Anxiety Disorder
Case #3: Johnny, middle school student: exposed to domestic violence at home, disengaging in previously preferred classes and activities, more withdrawn and isolating behaviors	Likely diagnosis: Posttraumatic Stress Disorder Differential diagnosis may include: Adjustment Disorder
Case #4: Ariela, high school student: new to school district, "extreme overwhelm" with multiple physical symptoms (shakiness, sweating, and chest pain), events are distressing, and she has taken steps to avoid these events	Likely diagnosis: Panic Disorder Differential diagnosis may include: Other Anxiety Disorder with Panic Attacks
Case #5: Marina, 8 year-old: recently involved in MVC and broke arm, changes in behavior at school (irritability, tearfulness, concentration difficulties, and seeking reassurance of mother's safety) and home (sleep disturbance and nightmares)	Likely diagnosis: Acute Stress Disorder Differential diagnosis may include: Adjustment Disorder and Posttraumatic Stress Disorder
Case #6: Jackson, 7th grade student: withdrawn, avoids peer interactions, denies having friends, fears of negative evaluation by peers, sleep disturbance	Likely diagnosis: Social Anxiety Disorder Differential diagnosis may include: Generalized Anxiety Disorder and Major Depressive Disorder

4. If left untreated, individuals with anxiety-related disorders may turn to substance use, disordered eating patterns, or self-harm to ease more severe anxiety symptoms.

References

1. Kowalchuk A, Gonzalez SJ, Zoorob RJ. Anxiety disorders in children and adolescents. Am Fam Physician. 2022;106(6):657–64.
2. Felitti VJ, Anda RF, Nordenberg D, et al. Relationship of childhood abuse and household dysfunction to many of the leading causes of death in adults. The Adverse Childhood Experiences (ACE) Study. Am J Prevent Med. 1998;14(4):245–58. https://doi.org/10.1016/s0749-3797(98)00017-8.

3. Menschner C, Maul A. Key ingredients for successful trauma-informed care implementation. Center for Health Care Strategies, Inc; 2016. https://www.chcs.org/media/ATC-whitepaper-040616-rev.pdf
4. Raja S, Hasnain M, Hoersch M, et al. Trauma informed care in medicine: current knowledge and future research directions. Fam Community Health. 2015;38(3):216–26. https://doi.org/10.1097/FCH.0000000000000071.
5. Cisler JM, Herringa RJ. Posttraumatic stress disorder and the developing adolescent brain. J Biol Psychiatry. 2021;89:114–51.
6. Weems CF, Russell JD, Neill EL, McCurdy BH. Annual research review: Pediatric post-traumatic stress disorder from a neurodevelopmental network perspective. J Child Psychol Psychiatry. 2019;60(4):395–408.
7. Neal AM. Somatic interventions to improve self-regulation in children and adolescents. J Child Adolesc Psychiatr Nurs. 2021;34:171–80.
8. American Psychiatric Association. Diagnostic and statistical manual of mental disorders text revision. 5th ed. American Psychiatric Publishing; 2022.
9. Gottschalk MG, Domschke K. Genetics of generalized anxiety disorder and related traits. Dialogues Clin Neurosci. 2017;19(2):159–68. https://doi.org/10.31887/DCNS.2017.19.2/kdomschke.
10. Bloomfield D. Pediatric mental health minute series: screening tools. American Academy of Pediatrics. https://www.aap.org/en/patient-care/mental-health-minute/screening-tools/.

Chapter 69
Autism Spectrum Disorder

Andrew Yeich and Sneha Jadhav

Case 1 **A 6-year-old boy named Aiden is brought to your office by his parents after his kindergarten teacher called them to discuss concerns about his behavior. His teacher reports that Aiden does well in structured class lessons and excels in math but seems to have difficulty integrating into the class's social environment. During lunch and recess, Aiden runs from classmate to classmate trying to play with everyone without regard for the friend groups that his teacher observes amongst the class. During group work assignments, Aiden has been ostracized within his assigned group after misinterpreting jokes made amongst his classmates. Aiden observes instruction and completes worksheets without issue, but often when called on to discuss a question he will change subjects to describe his favorite game, Minecraft. In your office, Aiden seems calm but very shy. He is looking down at his shoes and squeezing his left thumb with his right hand. What parts of Aiden's presentation suggest ASD?**

69.1 Evaluation and Diagnosis of ASD

Diagnosis for ASD depends on a combination of expert evaluation and contribution from the patient's caregivers. Initial evaluation can be based around the current guideline criteria which are displayed in Table 69.1 [1]. It is important to understand that while these typical patterns have been established in many ASD patients, they

A. Yeich (✉)
Penn State College of Medicine, Hershey, PA, USA
e-mail: ayeich@pennstatehealth.psu.edu

S. Jadhav
Johns Hopkins School of Medicine, Baltimore, MD, USA
e-mail: jadhav@kennedykrieger.org

R. P. Olympia, J. Brady-Olympia (eds.), *Clinical Considerations in School-based Health*, https://doi.org/10.1007/978-3-031-85765-2_69

Table 69.1 Diagnostic criteria for autism spectrum disorder (DSM V [1])

Domain 1: Social Communication & Interaction	Deficits in Social Reciprocity: 1. Abnormal back-and forth conversation 2. Reduced sharing of interest, emotions, and affect 3. Failure to initiate or respond to social interactions	Deficits in Nonverbal Communication: 1. Abnormal eye contact, body language, use and understanding of gestures 2. Lack of facial expressions and nonverbal communication	Deficits in Relationships: 1. Difficulty adjusting behavior for various social contexts 2. Difficulties sharing imaginative play or making friends 3. Absence of interest in peers	
Domain 2: Restrictive, Repetitive Behaviors	Stereotyped or repetitive motor movements, use of objects, or speech	Insistence on sameness, inflexible adherence to routines, or ritualized patterns of verbal or nonverbal behavior	Highly restricted, fixated interests abnormal in intensity or focus	Hyper/ hypoactivity to sensory input or an unusual interest in sensory aspects of the environment

present very differently depending on age, cognitive ability, and social factors. Symptoms can improve and worsen as a child develops, is placed in a new environment, or receives treatment. This typically occurs around 4 years of age in the U.S., and parents often identify abnormalities before 18 months. However, the variability in ASD behavioral profiles presents a diagnostic challenge to the healthcare system and necessitates involvement from school-based providers to prevent students from falling through the cracks [2].

The full ASD criteria for the 5th edition of the Diagnostic and Statistical Manual of Mental Disorders (DSM V) requires persistent deficits occurring during early development in all three aspects of the social communication and interaction domain, as well as one aspect in the restrictive, repetitive behavior domain [1]. This requirement should not limit initial clinical suspicion for ASD in students presenting with symptoms resembling only a few criteria until a full evaluation by a developmental pediatrician can be obtained. When ASD is identified as a possible diagnosis in a school setting, the next steps involve documenting the academic and social differences present in the school setting through collaboration with the child's teachers, presenting information and education to parents and care givers in a supportive manner, and ultimately seeking expert referral for diagnostic evaluation and intervention services [3]. In most cases, however, parents will already be aware of their child's diagnosis, and the role of a school health provider will involve advocacy within and outside of the school.

Case 2 A 13-year-old girl named Emily has just transferred to your middle school. Her parents ask to meet with you and relay that she was diagnosed with ASD when she was 3 years old. She had been receiving comprehensive ASD services before moving, but it was mostly coordinated through the previous school's health office as her parents work long hours and have several other children to care for. At present, Emily now only attends speech therapy. Her parents are trying to enroll her in a pediatrician's office but are having difficulty finding one with availability. After evaluating Emily and speaking with your parents, you decide that she has significant social and behavioral impairment, as well as possible symptoms of generalized anxiety disorder. What further interventions would benefit Emily within and outside the school setting?

69.2 Management of ASD

In the school health setting, the first step of ASD care involves developing common understanding and communication between the child's school, parents or caregivers, and primary care provider. Referral for a diagnostic evaluation by a developmental pediatrician is paramount in children who have yet to receive one. Following diagnosis, even if care is not coordinated through the school, school health providers can monitor the child's progress and ensure their needs are adequately met. ASD children with socioeconomic disadvantages are less likely to receive proper treatment, and developmental disorders may be understood differently between cultures [4, 5]. Because parental involvement in ASD care strongly impacts a child's long-term outcomes, it is crucial to identify and intervene in cases where a family seems overwhelmed or does not appear to be able to provide needed support. Even in situations of high parental involvement and support, school-based health services are typically preferred over outside interventions to ensure continuity within the school setting. Particular care must be given to transition points, including grade transitions, school transfers, family changes, and graduation.

Every patient with ASD faces unique challenges, and as such ideal management is tailored to their individual needs. Table 69.2 provides an overview and brief description of common evidence-based treatments. There are many different forms of early intensive behavioral interventions that broadly take the form of a teacher or therapist working individually with the child to develop the skills used in play, social interaction, communication, language, and cognitive tasks. When utilized adequately as an early intervention (15 or more hours per week), these treatments have improved adaptive skills, cognition, and language development. Speech and occupational therapy interventions are also common; current U.S. law mandates that schools provide occupational therapy services to students with ASD. Unfortunately, the quality and access of these required services vary school-to-school. Sensory-integration approaches with occupational therapists can involve music therapy, environmental stimulation, weighted blankets, swings, and massages. High rates of comorbid anxiety disorders in ASD children can be addressed

Table 69.2 Common interventions for autism spectrum disorder

Intervention name	Description	Supporting evidence
Early intensive behavioral interventions	Frequent 1-on-1 behavioral training using natural consequences to teach developmental skills	Significant improvements in adaptive skills, language skills, and cognition [6]
Parent-mediated interventions	Helps parents learn to interact with their ASD child; establishes joint engagement and relationship building between parent and child	Significant improvements in social behaviors and communication [7]
Speech therapy	Communication skills training with a speech therapist, can involve alternative modes of communication for limited or non-verbal patients	Limited evidence is available due to the variability of speech therapy protocols [8]
Sensory integration therapy	Addresses occupational performance by increasing ability to process sensory information	Significant improvements in occupational performance scales [9]
Mental health care	Specialized treatment for comorbid psychiatric disorders that commonly afflict children with ASD	Significant benefits for anxiety disorders [10]

through targeted cognitive behavioral therapy. Strong evidence supports these interventions in mitigating anxiety symptoms. All of the above interventions may be started as part of a coordinated Individual Education Program (IEP), which formally outlines the educational goals and services to instruct a student with specific needs. Another coordination option for ASD services is the 504 service agreement, which is a less structured version of the IEP. Both tools are created by a team, commonly composed of a vice principle or another representation of the school administration, the child's teacher(s), a school counselor, the school-based healthcare provider, and a behavioral specialist. Outside of the school, there are numerous federal and state agencies and programs that provide support services or advocacy for children with ASD and their families, including the Interagency Autism Coordinating Committee, the Children's Health Insurance Program, the U.S. Department of Housing and Urban Development, and Social Security Income benefits.

Case 3 On the first day of a new school year, you receive a phone call from 9-year-old Michael's homeroom teacher. She reports that Michael, whose ASD care you have been coordinating for several years now, is visibly upset and won't stop pacing back and forth by her desk. Michael's teacher says she is unsure what upset him; it's hard to hear her through the loud noises of her excited classroom. After helping Michael leave the environment, he is sitting calmly in your office. You notice both the sides of his head and the knuckles of his hands are red. What steps can you take to help both Michael and his teachers in the future?

69.3 Complications of Autism Spectrum Disorder in the School Setting

Disruptive behaviors, aggression, and self-injury can be common in children with ASD. These episodes can be particularly concerning in the school setting among peers and teachers who have limited experience with ASD or do not know the student well. The most effective approach to handling these behaviors is prevention through providing a structured school day, an appropriate level of support, adequate communication, and the use of behavioral therapy principles. For a patient experiencing a first-time event, or a new student entering your care with a history of such problems, it can be helpful to create a Behavioral Intervention Plan to guide future action. This involves analyzing the child's behaviors to identify any triggers that may have prompted their agitation. Learning the purpose and motivation of such episodes and equipping teachers and school staff with de-escalation tactics can support the student in returning to the learning environment. Examples of these techniques may include assisting the child in leaving a distressing environment, respecting personal space, identifying their needs and wants, and offering clear choices with optimism [11, 12]. Verbal redirection should be clear and simple in nature. The agitated student should be given ample time to consider the instructions, which may have to be repeated. Food, toys, and somatosensory items may facilitate conflict resolution [13, 14].

Unfortunately, students with ASD tend to be particularly vulnerable to bullying due to difficulties with communication, social reciprocity, and peer-to-peer interactions that characterize the disorder. Exposing ASD students to inclusive environments (those with non-ASD student peers) without adequate behavioral preparation limits the acquisition of social skills and facilitates victimization. Rather, it is crucial to provide peer-mediated interventions against bullying and disability awareness education to those interacting with ASD students. Increased supervision of peer interactions within and outside the classroom may be warranted [15].

As discussed in the previous section, there are several psychiatric and medical comorbidities common in children with ASD. Separate from the social and behavioral deficits that characterize ASD, attention deficit-hyperactivity disorder, anxiety disorders, sleep disorders, and obsessive-compulsive disorder are more common in children with ASD. Medically, these children are more likely to experience pre-term birth and perinatal hypoxia, enuresis, encopresis, Tourette syndrome and tic disorders, motor delay and seizure disorders. There may also be delays in acquiring self-help skills such as dressing, toileting, and general hygiene, as well as feeding and nutrition problems. Maintaining a high index of suspicion for these conditions in ASD children can reduce the time it takes them to receive adequate treatment [16].

Extra-Credit Points

1. Most children with ASD have normal IQ and excel in structured environments but possess underlying social and behavioral deficits that are exposed in more unstructured environments.

2. Early intensive intervention provides lasting long-term benefits for children with ASD. These services are ideally coordinated through the child's school using formal guidelines like a comprehensive IEP or a 504-service agreement.
3. In addition to the common symptoms of ASD, there are multiple psychiatric and medical comorbidities that need to be identified and managed if present in a child with ASD.
4. Referral to the emergency room should be considered in cases of severe and persistent changes in mood or behavior, threats or attempts of serious self-harm, unsafe behaviors that cannot be contained, and the usual indications applicable to the general population.
5. Helpful resources: https://www.autismspeaks.org; https://carolgraysocialstories.com/social-stories/what-is-it

References

1. Diagnostic and statistical manual of mental disorders. DSM-5. 5th ed. Washington D.C.: American Psychiatric Association; 2013.
2. Zwaigenbaum L, Bauman ML, Stone WL, et al. Early Identification of autism spectrum disorder: recommendations for practice and research. Pediatrics. 2015;136:S10–40.
3. Lipkin PH, Macias MM. Promoting optimal development: identifying infants and young children with developmental disorders through developmental surveillance and screening. Pediatrics. 2020;145:e20193449.
4. Golson ME, Haverkamp CR, McClain MB, et al. Influences of student race/ethnicity and gender on autism special education classification considerations. Autism. 2022;26:1423–35.
5. Donohue MR, Childs AW, Richards M, et al. Race Influences Parent report of concerns about symptoms of autism spectrum disorder. Autism. 2019;23:100–11.
6. Reichow B, Hume K, Barton EE, et al. Early intensive behavioral intervention (EIBI) for young children with autism spectrum disorders (ASD). Cochrane Database Syst Rev. 2018:5;CD009260.
7. Weitlauf AS, McPheeters ML, Peters B, et al. Therapies for children with autism spectrum disorder: behavioral interventions update. AHRQ Comparative Effectiveness Reviews. 2014;14:EHC036-EF.
8. Adams C, Lockton E, Freed J, et al. The social communication intervention project: a randomized controlled trial of the effectiveness of speech and language therapy for school-age children who have pragmatic and social communication problems with or without autism spectrum disorder. Int J Lang Commun Disord. 2012;47:233–44.
9. Kashefimehr B, Kayihan H, Huri M, et al. The Effect of sensory integration therapy on occupational performance in children with autism. OTJR: Occupation, Participation and Health. 2018;38:75–83.
10. Reaven J, Blakely-Smith A, Culhane-Shelburne K, et al. Group cognitive behavior therapy for children with high-functioning autism spectrum disorders and anxiety: a randomized trial. J Child Psychol Psychiatry. 2012;53:410–9.
11. Bone ME, Leppert ML. Autism spectrum disorder at home and in school. Pediatr Clin North Am. 2024;71:223–39.
12. Richmond JS, Berlin JS, Fishkind AB, et al. Verbal De-escalation of the Agitated Patient: Consensus Statement of the American Association for Emergency Psychiatry Project BETA De-escalation Workgroup. West J Emerg Med. 2012;13:17–25.

13. Sandbank M, Bottema-Beutel K, Crowley LS, et al. Autisim intervention meta-analysis of early childhood studies (Project AIM): updated systematic review and secondary analysis. BMJ. 2023;383:e076733.
14. Trembath D, Varcin K, Waddington H, et al. Non-pharmacological interventions for autistic children: An umbrella review. Autism. 2023;27:275–95.
15. Park I, Gong J, Lyons GL, et al. Prevalence of and factors associated with school bullying in students with autism spectrum disorder: a cross-cultural meta-analysis. Yonsei Med J. 2020;61:909–22.
16. Khachadourian V, Mahjani B, Sandin S, et al. Comorbidities in Autism spectrum disorder and their etiologies. Trans Psychiatry. 2023;13:71.

Chapter 70
Bipolar Disorder

Paige Chardavoyne

Bipolar disorder has two main types, bipolar I disorder and bipolar II disorder. In short, bipolar I disorder requires one or more lifetime episodes of mania. Bipolar II disorder requires at least 1 episode of hypomania (a less severe elevated mood state) and at least 1 major depressive episode. With manic, hypomanic, and major depressive episodes, symptoms are not attributable to the psychological effects of a substance (illicit or prescribed), treatment, or another medical/psychiatric condition [1]. As a primer for this chapter, below are some "fast facts" about bipolar disorders (Table 70.1). Much of this material will be covered in more detail throughout the chapter.

Bipolar disorders are very rare in children (age 12 or younger) and rare in adolescents (age 13–17). Meta-analyses have reported prevalence rates of zero or near-zero in children and around 3% or less in adolescents [5]. Bipolar disorders are complex and can be challenging to accurately diagnose. Below are the abridged diagnostic criteria for bipolar I and bipolar II disorders from the Statistical Manual of Mental Disorders Fifth Edition Text Revision (DSM-5-TR) (Table 70.2) [1].

When reviewing the DSM-5-TR criteria for bipolar disorders, one might notice overlapping symptoms between the bipolar disorders and other psychiatric conditions, such as ADHD, substance use disorders, disruptive mood dysregulation disorder (DMDD), oppositional defiant disorder (ODD), and intermittent explosive disorder (IED) [3, 6]. To illustrate this point, look at the cases below (Table 70.3) and consider which symptoms may be consistent with a bipolar disorder, which symptoms may be consistent with another psychiatric condition, and how to best help the child.

P. Chardavoyne (✉)
Medical College of Wisconsin, Milwaukee, WI, USA
e-mail: pchardavoyne@mcw.edu

R. P. Olympia, J. Brady-Olympia (eds.), *Clinical Considerations in School-based Health*, https://doi.org/10.1007/978-3-031-85765-2_70

Table 70.1 Bipolar disorder "fast facts"

Fact 1: Bipolar disorders are frequently comorbid with other mental health conditions, such as substance use disorders and attention-deficit/hyperactivity disorder (ADHD), but are very rare in children and rare in adolescents [2].
Fact 2: Episodes of mania and hypomania are distinct from day-to-day or within a single day changes in mood [3].
Fact 3. Episodes of mania and hypomania are often unprovoked versus being triggered by a psychosocial stressor or interpersonal interaction [3].
Fact 4: Bipolar disorders are highly heritable. Though exact estimates vary, studies suggest that heritability may be around 60–90% [2].
Fact 5: Earlier age of bipolar disorder onset has been associated with increased time to treatment and substance use [4].

Table 70.2 Abridged DSM-5-TR criteria for bipolar disorders

Bipolar I Disorder	A. Criteria have been met for at least 1 lifetime manic episode: 1. A distinct period of abnormally and persistently elevated, expansive, or irritable mood and abnormally and persistently increased activity or energy, lasting at least 1 week and present most of the day, nearly every day (or any duration if hospitalization is necessary). 2. During the period of mood disturbance and increased energy or activity, three (or more) of the following symptoms (four if the mood is only irritable) are present to a significant degree and represent a noticeable change from usual behavior: i. Inflated self-esteem or grandiosity. ii. Decreased need for sleep. iii. More talkative than usual or pressure to keep talking. iv. Flight of ideas or subjective experience that thoughts are racing. v. Distractibility, as reported or observed. vi. Increase in goal-directed activity or psychomotor agitation. vii. Excessive involvement in activities that have a high potential for painful consequences. 3. The mood disturbance is sufficiently severe to cause marked impairment in social or occupational functioning or to necessitate hospitalization to prevent harm to self or others, or there are psychotic features.

Table 70.2 (continued)

Bipolar II Disorder	A. Criteria have been met for a current or past hypomanic episode: 1. A distinct period of abnormally and persistently elevated, expansive, or irritable mood and abnormally and persistently increased activity or energy, lasting at least 4 consecutive days and present most of the day, nearly every day. 2. During the period of mood disturbance and increased energy and activity, three (or more) symptoms of mania have persisted (four if the mood is only irritable), represent a noticeable change from usual behavior, and have been present to a significant degree. 3. The episode is associated with an unequivocal change in functioning that is uncharacteristic of the individual when not symptomatic and the change in mood and function is observable by others. 4. The episode is not severe enough to cause marked impairment in social or occupational functioning or to necessitate hospitalization. B. Criteria have been met for a current or past major depressive episode: 1. Five (or more) of the following symptoms have been present during the same 2- week period and represent a change from previous functioning; at least one of the symptoms is either (1) depressed mood or (2) loss of interest or pleasure. Symptoms clearly attributable to a medical condition are excluded. i. Depressed mood most of the day, nearly every day, as indicated by either subjective report or observation made by others. (Note: In children and adolescents, can be irritable mood.) ii. Markedly diminished interest or pleasure in all, or almost all, activities most of the day, nearly every day (as indicated by either subjective account or observation). iii. Significant weight loss when not dieting, weight gain, or change in appetite nearly every day. (Note: In children, consider failure to make expected weight gain.) iv. Insomnia or hypersomnia nearly every day. v. Psychomotor agitation or retardation nearly every day (observable by others, not merely subjective feelings of restlessness or being slowed down). vi. Fatigue or loss of energy nearly every day. vii. Feelings of worthlessness or excessive or inappropriate guilt (which may be delusional) nearly every day (not merely self-reproach or guilt about being sick). viii. Diminished ability to think or concentrate, or indecisiveness, nearly every day (either by subjective account or as observed by others). ix. Recurrent thoughts of death (not just fear of dying), recurrent suicidal ideation without a specific plan, or a suicide attempt or a specific plan for committing suicide. 2. The symptoms cause clinically significant distress or impairment in social, occupational, or other important areas of functioning. C. The symptoms of depression or the unpredictability caused by frequent alternation between periods of depression and hypomania causes clinically significant distress or impairment in social, occupational, or other important areas of functioning.

Table 70.3 Case presentations

Case #1: Travis is a 16-year-old male with history of anxiety. Within the last few months, Travis has exhibited changes in behavior. He has been more distractable and irritable. It has also been more difficult to engage in conversation with him, as he has been more talkative and difficult to interrupt. Within the last few months, there have also been concerns that Travis is using substances.
Case #2: Ricky is a 7-year-old male without known medical history. Ricky is new to this school this year. Ricky's teachers have been struggling to manage his behavior, which continues to escalate. Ricky frequently struggles to stay engaged with classroom lessons, particularly during less structured activities. Today, he threw a pencil at a peer because he thought they were making fun of him. At times, it seems that his mood switches "out of the blue" and he acts impulsively.
Case #3: Allie is a 17-year-old female with history of major depressive disorder, single episode. School staff and peers have noticed a change in Allie's behavior the last couple of days. Allie reported she has not been sleeping as she has not felt tired recently. Instead of sleeping, she has begun a variety of school-based tasks, none of which it seems she will be able to complete. She also reports using this time to "uncover my secret powers" she believes she has. She reported she has been hearing spirits and has been talking to herself during school. Family, friends, and school staff are unaware of anything that might have precipitated this change.

To aid in formulating a diagnostic impression, it can be essential to obtain collateral information. School-based health providers are uniquely poised to gather this additional information from school staff (such as teachers) and those who know the child outside of school (such as family members). Bipolar disorders are highly heritable, so obtaining a family psychiatric history can be helpful. Additionally, review medical history, changes to medication or treatment, and substance use history.

Early diagnosis is important to triage the child to appropriate care. It is important to recognize that manic episodes can be associated with increased risk-taking behavior and risk for suicide [3]. If at any point there are concerns about the child's safety (risk of dangerousness to self/others), this would be a reason to present to the nearest emergency department (ED). ED's may have access to psychiatry consultation through in-house emergency/consult-liaison psychiatrists, telepsychiatry, or behavioral health liaisons. These providers can aid in triaging the child to the appropriate level of care (inpatient psychiatric hospitalization, partial hospitalization program, intensive outpatient program, or outpatient) and aid in legal processes if involuntary treatment needs to be pursued (legal processes for involuntary psychiatric treatment vary by state).

Once connected to care, children are typically treated with pharmacologic and non-pharmacologic interventions. Regarding pharmacologic management, bipolar disorders are treated with mood stabilizing medications, which can include lithium, antiepileptic agents (such as valproic acid), and antipsychotic medications (such as aripiprazole, olanzapine, and risperidone). Children with bipolar disorder are typically managed by child psychiatrists due to symptom and medication complexity. Different medications may be used in combination and the aforementioned medications require routine monitoring for side effects. This can include lipid panel to monitor for hyperlipidemia, hemoglobin A1c to monitor for hyperglycemia (diabetes), electrocardiogram (ECG) to monitor for prolonged QTc interval, and abnormal involuntary movement scale (AIMS) examination to monitor for dyskinesias. However, in areas where access to child psychiatry is minimal or there is a long wait to establish with child psychiatry, primary care providers may need to aid in filling prescriptions and monitoring for medication side effects. If you find yourself with diagnostic uncertainty or in the position where you need to provide psychiatric care in this way (and it feels out of your scope), consider seeing if you have access to a phone consultation service with a child and adolescent psychiatrist in your state of practice.

In addition to pharmacologic treatment, adjunctive psychotherapy is considered an essential part of the management of pediatric bipolar disorder [7]. Below is an overview of some of the psychotherapy techniques which can be used in pediatric bipolar disorder (Table 70.4) [7, 9].

Additional ways to support children with bipolar disorders and their families include considering school accommodations, resources for children and their families, and specialty clinics. If school is challenging due to psychiatric symptoms or medication side effects, the student may be eligible for a 504 plan or Individualized Education Program (IEP) [10]. Several organizations exist to support children with bipolar disorders and their families. Organizations such as the National Institute of Mental Health (www.nimh.nih.gov), the Depression and Bipolar Support Alliance (www.dbsalliance.org), and the National Alliance on Mental Illness (www.nami.org) can serve as sources for advocacy, education, and support [7]. Lastly, multidisciplinary treatment programs exist for adolescents and young adults with psychotic symptoms as part of bipolar I disorder. These clinics can encompass psychiatry, psychology (for individual and family psychotherapy), social work, and peer support. The Early Psychosis Intervention Network (EPINET) website (https://nationalepinet.org/epinet-clinics/) has a list of clinics providing care for individuals with early psychosis [11]. This clinic model focuses on early detection and treatment during the first few years of psychotic symptoms and has been shown to improve clinical and functional outcomes [12].

With additional knowledge from this chapter, let's look back at the clinical cases considering diagnostic impression and treatment recommendations (Table 70.5).

Extra Credit Points

1. Bipolar disorders are overall uncommon in the pediatric population.
2. Symptoms of bipolar disorder overlap with other more common pediatric psychiatric diagnoses.
3. Early diagnosis and treatment improves outcomes for individuals with bipolar disorder, though it is important that this diagnosis is correctly made.
4. Treatment of bipolar disorder is multimodal and involves pharmacologic and non-pharmacologic interventions.
5. Additional resources are available for children with bipolar disorders, their families, and providers who work with them.

Table 70.4 Basic overview of psychotherapy techniques

Psychotherapy type	Basic goal	Treatment aspects, advantages, and disadvantages
Cognitive behavioral therapy (CBT)	Identify and challenge negative thought processes	• Evidenced-based for several psychiatric conditions, including depression, substance use disorders, and anxiety. • Most effective when the child is motivated (as out of session work is traditionally involved) and has insight into their thoughts. If a child is lacking motivation, insight, or is too symptomatic to engage, this could be a barrier. • Therapist Aid has free CBT worksheets, which can be utilized (https://www.therapistaid.com/therapy-worksheets/cbt) [8].
Dialectical behavioral therapy (DBT)	Focuses on interpersonal effectiveness, mindfulness, emotion regulation, and distress tolerance	• Most effective when the child is motivated (as out of session work is traditionally involved) and has insight. If a child is lacking motivation, insight, or is too symptomatic to engage, this could be a barrier. • Requires time commitment from children and therapists. • DBT programs may have a minimal age requirement for participation given that concepts can be challenging to understand. • Additional training is required to be a certified DBT therapist.
Family therapy	Focuses on the family unit to address concerns for the family and individual	• Requires participation from the child and members of the family unit. • Views the family as a key part to improving the child's mental health. • May require less insight from the child and be a way to meet the child and family where they are at. • Can provide the family with psychoeducation about the bipolar disorder diagnosis, medications, and symptom management. • Additional training is required to be a certified family therapist.
Motivational interviewing (MI)	Used to help identify and change maladaptive behaviors	• Has a variety of indications, including for substance use disorders and to increase adherence to medical treatments. • Way to meet the child where they are at with insight and desire to change/address their mental health symptoms. • Number of sessions can vary and is less time-intensive than other techniques which follow specific protocols and are less flexible. • Does not traditionally require out of session work.

Table 70.5 Case presentations: diagnostic impression and treatment recommendations

Case #1: Travis is a 16-year-old male with history of anxiety. Within the last few months, Travis has exhibited changes in behavior. He has been more distractable and irritable. It has also been more difficult to engage in conversation with him, as he has been more talkative and difficult to interrupt. Within the last few months, there have also been concerns that Travis is using substances.	• Distractibility, irritability, and pressured speech can all be symptoms of bipolar disorder. • Travis is an adolescent so his likelihood of having bipolar disorder is higher than a child's. • Travis's recent substance use raises concern that he may be experiencing a substance-induced bipolar disorder and a substance use history should be obtained. • If Travis's symptoms are attributed to substance use, he may benefit from pharmacologic treatment and non-pharmacologic treatment for substance use disorders, which is often multimodal and includes psychotherapy, such as CBT and family therapy [13].
Case #2: Ricky is a 7-year-old male without known medical history. Ricky is new to this school this year. Ricky's teachers have been struggling to manage his behavior, which continues to escalate. Ricky frequently struggles to stay engaged with classroom lessons, particularly during less structured activities. Today, he threw a pencil at a peer because he thought they were making fun of him. At times, it seems that his mood switches "out of the blue" and he acts impulsively.	• Distractibility, changes in mood, and irritability can be symptoms of bipolar disorder. • Ricky is a child and bipolar disorder in this population is very uncommon. • Ricky's distractibility may also be a symptom of another psychiatric condition, such as ADHD. • Ricky's impulsivity may also be a symptom of ADHD. • To explore a diagnosis of ADHD further, providers should obtain further history (utilizing screening tools as needed), compare the child's presentation to DSM-5 TR criteria, screen for comorbid conditions (psychiatric and other medical diagnoses), and consider pharmacologic and non-pharmacologic interventions [14].

(continued)

Table 70.5 (continued)

Case #3: Allie is a 17-year-old female with history of major depressive disorder, single episode. School staff and peers have noticed a change in Allie's behavior the last couple of days. Allie reported she has not been sleeping as she has not felt tired recently. Instead of sleeping, she has begun a variety of school-based tasks, none of which it seems she will be able to complete. She also reports using this time to "uncover my secret powers" she believes she has. She reported she has been hearing spirits and has been talking to herself during school. She has never had symptoms like this before. Family, friends, and school staff are unaware of anything that might have precipitated this change.	• Decreased need for sleep, increased goal-directed behavior, auditory hallucinations, and potential delusions can be symptoms of mania with psychosis. • Allie is an adolescent so her likelihood of having bipolar disorder is higher than a child's. • Allie has a history of major depressive disorder and may be on an antidepressant, which can cause a "manic switch", meaning it can precipitate a manic episode. • It appears this might be Allie's first episode of psychosis and further history taking, examination, and workup are indicated. The differential for first episode psychosis is broad but recommended laboratory tests to rule in/out etiologies include: urine drug screen (UDS), urinalysis (UA), HIV, complete blood count (CBC) with differential, complete metabolic panel (CMP), thyroid stimulating hormone (TSH) with reflex, antinuclear antibody (ANA), ceruloplasmin, vitamin D, vitamin B9, and vitamin B12/methylmalonic acid [15]. • If a bipolar disorder diagnosis is made, consider implementing the interventions discussed in this chapter.

References

1. Bipolar and related disorders. Diagnostic and statistical manual of mental disorders. 5th ed., text rev. American Psychiatric Association; 2022, p. 350–71.
2. O'Connell KS, Coombes BJ. Genetic contributions to bipolar disorder: current status and future directions. Psychol Med. 2021;51(13):2156–67.
3. Bipolar disorder in children and teens. National Institute of Mental Health. https://www.nimh.nih.gov/health/publications/bipolar-disorder-in-children-and-teens. Accessed 4 May 2024
4. Joslyn C, Hawes DJ, Hunt C, et al. Is age of onset associated with severity, prognosis, and clinical features in bipolar disorder? A meta-analytic review. Bipolar Disord. 2016;18(5):389–403.
5. Parry P, Allison S, Bastiampillai T. "Pediatric bipolar disorder" rates are still lower than claimed: a re-examination of eight epidemiological surveys used by an updated meta-analysis. Int J Bipolar Disord. 2021;9(1):21.
6. Bipolar disorder. National Alliance on Mental Illness (NAMI). https://www.nami.org/About-Mental-Illness/Mental-Health-Conditions/Bipolar-Disorder/?tab=overview. Accessed 5 May 2024
7. Axelson D, Brent D, Solomon D. Pediatric bipolar disorder: efficacy and core elements of adjunctive psychotherapy. UpToDate. https://www.uptodate.com/contents/pediatric-bipolar-disorder-efficacy-and-core-elements-of-adjunctive-psychotherapy. Accessed 5 May 2024
8. CBT worksheets. Therapist aid. https://www.therapistaid.com/therapy-worksheets/cbt. Accessed 23 May 2024

9. Lebow J. Overview of psychotherapies. UpToDate. https://www.uptodate.com/contents/overview-of-psychotherapies. Accessed 23 May 2024
10. Accomodations for students with bipolar disorder and related disabilities. International Bipolar Foundation. https://ibpf.org/articles/accommodations-for-students-with-bipolar-disorder-and-related-disabilities/. Accessed 8 May 2024
11. Early Psychosis Intervention Network (EPINET) Clinics. Early Psychosis Intervention Network (EPINET). https://nationalepinet.org/epinet-clinics/. Accessed 8 May 2024
12. Kane JM, Robinson DG, Schooler NR, et al. Comprehensive versus usual community care for first-episode psychosis: 2-year outcomes from the NIMH RAISE early treatment program. Am J Psychiatry. 2016;173(4):362–72.
13. Fadus MC, Squeglia LM, Valadez EA, et al. Adolescent substance use disorder treatment: an update on evidence-based strategies. Curr Psychiatry Rep. 2019;21(10):96.
14. Wolraich ML, Hagan JF, Allan C, et al. Subcommittee on Children and Adolescents with Attention-Deficit/Hyperactive Disorder. Clinical Practice Guideline for the Diagnosis, Evaluation, and Treatment of Attention-Deficit/Hyperactivity Disorder in Children and Adolescents. Pediatrics. 2019;144(4):e20192528.
15. Skikic M, Arriola JA. First episode psychosis medical workup: evidence-informed recommendations and introduction to a clinically guided approach. Child Adolesc Psychiatr Clin N Am. 2020;29(1):15–28.

Chapter 71
Bullying

Sundeep Singh Randhawa

Case 1 While returning from recess, 14-year-old Atlas is seen being repeatedly pushed by two students while a third student is calling her various derogatory names and taunting her while recording the entire encounter on her phone. The entire time, Atlas is making attempts to gather her things and walk away but is unable to. The other students run off when they see the vice-principal in the vicinity, as they exit, one student shouts, "you better not be a snitch Atlas, otherwise you know what will happen." As the school nurse and hallway monitor, this is the first time you observe this. As you attempt to intervene and ask if she is ok, Atlas quickly states, "Nothing happened, it's fine, just leave me alone. I'm fine" and rapidly walks off with her head down as she appears to wipe away tears. What do you do next? Should his parents be contacted immediately?

Bullying among school-aged youth is a pervasive issue that significantly impacts the physical, emotional, and academic well-being of students. Surveys [1] indicate that as many as half of all children are bullied at some time during their school years, and at least 10% are bullied on a regular basis. Nearly half (45%) of middle school students are bullied on school property and nearly two-thirds of children who are bullied never report it [2]. The impact of bullying extends beyond the immediate distress experienced by victims. Whether the individual is a victim or the perpetrator, bullying behavior can lead to serious consequences, such as poor social-emotional adjustment, behavioral changes, withdrawal from social activities, decline in academic performance and mental health symptoms such as depression, psychotic symptoms and even suicide [3].

Bullying is the intentional, individual, or collective aggressive behaviors that intimidate and cause the physical or psychological discomfort of another individual or group [4]. This behavior can manifest in various forms, each with distinct

S. S. Randhawa (✉)
Child & Adolescent Psychiatry, RUSH University Medical Center, Chicago, IL, USA
e-mail: SSRandhawa@GRHG.org

R. P. Olympia, J. Brady-Olympia (eds.), *Clinical Considerations in School-based Health*, https://doi.org/10.1007/978-3-031-85765-2_71

characteristics and impacts on the victim(s). Understanding these forms is crucial for effective identification and intervention in a school-based health setting. Table 71.1 described the types of bullying that students may be exposed to.

The majority of students do not report bullying due to the fear of retaliation, embarrassment or other various social/personal reasons [5]. Being aware of signs can help facilitate proper identification and timely intervention. Table 71.2 delineates the types of signs, symptoms, indicators, and cues commonly seen in victims of bullying. It is important to note that signs and symptoms in victims will vary from case-to-case.

Case 2 Several weeks after the last observed encounter, 14-year-old Atlas was referred to the school-based health clinic by her homeroom teacher due to noticeable changes in her behavior and academic performance. Atlas, previously an engaged and high-achieving student, had become withdrawn, her

Table 71.1 Types of bullying

Types	Definition	Example
Physical bullying	This involves the use of physical force to intimidate or harm another individual. It may also involve damaging or stealing the victim's belongings. Physical bullying is often the most visible form and can result in immediate physical injuries, making it somewhat easier to identify.	• A student repeatedly pushes another student against lockers. • Hitting, kicking, pushing, or any other form of physical assault.
Verbal bullying	This includes the use of words to harm others. Verbal bullying can be just as damaging as physical bullying, leading to significant emotional and psychological distress. It often occurs in the presence of others, which can exacerbate the victim's feelings of humiliation and isolation.	• A group of students consistently calls a peer, derogatory name(s) and makes fun of their appearance. • Name-calling, insults, teasing, intimidation, or verbal threats.
Relational bullying "Social Bullying" "Emotional bullying"	Involves harming someone's social relationships or reputation. Relational bullying is often covert and can be difficult to detect, but its impact on the victim's mental health and social well-being can be profound.	• A student spreads false rumors about a classmate, leading to their exclusion from friend groups and after school activities.
Cyberbullying	The use of digital technologies, such as social media, text messages, and websites, to harass, threaten, or humiliate someone. This form of bullying can occur 24/7 and can reach a wide audience quickly, often done anonymously.	• A student creates a fake social media profile to post embarrassing photos and comments about a peer, leading to widespread ridicule. • Sending mean texts or emails, posting hurtful messages or images online to intentionally embarrass someone.

Table 71.2 Signs, symptoms, indicators, and cues seen in victims of bullying

Signs		Examples
Academic signs	Declining grades	A drop in academic performance can be a result of the stress and distraction caused by bullying. Victims may find it difficult to concentrate on their studies.
	Loss of interest in school	A general disinterest in school activities, reluctance to attend school, or frequent requests to stay home can indicate bullying.
	Increased absenteeism	Frequent absences from school, often with vague or unconvincing excuses, can be a sign that a student is trying to avoid a bullying situation.
Social indicators and signs	Loss of personal items	Victims may frequently lose or have their personal belongings damaged or stolen. This can include school supplies, clothing, or electronic devices.
	Avoidance of social situations	Reluctance to participate in group activities, avoidance of certain places within the school, or a preference for isolation can be indicative of bullying.
	Changes in peer relationships	Sudden changes in friendships, such as a loss of friends or avoidance by peers, can be a sign that a student is being bullied or ostracized.
Physical signs and symptoms	Unexplained injuries	Victims of bullying may present with bruises, cuts, or other injuries that they cannot or are unwilling to explain.
	Frequent headaches or stomach aches	Psychosomatic symptoms such as headaches or stomach aches are common in children experiencing stress or anxiety due to bullying.
	Changes in eating habits	Sudden changes in appetite, such as skipping meals or binge eating, can be a response to bullying. Some children may come home from school hungry because they avoided eating lunch to escape their bullies.
Communication signs and cues	Avoidance or minimization	Individual provides minimal details or makes attempts to "brush it off" so incident appears normal or mundane.
	Bargaining or pleading	Statements that indicate the individual dose not want anything to be shared with their parent or caregiver.
	Self-blame	Statements in which the individual describes themselves as the victim, deserving the punishment and therefore does not need any additional resources.
	Expressions of fear or helplessness	Statements that indicate fear of going to school, fear of specific individuals, or feelings of helplessness should be taken seriously.
	Talk of self-harm or suicidal ideation	Any mention of self-harm, suicidal thoughts, or behaviors should be addressed immediately and with urgency, as these are critical signs of severe distress.
Emotional and behavioral signs	Anxiety and depression	Increased levels of anxiety, persistent sadness, or signs of depression, such as a lack of interest in previously enjoyed activities, can indicate bullying.

(continued)

Table 71.2 (continued)

Signs		Examples
	Changes in sleeping habits	Difficulty sleeping, nightmares, or frequent waking can be signs of distress related to bullying.
	Withdrawal from social activities	A noticeable withdrawal from friends, family, and social activities can be a red flag. Victims may avoid social situations to escape their bullies.
	Decreased self-esteem	Victims often exhibit low self-esteem, feelings of worthless and helpless. They may express negative self-talk or lack of confidence.
	Behavioral changes	Sudden changes in behavior, such as increased irritability, aggression, or defiance, can be a response to bullying. Conversely, some children may become unusually passive or complaint.

grades had declined, and she frequently was absent from school in the last month. Atlas had routinely visited the school clinic during 5th period. During an assessment, the school nurse observed several bruises on her arms that appeared to be very recent. When asked how she got them, Atlas repeatedly hesitates, unable to provide an explanation. Atlas is informed that her parents may be contacted for safety concerns if she is unable to recall how she got the bruises; Atlas suddenly grabs her belongings and states, "NO! My parents don't need to know, PLEASE, PLEASE, PLEASE DON'T CALL THEM. I don't want to get in trouble or have anyone find out. The bruises were my fault, I mean they were just an accident." What should you do next? What are the various tools and approaches that can be taken?

When addressing bullying incidents in a school-based health setting, immediate response strategies are crucial to ensure the safety and well-being of the affected student. It is important to not be judgmental or force the student to share their experience; instead, allow them to give details at their own pace. Forcing them to share when they are not ready can negatively impact them and their trust in you. Table 71.3 (Immediate Triage and Support) and Fig. 71.1 (Triage and Follow up Assessment) outlines the key aspects for school-based health providers to manage these situations effectively.

Case Conclusion The nurse conducted a private and supportive conversation with Atlas, ensuring a safe and confidential environment. Atlas eventually disclosed that she had been experiencing bullying from a group of peers. The bullying included verbal taunts, social exclusion, and physical aggression, especially in 5th period. Atlas described feeling isolated and fearful, which contributed to her reluctance to attend school and participate in social activities. Over time, with consistent support and intervention, her emotional well-being improved, and she began to re-engage with her academic and social activities. She thanked the nurse for talking to her parents and felt confident and safe being in the school setting.

Table 71.3 Immediate triage and support

Ensure immediate safety	The initial priority is to ensure that the victim is not in acute danger. Immediate safety measures should be taken to prevent further harm.
Gather information	Conduct a thorough initial assessment to document the details of the bullying incident. This includes identifying the involved parties, understanding the context and nature of the bullying, and noting any physical or emotional signs observed. Accurate documentation is essential for further investigation and follow-up. Do not push the student to provide details if they appear uncomfortable or hesitant; it is important to allow the victim to express themselves at their own pace.
Provide emotional support	Offer immediate emotional support to the victim. This includes listening empathetically, validating their feelings, and reassuring them that they are not at fault. Creating a supportive environment helps to alleviate the initial emotional distress and builds trust between the student and the health provider.
Initial assessment and documentation	Use structured tools and protocols to assess the severity of the incident. This may involve direct observations and interviews with the victim, witnesses, and if appropriate, the perpetrator. Detailed documentation should include the time, location, and nature of the bullying, as well as any immediate actions taken.

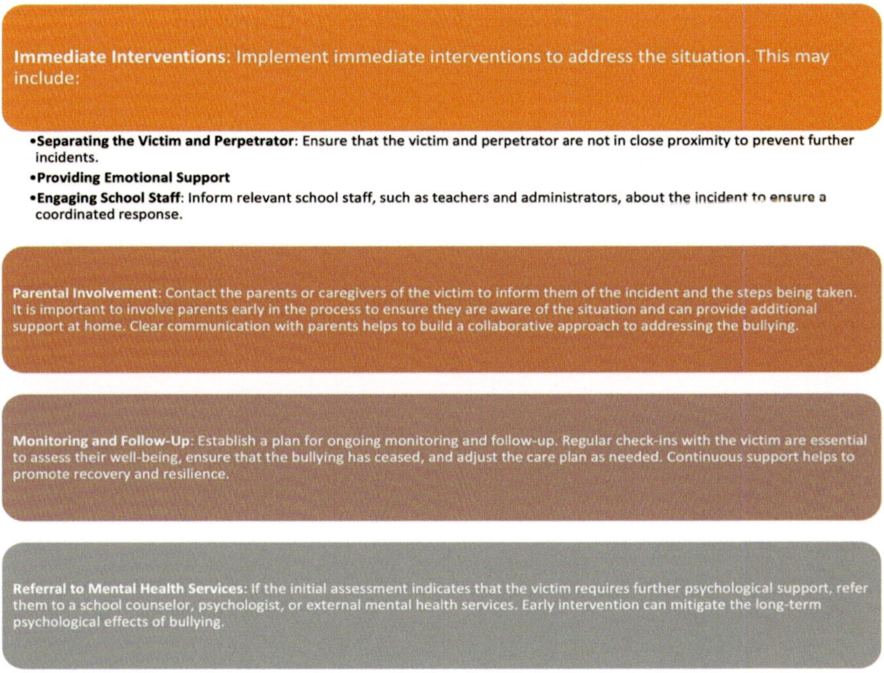

Fig. 71.1 Triage and follow up assessment

Extra Credit Points

1. Be aware and up-to-date with the types of bullying related signs and symptoms.
2. Create a supportive environment that is inviting and judgement free.
3. Involve Parents and Caregivers after assessing and supporting the student.
4. Monitor and routinely check-in to ensure students are feeling safe and that bullying hasn't returned.

References

1. AACAP. Bullying. April 2017. [Online]. https://www.aacap.org/AACAP/Families_and_Youth/Facts_for_Families/FFF-Guide/Bullying-080.aspx?WebsiteKey=a2785385-0ccf-4047-b76a-64b4094ae07f.
2. National Center for Bullying Prevention. www.psychiatry.org. 18 October 2019. [Online]. Available: https://www.psychiatry.org/news-room/apa-blogs/one-in-three-students-impacted-by-cyberbullying. Accessed 2024.
3. AACAP. aacap.org. June 2011. [Online]. https://www.aacap.org/App_Themes/AACAP/docs/resource_centers/resources/fact_sheets/Bullying_Fact_Sheet_2010.pdf.
4. AACAP. aacap.org. October 2023. [Online]. https://www.aacap.org/AACAP/Policy_Statements/2023/Prevention_Bullying.aspx.
5. National Center for Bullying Prevention. psychiatry.org. 18 October 2019. [Online]. https://www.psychiatry.org/news-room/apa-blogs/one-in-three-students-impacted-by-cyberbullying.

Chapter 72
Child Abuse (Physical and Sexual) and Neglect

Katharine Doughty and Catherine M. Huber

According to the National Child Abuse and Neglect Data System (NCANDS) report for 2022 [1], there were over four million reports to Child Protective Services (CPS) alleging maltreatment, involving approximately 7.5 million children in the United States. In 2022, the majority of victims were neglected (74.3%); 17% were physically abused; about 10% were sexually abused; and 6.8% were victims of psychological maltreatment. The Child Abuse Prevention and Treatment Act (CAPTA) defines child abuse and neglect as: "Any recent act or failure to act on the part of a parent or caretaker which results in death, serious physical or emotional harm, sexual abuse or exploitation; or an act or failure to act, which presents an imminent risk of serious harm [1]."

Case 1 Johnny is an 8-year-old male who presents to your school-based clinic for a well-child visit. He is new to the school district and parents have signed a release that allows him to receive medical care. Caregivers are not present and did not answer your phone call prior to beginning the appointment. The child presents with torn jeans, dirty fingernails, lice/nits visible in his hair, and complains of mouth pain. He does not recall how old he was the last time he saw a medical provider but remembers getting a lot of shots. Upon examination, he has visible tooth decay without signs of secondary infection; lice to the hair on his head; and no other abnormalities or signs of injury. Beyond the concern for dental neglect, are there other reasons to involve CPS?

Neglect can manifest in many different forms, from educational to nutritional and even medical. Determining if a family has everything necessary to provide a safe care environment for their child is difficult to do in a brief medical encounter.

K. Doughty · C. M. Huber (✉)
Nationwide Children's Hospital, Columbus, OH, USA
e-mail: Katharine.doughty@nationwidechildrens.org; Catherine.huber@nationwidechildrens.org

R. P. Olympia, J. Brady-Olympia (eds.), *Clinical Considerations in School-based Health*, https://doi.org/10.1007/978-3-031-85765-2_72

Teasing out the details regarding social determinants of health from a pediatric patient can be even more challenging [2].

When there is an issue surrounding medical neglect for a child, multiple factors need to be considered before making that diagnosis and determination [3].

- Was the child harmed or at risk of sustaining harm because of the lack of medical care?
- Were the recommendations made by medical providers going to offer significant benefit to the child?
- Was that benefit greater than its morbidity, such that a reasonable caregiver would choose the recommended treatment rather than not treating?
- Was there access to health care which was then not used?
- And finally, did the caregiver understand the medical recommendations given?

If there is a lack of understanding regarding the importance of the recommendations or an inability to access care, this would not meet the threshold for medical neglect or reporting to CPS. Other steps should be taken by the medical providers with the caregivers to create a reasonable treatment plan for the child before involving other parties.

Case 2 Ashley is a 10-year-old female who was sent to your office by her teacher after she repeatedly was leaving the classroom all day to use the bathroom. Patient stated that she was having dysuria so the teacher sent her to you. When asked about her discomfort, the child said, "Maybe it hurts because that's where Uncle Tommy touches me." What should you do next?

Sexual abuse of children and adolescents is a growing problem that requires care and support in the immediate time frame after disclosure, as well as ongoing support of the child's physical and psychological health. By age 18, 27% of people born female and 5% of people born male in the United States are estimated to have experienced contact sexual abuse [4, 5]. Working in the school setting provides a unique advantage for healthcare professionals to build continuous, trusting relationships with students. For this reason, students who have experienced sexual abuse may feel comfortable disclosing their abuse in the school setting. This is especially important given the child's verbal history is many times the presenting critical piece, as most children will have a normal physical examination [4].

Healthcare providers play an important role at the time of initial disclosure by obtaining a limited history to further understand the concern of sexual abuse and determine next steps. The way in which the provider talks to the patient regarding possible abuse is very important. Practice guidelines advise healthcare providers to conduct "minimal facts" history-taking and ask "open-ended" questions, keeping in mind that a question should never be suggestive of an answer [4, 5]. It is important to remember that this history taking is to acquire just enough information to make appropriate diagnostic and treatment decisions as well as to make appropriate reports and referrals [5]. In younger children, if the disclosure is spontaneous, it is important for the provider to document word for word what the child stated. Any descriptions of abuse the child gave should be documented exactly how they were said, using the child's own language. In the event a child makes a concerning statement and does not want to give additional information, they should not be coerced into talking about this more. Multiple interviews of the child should be avoided, as in many cases, the child will undergo a forensic interview conducted by a trained professional as part of the overall investigation [4]. Depending on the resources available in one's geographic area, the forensic interview would be conducted by this professional in association with a facility where child abuse is routinely evaluated, such as a pediatric emergency department or child advocacy center.

There are important considerations one must address when working with children and abuse is a concern. The first consideration is the child's safety: Will the child be safe if sent home after school? Will the alleged perpetrator have continued access to the child, potentially creating additional harm? Are there concerns that the non-offending caregiver will not be supportive and protective? If the alleged perpetrator is providing resources (financial, housing, food) to the family, the disclosure of alleged abuse can create a new stressor in the family. Is the child at risk for being harmed or punished due to this disclosure? Will the child be coerced into recanting [4, 5]? Gathering the appropriate information from the child, and when possible, the non-offending caregiver, about safety will help guide safe discharge plans and will be important for investigative agencies.

Considering a report to CPS may be a part of the safety determination process. Healthcare providers may worry about the stress a report to CPS could cause a family when involving such agencies. These concerns should not stop a healthcare provider from protecting a child. In every state, it is mandated that professionals, including healthcare professionals, report suspected child abuse and neglect to appropriate agencies (CPS and law enforcement (LE) agencies, including tribal agencies) [5]. It is important for providers to understand their state laws regarding mandated reporting in cases of suspected child abuse as well as understand which agencies they should report to as this varies by state.

From a medical evaluation standpoint, determining which cases warrant an immediate assessment and which cases merit a referral to a child abuse pediatrician or child advocacy center is a critical step to make at the time of initial disclosure. The clinical examination of a child where sexual abuse is a concern depends on several factors including the healthcare provider's scope of practice. For school nurses, priority interventions should include gathering preliminary, limited information regarding the following:

1) Timeframe of alleged abuse
2) Information about the alleged perpetrator
3) Any medical concerns the child has reported.

For the provider (physician, advanced practice nurse, or physician's assistant) working in a school-based health clinic, the above information should be obtained as well as completing a general physical examination and considering obtaining sexually transmitted infection (STI) testing. A thorough exam is important to assess for possible trauma sustained throughout the body. However, regarding the anogenital exam, the provider should consider if the patient will be referred to another facility that specializes in this type of evaluation. The referral location will depend on the timeframe in which the alleged abuse is thought to have occurred. If the timeframe is acute, generally if alleged abuse occurred within a 72- or 96-hour window, depending on the age of the child, a forensic evidence collection kit will be obtained. Unnecessary, repeated anogenital exams should be avoided as this could retraumatize the child and contaminate evidence.

Testing for sexually transmitted infections (STIs) is another consideration the healthcare provider must address. Knowing that sexually abused adolescents are at a higher risk for STI's, these patients should be screened for all infections, as should any sexually active adolescent presenting to the clinic [5]. Additionally, emergency contraception should be offered if the alleged abuse occurred within the window of the medication's effectiveness. STI's occur less frequently in prepubescent children, therefore each case should be evaluated individually for the appropriate testing [5]. In cases where the patient will be referred to a tertiary care center, the primary care provider should discuss the plan for STI testing with the receiving facility to ensure all proper testing will be completed.

Finally, the patient's current mental health status is another issue the provider should assess at the time of disclosure. Children and adolescents may exhibit a wide range of mental health symptoms during the disclosure process. Some may initially show clear symptoms of distress while others may not. Symptoms of a mental health concern, such as depression or post-traumatic stress disorder (PTSD), may have already developed or may develop later [5]. The initial support and validation a medical provider shows to the student is important not only during the immediate period of disclosure, but also will help establish a trusting provider-student relationship, one where a student feels comfortable sharing ongoing mental health challenges they are experiencing. If there are immediate mental health concerns, the provider should involve the appropriate school personnel to help ensure the student's safety and well-being. Resources from both the school and the school-based health clinic should be used in tandem to ensure the best possible care for the student.

Case 3 Sam is a 6-year-old male who comes to you after recess complaining of headache. He states it hurt this morning but now it is worse. When performing your exam, you see linear patterned bruising to his left cheek and bruising to his left ear. When asked if anything happened to his face to cause the injury, the child responds, "I don't know." Now what?

Bruising is the most common injury sustained by children. It can be caused by accidental or non-accidental mechanisms, be related to underlying medical conditions, or the purple-blue-red mark seen might not even be a bruise. For example, many children have blue-gray patches to their skin that are birth marks and can look like bruising. These are known as congenital dermal melanocytosis and though they can slowly change color over time, they would essentially be the same on a repeat exam one to two weeks later, while bruises should completely heal and resolve in most children. Healthy, normal, active children sustain bruises often. However, there are particular locations that one anticipates seeing bruising from playful, accidental mechanisms in mobile children and other locations that raise the concern for inflicted injury. TEN-4 FACES-P is a clinical decision rule that was created to help medical providers remember these concerning locations and therefore consider physical abuse as the cause of them for children under 4 years of age (Table 72.1) [6, 7].

When children are active and mobile, they often obtain bruising to the bony prominences of their body, for example the knees/shins of the lower legs, the chin and forehead of the face, and the elbows of the arms. It is rare and atypical for them to sustain bruising to the torso, ears, and neck from accidental mechanisms. If a medical provider comes across bruising to these locations or any of the FACES spots of the head during a physical examination, more questions should be asked of the child and additional medical work-up should be pursued. This may involve referring the student to the local tertiary care center for a more complete evaluation that cannot be performed in the school-based health clinic.

Despite many beliefs to the contrary, bruising cannot be dated by the naked eye. No matter the color, from purple-blue to red to brown-green, there is no way to tell if a bruise is 'old' or 'fresh' just from looking at it. Many factors are involved to create a bruise's appearance, from the underlying health status of the person to where on the body the injury is located; from how much force was used by the opposing object to what that object is made of. Every body is different, as is every bruise! The important thing to remember is the history provided for the injury. Older, verbal children should be able to provide a history of present illness for whatever their chief complaint might be, including for injuries. If they do not or seemingly will not, it does not mean they are lying or trying to be deceptive as they truly may not remember. Disclosure is a process. A child may not be comfortable talking about their body and what happened to it, even to a medical provider. Letting the child know that your job is to keep them healthy and safe provides reassurance that you are there to help them and continues to build upon the trusting healthcare provider-student relationship that children need.

Assessing the child's medical status is within the school-based healthcare provider's scope of practice and is their medical responsibility. If the child is complaining of pain, could they have sustained trauma and therefore, could it be from non-accidental trauma or abuse? Does the patient have any injuries that warrant care that cannot be provided in the current medical setting? Is there strong suspicion of underlying injuries that would need additional evaluation, like radiological studies or subspecialty consultation? Oftentimes, the older verbal child can participate in a

Table 72.1 Clinical decision rule for bruising in children under 4 years of age

TEN	4	FACES-P
Torso	Infants 4 months and younger with any bruise, anywhere	Frenulum
		Angle of Jaw
Ears		Cheeks
		Eyelids
Neck		Subconjunctival
		Pattern

head-to-toe physical examination and express if there are any locations that are painful and may have an occult injury. A thorough skin evaluation is important to assess for any signs of injury, no matter the cause. There are situations when a child would require transfer to another medical facility for further treatment, but oftentimes, cases can be managed in the primary care setting. Knowing your local resources, like a children's hospital with access to child abuse pediatricians, is important as this can provide additional support and guidance during these difficult encounters.

As stated previously, reports to CPS and/or LE are indicated when there are concerns for abuse or neglect. There does not need to be "proof" that this has occurred, only a reasonable suspicion to make the report in good faith. An "alleged perpetrator" is not necessary either; further determination of that component is part of CPS/LE's role. However, if the child has disclosed who harmed them, this information should be passed along to investigators. Always remember that pediatric medical providers play a critical role in the protection and well-being of children.

Case Resolutions After discussing your concerns with Johnny's caregivers, you were able to refer him to a nearby dental clinic and parents were able to have his teeth treated; CPS was not involved.

- After hearing Ashley's disclosure, as a mandated reporter, you contacted CPS and LE with these concerns. You then refer Ashley to the local Child Advocacy Center for forensic interview and comprehensive medical evaluation.
- After examining Sam, you determine that he does not require head imaging but would benefit from more monitoring throughout the day. You decide to keep him in clinic for observation and then make reports to CPS regarding the concern for physical abuse.

Extra Credit Points

1. When concerned about abuse/neglect, the provider should attempt to gather limited information from the child through open ended questions, in order to decrease the number of individuals who speak to the child regarding the concern.
2. Considerations that impose an immediate safety concern for the child from both a social and medical perspective include many factors and should be considered in respect to the timing of a CPS report.
3. If there are no acute concerns, the anogenital exam should be deferred until seen by a specialist.
4. TEN-4-FACESP is a clinical decision rule created to help medical providers determine concern for physical abuse in children under the age of 4 years.
5. Neglect is multifactorial and related to social determinants of health. It is important to assess if the family has access to necessary resources to keep children safe and healthy.
6. A child should be referred to a child abuse medical provider or child advocacy center when abuse and/or neglect is suspected, whether the abuse occurred recently or historically.

7. A child should be referred to the emergency department when it is not possible to refer to a child abuse medical provider or child advocacy center and the concern is recent. A referral to the emergency department should also be made when there is an immediate concern of safety or increased severity of the child's health status.

References

1. U.S. Department of Health & Human Services, Administration for children and families, administration on children, youth and families, children's bureau. Child maltreatment 2022. (2024).
2. Dubowitz H. Neglect in children. Pediatr Ann. 2013;42(4):73–7.
3. Jenny C. Recognizing and responding to medical neglect. Pediatrics. 2007;120:1385–9.
4. Dubowitz H, Finkel M, Feigelman S, et al. The initial medical assessment of possible child sexual abuse: history, history, history. Acad Pediatr. 2024;24(4):562–9.
5. Jenny C, Crawford-Jakubiak JE. The evaluation of children in the primary care setting when sexual abuse is suspected. Pediatrics. 2013;132:558–67.
6. Pierce MC, Kaczor K, Aldridge S, et al. Bruising characteristics discriminating physical child abuse from accidental trauma. Pediatrics. 2010;125:67–74.
7. Pierce MC, Kaczor K, Lorenz DJ, et al. Validation of a clinical decision rule to predict abuse in young children based on bruising characteristics. JAMA Network Open. 2021;4(4):1–12.

Chapter 73
Labor Trafficking and Commercial Sexual Exploitation

Kanani E. Titchen

Human trafficking (HT) in the United States is the exploitation of a person for sex or labor by means of force, fraud or coercion. Despite its name, the crime does not require movement. Children (under 18 years) who are engaged in sex for something of monetary value are *de jure* victims of trafficking per federal law: no coercion, force, or trickery need be present. By contrast, force, fraud, or coercion must be proven in cases of labor trafficking, no matter the victim's age.

In general, youth is a risk factor for human trafficking due to the innate dependence of children on adults, their propensity for trusting others and looking to others for guidance, and myriad other factors. More specifically, adolescence with its emphasis on separation and individuation from family and caregivers presents risk for exploitation, with some youth more vulnerable than others. A number of biopsychosocial factors are associated with creating and deepening these vulnerabilities.

A mixed methods study in 2016 found that 100% of 20 participating schools in San Diego County reported that recruitment for sex trafficking was occurring on their campuses, and 90% endorsed documented cases of sex trafficking victims [1]. The National Association of School Nurses in 2021 highlighted the pivotal roles that school nurses and educators play in identifying youth at risk for trafficking, those being groomed or recruited for human trafficking, and those who are actively being trafficked [2] (Table 73.1).

Many indicators of labor and sex trafficking among youth are nonspecific and could be attributed to a variety of causes (Fig. 73.1). However, a constellation of signs may suggest human trafficking and demands consideration by education and healthcare professionals. If there is suspicion of child labor or sex trafficking, it is rarely wrong to report this suspicion to Child Protective Services, and this is the

K. E. Titchen (✉)
University of California San Diego, San Diego, CA, USA

Rady Children's Health, San Diego, CA, USA
e-mail: ktitchen@health.ucsd.edu

R. P. Olympia, J. Brady-Olympia (eds.), *Clinical Considerations in School-based Health*, https://doi.org/10.1007/978-3-031-85765-2_73

Table 73.1 Pivotal roles of school nurses in addressing human trafficking in schools

Ensure patients' physical, cultural, and emotional safety within school health clinics
Recognize signs of human trafficking
Identify children at risk for human trafficking
Intervene on behalf of children suspected of being victims of human trafficking by coordinating with child protective services, law enforcement, social services, and community-based service providers
Address medical consequences of human trafficking
Promote universal education about human trafficking among students, teachers, school staff, and parents
Assist in development of school district protocols to address child trafficking
Mobilize key values of leadership in community and public health

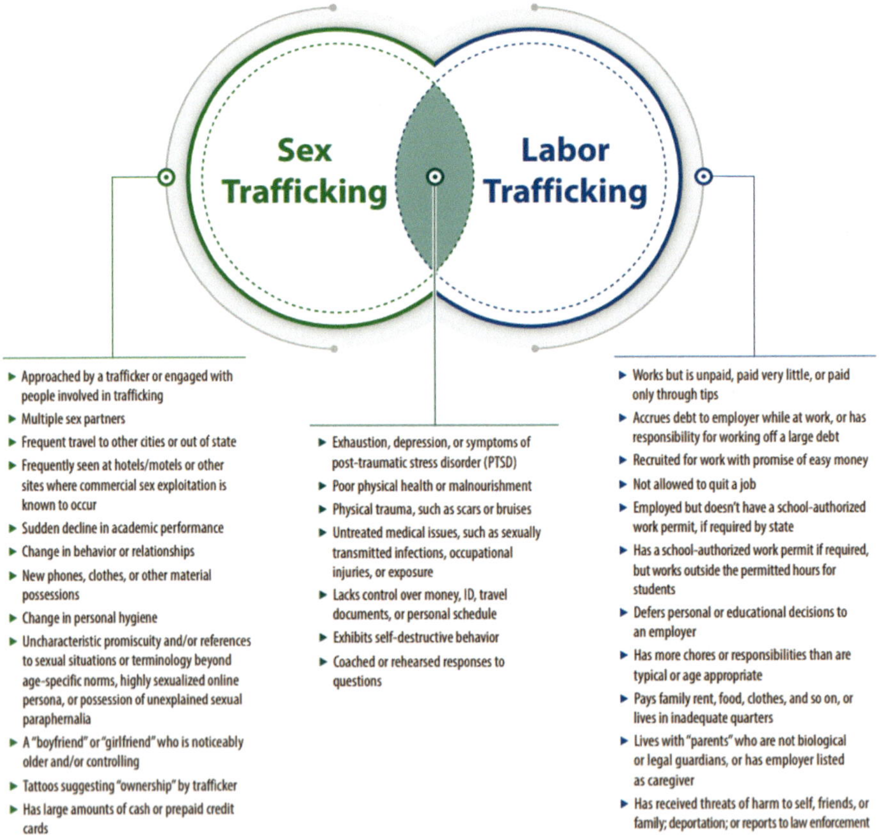

Fig. 73.1 Indicators of child labor and sex trafficking

recommended action for all mandated reporters. Unfortunately, it often takes multiple reports of exploitation for any action to be taken. Reporting could undermine trust in the authority figure, and there are risks for victims due to their vulnerabilities [3]: how such suspicions are reported is a delicate issue and will be covered in the following case study. Certainly, if there is a concern for the immediate safety of the child due to threats, suicidality, or physical injury, a referral and transfer to the nearest emergency department should be made.

Case Marta is a 13-year-old South Bay Middle School 8th grader. After enduring physical and sexual abuse as a child, Marta now lives with a foster family. She has an Individualized Education Plan (IEP) to accommodate her learning disabilities and was a successful student and peer leader prior to this year. Lately, however, her grades have faltered. Her teachers note new, concerning behaviors: unfinished assignments, sleeping in class, and unexplained absences especially after weekends [4].

Monday morning Marta reports to the school clinic for abdominal pain, dizziness, and headache. Teachers have noted that she is falling asleep in class. Marta appears tired and slurs her speech. She avoids eye contact as you obtain vital signs, preferring to respond to alerts on her new smart watch, including an inappropriate outburst of laughter and expletives after checking a message despite your instructions otherwise while taking blood pressure. After reassessing, her vitals are: temperature 98.3°F, HR 106 beats per minute, RR 16 breaths per minute, BP 92/54.

You invite Marta into a private exam room away from other waiting students. Your next action is to:

A. Insist Marta hand over her smart watch. South Bay Middle School has a strict policy prohibiting devices on campus.
B. Conduct a urine drug test and ask her about substance use. Her behavior in clinic is most likely due to substance use.
C. Inquire if Marta is having sex for money. You recognize signs of trafficking described in an online training you recently completed.
D. Ask Marta about her nutrition and hydration. While concerned about more serious issues, you opt to focus on the reasons she came to clinic.

A. You insist that she hand over her smart watch.

Upset, Marta pleads she "needs the watch" and promises to stop using it. When you insist on confiscation, she immediately removes the device from her wrist and hides it in her backpack. She attempts to leave the exam room, but you protest and ask her to sit down. Ignoring your request, Marta yells, "I'm going back to class!" She rushes out and slams the door.

Child trafficking begins with grooming. Tactics—like gifted cell phones or smart watches—exploit Marta's need for love and safety, thereby forging trust between victim and trafficker. However, these resources may also be used to exert control over Marta by creating a debt bondage she cannot repay. Additionally, traffickers use gifted devices to track victim movement and facilitate exploitation. Therefore, if Marta loses her smart watch, she could face extortion or physical abuse from her trafficker. At a minimum, you've threatened Marta's sense of security by attempting to take an object she feels she needs.

B. You conduct a urine drug test and ask her about substance use

After expressing concern about her teachers' reports, declining grades, and abnormal vitals, you ask about recent drug history. She denies substance use and blames her symptoms on the flu. When pressed again about the issue, Marta asks, "When can I go?" You respond, "What about your headache, dizziness, and belly pain?" You tell Marta you must collect a urine sample before she can leave. She takes the cup to the restroom and returns it. The specimen is clear, and you suspect she filled the cup with water.

Conducting a drug test for any adolescent without their knowledge and assent is unethical unless there are strong medical or legal reasons to do so: undisclosed drug testing violates adolescents' rights to consent, confidentiality, and autonomy. It would be in Marta's best interest to involve her in medical decision making [5].

Marta denies using any substances. She says that she thinks she just has a flu. She asks how long it will be before she can go back to class. You express that you're concerned about her and that her vital signs are a bit off. You ask her again about substances. She again denies any substance use and says, "I'm fine. I just want to go back to class." You give her a pass to return to class.

Marta already has stated that she is not using any substances. To continue to focus on possible substance use undermines Marta. In the absence of labs or further information from history or physical exam, the differential diagnosis for Marta's symptoms and behaviors remains broad. A trauma-informed approach involves partnering with and listening to our patients nonjudgmentally, and allowing room for but not forcing disclosure [6].

C. You talk to her about human trafficking.

You share with Marta privately that you're concerned that she's "being trafficked." She says she doesn't know what that means. You ask if she is being made to work against her will or have sex for money. She says no, absolutely not. You ask, "If something bad were happening to you, would you tell me?" She looks at you intently before replying softly, "No." She asks for Advil and some water. You share that you can give her water and an ice pack. She thanks you for the water and ice pack and remains quietly texting on her watch before she heads back to class.

This encounter could prove a turning point for Marta: you've provided universal education about human trafficking, and you've provided for Marta's immediate needs—namely, a quiet place to talk, water, and a pain reliever. However, Marta may never perceive that she's being forced to do anything against her will: in fact, many victims of human trafficking do not identify as victims [7]. *Nonetheless, because of your kindness in not forcing disclosure, Marta is likely to return.*

D. You ask her about nutrition and hydration.

Marta shares that she skips breakfast and lunch and drinks coffee to stay awake in class. You ask Marta what makes it difficult for her to eat, and she shrugs. "I don't have time in the morning, and I don't like the school lunch. My mom works nights, so I feed my little sister and get her to bed." You offer her some water, and she accepts. You ask Marta if she would like some assistance in getting nutrition at school, if she needs a private space to eat, or if she'd like you to connect her to resources for her family. She is quiet, and then she gives you a puzzled look with tears in her eyes. She finally says, "No, but thank you," and she asks if she can go back to class. You say of course if she's feeling better.

By addressing Marta's immediate concerns and asking only relevant questions (in order to prevent re-traumatization,) you've now aligned your goals with Marta's. She offers you more information about her personal life, which provides you with insight about possible causes for her symptoms and behaviors. More importantly, you've made it clear to Marta that you're a person who can be trusted to address her short-term and potentially her (yet undiscovered) long-term needs and safety goals [6]

73.1 Beneath the Surface

What's really happening to Marta? Is she experiencing bullying, normal middle school friendship conflicts, or something as sinister as labor or sex trafficking? Is she using illicit substances? If she is being victimized, does she recognize this? Is there food insecurity? Or is it possible that a trafficker is controlling her food intake or demanding that she conform to a certain physique? Is the smart watch significant?

Up to 84% of victims of human trafficking engage in substance use, sometimes as a means of coping with trauma from exploitation, but some traffickers also supply illicit substances to their victims to induce a habit, to control victims, to punish them, or to criminalize them [8, 9]. In one urban study in 2019, 70% of female sex workers were found to use opioids daily [10]. In another study, 66% of victims of human trafficking reported that their substance use disorder led to human trafficking, while only 4.5% reported that human trafficking led to their substance use disorder [11, 12]. Disordered eating has been reported in cases of human trafficking, especially among women, many of whom report diminished appetite, abdominal pain, and weight loss [13]. Online recruitment of minors through cell phones and other devices to provide sexually explicit photos, videos, and media content has been reported [14, 15].

73.2 Menstruation Offers an Opportunity

Marta returns to the clinic two weeks later. She has been given a pass to the nursing office simply for "period," and she asks you for a menstrual pad, but then she lingers in the waiting room. You invite her back to a clinic room, and you ask her if she'd like some water and a hot pack for her cramps. Marta looks down quietly, and you then see she's crying. You hand her tissues and share that you're concerned. Marta dabs her eyes, and she takes a deep breath. "I'm on my period," she says by way of explanation. "Sure," you reply, "periods can really mess with our emotions. Still, I wonder if you're getting enough to eat and sleep, and if you're still having headaches and belly pain and dizziness?"

She looks at you, maybe surprised that you remembered?

Marta shares that she's still having those symptoms and still not eating much. You extend an offer that she have lunch in the nursing office. To your surprise, she accepts. You ask her if she'd also like a list of resources for food for her family: she declines but agrees to come tomorrow at lunch. As she's leaving, she spontaneously hugs you quickly and then rushes out the door.

Patient care needs to be "attentive to the various ways people from diverse backgrounds experience and express illness." [6] *We need to determine what services might address the emotional, physical, and cultural needs of our patients. Research into adjuvants to Trauma-Focused Cognitive Behavioral Therapy is underway and includes peer support, psychoeducation, and psychodrama* [4, 16].

Marta begins to spend time in your clinic waiting room during the lunch hour. You make it a point to check in with her daily, even if you're busy seeing other students. You notice that she's still not eating much during that time, but she seems to like being in the clinic.

73.3 Pre-syncopal Distress

After another week, Marta appears with a pass for pre-syncope at PE. Her heart rate is 116 beats per minute, and blood pressure 89/46. She endorses lightheadedness with visual changes upon standing. She looks cold, so you bring her a blanket. Although her orthostatic blood pressure changes are within normal limits, her standing blood pressure is hypotensive to 88/43, and her heart rate increases from 48 supine to 124 beats per minute upon standing. You express concern to Marta and let her know that her heart muscle is showing signs of distress. You inform her that you might need to have her hospitalized.

To your surprise, Marta appears relieved.

While doing a trauma-sensitive physical exam [17], you notice a small mark on Marta's lower abdomen—a non-descript tattoo. You don't remember seeing that when you previously examined Marta initially a few weeks ago, and you ask her where she got it. She begins to cry. You ask her gently why she's crying. She answers, "I just want my mommy." You share that you'll absolutely reach out to her mom right now.

You decide this is the right time to be compassionately candid with Marta and share that with this new tattoo, her smartwatch, her chronic abdominal pain and headaches, her low nutrition, and now alarming vital signs, you're wondering if there's someone else in her life who has pressured or convinced her to do things that might be interfering with her health and education and her peace of mind. You share that you've seen many kids from different backgrounds who are sometimes forced to work or have sex, and you ask her if she's heard of this. She nods.

You ask her if something like this is happening to her. She nods and continues to cry.

73.4 Partnering with the Patient

You inform Marta that your job is to find her help and support her, so you'll call the hospital, and you inform her that you also need to call for other support from Child Protective Services (CPS).(4) She nods and continues to cry and asks if she's going to go to jail or if she is going to be taken away from her mom, who doesn't know about any of this. You ask her why she thinks she might go to jail. She says that she knows she's been doing "illegal stuff" for her boyfriend. He bought her the watch. He put the tattoo on her. He told her to try to get friends to join them [4]. He told her that if she got caught or told anyone about what they were doing ("prostituting," she said,) she'd go to jail, and "they'd put my sister in the system." [18]

You thank her for telling you this. You share that you'll let CPS know this, and you reassure her that kids in her position don't go to jail: they receive help. You reiterate that you're attempting to get her and her family support. You inform her that CPS will have more questions, and you ask her if she'd like to be with you when you call them, or if she'd like to tell them herself what's been going on. She says, no, she wants you to do it. You tell her you're going to call the hospital and her mom right now, and she nods. You prepare for your meeting with her mom by compiling resources for Marta and her family (Table 73.2).

Extra Credit Points

1. Indicators of labor and sex trafficking can be nonspecific: keep child trafficking on the list of differential diagnoses when considering a constellation of concerning signs and symptoms.
2. It often takes multiple reports of suspicion of abuse/trafficking to Child Protective Services for appropriate action to be taken.
3. Avoid the rescue fantasy: the goal is to form a trusting relationship with the child rather than to force disclosure.
4. Provide universal education about labor and sex trafficking in your school health clinic and throughout the school in the form of posters, QR codes, fliers, and by advocating for district-wide education of students, parents, and education professionals.
5. Advocate for development of a trauma-informed protocol for reporting human trafficking through collaboration with child welfare services, law enforcement, social services, legal advocates, and community nonprofits.

Table 73.2 Resources for the school health practitioner

Resource	Website
National Education Association Toolkit	https://www.nea.org/resource-library/combating-human-trafficking
SOAR Online to Health and Wellness: Foundational Human Trafficking Trainings for School Based Professionals	https://nhttac.acf.hhs.gov/soar/soar-for-individuals/soar-online
Human Trafficking School Safety Protocol Toolkit	https://nhttac.acf.hhs.gov/resource/human-trafficking-school-safety-protocol-toolkit
Addressing Human Trafficking in America's Schools (webinar series)	https://safesupportivelearning.ed.gov/human-trafficking-webinar-series
Staff Development Series: Addressing Human Trafficking in America's Schools	https://safesupportivelearning.ed.gov/addressing-human-trafficking-americas-schools-staff-development-series
Policy and Protocol Development	https://safesupportivelearning.ed.gov/human-trafficking-americas-schools/school-policies-protocols-to-combat-trafficking
Human Trafficking and Health Care Providers: Legal Requirements for Reporting and Education	https://healtrafficking.org/2021/01/legal-requirements-for-reporting-and-education/

Acknowledgments Thank you to Dr. Rachel Hartsell for her preliminary research and initial editing.

References

1. Carpenter A, Gates J. The nature and extent of gang involvement in sex trafficking in San Diego County. [Internet]. San Diego, CA: Univ San Diego Point Loma Nazarene Univ.; 2016. Report No.: 249857. https://www.ojp.gov/pdffiles1/nij/grants/249857.pdf
2. National Association of School Nurses. Human trafficking [Position Statement]. Silver Spring, MD; 2021.
3. English A. Mandatory reporting of human trafficking: potential benefits and risks of harm. AMA J Ethics. 2017;19(1):54–62.
4. U.S. Department of Education. Human trafficking in America's schools: What schools can do to prevent, respond, and help students to recover from human trafficking. (2nd ed.) [Internet]. U.S. Department of Education, Office of Safe and Supportive Schools.; 2021 [cited 2024 Oct 20]. https://www.ed.gov/sites/ed/files/documents/human-trafficking/human-trafficking-americas-schools.pdf
5. American Academy of Pediatrics Committee on Substance Abuse. Testing for drugs of abuse in children and adolescents. Pediatrics. 1996;98(2 Pt 1):3305–7.
6. Hemmings S, Jakobowitz S, Abas M, Bick D, Howard LM, Stanley N, et al. Responding to the health needs of survivors of human trafficking: a systematic review. BMC Health Serv Res. 2016;16(1):320.

7. Murdock L, Hodge-Williams C, Hardin K, Rood CJ. Youth survivor perspectives on healthcare and sex trafficking. J Pediatr Nurs. 2022;66:95–103.
8. Lederer L, Wetzel CA. The health consequences of sex trafficking and their implications for identifying victims in healthcare facilities. Annals Health L. 2014;23(1):61–91.
9. Forget J. Violent drug organizations use human trafficking to expand profits. [Internet]. 2021 [cited 2024 Oct 20]. https://www.dea.gov/stories/2021/2021-01/2021-01-28/violent-drug-organizations-use-human-trafficking-expand-profits
10. Footer KHA, Park JN, Allen ST, Decker MR, Silberzahn BE, Huettner S, et al. Police-related correlates of client-perpetrated violence among female sex workers in Baltimore City, Maryland. Am J Public Health. 2019;109(2):289–95.
11. The intersection of human trafficking and addiction. In Providence, RI; 2016 [cited 2024 Oct 20]. https://2017-2021.state.gov/wp-content/uploads/2020/10/TIP_Factsheet-The-Intersection-of-Human-Trafficking-and-Addiction-1-508.pdf
12. Aljadeff G, Titchen K. Hooked: how human traffickers leverage substance use for control. Pediatr Rev. 2024;45(6):366–8.
13. Oram S, Ostrovschi NV, Gorceag VI, Hotineanu MA, Gorceag L, Trigub C, et al. Physical health symptoms reported by trafficked women receiving post-trafficking support in Moldova: prevalence, severity and associated factors. BMC Womens Health. 2012;12:20.
14. Baird K, Connolly J. Recruitment and entrapment pathways of minors into sex trafficking in canada and the united states: a systematic review. Trauma, Violence, Abuse. 2023;24(1):189–202.
15. Gezinski LB, Gonzalez-Pons KM. Sex trafficking and technology: a systematic review of recruitment and exploitation. J Hum Traffick. 2024;10(3):497–511.
16. Hopper EK, Azar N, Bhattacharyya S, Malebranche DA, Brennan KE. STARS experiential group intervention: a complex trauma treatment approach for survivors of human trafficking. J Evid Inf Soc Work. 2018;15(2):215–41.
17. Elisseou S, Puranam S, Nandi M. A Novel, Trauma-informed physical examination curriculum for first-year medical students. MedEdPORTAL. 2019;15:10799.
18. Thulander S, Benjamin C. In Harm's way: How systems fail human trafficking survivors. Polaris Project. 2023;

Chapter 74
Depression and Suicide

Jasmin Gange Lagman and Nungshitombi Chongtham

74.1 Depression

Case 1 Joseph, a 13 year old honor student was referred to you by the homeroom teacher due to his grades declining significantly in this past grading period. He seems tired most of the time and less engaged in class. His usual group of friends often find him irritable and angry since he broke up with his girlfriend two months ago. He no longer joins the baseball practices he used to enjoy, stating he is not good enough. His parents shared that he has been withdrawing to his bedroom and is reluctant to talk to them. What should you do?

One of the most common psychiatric disorders in children and adolescents is depressive disorder [1]. Depression can impact a child's development negatively and can affect school attendance, school performance, and/or social interactions with peers and teachers [2]. It can present in a wide range, from subsyndromal symptoms to severe with psychosis in rare cases [1]. As children and adolescents spend a significant amount of their time in school, school health providers can play a role in supporting students with mental health problems, providing a safe, non-stigmatizing, and supportive natural environment [2].

The two most common types include Major Depressive Disorder (MDD) which includes symptoms of depressed mood or loss of interest most of the time for at least two weeks that interfere with daily activities and Persistent Depressive Disorder (PDD) which consists of less severe depression symptoms but lasts much longer, usually for at least two years [3, 4]. As with the Diagnostic and Statistical Manual fifth edition (DSM-5-TR) criteria, MDD is characterized by a discrete episode of at least two weeks duration of changes in mood, interest or pleasure, cognition, and

J. G. Lagman (✉) · N. Chongtham
Penn State Hershey Medical Center, Hershey, PA, USA
e-mail: jlagman@pennstatehealth.psu.edu; nchongtham@pennstatehealth.psu.edu

R. P. Olympia, J. Brady-Olympia (eds.), *Clinical Considerations in School-based Health*, https://doi.org/10.1007/978-3-031-85765-2_74

neurovegetative functions and must be present most of the day or nearly every day with significant distress or functional impairment [1]. The widely known mnemonic for symptoms of depression is as follows:

SIG-E-CAPS stands for [5]:

- **S**leep changes (either increased or decreased sleep);
- **I**nterest deficit (anhedonia);
- **G**uilt (worthlessness, hopelessness, regret);
- **E**nergy deficit;
- **C**oncentration deficit;
- **A**ppetite disorder (either decreased or increased);
- **P**sychomotor retardation or agitation; and
- **S**uicidality.

Depression is considered with the presence of four SIGECAPS symptoms and one of the two cardinal signs: depressed mood or anhedonia [5].

74.2 Screening

With depression as the leading cause of disability in the US, the United States Preventive Services Task Force (USPSTF) recommends screening for major depressive disorder (MDD) in adolescents aged 12–18 years old with adequate systems in place, so accurate diagnosis, effective treatment, and appropriate follow-up are ensured [3]. Psychometrically sound and freely available screening instruments can be used such as the Patient Health Questionnaire-9 (PHQ-9) (https://www.apa.org/depression-guideline/patient-health-questionnaire.pdf) for initial screening for adolescents 12–18 years old. For younger children less than 12 years old, the use of Pediatric Symptom Checklist (appropriate for ages 3 to 17 years) (https://www.massgeneral.org/psychiatry/treatments-and-services/pediatric-symptom-checklist) and Strengths and Difficulties Questionnaire (appropriate for ages 2 to 17 years) (https://www.sdqinfo.org/) can be used.

74.3 Management

After screening and stratification of symptoms is completed, a decision to monitor, treat, or refer the patient will be made. Table 74.1 shows indications for initial treatment, therapy, and pharmacotherapy based on category of depression, taken from AACAP and GLAD-PC recommendations [1, 6–8]

If pharmacotherapy is needed, a Serotonin Selective Reuptake Inhibitor (SSRI) is recommended as the first line option for depression [1, 8]. Fluoxetine is approved by the Food and Drug Administration (FDA) for MDD for patients eight years old and above, while Escitalopram is FDA approved for patients 12 years old and above.

Table 74.1 Treatment for mild, moderate, and severe depression

	Mild depression	Moderate depression	Severe depression
PHQ-9 score	5–9	10–19	≥20
Definition per DSM-5-TR	Closer to 5 symptoms which are distressing but manageable. Functional impairment is mild.	The symptoms, intensity and degree of impairment are between mild and severe depression.	Closer to 9 symptoms which are seriously distressing and unmanageable. The symptoms markedly interfere with the degree of functional impairment.
Initial Treatment	Support and monitoring every 1–2 weeks for 6–8 weeks.	Consider referral to a mental health specialist.	Recommend referral to a mental health specialist.
Therapy	Supportive therapy	+/− CBT/IPT	CBT/IPT
Pharmacotherapy - SSRI		+/−	+

Abbreviations: CBT (Cognitive Behavioral Therapy), IPT (Interpersonal Therapy), SSRI (Selective Serotonin Reuptake Inhibitor)

Do not use an SSRI together with a Monoamine oxidase inhibitor (MAOI), as this may lead to increased serotonin levels and serotonin syndrome (agitation, pressured speech, tachycardia, diarrhea, shivering, diaphoresis, mydriasis, clonus, hyperreflexia, tremors, seizures, delirium, hypertension, hyperthermia, muscle rigidity). If a student presents with psychotic symptoms or suicidal/homicidal thoughts, refer to crisis or an emergency department [7].

74.4 SSRI Recommendations [8]

- First Line
  - Fluoxetine – 10–60 mg with 10 mg increments.
- Second Line:
  - Escitalopram (First line for 12 years and older) – 5–20 mg with 5 mg increments.
  - Citalopram – 10–40 mg with 10 mg increments.
  - Sertraline – 25–200 mg with 12.5–25 mg increments.
- Side Effects:
  - Common side-effects may include headaches, gastrointestinal upset, insomnia.
  - May cause increased anxiety and agitation
  - FDA black box warning of increased suicidal thoughts for patients less than 24yo.

- When to change medication:
  - Use a different SSRI if the maximum dose of the current medication has been reached, with no improvement in target symptoms after 4–6 weeks, or with major side-effects.
  - Use a second-line medication if with two failed SSRI trials with CBT/IPT
  - If with three failed trials, reevaluate diagnosis, consider medication combinations and refer to a mental health specialist.

74.5 Suicide

Case 2 Allana, a 16-year-old female was sent to the school nurse after a classmate saw multiple superficial cuts on her arms. In your office, Allana is crying and tells you that she had an argument with her mother this morning and made cuts on her arm using a razor blade. She wishes she was dead and she does not know if she can keep herself safe. What should you do?

Suicide in children and adolescents have been steadily increasing in the past decade with significantly higher than expected rates during the COVID-19 pandemic [9]. It is the second most common cause of death in youth ages 10–24 years and the tenth most common cause of death among 5-9-year-old [10]. In 2021, CDC reported more than 1 in 5 (22%) high school students seriously considered attempting suicide and 1 in 10 (10%) actually attempted suicide [10]. Schools play an important role in suicide prevention given the opportunity to engage most children and adolescents who are already enrolled for education. It is essential that school staff are familiar with identifying students who are at risk of suicide, recognize the warning signs and have knowledge about available mental health resources.

74.6 Definitions

- Suicide: death caused by self-directed injurious behavior with intent to die as a result of the behavior
- Suicide attempt: non-fatal, self-directed, potentially injurious behavior with intent to die as a result of the behavior. A suicide attempt might not result in injury
- Suicidal ideation: thinking, considering, or planning to kill self

74.7 Risk Factors for Suicide

A previous suicide attempt is the leading risk factor of suicide. However, many risk factors which are common across all ages, race and sex can contribute to suicide (Table 74.2).

Table 74.2 Individual, relationship, and community/societal risk factors for suicide [10]

Individual factors	Relationship factors	Community/Societal factors
• Previous suicide attempt • History of depression and other mental illnesses • Serious illness such as chronic pain • Criminal/legal problems • Job/financial problems or loss • Impulsive or aggressive tendencies • Substance use • Current or prior history of adverse childhood experiences • Sense of hopelessness • Violence victimization and/or perpetration	• Bullying • Family/loved one's history of suicide • Loss of relationships • High conflict or violent relationships • Social isolation	• Lack of access to healthcare • Suicide cluster in the community • Stress of acculturation • Community violence • Historical trauma • Discrimination • Stigma associated with help-seeking and mental illness • Easy access to lethal means of suicide among people at risk • Unsafe media portrayals of suicide

Table 74.3 Warning signs of suicide

• Talking about or making plans for suicide • Expressing hopelessness about the future • Displaying severe/overwhelming emotional pain or distress
• Showing worrisome behavioral cues or marked changes in behavior, particularly in the presence of the warning signs above. Specifically, this includes significant: – Withdrawal from or changing in social connections/situations – Changes in sleep (increased or decreased) – Anger or hostility that seems out of character or out of context – Recent increased agitation or irritability
• Risk is greater if the warning sign is: – new and/or – has increased and – possibly related to an anticipated or actual painful event, loss, or change.
• **Acute warning signs:** These are not always communicated directly or outwardly: – Threatening self-harm or suicide, or talking of wanting to self-harm or attempt suicide; and/or, – Seeking access to firearms, available pills, or other means; and/or, – Talking or writing about death, dying or suicide, when these actions are out of the ordinary.

Source: American Association of Suicidology: Youth Warning Signs

A higher risk of suicide is also reported in those exposed to violence including sexual and physical abuse, bullying and domestic violence. Those with intellectual and learning disabilities, immigrants, minority race, in rural areas, in foster care or juvenile justice system, LGBTQ and gender non-conforming youths are also vulnerable to increased risks of suicide [10]. Some association with increased social media use and suicidal behavior trends have been reported but role of other factors may be contributing to both [11, 12]. Suicide attempts are more common among females but more lethal among males. The most common methods of youth suicide are firearms, suffocation, and overdose/poisoning. Table 74.3 lists common warning signs of suicide in children and adolescents.

74.8 Warning Signs of Suicide

If risks for suicide are identified, the student should be evaluated by a trained mental health crisis response personnel in the school who can be a school counselor, school psychologist, school nurse or a school physician. If trained mental health crisis response personnel are not available in your school, teachers can provide support and ask directly about suicidal thoughts. Parents or legal guardians of the student should be notified and appropriate referrals for mental health care should be made. Students in acute crisis with suicidal ideations who are deemed to be at imminent risk of suicide due to presence of clear intent or plan of suicide or when there has been an actual self-harm attempt with intent to be dead (regardless of severity) should be referred immediately to crisis or an emergency department. It is recommended not to use 'no suicide contracts' or 'contracting for safety' agreements as there is little evidence in its usefulness [13].

74.9 Suicide Screening Tools

There are evidenced-based, validated tools which are publicly available for use to detect suicidal ideations and behaviors in children and adolescents, including the following [11]:

- Ask Suicide-Screening Questions (ASQ) (https://www.nimh.nih.gov/sites/default/files/documents/research/research-conducted-at-nimh/asq-toolkit-materials/asq-tool/screening_tool_asq_nimh_toolkit_1.pdf)
- Suicide Behavior Questionnaire-Revised (SBQ-R) (https://youthsuicideprevention.nebraska.edu/wp-content/uploads/2019/09/SBQ-R.pdf)
- Columbia Suicide Severity Rating Scare (C-SSRS) (https://cssrs.columbia.edu/the-columbia-scale-c-ssrs/about-the-scale/)

Case Resolutions **Case 1** – Joseph presents with symptoms of depression such as declining grades (decreased concentration), decreased energy, less engaged, more irritable, with increased guilt. Screening with PHQ-9 can be done and evaluated clinically. ASQ screening tool is administered to assess for suicidality and it indicates no risk. He may benefit from individual therapy and possible referral to his family doctor, pediatrician or psychiatrist for further evaluation and treatment.

Case 2 – Allana presented with suicidal ideation along with impulsive tendency of self-harming. She has ongoing conflict with family and is unsure if she can keep herself safe. She needs to be evaluated by crisis or referred to an emergency department.

Extra Credit Points

1. Symptoms of depression in children and adolescents can present differently depending on their developmental stage.

2. Therapy and/or medication management is indicated for moderate to severe depression.
3. Patients presenting with severe depression who have psychotic symptoms or threats of suicide will need further evaluation by crisis or emergency resources.

References

1. Walter HJ, Abright AR, Bukstein OG, et al. Clinical practice guideline for the assessment and treatment of children and adolescents with major and persistent depressive disorders. J Am Acad Child Adolesc Psychiatry. 2023;62(5):479–502. https://doi.org/10.1016/j.jaac.2022.10.001.
2. American Academy of Pediatrics. Supporting students with depression in school. https://www.aap.org/. Accessed 31 May 24.
3. US Preventive Services Task Force, Mangione CM, Barry MJ, et al. Screening for depression and suicide risk in children and adolescents: US preventive services task force recommendation statement. JAMA. 2022;328(15):1534–42. https://doi.org/10.1001/jama.2022.16946.
4. National Institute of Mental Health. Depression.2024. https://www.nih.gov/. Accessed 31 May 24
5. Maurer DM, Raymond TJ, Davis BN. Depression: screening and diagnosis. Am Fam Physician. 2018;98(8):508–15.
6. American Psychiatric Association. Diagnostic and statistical manual of mental disorders. 5th ed. Washington, DC: American Psychiatric Association; 2013. p. 160–1.
7. Zuckerbrot RA, Cheung A, Jensen PS, Stein REK, Laraque D, GLAD-PC STEERING GROUP. Guidelines for Adolescent Depression in Primary Care (GLAD-PC): Part I. Practice preparation, identification, assessment, and initial management. Pediatrics. 2018;141(3):e20174081. https://doi.org/10.1542/peds.2017-4081.
8. Cheung AH, Zuckerbrot RA, Jensen PS, Laraque D, Stein REK, GLAD-PC STEERING GROUP. Guidelines for Adolescent Depression in Primary Care (GLAD-PC): Part II. Treatment and Ongoing Management. Pediatrics. 2018;141(3):e20174082. https://doi.org/10.1542/peds.2017-4082.
9. Bridge JA, Ruch DA, Sheftall AH, et al. Youth suicide during the first year of the COVID-19 pandemic. Pediatrics. 2023;151(3):e2022058375. https://doi.org/10.1542/peds.2022-058375.
10. Centers for Disease Control. Facts about suicide. 2024. Accessed 1 Jun 2024
11. American Academy of Pediatrics. Screening for suicide risk in clinical practice. 2023. https://www.aap.org/. Accessed 1 Jun 2024.
12. Leventhal AM, Cho J, Keyes KM, Zink J, Riehm KE, Zhang Y, Ketema, Digital media use and suicidal behavior in U.S. adolescents, 2009–2017, Prev Med Rep. 2021;23. https://doi.org/10.1016/j.pmedr.2021.101497
13. Garvey KA, Penn JV, Campbell AL, Esposito-Smythers C, Spirito A. Contracting for Safety with patients: clinical practice and forensic implications. J Am Acad Psychiatry Law. 2009;37(3):363–70.

Chapter 75
Disordered Eating

Caroline Shank and Khalida Itriyeva

Despite their high prevalence, eating disorders (EDs) in adolescents often go undiagnosed until medical complications develop, particularly in individuals with "normal" or higher body mass indices (BMIs) and those from historically minoritized communities. As the peak age of onset for EDs is between 13–18 years old, screening in this patient population is critically important [1]. EDs may present differently based on age: binge-purge behaviors are more common in later adolescence, and preteens often present earlier due to rapid weight loss, and the existence of premorbid psychopathology [2]. Medical providers at school-based health centers (SBHCs) are in a unique position to detect EDs early to interrupt their progression and to provide timely referral to treatment. Therefore, SBHC providers should be aware of the common presenting signs and symptoms of EDs. Table 75.1 summarizes the ED diagnoses that will be referenced throughout this chapter.

75.1 Cases for Discussion

Case 1 15-year-old Leah presents for her sports clearance physical just before the soccer season starts. She arrives in an oversized sweatshirt and sweatpants despite the warm weather outside. Her vital signs are as follows: pulse 46 beats per minute, blood pressure 90/60 mmHg, height 5′2″, weight 95 pounds (43

C. Shank (✉)
Cohen Children's Medical Center, Hempstead, NY, USA
e-mail: cshank@northwell.edu

K. Itriyeva
Cohen Children's Medical Center, Zucker School of Medicine at Hofstra/Northwell, Hempstead, NY, USA
e-mail: kitriyeva@northwell.edu

R. P. Olympia, J. Brady-Olympia (eds.), *Clinical Considerations in School-based Health*, https://doi.org/10.1007/978-3-031-85765-2_75

Table 75.1 ED Diagnoses

Anorexia nervosa (AN): characterized by restrictive intake leading to significantly low body weight, fear of gaining weight, and body dysmorphia
Bulimia nervosa (BN): characterized by repeated episodes of binge eating and compensatory behaviors for the prevention of weight gain, such as self-induced vomiting and laxative use
Binge-eating disorder (BED): recurrent binge eating episodes not associated with use of compensatory behaviors
Avoidant/restrictive food intake disorder (ARFID): disrupted eating patterns leading to failure to meet nutritional requirements by limiting the quantity or variety of foods consumed, but not related to body dysmorphia. Examples include avoidance based on sensory qualities of food, concern about unpleasant consequences of eating (e.g.—choking, vomiting)
Other specified feeding or eating disorders (OSFED):
Atypical AN: all of the criteria for AN are met yet the individual's weight is within or above the normal range despite significant weight loss
BN (of low frequency and/or limited duration): all of the criteria for BN are met, but on average, the binge eating and compensatory behaviors occur less than once a week and/or for <3 months
BED (of low frequency and/or limited duration): All of the criteria for BED are met, but on average, the binge eating occurs less than once a week and/or for <3 months
Purging disorder: recurrent purging behavior (e.g. self-induced vomiting, misuse of laxatives, diuretics, or other medications) in the absence of binge eating with the intent to influence weight or body shape

Adapted from the Diagnostic and Statistical Manual of Mental Disorders (5th ed.), American Psychiatric Association [3]

kilograms). She becomes distressed upon standing on the scale. Her last menstrual period was 3 months ago. Leah is anxious to finish her physical because she is eager to return to class for an exam.

Case 2 17-year-old Arielle presents for complaints of heartburn and abdominal pain. Her vital signs are as follows: pulse 105 beats per minute, blood pressure 125/80 mmHg, height 5′3″, weight 130 pounds (59 kilograms). The SBHC social worker who has been seeing her for individual psychotherapy pulls you aside and mentions that Arielle has a history of self-harm, and recently disclosed to her that she has been binging and purging at home.

Case 3 13-year-old Leo presents with a chief complaint of inability to swallow. His vital signs are as follows: pulse 101 beats per minute, blood pressure 115/75 mmHg, height 5′1″, weight 110 pounds (50 kilograms). He relays that last week he choked on a piece of broccoli in the school cafeteria, requiring a school staff member to administer the Heimlich maneuver. Since then, he has been unable to tolerate solids as he fears he will choke again but has been drinking plenty of liquids including nutritional supplements that his mother has been giving him.

Sports physicals are a key access point to medical providers for teenagers in both the primary care setting and at SBHCs, as seen in Case 1. A brief review of her vital

Table 75.2 History taking

Weight history: Highest weight and when, lowest weight and when
Body image: What do you think your weight should be? Do you do any body checking (e.g. weighing, body pinching, mirror checking?)
Diet history: 24-hour food recall. Do you count calories? What is your daily calorie goal? Do you avoid any specific foods? Do you feel guilty about eating, and if so, how do you deal with that guilt (exercising, purging, and eating less)?
Exercise history: How often, what activities? Do you have stress when you are unable to exercise?
Binge eating and purging: Do you ever binge? How often, which foods, any triggers? Do you vomit? How often? How soon after eating? Do you use laxatives, diuretics, diet pills, caffeine?
Menstrual history: Age at menarche? Frequency of menses? Last menstrual period (LMP)? Weight at time of LMP?
Family history: Any family history of dieting or an eating disorder? Anyone on special diets (vegetarian, gluten-free)? Family history of psychiatric disorders (depression, anxiety, bipolar disorder, obsessive-compulsive disorder, substance abuse, or other psychiatric illnesses?) Is there any difficulty obtaining food at home (screening for food insecurity)?
Review of systems: Dizziness, syncope, weakness, or fatigue? Pallor, easy bruising or bleeding, cold intolerance? Hair loss, lanugo, dry skin? Constipation, diarrhea, early fullness, bloating, abdominal pain, heartburn? Palpitations, chest pain? Muscle cramps, joint pains? Excessive thirst and voiding?

Adapted from AAP: Identification and Management of Eating Disorders in Children and Adolescents [4]

signs and history reveals bradycardia and secondary amenorrhea, defined as the absence of three consecutive menstrual cycles. AN should be suspected in this patient and additional history pertaining to weight loss and degree of weight loss to assess risk and severity. Table 75.2 provides ED history-taking questions. Although students typically present to SBHCs alone, providers should always contact the patient's parent or guardian to obtain a thorough history, as the adolescent may not be forthcoming about this sensitive topic. Additionally, providers can consider using developed screening questionnaires. For example, the Sick, Control, One, Fat and Food (SCOFF) questionnaire for DSM-5 EDs was developed in 1999 and is the most widely used screening tool for EDs. The SCOFF questionnaire consists of the following questions: (1) Do you make yourself sick because you feel uncomfortably full? (2) Do you worry you have lost control over how much you eat? (3) Have you recently lost one stone (14 pounds) in a 3-month period? (4) Do you believe yourself to be fat when others say you are too thin? (5) Would you say that food dominates your life? [4]. Positive responses to at least two of the five questions warrants close follow up with the student's primary care provider or referral to an eating disorder specialist.

A comprehensive physical examination, including close attention to growth parameters and vital signs, allows the provider to assess for signs of medical compromise and symptoms of ED behaviors, findings that may be subtle and are often overlooked [5]. For the patient in Case 1, it is essential that orthostatic vital signs and a resting pulse are obtained with her vital signs. Her skin should be assessed to evaluate for acrocyanosis and lanugo. Table 75.3 lists the physical examination

Table 75.3 Physical examination findings in children and adolescents with EDs

Features related to inadequate energy intake or malnutrition
Growth trajectory deviations (height, weight, BMI); weight loss or crossing percentiles
Abnormal vital signs: low resting HR or BP, orthostatic increase in HR (>20 beats per minute) or decrease in BP (<10 mmHg), hypothermia
Flat or anxious affect
Pallor, dry sallow skin, carotenemia
Cachexia (facial wasting, decreased subcutaneous fat, decreased muscle mass)
Dull, thin scalp hair, or lanugo
Cardiac murmur (1/3 with mitral valve prolapse), cool extremities; acrocyanosis, poor perfusion
Stool mass left lower quadrant
Delayed or interrupted pubertal development
Small breasts, vaginal dryness
Small testes
Features related to purging:
Abnormal vital signs: orthostatic increase in HR (>20 bpm) or decrease in BP (<10 mmHg)
Angular stomatitis, palatal scratches, dental enamel erosions
Russell's sign (abrasion or callous on knuckles from self-induced emesis)
Salivary gland enlargement (parotid and submandibular)
Epigastric tenderness
Bruising or abrasions over the spine (excessive exercise/sit-ups)
Features related to excessive energy intake:
Deviation from growth trajectory (height, weight, BMI); rapid increase in weight
Obesity
Elevated blood pressure or hypertension
Acanthosis nigricans, acne, hirsutism
Hepatomegaly
Premature puberty
Musculoskeletal pain

Adapted from AAP: Identification and Management of Eating Disorders in Children and Adolescents [4]

findings that may be seen in patients with restrictive eating leading to malnutrition. For a patient with a history of purging, as shown in Case 2, callouses on the knuckles (Russell's sign), salivary/parotid gland enlargement, and dental caries may also be observed.

75.2 Laboratory Evaluation

Initial laboratory evaluation is necessary to rule out other diagnoses that may present similarly and to screen for medical complications of EDs [5]. See Table 75.4 for the differential diagnosis of EDs.

Table 75.4 Differential diagnosis for EDs according to presentation

Weight loss	
	Gastrointestinal: inflammatory bowel disease, celiac disease
	Endocrine: hyperthyroidism, diabetes mellitus, adrenal insufficiency
	Infectious: chronic infections, such as tuberculosis or human immunodeficiency virus
	Psychiatric: depression, psychosis, anxiety or obsessive-compulsive disorder
	Other: neoplasm, superior mesenteric artery syndrome
Vomiting	
	Gastrointestinal: gastroesophageal reflux
	Neurologic: increased intracranial pressure, migraines
	Other: food allergy
Binge eating or unexplained weight gain	
	Endocrine: hypothyroidism, hypercortisolism
	Psychiatric: depression
	Iatrogenic: medication side effect
	Genetic: Prader Willi syndrome; Kleine-Levin syndrome

Adapted from AAP: Identification and Management of Eating Disorders in Children and Adolescents [1]

Initial screening laboratory evaluation for EDs includes a complete blood cell count with differential, serum electrolytes, liver transaminases, urinalysis, and thyroid studies. A screening for vitamin deficiencies may also be considered based on the patient's history and severity of malnutrition, as well as their eating behaviors (e.g.—very limited/picky diet). Importantly, laboratory studies are often normal in patients with AN unless they are partaking in compensatory behaviors such as purging or laxative use. However, normal laboratory results do not preclude the need for hospitalization for medical stabilization in cases where it is otherwise appropriate (e.g.—in patients with bradycardia or food refusal) [5]. A pregnancy test and reproductive hormone levels are indicated if the patient is amenorrheic, as in the patient in Case 1. Typical laboratory evaluation for patients with amenorrhea includes serum prolactin, luteinizing hormone (LH), follicle stimulating hormone (FSH), and estradiol levels. A serum estradiol level may serve as a baseline for reassessment during recovery. In patients with malnutrition and hypothalamic amenorrhea, LH, FSH, and estradiol levels are all suppressed. Additionally, for those patients who have not had a period in >12 months, bone densitometry may be considered to evaluate bone health, which may be negatively impacted by malnutrition and the resultant hypoestrogenic state. In addition to a laboratory evaluation, an electrocardiogram should be obtained to evaluate for bradycardia and the presence of arrhythmias. To rule out other diagnoses that may present similarly to EDs, celiac studies, inflammatory markers (e.g.—erythrocyte sedimentation rate), stool studies, serum cortisol concentrations, or radiographic imaging of the brain or gastrointestinal tract may also be considered. EDs can affect every organ system with potentially serious medical complications that develop because of malnutrition, weight changes, or purging [1, 5].

Table 75.5 Medical complications of EDs

ED behaviors
Related to dietary restriction or weight loss:
Fluids and electrolytes: dehydration; electrolyte abnormalities: hypokalemia, hyponatremia
Psychiatric: depressed mood or mood dysregulation; obsessive compulsive symptoms; anxiety
Neurologic: cerebral cortical atrophy; cognitive deficits; seizures
Cardiac: decreased cardiac muscle mass; right axis deviation; low cardiac voltage; cardiac dysrhythmias; cardiac conduction delays; mitral valve prolapse; pericardial effusion; congestive heart failure; edema
Gastrointestinal: delayed gastric emptying; slowed gastrointestinal motility; constipation; superior mesenteric artery syndrome; pancreatitis; elevated transaminases; hypercholesterolemia
Endocrinologic: growth retardation; hypogonadotropic hypogonadism; amenorrhea; testicular atrophy; decreased libido; sick euthyroid syndrome; hypoglycemia/hyperglycemia; impaired glucose tolerance; hypercholesterolemia; deceased bone mineral density
Hematologic: leukopenia; anemia; thrombocytopenia; elevated ferritin; depressed erythrocyte sedimentation rate
Related to vomiting
Fluids and electrolytes: electrolyte disturbances: hypokalemia, hypochloremia, metabolic alkalosis
Dental: enamel erosion
Gastrointestinal: gastroesophageal reflux; esophagitis; Mallory-Weiss tears; esophageal or gastric rupture
Related to laxative use
Fluids and electrolytes: hyperchloremic metabolic acidosis; hypocalcemia
Gastrointestinal: laxative dependence
Related to binge eating
Obesity with accompanying complications; gastric rupture
Related to refeeding
Night sweats; polyuria; nocturia; refeeding syndrome: electrolyte abnormalities, edema, seizures, congestive heart failure (rare)
Seen among all ED behaviors
Suicide

Adapted from AAP: Identification and Management of Eating Disorders in Children and Adolescents [1]

The patient in Case 2 fits the description of a patient with recurrent binge-purge episodes, and her height and weight indicate a normal BMI, which is often seen in patients with bulimia nervosa. It is imperative to obtain serum electrolytes for this patient. Hypokalemia, hypochloremia and metabolic alkalosis are electrolyte derangements that may be seen in patients who are purging via self-induced vomiting. If there is laxative abuse, hyperchloremic metabolic acidosis may be seen. Hypokalemia may also indicate diuretic abuse. Table 75.5 lists the common medical complications of EDs. Of note, Arielle in Case 2 also has a history of self-harm, and it is well-established that EDs may worsen pre-existing mental health conditions [1].

Case 3 describes a teenager who had a traumatic event (choking on a piece of broccoli) and is now unable to swallow solid food. After additional history is obtained and other medical causes of dysphagia are ruled out, this patient can be diagnosed with avoidant/restrictive food intake disorder (ARFID) and will likely need a multidisciplinary approach to treatment involving both therapy and psychiatry, as well as medical follow-up to ensure nutritional goals are met. ARFID comprises a variety of restrictive eating behaviors that do not involve a fear of weight gain or distorted cognitions related to weight or body image, but lead to significant physical and emotional impairment.

75.3 Treatment

The ultimate goals of care in ED treatment include refeeding/nutritional rehabilitation and weight restoration for individuals who have lost weight in the setting of their disordered eating behaviors, normalizing eating habits/patterns, and re-establishing a healthy relationship with food and body image. Several pharmacologic agents have been evaluated for the treatment of EDs, particularly AN, BN, and BED, and continue to be an area of research. While there are no FDA-approved medications for the treatment of anorexia nervosa, two medications have been approved for the treatment of BN and BED [6]. Olanzapine has been used with some success off-label for weight gain in anorexia nervosa [6] Cyproheptadine has also been studied as an appetite stimulant for patients with EDs, but there is insufficient evidence for use in anorexia nervosa compared with placebo [7]. Fluoxetine is FDA-approved for BN treatment, and lisdexamfetamine is FDA-approved for BED treatment [6]. Selective serotonin reuptake inhibitors (SSRIs) are commonly used medications for patients with EDs, as they treat the frequently comorbid conditions of anxiety, depression, and obsessive-compulsive disorder [8]. An additional exciting area of study is the potential role of ketamine and psilocybin in the treatment of EDs [8].

Multiple therapeutic modalities exist for the treatment of EDs, including family-based treatment (FBT), cognitive behavioral therapy (CBT), and dialectical behavioral therapy (DBT). FBT is often considered the gold standard treatment, particularly for young individuals with anorexia nervosa, and focuses on weight restoration, reducing blame, and empowering caregivers to care for their child [1, 5].

75.4 Role of School-Based Health Centers in ED Evaluation and Treatment

Once an ED has been diagnosed, prompt referral to both medical and psychiatric care is essential. Medically unstable patients need urgent referral to a hospital. Table 75.6 lists the indications for medical hospitalization in patients with EDs [5]. Based on these recommendations, if the patient in Case 1 has a heart rate that is <50 while awake, she would meet criteria for inpatient hospitalization. For the patient in Case 2, if she has electrolyte abnormalities, she would need an urgent hospital referral. For the patient in

Table 75.6 Indications for Hospitalization for EDs

≤75% median BMI for age and sex
Dehydration
Electrolyte disturbance (hypokalemia, hyponatremia, hypophosphatemia)
EKG abnormalities (prolonged QTc or severe bradycardia)
Physiologic instability
Severe bradycardia <50 bpm while awake, <45 bpm at night
Hypotension (90/45 mmHg)
Hypothermia (body temperature < 96 degrees Fahrenheit)
Orthostatic increase in pulse (>20 bpm) or decrease in BP (>20 mmHg systolic or > 10 mm Hg diastolic)
Arrested growth and development
Failure of outpatient treatment (defined as weight loss or inability to progress with weight gain)
Acute food refusal
Uncontrollable binge eating and purging
Acute medical complications of malnutrition
Comorbid psychiatric or medical condition that prohibits or limits appropriate outpatient treatment (e.g.—suicidality)

Adapted from Society for Adolescent Health and Medicine position paper [10]

Case 3, referral to the emergency department would be necessary if the patient presented with complete food refusal due to the severity of his ARFID.

Patients with mild illness may be managed in the outpatient setting with close coordination from the medical provider, nutritionist, and mental health professional. Most patients with EDs can be treated in an outpatient setting, with FBT as the gold standard therapy. Timely referral to a specialized multidisciplinary team is preferred when access is available [1, 9]. FBT has the largest evidence base of any treatment for the adolescent and young adult AN population, with multiple clinical trials. Practical implementation of FBT is limited by a paucity of qualified practitioners as well as limited insurance coverage. For patients who do not improve with outpatient care (e.g.—failure to make progress with weight gain, persistence of disordered eating behaviors, etc.), higher levels of care such as intensive outpatient programs, partial hospitalization programs, residential programs, and inpatient programs should be considered (Table 75.7). Goal weights are often predicted as treatment goals, and depend on the patient's premorbid growth trajectory, age, height, pubertal stage, and menstrual history, as children and adolescents continue to grow and develop throughout puberty and into young adulthood [1, 9].

Extra-Credit Points

1. SBHC providers should be knowledgeable about the early signs and symptoms of EDs to provide timely referral to treatment.
2. When an ED is suspected, SBHC providers should initiate a comprehensive evaluation of the patient that includes both medical and psychological assessments.

Table 75.7 Levels of Care for EDs

Family-Based Treatment:
Caregivers are empowered to refeed their child back to health.
Progresses through 3 phases that target the goals of treatment in children and adolescents with EDs: physical, behavioral, and psychological recovery.
Typically conducted over a 6- to 12- month time period [1].
Partial Hospitalization Programs:
Also referred to as "day treatment programs."
Provide an intermediate level of care for patients with EDs who are medically stable and do not require 24-hour supervision but need more than outpatient care [5].
Can be a step-down from inpatient or residential levels of care.
Often employ FBT principles.
Typically 4–7 days per week, duration of treatment between 3–18 weeks.
Can be virtual or in-person [8].
Residential Programs:
May be necessary for a minority of medically stable patients with EDs.
Indications include poor motivation for recovery, need for structure and supervision, lack of supportive family environment, absence of outpatient treatment in the patient's locale, or outpatient treatments having been unsuccessful.
Provide 24 hour per day supervision, medical oversight, group-based therapy, nutritional counseling, and family therapy.
Length of stay can be weeks to months, depending on illness severity and financial resources [5].
Insurance coverage can be a limiting factor.
Psychiatric Inpatient ED Programs:
Indicated for patients who have required nasogastric tube placement, difficulty finishing meals during inpatient medical hospitalization, or need considerable weight gain prior to outpatient treatment.
Length of stay varies from weeks to months depending on patient progress.
Insurance coverage can be a limiting factor.

3. It is imperative to involve the patient's parent or guardian in the discussion as they might provide important collateral information that the adolescent may not share. Most patients with EDs can be treated in the outpatient setting, however some patients with medical complications will meet the criteria for inpatient hospitalization.

References

1. Campbell K, Peebles R. Eating disorders in children and adolescents: state of the art review. Pediatrics. 2014;134(3):582–92.
2. Peebles R, Wilson JL, Lock JD. How do children with eating disorders differ from adolescents with eating disorders at initial evaluation? J Adolesc Health. 2006;39(6):800–5.
3. American Psychiatric Association. Diagnostic and statistical manual of mental disorders. 5th ed; 2013.

4. Kutz AM, Marsh AG, Gunderson CG, Maguen S, Masheb RM. Eating disorder screening: a systematic review and meta-analysis of diagnostic test characteristics of the SCOFF. J Gen Intern Med. 2020;35(3):885–93. https://doi.org/10.1007/s11606-019-05478-6.
5. Hornberger LL, Lane MA, COMMITTEE ON ADOLESCENCE. Identification and management of eating disorders in children and adolescents. Pediatrics. 2021;147(1):e2020040279.
6. Muratore AF, Attia E. Psychopharmacologic Management of Eating Disorders. Curr Psychiatry Rep. 2022;24(7):345–51. https://doi.org/10.1007/s11920-022-01340-5.
7. Fitzpatrick KK, Lock J. Anorexia nervosa. BMJ Clin Evid. 2011;2011:1011. Published 2011 Apr 11
8. Calder A, Mock S, Friedli N, Pasi P, Hasler G. Psychedelics in the treatment of eating disorders: rationale and potential mechanisms. Eur Neuropsychopharmacol. 2023;75:1–14. https://doi.org/10.1016/j.euroneuro.2023.05.008.
9. Herpertz-Dahlmann B. Intensive treatments in adolescent anorexia nervosa. Nutrients. 2021;13(4):1265. Published 2021 Apr 13. https://doi.org/10.3390/nu13041265.
10. Society for Adolescent Health and Medicine, Golden NH, Katzman DK, Sawyer SM, Ornstein RM, Rome ES, Garber AK, Kohn M, Kreipe RE. Position paper of the Society for Adolescent Health and Medicine: medical management of restrictive eating disorders in adolescents and young adults. J Adolesc Health Off Publ Soc Adolesc Med. 2015;56(1):121–5.

Chapter 76
Disruptive Behavior Disorders

Stephanie Harvison, Tara Kelly, and Alexis Steefel

Experiencing anger and frustration are normal feelings for an individual of any age to experience, and as children learn skills to manage these feelings, becoming argumentative and acting out may be expected. However, when these behaviors persist over time and become more severe, they may manifest into a disruptive behavior disorder. If left untreated, disruptive behavior disorders create long-term social and health effects and outcomes that impact interpersonal relationships and their communities. [1] These outcomes may include additional challenges such as mood or anxiety disorders, substance abuse, inability to maintain lasting relationships, dropping out of school, and increased involvement in the legal system.

Data from the National Survey of Children's Health revealed that 7.4% of children aged 3–7 years had a diagnosed behavioral or conduct this disorder [2]. Of these children, only 53.5% received treatment. It is anticipated that males are twice as likely to be diagnosed with a disruptive behavior disorder than females [3]. Additionally, children that have difficult temperaments, challenges with caregiving, and sociodemographic characteristics are often found to be at higher risk for developing a disruptive behavior disorder [4]. Disruptive behavior disorders are associated with negative outcomes including impacts on family functioning, mental health, education and employment during adolescence and adulthood. Therefore, early intervention is crucial for modifying the child's behavior [5]. Consider these 4 students with potential disruptive behavior disorders (Table 76.1).

Since early intervention is key to the successful treatment of disruptive behavior disorders, recognizing key characteristics of these disorders is vital (Table 76.2) [6].

Fortunately, when interventions are implemented early and family is involved in the treatment process to learn skills that can support behavioral modifications,

S. Harvison · T. Kelly (✉) · A. Steefel
Penn State Hershey Medical Center, Hershey, PA, USA
e-mail: sharvison@pennstatehealth.psu.edu; tkelly3@pennstatehealth.psu.edu; asteefel@pennstatehealth.psu.edu

R. P. Olympia, J. Brady-Olympia (eds.), *Clinical Considerations in School-based Health*, https://doi.org/10.1007/978-3-031-85765-2_76

Table 76.1 Four Student Presentations: Disruptive Behavior Disorder Diagnosis

Case #1:	Ryan is 7-year-old-male who has been demonstrating impulsive, aggressive behaviors in the form of temper tantrums and verbal altercations. He has had many outbursts at home and at school and seems to show signs of anger during these moments. Rarely does it feel like an event precipitates these behaviors; making the response seem out of proportion to any activity he is engaging in at the time. This anger and aggression is directed towards a wide range of individuals in his life, including his two pet dogs. Fortunately, no one has been physically injured, but his parents and schoolteachers have begun to worry about the safety of others. Outbursts occur multiple times a week and they have been happening for approximately 4 months.
Case #2:	Jacob is a fourth grader who recently moved to a new school. His teacher reported difficulty during this transition and often lost his temper easily. During parent/teacher conferences, his teacher shared her observations as well as concerns that Jacob seemed to be having difficulty sustaining attention in the classroom. She reached out to Jacob's art, music, and gym teacher for any consistencies in his behavior. However, they only reported that Jacob seems to get easily annoyed, specifically surrounding rules and instructions he is asked to follow. He will frequently get into arguments with them when asked to follow the rules. In one such instance, he reportedly grabbed a kickball from his gym teacher and threw it to the other side of the gym. During this meeting, Jacob's parents shared similar concerns regarding the time Jacob spends at home, many of which had been going on prior to their move, which was approximately 9 months ago. They reported he has begun to ignore them and there have been several instances where he has blamed siblings and neighborhood friends for items broken in their home. Parents have tried to address his behavior through corrective measures, but he refuses to comply, and they are connecting with a mental health professional for more support.
Case #3:	Kevin is a 17-year-old male who has begun to volunteer his time after school at the local fire department. As a child, he enjoyed helping his father make bonfires in their backyard, and always found seeing responses to fire as fascinating. Now that he is an adolescent, he has identified a feeling of pleasure associated with fire activity and has even begun setting fires intentionally without reason or purpose to do so. As his fascination with this activity has progressed, his actions have become riskier and have led to more property destruction.
Case #4:	Robert is a sophomore and has struggled in recent years in school, home, and his community. He is frequently labeled as a "bully" and has been suspended on several occasions for initiating fights with other students. Robert has been confronted by local police on many occasions due to accusations of destroying school property, breaking and entering, and setting fires in his neighborhood. Additionally, his parents have reported that bottles of alcohol in their home are depleted, and that the school has called with concerns that Robert is arriving late on several occasions and appears impaired as he sleeps through many of his classes. His parents are concerned for the well-being of other members of their family as Robert does not seem remorseful for his actions or seem motivated to make any changes. In the past 6 months, his parents have been unable to locate him at night. When confronted about his whereabout, he has been caught telling lies and coerced his siblings to hide his actions for him.

Table 76.2 Defining Characteristics of the Most Commonly Diagnosed Disruptive Behavior Disorders

Oppositional Defiant Disorder	Pattern of angry/irritable mood, argumentative/defiant behavior, or vindictiveness lasting at least 6 months Mood symptoms may include: low frustration tolerance, losing temper, angry and resentful Defiant behaviors may include: arguing with authority figures or adults, actively defies rules or refuses to comply with request from authority figures, deliberately annoying others, blaming other for mistakes or behaviors
Intermittent Explosive Disorder	Recurrent behavioral outbursts representing a failure to control aggressive impulses Verbal aggression or physical aggression toward property, animals, or individuals, occurring on average twice weekly over a minimum of 3 months and/or three behavioral outbursts involving damage or destruction to property and/or physical injury against animals or individuals within a 12-month period
Conduct Disorder	Repetitive and persistent pattern of behavior in which the basic rights of others or major societal norms/rules are violated Symptom categories include: aggression toward people and animals, destruction of property, deceitfulness or theft, and serious violations of rules (runaway or truancy)
Pyromania	Deliberate and purposeful fire setting on more than one occasion Fascination with fire and its situational contexts Pleasure, gratification, or relief when setting fires or witnessing its aftermath
Kleptomania	Recurrent failure to resist impulses to steal objects that are not needed for personal use Increasing sense of tension immediately before committing theft Pleasure, gratification, or relief at the time of committing theft

outcomes can be effective and allow children to grow into functioning members of society [7]. Parent management training programs, the most studied and the most impactful form of treatment found for disruptive behavioral disorders, aims at decreasing externalized problem behaviors while increasing positive and prosocial behaviors [5]. Although full participation for the child and family is crucial to seeing behavioral changes with this method of treatment, it is often found that full commitment is difficult for various reasons. However, peer support and/or group-based models for interventions have evidenced an increase in engagement with treatment. These interventions necessitate a trained practitioner. Please seek out a mental health provider to receive an appropriate referral for services. Table 76.3 describes case resolutions for our 4 students with disruptive behavior disorders.

Table 76.3 Four Student Presentations: Disruptive Behavior Disorder Diagnosis—Case Resolutions

Case #1: Ryan, 7 years old: temper tantrums, verbal altercations, outbursts occurring at home and school multiple times per week for last 4 months	Likely diagnosis: Intermittent Explosive Disorder Differential diagnosis may include: Disruptive Mood Dysregulation Disorder, Attention-Deficit/Hyperactivity Disorder, and Oppositional Defiant Disorder	If outbursts result in self-harm or a self-harm attempt, it would be appropriate to encourage follow up with mental health providers. If outbursts result in statements of contemplating or planning suicide, further evaluation at the emergency department is warranted.
Case #2: Jacob, fourth grade student: new to district, low frustration tolerance, concentration difficulties, arguing with teachers and parents, refusing to follow rules or requests, blames others for behaviors	Likely diagnosis: Oppositional Defiant Disorder Differential diagnosis may include: Adjustment Disorder, Attention-Deficit/Hyperactivity Disorder, and Disruptive Mood Dysregulation Disorder	If episodes result in significant disruption to the classroom, student may benefit from connection with outpatient mental health providers by encouraging discussion with primary care provider.
Case #3: Kevin, 17-year-old: volunteers at local fire department, intentionally setting fires causing property destruction, identified feeling "pleasure" with fire activity	Likely diagnosis: Pyromania Differential diagnosis may include: Conduct Disorder	Referral for emergency department evaluation may be appropriate if the student is engaging in unsafe behaviors or threatening the safety of other students at school.
Case #4: Robert, tenth grade student: disciplinary action due to fighting at school, police involvement due to destruction of property and fire setting, concern for alcohol use	Likely diagnosis: Conduct Disorder Differential diagnosis may include: Oppositional Defiant Disorder, Major Depressive Disorder or Bipolar Disorder, and Substance Use Disorder	Unless there is a concern for an acute mental health crisis or acute intoxication, these concerns are quite often more appropriately addressed by legal authorities instead of a referral to the emergency department.

Extra-Credit Points

1. If left untreated, disruptive behavior disorders create long-term social and health effects and outcomes that impact interpersonal relationships and their communities.
2. Early intervention is key to the successful treatment of disruptive behavior disorders; therefore, recognizing key characteristics of these disorders is vital.
3. Parent management training is the most studied and the most impactful form of treatment for disruptive behavioral disorders.

References

1. Colman I, Murray J, Abbott RA, et al. Outcomes of conduct problems in adolescence: 40 year follow-up of national cohort. BMJ. 2009;338:a2981. https://doi.org/10.1136/bmj.a2981.
2. Ghandour RM, Sherman LJ, Vladutiu CJ, et al. Prevalence and treatment of depression, anxiety, and conduct problems in US children. J Pediatr. 2019;206:256–67. https://doi.org/10.1016/j.jpeds.2018.09.021.
3. Erskine HE, Ferrari AJ, Polanczyk GV, et al. The global burden of conduct disorder and attention-deficit/hyperactivity disorder in 2010. J Child Psychol Psychiatry. 2014;55(4):328–36. https://doi.org/10.1111/jcpp.12186.
4. Trentacosta CJ, Goodlett BD. Longitudinal prediction of disruptive behavior disorders in adolescent males from multiple risk domains. Child Psych Human Dev. 2013;44:561–72.
5. Acri M, Chacko A, Gopalan G, McKay M. Engaging families in treatment for child behavior disorders: a synthesis of the literature. In: Lochman JE, Matthys W, editors. The Wiley handbook of disruptive and impulse-control disorders. Wiley; 2018. p. 393–410.
6. American Psychiatric Association. Diagnostic and statistical manual of mental disorders text revision. 5th ed. American Psychiatric Publishing; 2022.
7. Kaminski JW, Claussen AH. Evidence base update for psychosocial treatments for disruptive behaviors in children. J Clinical Child Adol Psych. 2017;46(4):477–99.

Chapter 77
Early Psychosis

Apurva Bhatt and Zhanna Elberg

Case 1 Saira is an 8-year-old South Asian female with Attention Deficit Hyperactivity Disorder (ADHD) who is brought to you for evaluation of new onset hallucinations. This morning Saira's teacher noticed a sudden change in her behavior, noticing Saira staring at the corner of the classroom ceiling, appearing scared and anxious, and not behaving like herself.

Psychosis is defined by the Diagnostic and Statistical Manual of Mental Disorders as a set of symptoms including hallucinations, delusions, disorganized speech, disorganized behavior, and negative symptoms (Table 77.1) [1].

These experiences can occur on a spectrum, ranging from within cultural norms and not causing any distress or functional impairment, to full threshold psychosis that causes significant distress and impairment in functioning (Fig. 77.1).

Medical conditions must be ruled out in children presenting with psychosis symptoms because certain physical illnesses can mimic psychotic symptoms (Table 77.2).

Hallucinations and other psychotic experiences (PE's) have a prevalence of 12–17% in children and 9–12% percent in adolescents [2]. Although PE's occurring in adolescence are associated with more concerning psychopathology, these experiences can still be distressing in childhood [3]. Children may hesitate to share their experiences with PE's due to stigma. If they do, it's crucial to explore and understand these experiences to determine the right intervention. Using a structured, developmentally appropriate tool to assess hallucinations and PEs is essential. In speaking with Saira, you use the SOCRATES Assessment of Perceptual

A. Bhatt (✉)
Stanford University, Stanford, CA, USA
e-mail: apbhatt@stanford.edu

Z. Elberg
University at Buffalo Jacobs School of Medicine and Biomedical Sciences, Buffalo, NY, USA
e-mail: zelberg@buffalo.edu

R. P. Olympia, J. Brady-Olympia (eds.), *Clinical Considerations in School-based Health*, https://doi.org/10.1007/978-3-031-85765-2_77

Table 77.1 Psychosis symptom definitions

Hallucinations: Perceptions in the absence of a stimulus. Can be visual, auditory, olfactory, tactile, somatic. Can be exaggerations in normal human experiences (thoughts, sensory experience) that are not tied to reality, held with conviction (even if there is opposing evidence)
Delusion: A rigid, unshakeable belief, inconsistent with common/cultural experience.
Disorganized speech: speech that is difficult to understand, incomprehensible or incoherent
Disorganized behavior: unusual behavior, including catatonia
Negative symptoms: anhedonia, avolition, apathy, asociality, alogia, reduced eye contact and intonation of speech

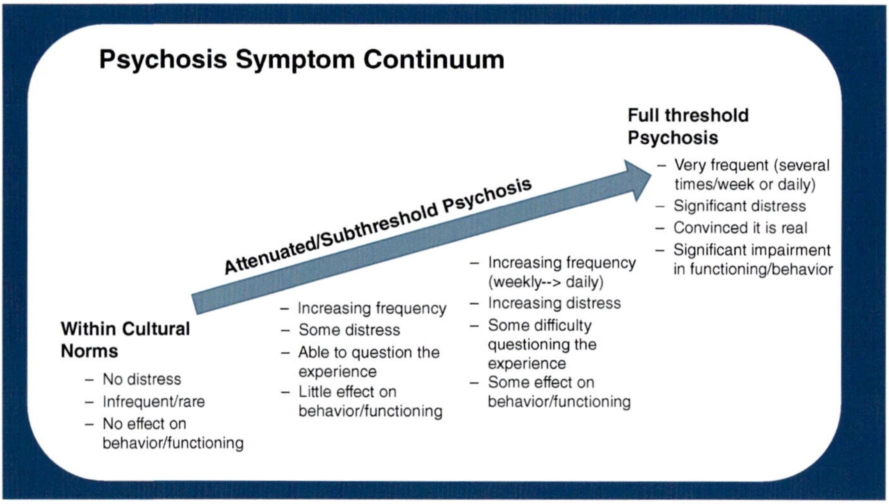

Fig. 77.1 The psychosis symptom continuum

Abnormalities and Unusual Thought Content [4], a structured tool, to better assess and characterize her experiences (Table 77.3).

Other screening questionnaires include the Psychosis Risk Screening with the Prodromal Questionnaire—Brief Child version (PQ-BC) [5] or PRIME screen [6, 7], which can be completed by a school psychologist or primary care provider. Youth with psychosis and psychotic-like experiences are at increased risk for suicide, so it is also important to conduct a suicide risk screening and assessment. Given all students voicing psychosis symptoms that are new or recent onset require a medical evaluation and work up to rule out medical causes (Table 77.2), they should be directed to go to the emergency department as next steps.

Back to the Case Saira reports beginning this morning she began seeing a shadowy gray figure that is scary and distracting, and began hearing a loud, scary muffled voice. She wants it to stop and wants to go home. She appears anxious but denies thoughts of harming herself or others, and denied suicidal thoughts. Given the acute onset of these hallucinations, you send her to the emergency department where a medical investigation [medical physical exam, neurological exam, basic

Table 77.2 Non-psychiatric conditions associated with acute psychosis in children

Substrate deficiencies: Hypoglycemia Cerebral hypoxia	**Drug overdose or abuse** Cannabis and synthetic cannabinoids Hallucinogens Sympathomimetic agents (cocaine, methamphetamine, ecstasy, bath salts) Anticholinergic agents Salvia divinorum
Central nervous system abnormalities Brain tumor Brain abscess Intracranial injury (head trauma) Central nervous system infection (meningitis, encephalitis) Stroke Interictal psychosis Temporal lobe epilepsy Landau-Kleffner syndrome Subacute sclerosing panencephalitis	**Drug related syndrome** Baclofen withdrawal Benzodiazepine withdrawal Alcohol withdrawal syndrome (delirium tremens) Neuroleptic malignant syndrome (due to antipsychotic medication exposure) Serotonin syndrome
Autoimmune conditions Systemic lupus erythematosus N-methyl-D-aspartate-receptor encephalitis Pediatric Acute-onset Neuropsychiatric Syndrome (PANS) Pediatric Autoimmune Neuropsychiatric Disorders Associated with Streptococcal Infections (PANDAS)	**Medication-induced psychosis** Stimulant medications Antibiotic-induced mania Antiseizure medications Corticosteroids Isoniazid
Metabolic disease Urea cycle defect Acute intermittent porphyria Wilson Disease	**Other** Hypo- or hypernatremia, hypocalcemia, hypomagnesemia Hepatic Failure Uremia Postpartum psychosis Hashimoto thyroiditis, Thyroid storm Antiphospholipid syndrome

Table 77.3 SOCRATES Assessment of Perceptual Abnormalities and Unusual Thought Content [4]

SOURCE — Did the voice(s) sound like it/they were inside your head or outside?
ONSET, FREQUENCY, DURATION — When did it start? How often? How long?
CONTENT/CHARACTER — What does it/do they say? Who is it? What's it like?
REALITY TESTING — What do you think is causing these experiences?
ATTRIBUTION — Related to above, why/how might it be happening?
TIMING — Do you hear it at certain times? When? What else is occurring?
EFFECTS on FUNCTIONING — Have these experiences changed how you act? Interrupted your ability to carry out day-to-day tasks?
SEVERITY of DISTRESS — Is it distressing? On a 1–10 scale, how distressing?

laboratory tests including but not limited to comprehensive metabolic panel, complete blood count, thyroid stimulating hormone with reflex to free T4, urine drug screen, erythrocyte sedimentation rate, antinuclear antibody, an electroencephalogram (EEG) and Magnetic Resonance Imaging (MRI) Brain] and psychiatric assessment is completed. All of her labs, EEG and MRI brain return normal, except for her urine drug screen which shows evidence of taking prescribed stimulant medication. It is determined that Saira experienced a rare side effect of her stimulant medication, and once the medication wore off later in the evening, all her psychosis symptoms completely abated. The medication was stopped and she was referred to an outpatient child and adolescent psychiatrist for further evaluation and care.

Case 2 Justin is a 16 year old male who was recently hospitalized for a first episode psychosis and diagnosed with Schizophrenia Spectrum Disorder. He used to be a good student but over the past 6 months has withdrawn from his extracurricular activities and struggled in completing his school work. He was often seen mumbling to himself and often appeared lost in his thoughts. His hygiene declined and he lost a significant amount of weight. He disclosed to his guidance counselor that the cafeteria workers were poisoning the food and tried to warn other students. After discharge from the hospital, he seems more tired and is often seen falling asleep in class.

The differential diagnosis of first episode of psychosis (FEP) can be seen in Table 77.4. Many individuals living with psychosis recover as newer treatment models for the first episode of psychosis have emerged over the last 20 years. Early psychosis intervention efforts have focused on decreasing the length of untreated psychosis (DUP) (length of time between onset of psychosis symptoms and receiving evidence-based treatment) and have shown promise of recovery.

Coordinated specialty care (CSC) programs for first episode psychosis are evidence based treatment models that have been shown to help young adults return to their developmental trajectory and achieve their personal goals. CSC programs involve multidisciplinary teams all collaborating to support individuals living with psychosis (Table 77.5). The core values of CSC are described below (Table 77.6). It is important to ensure students experiencing FEP are referred to a local CSC program (if available in their region). A directory of early psychosis programs is available here: https://med.stanford.edu/peppnet/interactivedirectory.html

Well established evidence-based guidelines for treatment of psychosis related to schizophrenia spectrum disorders include the use of antipsychotics [9]. The goal of

Table 77.4 Differential Diagnosis of First Episode Psychosis

Schizophrenia spectrum disorder	Schizoaffective Disorder
Schizophreniform Disorder	Bipolar Disorder with Psychotic Features
Major Depressive Disorder with Psychotic Features	Substance Induced Psychosis
Delusional Disorder	

Table 77.5 Program Components of Coordinated Specialty Care [8]

Team Leadership	Oversees all aspects of team functioning and provides administrative and clinical oversight
Psychotherapist/Clinician	Conducts assessments and offers psychotherapy for FEP based on cognitive and behavioral principles and emphasizes resilience training, helps process trauma, reduces feelings of stigma focuses on illness and wellness management and works to improve general coping skills.
Supported education and employment (SEE)	The SEE Specialist supports each client's return to work or school as well as attainment of expected vocational and educational milestones. The SEE Specialist strives to integrate vocational and mental health services, is the CSC team liaison with outside educators and employers, and frequently works with the client in the community to enhance school or job performance.
Family education and support	Family education and support specialists educate family members about psychosis and its treatment and strengthen their capacity to aid in the client's recovery by reducing family stress through improved communication and problem-solving skills.
Case management	Case managers assist clients with problem solving to ensure that their immediate practical needs are met
Peer support	Peer specialists have lived experience and work with program participants and family members to support and advocate for the participant within the context of the team. The Peer Specialist uses his/her personal recovery story to instill hope, promote engagement and demonstrate goal attainment.
Prescriber Services, Pharmacotherapy and Coordination with Primary Care	Psychiatry providers monitor symptoms, side effects (especially cardiometabolic risk) and address attitudes towards medication treatment at each visit. Prescribers maintain close contact with primary care providers to assure optimal medical treatment for risk factors

Table 77.6 Core values of CSC (Coordinate Specialty Care Programs)

Person Centered Care	Attend to the individual's values and what's important to them
Team Based Approach	A multidisciplinary team with special training or lived experience of psychosis works together in supporting individuals experiencing psychosis
Recovery Oriented Services	Offer hope that things will get better; Foster self-efficacy and empowerment.
Shared Decision Making	Individuals and their support persons are partners in recovery. They are informed they have choices and are actively involved and supported in the treatment decision-making process.

treatment is remission since more than 50% of young adults with FEP will experience recovery. Pharmacological treatment includes the use of oral medications such as antipsychotics and Long Acting Injectable (LAI) medications which have been shown to improve treatment adherence and outcomes [9]. These medications, although efficacious at treating positive symptoms of psychosis, such as delusions

Table 77.7 Potential Side Effects of Antipsychotics

Sedation	Weight gain	Akathisia
Menstrual irregularities	Extrapyramidal side effects: dystonia/muscle stiffness/twitches	Decreased sex drive/decreased sexual arousal
Gynecomastia	Galactorrhea	Dry mouth
Orthostatic hypotension	Constipation	Metabolic syndrome

and hallucinations, do pose risk of side effects that can be functionally impairing. The choice for the initial pharmacological agent is often driven by the side effect profile (Table 77.7) and not concerns about efficacy since most individuals with FEP tend to respond similarly to different antipsychotics.

Suicide Risk Youth with FEP are at increased risk for suicide, especially in the first year after diagnosis. Tools such as the Columbia Suicide Severity Rating Scale (CSSRS) (https://cssrs.columbia.edu/the-scale-in-action/schools/) may be useful in systematically assessing and managing suicide risk [10].

Back to the Case You refer Justin to a local CSC program and communicate with his current psychiatrist your observation about daytime sedation. Justin's medication is moved to bedtime and the school team adjusts Justin's school start time to later in the morning which leads to improvement in his ability to participate in class.

Extra Credit Points

1. Recovery from FEP is highly personal, and with support individuals can return to an expected developmental trajectory including returning to school and other activities.
2. Youth experiencing psychosis benefit from a non-stigmatizing, recovery-oriented approach
3. School staff should make every effort to explore what accommodations/interventions can best support an individual student living with psychosis.

References

1. American Psychiatric Association. Diagnostic and statistical manual of mental disorders. American Psychiatric Association Publishing; 2022.
2. Kelleher I, Connor D, Clarke MC, et al. Prevalence of psychotic symptoms in childhood and adolescence: a systematic review and meta-analysis of population-based studies. Psychol Med. 2012;42(9):1857–63. https://doi.org/10.1017/S0033291711002960.
3. Maijer K, Begemann MJH, Palmen SJMC, et al. Auditory hallucinations across the lifespan: a systematic review and meta-analysis. Psychol Med. 2018;48(6):879–88. https://doi.org/10.1017/S0033291717002367.
4. Kelleher I, Cannon M. SOCRATES assessment of perceptual abnormalities and unusual thought content. Royal College of Surgeons in Ireland; 2021. https://doi.org/10.25419/RCSI.10795397.V2.

5. Karcher NR, Barch DM, Avenevoli S, et al. Assessment of the prodromal questionnaire-brief child version for measurement of self-reported psychotic like experiences in childhood. JAMA Psychiatry. 2018;75(8):853–61. https://doi.org/10.1001/jamapsychiatry.2018.1334.
6. Psychosis screening. Accessed 31 May 2024. https://www.psychosisscreening.org/.
7. Miller TJ, Cicchetti D, Markovich PJ, et al. The SIPS screen: a brief self-report screen to detect the schizophrenia prodrome. Schizophr Res. 2004;70:78.
8. Recovery After an Initial Schizophrenia Episode (RAISE). National Institute of Mental Health (NIMH). Accessed 1 June 2024. https://www.nimh.nih.gov/health/topics/schizophrenia/raise/evidence-based-treatments-for-first-episode-psychosis-components-of-coordinated-specialty-care.shtml.
9. American Psychiatric Association. The American Psychiatric Association practice guideline for the treatment of patients with schizophrenia. American Psychiatric Association Publishing; 2020.
10. Bornheimer LA. Suicidal ideation in first-episode psychosis (FEP): examination of symptoms of depression and psychosis among individuals in an early phase of treatment. Suicide Life Threat Behav. 2019;49(2):423–31. https://doi.org/10.1111/sltb.12440.

Chapter 78
Gender Dysphoria and Incongruence in Adolescents

Rosemary Claire Roden

In this chapter, we will discuss the concept of gender dysphoria, the gendered sense of self, and appropriate language for discussing these matters in a professional and respectful way. This chapter is not comprehensive and is a very superficial overview of the topic. The standards of medical care and the ethics of medical management of gender dysphoria are beyond the scope of this chapter. Additionally, we understand that, as we write this book, the legal status of transgender adolescents varies state by state, and is likely to change even between finishing writing and final publication, so before taking any actions related to gender incongruence or dysphoria with any particular student we recommend that school staff be familiar with current local laws and regulations.

78.1 History

Gender Incongruence or *Dysphoria* is the experience of having a gender that does not align with the sex assigned at birth (Table 78.1). This concept has existed as long as written history. Some examples of individuals that might experience something we understand today as gender incongruence include the pharaoh Hatshepsut and Roman emperor Elagabalus. Hatshepsut was female-bodied pharaoh who ruled Ancient Egypt 1478–1458 BCE. This individual was depicted in masculine stances and attire of the time, and used the male title "pharaoh." Elagabalus ruled from 218–222 CE, during which the emperor was known for using makeup, women's clothing, and female mannerisms, as well as reportedly seeking a surgeon who could create a vulva and vagina in place of a penis [1].

R. C. Roden (✉)
Penn State Children's Hospital, Hershey, PA, USA
e-mail: rroden@pennstatehealth.psu.edu

R. P. Olympia, J. Brady-Olympia (eds.), *Clinical Considerations in School-based Health*, https://doi.org/10.1007/978-3-031-85765-2_78

Table 78.1 Appropriate verbiage in gender health spaces as of Spring, 2024; *indicates offensive or insulting

Term	Meaning	Outdated term
Assigned female at birth (AFAB)	Individual with a vulva +/− without internal gonads	Biological female*, born female*, really a girl/woman*
Assigned male at birth (AMAB)	Individual with a phallus +/− without external gonads	Biological female*, born female*, really a boy/man*
Cisgender/ Non-Transgender	Adjective; experiencing a gender congruent with the sex assigned at birth	
Drag	Adopting the clothing and mannerisms of another sex purely for performances	Transvestite*, Cross-Dressing*, Tranny** (very offensive, do not use)
Gender Affirmation	The act of respecting an individual's stated, experienced gender	
Gender Affirming Healthcare	Healthcare that aims to improve or relieve distress related to physical aspects that are not congruent with an individual's gendered experience	
Gender Dysphoria	Experiencing of a gender different from the sex assigned at birth; a *diagnosis* that requires *distress*	Gender Identity Disorder* and Transsexualism are not in the DSM-5
Gender Incongruence	Experiencing of a gender different from the sex assigned at birth; this does not imply *distress*	
Gender Role	The traits and behaviors that, in a particular time and place, denote appropriate behavior for men and women	
Intersex	Congenital conditions where the gonads, genitals, chromosomes, and hormonal milieu do not align with a single sex	Use of either Intersex or Differences of Sexual Development (DSD) may be appropriate given context; hermaphrodite*
Nonbinary	The state of having a gender that is neither male nor female in a very broad sense; terms "agender" or "genderfluid" are related, but distinct, concepts	
Sex	Biological traits incurring "maleness" or "femaleness," includes chromosomes, hormones, gonads, genital structures, and secondary sex characteristics	
Transgender	Adjective; experiencing a gender different from the sex assigned at birth	Use of "transgender" as a noun ("He's a transgender.") or a verb ("He's transgendered.")
Transgender Man, Trans-man	A man who was assigned female at birth	

(continued)

Table 78.1 (continued)

Term	Meaning	Outdated term
Transgender Woman, Trans-Woman	A woman who was assigned male at birth	
Transition	Use of social, medical, and/or procedural intervention to achieve a body congruent with the experienced gender	Sex change*, sex change operation*, sex reassignment, gender reassignment

78.2 The Gendered Sense of Self

The gendered sense of self generally develops around age 3 years in most children [2]. For those who experience incongruence, this feeling may begin as early as one is able to state what gender they are or may start later, most commonly in puberty or late adolescence [3]. Gender incongruence is relatively uncommon, though the incidence is increasing with younger ages [4]. The most generous estimates of gender incongruence are about 1.5% of the total population of the United States, and most place it far lower; this is also lower than the estimated prevalence of intersex conditions or differences of sexual development at 2% of the general population of the United States (see Table 78.1) [5].

There are many tools that aid in understanding gender identity. A favorite is The Gender Unicorn, which is a worksheet that assists the user in understanding their own gendered self (Fig. 78.1).

Filling out your own Gender Unicorn worksheet, either in private or in a group, can be a useful exercise for understanding these different domains and how they interact in unique combinations for all people. For some, this may be a difficult exercise, and for others it might be quite straightforward.

Some young people may experience intense distress related to the experience of gender incongruence, but this is not a universal feeling [7]. Expert consultation, such as referral to a pediatrician or mental health provider, may be necessary if there is *dysphoria* or distress related to gender incongruence. Referral to a gender care specialist should only be completed with parental knowledge, involvement, and agreement. Referral for problems like eating disorder or depression that might be related to gender incongruence should be made as they would be for any child regardless of gender.

78.3 Language

The nomenclature surrounding gender dysphoria is constantly changing (Table 78.1), so the contents of this table may be out of date by the time this book is in press. For that reason, we suggest that instead of strictly adhering to the recommended terms

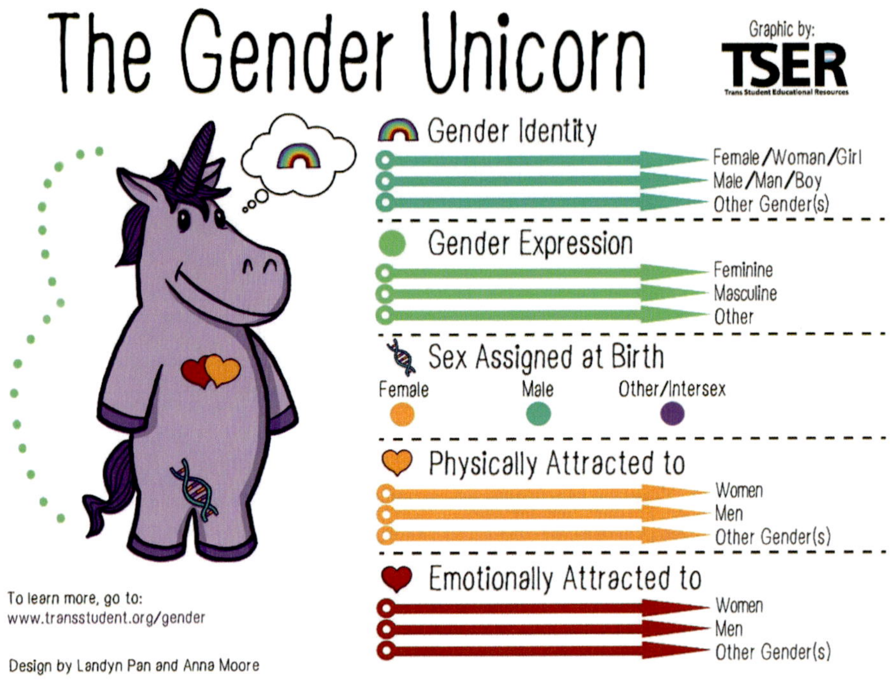

Fig. 78.1 The Gender Unicorn [6]

here, the best way to use the "correct" word in a given situation is to ask a person what words should be used when talking to them. For example, may individuals prefer the term "Transsexual" as a label for their identity, regardless of its designation of offensive or outdated here. If a person states that they prefer the word "transsexual," then that is the word that should be used when describing that individual or discussing their care.

It may be difficult for cisgender individuals to understand the transgender experience, and similarly it may be difficult for transgender individuals to understand a cisgender experience. In either case, understanding the exact nuances of why a person feels the way do is not as important as understanding that the individual, gendered sense of self is deeply personal. Transgender individuals are at higher risk for various mental health conditions, including depression, anxiety, eating disorders, and substance use disorders, though for children who are raised in homes where their asserted gender identity is honored—by using the correct names, correct pronouns, etc.—these risks melt away to no greater than that of the general population [8]. As a result we recommend that transgender youth are treated with the same respect offered to all other students; to do otherwise is rude.

78.4 Manners, or, Treat Others How You Want to Be Treated

The author recognizes that there is a good deal of social and political focus on the concept of gender incongruence in children and adolescents. It is not reasonable to expect that all readers of this book are familiar with the concept of gender dysphoria and incongruence as it is laid out here, nor to expect that everyone who might find themselves in need of a quick reference is comfortable with what we have discussed. Instead, we would like to focus on the more straightforward basics of the golden rule: treat others as they want to be treated. Table 78.2 provides some cases of conversational use of terms that may feel unfamiliar, but are ultimately comfortable for most native speakers of English.

Extra Credit Points

1. Gender is a complex bio-psycho-social phenomenon that is both deeply personal and public facing, where no two individuals experience or express the gendered self in exactly identical ways. Just as students may be exploring other parts of their lives and identities, they may explore their gender.
2. Gender incongruence itself is not a disease and is not necessarily a problem. Most of the adverse mental health outcomes relate to other people being unkind or lacking understanding and patience for individuals who experience incongruence [8]
3. Before discussing a student's possible gender incongruence with other people, first discuss it with the child and what they want you to do with that information
4. Be aware of your state and local statutes regarding the legal status of gender affirming care for minors before approaching parents or students about possible gender incongruence [7]
5. All students are, as of this writing, legally able to use the bathroom or locker room of their choice in public schools throughout the United States, though this may change in the future [9]

Table 78.2 Examples of possible scenarios where gender incongruence or dysphoria may intersect with the school environment

Cases	Response	Rationale
A student requests to be called something other than their legal first name	Use the name the student requests	Individuals may request to be called something other than the legal first name for many reasons, including[a]: Preference for a nickname in all environments Use of middle name in all environments Preference of use of first name only in intimate environments Finding that others find their first name difficult to pronounce
A student uses the pronouns "they/them"	Use "they/them" pronouns for the student, or for situations where the pronouns aren't known	In informal, spoken English, the pronouns "they" and "them" commonly refer to an unidentified third party. Examples include: "That's what they say" "Oh no! I hope they are ok." "What do they want?"
One student is asking another student about if they are "really a boy or a girl"	Separate the students and remind the inquisitive one that it is rude to talk about private matters in public	Under no circumstances should children be made to disclose matters about their personal health or anatomy to other students, especially not under duress.
Parents are unaware of a preferred name or pronouns in the school environment	Discuss the preferred name and/or pronouns privately with the student, and under what context it may be used.	Children and adolescents may frequently try new identities and names in the school environment as opposed to the home environment related to cognitive and psychosocial development; please see chapter on "Adolescent Growth and Development" in this volume
Parents of other students are asking about the gender and sex assigned at birth status of another student that is not their child	Do not disclose private health information to individuals outside of the student's legal guardians without explicit, written permission from parents to do so.	Under no circumstances should disclosures about unrelated children's personal health or anatomy be made to individuals who are not that child's legal guardians.
An individual accidentally uses the wrong name or pronouns	Quickly apologize, self-correct, and continue the conversation	Mistakes happen. The important thing is to apologize when they do and correct them.
A student is being bullied for appearing to be transgender because they use the "wrong" bathroom	Discipline aggressor students as one would typically discipline students who bully based on gender or gender roles	Discrimination based on gender is explicitly prohibited in public schools in the United States, in particular transgender children may use the bathroom of their choice in a school environment [9]

[a]The author notes that she has always used her middle name in all environments since early childhood

References

1. Poteat T, Rachlin K, Lare S, et al. History and prevalence of gender dysphoria. Contemp Endocrinol. 2019:1–24.
2. Scharf RJ, Scharf GJ, Stroustrup A. Developmental milestones. Pediatr Rev. 2016;37:25–38.
3. Coleman E, Radix AE, Bouman WP, et al. Standards of care for the health of transgender and gender diverse people, version 8. Int J Transgender Heal. 2022;23:1–259.
4. Morandini JS, Kelly A, de Graaf NM, et al. Shifts in demographics and mental health co-morbidities among gender dysphoric youth referred to a specialist gender dysphoria service. Clin Child Psychol Psychiatry. 2022;27(2):480–91. https://doi.org/10.1177/13591045211046813.
5. Roden RC, Billman M, Francesco A, et al. Treatment goals of adolescents and young adults for gender dysphoria. Pediatrics. 2024;153:1–6.
6. Trans Student Educational Resources. The Gender Unicorn. Available at: http://www.transstudent.org/gender. Accessed 12 May 2024.
7. James SE, Herman JL, Durso LE, et al. Early insights: a report of the 2022 U.S. Transgender survey. 2024.
8. Rafferty J, Yogman M, Baum R, et al. Ensuring comprehensive care and support for transgender and gender-diverse children and adolescents. Pediatrics. 2023;142(4):e20182162.
9. Doumar JRG, Miller MJTE. G.G, by his next friend and mother, Deirdre Grimm v. Gloucester County School Board Statement of Interested of the United States. vol. 4. 2015.

Chapter 79
Global Developmental Delay

Lauren Misik and Elizabeth W. Barnhardt

Case 1 Billy is a 4 year old who presents to your clinic due to concerns for constipation. In interacting with Billy, he is speaking in 2–3 word phrases and is very social. Per review of his Individualized Education Plan, you note he is receiving speech, physical, and occupational therapies. You also notice on exam that the child has significant hypotonia, puffiness around his eyes, full cheeks, prominent lips, a wide mouth, and short stature. You are concerned that the child may have an underlying genetic syndrome. What could be your next steps?

Global Developmental Delay (GDD) is defined as a significant delay in 2 or more developmental domains, including gross or fine motor, speech/language, cognitive, social/personal, and activities of daily living [1]. A diagnosis of GDD is an important diagnosis to recognize as it is thought to predict a future diagnosis of intellectual disability (ID) [2]. This diagnosis is typically given to children younger than 5 years of age whereas a diagnosis of intellectual disability can only be established for children in whom IQ testing is both valid and reliable, typically corresponding to an age of 5 years and older [1]. Delays in development in younger children are more amenable to change, especially through the receipt of appropriate intervention, due to the brain's significant neuroplasticity. The prevalence of GDD. is estimated to be 1–3% [1]. Although not all children with GDD go on to meet criteria for an intellectual disability diagnosis it is prudent that school-based health clinicians are aware of this risk. Co-location within the school allows for

L. Misik
Fellow, Developmental and Behavioral Pediatrics, Nationwide Children's Hospital, Columbus, OH, USA
e-mail: lauren.misik@nationwidechildrens.org

E. W. Barnhardt (✉)
Division of Developmental and Behavioral Pediatrics, Nationwide Children's Hospital/The Ohio State University, Columbus, OH, USA
e-mail: elizabeth.barnhardt@nationwidechildrens.org

R. P. Olympia, J. Brady-Olympia (eds.), *Clinical Considerations in School-based Health*, https://doi.org/10.1007/978-3-031-85765-2_79

Table 79.1 Developmental Screening Tools for School-based health clinicians [3]

Name of Tool	Description	Age Range	Administration Time	Availability
ASQ (Ages and Stages Questionnaire)	Parent-completed, covers communication, social-emotional skills, gross & fine motor, problem-solving, and adaptive skills	2–60 months, Social-Emotional Questionnaire available for ages 1–72 months	10–15 minutes	Cost associated, electronic and paper versions available
PEDS (Parents' Evaluation of Developmental Status)	Parent interview, surveillance +screening tool available	0–8 years old	4–6 minutes	Cost associated, electronic and paper versions available
SWYC (Survey of Well-being of Young Children)	12 age-specific forms, includes cognitive, language, motor skills	1–65 months, Preschool	5 minutes	Free for download online
Pediatric Symptom Checklist	Parent-completed questionnaire to assess social-emotional development	6–12 years	5–10 minutes	Free for download online
Preschool Pediatric Symptom Checklist	Parent-completed questionnaire to assess social-emotional development	18–60 months	5 minutes	Free for download online
Social Communication Questionnaire	Parent-completed questionnaire used to screen for autism spectrum disorders	4+ years	5–10 minutes	Cost associated

direct communication with a child's teachers and therapists and access to documentation from their Individualized Education Plans (IEPs) and Evaluation Team Reports (ETRs).

Children with GDD are often identified in the medical home. The American Academy of Pediatrics recommends routine developmental screening at the 9, 18, and 30 month well child checks [3]. Pertinent to school-based health clinicians is the recommendation that close attention be paid to children at ages 4–5 (typically the age of school entry) as this is the age at which many children present with more subtle developmental or learning difficulties. School-based health clinicians can consider screening for developmental delays in kindergarten and preschool-aged children using one of the tools shown below (Table 79.1).

79.1 The Evaluation of Children with Global Developmental Delay

There are several notable aspects of the evaluation of children with GDD school-based health clinicians should consider.

79.1.1 Clarify the Etiology

Identifying an etiology for a GDD diagnosis allows for the identification of prognostic information, the creation of appropriate academic and therapeutic goals, and the opportunity to screen for comorbid medical conditions. Families commonly cite understanding the etiology of their child's developmental delays as being important for their overall wellbeing [1].

A school-based health clinician evaluating a child with GDD should ask questions regarding the child's birth history, in utero environment, medical history, social history and family history. It is also important to ascertain the child's developmental trajectory, paying special attention to any history of regression in their developmental skills. The clinician should also evaluate potential environmental or genetic risk factors for delays. Table 79.2 below provides an overview of risk factors to consider.

Regressions in speech development are sometimes seen in children with autism spectrum disorder (ASD) and developmental regressions across multiple domains

Table 79.2 Risk factors for developmental delays

Environmental	Parental health and behaviors during pregnancy, in utero alcohol/drug/tobacco exposures
	Complications during birth including prematurity, hypoxia, low-birth weight
	Exposure of mother or child to high levels of environmental toxins (ex: lead)
	Maternal medications during pregnancy
	Maternal TORCH infections during pregnancy (Toxoplasma, Others- HBV and HIV, Rubella, CMV, and Herpesvirus)
Family-Level Factors	Poor nutrition
	Abuse and neglect
	Low maternal education
	Large family size
	Short spacing between births
	Poverty
	Family history of developmental delays
Genetic Considerations	Chromosomal disorders
	Inborn errors of metabolism
	Male gender
Medical Risk Factors	Vision Impairment
	Hearing Impairment
	Prolonged illness/hospitalization
	Congenital heart disease

are more concerning for a potential inborn error of metabolism or underlying neurological process.

A detailed physical exam is also incredibly important. A physical exam should include a detailed skin examination looking for evidence of neurocutaneous stigmata, an evaluation of facial features, a full neurological examination, and a musculoskeletal exam. Patterns of abnormal growth may also hint at an underlying genetic diagnosis.

For any child diagnosed with either GDD, ID, or ASD, genetic testing with consideration of testing for inborn errors of metabolism is recommended [4]. School-based health clinicians can refer to a medical geneticist to complete recommended testing. The first tier of testing typically includes a chromosomal microarray and testing for Fragile X with recent evidence pointing towards the utility of whole exome sequencing as a first-tier test [5]. If a genetic etiology is not identified after a detailed evaluation, neuroimaging may be reasonable [1]. For children with gross motor delays and associated hypotonia, muscular weakness or developmental regression, school-based health clinicians could consider ordering thyroid studies (thyroid stimulating hormone and thyroxine) as well as a blood creatine kinase (CK) to rule out congenital hypothyroidism and muscular dystrophy, respectively [6].

Case 1 Follow-Up The presence of Billy's dysmorphic features and multiple developmental delays should raise suspicion for an underlying genetic syndrome. Thus, a reasonable next step in this case could be to review his developmental testing completed as part of his Evaluation Team Report. In reviewing his testing, you confirm your suspicions that the child has significant developmental delays in several areas, namely his speech, gross motor, and fine motor skills. You appropriately refer to Genetics for additional evaluation. A chromosomal microarray is completed which reveals a deletion at chromosome band 7q11.23 involving the elastin gene, consistent with Williams syndrome. Subsequently, you then access guidelines for the health supervision of children with Williams syndrome [7] and monitor for common comorbidities.

Case 2 Ruby is a 7-year-old girl who is presenting to your school-based health clinic with behavioral concerns. Ruby struggles to stay on task and contain her body during quiet activities. She is behind in all academic subjects and frequently loses interest or gets frustrated with her work. She has a noticeable delay in speech when compared to her peers, and her teachers note she struggles with pencil grip. She does not have an IEP or 504 plan in place, but her teachers notice that she needs more prompting and supervision when compared to peers. Concerns for a potential diagnosis of Attention –Deficit/Hyperactivity Disorder (ADHD) have been brought up to Ruby's parents and teachers. Based on this information, you request a meeting with Ruby's parents to share your suspicions for a diagnosis of GDD.

79.1.2 Assess for Comorbidities

Children with GDD may be at risk for several comorbid conditions. Table 79.3 provides an overview of conditions which are more common in children with GDD. Specific genetic syndromes may also have published screening guidelines related to the medical comorbidities present for a given condition, such as was the case for Billy.

79.1.3 Connect Child to Appropriate Resources

For children with GDD, school-based health clinicians are uniquely positioned to ensure that their patients are receiving both appropriate school-based and community-based supports. In addition to receiving services like speech, occupational, and physical therapy at school, many children also benefit from the receipt of private developmental therapies. When caring for children with GDD, clinicians should be knowledgeable about state and regional resources for children with intellectual and developmental disabilities. There may be additional funding to support families with children with GDD, such as that available through the federal Supplemental Security Income (SSI) program.

79.1.4 Provision of Family Support

To effectively support a child with GDD, their family must also be adequately supported [8]. For many genetic conditions or other conditions contributing to developmental impairment, there are increasingly more opportunities for peer support and resources. For example, in the case of Billy, our child newly diagnosed with Williams syndrome, you might consider connecting them to the Williams Syndrome Association which provides several fantastic supports and resources for families as well as opportunities for parents to connect.

Table 79.3 Common Comorbidities in children with GDD

Constipation and toileting difficulties
Sleeping difficulties
Behavioral difficulties including attention deficit hyperactivity disorder (ADHD), Oppositional defiant disorder (ODD)
Autism spectrum disorder
Feeding difficulties
Epilepsy
Sensory deficits (hearing or vision)

79.1.5 Collaborate with Other Health Professionals

Children with GDD often have complex medical, developmental, and behavioral needs. Communication between the school team, medical team, and community support team members is of the utmost importance. School-based health clinicians can consider involving a Developmental Behavioral Pediatrician to evaluate for common medical comorbidities. Either a Developmental Behavioral Pediatrician or a Child Psychiatrist could be consulted to provide diagnostic clarification regarding comorbid mental health diagnoses or to provide support for medication management of behavioral issues.

Case 2 Follow-Up After talking with Ruby's school-based health clinician, Ruby's parents request an IEP evaluation to be completed for Ruby. During testing obtained to formulate her evaluation team report, Ruby's FSIQ is determined to be 68. Her adaptive skills are found to be "extremely low". With careful history taking, her school-based health clinician determines that Ruby would have met criteria for a global developmental delay diagnosis at as young as 2 years of age. Ruby is provided with an IEP under the "intellectual disability" classification. Given this information, it is determined that a diagnosis of ADHD would not be appropriate for Ruby as her attention span is consistent with her overall developmental level, as is her social development. With the implementation of her IEP and working towards goals consistent with her current abilities, Ruby makes progress and has significantly fewer behavioral outbursts in the classroom related to schoolwork. Her school-based clinician provides a "warm hand-off" to Ruby's pediatrician, who schedules a follow-up visit with Ruby and her family to discuss next steps, including referrals to private speech and occupational therapies to supplement her school-based therapies and genetic testing.

Extra Credit Points

1. Consider a diagnosis of Global Developmental Delay (for children less than 5) or Intellectual Disability (for children older than 5) who are receiving multiple developmental therapies at school as part of their Individualized Education Plan
2. School based clinicians should consider discussing cognitive re-evaluation at ~5 years of age for children with a history of GDD.
3. School-aged children with previously unidentified developmental delays may present with challenging behaviors in the school environment.
4. Children with GDD are more likely to have several significant medical and behavioral challenges.
5. School-based health clinicians can assist in helping parents of children with GDD navigate complex systems of care.

References

1. Moeschler JB, Shevell M, Committee on Genetics. Comprehensive evaluation of the child with intellectual disability or global developmental delays. Pediatrics. 2014;134(3):e903–18. https://doi.org/10.1542/peds.2014-1839.
2. Shevell M, Ashwal S, Donley D, et al. Practice parameter: evaluation of the child with global developmental delay: report of the quality standards subcommittee of the American Academy of Neurology and The Practice Committee of the Child Neurology Society. Neurology. 2003;60(3):367–80. https://doi.org/10.1212/01.wnl.0000031431.81555.16.
3. Lipkin PH, Macias MM, COUNCIL ON CHILDREN WITH DISABILITIES, SECTION ON DEVELOPMENTAL AND BEHAVIORAL PEDIATRICS, Norwood KW, Brei TJ, Davidson LF, Davis BE, Ellerbeck KA, Houtrow AJ, Hyman SL, Kuo DZ, Noritz GH, Yin L, Murphy NA, Levy SE, Weitzman CC, Bauer NS, Childers DO Jr, Levine JM, Peralta-Carcelen AM, Smith PJ, Blum NL, Contompasis SH, Korb DR, McGuinn LJ, Voigt RG. Promoting optimal development: identifying infants and young children with developmental disorders through developmental surveillance and screening. Pediatrics. 2020;145(1):e20193449. https://doi.org/10.1542/peds.2019-3449.
4. Hyman SL, Levy SE, Myers SM, COUNCIL ON CHILDREN WITH DISABILITIES, SECTION ON DEVELOPMENTAL AND BEHAVIORAL PEDIATRICS. Identification, evaluation, and management of children with autism spectrum disorder. Pediatrics. 2020;145(1):e20193447. https://doi.org/10.1542/peds.2019-3447.
5. Manickam K, McClain MR, Demmer LA, et al. Exome and genome sequencing for pediatric patients with congenital anomalies or intellectual disability: an evidence-based clinical guideline of the American College of Medical Genetics and Genomics (ACMG). Genet Med. 2021;23(11):2029–37. https://doi.org/10.1038/s41436-021-01242-6.
6. Noritz GH, Murphy NA, Neuromotor Screening Expert Panel. Motor delays: early identification and evaluation [published correction appears in Pediatrics. 2017 Sep;140(3)]. Pediatrics. 2013;131(6):e2016–27. https://doi.org/10.1542/peds.2013-1056.
7. Morris CA, Braddock SR, COUNCIL ON GENETICS, Chen E, Trotter TL, Berry SA, Burke LW, Geleske TA, Hamid R, Hopkin RJ, Introne WJ, Lyons MJ, Scheuerle AE, Stoler JM. Health care supervision for children with Williams syndrome. Pediatrics. 2020;145(2):e20193761. https://doi.org/10.1542/peds.2019-3761.
8. Pickles DM, Lihn SL, Boat TF, Lannon C. A roadmap to emotional health for children and families with chronic pediatric conditions. Pediatrics. 2020;145(2):e20191324. https://doi.org/10.1542/peds.2019-1324.

Chapter 80
Learning and Intellectual Developmental Disorders

Nikhil Rao

Case 1 Since entering third grade, Bobby has gradually become more irritable and disinterested in school, engaging in outright refusals and anger outbursts, especially in language arts class. At home and in sports, he remains his typical good-natured self. Formerly known as an affable, eager student, this change has worried his teacher and parents. As the school therapist, you have been asked to weigh in on mental health concerns.

Learning disorders are common, affecting an estimated 5–15% of school age children [1]. Though considered innate to the child and lifelong in nature, signs may not be evident before elementary school or even later depending on compensatory ability. The DSM-5 now classifies Specific Learning Disorder (SLD) as a single diagnosis, with specifiers for Reading (dyslexia), Written Language (dysgraphia), and Math (dyscalculia).

Educational struggles may result in a variety of psychological reactions, from anxious withdrawal and low self-esteem, to irritability and other externalizing behaviors. When these are particularly notable in school or especially a specific class compared to other environments, this may herald that a youth has an unidentified SLD [2]. Of course, the most common sign is lower than expected performance in a specific discipline.

The current approach to youth performing below grade level is known as Response to Intervention (RtI), which consists of three phases [3]. Tier 1 encompasses the general educational environment. Youth performing below expectation are referred to interventional classes involving specific skill acquisition (Tier 2). Those who fail to respond will proceed to the more intensive Tier 3 intervention such as one-on-one instruction. Many will show improved performance and return to Tier 1 or 2, while others will show persistent deficits in proficiency.

N. Rao (✉)
Oregon Health and Sciences University, Portland, OR, USA

R. P. Olympia, J. Brady-Olympia (eds.), *Clinical Considerations in School-based Health*, https://doi.org/10.1007/978-3-031-85765-2_80

Throughout this process, the school-based health team should consider medical, neurodevelopmental, and mental health contributors to learning challenges. Medically, these include sensory (vision and hearing), motor (fine motor, tremor), and vestibular (head posture, gaze, and coordination) components.

Roughly half of all children with SLD will have another neuropsychiatric concern. Anxiety and other internalizing problems are substantially more common, with bidirectional effects, as learning struggles exacerbate negative self-image and vice versa. Neurodevelopmental disorders are highly comorbid with each other, and this holds true for Specific Learning Disorder, with a second learning domain being the most common comorbidity, followed by ADHD, then ASD [4]. Early recognition may allow a youth to respond to intervention and return to age-typical or expected performance based on capacity.

For those who do not respond to 6 months of intervention and/or comorbidity management, further investigation is indicated (Table 80.1). Testing should include both assessment of intelligence as well as academic achievement [5]. One should be careful in interpreting the full-scale IQ (FSIQ) too closely, as SLDs (e.g. Reading Disorder and Verbal Comprehension) and common comorbidities (e.g. ADHD and Cognitive Performance Index [CPI]) will artificially depress the score. In these cases, alternate indices such as the Generalized Ability Index (GAI) may prove to be better estimates of a youth's underlying cognitive capacity while low scores in ancillary and complementary indices (such as the Quantitative Reasoning Index in Math Disorder) may illuminate areas of specific concern [6].

In formalizing the diagnosis of Specific Learning Disorder, one should consider age-typical performance, general cognitive abilities, response to intervention, and interdependent neuropsychiatric concerns.

Case 2 Stephen is a 10 year old boy with an IQ score of 62 who has recently transferred to your school from another district. Your team is just getting to know him, but his emotional and behavioral challenges, as well as learning difficulties, seem in excess of what is expected given his cognitive scores.

Intellectual Developmental Disorder (Intellectual Disability or IDD) is defined by the DSM-V as having an IQ lower than 70 in addition to substantial challenge in two or more areas of adaptive functioning, including conceptual, social, and practical domains [7]. Severity of IDD is no longer based strictly on IQ but on impact of adaptive functioning deficits on ability to perform at an age-typical level.

Mental age, though no longer used as a formal metric, nevertheless retains strong clinical utility in understanding the youth with IDD:

$$MentalAge = \frac{ChronologicalAge \times IQ}{100}.$$

In Stephen's case, we would thus expect him to present with the cognitive and adaptive capacities of a 6 year old. However, it should be remembered that the IQ is not a monolithic score, and that strengths or challenges in subscales may distort it. Stephen presents with a much lower CPI than his FSIQ and thus his GAI of 74 would be more representative [8].

Table 80.1 Psychoeducational Testing

Domain	Examples	Example Subscores	Webinar
Intelligence	Wechsler Intelligence Scale for Children (WISC-V)	Cognitive Performance Index—Processing speed, working memory. Heavily influenced by NDD General Ability Index—Logical reasoning. Less influenced by LD and ADHD	https://youtu.be/i-suBVVrEN0
Educational Achievement	Wechsler Individual Achievement Test (WIAT-4) Wide Ranging Achievement Test Kaufman Test of Educational Achievement	Multiple components within reading, math, and writing. Within-subject component subscores may reveal SLD deficits	https://youtu.be/WCldK30maV0
Adaptive Functioning	Vineland Adaptive Behavior Scales (Vineland 3) Adaptive Behavior Assessment Scale (ABAS-3)	Conceptual (learning) Social (including emotion regulation) Practical (self-care)	https://youtu.be/XHqVZGXfCdY
Autism	Autism Diagnostic Observation Scale (ADOS-2)	Social Affect Repetitive and Restricted Behavior	https://youtu.be/So05QaAjkKw?feature=shared
Comprehensive Behavioral	Behavioral Assessment System for Children (BASC-3)	Externalizing Problems Internalizing Problems Behavioral Symptoms Adaptive Skills	https://youtu.be/du_6zGRy4x0

The above provides some insight into Stephen's learning challenges, as that pattern (CPI<GAI) is often a marker of ADHD or other processing difficulty. Further exploration of his adaptive functioning scores (e.g. BASC, Vineland, or ABAS) reveals that while his conceptual (learning) performance is closer to his estimated mental age, he has significant variance in both social and practical (activities of daily living) domains.

In speaking with his parents and teachers, it becomes clear that Stephen decompensates in stimulating environments with both overwhelm and distractibility. Unexpected schedule changes have resulted in major blowouts and he struggles during transition time. Stephen also has more challenges in the afternoon. Socially,

Table 80.2 Objective and Observer-Report Measures for Psychiatric Symptoms

Domain	Test
ADHD	NICHQ Vanderbilt Assessment Scales
Sensory Sensitivity	Parent Glasgow Sensory Questionnaire (GSQ-P)
Aggression	Modified Overt Aggression Scale (MOAS)
Anxiety	Screen for Childhood Anxiety Related Disorders (SCARED)
Depression	Mood and Feelings Questionnaire (MFQ-P)

GSQ-P form and validation study available at: https://eprints.gla.ac.uk/300281/2/300281.pdf
All others available at: https://www.aacap.org/AACAP/Member_Resources/AACAP_Toolbox_for_Clinical_Practice_and_Outcomes/Forms.aspx

Stephen shows limited social approach and poor eye contact, and becomes overwhelmed with peer engagement, either becoming escalated or withdrawing. Many if not all of these challenges would not be surprising in a 3–4 year old, but from the perspective of either Stephen's chronological (10) or mental (7) age, these are striking. Further neuropsychiatric evaluation (Table 80.2) including the ADOS-2 reveals diagnoses of ASD and ADHD which provide substantial explanatory power and treatment guidance for his challenges.

The differential for comorbid NDD or mental illness in IDD is broad, as a preponderance of other diagnoses are more common in these youth, including not just ADHD and ASD, but also anxiety, mood, and psychotic disorders, with frequency of these comorbid diagnoses estimated at 25–50%, compared to 6–7% for the general population [9]. ADHD and ASD are the most common comorbid disorders, with anxiety disorders closely following. It should be kept in mind that youth with IDD are at increased risk for trauma and neglect as well [10]. Unfortunately, these symptoms are often misattributed to general effects of IDD, precluding appropriate management and leading to worsened outcomes.

Anxiety and mood disturbance may be symptoms of ADHD and ASD rather than distinct diagnoses. This also holds true for other symptoms such as repetitive behaviors, which are seen in both ASD and OCD. These distinctions become important as interventions that are effective for one disorder may be ineffective or even harmful for another despite the overlap in symptoms (e.g. SSRIs in anxiety disorders vs IDD/ASD) [11].

Behavioral interventions and psychotherapy should be considered first line in children with neuropsychiatric comorbidity, with the exception of ADHD in which pharmacotherapy is typically necessary for significant clinical response [12]. The role of behavioral intervention is especially clear in the case of behaviors with functional or sensory components. This often looks like elopement during times of transition or sensory overwhelm, or tantrums and property destruction in response to frustration in a particularly challenging class. One

Table 80.3 Common Medications, Indications, and Drawbacks

Medication Class	Indications	Efficacy	Risk	Side Effects
Stimulants	Concentration Hyperactivity Impulsivity Aggression	High	Low-Medium	Irritability, appetite suppression, insomnia. Rebound—Irritability/agitation worse than baseline *as medication wears off*
Alpha Agonists	Impulsivity Hyperactivity Anxiety Aggression Insomnia	Medium	Low	Sedation, Orthostatic hypotension. Dizziness
Antipsychotics	Impulsivity Aggression Psychosis	High	High	Sedation, weight gain, dyslipidemia, diabetes Akathisia—restlessness, tics, irritability, aggression Extrapyramidal Symptoms—Tremor and spasticity Tardive Dyskinesia—Often irreversible. Writhing motions of small muscles of tongue and fingers.
Antidepressants	Anxiety Depression	Low	Medium	GI distress, headache, cognitive dulling SSRI Activation Syndrome—anxiety, tremor, restlessness, insomnia, irritability and impulsivity
Mood Stabilizers	Impulsivity Aggression Mania	Medium	High	psychiatric and cognitive symptoms, rash, weight gain, liver injury, kidney injury, pharmacodynamic interactions

should also consider sensory needs such as a youth who benefits from fidget or movement, or who may become overwhelmed in an environment with many auditory stimuli (such as many children talking in a crowded lunchroom). Additionally, assisting the youth in developing coping skills and the ability to take space play a substantial role in aiding them in successfully remaining a part of the classroom. Last, the role of impaired communication in sustaining externalizing behaviors cannot be understressed. Improving the youth's ability to recognize and relay their needs is imperative. The school-based health team should involve occupational therapists, speech language pathologists, and positive behavior specialists from the special education team and collaborate to develop appropriate communication, sensory, and coping strategies [13].

Unfortunately, rates of psychotropic prescribing in IDD youth with behavioral concerns are extremely high, with a plurality on three or more agents (Table 80.3), despite significant risk of sequelae [14]. Youth with IDD may have reduced ability to communicate response to medication as well as emergence of side effects. Thus, objective measurement and observation becomes important as many of these side effect syndromes may in fact mimic or escalate the target behavior. Examples include:

- Stimulants worsening hyperactivity or aggression either during peak effect or as plasma concentration drops below the therapeutic window [15].
- SSRI activation syndrome, which presents as restlessness, impulsivity, and insomnia, much like the anxiety it is intended to treat [16].
- Antipsychotic-induced akathisia, generally associated with antipsychotics, in which the youth suffers from increased restlessness or repetitive movements, even aggression [17].

Atypical antipsychotics are increasingly prescribed in these youth, often for aggression and impulsivity, with or without a clear indication such as ASD or psychosis [18]. Yet, they entail high risk for myriad side effects and long-term health consequences, most notably obesity, diabetes, and dyslipidemia, but also neurologic sequelae including permanent consequences such as tardive dyskinesia. The provider should consider antipsychotic-sparing strategies when possible, keeping in mind that stimulants are highly effective in aggression management in this population and that alpha agonists (e.g. clonidine and guanfacine) have broad efficacy across aggression, impulsivity, hyperactivity, and anxiety symptom clusters while having minimal risk, with sedation and orthostasis being the most common side effects [19]. It is paramount to optimize behavioral strategies, environmental supports, and lower morbidity medications before resorting to a medication class that *will*, rather than may, have lifelong consequences.

Case 3 Nina is a 6 year old female with an FSIQ of 48. Staff have noted somnolence, incontinence, and limited attention span, but today have referred to you the school nurse due to suddenly worsening irritability and striking herself in the head repeatedly with her fists.

Medical comorbidity is high in IDD (Table 80.4). Genetic, metabolic, and CNS syndromes, including epilepsy and congenital CNS malformation, are substantially more common in this population, with 10–15% prevalence, and increasing incidence with severity of IDD [20, 21]. Even outside of these often multi-organ syndromic etiologies, many common acute and chronic disorders are more pervasive in these youth [22]. Yet, due to reduced body awareness and communication deficits, they may not present typically. Indeed, change in behavior including both internalizing and externalizing symptoms such as clinginess, anxiety, or acting out behaviors may herald a medical rather than neuropsychiatric concern [23].

The child with IDD with a sudden change in behavior should be assessed for acute infections including upper respiratory infection, acute otitis media, and

Table 80.4 Medical Comorbidities in Developmental Disorders

Acute	Chronic	Screening Considerations
Infection	Epilepsy	Vision and Hearing
Physical injury	Asthma	Sleep Disordered Breathing
Hypersensitivity	Allergy	Nutrition and Obesity
Dental pain	Metabolic Disease	Constipation
Sleep Disturbance	Cancer (hematologic)	Thyroid Disease

gastrointestinal (GI) infection in addition to physical injury with careful physical examination. Acute exacerbations of chronic illnesses should also be considered, especially epilepsy (post-ictal state), asthma, and allergy. Dental issues, given known challenges with oral hygiene in children with IDD, should also remain in the differential. In Nina's case, inflamed tympanic membranes are immediately visible on otoscopy.

Morbidity and mortality from medical causes are dramatically higher in individuals with IDD, often due to delayed detection and inadequate management of treatable conditions [24]. Aside from syndrome-specific medical concerns that should be identified by the standard genetic and imaging workup as recommended by AAP [20], common pathologies should be screened for and monitored regularly.

Respiratory disorders including allergy, asthma, and pediatric obstructive sleep apnea occur at higher rates in the IDD population. Notably, each of these conditions when under-treated have significant negative consequences to neuropsychiatric function which can be reversed with treatment [25, 26]. Constipation is common in IDD and the severe and chronic nature is associated with major GI complications such as diverticulitis and nausea, as well as negative CNS effects including worsening frequency of epileptiform events and changes to mood and anxiety [27].

Nutrition is also important to consider given the wide range of disordered eating patterns in youth with NDD, including Binge Eating Disorder and Avoidant/Restrictive Food Intake Disorder [28, 29]. Failure to thrive secondary to ARFID should be monitored. Whether via binge eating or underlying metabolic influences, obesity and related illnesses occur at a much higher rate and contribute significantly to morbidity and mortality [24]. Bodyweight and appetite management may require both behavioral and medication strategies. Even in normal bodyweight youth, selective eating may result in significant micronutrient deficiency [30].

Extra Credit Points

1. Look for discrepancies in performance between subjects (math vs reading) or modes of learning (oral vs written) to spot specific learning disorders. Explore and rule out other contributors, such as hearing and vision problems, auditory or visual processing differences, or developmental coordination disorder.
2. Youth with IDD have higher rates of medical illness and difficulty communicating and recognizing physical sources of distress. Changes in behavior should always be considered within this context, with constipation, asthma/allergy, and infection being common. Many chronic and acute medical conditions are more common in individuals with IDD and undertreatment remains a major contributor to their higher morbidity than the general population.
3. Neurodevelopmental disorders often co-occur, and many youth with IDD will also have ADHD, ASD, or another LD. Mental health disorder burden is likewise higher, and may present atypically. Be careful in over-ascribing a youth's challenges or needs to cognitive or learning differences.
4. Adaptive functioning is not wholly determined nor limited by neurocognitive capacity, and ultimately of greater import in our youths' abilities to reach their potential. Consider how the school environment and mental health supports can improve a youth's ability to cope and navigate the world around them.

References

1. McDonough EM, Flanagan DP, Sy M, Alfonso VC. Specific learning disorder. In: Goldstein S, DeVries M, editors. Handbook of DSM-5 disorders in children and adolescents. Springer International Publishing; 2017. p. 77–104.
2. Diakakis P, Gardelis J, Ventouri K, et al. Behavioral problems in children with learning difficulties according to their parents and teachers. Pediatrics. 2008;121(Supplement_2):S100–1.
3. Shinn MR. Identifying students at risk, monitoring performance, and determining eligibility within response to intervention: research on educational need and benefit from academic intervention. School Psychol Rev. Published online December 1. 2007; https://doi.org/10.1080/02796015.2007.12087920.
4. Margari L, Buttiglione M, Craig F, et al. Neuropsychopathological comorbidities in learning disorders. BMC Neurol. 2013;13(1):198.
5. Shah HR, Sagar JKV, Somaiya MP, Nagpal JK. Clinical practice guidelines on assessment and management of specific learning disorders. Indian J Psychiatry. 2019;61(Suppl 2):211–25.
6. Maccow G. Advanced interpretation of the WISC-V. Powerpoint Slideshow February 5, 2015. Accessed 9 May 2024. https://pdfs.semanticscholar.org/5621/25aed484a9ccfb88cf46df8cdef3ce89a1e6.pdf.
7. Patel DR, Cabral MD, Ho A, Merrick J. A clinical primer on intellectual disability. Transl Pediatr. 2020;9(Suppl 1):S23–35.
8. Russo N, Kaplan-Kahn EA, Wilson J, Criss A, Burack JA. Choices, challenges, and constraints: a pragmatic examination of the limits of mental age matching in empirical research. Dev Psychopathol. 2021;33(2):727–38.
9. Boat TF, Wu JT, Disorders C to E the SSIDP for C with M, et al. Clinical characteristics of intellectual disabilities. In: Mental Disorders and disabilities among low-income children. National Academies Press (US); 2015.
10. Marcal S. A trauma-informed toolkit for providers in the field of intellectual & developmental disabilities. Center for Disability Services New York. White Paper Accessed 11 May 2024. https://www.pacesconnection.com/fileSendAction/fcType/0/fcOid/468137553002812476/filePointer/468137553002812517/fodoid/468137553002812512/IDD%20TOOLKIT%20%20CFDS%20HEARTS%20NETWORK%205-28%20FinalR2.pdf.
11. Sohanpal SK, Deb S, Thomas C, Soni R, Lenôtre L, Unwin G. The effectiveness of antidepressant medication in the management of behaviour problems in adults with intellectual disabilities: a systematic review. J Intellect Disabil Res. 2007;51(10):750–65.
12. 2019 autism spectrum disorder & intellectual developmental disorder: Florida best practice psychotherapeutic medication recommendations for target symptoms in children and adolescents.
13. Doehring P, Reichow B, Palka T, Phillips C, Hagopian L. Behavioral approaches to managing severe problem behaviors in children with autism spectrum and related developmental disorders: a descriptive analysis. Child Adolesc Psychiatr Clin N Am. 2014;23(1):25–40.
14. McLaren JL, Lichtenstein JD, Metcalfe JD, Charlot LR, Drake RE, Beasley JB. Psychotropic use among youths with intellectual and developmental disabilities. Psychiatr Serv. 2021;72(9):988–97.
15. Carlson GA, Kelly KL. Stimulant rebound: how common is it and what does it mean? J Child Adolesc Psychopharmacol. 2003;13(2):137–42.
16. Luft MJ, Lamy M, DelBello MP, McNamara RK, Strawn JR. Antidepressant-induced activation in children and adolescents: risk, recognition and management. Curr Probl Pediatr Adolesc Health Care. 2018;48(2):50–62.
17. Forcen FE, Radwan K, Arauz A, et al. Drug-induced akathisia in children and adolescents. J Child Adolesc Psychopharmacol. 2017;27(1):102–3.
18. Park SY, Cervesi C, Galling B, et al. Antipsychotic use trends in youth with autism spectrum disorder and/or intellectual disability: a meta-analysis. J Am Acad Child Adolesc Psychiatry. 2016;55(6):456–468.e4.

19. Naguy A. Clonidine use in psychiatry: panacea or panache? Pharmacology. 2016;98(1–2):87–92.
20. Moeschler JB, Shevell M, COMMITTEE ON GENETICS, et al. Comprehensive evaluation of the child with intellectual disability or global developmental delays. Pediatrics. 2014;134(3):e903–18.
21. Murias K, Moir A, Myers KA, Liu I, Wei XC. Systematic review of MRI findings in children with developmental delay or cognitive impairment. Brain Dev. 2017;39(8):644–55.
22. Liao P, Vajdic C, Trollor J, Reppermund S. Prevalence and incidence of physical health conditions in people with intellectual disability—a systematic review. PLoS One. 2021;16(8):e0256294.
23. King BH, de Lacy N, Siegel M. Psychiatric assessment of severe presentations in autism spectrum disorders and intellectual disability. Child Adolesc Psychiatr Clin N Am. 2014;23(1):1–14.
24. Weitzman C, Nadler C, Blum NJ, Augustyn M. Supporting access for everyone consensus panel. Health care for youth with neurodevelopmental disabilities: a consensus statement. Pediatrics. 2024;153(5):e2023063809.
25. Sastre J, Crespo A, Fernandez-Sanchez A, et al. Anxiety, depression, and asthma control: changes after standardized treatment. J Allergy Clin Immunol Pract. 2018;6(6):1953–9.
26. Esbensen AJ, Schwichtenberg AJ. Sleep in neurodevelopmental disorders. Int Rev Res Dev Disabil. 2016;51:153–91.
27. Wagenaar MC, Van Der Putten AAJ, Douma JG, Van Der Schans CP, Waninge A. Definitions, signs, and symptoms of constipation in people with severe or profound intellectual disabilities: a systematic review. Heliyon. 2022;8(5):e09479.
28. Pruccoli J, Guardi G, La Tempa A, Valeriani B, Chiavarino F, Parmeggiani A. Food and development: children and adolescents with neurodevelopmental and comorbid eating Disorders—a case series. Behav Sci. 2023;13(6):499.
29. Dinkler L. Restrictive eating disorders: aetiological, epidemiological and neurodevelopmental aspects; 2020. Accessed 10 May 2024. https://gupea.ub.gu.se/handle/2077/66196.
30. Samuel TM, Musa-Veloso K, Ho M, Venditti C, Shahkhalili-Dulloo Y. A narrative review of childhood picky eating and its relationship to food intakes, nutritional status, and growth. Nutrients. 2018;10(12):1992.

Chapter 81
Obsessive Compulsive Disorder

Ulrick Vieux

As the child and adolescent psychiatrist who is providing consultation-liaison services in a school-based clinic, the school counselor requests that you see students who are engaging in behavior that is preventing them from reaching their full potential despite a desire to do well in school. A concern is that these students may be suffering from (OCD). This observation was made after a faculty development presentation by the school-based child and adolescent psychiatrist, wherein the presenting signs of OCD were reviewed. OCD is a debilitating condition that affects 1–4 percent of the child, adolescent, adult population, as well as, 8 percent of college athletes. Up to 25 percent of elite high school and professional athletes experience subthreshold obsessive-compulsive symptoms [1, 2]. A thorough clinical interview ideally by a child and adolescent psychiatrist is the gold standard of making a diagnosis of OCD. Semi-structured scales such as the children's Yale-Brown obsessive-compulsive scale (C-YBOCS) can be used as a tool to assess the severity of the illness. Treatment modalities such as non-pharmacological treatments include cognitive behavioral therapy (CBT), behavior therapy (BT), motivational enhancement treatment; and pharmacological modalities such as SSRI's and D-cycloserine [3].

Obsessive compulsive disorder is an underdiagnosed and undertreated disorder, often manifested as a cycle of Obsession-Anxiety-Compulsion-Temporary Relief (Fig. 81.1). This disorder manifests as either obsessive (worries) or compulsions (rituals) behavior even though both may be present (Table 81.1). This disorder begins in childhood and is a chronic remitting relapsing condition that can persist into adulthood [1]. Treatment of this disorder is paramount to prevent adverse sequalae of this disorder (Table 81.2). Medication treatments include selective serotonin reuptake inhibitors like Zoloft (sertraline), Prozac (fluoxetine), Paxil

U. Vieux (✉)
Hackensack University Medical Center, Hackensack, NJ, USA
e-mail: ulrick.vieux@hmhn.org

R. P. Olympia, J. Brady-Olympia (eds.), *Clinical Considerations in School-based Health*, https://doi.org/10.1007/978-3-031-85765-2_81

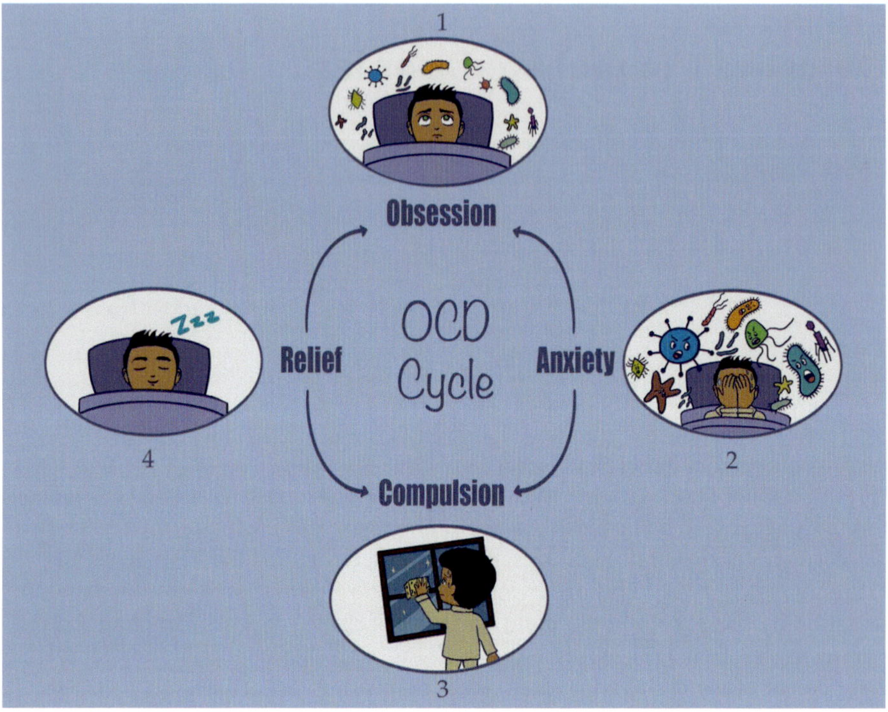

Fig. 81.1 OCD Cycle

Table 81.1 Obsessions and compulsions associated with OCD

Obsessions (Worries)	Compulsions (Rituals)
Fear of germs from people or the environment	Cleaning
Fear of forgetting or losing things	Repetitive hand washing
Intrusive thoughts of violent, sexual, or religious themes	Mental counting rituals
Fear of making mistakes	Arranging objects in a specific order
Fear of catastrophic family event or loss	Repetitive checking

(paroxetine), Lexapro (escitalopram) and tricyclic antidepressants (TCAs) such as clomipramine. Non-pharmacological interventions include cognitive behavioral therapy (CBT) and other forms of psychotherapy [4]. A challenge in diagnosis is that the symptoms of OCD tend to present internally and oftentimes children may not possess the necessary verbal skills to describe their symptoms and may minimize them because of feelings of shame. Only 40 percent of patients identified with OCD will receive OCD-specific therapy and less than 10% receive evidence-based treatment. The World Health Organization places OCD in the top ten of debilitating disorders: approximately 8 in 10 of those who develop OCD will develop it prior to the age of 18 [1].

Table 81.2 Treatment for OCD

Treatment modalities and medications	Exposure and response prevention (ERP) therapy
	Be willing to accept uncertainty
	Avoid seeking reassurance
	Mindfulness meditation
	Medication- SSRI and Tricyclic

Case 1 Gabriel is a 15 year-old tenth grade student who is the star basketball player on the varsity team. He is already being recruited by Division 1 programs. He is a solid A student and despite being one of the younger players on the basketball team, he is regarded as a well-respected leader. He has not been subject to bullying as other precocious young athletes have faced when playing with older teammates. Despite the outward appearance of success and being well adjusted, his basketball coach (with permission of his parents) requested a consult due to concerns that the patient is struggling in manners that are not noticeable among some of his teachers and peers. During the interview, Gabriel mentioned that he engages "in rituals' that he needs to complete in order to "feel right." His coach requested the consult based on a faculty development presentation that was done by the school-based child and adolescent psychiatrist, who was concerned that behavior such as over responsibility, perfectionism, secrecy, calorie obsession, body hyperfocus, superstitions and rituals can all mask symptoms of OCD. In addition, the coach noticed that the student's parents were reinforcing Gabriel's rituals by providing reassurance and accommodating Gabriel's fears and his desire to avoid uncomfortable situations [2]**.**

Case 2 Denise is a 16 year-old 11th grade student who is in advanced placement honors. She was born full term, C-section with all developmental milestones met without any delays. She was diagnosed with pediatric autoimmune neuropsychiatric disorders associated with streptococcus (PANDAS) when she was 6 years old. Her mother said that at age 5 she had a group A Streptococcus infection and almost immediately her behavior changed. Significant family history includes mother being diagnosed with anxiety as an adult but was under-diagnosed as a child and adolescent and not treated. Mother felt that her daughter's anxiety led to her not completing college, despite being an A student with the dream of becoming a physician. Mother would like her daughter to be treated and is seeking guidance on the ideal modality. Mother reported Denise had a two-week course of oral antibiotics when OCD symptoms first presented due to a differential diagnosis of PANDAS. Teacher reports that the patient is very motivated to excel; however, she tends to perseverate over things [3]**. Denise recently had the SARS-COV2 (Covid) virus and mother is concerned that Covid will exacerbate her OCD symptoms** [5, 6]**.**

Case 3 Cassandra is a 14 year old female ninth grade student who is in regular education. She has been tardy several times which affects her attendance. However, when she is in school she is able to complete the entire day. Referred to you because her homeroom teacher feels that her tardiness is not due to oppositional behavior and not due to properly preparing for school. During the interview, the patient mentioned that she wants to go to school on time. She enjoys school as a B student with plans on going to college. She states that she wakes up at 6 am in preparation for class that starts at 8:20 am. As the consulting school based psychiatrist you are asked to see Cassandra. Initial session with Cassandra after lunch period at around 1 pm. She acknowledged that she missed the first period and was able to come in at 9 am for the start of the second period. She is embarrassed by constantly missing the first period. She takes pride in her intelligence and has a goal to go to college. She shares that the reason why she is tardy for her first class is that she will leave home and on the subway ride to her school she will think that she has not locked the front door of her apartment. The thoughts are so overwhelming that she will make it to school on time but will be unable to enter the school and instead go back to her apartment to ensure that the front door was locked hence the reason for her consistently missing the first period.

Case 4 Jose is an 8 year old male third grade student who has an IEP with accommodations of increased time for test taking, sitting in the front row. Collateral information obtained from parents provided that Jose was a full term, C-section delivery. All developmental milestones were met on time. Jose symptoms occurred suddenly after a streptococcal infection. Parents shared it felt like overnight Jose presented with obsessive-compulsive symptoms, restricted food intake, anxiety and mood lability. Family denies any family history of mental illness. Patient treatment included a 6 week course of antibiotics. Symptom improvement was observed. Family is in consultation with their pediatricians and is considering an intravenous immunoglobulin (IVIG) trial [6–9].

Exposure and response prevention (ERP) therapy is the first-line, evidence-based treatment for OCD. The goal of ERP is to alleviate the discomfort associated with distress and establish skills that enable the individual to function with the discomfort. This cognitive behavioral therapy (CBT) modality utilizes psychoeducation and can use *in vivo* exposure, imaginal exposure and/or interoceptive exposure to help patients minimize urges to perform compulsions and obsessions. It was found that 80% of clients respond to ERP [10]. Mindfulness meditation is utilized to help accept the discomfort of a negative thought thus minimizing the desire to react thereby minimizing the OCD presentation [11].

Obsessive compulsive disorder is a debilitating disease. Early diagnosis and treatment that can minimize the adverse sequelae of the disorder. It is often undiagnosed and undertreated, and without treatment the disorder can be debilitating. Like the many mental illnesses, the initial presentation is often during childhood and adolescence. Approximately 8 in 10 of those with OCD presented with symptoms prior to the age of 18 and 4 in 10 with OCD will have it as a chronic condition [1]. PANDAS can present with OCD symptoms (for example, tics, obsessions, and compulsions) other due to immune system alterations that are triggered by group A streptococcal (GAS) infections and stress [4, 6]. This provides a greater context of the complexity of this disorder. It is vital to note that 60–80% of OCD cases have a comorbidity which makes comorbidity the rule rather than an exception. Common comorbid diagnoses include attention deficit hyperactivity disorder (ADHD), tics, autism spectrum disorder, food allergies, eating disorder, sport and specific learning disorder (SLD) [3].

Extra Credit Points

1. High school athletes can mask OCD symptoms. Traits that are encouraged such as hyperfocus, perfectionism, secrecy and superstition can all be symptoms of OCD.
2. One of the challenges of treating OCD is that it is often under-diagnosed and is associated with poor insight from patients and a substantial amount of family support that accommodates the disorder.
3. For mild to moderate child and adolescent OCD cases CBT (Cognitive-Behavioral Therapy) is the gold standard treatment modality. Studies have shown CBT to be comparable and some studies have shown superior results to medication management.
4. For more severe presentations, SSRI are the first-line medications for any age. Preferred SSRIs include fluoxetine, fluvoxamine, sertraline and paroxetine. Clomipramine which is a TCA can also be used [7].
5. Co-morbid diagnosis is the norm with OCD with disorders such as autism spectrum disorder and attention deficit/hyperactivity disorder the most common co-morbid diagnosis with OCD [1].

References

1. Nazeer A, Latif F, Mondal A. Obsessive-compulsive disorder in children and adolescents: epidemiology, diagnosis and management. Transl Pediatr. 2020;9(Suppl 1):S76–93.
2. Cromer L, Kaier E, Davis J, et al. OCD in college athletes. Am J Psychiatry. 2017;174:6. https://ajp.psychiatryonline.org/doi/10.1176/appi.ajp.2017.16101124
3. Avasthi A, Sharma A, Grover S. Clinical practice guidelines for the management of obsessive-compulsive disorder in children and adolescents. Indian J Psychiatry. 2019;61(Suppl 2):306–16. PMID: 30745705; PMCID: PMC6345139. https://doi.org/10.4103/psychiatry.IndianJPsychiatry_554_18.
4. Marazziti D, Mucci F, Fontenelle L. Immune system and obsessive-compulsive disorder. Psychoneuroendocrinology. 2018;93:39–44.
5. Della Vecchia A, Marazziti D. Back to the future: the role of infections in psychopathology. Focus on OCD. Clin Neuropsychiatry. 2022;19(4):248–63.
6. La Bella S, Scorrano G, Rinaldi M, et al. Pediatric autoimmune neurospsychiatric disorders associated with streptococcal infections (PANDAS): myth or reality? The state of the

art on a controversial disease. Microorganisms. 2023;11:2549. https://doi.org/10.3390/Microorganisms11102549.
7. Del Casale A, Sorice S, Padovan A, et al. Psychopharmacological treatment of obsessive-compulsive disorder (OCD). Curr Neuropharmacol. 2019;17(8):710–36.
8. Wilbur C, Bitnun A, Kronenberg S, et al. PANDAS/PANS in childhood: controversies and evidence. Paediatr Child Health. 2019;24(2):85–91.
9. Goodman W, Storch E, Sheth S. Harmonizing the neurobiology and treatment of obsessive-compulsive disorder. Am J Psychiatry. 2021;178:17–29. https://doi.org/10.1176/appi.ajp.2020.20111601.
10. Law C, Boisseau CL. Exposure and response prevention in the treatment of obsessive-compulsive disorder: current perspectives. Psychol Res Behav Manag. 2019;12:1167–74. https://doi.org/10.2147/PRBM.S211117. PMID: 31920413; PMCID: PMC6935308
11. Lee SM, Suh HW, Kwak HY, Kim JW, Chung SY. Meditation-based intervention for obsessive-compulsive disorder: a PRISMA-compliant systematic review and meta-analysis. Medicine (Baltimore). 2022;101(30):e29147. https://doi.org/10.1097/MD.0000000000029147. PMID: 35905202; PMCID: PMC9333541

Chapter 82
Psychosomatic Disorders

Paige Chardavoyne and Anum Khan

From the roots "psyche" meaning the mind and "soma" meaning the body, psychosomatic disorders are a group of conditions characterized by one or more bodily symptom(s) with significant functional impairment [1]. Psychosomatic disorders have been described as an issue with the body's software versus the body's hardware as in organic disease patterns [2, 3]. Psychosomatic disorders include somatic symptom disorder and functional neurological symptom disorder/conversion disorder, both of which have diagnostic criteria included in the Diagnostic and Statistical Manual of Mental Disorders Fifth Edition Text Revision (DSM-5-TR) (Table 82.1) [4].

Somatic symptomatology in somatic symptom disorder may or may not be clearly medically explained but the hallmark of this diagnosis is the accompanying abnormal thoughts, emotions, and behaviors in response to these symptoms. Common somatic symptoms in children include abdominal discomfort, fatigue, and pain [2]. In functional neurological symptom disorder, functional impairment is also present but there is a disconnect between reported symptoms and recognized pathophysiology. Potentially affected neurological processes include speaking, walking, and swallowing [2, 4]. Functional neurological symptom disorder encompasses nonepileptic seizures (as discussed in Chap. 48) and functional movement disorders. Related conditions include functional chronic pain syndromes, functional fatigue syndromes, functional gastrointestinal disorders, functional respiratory symptoms, and functional cardiac symptoms [2]. Common amongst the psychosomatic disorders is functional impairment, which may present in the school setting as declining grades/poor scholastic performance, increased isolation/withdrawing

P. Chardavoyne (✉)
Medical College of Wisconsin, Milwaukee, WI, USA
e-mail: pchardavoyne@mcw.edu

A. Khan
UW Health Swedish American Hospital, Rockford, IL, USA

R. P. Olympia, J. Brady-Olympia (eds.), *Clinical Considerations in School-based Health*, https://doi.org/10.1007/978-3-031-85765-2_82

Table 82.1 DSM-5-TR criteria for somatic symptom disorder and functional neurological symptom disorder

Somatic Symptom Disorder	A. One or more somatic symptoms that are distressing or result in significant disruption of daily life. B. Excessive thoughts, feelings, or behaviors related to the somatic symptoms or associated health concerns as manifested by at least one of the following: 1. Disproportionate and persistent thoughts about the seriousness of one's symptoms. 2. Persistently high level of anxiety about health or symptoms. 3. Excessive time and energy devoted to these symptoms or health concerns. C. Although any one somatic symptom may not be continuously present, the state of being symptomatic is persistent (typically more than 6 months).
Functional Neurological Symptom Disorder	A. One or more symptoms of altered voluntary motor or sensory function. B. Clinical findings provide evidence of incompatibility between the symptom and recognized neurological or medical conditions. C. The symptom or deficit is not better explained by another medical or mental disorder. D. The symptom or deficit causes clinically significant distress or impairment in social, occupational, or other important areas of functioning or warrants medical evaluation.

from friends and staff, and school avoidance/refusal. Thus, features obtained from the history and physical examination can be key in elucidating whether a psychosomatic disorder is present. Some general features of psychosomatic disorders include:

- Abrupt onset versus gradual onset of symptoms
- Episodic symptoms which may resolve with distraction.
- Ability to provide an exact date/time of symptom onset
- Symptoms change over time or are variable in presentation

With this in mind, look at the following clinical cases and identify which features may be consistent with a psychosomatic disorder (Table 82.2).

Given the medical symptoms and concern for underlying medical etiologies, it is not surprising that children with psychosomatic disorders, such as those in the cases above, can be difficult to appropriately triage and are most likely to present to other medical professionals than mental health professionals when symptoms first develop [4]. During initial symptom onset, children may be triaged to emergency departments or urgent care facilities depending on the perceived acuity, anticipated medical work-up, and potential treatment. For example, Gina from case #1 may have initially been seen at an emergency department due to concern for seizure and Leo

Table 82.2 Case presentations and features which may be consistent with a psychosomatic disorder

Case #1: Gina is a 13-year-old girl who presents with new onset seizures. You witness a seizure episode. Hip thrusting is present and her eyes appear squeezed shut. She does not bite her tongue during the episode and does not have urinary incontinence. After the episode resolves, she does not have alteration of mental status. She was recently admitted to the hospital where medical workup was unremarkable. Notably, an episode was observed while she was on electroencephalography (EEG) and no epileptiform activity was observed. You learn that she has been under increased psychosocial stress lately involving family conflict. She has been missing classes due to these events and has been isolating.	Atypical symptoms for a seizure Symptoms present: hip thrusting, eyes squeezed shut Symptoms absent: tongue biting, urinary incontinence, post-ictal state Episode without epileptiform activity EEG correlate Recent psychosocial stress and symptoms (such as isolation) which may be consistent with a psychiatric condition, such as depression

(continued)

Table 82.2 (continued)

Case #2: Leo is an 8-year-old boy who presents with abdominal pain. This pain has been going on since the first day of this school year. He reported that the pain "comes and goes" and often differs in intensity (sometimes sharp and other times dull) and exact location. Days when he is busiest at school tend to be more symptom free. Abdominal imaging and laboratory tests were recently obtained and unremarkable.	Symptoms atypical for known abdominal pathology and medical workup is negative to this point Abrupt onset of symptoms where the exact date is known Symptoms are episodic in nature and resolve during busy periods (when distracted) Symptoms vary in intensity and location
Case #3: Kathleen is a 16-year-old girl who presents with trouble swallowing. She reported being in her normal state of health until a week ago when, at the end of the night while watching a movie, she felt a piece of popcorn get stuck in her throat that she had to cough up. Since then, she has not eaten solid food for fear of being unable to swallow. Upon gross examination of her throat no abnormalities are present and a recent swallow study was unremarkable. Thinking about eating solid food again is a source of distress.	Abrupt onset of symptoms where the date and time of initial onset are known Significant distress accompanies the child's presentation and an underlying psychiatric condition, such as an anxiety disorder, may be present Presentation is medically unexplained after physical examination and swallow study

from case #2 may have initially been seen at an urgent care facility due to concern for abdominal pain. When considering medical work-up, it is recommended to be clinically conservative in these cases and only order labs or place referrals that may be clinically necessary to rule out potential medical causes of illness. If symptom report, physical exam, and medical work-up are more consistent with a psychosomatic disorder, similar subsequent episodes may be able to be managed in the outpatient setting. However, during an episode, appropriate triage can remain difficult to determine (as noted above, symptoms may change over time or vary in presentation), and children may be sent back to emergency departments or urgent care facilities for evaluation. Appropriate triage can be even more challenging if an individual has a history of a known disease process with similar presenting symptoms. For example, imagine if Gina from case #1 had a history of epilepsy and was now presenting with these seizure-like episodes more consistent with a psychogenic non-epileptic event.

If symptoms persist or cause impairment and the child is ready to engage with mental health, a referral to psychology may be an appropriate starting point. In psychotherapy, children can discuss a variety of topics, including distress and underlying psychosocial stressors which may be leading to or exacerbating their physical symptoms. If there are concerns for a co-morbid psychiatric condition, such as depression or anxiety, and thoughts that the child would benefit from medication, this can be discussed with the patient's primary care provider (PCP) or a child psychiatrist. Indications for a child psychiatry referral can include complex presentation and medication regimen. If a child psychiatrist is not available, which could be due to long wait times or lack of a child psychiatrist in your area, provider consultation with a child psychiatrist in your state of practice may be available.

As alluded to in the last paragraph, biological, psychological, and social factors can predispose and precipitate psychosomatic disorders [2, 4]. Biological factors include gender (as these conditions are more common in females than males) and family history of psychiatric conditions which may be comorbid (such as depressive disorders and anxiety disorders). Psychological factors include comorbid medical illness, mood symptoms (such as anxiety and depression), limited/maladaptive coping skills, and personal history of trauma/stressful life events. Regarding the latter, data suggests that history of trauma may be present in around 30% of children with psychosomatic disorders, though this value is challenging to approximate [5]. What appears clearer is that history of trauma can lead to more challenging clinical course, increased psychiatric comorbidity, and worse outcomes. Psychologically, the theory is that the increased awareness and hyperarousal that can be seen after trauma is also directed towards a child's somatic symptoms [6]. Social factors include family factors (such as reinforcing seeking medical attention).

Due to these biopsychosocial factors, when assessing for a psychosomatic disorder, it is important to gather a psychiatric history and assess for stressors. Screening for general physical and emotional symptoms which may be impairing function can be completed with the longstanding, well-established Pediatric Symptom Checklist, which is completed by parents, or the Pediatric Symptom Checklist - Youth Report, which is completed by the child [7, 8]. Both checklists are available at https://www.massgeneral.org/psychiatry/treatments-and-services/pediatric-symptom-checklist [7]. The website also includes information about checklist administration, interpretation, and next steps. To assess for adverse childhood experiences (ACEs), screening tools such as the Pediatric ACEs and Related Life-events Screener (PEARLS) may be used and is available at https://www.acesaware.org/learn-about-screening/screening-tools/ [9]. Another commonly used tool is the ACE Questionnaire, which has been adapted for use in the pediatric population [10].

Once the diagnosis has been made or is highly suspected, it is important to share your thoughts and provide psychoeducation about the condition with the child, family supports, and school personnel. Great care should be taken when discussing psychosomatic disorders. It is important to validate the child's experience. The symptoms are subconscious, non-intentional, uncontrollable, involuntary, and are a reality to the child whether or not they are medically explained. On the other hand, it is also important that family, providers, and school personnel avoid reinforcing somatic symptoms when working with a child. Below are some guidelines for effectively communicating a diagnosis of a psychosomatic disorder with a child [2, 11].

- Discuss how the clinical history and physical exam findings led to the diagnosis.
- Point out any observed examination findings and explain how these may vary from typical disease patterns.
- Discuss the connection between biopsychosocial factors and current presentation. Children may be more receptive to understanding how the "brain and body" are highly linked in times of distress.
- Involve family and other social supports in conversations where appropriate.

Communicating the diagnosis is essential for facilitating appropriate treatment. As with many medically explained presentations, psychosomatic disorders have effective treatment modalities. An element about psychosomatic disorders that is notable is that full and complete recovery is possible. Treatment for psychosomatic disorders is multifactorial and can include the following, some of which has been discussed in more detail earlier in the chapter [2, 11]:

- Assess for and treat any comorbid medical conditions (psychiatric and non-psychiatric).
- Screen for trauma history and, if present, consider referral to trauma-focused specialists.
- Provide psychoeducation about the psychosomatic disorder to the child and their family supports.
- Refer to physiotherapy targeted to symptomatology when physical symptoms are impairing function.
- Refer to mental health (psychotherapy and psychiatry) when the individual is ready to engage and consider having the child establish with long-term mental health providers.
- Consider involving wraparound services if the child needs additional community support, if the child is struggling to attend school, if safety concerns are present, and if the child is having ongoing mental health symptoms impairing function.
- In instances, it may be helpful to create or alter individualized education program (IEP) plans or 504 plans for students who are struggling with physical symptoms and/or their psychological impact in the classroom setting.

Extra Credit Points

1. Psychosomatic disorders are conditions which impair an individuals' ability to function and may cause significant distress.
2. It is paramount for individuals working with this population to not perpetuate the stigma that has often been associated with this group of conditions.
3. Whether or not symptoms have a medical explanation or are part of a recognized pathophysiology, the symptoms are real, unintentional, subconscious, and not "in the head".
4. History and physical examination findings can rule in this diagnosis. Medical workup should be limited to what is clinically necessary.
5. Early multifactorial treatment is important and can lead to full recovery.

References

1. Psychosomatic. APA dictionary of psychology. American Psychological Association; 2018. Accessed 2 Apr 2024. https://dictionary.apa.org/psychosomatic.
2. Sunde KE, Hilliker DR, Fischer PR. Understanding and managing adolescents with conversion and functional disorders. Pediatr Rev. 2020;41(12):630–41.
3. Stone J. Functional neurological disorder (FND). Accessed 5 Apr 2024. https://neurosymptoms.org/en/.
4. Somatic symptom and related disorders. Diagnostic and statistical manual of mental disorders. 5th ed., text rev. American Psychiatric Association; 2022. p. 350–71.
5. Thomson K, Randall E, Ibeziako P, et al. Somatoform disorders and trauma in medically-admitted children, adolescents, and young adults: prevalence rates and psychosocial characteristics. Psychosomatics. 2014;55(6):630–9.
6. Malas N, Ortiz-Aguayo R, Giles L, et al. Pediatric somatic symptom disorders. Curr Psychiatry Rep. 2017;19:1–11.
7. Pediatric symptom checklist. Massachusetts General Hospital. Accessed 24 May 2024. https://www.massgeneral.org/psychiatry/treatments-and-services/pediatric-symptom-checklist.
8. Jellinek MS, Murphy JM, Robinson J, et al. Pediatric symptom checklist: screening school-age children for psychosocial dysfunction. J Pediatr. 1988;112(2):201–9.
9. Screening tools. ACEs aware. Accessed 24 May 2024. https://www.acesaware.org/learn-about-screening/screening-tools/.
10. Watson P. How to screen for ACEs in an efficient, sensitive, and effective manner. Paediatr Child Health. 2019;24(1):37–8.
11. O'Neal MA, Dworetzky BA, Baslet G. Functional neurological disorder: engaging patients in treatment. Epilepsy Behav Rep. 2021;16:100499.

Chapter 83
School Refusal

Richard E. Mattison

Case 1 After an uneventful first grade year, 8-year-old Beth started to show SR symptoms early in second grade. She began to attend school erratically, or often ended up in the nurse's office feeling ill and wanting to go home. Her teacher thought she often looked tense, had become less interactive with her couple friends, and was less focused on her work. When contacted, her mother noted that that their family had recently been dealing with stress.

School absenteeism has been receiving increased attention (**www.attendance-works.org**) since the COVID pandemic of 2021, especially because of growing chronic school absenteeism (defined as 10% of the 180 days in a school year). Of particular concern are those students who have a continual trajectory of high absenteeism from kindergarten through eighth grade (8% of a national study) and are subsequently at high risk for dropping out [1]. Thus, school attendance teams (SAT) have become increasingly established especially in larger secondary school programs (which may already have School Based Health Clinics [SBHC]), and are showing promising effectiveness in decreasing SR [2]. Programmatically, they may meet every 2 weeks to identify and closely track at-risk students (e.g., 25% absences over 2 weeks). They are typically multi-disciplinary and can include the school's nurse (who is at the front line with SR), psychologist, social worker [SW], and/or guidance counselor [GC], plus mental health (MH) professionals who are already part of the SBHC staff. (Note that while SATs are the school staff of primary focus in this chapter, the same discussion can also apply to the single school staff member, e.g., the school nurse, in smaller schools who may be designated to oversee school attendance.)

Interventions for students with absenteeism of concern are often delivered using the Multi-tiered System of Supports (MTSS) approach which schools often employ

R. E. Mattison (✉)
Penn State Hershey Medical School, Hershey, PA, USA
e-mail: rmattison@pennstatehealth.psu.edu

R. P. Olympia, J. Brady-Olympia (eds.), *Clinical Considerations in School-based Health*, https://doi.org/10.1007/978-3-031-85765-2_83

to address the various academic, attendance, behavioral, and emotional problems of students [3]. For example, Tier 1 focuses on the majority of students (75–90%) who benefit from the general supports for attendance that schools already have in place. Tier 2 monitors students who show more attendance problems (10–25%), especially at-risk students who are vulnerable for above-average absenteeism because of known chronic diseases like asthma. These students may need, for example, smaller group help to keep up academically. Finally, Tier 3 centers on supports for those students whose absenteeism doesn't respond to the previous interventions and requires more individual support (<10%), such as students whose families may be homeless or who may require more comprehensive MH support both within and outside of school. This chapter will provide suggestions to help school and SBHC staff work together in the identification and support/treatment of students with SR (one type of school absenteeism for whom Tier 3 support often becomes necessary.)

The most common types of school absenteeism are school refusal (SR; the focus of this chapter) and truancy. SR is a symptom complex [3] of strong emotionality to avoid school which has been found to occur in 1–5% of students, presents especially during transitions between school levels, appears more commonly in adolescents, and occurs equally between genders. SR presents with characteristic symptoms: reluctance or refusal to attend school, desire to remain close to parents (symptoms may show early at home but parents say nothing), emotional distress at the prospect of going to school, and no antisocial behaviors. The distress can show as intense emotions (not unlike a fight or flight response), physical symptoms (from stomach-aches to vomiting), meltdowns (screaming tantrums to threats of hurting oneself), active avoidance of school (from begging not to go to hiding), and/or disrupted sleep from worry. If the child goes to school, they may then frequent the nurse's office or want to call home. Prolonged SR symptoms can gradually cause secondary disruption socially (absences lead to losing friends and impaired growth of social skills) and academically (falling behind in school and increased fear of failing), plus worsen anxiety and/or depressive symptoms to the point of becoming disorders that require specific treatments. Impaired relationships with teachers and parents can also accumulate. General variables which have been found to significantly worsen absenteeism are lower socio-economic status, parental divorce, and comorbid educational disabilities. Associated school factors include ineffective school attendance policies, poor record keeping, unsafe school environments, and inadequate identification of special education needs.

When any student with possible SR presents to a SAT, basic information is necessary and can be ideally gathered with permission by protocols that SATs and SBHC staff have developed together, for example, (Table 83.1). SATs must begin with the paramount inquiry into acute issues such as medical or abusive situations, suicidal talk, or bullying in school. Such "emergencies" should then be handled according to protocols that have already been established. Ideally, SAT and/or SBHCs will include a consultant child psychiatrist who can help teams create such acute plans, as well as regularly be available for consultation concerning students with problematic school attendance, as well as helping to arrange collaborative treatment in the community.

Table 83.1 School information necessary for thorough evaluation of students with potential SR

Source + Measure [4]	School information
Teacher:	
Recent serious events	Medical crisis, abuse, suicidal talk, bullying
Report cards—impairment	Grade-point average and subject failures, disciplinary referrals and suspensions, absences (excused/unexcused, tardy, home early), and teacher comments
School records	Teacher comments, cognitive/achievement testing, school services
PSC-17	Brief standardized survey of general MH concerns such as attention, externalizing, and internalizing problems
Student:	
Recent serious events	Same as above
PHQ-9 and SCARED	Types and severity of anxiety and depressive symptoms
	(Including suicidality)
Psychiatric interview	To include discussion of school and mental state exam (especially mood assessment)
Parent:	
Recent events, PSC, PHQ	Same as above
SRAS	Types and severity of SR symptoms
Adverse Childhood Experiences	Checklist for expanded history of serious stresses
Psychiatric interview	To complement student's above psychiatric interview

Abbreviations: *PHQ-9* Patient Health Questionnaire, *PSC-17* Pediatric Symptom Checklist, *SCARED* Screen for Anxiety Related Emotional Disorders, *SRAS* School Refusal Assessment Scale

Next the SAT can review standard school information that exists in every student's file, to especially identify any changes between a student's past and current impairment, as well as uncovering other teacher concerns. Then a brief but comprehensive screening can include a battery like the Pediatric Symptom Checklist (PSC-17), Patient Health Questionnaire (PHQ-9), and Screen for Anxiety Related Emotional Disorder (SCARED) [4], which can be completed by students, parents, and/or teachers. In the case of SR, the School Refusal Assessment Scale (SRAS) [5] can be added to further clarify the occurrence and severity of SR symptoms, as well as the main areas that are commonly involved in SR (such as school situations of distress [can't keep up], painful social situations [gym or reading out loud], needs for attention from parents, and enjoyable cocooning at home (movies or video games).

Finally, if a student remains of sufficient concern after the above initial SAT inquiry, a more extended MH portion of the protocol can be administered by SBHC staff (Table 83.1). This can include a full psychiatric interview of the student (including a mental state exam), as well as full history from the parent. Additional objective measures can also be used to expand any information from the initial screening instruments.

Such above targeted gathering of appropriate information helps the SAT and SBHC to determine the student's current diagnostic picture, degree of functional impairment, and types and level of interventions that are needed. For example, Case 1 could demonstrate the common presentation of acute SR in an otherwise normal developing little girl, who then may respond to early straight-forward interventions by mainly the SAT. These might include the school SW/GC coordinating teachers' understanding of and practical responses to the situation, e.g., being alert to signs that the girl needs to talk to the SW/GC, ensuring normal peer group interactions, and helping the family to obtain necessary therapeutic interventions to deal with the new stresses at home. The SAT (led by the school nurse) should monitor the little girl's response closely over at least one school marking period, and SBHC staff should remain available to help the SAT re-evaluate any changes. Thus, comprehensive understanding, practical interventions at school, and sustained monitoring could prevent this case from worsening. Details of the case should subsequently appear in the girl's cumulative file in case of later relapse.

Case 2 Charlie is a 13-year-old boy who started middle school in sixth grade this year and just finished his first marking period. Elementary school records show that he had never been a discipline problem, was well-liked, and was good at sports. However, in third grade and fourth grade he had received some small group help for an academic deficit in word recognition identified during routine group reading testing. Last year in fifth grade he missed 14 days of school scattered throughout the year and looked less cheerful in class as the year progressed. The ongoing reading problem appeared to bother him at times, though his GPA was "C." During the summer his parents didn't think he was his usual active self although he did appear to enjoy the annual family shore vacation. They are now increasingly worried about him both at home and school, and have reached out to the school nurse and SAT. They note that he did not go out for sports this year because he felt he wasn't good enough, now complains about school being too hard, and is starting to miss school, i.e., some mornings becoming so distressed that he pulls the bed covers over his head and then screams/sobs to be left alone. The family has not seen any suicidality which was on their mind because the father had a younger sib who tried unsuccessfully during college.

Charlie represents a more complicated yet common presentation of SR. The SAT quickly executed the Table 83.1 protocol for new SR (no recent acute stressful events found) and expedited his referral to the SBHC (and subsequently their child psychiatrist consultant). The team eventually hypothesized that although Charlie functioned better in grade school with reading help, he had a lingering and broader learning disability in reading that was growing more impactful in general. His clinical picture and impairment had thus changed, and he now needed thorough re-evaluation for possible intensive Tier 3 services, including SBHC reassessment for an evolving comorbid Depressive Disorder (Table 83.2).

Table 83.2 Comorbid diagnoses often associated with SR

Diagnosis	Presentation
Anxiety disorder	Anxiety symptoms consistent with a specific disorder, such as generalized anxiety (GAD), fear triggered at school by loud arguing or any fighting (PTSD), or increased shyness in the presence of staff and peers (SAD)
Depressive disorder	Increased sadness even in happy school situations, more isolative during cafeteria/gym, less productive in work, early suicidal ideation
Neurodevelopmental disorders	Disruptive cognitive/achievement deficits (ADHD-I/LangD/LD) that may become more apparent over time
Autism Spectrum Disorder	More apparent deficits in social interaction skills, more restricted interests
Substance use disorders	General impairment

Abbreviations: *ADHD-I* Attention-Deficit Hyperactivity Disorder, predominantly inattentive presentation, *LangD* Language Disorder, *LD* Specific Learning Disorder, *GAD* Generalized Anxiety Disorder, *PTSD* Posttraumatic Stress Disorder, *SAD* Separation Anxiety Disorder

More intensive reassessment by the team indeed revealed that Charlie has a chronic Language Disorder which over time had also been affecting his Reading Comprehension. Furthermore, another neurodevelopmental deficit was more evident that often accompanies this clinical scenario—ADHD—Inattentive type. Such a complicated, evolving presentation is not uncommon in secondary school students who show Charlie's history [6], where the increasing academic stress of secondary school can then cause a student engage in more negative thinking, alienation from peers, and diminished enthusiasm for school. Charlie now needs broader school interventions to help him with his various neurodevelopmental deficits (Tier 3 specific interventions and strategies), cognitive behavioral therapy (CBT) to also help him and important others understand and adjust to his academic and mood disorders, plus possible medications to help his ADHD-I (e,g, long-acting methylphenidate) and his depressive disorder with chronic anxiety symptoms (e.g., sertraline).

His new treatment plan will require the coordinated participation of Charlie, his teachers, his parents, the SAT and SBHC staff, and likely MH staff in the community (such as a child psychiatrist to provide any indicated medications, unless only a pediatrician is available in smaller communities). "Collaboration" must be stressed, for example, especially to ensure as much as possible the delivery of a similar CBT approach (which will increase the chances that the CBT will succeed), including school personnel. Thus, very importantly, a designated, experienced leader will be required to coordinate and monitor the multimodal treatment. This leadership role likely will fall into the hands of the SBHC staff with the most MH experience, working closely with an SAT leader with the strongest MH background.

Extra-Credit Points

1. Early targeted evaluation and treatment of SR with subsequent close monitoring appears to often be an effective treatment.
2. SR can often be related to anxiety, depressive, and/or learning disorders.

3. CBT appears to be an especially helpful therapy for SR when used in concert by teachers, parents, and SAT/SBHC staff.
4. Coordination of a multimodality treatment plan is vital, and will often depend on SBHC leadership to ensure multi-discipline collaboration.

References

1. Simon O, Nylund-Gibson K, Gottfried M, Mireles-Rios R. Elementary absenteeism over time: a latent class growth analysis predicting fifth and eighth grade outcomes. Learn Individ Diff. 2020;78:1–12.
2. Lim C, Cung PJ, Biely C, et al. School attendance following receipt of care from a school-based health center. J Adolesc Health. 2023;73:1125–31.
3. Ingul JM, Havik T. Emerging school refusal: a school-based framework for identifying early signs and risk factors. Cog Behav Pract. 2019;26:46–22.
4. Trafalis S, Giannini C, Joves J, et al. A pediatrician-friendly review of three common behavioral health screeners in pediatric practice: findings and recommendations. Pediatr Investig. 2021;5(1):58–64.
5. Kearney CA. Identifying the function of school refusal behavior: a revision of the school refusal assessment scale. J Psychopath Behav Assess. 2002;24(4):235–45.
6. Benner GJ, Mattison RE, Nelson RJ, Ralston NC. Types of language disorders in students classified ED: prevalence and association with learning disabilities and psychopathology. Educ Treat Child. 2009;32:631–53.

Chapter 84
Sleep Disorders in Children and Adolescents

Rebecca V. Taylor

Sleep is arguably the most important thing we can do to promote our health. On average, a person spends roughly 1/3 of their life asleep and missing quality sleep can have major detriments. Sleep is a relatively poorly understood construct that is the result of a complex interplay of internal systems, hormones, and neurotransmitters. Sleep architecture consists of REM and non-REM sleep, each with distinct physiological, EEG, and neurological features. The NREM portion of sleep is responsible for rest and restoration and is separated into 3 stages, with each one being deeper than the last. The REM phase of sleep, named for the occurrence of rapid eye movements, is responsible for memory consolidation, as well as development, and dreams; it is in this phase that nightmares occur. A complete cycle of NREM and REM sleep occurs every 90–110 minutes of the night [1]. A review and consensus by the American Academy of Sleep Medicine in 2016 highlighted research and impacts of chronically poor sleep, including difficulties with emotional regulation, irritability, tantrums, attention, relationships, impulsivity, substance use, suicidal thoughts, falls, cortisol production (immunity), academic achievement, memory and difficulties with development of language, and executive functions [2, 3].

84.1 Sleep Requirements (Table 84.1)

As we age, our need for sleep decreases. Newborns spend roughly 80% of their day asleep, and are obtaining long stretches of sleep by 6 months of age when melatonin has become a more stable influence. This is the generally accepted age when a

R. V. Taylor (✉)
Duke University School of Medicine, Durham, NC, USA
e-mail: Rebecca.v.taylor@duke.edu

R. P. Olympia, J. Brady-Olympia (eds.), *Clinical Considerations in School-based Health*, https://doi.org/10.1007/978-3-031-85765-2_84

Table 84.1 Sleep requirements by age

Age	Total sleep (hours)	Naps	Misc.
Newborn—2 months	14–17		Concerns if <12 hours, >18 hours/day REM sleep compromises majority of sleep.
3 months—11 months (infant)	12–16	2–4	Stage 3 NREM sleep seen at 3–6 months. Sleeping through the night occurs at 6 months.
12 months—36 months (toddler)	11–14	1–2	At 1 year of age, REM sleep is roughly 25–40% Concerns if <10 hours, >16 hours/day
3 years—5 years (preschool)	10–13	1	Concerns if <10 hours, >14 hours/day
6 years—12 years (school age)	9–12	0	Sleep architecture is similar to adults by age 12. Concerns if >13 hours/day
13 years—18 years (teenager)	8–10	0	Concerns if <8 hours, > 10 hours/day

Adapted from Paruthi et al. [3] and Zandieh et al. [4]

regular bedtime routine should be introduced. By a year of age, sleep occupies only 50% of the day [1].

84.2 Sleep Disorders

84.2.1 Psychiatric Conditions

Case 1 B is a 15-year-old previously healthy female who has had concerns for worsening grades in the past 2–3 months. Teachers have noted she pays less attention in class and is less engaged. She is sent to the counselor after falling asleep during class. She discloses to the counselor that she is having difficulty falling asleep for the last month, and is only sleeping 4 hours a night, despite being tired. Her mood has been more withdrawn, and things just seem less enjoyable than they used to be. She is diagnosed by PCP with depression and started on medications and therapy for Major Depressive Episode.

Insomnia is the most common term associated with sleep issues, and is simply a difficulty with quality of sleep along with difficulty falling asleep, staying asleep, or waking up too early that occurs at least 3 nights a week. There are a number of environmental factors that influence sleep, and this is one of the first things to assess when discussing sleep habits. There are also many psychiatric conditions associated

Table 84.2 Psychiatric conditions associated with sleep difficulties

Psychiatric Condition	Impact on sleep	Other
Autism Spectrum Disorder (ASD)	Difficulty falling asleep, staying asleep	Experienced by up to 50% of patients with ASD
ADHD	Difficulty settling down and falling asleep	Previously a criterion for diagnosis; experienced by up to 50% of patients with ADHD
Depressive Disorders	Quality and quantity of sleep impacted	Criteria for diagnosis is disrupted sleep, either falling asleep, staying asleep, or oversleeping
Bipolar Disorders	Reduction in sleep quantity	Criteria for mania and hypomania are a decreased need for sleep
Anxiety Disorders	Quality and quantity of sleep impacted	Often reported as a symptom before anxiety is able to be articulated by young patients
Post Traumatic Stress Disorder (PTSD)	Fragmented sleep, often due to nightmares	Nightmares and sleep disruption are criteria for the diagnosis of PTSD

Adapted from Alfano et al. [5], Ramtekkar and Ivanenko [7]

with sleep difficulties, either as a criterion of the disorder, or as a common feature (Table 84.2). Poor sleep is now known to be a risk factor for development of these disorders, as well as a perpetuating factor, solidifying the idea that sleep and psychiatric disorders have a bidirectional relationship [5–7].

84.2.2 Sleep Parasomnias

Case 2 R is a 12-year-old who complains of being tired in class for the last few weeks, and has seemed more irritable with peers and teachers. The school nurse calls the family to discuss and parents report that sleep has been very fitful most nights for the past few weeks. They have seen random movements and jerking of limbs, and there has been at least 3 episodes of enuresis. They are able to see PCP who is concerned about nocturnal epilepsy and refers to neurology, who diagnoses sleep related hypermotor epilepsy (SHE) and starts on antiseizure medications.

Several sleep related disorders occur either in NREM or REM sleep, with distinguishing features of each condition that helps to identify them (Table 84.3). Many are self-limiting and do not require treatment only psychoeducation and implementation of safety parameters at home [8, 9]. In the case of SHE, further evaluation by a specialist is required [9].

Table 84.3 Sleep related disorders

Parasomnia	Symptoms	Stage of Sleep
Confusional states	Confusion, open eyes, unable to be woken	NREM
Night Terrors	Agitated, flushed face, sweating, unresponsive, no memory of event	NREM
Sleepwalking	Movement and walking while asleep; can lead to injuries and concern if going outside while in this state	NREM
Nocturnal Seizures (SHE)	Disorganized body movements, unresponsive, confused, enuresis, tongue injury; several genetic variants identified	NREM
Nightmare Disorder	Recurrent nightmares and awakenings with anxiety, fear	REM
REM Sleep Behaviour Disorder	Aggressive behaviours in REM sleep due to acting out dreams from lack of atonia	REM
Sleep Paralysis	Experience of waking without being able to move, due to atonia persisting past REM sleep	REM

Adapted from Krishna et al. [8] and Morse [9]

84.2.3 Other Sleep Disorders

Case 3 S is an 8-year-old who complains of daily headaches, fatigue for weeks. His teacher heard him snoring in class when he fell asleep one day. The school nurse is alerted, and encouraged the family to talk to the pediatrician about possibility of a breathing related sleep disorder such as obstructive sleep apnea (OSA). The nurse notes other symptoms including mouth breathing, and mild obesity. Family is able to be evaluated and S is referred for removal of adenoids and tonsils given the diagnosis of OSA.

Some sleep disorders are related to disruptions, including the sleep apneas, hypoventilation syndromes, and hypoxemia. Other sleep disorders are related to hypersomnolence and excessive sleeping. All of these conditions can lead to excessive daytime sleepiness (EDS), defined as difficulty staying awake and irrepressible need for sleep. These all warrant further investigation for targeted treatment (Table 84.4).

84.3 Evaluation

Any concerns for sleep or sleep-related disorders should be brought to the attention of the pediatrician. The first step in evaluating sleep is keeping a 1–2 week sleep diary of sleeping hours, waking hours, time to fall asleep, nighttime awakenings, naps, and rating the quality of sleep. A medical evaluation will further investigate sleep habits and history. Several questionnaires are designed to assist with screening for sleep issues in this population, including The Children's Sleep Habit Questionnaire (CSHQ), and the BEARS (bedtime issues, excessive daytime

Table 84.4 Miscellaneous sleep disorders

Sleep Disorder	What is it?	Symptoms	Evaluation/Treatment
Obstructive Sleep Apnea (OSA)	Partial or complete obstruction of airway with oxygen deprivation	Snoring, mouth breathing, obesity, enuresis, headaches, attention issues	Sleep study Adenotonsillectomy CPAP
Delayed Sleep Phase Disorder (DSPD)	Circadian rhythm disruption of sleep period	Shifting of sleep period by more than 2 hours for 3 months	Correction of sleep period, sleep hygiene
Nocturnal Enuresis	Primary when never attained continence, secondary is a regression	Can be its own isolated issue or symptom of OSA or SHE	Behavioural interventions
Restless Leg Syndrome (RLS)	Sensorimotor condition, can be related to ADHD, kidney disease	Unpleasant experience in legs only alleviated by movement	Evaluate ferritin, treat if <50 with iron; treat related conditions [3]
Periodic Limb Movement Disorder (PLMD)	Less volitional involvement, can be related to ADHD	Stereotypic, repetitive movements of the limbs	Evaluate ferritin, treat if <50 with iron; treat related conditions [3]
Narcolepsy	Constellation of symptoms impacting quality sleep at night	EDS, cataplexy, sleep attacks, hypnagogic hallucinations, sleep paralysis, confusion	MSLT or CSF hypocretin-a level, stimulant medications
Idiopathic hypersomnia	Excessive sleeping	Excessive sleeping for more than 3 months	Evaluate for other causes such as narcolepsy
Klein-Levine Syndrome	Rare syndrome of cyclical symptoms	Hypersomnia, hyperphagia, hypersexuality	Limited treatment; cycles often resolve

Adapted from Ramtekkar and Ivanenko [7], Krishna et al. [8], and Kansagra et al. [10]

sleepiness, night awakenings, regularity, duration of sleep, and snoring) and are readily available [11]. Following evaluation, a polysomnography with EEG and oxygen monitoring or the multiple sleep latency test (MSLT) may be ordered for a more detailed evaluation of sleep [5, 8, 12].

84.4 Treatment Options

Sleep Hygiene is a mainstay of treatment for improving sleep, regardless of the etiology or age (Table 84.5). These are supplied as a list of interventions, along with recommending parental engagement and a sleep diary for assessment and tracking of sleep habits and improvements [12, 13].

Cognitive Behavioral Therapy for Insomnia (CBT-i) is a brief therapy intervention that includes behavioral aspects (sleep hygiene) and cognitive therapy aimed at improving sleep, with the goal of sustained improvement over time. It has robust

Table 84.5 Sleep hygiene tips

Sleep Hygiene Tips	
Regular bedtime	Bedroom is cool, comfortable, dark
Regular wake up time	Only use bed for sleep
Regular routine before bed	Do not stay in bed if not asleep >30 min
No screens 1 hour before bed	Relaxing activity before sleep

Adapted from CHOC Sleep Hygiene Tips [14, 15]

data in the adult population and while research is less among children and adolescents, it has proven to be safe and effective, especially when parents are engaged. Behavior therapy and CBT-i both include faded bedtimes, graduated extinctions, as well as motivational interviewing, and thought challenges [13, 16]. While these interventions are effective regardless of etiology, targeted treatments for identified underlying conditions is warranted [3].

84.5 Medications

There are no approved medications for insomnia in pediatric patients, however several medications have been utilized when appropriate (Table 84.6). Medications should be aimed at underlying etiologies that can improve sleep as a byproduct. There are however several medications which may impact sleep negatively, including antihistamines, SSRIs, SNRIs, bupropion, and stimulant medications. Any medication recommendation or prescription should be given with recommendations for sleep diary, sleep hygiene, and psychoeducation about sleep. In addition, medications need to be administered and monitored by families given the risk of overuse and overdose [17, 18].

Extra Credit Points

1. Restful sleep is vital for all persons, and amount of sleep needed changes with age. Deficiencies in sleep can have impacts on attention, memory, mood, among many others.
2. The causes of sleep issues can be large and requires a thoughtful, thorough workup. A sleep diary is important for assessment and tracking of sleep.
3. A thorough assessment for mental health concerns is warranted.
4. Sleep hygiene and CBT-i are first line and effective for all ages; medication options are limited.

Table 84.6 Common medications for sleep disorders

Medication	Info	Dosing and Notes
Melatonin	Over the counter. Data for use in neuroatypical (ADHD, ASD) and DSPD patients	3-5 mg 30 min before bed No concerning side effects
Ramelteon	Prescription that targets melatonin receptor agonism	Not approved in peds No concerning side effects
Antihistamines	Diphenhydramine, doxylamine (OTC), hydroxyzine; can worsen sleep for many	No more effective than placebo; sedating effect wears off
Herbal supplements	Valerian root	No data to establish safety or efficacy
Clonidine	FDA approved for ADHD	QHS dosing can help with insomnia related to ADHD
Antidepressants	TCAs, mirtazapine; TCAs generally avoided due to overdose toxicity risk	No established data for use in peds.
Antipsychotics	FDA indication in schizophrenia, bipolar disorder: olanzapine, quetiapine	Can be utilized for insomnia associated with these conditions
Gabapentin	Data for use in sleep maintenance, RLS, but no FDA indication	5-15 mg/kg for dosing
Benzodiazepine (BZD), non-BZD agonist	High side effect risk (daytime sedation, amnesia, dizziness).	Not approved in peds. Low dose Clonazepam benefit NREM disorders

References

1. Bathory E, Tomopoulos S. Sleep regulation, physiology and development, sleep duration and patterns, and sleep hygiene in infants, toddlers, and preschool-age children. Curr Probl Pediatr Adolesc Health Care. 2017;47(2):29–42. https://doi.org/10.1016/j.cppeds.2016.12.001.
2. Owens J, Chervin R, Eichler A. Cognitive and behavioral consequences of sleep disorders in children. UpToDate. 2023. https://www.uptodate.com/contents/cognitive-and-behavioral-consequences-of-sleep-disorders-in-children. Published Feb 2023. Accessed Feb 2024.
3. Paruthi S, Brooks LJ, D'Ambrosio C, Hall WA, Kotagal S, Lloyd RM, Malow BA, Maski K, Nichols C, Quan SF, Rosen CL, Troester MM, Wise MS. Consensus statement of the American Academy of sleep medicine on the recommended amount of sleep for healthy children: methodology and discussion. J Clin Sleep Med. 2016;12(11):1549–61. https://doi.org/10.5664/jcsm.6288.
4. Zandieh SO, Johnson S, Katz ES. Sleep from infancy through adolescence. Sleep Med Clin. 2023;18(2):123–34. https://doi.org/10.1016/j.jsmc.2023.01.007.
5. Alfano CA, Gamble AL. The role of sleep in childhood psychiatric disorders. Child Youth Care Forum. 2009;38(6):327–40. https://doi.org/10.1007/s10566-009-9081-y.
6. Himelfarb M, Shatkin JP. Pediatric Insomnia. Child Adolesc Psychiatr Clin N Am. 2021;30(1):117–29. https://doi.org/10.1016/j.chc.2020.08.004.
7. Ramtekkar U, Ivanenko A. Sleep in children with psychiatric disorders. Semin Pediatr Neurol. 2015;22(2):148–55. https://doi.org/10.1016/j.spen.2015.04.004.
8. Krishna J, Kalra M, McQuillan M. Sleep disorders in childhood. Pediatr Rev. 2023;44(4):189–202. https://doi.org/10.1542/pir.2022-005521.

9. Morse, A, Kotagal S, Chervin R, Hoppin A. Parasomnias of childhood, including sleepwalking. UpToDate. 2023. https://www.uptodate.com/contents/parasomnias-of-childhood-including-sleepwalking. Published Oct 2023. Access Feb 2024.
10. Kansagra S. Sleep disorders in adolescents. Pediatrics. 2020;145(Suppl 2):S204–9. https://doi.org/10.1542/peds.2019-2056I.
11. Zinner S. Screening and surveillance. Published 11/2020. Accessed 04/2024. http://depts.washington.edu/dbpeds/Screening%20Tools/ScreeningTools.html#section4_textarea22_heading.
12. Dewald-Kaufmann J, de Bruin E, Michael G. Cognitive Behavioral therapy for insomnia (CBT-i) in school-aged children and adolescents. Sleep Med Clin. 2019;14(2):155–65. https://doi.org/10.1016/j.jsmc.2019.02.002.
13. Hall WA, Nethery E. What does sleep hygiene have to offer children's sleep problems? Paediatr Respir Rev. 2019;31:64–74. https://doi.org/10.1016/j.prrv.2018.10.005.
14. Sleep Hygiene for Children. Children's Hospital of California (CHOC). https://www.choc.org/wp/wp-content/uploads/2016/04/Sleep-Hygiene-Children-Handout.pdf. Accessed Feb 2024.
15. Sleep Hygiene for Teens. Children's Hospital of California (CHOC). https://www.choc.org/wp/wp-content/uploads/2016/04/Sleep-Hygiene-Teen-Handout.pdf. Accessed Feb 2024.
16. Ma ZR, Shi LJ, Deng MH. Efficacy of cognitive behavioral therapy in children and adolescents with insomnia: a systematic review and meta-analysis. Braz J Med Biol Res. 2018;51(6):e7070. https://doi.org/10.1590/1414-431x20187070.
17. Ekambaram V, Owens J. Medications used for pediatric insomnia. Child Adolesc Psychiatr Clin N Am. 2021;30(1):85–99. https://doi.org/10.1016/j.chc.2020.09.001.
18. Deshpande P, Salcedo B, Haq C. Common sleep disorders in children. Am Fam Physician. 2022;105(2):168–76.

Chapter 85
Speech and Language Impairments

Nandini Sarkar and Robert P. Olympia

Case 1 Esperanza is a 5-year-old girl raised in a bilingual household, where both English and Spanish are regularly spoken. Recently, her preschool teacher has expressed concern because Esperanza often responds to classroom questions using non-English words, especially when she is excited or unsure about the correct English terms. Although Esperanza actively participates in group discussions and communicates well with peers, her occasional use of non-English words led her teacher to wonder if there may be an underlying issue with her language development. She refers Esperanza to the nurse's office for further evaluation. As the school nurse, how should you proceed?

85.1 Normal Speech/Language Development

Speech and language development varies among children but typically follows a set of developmental milestones [1–4]. By the age of 5, most children have grasped the fundamentals of language and can use thousands of words with complex grammar. Monolingual and bilingual development differ in early stages of language acquisition but tend to converge after a few years. Children who switch between two

N. Sarkar
Penn State College of Medicine, Hershey, PA, USA
e-mail: nsarkar@pennstatehealth.psu.edu

R. P. Olympia (✉)
Department of Emergency Medicine and Pediatrics, Penn State College of Medicine
Attending Physician, Hershey, PA, USA

Division of Pediatric Emergency Medicine, Department of Emergency Medicine, Penn State
Milton S. Hershey Medical Center, Hershey, PA, USA
e-mail: rolympia@hmc.psu.edu

R. P. Olympia, J. Brady-Olympia (eds.), *Clinical Considerations in School-based Health*, https://doi.org/10.1007/978-3-031-85765-2_85

languages often have distinct phonological systems for each; essentially, a child's pronunciation in both languages is similar to that of a native-speaking child [5]. During language development, virtually all bilingual children engage in 'code-mixing,' or using two languages within a single utterance or conversation. However, they usually learn to differentiate between them over time and achieve proficiency in both languages by the time they are 5 years old [4, 5]. Both monolingual and multilingual children are expected to demonstrate mature speech patterns by the age of 8 [4]. A guideline to estimate if a child's language skills are progressing normally is the following formula: *Mean # of words used per sentence = (age of child in years) + 1*. Referral to a speech-language pathologist may be indicated if a child consistently fails to meet developmental milestones.

85.2 Common Abnormalities in Speech/ Language Development

Speech/language impairments can affect a child's articulation, fluency, voice, language, or some combination of the above (Table 85.1) [6–10].

These conditions can be primary, where delays in language acquisition occur independently of other conditions, or secondary, where impairments arise due to underlying health or neurodevelopmental issues (i.e. autism spectrum disorders, intellectual disabilities, hearing impairments, etc.). Speech and language impairments can further be divided into receptive and expressive disorders. Children with *receptive* disorders struggle to understand what they hear and read, while those with *expressive* disorders find it difficult to communicate their thoughts and feelings. Many children experience both disorders simultaneously, also known as *mixed* disorders. Table 85.2 outlines common categories of speech and language impairments.

Case 2 Arthur is a 7-year-old boy whose speech is frequently interrupted by repetitions of syllables and whole words, along with noticeable prolongations. At times, he gets "stuck" while speaking and slaps himself on the face to force the words out. These disfluencies become more pronounced when he is anxious, excited, or speaking in front of a group. Arthur is aware of his stuttering and

Table 85.1 Characteristics of Speech/Language Impairments

Articulation	Difficulty producing certain sounds; may be removed, added, changed, or distorted.
Fluency	Disruption in the flow of speech, often with abnormal number of repetitions, hesitations, prolongations, or disturbances.
Voice	Problems with pitch, loudness, resonance, or quality of the voice.
Language	*Expressive*—difficulty expressing ideas *Receptive*—difficulty understanding others *Mixed*—both expressive and receptive

Table 85.2 Categories of common speech and language impairments in children

Impairment	Clinical Pearls
Speech Delay	Follows normal developmental pattern, but at a slower rate Clinically relevant delays are <75% of expected age (i.e. 36-month child does not have skills expected at 27 months) Usually normal intelligence, comprehension, hearing, articulation Many children catch up to their peers by age 5 years Example: https://youtu.be/uFC4UK5rk4E?si=Xz9-DGdFqVOH2sYn&t=36
Receptive Language Disorder	Usually have difficulties with syntax (i.e. forming sentences) Speech may be delayed and indistinct with incorrect grammar Low comprehension—child may not look or point at named objects Normal response to nonverbal stimuli
Expressive Language Disorder	Variable, but commonly difficulties with syntax +/− delayed speech Usually normal intelligence, comprehension, hearing, articulation, etc. May be difficult to distinguish from developmental delays
Stuttering	Fluency disorder with repetition of speech, abnormal pauses, excessive filler words, and actions to get words out (i.e. self-slapping) Different from developmental dysfluency, where entire words or phrases are repeated because child thinks faster than they can speak Example: https://www.youtube.com/watch?v=rysVhDb3qKM
Articulation Disorders	Motor speech disorder Presents with difficulty producing specific sounds correctly Mild disorders not disrupting socialization are common Example: https://www.youtube.com/watch?v=PYxM229pAzw
Dysarthria	Muscle movement disorder affecting speech production Typically occurs after brain trauma—ranges from mild to severe depending on severity of injury Example: https://www.youtube.com/shorts/K-YO7cmQUc8
Childhood Apraxia of Speech	Neurological motor planning disorder Difficulty coordinating movements to produce sound Children commonly have unintelligible speech, delayed onset of babbling, difficulty with long words/sentences, inability to regulate loudness/rhythm Also associated with reading and spelling impairment Example: https://www.youtube.com/watch?v=szjfC9K190U
Intellectual Disability	Speech/language delay often first sign of global developmental delay Suspect if other skill deficits accompany speech/language delay Low comprehension—child may not look or point at named objects
Autism Spectrum Disorders	Criteria: social interaction deficits + repetitive/restrictive behaviors Children typically have speech/language skill delay or regression Example: https://www.youtube.com/watch?v=o_NbDdBq0pU

often shows signs of frustration and embarrassment, which sometimes leads to him avoiding speaking situations altogether. Having noticed this, his teacher brings him into the school nurse's office to see you. How should you proceed?

85.3 Screening for Speech/Language Impairment

Approximately 15% of children exhibit delays when first learning language, but only half of them continue to experience persistent difficulties in language acquisition [4]. Table 85.3 lists risk factors and "red flags" for speech and language

Table 85.3 Risk factors and "red flags" for speech and language impairments

Risk Factors	Red Flags
Pre-existing health or neurodevelopmental condition	Lack of participation in social settings
Childhood illness	Regression in previously held skills or milestones
Family history	Inability to meet milestones[a]
Poor language environment	
Socioeconomic status	
Parental education level	

[a]*Milestones have different criteria at different months—follow US guidelines to determine if inability to meet a milestone is a cause for concern*

Table 85.4 Developmental Screening Tools

Parents' Evaluation of Developmental Status-Revised (PEDS-R)	Evidence-based tool helps identify children with developmental/behavioral disabilities Parents fill out 12 short questions in <2 min Used for children from birth to 8 years of age https://pedstest.com/introduction-to-peds/
Denver II	Assesses child performance on age-appropriate tasks as compared to other children in their age group Free PDF consists of 125 tasks to complete as well as guide to interpreting results https://occupationaltherapyinsights.libsyn.com/denver-2-assessment
Ages and Stages Questionnaire (ASQ)	Screens development of children 1 month – 5.5 years Parent-centric and easy-to-use, taking 15 min for parents to complete and 3 min for professionals to score Available in multiple languages Free sample questionnaire available https://agesandstages.com/products-pricing/asq3/
Language Development Survey (LDS)[a]	Vocabulary checklist screening for language delays Parent-centric assessment https://pubs.asha.org/doi/10.1044/jshd.5404.587
MacArthur-Bates Communicative Development Inventory (CDI)[a]	Child vocabulary checklist, including comprehension and production of speech Online version available (Web-CDI), but expensive Short form is free, while long CDI form is available for purchase; both appropriate for child 8–18 months https://mb-cdi.stanford.edu/forms.html

[a]LDS and CDI specifically screen for speech/language skills

impairments [11–16]. Students displaying developmental red flags should be referred to a pediatrician and speech-language pathologist for evaluation.

History, physical and neurological examinations, and developmental screenings should be performed at all routine well-child visits to potentially detect speech and language impairments. Validated tools to screen for developmental issues are listed in Table 85.4.

85.4 Diagnostic Approach to Speech/Language Impairments

1. Take a thorough history and physical to evaluate for underlying causes
   (a) History-taking should include any concerns parents have about their child's development, age of onset of the specified problem, any difficulties with listening or hearing, issues with oromotor function, and developmental milestones. A comprehensive history should also cover the child's past medical history, family history, and social history.
   (b) Physical exam should assess the child's height, weight, head circumference, milestones, and behavior.
      (i) HEENT (Head-Eyes-Ears-Nose-Throat) exam should be conducted to check for auditory issues and any abnormal structure or function in the oromotor region (i.e. cleft palate or cleft lip).
      (ii) Neurological exam should be performed to assess for structural issues (i.e. motor reflexes and muscle tone).
2. Assess if the impairment is isolated or due to a global developmental delay.
   (a) Rate the magnitude of the impairment using the American Speech-Language-Hearing Association's list of developmental milestones [2, 3]. Clinically relevant delays are where the child's developmental ability is less than 75% of what they should be able to do at their current age.
3. Evaluate for hearing loss to rule out auditory impairment.
4. Refer child to a speech-language pathologist.
5. Refer child to psychometric testing to determine if the impairment is due to a global developmental delay or intellectual disability.

Above all else, referral for assessment by a speech-language pathologist is essential for diagnosis and treatment of speech/language impairments.

85.5 Treatment Options

Treatments for primary disorders primarily focus on speech and language therapy but can also include educating parents and guardians on creating a language-enriching environment for their children [10]. Examples of how to do so include limiting screen time, speaking to infants with "baby talk" and exaggerated tones, and increasing the amount of time spent conversing with children every day [17, 18]. Moreover, school-aged children should be referred to special education programs at their schools, if available. Secondary disorders are treated slightly differently, with a focus on treating or managing the underlying cause. For instance, children with hearing loss should be referred to an audiologist for evaluation and may be recommended to learn sign language, depending on the severity of their hearing deficit. For speech/language impairments caused by intellectual disability or autism spectrum disorders, first-line management includes special education or early intervention school programs that offer specific speech/language services that encourage children to communicate more. Treatment for motor speech disorders, such as dysarthria or childhood apraxia of speech, involves motor learning therapy techniques aimed at improving speech clarity [4, 17]. Overall, speech/language therapy, as well as early intervention or special education programs in schools, are essential in supporting children with speech/language impairments. For reference, potential speech/language strategies employed by these programs are listed below.

- Encourage children to practice undeveloped speech/language skills
- Incentivize communication and limit screen time
- Support active engagement of children by developing trusting relationships with them
- For motor speech disorders, practice motor speech patterns and tongue/lip placements
- Educate children on assistive devices or modalities if needed (i.e. sign language)

Children with speech/language impairments should be regularly monitored for their continued developmental pattern, additional associated conditions (i.e. attention deficit hyperactivity disorder), and overall health.

Extra Credit Points

1. When suspecting speech/language impairment in a child, immediately refer them to a speech-language pathologist.
2. Rule out underlying or secondary causes (i.e. hearing loss or intellectual disability) when evaluating speech-language impairments.
3. Consult the American Speech-Language-Hearing Association's developmental milestones to assess whether a child is developmentally on-track for their age.
4. Watch out for speech/language impairment "red flags" like regression in skills or avoidance of social interactions.
5. Conducting a thorough history and physical exam is essential for detecting speech/language impairments.

References

1. Wolraich ML, Dworkin PH, Drotar DD, Perrin EC. Developmental-Behavioral Pediatrics: evidence and practice. Elsevier Mosby; 2007.
2. Communication Milestones: Age Ranges. American Speech-Language-Hearing Association. https://www.asha.org/public/developmental-milestones/communication-milestones/.
3. Preschool Language Disorders. American Speech-Language-Hearing Association. https://www.asha.org/public/speech/disorders/preschool-language-disorders/#signs.
4. DynaMed. Speech and language disorders. EBSCO Information Services. Accessed 20 Sept 2024
5. Nicoladis E, Genesee F. Language development in preschool bilingual children. J Speech Lang Pathol Audiol. 1997;21(4) https://doi.org/10.7939/r3348gw0n.
6. Duffy JR. Functional speech disorders: clinical manifestations, diagnosis, and management. Handb Clin Neurol. 2016;139:379–88. https://doi.org/10.1016/B978-0-12-801772-2.00033-3.
7. Berkman ND, Wallace I, Watson L, et al. Screening instruments for speech and language delays and disorders in children age 5 years and younger. www.ncbi.nlm.nih.gov. Published 1 July 2015. https://www.ncbi.nlm.nih.gov/books/NBK305678/table/ch3.t4/.
8. Assessment and Evaluation of Speech-Language Disorders in Schools. American Speech-Language-Hearing Association. Published 2010. https://www.asha.org/SLP/Assessment-and-Evaluation-of-Speech-Language-Disorders-in-Schools/.
9. Carter J, Musher K. Speech and language impairment in children: evaluation, treatment, and prognosis. In: Duryea TK, Augusten M, Tehrani N, editors. UpToDate. Published online 22 Aug 2024.
10. Law J, Dennis JA, Charlton JJV. Speech and language therapy interventions for children with primary speech and/or language disorders. Cochrane Database Syst Rev. 2017;2017(1):CD012490. Published 2017 Jan 9. https://doi.org/10.1002/14651858.CD012490.
11. Naqvi Y, Winters R. Speech assessment. PubMed. Published 2020. https://www.ncbi.nlm.nih.gov/books/NBK559025/.
12. US Preventive Services Task Force. Screening for speech and language delay in preschool children: recommendation statement. Pediatrics. 2006;117(2):497–501. https://doi.org/10.1542/peds.2005-2766.
13. Zorowka PG. Disorders of speech development: diagnostic and treatment aspects. J Neural Transm Suppl. 2005;69:37–49. https://doi.org/10.1007/3-211-31222-6_3.
14. Feldman HM. How young children learn language and speech. Pediatr Rev. 2019;40(8):398–411. https://doi.org/10.1542/pir.2017-0325.
15. Feltner C, Wallace IF, Nowell SW, et al. Screening for speech and language delay and disorders in children 5 years or younger: evidence report and systematic review for the US preventive services task force. JAMA. 2024;331(4):335–51. https://doi.org/10.1001/jama.2023.24647.
16. McLaughlin MR. Speech and language delay in children. Am Fam Physician. 2011;83(10):1183–8.
17. O'Hare A, Bremner L. Management of developmental speech and language disorders: part 1. Arch Dis Child. 2016;101(3):272–7. https://doi.org/10.1136/archdischild-2014-307394.
18. Qu G, Hu W, Meng J, et al. Association between screen time and developmental and behavioral problems among children in the United States: evidence from 2018 to 2020 NSCH. J Psychiatr Res. 2023;161:140–9. https://doi.org/10.1016/j.jpsychires.2023.03.014.

Chapter 86
Teen Dating Violence

Aliza Grossberg

According to the Centers for Disease Control and Prevention (CDC), teen dating violence (TDV) can occur in person or electronically and includes physical violence, sexual violence, psychological aggression, and stalking [1]. Teen dating violence includes a pattern of behaviors utilized to obtain power and control over a partner. According to the CDC's 2019 Youth Risk Behavior Survey, 1 in 12 high school students who dated in the 12 months prior to the survey experienced physical dating violence and 1 in 12 were victims of sexual dating violence [2]. It is also important to note that teen girls and LGBTQ+ adolescents are at a greater risk of experiencing teen dating violence compared to their male or heterosexual and cisgender counterparts [3]. Directly and privately screening adolescents ages 13 and older for teen dating violence is recommended [4]. Speaking to youth about healthy relationships and about signs of unhealthy relationships, as well as resources to seek help if they are worried about themselves or a peer, are some of the ways that school-based providers can respond to, mitigate, and prevent teen dating violence.

Case 1 There have been students vaguely talking about a social media post in the hallways and in conversation with one another. One student, Lisa, comes to your office because she is worried about her friend, Xander. Sara explains that Mark and Xander have been dating for four months and that last night, they got into a fight publicly at a party. Mark then posted a video of Xander on Tik Tok that shows Xander throwing up while others are laughing at, making fun of, and neglecting to help Xander because their friends have sided with Mark.

A. Grossberg (✉)
New York University Grossman School of Medicine, New York, NY, USA
e-mail: aliza.grossberg@nyulangone.org

R. P. Olympia, J. Brady-Olympia (eds.), *Clinical Considerations in School-based Health*, https://doi.org/10.1007/978-3-031-85765-2_86

Since the posting of the video, Xander has been coming late to school and has been responding to Lisa's texts with one-word responses. You decide to bring Xander to your office to speak to Xander privately about the situation. When you ask Xander about the video, Xander consistently explains that it is "no big deal" and that they are "fine," denying that the video had any impact on them. You continue to be worried about Xander and suspect they are minimizing the incident and its effect. Eventually, Xander breaks down crying in your office. What do you do?

The video that was posted was done so without Xander's consent. It is important to meet with Xander privately and support them through navigating the challenges of what they have experienced. Moreover, having conversations with Xander's parents about the incident and about ways to support Xander are also crucial. Referring Xander to local or virtual resources or support groups can help them cope during this difficult time and ensuring they have sufficient ongoing support, whether through school counseling, or through resources outside of school, is also necessary. It is also imperative to speak with Mark and Mark's guardian(s) about the situation and to provide psychoeducation on the harmful effects of posting content, or engaging in behaviors, without someone's consent. If you have acute safety concerns, such as concerns about suicidality, you must refer the youth to the emergency room. Additionally, as a mandated reported, if you suspect or learn of physical or sexual abuse, you must make a report immediately and inform the child's guardian of this report.

In order to identify and respond to students at risk for or impacted by teen dating violence, school health providers or nurses can utilize the acronym **RADAR** (Table 86.1).

It becomes apparent that Mark posted this video in response to being mad at Xander. Discussing healthy communication is vital to ensure that situations like this do not happen again. Moreover, it would be helpful to provide this psychoeducation to classes at large before similar incidents occur. This information should be delivered by experts, whether from a local agency, or from school-based providers, who can field questions and refer students to available resources. The National Association of School Nurses suggest that a "comprehensive, developmentally appropriate, and evidence-based health education program be implemented for all students" [7]. Promoting healthy relationships is an important part of comprehensive health education (Table 86.2).

Case 2 Diane comes to your office one day crying. She says that she and her boyfriend, Sean, were up late texting last night, and that during their texting conversation, Sean asked Diane what she was wearing and asked her to send explicit pictures of herself. Diane said she stopped responding and is not sure what to do. When you non-judgmentally ask Diane questions about her relationship, you also learn that Sean will often yell at her, blame her for things that happen to him, and call her stupid. What are your next steps?

Table 86.1 RADAR acronym [5]

	Important Considerations [6]	Examples [6]
R: Routine Universal Screening	"Ask privately, look at and listen to the student Mirror the patient's language Respond with empathy"	"There are good and bad aspects to every relationship. What are three things you like most about your partner/relationship and three things you like least?" "How would you describe your relationship with your partner?" "All couples disagree. How do you and your partner handle disagreements or fights?" "What sorts of things do you and your partner do for fun?"
A: Ask Direct Questions	Same as above	"Do you ever feel forced to do things you don't want to do?" "Do your fights ever become physical?" "Does your partner put you down or make fun of you?" "Has your partner posted things to social media about you that you didn't want posted?" "Has your partner ever pressured/forced you to have sex or perform sexual acts when you did not want to?" "Does your partner want you to get pregnant? How do you feel about this?" "Do you feel like you partner hears and respects your concerns/requests?"
D: Document Screening	"Document that you asked, even with a negative screen Document patient's exact words in quotes and avoid terms that cast doubt Document any observed injuries; include photos if possible Describe safety and follow-up plans Document resources provided/discussed"	

(continued)

Table 86.1 (continued)

	Important Considerations [6]	Examples [6]
A: Assess Readiness and Safety	"Student may not be ready to recognize/disclose Intimate Partner Violence [IPV] Patient may not be ready for change Be patient Don't judge Primary goal is always safety"	
R: Review, Respond, Refer	"Thank them for their trust Offer options Co-create a follow up plan Know when and where to refer Strongly encourage family/adult involvement Refer for trauma-focused treatment"	"Thank you for sharing with me. I know it can be really difficult to talk about something so personal." "I care about you and your safety. Do you think it would be helpful for us to check in about this next time I see you?"

In this scenario, Sean has initiated a sexting conversation with Diane. Sexting is often defined as "behaviors such as [the] sending, receiving, or forwarding of nude or partially nude images via cell phones [or other electronic media]" [9]. Engaging in sexting can lead to shame, embarrassment, and guilt for youth. State laws differ with regards to sexting; however, some states consider sending, possessing, or taking a nude picture of someone to be crimes. In order to support Diane, it is important to affirm her emotions in response to this situation and explain that this is not her fault. It is also necessary to speak to Sean about the texting conversation and about his outbursts and emotional abuse in an open and non-judgmental environment and to talk with him about the seriousness, consequences, and harmful effects of his actions.

It can be helpful to provide youth with knowledge regarding their experiences of teen dating violence. The Teen Power and Control Wheel [4] (Fig. 86.1) demonstrates different types of unhealthy behaviors that can exist between teens. Some examples include physical violence, sexual violence, emotional abuse, peer pressure, threats (such as threats to harm someone or threats to die by suicide), denying or minimizing abusive behavior, blaming the person being mistreated, and controlling who someone sees or talks to. It shows that often times these forms of unhealthy behaviors in teen relationships are not isolated and frequently represent a pattern of behaviors. This tool can help with ensuring student safety, providing students with power and agency regarding their experiences, and helping to guide conversations about healthy relationships amongst teens.

Table 86.2 Characteristics of healthy & unhealthy relationships [8]

Healthy Relationships	Unhealthy Relationships
Mutual respect. Respect means that each person values who the other is and understands the other person's boundaries.	*Control.* One dating partner makes all the decisions and tells the other what to do, what to wear, or who to spend time with. He or she is unreasonably jealous, and/or tries to isolate the other partner from his or her friends and family.
Trust. Partners should place trust in each other and give each other the benefit of the doubt.	*Hostility.* One dating partner picks a fight with or antagonizes the other dating partner. This may lead to one dating partner changing his or her behavior in order to avoid upsetting the other.
Honesty. Honesty builds trust and strengthens the relationship.	*Dishonesty.* One dating partner lies to or keeps information from the other. One dating partner steals from the other.
Compromise. In a dating relationship, each partner does not always get his or her way. Each should acknowledge different points of view and be willing to give and take.	*Disrespect.* One dating partner makes fun of the opinions and interests of the other partner or destroys something that belongs to the partner.
Individuality. Neither partner should have to compromise who he/she is, and his/her identity should not be based on a partner's. Each should continue seeing his or her friends and doing the things he/she loves. Each should be supportive of his/her partner wanting to pursue new hobbies or make new friends.	*Dependence.* One dating partner feels that he or she "cannot live without" the other. He or she may threaten to do something drastic if the relationship ends.
Good communication. Each partner should speak honestly and openly to avoid miscommunication. If one person needs to sort out his or her feelings first, the other partner should respect those wishes and wait until he or she is ready to talk.	*Intimidation.* One dating partner tries to control aspects of the other's life by making the other partner fearful or timid. One dating partner may attempt to keep his or her partner from friends and family or threaten violence or a break-up.
Anger control. We all get angry, but how we express it can affect our relationships with others. Anger can be handled in healthy ways such as taking a deep breath, counting to ten, or talking it out.	*Physical violence.* One partner uses force to get his or her way (such as hitting, slapping, grabbing, or shoving).
Fighting fair. Everyone argues at some point, but those who are fair, stick to the subject, and avoid insults are more likely to come up with a possible solution. Partners should take a short break away from each other if the discussion gets too heated.	*Sexual violence.* One dating partner pressures or forces the other into sexual activity against his or her will or without consent.
Problem solving. Dating partners can learn to solve problems and identify new solutions by breaking a problem into small parts or by talking through the situation.	

(continued)

Table 86.2 (continued)

Healthy Relationships	Unhealthy Relationships
Understanding. Each partner should take time to understand what the other might be feeling.	
Self-confidence. When dating partners have confidence in themselves, it can help their relationships with others. It shows that they are calm and comfortable enough to allow others to express their opinions without forcing their own opinions on them.	
Being a role model. By embodying what respect means, partners can inspire each other, friends, and family to also behave in a respectful way.	
Healthy sexual relationship. Dating partners engage in a sexual relationship that both are comfortable with, and neither partner feels pressured or forced to engage in sexual activity that is outside his or her comfort zone or without consent.	

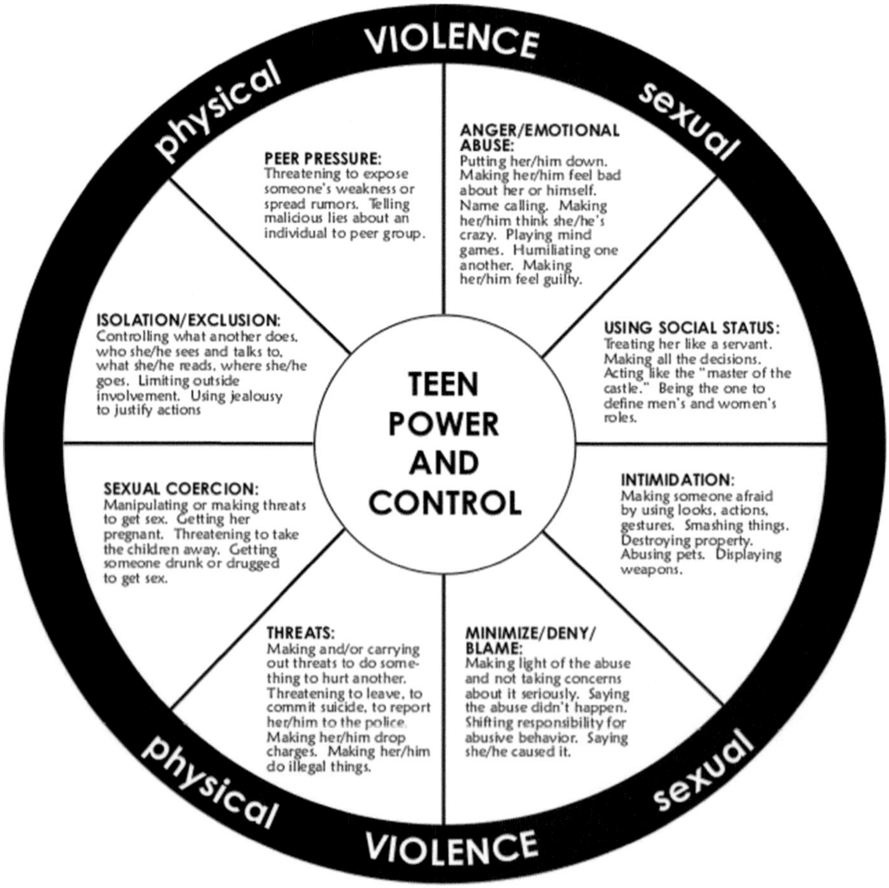

Fig. 86.1 The Teen Power and Control Wheel (Developed by the Domestic Abuse Intervention Project)

Extra Credit Points

1. Teen dating violence can impact any youth and teen girls and LGBTQ+ youth are at a higher risk of teen dating violence.
2. Teaching about healthy relationships and providing comprehensive health education can help to prevent incidents of teen dating violence.
3. Screening for teen dating violence is recommended for anyone 13 years or older.
4. When approaching a student with questions or conversations about teen dating violence, it is necessary to speak to the student alone and with a non-judgmental approach.
5. When discussing teen dating violence, speak to the student privately, be empathetic, and mirror their language throughout the conversation.

References

1. CDC. About teen dating violence. Intimate partner violence prevention. Published 22 May 2024. https://www.cdc.gov/intimate-partner-violence/about/about-teen-dating-violence.html.
2. Basile KC, Clayton HB, DeGue S, Gilford JW, Vagi KJ, Suarez NA, et al. Interpersonal violence victimization among high school students—youth risk behavior survey, United States, 2019. MMWR Suppl. 2020;69(1):28.
3. Walls NE, Atterberry-Ash B, Kattari SK, Peitzmeier S, et al. Gender identity, sexual orientation, mental health, and bullying as predictors of partner violence in a representative sample of youth. J Adolesc Health. 2019;64(1):86–92. https://doi.org/10.1016/j.jadohealth.2018.08.011.
4. Murray A, Azzinaro I. Teen dating violence: old disease in a new world. Clin Pediatr Emerg Med. 2019;20(1):25–37. https://doi.org/10.1016/j.cpem.2019.02.001. Developed from Domestic Abuse Intervention Project
5. Alpert E. 6th Edition Massachusetts Medical Society Committee on violence intervention and prevention intimate partner violence the clinician's guide to identification, assessment, intervention, and prevention. https://www.massmed.org/Patient-Care/Health-Topics/Violence-Intervention-and-Prevention/Intimate-Partner-Violence-(pdf)/.
6. Recognizing & responding to teen dating violence in the clinical setting. 2021. https://violence.chop.edu/sites/violence.chop.edu/files/documents/TDV%20Webinar%20Slides%20Final%20 5.19.21%20-%20download.pdf.
7. National Association of School Nurses. Comprehensive health education in schools [Position Statement]. 2022.
8. Youth.gov. Characteristics of healthy & unhealthy relationships. Youth.gov. Published 2011. https://youth.gov/youth-topics/teen-dating-violence/characteristics.
9. Ahern NR, Mechling B. Sexting: serious problems for youth. J Psychosoc Nurs Ment Health Serv. 2013;51(7):22–30. https://doi.org/10.3928/02793695-20130503-02.

Chapter 87
Visual and Hearing Impairments

Caroline Hayley Lee and Robert P. Olympia

87.1 Visual Impairments

Case 1 An 8-year-old boy presents with sudden vision loss in the left eye, described as a "dark curtain," along with flashes of light and shadows. He denies pain, redness, injury, or family history of eye issues. Examination shows reduced visual acuity, a relative afferent pupillary defect, and a pale retina in the left eye. Extraocular movements are intact. What is the most likely diagnosis and appropriate treatment?

Case 2 A 5-year-old boy complains about his ability to distinguish certain colors in class. His parents first noticed the issue when he had trouble identifying red and green objects during school activities. His teacher also reported that he struggles with color-based tasks, such as identifying traffic light colors during safety lessons. He has no vision complaints, eye pain, or headaches, and his development is otherwise normal. A family history of color vision deficiency is noted, as the maternal grandfather has similar difficulties. On examination, his visual acuity is 20/20 in both eyes, and the Ishihara test confirms red-green color deficiency. Fundoscopic exam is normal. What is the most likely diagnosis and appropriate treatment?

C. H. Lee
Penn State College of Medicine, Hershey, PA, USA
e-mail: clee14@pennstatehealth.psu.edu

R. P. Olympia (✉)
Department of Emergency Medicine and Pediatrics, Penn State College of Medicine
Attending Physician, Hershey, PA, USA

Division of Pediatric Emergency Medicine, Department of Emergency Medicine, Penn State
Milton S. Hershey Medical Center, Hershey, PA, USA
e-mail: rolympia@hmc.psu.edu

R. P. Olympia, J. Brady-Olympia (eds.), *Clinical Considerations in School-based Health*, https://doi.org/10.1007/978-3-031-85765-2_87

Children with visual impairment can present in multiple ways, which often depends on age and developmental stage. Much younger children may not have the skills or vocabulary to adequately express this problem. In this case, parents may notice behavioral changes including increased clumsiness, squinting, or avoidance of certain activities [1–3]. Older children may be better able to articulate and describe vision changes including blurry vision, double vision, or location in certain areas. They may be able to better report associated symptoms such as pain, sensitivity to light, headache, or neurological changes [1–3]. Despite the type of visual impairment, any issues with vision can significantly impact a child's daily activities, social interactions, and academic performance. Parents or teachers are often the first to notice changes associated with impaired vision. Understanding these presentations and being vigilant for signs of visual impairment are crucial for early diagnosis and intervention [1–3].

When encountering a student with acute visual impairment (vision loss or change in visual acuity), eye pain, or eye redness, a focused history and physical examination is an important first step (Table 87.1) [1–3]. Disposition and focused interventions are often based on your differential diagnosis (Tables 87.1 and 87.2) [1–3]. In general, a student with vision loss associated with trauma (Chap. 110), acute vision loss, complete vision loss, complaints of "flashers" or "floaters" (consistent with possible retinal detachment), significant eye pain, or vision impairments associated with other neurologic findings (severe headache, weakness or numbness or paresthesia, unsteady gait, etc.) should be evaluated in an emergency department with ophthalmology consultation services [4–6]. Table 87.3 lists behaviors in students that may indicate vision changes requiring non-emergent ophthalmology referrals [7, 8]. In students with chronic visual impairments, school health providers should be aware of their baseline vision ability and vision aiding devices utilized by these students (Table 87.4) [1–3, 9, 10]; changes in baseline vision ability should prompt an ophthalmology referral. A multidisciplinary approach involving parents, educators, and healthcare providers can help ensure timely and effective management of vision impairment in children.

Case 1 Resolution Retinal detachment of the left eye. Acute vision loss may be less common in children but is considered an ophthalmologic emergency. Concern for a retinal detachment requires prompt intervention to prevent permanent vision impairment with surgical treatment. Consequently, any child presenting with acute painless loss of vision in one eye should be taken to the emergency department for evaluation. Following treatment, patient should be monitored in multiple settings by school for vision changes.

Table 87.1 Focused history, assessment, and intervention of visual impairment in children [3–6]

Focused History	Focused Assessment	Focused Intervention
Onset of vision loss Duration of vision loss Unilateral or bilateral presentation Description of vision loss (entire vs. partial field, near vs. far vision loss, "blurry", color loss) Presence and location of pain Presence of any vision devices (glasses, contact lens) Presence of any specific eye symptoms (double vision, eyelid swelling, squinting, drainage, photophobia, itching, grittiness, photopsia) Presence of sick contacts Presence of allergies with specification of reaction History of treatment with eye drops recently History of visual impairment History of similar eye complaints (herpes simplex keratitis, allergic conjunctivitis, uveitis, corneal erosions) History of head or eye trauma History of poor academic performance or academic concerns History of unmet developmental milestones or concerns Family history of vision loss or associated syndromes Surgical history of cataract extraction, muscle surgery, glaucoma, or retina surgery Past medical history of sickle cell disease, thrombotic disorders, migraine headaches, partial seizures, and psychiatric illness	Vital signs Basic Vision Screening (object/pattern recognition, field of vision, contrast testing) Assessment of visual reflexes and red reflexes Assessment of visual motor ability Assessment of ocular motility Assessment of basic neurological status Direct funduscopic examination Presence of blood (hyphemia) or pus (hypopyon) in the anterior chamber Presence of proptosis Presence of conjunctival injection Presence of homonymous visual field abnormalities Presence of periorbital swelling or trauma Consultation with teacher/parents for observations of child in multiple settings	Sharing vision screening results with parents Suggest further evaluation by healthcare provider, primary care physician, Pediatric Ophthalmologist, Developmental-Behavioral Pediatricians, Low Vision Specialists Request follow up and directions/guidance from provider Adaptation of environmental factors to optimize vision in the classroom Provide appropriate lighting Provide orientation and mobility instruction and scanning techniques to help child navigate the classroom Keep sharp or harmful objects in an enclosed container Create a safe classroom environment with without floor clutter and free space to move around, can place tape to provide high contrast Implement sound and auditory cues to help children with vision impairments to help signal or transition student Implore technology with low vision optical devices Use braille resources/books, magnifies, and audio Directly supervising children by sight and sound

Table 87.2 Traumatic vs. non-traumatic causes of acute vision impairment in children [1–6]

Traumatic	Non-Traumatic
Periorbital: Eyelid Hematoma, Edema from Trauma	**Periorbital:** Orbital/Periorbital Cellulitis, Tumor, Allergic Edema
Cornea/Conjunctiva: Chemical Burns, Thermal Burns, UV or Infrared Burns, Laceration of Cornea	**Cornea/Conjunctiva**: Conjunctivitis (Bacterial, Viral, Fungal)
Anterior Chamber: Traumatic Iritis, Hyphemia, Post-Traumatic Cataract, Dislocation of Lens, Glaucoma	**Anterior Chamber:** Acute Iritis, Glaucoma, Uveitis
Posterior Chamber: Vitreous Hemorrhage	**Posterior Chamber**: Endophthalmitis
Retina: Severed Retinal Artery, Retinal Tears or Detachment, Commotio Retinae	**Retina:** Retinal Vein/Artery Obstruction
Cortex: Head Trauma	**Cortex:** Optic Neuritis, Toxins, Hysteria, Hypoglycemia, Leukemia, Cerebrovascular Accidents, Migraine, Multiple Sclerosis, Acute Disseminated, Encephalomyelitis, Meningitis, encephalitis, Seizures, Cerebral Venous Sinus Thrombosis, Idiopathic Intracranial Hypertension, Posterior Reversible Encephalopathy Syndrome
Other: Carotid Artery Trauma	**Other:** Poisoning, Ventricular Shunt Malfunction, Vitamin A Deficiency, Measles, Neoplasm

Table 87.3 Behaviors in children requiring ophthalmology referral due to possible visual impairment [7, 8]

Falls or Unintentional Injury: Children with vision impairments are at a greater risk for these injuries
Decreased Distance: Needs to have book/phone close to read or sits close to TV/screen
Reading Difficulty: Difficulty with reading and/or speech concerns
Abnormal Eye Movements: Eyes that move independently or uncoordinated
Light Sensitivity: Avoids bright lights or requiring certain light levels to complete tasks
Rubbing or Squinting Eyes Frequently: Rubbing or touching eyes frequently
Eye Contact Changes: Avoiding eye contact with others and situations that require high level of eye contact
Behavioral Changes: Increased frustration from tasks associated with visual difficulty and compensation

Case 2 Resolution Red-green color vision deficiency. Color vision deficiency typically does not require medical treatment but may require support in adapting to specific tasks, particularly in educational settings. Management strategies can include education on coping strategies for distinguishing colors, such as relying on labels, context, or patterns. Recommendation for non-color-based learning tools may help with some students.

Table 87.4 Vision aiding devices and technology [9, 10]

Vision Aiding Technology	Indication	Function
Magnifiers 1. Refracted Glasses 2. Spectacles 3. Stand Magnifiers 4. Hand-Held Magnifiers	**Any persons with visual impairment**	Devices that make objects appear larger and clearer
Braille Devices	**Any persons with visual impairment**	Tactile code used by visual impaired to read and write
Screen Readers 1. Computer Programs: Nonvisual Desktop Access (NVDA) & Job Access with Speech (JAWS) 2. Smart Phone Programs: TalkBack on Android & Voiceover on IOS	**Any persons with visual impairment** Particularly helpful for those who do not use Braille	Technology that converts text on screens into Braille or synthetic speech
White Canes 1. Long Canes 2. Identification Canes 3. Support Canes	**Any persons with visual impairment** **Long Canes:** Those who need to probe obstacles ahead on the ground to create a path **Identification Canes:** Those who do not always need to probe ahead, but want others to be aware of their visual impairment **Support Canes:** Designed for those who require extra stability, similar to walker	Allows person with visual impairment to act independently

87.2 Hearing Impairment

Case 3 A 7-year-old boy presents with sudden-onset ear pain and hearing loss after swimming. He reports worsening pain, ear discharge, and sensitivity when his ear is touched. He has a history of frequent ear infections and cerumen impactions. On examination, his outer ear is tender to touch, with redness, swelling, and yellow discharge in the ear canal obscuring the tympanic membrane. There is no fever or other systemic symptoms. What is the most likely diagnosis and appropriate treatment?

Case 4 A 10-year-old girl complains of a pounding headache and sensitivity to noise in the classroom. Her parents and teachers report ongoing difficulties with listening, following instructions, and understanding spoken language in noisy environments. She has a history of dyslexia and asthma but met developmental milestones. Hearing tests show normal hearing, while speech and language examinations reveal difficulty with auditory discrimination and following complex verbal instructions. What is the most likely diagnosis and appropriate intervention?

Acute hearing loss can be broken down into two main types, conductive and sensorineural. Conductive hearing loss typically occurs from dysfunction of the outer or middle ear, preventing the transmission of sound waves to the inner ear. This type of hearing loss affects the ability to hear faint sounds and interpret the loudness of sound, also known as the amplitude [1–3, 11, 12]. The most common cause of conductive hearing loss involves acute or chronic middle ear effusion from otitis media. Chronic or recurrent otitis media can also result in cholesteatoma, an epidermal inclusion cyst of the middle ear, which can cause a slowly progressive conductive hearing loss [1–3, 11, 12]. Other common causes seen in children include impacted cerumen, otitis externa, a foreign body located in the external ear canal, and perforation of the tympanic membrane from self-inflicted injury from objects like cotton swabs [1–3, 11, 12]. Acute head injury, such as basilar skull fractures, can also present with conductive hearing loss caused by hemotympanum, rupture of tympanic membrane, or disruption of inner ear ossicles [1–3, 11, 12]. Conductive hearing loss is rarely related to congenital malformations of the external or middle ear. This type of hearing loss is commonly responsive to amplification measures, such as hearing aids [1–3, 11, 12].

Sensorineural hearing loss is the other primary type of hearing loss and be further divided into congenital and acquired causes (Table 87.5) [1–3, 11, 13]. It occurs from dysfunction of the inner ear or auditory nerve, preventing neuronal transmission of auditory information to the brain. This type of hearing loss most commonly

Table 87.5 Causes of sensorineural hearing loss [1, 13]

Congenital or Neonatal	Acquired
Anatomic Abnormalities: Aplasia of Inner Ear, Abnormal Cochlear Development	**Bacterial Meningitis:** Streptococcus pneumoniae, Hemophilus influenzae, Neisseria meningitidis
Genetic Syndromes: Waardenburg Syndrome, Jervell and Lange Nielsen Syndrome, Usher Syndrome, Alport Syndrome	**Viral Labyrinthitis:** Measles, Mumps, Parainfluenza, Adenovirus, Herpes Simplex, CMV, Rubella, Rubeola
Chromosomal Abnormalities: Trisomy 13–15, Trisomy 18, Trisomy 21	**Intrauterine Infections:** CMV, Rubella, Syphilis, Toxoplasmosis, Herpes Simplex
Infections: TORCH, Congenital Syphilis	**Trauma:** Temporal Bone Fractures, Nose Induced Injury (Acute >120 dB, Chronic 80–100 dB), Barotrauma, Perilymphatic Fistula, Lightning Injury
Metabolic Causes: Hypothyroidism, Storage Disorders	**Tumor:** Acoustic Neuroma, CNS Tumors, Leukemic Infiltrates, Vestibular Schwannomas/Neurofibromatosis Type 2
Neonatal Causes: Birth Asphyxia, Extreme Prematurity, Kernicterus, Use of Ototoxic Drugs	**Miscellaneous:** Kawasaki Disease, Hypothyroidism, Hypoparathyroidism, Ototoxic Drugs, Hyperlipidemia, Hyperbilirubinemia, Acute Otitis Media, Autoimmune Disease, Functional Hearing Loss, Idiopathic

presents with difficulty understanding speech and distinguishing pitch, also known as frequency of sound. Frequency is measured in Hz, vowels have low frequency but a higher intensity than consonants, which are usually of a higher frequency and lower intensity [1–3, 11, 13]. Consequently, those with sensorineural hearing loss have may have difficulty comprehending only certain parts of words [1–3, 11, 13]. Congenital sensorineural hearing loss arises from genetic disorders, chromosomal abnormalities, metabolic and storage diseases, and abnormal development of auditory apparatus [1]. Approximately half of congenital sensorineural hearing loss is linked to a genetic cause and about one-third is considered syndromic [1]. More than 300 syndromes have been implicated including Branchio-Oto-Renal (BOR) Syndrome, CHARGE Syndrome, Waardenburg Syndrome, Jervell and Lange-Nielsen Syndrome, Usher Syndrome, and chromosomal disorders caused by trisomies (13 to 15, 18,21) [1]. Hearing loss can be present at birth or develop over time. Acquired sensorineural hearing loss is less common than congenital pathology (Table 87.5) [1–3, 13]. The absence of associated symptoms can make it a more difficult diagnosis. It typically presents in late childhood and can result from different causes including inner ear infections, autoimmune disorders, trauma, or tumors [1–3, 13]. Mixed hearing loss may also occur with components of both sensorineural and conductive hearing loss. With this presentation, the outer, middle, and inner ear are most likely affected [1–3, 13].

Regardless of the underlying cause, early identification of hearing impairment is crucial for a student's ability to communicate effectively and achieve academic success. Even mild hearing impairments can have significant educational and medical implications. Mild to moderate hearing loss in young students is often subtle and can easily go unnoticed, as its effects may not always manifest as clear language delays [1–3]. Instead, students may display other signs of hearing loss, such as hypersensitivity to sound, frequent complaints about classroom noise, or headaches. School health providers are often the first to encounter students experiencing sudden hearing loss or a gradual decline in hearing ability. Many school nurses are trained to perform initial screenings and can play a key role in early detection. By identifying hearing impairments early, school nurses can advocate for timely referrals to primary care physicians, pediatric otolaryngologists, audiologist, speech language therapies, education specialists, and interventions, helping to address and remediate these issues effectively [1–3, 11].

When encountering a student with acute hearing impairment, a focused history and physical examination is an important first step (Table 87.6) [3]. Disposition and focused interventions are often based on your differential diagnosis (Table 87.6) [1, 11–13]. In general, a student with hearing loss associated with trauma or hearing impairments associated with other neurologic findings (severe headache, weakness or numbness or paresthesia, etc.) should be evaluated in an emergency department. Table 87.7 lists behaviors in children requiring non-emergent otolaryngology/audiology referral due to possible hearing impairment. In students with chronic hearing impairments, school health providers should be aware of their baseline hearing ability and hearing loss technology utilized by these students (Table 87.8); changes in baseline hearing ability

Table 87.6 Focused history, assessment, and intervention of hearing impairment in children [3, 11–13]

Focused History	Focused Assessment	Focused Intervention
Onset of hearing loss Duration of hearing loss Unilateral or bilateral presentation Description of hearing loss (muffled, ringing, popping sounds) Presence and location of pain Presence of fever and otalgia (acute otitis media or externa) Presence of tinnitus, vertigo, dizziness (inner ear disease or central nervous system involvement) Presence of headache (tumor of central nervous system or middle ear infection) Presence of any hearing devices History of otitis, hearing loss, cerumen, upper respiratory infection History of barotrauma (e.g. scuba diving, plane, peri lymphatic fistula) History of noise exposure at school or play; use of ear buds for listening to music History of birth asphyxia, prematurity, hyperbilirubinemia, or maternal infection History of head trauma History of poor academic performance or academic concerns History of unmet developmental milestones or concerns Family history of hearing loss or associated syndromes Surgical history of myringotomy tubes Medication history	Vital signs Review of Systems: dizziness, neurological deficits, impaired balance, tinnitus, vision impairment, headache, cough, shortness of breath, nasal congestion, or sinus pressure/pain Ear Assessment: trauma, external ear canal drainage/bleeding, foreign body, cerumen, tenderness of mastoid/external ear, or swelling/redness Otoscopic examination: middle ear effusion, perforated tympanic membrane, foreign body, impacted cerumen, external auditory canal effusion, or abnormality of tympanic membrane Basic Hearing Screening Consultation with teacher and observation of student in classroom setting- tilting of head towards speaker, frequent request to repeat questions	Sharing hearing screening results with parents Speech, language, and auditory training Suggest further evaluation by healthcare provider or audiologist Captioned films, videos, and DVDs Request follow up and directions/guidance from provider (Audiologist, Otolaryngology, primary care physician) Arrange classroom accommodations such as preferential seating to facilitate lip reading, decreased ambient noise, note taker Educate students about how noise and personal listening devices can affect ability to hear, volume should be audible but not loud Discuss sources of loud noise at home, school, or work, and how to protect against Initiate measures to address noise in the school, such as gym, machinery or band Counseling services Alternative communication methods and devices Interpreter services for students using sign language

Table 87.7 Behaviors requiring otolaryngology/audiology referral due to possible hearing impairment [14, 15]

Speech Delays: Delayed language skills, abnormal speech, speech milestones unmet
Attention Issues: Difficulty paying attention/concentration, inattentiveness, distractibility
No Response to Name: No or delayed response to calling child's name
Background Noise: Difficulty hearing over background noise or talking on phone
Increased Volume: Listening to music or TV at very high volume
Communication Breakdown: Easy frustrated, or falling behind in communication skills, difficulty keeping up with group conversations

should prompt an otolaryngology/audiology referral [1–3, 14–20]. A multidisciplinary approach involving parents, educators, and healthcare providers can help ensure timely and effective management of hearing impairment in children.

Case 3 Resolution Otitis Externa. Start with immediate care of ear by cleaning out ear canal to remove excess discharge and debris if possible. Can consider applying a warm compress to alleviate pain and swelling. Treat patient with topical antibiotic drops (Ofloxacin, Ciprofloxacin) and recommend over the counter pain relievers such as Ibuprofen. Advise follow up with his primary care physician in 1–2 weeks to assess improvement and ensure resolution of infection. Also advise him to keep his ear dry, avoid inserting objects into the ear canal while recovering, and thoroughly dry his ear after swimming in the future.

Case 4 Resolution Auditory Processing Disorder (APD). Her difficulties with understanding and processing spoken language, despite normal hearing, are suggestive of APD. APD is characterized by challenges in the processing of auditory information in the central nervous system. This can lead to issues with distinguishing sounds, following directions, and understanding speech in noisy environments.

Extra-Credit Points

1. When encountering a student with acute visual or hearing impairment, a focused history and physical examination is an important first step.
2. Acute vision loss in a child may be related to traumatic and non-traumatic causes.
3. Acute hearing loss can be broken down into two main types, conductive and sensorineural.
4. A multidisciplinary approach involving parents, educators, and healthcare providers (including ophthalmologists, otolaryngologists, and audiologists) can help ensure timely and effective management of visual and hearing impairment in children.

Table 87.8 Hearing loss devices and technology [1–3, 16–20]

Hearing Aiding Technology	Indication	Function
Hearing Aids 1. Behind-the-ear (BTE) 2. In-the-ear (ITE) 3. Receiver-in-the-ear (RITE) 4. In-the-canal (ITC) 5. CROS/BiCROS	**Mild-Severe Sensorineural Hearing Loss** 1. **BTE:** Often for young children since it can accommodate various ear mold tubing, also study and easy to clean 2. **ITE:** Larger aids, may be easier to handle compared to smaller aids 3. **RITE:** Typically, smaller in size, can reduce occlusion effect with increased comfort 4. **ITC:** Smallest aids available, but small size makes them hard to handle and adjust for some	Amplifies sound using built in microphone with receiver that delivers amplified sound into ear canal Improved tinnitus Improved hearing clarity Improve speech comprehension
Cochlear Implant 1. External Sound Processer Behind Ear 2. External Sound Processer Over Ear 3. External Sound Processer on Scalp	**Severe-Profound Sensorineural Hearing Loss** Typically, those who do not benefit from traditional hearing aids Often put in both ears at the same time in children with hearing loss to prevent speech/developmental delays Cochlear implants work better often in patients who knew how to read/speak before hearing loss	Surgically implant device that directly stimulates auditory nerve Improved tinnitus Improved hearing clarity
Cochlear Hybrid Hearing	**Severe-Profound High Frequency Hearing Loss** with Normal-Moderate Low Frequency Hearing Loss Also referred to as “Ski Slope” hearing loss	Combination of hearing aid and cochlear implant, amplification of natural low-frequency hearing Improvement in understanding consonants Improvement of hearing clarity Improvement of high-frequency sounds
Electro-Acoustic Stimulation (EAS)	**Severe-Profound High Frequency Hearing Loss** Similar to Cochlear Hybrid Hearing	Combination of hearing aid and cochlear implant Improved high- and low-pitched sounds Improved sound localization Reduced listening efforts

(continued)

Table 87.8 (continued)

Hearing Aiding Technology	Indication	Function
Bone-Anchored Auditory Implant (BAI) 1. Surgical Implantable Bone Anchored Hearing Aids (BAHA) 2. Nonsurgical Bone Conduction Hearing Aids (BCHA)	**Conductive Hearing Loss** or **Single-Sided Deafness** Restore partial hearing in those that aren't good candidates for hearing aids Does not require any device in the ear canal **BAHA:** Processer can be removed as desired **BCHA:** Recommended typically for children under 5 years old and those who do not wish surgery	Surgically implanted device that sends sound as vibrations directly to best functioning ear Improved hearing clarity
Assistive Listening Devices 1. FM Systems 2. Infrared Systems 3. Audio Induction Loops 4. Personal Amplified Systems 5. Bluetooth Systems	**Anyone with hearing assistive devices**, allows better adaptability of technology to acoustics of different environments	Assistive listening systems and devices used to eliminate effects of distance, background noise, and reverberation in those with hearing technology
Telecommunication Products & Services	**Anyone with hearing or speech difficulties** requiring assistance placing or receiving telephone calls	Enable students with hearing loss to type phone messages over a telephone network known as Telecommunication Relay Services to connect with a communication assistant to help with phone call communication
Speech-To-Text-Reporters	**Anyone with hearing difficulties** requiring communication support	Service that transcribes spoken words into written text, text appears in real time on technology to be read

References

1. Shaw KN, Bachur RG, Chamberlain JM, Lavelle J, Nagler J, Shook JE. Fleisher & Ludwig's textbook of pediatric emergency medicine. Wolters Kluwer; 2021.
2. Donoghue EA, Kraft CA, American Academy of Pediatrics. Managing chronic health needs in child care and schools: a quick reference guide. American Academy of Pediatrics; 2019.
3. Selekman J, Shannon RA, Yonkaitis CF. School nursing: a comprehensive text. 3rd ed. F. A. Davis Company; 2019.
4. Sudden vision loss: common causes & treatments. Cleveland clinic. https://my.clevelandclinic.org/health/symptoms/24803-sudden-vision-loss.
5. Childhood Eye Diseases and Conditions. Childhood eye diseases and conditions. American Academy of Ophthalmology. Published November 2013. https://www.aao.org/eye-health/tips-prevention/common-childhood-diseases-conditions.

6. Vision Problems | Boston Children's Hospital. www.childrenshospital.org. https://www.childrenshospital.org/conditions/vision-problems.
7. Red Flags Vision Checklist. Child development programs. https://www.childdevelopmentprograms.ca/vision/program-information/red-flags-vision-checklist/.
8. Know the Red Flags and Risk Factors RED FLAGS: VISION. https://www.nationaldb.org/media/doc/M1L1_Red_Flags_Risk_Factors_a.pdf.
9. Low Vision Assistive Devices. Low vision assistive devices. American Academy of Ophthalmology. Published February 25, 2019. https://www.aao.org/eye-health/diseases/low-vision-assistive-devices.
10. Lewis V. A to Z of assistive technology for low vision. Perkins School for the Blind. https://www.perkins.org/resource/z-assistive-technology-low-vision/.
11. Zahnert T. The differential diagnosis of hearing loss. Deutsches Aerzteblatt Online. 2011;108(25) https://doi.org/10.3238/arztebl.2011.0433.
12. Sooriyamoorthy T, De Jesus O. Conductive hearing loss. PubMed. Published August 23, 2023. https://www.ncbi.nlm.nih.gov/books/NBK563267/.
13. Tanna RJ, Lin JW, De Jesus O. Sensorineural hearing loss. PubMed. Published August 23, 2023. https://www.ncbi.nlm.nih.gov/books/NBK565860/.
14. Marino B. Red flags for hearing loss in toddlers – Southwestern Hearing Centers. Southwestern Hearing. Published January 30, 2021. Accessed 13 Oct 2024. https://www.southwesternhearing.com/red-flags-for-hearing-loss-in-toddlers/.
15. 125395. Position Statement: Red Flags-Warning of Ear Disease. American Academy of Otolaryngology-Head and Neck Surgery (AAO-HNS). https://www.entnet.org/resource/position-statement-red-flags-warning-of-ear-disease/.
16. National Institute on Deafness and other Communication Disorders. Hearing Aids. NIDCD. Published October 11, 2022. https://www.nidcd.nih.gov/health/hearing-aids.
17. ASHA. Hearing Assistive Technology. Asha.org. Published 2009. https://www.asha.org/public/hearing/Hearing-Assistive-Technology/.
18. Hearing Loss Association of America. Hearing assistive technology – hearing loss Association of America. Hearing Loss Association of America. Published 2017. https://www.hearingloss.org/hearing-help/technology/hat/.
19. Cleveland Clinic. Hearing aids: uses & how they work. Cleveland Clinic. Published February 21, 2023. https://my.clevelandclinic.org/health/treatments/24756-hearing-aids.
20. Mayo Clinic. Cochlear implants – Mayo clinic. Mayoclinic.org. Published May 10, 2022. https://www.mayoclinic.org/tests-procedures/cochlear-implants/about/pac-20385021.

Part VI
Infectious Disease Emergencies

Chapter 88
Septic Shock

Sandra Schumacher, Sarah Meyers, and Jeffrey Campbell

There are four major types of shock: cardiogenic, obstructive, hypovolemic, and distributive (the most common type). There are three types of distributive shock, also known as vasodilatory shock: anaphylactic, neurogenic, and septic (the most frequent type of distributive shock). All types of shock are medical emergencies. In distributive shock, the blood vessels become extremely dilated, which lowers the blood pressure and decreases how much blood flows through vital organs such as the heart, brain, and kidneys. Often the capillaries become leaky as well, resulting in fluid loss into interstitial body spaces. Unless treated early, septic shock typically is fatal.

In compensated shock, an individual can maintain blood pressure by increasing the heart rate and contractility, and by constricting the peripheral blood vessels. However, as shock worsens, the body is unable to maintain perfusion of vital organs through these compensatory mechanisms. Decompensated shock includes falling blood pressure. Normal systolic blood pressure is above 90 mmHg for an older child. For a child 1–10 years old, the minimal systolic is determined by 70 + (2 × age [in years]) mmHg.

Case 1 Ramit is a high school junior who was sent to the school nurse's office after he asked his math teacher if he could be excused, saying, "I think I might be getting the flu." He tells you he was feeling "totally normal" this weekend, and even went on a long hiking trip with his brother, but suddenly was nauseated and vomited in the bathroom today. He endorses multiple abrasions during the hike. He also thinks he "must have gotten a little sunburned" on the

S. Schumacher (✉)
Boston Children's Hospital, Boston, MA, USA
e-mail: sandra.schumacher@childrens.harvard.edu

S. Meyers · J. Campbell
Boston Medical Center, Boston, MA, USA
e-mail: sarah.meyers@bmc.org; jeffrey.campbell@bmc.org

R. P. Olympia, J. Brady-Olympia (eds.), *Clinical Considerations in School-based Health*, https://doi.org/10.1007/978-3-031-85765-2_88

hike, since he has noticed a red rash developing across his body. Ramit's vital signs are notable for a temperature of 102.3 °F, pulse of 122, and blood pressure of 95/62. What would you do?

Toxic shock syndrome (TSS) is a life-threatening syndrome that results from infection with a superantigen toxin-producing strain of bacteria, usually *Staphylococcus aureus* or *Streptococcus pyogenes* (Group A Streptococcus), which causes severe inflammation leading to fever, rash, hypotension, and eventually multi-organ failure due to inadequate tissue perfusion [1]. Clinical findings that should raise suspicion for TSS include fever, hypotension, diffuse erythroderma (sunburn-like rash), vomiting, diarrhea, myalgias, and mucous membrane involvement [2]. Though TSS has classically been associated with tampon use, soft tissue infection, such as from an abrasion, is a common source [1].

Because toxic shock syndrome can initially present as an influenza-like illness [3], it is easily missed by providers; however, early recognition is crucial. The clinical features of TSS are like that of severe sepsis, Rocky Mountain spotted fever, leptospirosis, measles, Kawasaki disease, multisystem inflammatory syndrome in children (MIS-C), adenovirus, and drug reactions [3]. For cases of TSS in which the focus of infection is a foreign body (e.g., tampon, nasal packing, wound packing, intrauterine device), the foreign body should be promptly removed [3]. Empiric antibiotic therapy usually consists of a beta-lactam antibiotic with the addition of vancomycin for MRSA coverage and clindamycin for its ability to inhibit toxin production [4]. TSS can progress rapidly, so the school-based health professional must keep this diagnosis in mind for any student presenting with high fevers, flu-like illness, and diffuse rash.

Case 2 Stephen is a 6-year-old with sickle cell disease who presents to the school nursing office with cough and headache. You find that he is febrile at 102 °F, his pulse is 140, and his blood pressure is 80/30. He does not have a history of infections related to sickle cell. He has been appropriately vaccinated against *Streptococcus pneumoniae*, *Haemophilus influenza*, and *Neisseria meningitidis*. He took amoxicillin prophylaxis until he turned 5 years old. What are your next steps?

Stephen is presenting with sepsis from *Streptococcus pneumoniae* bacteremia. Sickle cell disease leads to immune dysfunction (primarily through splenic dysfunction early in childhood), and children with sickle cell disease are at increased risk of infection from bacteria and viruses. Before the introduction of vaccination and antibiotic prophylaxis, children with sickle cell disease were 400 times more likely to develop invasive pneumococcal disease than children without sickle cell disease [5]. *Streptococcus pneumoniae*, *Haemophilus influenzae*, *Salmonella* species, *Escherichia coli*, and *Staphylococcus aureus* are among the most common bacteria causing severe infections in children with sickle cell disease [6], and these children are also at increased risks of complications from viral infections including influenza, COVID-19, and parvovirus B19. Vaccination of children with sickle cell disease is critical to decrease the risk of vaccine-preventable illnesses. However, the risk of sepsis from bacteria and viruses remains elevated even in fully vaccinated children with sickle cell disease [7]. For these children, fever may be the only symptom of a severe infection that can quickly progress to sepsis and shock, and prompt evaluation and initiation of empiric antibiotics is critical for all children with sickle cell disease, regardless of vaccination status. Antibiotics should be administered after blood cultures have been obtained but ideally within 60 min of initial evaluation.

Children with sickle cell disease represent a fraction of the large population of children with immunocompromising conditions in the United States. An estimated 1/1200 people in the US have a primary (genetic) immunodeficiency [8], and up to 3% of adults in the United States are estimated to have either a primary or secondary immunodeficiency [9]. Children with immunodeficiencies are often able to participate in typical childhood activities and attend school. Thus, clinicians practicing in schools must be aware of these children's increased risk for infection incidence and severity. It is critical to recognize early signs of infection, sepsis, and shock in these children so that they can be quickly evaluated and started on appropriate antibiotic therapy. Table 88.1 lists some causes of immunodeficiency among children.

Case 3 Susan is a 16-year-old female who was in her usual healthy state until last night when she developed a headache. She woke up with a continued headache yet went to school, but during her first class she became very warm and was not able to focus on her studies. She went to the school's nursing office where she began vomiting, appeared to have a stiff neck, and seemed confused. Susan was febrile and tachycardic with a normal respiratory rate and somewhat lower blood pressure. The nurse was concerned about potential meningitis, so he immediately called for an ambulance. When the medical personnel

Table 88.1 Causes of immunodeficiency in children

Causes	Examples
Primary (genetic) immunodeficiencies	• Severe combined immunodeficiency (SCID) • Common variable immunodeficiency (CVID)
Infections	• HIV • Measles
Medications	• High dose/chronic steroids • Chemotherapy • Immunomodulators (e.g., for auto-immune disorders)
Conditions that impair immune function	• Cancers (e.g., leukemia) • Nutritional disorders (e.g., protein-losing enteropathy, malnutrition) • Nephropathy • Splenic dysfunction/splenectomy • Stress
Impaired barriers/opportunities for pathogens to enter and thrive	• Indwelling devices (e.g., long-term central lines, cardiac implanted devices) • Need for frequent intravenous medications • Burns • Severe diabetes

arrived to take Susan to the hospital, the nurse noticed Susan had developed a petechial rash on her legs as well.

Septic shock is associated with an infection. In Susan's case, she had meningitis with the classic triad of sudden fever, neck stiffness, and altered mental status. Specifically, she had *Neisseria meningitidis,* which can be associated with a petechial rash on the abdomen or legs that quickly disseminates, becoming purpuric (purpura fulminans) and even necrotic. Early, proper antibiotic treatment is crucial. According to the Centers for Disease Control and Prevention (CDC), even with treatment, about 10–15 out of 100 people with meningococcal disease will die from it. If meningococcal infection is suspected outside a hospital setting, many experts suggest giving intramuscular ceftriaxone if the patient cannot be transferred within an hour to the hospital. However, transfer to the hospital should never be delayed for antibiotic administration. Intravenous fluids and pressor support are needed to maintain perfusion.

Neisseria meningitidis is a gram-negative diplococcus bacterium with 13 serogroups (the most common being A, B, C, W, X, and Y) based on capsular type. Spread occurs by large respiratory droplets or direct contact with respiratory droplets. Up to 10% of the general population carries the bacteria in their nose and throat without any adverse effects. It is exclusively a human pathogen, and is the main cause of bacterial meningitis in children and young adults. The incubation period is usually 4 days, with a range of 1–10 days. *Neisseria meningitidis* has a world-wide distribution and is particularly prominent in the meningitis belt of sub-Saharan Africa. The annual incidence of meningococcal disease in the US is decreasing, with 210 cases in 2021 per CDC data, but we must remain vigilant of this seasonal disease that typically peaks in the winter months in the US. Living in crowded areas such as dormitories, household contacts, functional asplenia, and complement deficiencies are risk factors.

Vaccination is a key means of preventing *Neisseria meningitidis*. There are three types of meningococcal vaccines in the US: meningococcal conjugate or MenACWY vaccines, serogroup B meningococcal or MenB vaccines, and pentavalent meningococcal or MenABCWY vaccine. The CDC recommends:

1. Routine MenACWY vaccination for all teens at 11–12 years with a booster dose at 16 years old. Children and adults at increased risk for meningococcal disease should also receive this vaccine.
2. MenB vaccination for people 10 years or older at increased risk of meningococcal disease.
3. MenABCWY vaccination as an option for people 10 years or older who are getting MenACWY and MenB vaccines at the same visit [10].

88.1 Case Conclusions

Case 1 Ramit is transferred to the local emergency department, where he becomes hypotensive to 68/42, requiring aggressive fluid resuscitation. He is started on broad-spectrum antibiotics and admitted to the ICU. After a few days of treatment, his vital signs have stabilized, and he is able to be discharged home on oral antibiotics. A week after his initial presentation, he has returned to school, and returns to your office because "my skin is peeling." His vital signs are normal, and he is otherwise feeling well. You explain that desquamation, or peeling of the skin, is a common feature of toxic shock syndrome and can occur up to 1–2 weeks after the onset of acute illness.

Case 2 Stephen is quickly transferred to a local hospital, where he receives rapid fluid boluses and ceftriaxone, vancomycin, and azithromycin. A chest X-ray shows a right-sided consolidation and blood cultures grow Streptococcus pneumoniae. Blood cultures clear after 24 h, and Stephen's clinical status stabilizes. Vancomycin is stopped, and he completes a 7-day course of ceftriaxone for pneumococcal bacteremia, as well as a 5-day course of azithromycin for acute chest syndrome.

Case 3 Susan is emergently transferred to the intensive care unit of her nearby hospital and placed on standard and droplet precautions for the first day of antibiotic therapy to avoid potential infectious spread to others. She is treated with fluid resuscitation, pressure support with medications, and ceftriaxone for a week and gradually improves. Postexposure chemoprophylaxis is given to her household contacts. She is grateful to be alive thanks in part to your quick recognition of septic shock and meningitis.

Extra Credit Points

1. Septic shock is associated with an infection and is a medical emergency requiring antibiotics and often pressure support as soon as possible.
2. Toxic shock syndrome is associated with Staphylococcal and Streptococcal infections and should be considered especially in a child with fever, hypotension, and a sunburn-like rash. TSS was classically associated with high absorbency tampon use until these were taken off the market, and now is more common with soft tissue infection.
3. Immunocompromised individuals are most at risk of infection and septic shock. Sickle cell disease is an example of those who must be considered high risk for infection and treated conservatively and emergently with antimicrobials if infection is possible.
4. Meningococcal disease is a medical emergency requiring antibiotics. Vaccination can help prevent this life-threatening illness.

References

1. Wilkins AL, Steer AC, Smeesters PR, Curtis N. Toxic shock syndrome—the seven Rs of management and treatment. J Infect. 2017;74(Suppl 1):S147–52. https://doi.org/10.1016/S0163-4453(17)30206-2.
2. Centers for Disease Control and Prevention. Toxic shock syndrome (other than streptococcal) (TSS): 2011 case definition. 2011. https://ndc.services.cdc.gov/case-definitions/toxic-shock-syndrome-2011/. Last Accessed 29 Mar 2024.
3. Gottlieb M, Long B, Koyfman A. The evaluation and management of toxic shock syndrome in the emergency department: a review of the literature. J Emerg Med. 2018;54(6):807–14. https://doi.org/10.1016/j.jemermed.2017.12.048.
4. Gaensbauer J, Nomura Y. Infections: bacterial & spirochetal. In: Bunik M, Hay WW, Levin MJ, Abzug MJ, editors. Current diagnosis & treatment: pediatrics. 26th ed. New York: McGraw-Hill Education; 2022.
5. Overturf GD, Powars D, Baraff LJ. Bacterial meningitis and septicemia in sickle cell disease. Am J Dis Child. 1977;131(7):784–7. https://doi.org/10.1001/archpedi.1977.02120200066014.
6. Gaschignard J, Koehl B, Rees DC, Rincon-Lopez E, Vanderfaeillie A, Pascault A, et al. Invasive bacterial infections in children with sickle cell disease: 2014-2019. Pediatrics. 2023;152(4) https://doi.org/10.1542/peds.2022-061061.
7. Ochocinski D, Dalal M, Black LV, Carr S, Lew J, Sullivan K, et al. Life-threatening infectious complications in sickle cell disease: a concise narrative review. Front Pediatr. 2020;8:38. https://doi.org/10.3389/fped.2020.00038.
8. Boyle JM, Buckley RH. Population prevalence of diagnosed primary immunodeficiency diseases in the United States. J Clin Immunol. 2007;27(5):497–502. https://doi.org/10.1007/s10875-007-9103-1.
9. Harpaz R, Dahl RM, Dooling KL. Prevalence of immunosuppression among US adults, 2013. JAMA. 2016;316(23):2547–8. https://doi.org/10.1001/jama.2016.16477.
10. American Academy of Pediatrics Committee on Infectious Diseases, Kimberlin DW, Barnett ED, Lynfield R, Sawyer MH. Meningococcal infections. Red Book: 2021–2024 report of the committee on infectious diseases. American Academy of Pediatrics; 2021. p. 519–32.

Chapter 89
Meningitis and Encephalitis

James M. McCluskey III and Alice I. Sato

Case 1 During June, an otherwise healthy 8-year-old boy was brought to the school nurse for headache and making comments that did not make sense. The teacher noted he was not interested in his lunch and kept his head down. He had been disengaged throughout the morning lessons and had a new tremor when attempting to write. On examination, he had a fever of 101.3°F (38.5°C), but otherwise normal vital signs. In addition to noting his coarse bilateral hand tremor, he closed his eyes and pulled away when checking his pupillary reflex (photophobia). He had worsening of his headache and neck discomfort with touching his chin to his chest (nuchal rigidity). He had a faint maculopapular rash over his chest and upper back. The boy was slow to respond to questions and answered with only single words that weren't relevant to the question asked. He retreated to laying down on the cot and closing his eyes. What are the most important next steps of management for this student?

Triage The differential diagnosis for a headache in an otherwise healthy school aged child is broad, but quickly narrows in the presence of a fever, nuchal rigidity, photophobia, and rash—classic signs of **meningitis** (inflammation of the meninges surrounding the central nervous system [CNS]). The classic triad of fever, stiff neck, and a change in mental status occurs in less than half of patients with meningitis, and the use of other classic findings like Kernig and Brudzinski signs are falling out of favor [1]. However, this boy also has signs of inflammation of the brain parenchyma, (**encephalitis**), given his abnormal behavior and tremor. Combining the two, his symptomology is consistent with **meningoencephalitis**. All of these conditions are an emergency and should be triaged as such. This child should be sent to the closest emergency department (ED) for further evaluation, especially given his

J. M. McCluskey III (✉) · A. I. Sato
The University of Nebraska Medical Center, Omaha, NE, USA
e-mail: alice.sato@unmc.edu

R. P. Olympia, J. Brady-Olympia (eds.), *Clinical Considerations in School-based Health*, https://doi.org/10.1007/978-3-031-85765-2_89

encephalopathy. There are many complications that can develop from meningitis or encephalitis, including but not limited to seizures, vision or hearing issues, acute flaccid myelitis, and permanent cognitive impairments. Prompt specific antimicrobial treatment and support can save brain function, organ function and life. Emergency medical service activation may be needed.

Case 1 Continued *The school nurse contacts the child's care givers. They state that while he was fine yesterday, but this morning, he did seem especially tired. There were no known recent sick contacts, but family had just returned from a camping trip at a local state park the previous week. He is up to date on all recommended vaccinations for age. His care givers are nearby and will promptly take him to the ED.*

Precautions and Isolation After triaging the student, precautions should be considered. Meningitis and encephalitis are most frequently infectious in etiology and similar agents can be responsible for both conditions. Most are viral or bacterial infections, with fungal or parasitic occurring rarely (Table 89.1). Worldwide, the most common cause of meningitis is non-polio enteroviruses acquired via respiratory secretions or fecal-oral routes [3]. General precautions should be initiated, including mask wearing for those in close contact, hand washing, and the cleaning of surfaces that may contain fomites. If possible, the student should be placed in a room with the door closed and with enhanced ventilation and/or high efficiency particulate air (HEPA) filtration.

Vaccination Status Vaccination is a means of preventing selected types of meningitis and encephalitis. Vaccination history can help risk stratify not only the student, but also their contacts. Prior to 1990, one study suggested that *Haemophilus influenzae* (Hib) meningitis was a leading cause of postnatally acquired developmental disabilities [4]. Implementing vaccines against Hib in 1990, *Streptococcus pneumoniae* in 2000, and *Neisseria meningitidis* ACYW in 2005, have since significantly decreased cases. However, *S. pneumoniae* and *N. meningitidis* remain the leading causes of bacterial meningitis [1]. In Case 1, the student is up to date on all recommended vaccinations for his age, thus he is likely to be protected against Hib and *S. pneumoniae* as well as viral causes such as measles and varicella [2]. However, the two *N. meningitidis* vaccines (against serotypes ACYW-135 and B) are not typically recommended until 11–12 years of age, leaving him at risk [2, 5]. School vaccination records can assist in determining which students and school staff are at highest risk.

Case 1 Conclusion In the ED, lumbar puncture (LP) was performed prior to the child being admitted to the hospital. He gradually improved and was discharged on hospital day 5 after his cerebral spinal fluid (CSF) bacterial culture remained negative and his CSF IgM antibody testing for West Nile virus was positive. The patient returned to school the day following his discharge from the hospital. The teacher brought him to the school nurse again, stating that he was again complaining of a

Table 89.1 Clinically relevant characteristics of meningitis and encephalitis

Etiology	Examples of specific organisms	Route of transmission	Clinical signs and symptoms	Diagnostic testing	Treatment[a]
Bacterial	*Streptococcus pneumoniae*, *Neisseria meningitidis*, *Haemophilus influenzae type b (Hib)*	Respiratory droplets, secretions, or surfaces contaminated with these	Fever, headache, nuchal rigidity, photophobia, maculopapular rash that becomes petechial or purpuric (meningococcemia)	LP with culture, CSF analysis, CSF PCR	Ceftriaxone plus vancomycin with final antibiotic selection tailored to culture and susceptibility results **Duration**: *S. pneumoniae*: 10–14 days Hib: 7–10 days *N. meningitidis*: 5–7 days Dexamethasone for Hib meningitis.
Viral	Enteroviruses, Herpes Simplex Virus (HSV), Epstein-Barr virus (EBV), West Nile virus (WNV), Influenza	Respiratory droplet (HSV and EBV), fecal-oral (enteroviruses), Mosquito/ vector borne (WNV)	Fever, headache, nuchal rigidity, photophobia, maculopapular rash, vesiculopapular rash (HSV)	LP, CSF analysis, CSF PCR, MRI (temporal lobe involvement [HSE])	Supportive care Acyclovir for HSE (21 days)
Spirochete (Lyme)	*Borrelia burgdorferi*	Tick/vector borne	Fever, headache, nuchal rigidity, photophobia, erythema migrans, facial palsy	LP CSF analysis, CSF PCR and serology	Doxycycline or ceftriaxone for 14–21 days
Fungal	*Candida albicans*, *Cryptococcus neoformans*, *C. gattii*	Inhalation of spores	Fever, headache, nuchal rigidity, photophobia, seizures, confusion, lethargy, elevated opening pressure	LP with culture, CSF analysis, CSF PCR, and serology	**Induction**: Amphotericin B with flucytosine for ≥2 weeks **Consolidation**: Fluconazole for ≥8 weeks

CSF cerebrospinal fluid, *EBV* Epstein-Barr virus, *Hib Haemophilus influenzae*, *HSE* herpes simplex virus encephalitis, *HSV* herpes simplex virus, *IV* intravenous, *LP* lumbar puncture, *MRI* magnetic resonance imaging, *PCR* polymerase chain reaction, *WNV* West Nile virus

Information adapted from *Red Book: 33rd edition* [2]

[a] General guidance for typical treatments, however there may be other comorbidities and/or complications that lead to differing treatments

headache and was frequently "zoning out" during class. On this evaluation he had a completely normal physical examination but was endorsing a headache.

Return to School This student was ultimately diagnosed with West Nile virus (WNV) meningoencephalitis. WNV is an emerging cause of vector-borne viral meningitis or encephalitis and is found nationwide [2]. This student likely acquired his infection while camping when an infected female *Culex* mosquito had their bloodmeal from him. Fortunately for his classmates, WNV, like most other vector-borne viruses, does not spread person-to-person. Although this student is improving, he continues to experience symptoms that were not present prior to his infection. Returning to school for a student recovering from meningitis or encephalitis should have many considerations, for simplicity we will organize these into three categories: treatment, accommodations, and follow-up.

Treatment First is ensuring that students complete their recommended treatment. Many students with CNS infections will require antimicrobial therapy for 5–21 days or longer (Table 89.1). Fortunately, most viral meningitis cases require only supportive care, though there are exceptions. Students requiring longer intravenous (IV) therapy may return to school with a midline extended dwell catheter ("midline") or a peripherally inserted central catheter (PICC line), usually in the upper arm. These catheters are durable IV lines that can be used for prolonged periods, but they do not come without risks. Complications of midlines are most commonly line dysfunction, thrombophlebitis, or local infection around the catheter site. Midline complications are unlikely to be an emergency and can be managed by contacting the student's physician. However, PICC lines are central access, meaning they end deep in the central circulatory system. Common but serious complications of PICC lines include bloodstream infection and thrombus, which are emergencies (Chap. 60). Healthcare providers should monitor for fever, swelling, erythema around the site, or an increase in arm circumference, all of which require evaluation. Other care considerations for PICC or midlines include cleanliness, never submerging them, and avoiding lines being accidentally pulled out (See Chap. 60). For PICC lines more specifically, the student should not repeatedly lift or abduct the arm more than 90° or lift more than 10 pounds. Other recommendations for PICC care or troubleshooting can be found on various healthcare websites or Chap. 60 [5].

Accommodations Most patients with viral meningitis recover completely; however, fatigue, malaise, and weakness can linger for weeks or months. If a student experienced a severe complication, they more commonly have residual neurologic deficits [6]. A potentially frustrating aspect of meningitis or encephalitis cases for patients and their care givers is that the exact clinical course cannot be predicted, and limitations are less clear than other types of injury. There is concerning long-term data suggesting that cognitive and development outcomes can be compromised in meningitis and encephalitis survivors [6, 7]. In the absence of specific guideline recommendations, we recommend an approach similar to that taken for students returning to school after a concussion [8] (Chap. 109). For students experiencing headaches, trouble concentrating, or other neurologic or neuropsychiatric difficulties, schools in coordination with the student's physician could develop an individualized education program (IEP) or plan for graded re-entry to full-time schooling. Both academic and physical activity accommodations may be needed, particularly if the student is completing treatment via IV access. Social and emotional supports may also be needed, particularly for patients with severe sequelae.

Follow-Up All students should follow up with a primary care provider (PCP) to ensure that the student and the student's caregivers have an opportunity to discuss concerns they may have, and the student could be examined to ensure recovery. For those requiring prolonged therapy, follow-up with their PCP after hospital discharge and completion of therapy should be arranged. Audiologic screening is usually performed before hospital discharge but should also be repeated 1–3 months after discharge, and in some cases hearing aids or cochlear implants are needed [9]. Lastly, depending on the residual symptoms that the student may have, follow-up with physical, occupational, vestibular, and behavioral therapists can be helpful.

Case 2 (Inspired by a Case from the National Association of School Nurses [NASN] Blog) [10] In February, an otherwise healthy 17-year-old female came home from school complaining to her mother of body aches and fatigue. She developed a fever of 101°F (38.3°C). Her pediatrician recommended that she be seen the following morning if she failed to improve. The next morning the student awoke complaining of pain from her "eyelashes down to her toes" including intense back pain, where her mother noted a dark purple macular rash. She was rushed to the ED where she was promptly admitted to the intensive care unit, but shortly thereafter passed away. Later that day, the intensivist contacted the school nurse and informed them that the student's CSF polymerase chain reaction (PCR) results returned positive for *N. meningitidis*. What is the next most appropriate step for the school nurse to take?

Meningococcal disease, caused by the bacteria *N. meningitidis*, manifests as septicemia in about 40% of cases, meningitis in about 50%, and pneumonia in about 10% [2]. The onset of this invasive infection can be sudden, characterized by fever, chills, malaise, muscle and limb pain, and a rash that may start as macular or maculopapular but typically progresses to petechial or purpuric forms within hours [2].

Notify and Work with the Local Public Health Department Meningococcal disease is spread via respiratory droplets and is known for its epidemic potential and is thus a notifiable condition. Many times notification is done by the diagnostic laboratory or physician caring for the patient in the hospital.

Identification and Prophylaxis as Indicated for High Risk Contacts The school nurse should work with public health authorities to identify high risk contacts of the student. Meningococcal bacteria are spread via saliva or spit. Generally, it takes close or lengthy contact to spread these bacteria, for example, coughing, kissing, or household contacts. It is not spread through casual contact or by breathing air where someone with meningococcal disease has been. Prophylactic antibiotics are indicated in high risk contacts to the index patient in the preceding 7 days, and up to 24 h after antibiotics have started in the index patient [2]. Oral and intramuscular prophylactic options are available.

Information Dissemination Coordinate communication with school leadership and public health authorities to inform the school community about the situation without causing panic.

Vaccination Awareness Given the impact of this case, the school nurse should promote awareness about the availability and importance of meningococcal vaccination to students, parents, and staff. Expanded vaccine recommendations may also be given during outbreaks.

Extra Credit Points

1. Although headaches are common in school aged students, when they are accompanied by other symptoms like fever, neck stiffness, and certain rashes, they can be a sign of meningitis or encephalitis.
2. Since the development and distribution of *Haemophilus influenzae*, *Streptococcus pneumoniae,* and *Neisseria meningitidis* vaccinations in the US, case incidence and sequalae from meningitis and encephalitis have decreased substantially; however ongoing vaccination is key to maintaining this trend.
3. Given that most infectious agents that cause meningitis and encephalitis are spread via respiratory droplets or via the fecal-oral route, implementing precautions such as masking, hand hygiene, surface cleaning, and isolation are essential.
4. Important steps for students returning to school after cases of meningitis or encephalitis are: (a) treatment completion; (b) tailored reintegration plans; (c) ensuring appropriate follow-up.

References

1. Hasbun R. Progress and challenges in bacterial meningitis: a review. JAMA. 2022;328(21):2147–54.
2. American Academy of Pediatrics Committee on Infectious Diseases. Red Book. 33rd ed. American Academy of Pediatrics (AAP); 2024.
3. Kohil A, Jemmieh S, Smatti MK, Yassine HM. Viral meningitis: an overview. Arch Virol. 2021;166(2):335–45.
4. Centers for Disease Control and Prevention (CDC). Postnatal causes of developmental disabilities in children aged 3–10 years–Atlanta, Georgia, 1991. MMWR Morb Mortal Wkly Rep. 1996;45(6):130–4.
5. Government of Alberta. Peripherally inserted central catheter (PICC): care instructions. https://myhealth.alberta.ca/Health/aftercareinformation/pages/conditions.aspx?hwid=ug6122. Accessed 27 Apr 2024.

6. Roed C, Omland LH, Skinhoj P, Rothman KJ, Sorensen HT, Obel N. Educational achievement and economic self-sufficiency in adults after childhood bacterial meningitis. JAMA. 2013;309(16):1714–21.
7. Christie D, Rashid H, El-Bashir H, et al. Impact of meningitis on intelligence and development: a systematic review and meta-analysis. PLoS One. 2017;12(8):e0175024.
8. Halstead ME, McAvoy K, Devore CD, et al. Returning to learning following a concussion. Pediatrics. 2013;132(5):948–57.
9. Bower C, Reilly BK, Richerson J, Hecht JL, Committee on Practice & Ambulatory Medicine, Section on Otolaryngology–Head And Neck Surgery. Hearing assessment in infants, children, and adolescents: recommendations beyond neonatal screening. Pediatrics. 2023;152(3):e2023063288.
10. Wukovits P. There is not only one meningitis vaccine – two mothers tell their stories. National Association of School Nurses. Accessed April 27, 2024. https://www.nasn.org/blogs/patti-wukovits-rnbsn/2021/09/23/meningitisbvaccine.

Chapter 90
Pneumonia and Croup

Elena Petkovska and Selena Hariharan

Case 1 A 10-year-old otherwise healthy girl presents with cough, fever, and reported difficulty breathing. Her temperature is 37.0 °C, respiratory rate is 18 breaths/min, and oxygen saturation is 98% on room air. She appears to be comfortable and speaks in full sentences without any increased work of breathing. She has crackles in the right lower posterior chest. Other findings from her examination are normal. What is the most likely diagnosis?

Pneumonia is a lower respiratory tract infection associated with fever, respiratory symptoms, and evidence of parenchymal involvement by physical examination or infiltrates on chest radiography.

Pathologically, it represents an inflammatory process of the lungs. Radiologically, pneumonia is defined as an infiltrate on chest radiograph in a child with symptoms of an acute respiratory illness [1]. Pneumonia typically follows an upper respiratory tract infection that permits invasion of the lower respiratory tract by bacteria, viruses, or other pathogens that trigger an immune response and produce inflammation. The lower respiratory tract air spaces fill with white blood cells, fluid, and cellular debris [2–4].

Pneumonia in children remains a challenging diagnosis because the presenting symptoms are nonspecific and variable, depending on the patient's age, responsible pathogen, and severity of the infection. Fever and cough have traditionally been considered the hallmarks of pneumonia. However other findings, such as tachypnea, increased work of breathing, and hypoxia, while not diagnostic of pneumonia may precede the cough. Cough may not be a feature initially since the alveoli have few cough receptors. Cough begins when the products of infection irritate cough receptors in the airways. Unfortunately, there is no classic constellation of signs of

E. Petkovska (✉) · S. Hariharan
University of Cincinnati College of Medicine, Cincinnati, OH, USA
e-mail: elena.petkovska@cchmc.org; selena.hariharan@cchmc.org

R. P. Olympia, J. Brady-Olympia (eds.), *Clinical Considerations in School-based Health*, https://doi.org/10.1007/978-3-031-85765-2_90

symptoms that are clinically diagnostic of pneumonia, including auscultatory findings, length of illness, or reported dyspnea. The only findings that increased the likelihood of pneumonia were relative hypoxemia (<96%), objective increased work of breathing (flaring, grunting and retracting), and chest pain. Even though the clinical diagnosis of pneumonia may be subjective without these findings, the Infectious Disease Society of America recommends clinical diagnosis of community acquired pneumonia in a well child to minimize radiation exposure and unnecessary testing in children [3]. In the setting of hypoxemia, respiratory distress, and failed antibiotic therapy, chest radiographs, posteroanterior and lateral, should be obtained to verify the presence or absence of complications of pneumonia, including parapneumonic effusions, necrotizing pneumonia, and pneumothorax [5]. Alternatively, ultrasound is becoming increasingly common, especially with the increased use of point-of-care ultrasound. Reasons include increased ability to recognize parenchymal consolidation and infectious empyema with ultrasound [6].

In addition, children who are admitted should have a blood culture drawn as up to 7% of children with CAP and 15% of children with infectious empyema will have bacteremia, assisting to focus antibiotic therapy and improve antibiotic stewardship. In addition, if the empyema is sampled, a bacterial pathogen may be identified in up to 35% of patients [6].

Pneumonia is encountered commonly in daily practice, and otherwise healthy children typically do well with outpatient treatment. It is important to recognize those children with respiratory distress and those who are at risk for severe or complicated pneumonia.

90.1 Evaluation

When evaluating a child with cough and potential lower respiratory tract disease, the goal is to identify whether a child has bacterial pneumonia versus another clinical syndrome (e.g. bronchiolitis vs asthma) and assessing severity. Initial assessment should include the following (Table 90.1).

Children who are ill-appearing, dehydrated, or have signs of respiratory distress (tachypnea, hypoxemia, increased work of breathing, altered mental status) require prompt activation of the emergency response system as well as rapid and aggressive management [2, 4]. Children who have none of these features can be treated outpatient and should be referred to their primary care provider or an urgent care center as soon as possible. As this patient in Case 1 is clinically stable with no findings of respiratory distress, the child can be referred to a primary care provider or urgent care.

Case 2 A previously healthy, fully immunized 5-year-old girl presents with runny nose, cough, fatigue, and fast breathing. Temperature is 38.3 °C. Physical examination reveals a tired-appearing child with tachypnea and intercostal retractions. Lung examination reveals crackles over all lung fields bilaterally.

Table 90.1 Initial assessment of a student with possible pneumonia [1, 2]

General appearance	Demeanor
	Mental status
	Hydration
	Color (observe for cyanosis)
Vitals signs	Fever (although not specific for pneumonia, may be the only presenting sign)
	Tachypnea: Most sensitive and specific sign of pneumonia, found twice as frequently in children who have evidence of pneumonia on chest radiography
	Hypoxemia: Predictive of lower respiratory tract infection as a sign of significant disease
Lung exam	Respiratory status Increased work of breathing: Retractions, nasal flaring Impending respiratory failure from severe disease: Head bobbing, accessory muscle use, grunting
	Auscultation findings: Rales or crepitations Consolidated lung parenchyma: Decreased breath sounds Viral or atypical pneumonia: Wheezing

Patients with findings of lower respiratory tract infection and respiratory distress require emergent treatment. If the child appears to have impending respiratory failure, the child should be transported to the emergency department by EMS.

It is virtually impossible to clinically differentiate bacterial from viral pneumonia except that bacterial pneumonia might have a more abrupt and severe onset after days of symptoms of an upper respiratory tract infection. The patient may appear ill and sometimes experience toxic effects, with moderate to severe respiratory distress and localized chest pain.

S. pneumoniae (AKA pneumococcal pneumonia) is the most common cause of typical bacterial pneumonia in children younger than 5 years and a common cause in older children also. Pneumococcal pneumonia is typically a lobar pneumonia. Viral and atypical bacterial pneumonia have more gradual, insidious onset. The clinical presentation may be milder, and auscultatory findings are more likely to be diffuse. Wheezing is more frequent in viral than bacterial pneumonia [1]. Differential diagnosis for a student with fever and respiratory distress include the following (Table 90.2).

90.2 Treatment and Return to School

Uncomplicated bacterial pneumonia can be effectively treated in most children on an outpatient basis with oral antibiotics and supportive care. The causative agent of CAP is usually not identified, particularly in the outpatient setting; therefore, antibiotic treatment is generally targeted towards the most common bacterial organisms. For immunized infants and children of all ages, high-dose amoxicillin is recommended for children with mild-to-moderate CAP with presumed bacterial

Table 90.2 Differential diagnosis for fever and respiratory distress

	Disease processes	Sign and symptoms	Disposition	Treatment
Croup	Viral infection of the upper airway resulting with edema and narrowing of the subglottic portion of the larynx	Barking cough with fever and a hoarse cry or voice, with or without inspiratory stridor	Patients with increased work of breathing and stridor at rest need to be treated promptly in the ED Other patients can be managed at PCP's office or urgent care	Steroids recommended for all croup; Nebulized Epinephrine treatment reserved for moderate to severe croup
Asthma	Airflow obstruction in lower respiratory tract due to contraction of airway smooth muscle, thickening of the airway wall due to edema and mucus plugging in the airways	Cough, wheezing, shortness of breath, and chest tightness	Patients with distress: Emergent management in the ED Other patients: Evaluate at UC or PCP office	Acute exacerbation: Oral steroids and short acting beta agonist inhaler/ nebulized treatment
Pertussis	Bordetella adheres mucosal lining of the respiratory tract causing local inflammatory response while released toxins act locally and systemically	Paroxysms of coughing +/− inspiratory whoop, post tussive vomiting, cough with cyanosis	Patients with respiratory distress or signs of dehydration: Evaluate in the ED Other patients: Evaluate in UC or PCP office	Macrolide antibiotics started in the first 3 weeks of onset of cough can shorten duration of symptoms; supportive care as needed
Tuberculosis (TB) (active)	The inhaled mycobacterium is phagocytosed by the alveolar macrophages. If innate immunity is inadequate, bacilli continue to multiply inside macrophages and spread to interstitium of the lungs then transferred to regional lymph nodes as means of extrapulmonary spread [7]	Active TB: Chronic cough, fatigue, weight loss or failure to thrive, fever, night sweats Latent TB: Consider in asymptomatic patients with positive test, especially in immigrants	Clinically stable patients: Managed outpatient by PCP as they will require prolonged treatment and close follow up	Treatment: 4 drug anti-TB therapy for 6 months

origin. This regimen adequately covers Streptococcus pneumoniae, the most common bacterial cause of bacterial CAP in this age group. For children with amoxicillin allergy, alternative antibiotic regimens include second- or third generation cephalosporins, oral levofloxacin, or oral linezolid. The duration of therapy is typically 7–10 days. For school-aged children and adolescents, a macrolide, most commonly a 5-day course of azithromycin, may be added if there is suspicion for atypical pathogens, as Mycoplasma pneumoniae is more common in these age groups. Macrolide monotherapy does not provide sufficient coverage for S. pneumoniae and should not be routinely prescribed alone.

Indications for inpatient management include hypoxia, respiratory distress, dehydration, underlying comorbidities that may predispose patients to complications (e.g., cardiopulmonary disease, neurocognitive disorders, metabolic disorder, immunocompromised host) and failure of outpatient therapy (48–72 h with no response) [8]. In addition, even well appearing children with anything larger than a scant pleural effusion should be admitted. Once treatment is started, patients are encouraged to follow up with PCP closely to monitor for clinical improvement and assess respiratory status. Patients who are fever-free for at least 24 h, whose respiratory state is at baseline, and who can maintain hydration, may return to school as tolerated. Despite pathophysiologic improvement, children may continue to cough for several weeks. While this can be frustrating, it is not appropriate to exclude a student from school for weeks to months. Schools should have a protocol to manage the potential disruption and discuss with parents ahead of time ideas to control cough.

Case 3 A 5 year old child presents to the school nurse's office with barky cough and hoarse voice. There is no difficulty breathing or tachypnea, oxygen saturation is 99%. This is a typical presentation for which common infectious cause of upper airway obstruction in children?

Croup, also known as laryngotracheobronchitis, generally affects children between 6 months and 3 years of age, although it can occur in school age children as well [9]. When seen in older children it is often patients with congenital and acquired airway abnormalities. Croup is typically caused by a viral infection, with parainfluenza virus being the most common culprit, followed by respiratory syncytial virus (RSV). These viruses are prevalent during the fall and winter months, contributing to the seasonal nature of the condition [9].

The onset of croup is frequently preceded by symptoms resembling a common cold, including fever, congestion, and rhinorrhea, though the barky cough may be the first presenting symptom. As the infection progresses down the respiratory epithelium to the larynx and trachea causing subglottic narrowing, patients subsequently develop hoarseness and a distinctive barky cough. One of the hallmark features of croup that requires additional intervention is stridor, which is a harsh, high-pitched, inspiratory sound resulting from turbulent airflow through the narrowed airway. In more advanced cases of croup, the stridor can be biphasic, audible both during inspiration and expiration. Stridor, persistent spasmodic cough and respiratory distress typically develop in the evenings [10]. Another unique feature of croup is that symptoms worsen at night and improve during the day. The diagnosis is clinical, and imaging is not routinely recommended unless the patient has atypical presentation or when alternative diagnosis is considered [11].

90.3 Assessment of the Severity of Croup

When evaluating a child with suspected croup, it's essential to prioritize their comfort while carefully assessing the severity of their condition. Increased respiratory effort due to anxiety can exacerbate subglottic narrowing, so a calm and supportive approach is crucial [12].

The most used system for classifying the severity of croup is the Westley score ranging from 0 to 17 points divided by five factors: stridor, retractions, cyanosis, level of consciousness, and air entry (Table 90.3).

90.4 Management

The absence of stridor and respiratory distress, along with normal oxygen saturation, are consistent with mild croup. For this patient, it is appropriate to follow up with PCP or urgent care center for evaluation and possible dexamethasone (oral or intramuscular dexamethasone), while anticipating probable discharge for parents to provide supportive care at home. Supportive care includes antipyretics, encouragement of fluid intake, and exposure to cold air or mist. Caregivers should also be provided with guidance that if the child develops stridor at rest or signs of distress, they should seek emergency care.

Case 4 A 5-year-old girl was brought to the office for harsh cough and difficulty breathing. She developed a cold with a runny nose 3 days ago and has been feeling ill. When you call her mother, the mom said her daughter was awake most of the previous night with a barking cough and noisy breathing. The physical examination reveals persistent inspiratory stridor, respiratory rate of 40/min and suprasternal retractions at rest. There is no cyanosis and the rest of her physical exam is reassuring.

Table 90.3 Westley score for croup

Clinical feature	Associated score
Inspiratory stridor	0 (none); 1 (when agitated); 2 (at rest)
Retractions	0 (none); 1 (mild); 2 (moderate); 3 (severe)
Air entry	0 (Normal); 1 (decreased); 2 (markedly decreased)
Cyanosis	0 (none); 4 (when crying); 5 (at rest)
Level of consciousness	0 (alert); 5 (disoriented)

Mild croup: scores 1–2; Moderate croup: scores 3–8; Severe croup: scores >8; and a score greater than 12 indicates impending respiratory failure [13]

The patient in this scenario has moderate croup. Patients with stridor at rest and retractions suggestive of significant upper airway obstruction need prompt evaluation and treatment in the emergency department. These patients will require racemic epinephrine which treats airway edema and obstruction, providing acute symptoms relief.

When assessing patients with moderate or severe croup, it is essential to recognize the signs of respiratory distress that can lead to respiratory fatigue and impending respiratory failure, including decreased breath sounds with decreasing stridor, decreased retractions, dusky appearance, pallor or cyanosis, and any change in mental status like listlessness or fatigue [14]. If any of these findings is apparent, the child should be transported by emergency medical services as opposed to private vehicle.

Patients with pre-existing upper airway anomalies or a history of multiple intubations should also prompt expedient evaluation and treatment in PCP's office or ED, even if the initial presentation is mild, due to the increased risk for developing severe croup [9]. The differential diagnosis of a student with respiratory distress and possible upper airway obstruction include the following (Table 90.4).

90.5 Treatment and Return to School for Croup

Steroids are the mainstay of therapy for croup and are recommended for all patients with croup. Multiple trials have demonstrated that corticosteroids reduce the number and duration of intubations, decrease rate and duration of hospitalizations, and reduce the number of visits to a health care practitioner for persistent croup symptoms. Dexamethasone 0.6 mg/kg appears to be equally effective if given orally or parenterally. However, oral administration is preferred as it is generally less traumatic. Recent randomized clinical trials including doses of 0.15 mg/kg have concluded that lower doses (0.15 mg/kg) are equally effective, though sample sizes were small and none of the trials were designed to show non-inferiority. Symptoms improve within 1–3 h and the effect persists for 24–48 h after a single dose is administered [14].

Nebulized epinephrine is recommended for all patients with moderate to severe croup. Based on historical data, epinephrine administered to children with severe croup substantially reduces intubation. Epinephrine has been shown to substantially reduce respiratory distress within 10 min of administration and to last for more than an hour. The effects from epinephrine dissipate within 2 h after administration [14]. Past studies are recommending that patients who receive nebulized epinephrine should be observed for 3–4 h after the initial treatment [17], however, because the effect of nebulized epinephrine wanes over period of 2 h many institutions have adjusted their protocol to 2-h post treatment observation period. The need for additional intervention and/or admission to the hospital is determined

Table 90.4 Differential diagnosis of a student with respiratory distress and possible upper airway obstruction

	Disease process	Clinical signs and symptoms	Diagnostic tests	Treatment
Foreign body aspiration	Foreign object inhaled into the airway, leading to airway obstruction	Cough and stridor after episode of choking (choking episode may not be witnessed, especially in younger children)	First step: Chest X ray-may not prove useful in acute phase if aspirated object is radiolucent-lucent second step: CT or bronchoscopy	Rigid bronchoscopy is gold standard and most used tool for retrieval, but flexible bronchoscopy has diagnostic role [15]
Epiglottitis	Inflammation and swelling of the epiglottis, which can rapidly progress to airway compromise: Consider in unvaccinated pediatric populations and regions where immunization rates have declined	Sudden onset of respiratory distress, accompanied by anxiety, fever, and a muffled voice often with drooling and difficulty swallowing (dysphagia); children may adopt a distinct "tripod" position aimed at alleviating airway obstruction	Cherry-red, swollen epiglottis seen on exam is classic but diagnosis is clinical as examination or irritation of patient can prompt airway catastrophic airway obstruction	Emergent endotracheal intubation by most experienced provider; appropriate antibiotic therapy targeting the underlying bacterial infection Rapid recognition of this condition and activation of emergency response is essential [12, 13]
Retropharyngeal abscess	Infection and suppuration of retropharyngeal chains of lymph nodes, which drain the nasopharynx, paranasal sinuses, and adenoids	Fever, sore throat, dysphagia, odynophagia, neck pain, neck swelling, limited neck mobility and torticollis, usually with pharyngitis/ tonsillitis and cervical lymphadenitis on examination [16]	Enlargement of retropharyngeal/ prevertebral tissue seen on plain lateral neck radiographs; CT is most sensitive and imaging of choice [16]	Prompt treatment with IV antibiotics and possible surgical drainage, especially if exhibiting symptoms of airway obstruction

(continued)

Table 90.4 (continued)

	Disease process	Clinical signs and symptoms	Diagnostic tests	Treatment
Tracheitis	Result of bacterial superinfection of trachea that causes thick pus to develop within the lumen of the subglottic area causing ulcerations, pseudomembrane, microabscesses of the mucosal surface	Sudden worsening of symptoms following mild-to-moderate episode of croup—distinguished from croup by acute onset of high fever, toxic appearance, and poor response to epinephrine	Clinical and radiographic findings suggestive but only airway endoscopy can confirm diagnosis. Visualization of subglottis and trachea: Inflamed and irregular mucosa with pseudomembrane or thick, purulent secretions [13]	Broad-spectrum intravenous antibiotics with close monitoring of the airway, as intubation and respiratory support frequently required [14]
Allergic reaction/ anaphylaxis	Edema of the retropharynx and/or larynx	Sudden onset difficulty breathing, stridor or wheezing. Can involve other systems including facial swelling, rash, GI symptoms or altered mental status	Clinical diagnosis	Emergent administration of IM Epinephrine (first line medication); Adjunct medications based on associated symptoms H1 antagonists should be used only as adjunct therapy after epinephrine is administered, because it is not effective for airway edema or hypotension and is only proven beneficial for cutaneous manifestations

mainly by the response to therapy with glucocorticoids and nebulized epinephrine. Supportive care both in home and inpatient management should be focused on hydration and fever control. Once the patient clinically improves, is afebrile for minimum of 24 h and able to maintain hydration, the child can return to school as tolerated.

Extra Credit Points

1. Presenting symptoms of pneumonia are variable, depending on the patient's age, responsible pathogen, and severity of the infection.
2. Auscultation findings in patients with typical pneumonia may include crepitations and decreased breath sounds or exam may be totally normal.
3. Routine chest radiographs are not recommended for patients well enough to be treated in the outpatient setting.
4. The hallmark signs of croup are barky cough and stridor.
5. In both diagnoses, recognize the signs of respiratory fatigue and impending respiratory failure, as these patients will require emergent intervention.
6. In patients with rapid progression of symptoms consider other diagnosis including epiglottitis, RPA, foreign body aspiration or other respiratory emergencies.

References

1. Gereige RS, Laufer PM. Pneumonia. Pediatr Rev. 2013;34(10):438–56.
2. Durbin WJ, Stille C. Pneumonia. Pediatr Rev. 2008;29(5):147–60.
3. Shah SN, Bachur RG, Simel DL, Neuman MI. Does this child have pneumonia?: the rational clinical examination systematic review. JAMA. 2017;318(5):462–71.
4. Mani CS. Acute pneumonia and its complications. Principles and practice of pediatric. Infect Dis. 2018:238–49.e4.
5. Messinger AI, Kupfer O, Hurst A, Parker S. Management of pediatric community-acquired bacterial pneumonia. Pediatr Rev. 2017;38(9):394–409.
6. Pereda MA, Chavez MA, Hooper-Miele CC, Gilman RH, Steinhoff MC, Ellington LE, Gross M, Price C, Tielsch JM, Checkley W. Lung ultrasound for the diagnosis of pneumonia in children: a meta-analysis. Pediatrics. 2015;135:714–22.
7. Holmberg PJ, Temesgen Z, Banerjee R. Tuberculosis in children. Pediatr Rev. 2019;40(4):168–78.
8. Popovsky EY, Florin TA. Community-acquired pneumonia in childhood. In: Encyclopedia of respiratory medicine; 2022. p. 119–31.
9. Fitzgerald DA. The assessment and management of croup. Paediatr Respir Rev. 2006;7(1):73–81.
10. Bjornson CL, Johnson DW. Croup in children. CMAJ. 2013;185(15):1317–23.
11. Buttaravoli P. Chapter 31. Laryngotracheobronchitis. In: Buttaravoli P, editor. Minor emergencies. 2nd ed. Mosby; 2007. p. 131–4.
12. Virbalas J, Smith L. Upper airway obstruction. Pediatr Rev. 2015;36(2):62–72.
13. Cherry JD. Clinical practice. Croup. N Engl J Med. 2008;358(4):384–91.
14. Alberta Clinical Practice Guidelines Guideline Working Group. Guidelines for the diagnosis and management of croup. 2008.
15. Green SS. Ingested and aspirated foreign bodies. Pediatr Rev. 2015;36(10):430–6.
16. Tebruegge M, Curtis N. Infections related to the upper and middle airways. In: Long SS, Prober CG, Fischer M, editors. Principles and practice of pediatric infectious diseases. 5th ed. New York: Elsevier Saunders; 2018. p. 208.
17. Kunkel NC, Baker MD. Use of racemic epinephrine, dexamethasone, and mist in the outpatient management of croup. Pediatr Emerg Care. 1996;12(3):156–9.

Chapter 91
Appendicitis, Pancreatitis, and Cholecystitis

Lauren A. McNickle

Case 1 Penny is a 10 year old female student with past medical history of autism spectrum disorder and non-verbal, who presents to your office with sudden onset fever, vomiting, and diarrhea. She is actively vomiting in your office. Penny appears to feel ill but is non-toxic. She appears very uncomfortable and is holding her belly while hunched over. She has difficulty ambulating to the restroom due to her discomfort. What should you do next?

Appendicitis is one of the most common surgical conditions in children, leading it to be the fifth most common reason for hospitalization [1]. The peak age of incidence occurs in children between ages 9 and 12 years [2]. The appendix is a small outpouching of the large intestine. It is unclear exactly what its role is, but the thought is it may play a role in maintaining our normal gut flora. There are many beliefs as to the cause of appendicitis, but no specific etiology has been identified. Theories such as obstruction of the appendix from stool, appendicoliths, lymphoid hyperplasia, or neoplasm have been suggested [3]. If left untreated, there are concerns for perforation of the appendix which leads to increased morbidity and mortality. Perforation rarely develops before 12 h of symptoms but is common after 72 h [2]. Current management for perforated appendicitis involves percutaneous drainage of the abscess. Mesenteric adenitis, which involves inflammation of lymph nodes within the abdomen, often presents very similar to appendicitis however the management is supportive versus surgical. Appendicitis can present with vague symptoms such as abdominal pain, vomiting, diarrhea, fatigue, anorexia, and fever. Table 91.1 highlights some of the most common presentations of abdominal right sided pain and their dispositions/treatments.

As demonstrated in Table 91.1, common complaints that accompany abdominal pain can be vomiting and diarrhea. Vomiting and diarrhea are often associated with

L. A. McNickle (✉)
Penn State Hershey Medical Center, Department of Emergency Medicine, Division of Pediatric Emergency Medicine, Hershey, PA, USA

R. P. Olympia, J. Brady-Olympia (eds.), *Clinical Considerations in School-based Health*, https://doi.org/10.1007/978-3-031-85765-2_91

Table 91.1 Etiologies of right sided abdominal pain

Etiology	Presenting symptoms	Disposition and treatment
Appendicitis	Abdominal pain: **Periumbilical/ right lower quadrant** Vomiting Diarrhea Anorexia Fever Fatigue	Refer to ED Surgical removal
Cholecystitis	Abdominal pain: **Right upper quadrant** Vomiting Fever Fatigue	Refer to ED for laboratory testing and ultrasound Surgical removal
Mesenteric adenitis	Abdominal pain: **Periumbilical/ right lower quadrant** Vomiting Diarrhea Anorexia Fatigue	Refer to ED for labs and imaging Supportive care
Fitz Hugh Curtis	Abdominal pain: **Right upper quadrant** Fever Nausea Vomiting Fatigue	Refer to ED for sexually transmitted infection (STI) testing Antibiotic treatment
Liver laceration	Abdominal pain: **Right upper quadrant** History of trauma Dizziness	Refer to ED for labs and imaging Supportive care or surgical intervention
Ovarian cyst or torsion	Abdominal pain: **Right lower quadrant** Intermittent severe pain Nausea and/or vomiting	Refer to ED for ultrasound Supportive care (cyst) or surgical intervention (torsion)

ED Emergency Department

viral or bacterial gastroenteritis (Chap. 95). Studies have suggested that gastroenteritis is a common initial diagnosis in the case of missed appendicitis [4]. It can be helpful to determine if other members of the family are sick with similar symptoms. To aid in your diagnosis, there are specific exam maneuvers that are often positive when appendicitis is present. Table 91.2 highlights these key exam findings. If you cannot remember all the exam maneuvers, a simple quick test is having the patient jump up and down. Often, appendicitis causes peritoneal irritation which will be elicited when patients jump up and down, and often children with appendicitis are unable to complete the task without pain or discomfort.

In addition to physical exam maneuvers, various scoring systems have been developed to aid in diagnosing appendicitis. Two common scoring systems include the Alvarado Score (Table 91.3) and Pediatric Appendicitis Score (PAS) (Table 91.4). The Alvarado Score was implemented in 1986 and looks at symptoms, physical

Table 91.2 Classic physical exam maneuvers for appendicitis [3]

Name of sign	Exam maneuver
Rovsing	Pain in the right lower quadrant on palpation of the left side
Obturator	Pain on internal rotation of the right hip
Psoas	Pain on extension of the right hip, particularly found in retrocecal appendicitis
Rebound tenderness	Pain with release of pressure after deep palpation of the abdomen
Dunphy's	Pain with coughing
Markle	Pain with heel-drop

Table 91.3 Alvarado Score for diagnosing appendicitis [5]

Symptoms	Score
Migratory iliac fossa pain	1
Nausea/vomiting	1
Anorexia	1
Physical exam findings	
Tenderness in right iliac fossa	2
Rebound tenderness in right iliac fossa	1
Elevated temperature	1
Laboratory findings	
Leukocytosis	2
Shift to the left of neutrophils	1
Total	10

Table 91.4 Pediatric Appendicitis Score [6]

Symptoms	Score
Migration of pain to RLQ	1
Anorexia	1
Fever	1
Nausea or vomiting	1
Physical exam findings	
RLQ tenderness to coughing, percussion, or hopping	2
Tenderness over right iliac fossa	2
Laboratory findings	
Leukocytosis, WBC > 10,000	1
Neutrophilia, ANC > 7500	1
Total	10

exam findings, and laboratory findings [5]. The PAS was developed in 2002 and similarly looks at symptoms, physical exam findings and laboratory findings, although points are distributed slightly differently. The Alvarado and PAS stratifies patients in low, equivocal, or high risk. A score of ≤4 is considered low risk. An equivocal score of 4–6 should prompt further imaging and a surgical consult. A high-risk score of ≥7 would also prompt further imaging and warrant a surgical consult [6]. While these scores can be useful tools in stratification of risk, clinical judgement should also be implemented as various studies have demonstrated differing sensitivities and specificities for both scoring systems. Inflammatory markers, such as sedimentation rate and C-reactive protein, may be helpful to track trends in children or adolescents who have equivocal scores and when diagnostic imaging or surgery consultation is not readily available.

When your clinical suspicion is high for appendicitis, several imaging modalities are available to aid in diagnosis. Ultrasound is the gold standard for appendicitis as it prevents exposure to ionizing radiation in the pediatric population. It has a sensitivity of 80–92% with a specificity of 86–98%. Depending on the location of the appendix, it may be difficult to visualize on ultrasound therefore a CT scan may be warranted which increases sensitivity to 95% and sensitivity to 96%. In some institutions MRI may be available, which also prevents exposure to radiation and is reported to be equivocal to CT [2]. Some pediatric surgeons may be willing to take patients straight to the operating room if clinical presentation is highly suspicious for appendicitis [6].

Case 2 Emily is a previously healthy 5 year old female student presenting with concerns for abdominal pain, vomiting, and lethargy. She was in class when she started vomiting and her teacher noticed she was very sleepy. She is uncomfortable appearing and does not want to drink water when offered. She points to her mid-abdomen when asked where her abdominal pain is located. You call Emily's mom to come pick her up and she informs you Emily's dad started with similar symptoms around Emily's age. What should you do next?

A less common, but do not miss cause of abdominal pain in the pediatric population is pancreatitis. While often thought of as an adult pathology, the incidence of pancreatitis is growing in the pediatric population (10–15 cases per 100,000 children). Common presenting symptoms include epigastric or diffuse abdominal pain (80–95%), nausea and vomiting (40–80%), abdominal distension, fever, breathlessness, irritability, and impaired consciousness. Diagnosis must meet two out of three of the following criteria: abdominal pain, a serum amylase or lipase three or more times the upper limit of normal, and findings consistent with pancreatitis on abdominal imaging: CT, MRI or ultrasound. Common causes of pancreatitis include gallstones, medication induced, hypertriglyceridemia, and viral infections. Hereditary pancreatitis also exists and often presents with recurrent pancreatitis beginning in childhood or adolescence. Treatment frequently requires an inpatient admission where patients receive supportive care consisting of intravenous fluids, oxygen, analgesia, and proper nutrition. Patients with severe pancreatitis can require critical levels of care including endotracheal intubation, cardiac support and renal support [7]. While pancreatitis is less common in the pediatric population, always consider it on your differential as it has the propensity to cause critical illness.

Case 3 Olivia is a 14 year old female student with past medical history of Type II Diabetes Mellitus presenting to your office with abdominal pain after eating lunch. She is holding her right upper abdomen and complains of nausea. She is

also clammy and has a fever of 101.4 °F. She has had some fatigue recently but otherwise felt well. What should you do next?

The final do not miss abdominal pain diagnosis in the pediatric population is cholecystitis. While cholecystitis is a rare diagnosis in pediatrics, its incidence has been increasing. This diagnosis is often seen in females that are Caucasian and in late adolescence [8]. Cholecystitis commonly presents as right upper quadrant pain which may be accompanied by vomiting and/or fever. A hallmark physical exam finding is a positive Murphy Sign where the patient has pain when asked to take a deep breath in while the examiner palpates the right subcostal area. Diagnosis usually consists of right upper quadrant pain and/or positive Murphy Sign, signs of inflammation such as fever, elevated WBC and/or elevated neutrophil count, and imaging (often ultrasound) that is indicative of acute cholecystitis [9]. While the most cause of cholecystitis is often thought to be secondary to gallstones, in the pediatric population, about 50–70% of cholecystitis occurs without the presence of stones [10]. Acute acalculous cholecystitis is usually associated with systemic, non-infectious disease, such as Kawasaki's Disease in infants and young children and with systemic infectious disease such as Epstein Bar Virus in older children and adolescents [8]. With these etiologies in mind, the treatment approach is also much different than adults. Instead of jumping to removal of the gallbladder, often management consists of inpatient care with antibiotic therapy first [10]. As the etiologies of cholecystitis are much different in the pediatric population versus the adult population, it is key to keep an open mind when a pediatric patient is presenting with right upper quadrant abdominal pain.

91.1 Case Conclusions

Case 1 Penny's mom took her to the local emergency department where labs and imaging were immediately obtained. Her ultrasound was concerning for rupture, therefore a CT scan was obtained at the request of pediatric surgery which demonstrated acute appendicitis with signs of perforation. She was started on antibiotics and pediatric surgery took her to the operating room.

Case 2 Emily's dad took her to the local emergency department given his history of pancreatitis where labs and imaging were immediately obtained. Emily's lipase was found to be over 1000 and her CT scan of her abdomen demonstrated inflammation around her pancreas. She was admitted to the hospital for 3 days where she received intravenous fluids and pain control. She will be following up with genetics and pediatric gastroenterology as there is likely a familial component.

Case 3 Olivia was seen in the emergency department where additional information was obtained that she has had a recent severe sore throat. Labs and imaging were completed which demonstrated an active Epstein Bar infection along with elevated white blood cell count and inflammatory markers. An ultrasound was performed of her right upper quadrant which demonstrated the presence of acalculous cholecystitis. Olivia was admitted to the hospital for pain control and intravenous antibiotics.

Extra Credit Points

1. Appendicitis commonly presents as focal right lower quadrant pain or periumbilical pain that migrates to the right lower quadrant.
2. Common symptoms of appendicitis include: anorexia, nausea or vomiting, migration of pain, pain with cough, percussion, or hopping, periumbilical pain, right lower quadrant tenderness, and rebound abdominal pain
3. Two common scoring systems to aid in the diagnosis of appendicitis include the Alvarado Score (Table 91.3) and Pediatric Appendicitis Score (Table 91.4).
4. Pancreatitis, while rare, does occur in the pediatric population, and often presents with severe epigastric or left upper quadrant pain, vomiting, and sometimes lethargy.
5. Cholecystitis can present in the pediatric population, often presenting as right upper quadrant pain, nausea/vomiting, and/or fever.

References

1. Gil LA, Deans KJ, Minneci PC. Appendicitis in children. Adv Pediatr Infect Dis. 2023;70(1):105–22. https://doi.org/10.1016/j.yapd.2023.03.003.
2. Lipsett SC, Bachur RG. Chapter 16: abdominal emergencies. In: Fleisher and Ludwig's textbook of pediatric emergency medicine. 8th ed. Wolters Kluwer; 2021. p. 1290–312.
3. Rentea RM, Peter SDS, Snyder CL. Pediatric appendicitis: state of the art review. Pediatr Surg Int. 2017;33(3):269–83. https://doi.org/10.1007/s00383-016-3990-2.
4. Galai T, Beloosesky OZ, Scolnik D, Rimon A, Glatstein M. Misdiagnosis of acute appendicitis in children attending the emergency department: the experience of a large, Tertiary Care Pediatric Hospital. Eur J Pediatr Surg. 2017;27(2):138–41. https://doi.org/10.1055/s-0035-1570757.
5. Awayshih MMA, Nofal MN, Yousef AJ. Evaluation of Alvarado score in diagnosing acute appendicitis. Pan Afr Med J. 2019;34:15. Published 2019 Sep 6. https://doi.org/10.11604/pamj.2019.34.15.17803.
6. Becker C, Kharbanda A. Acute appendicitis in pediatric patients: an evidence-based review. Pediatr Emerg Med Pract. 2019;16(9):1–20.
7. Szatmary P, Grammatikopoulos T, Cai W, et al. Acute pancreatitis: diagnosis and treatment. Drugs. 2022;82(12):1251–76. https://doi.org/10.1007/s40265-022-01766-4.
8. Chandra S, Friesen C, Attard TM. Trends in the epidemiology of pediatric acute and chronic cholecystitis-related admissions in the USA: a nationwide emergency department and inpatient sample study. J Investig Med. 2019;67(8):1155–9. https://doi.org/10.1136/jim-2018-000948.
9. Yokoe M, Hata J, Takada T, et al. Tokyo guidelines 2018: diagnostic criteria and severity grading of acute cholecystitis (with videos). J Hepatobiliary Pancreat Sci. 2018;25(1):41–54. https://doi.org/10.1002/jhbp.515.
10. Poddighe D, Sazonov V. Acute acalculous cholecystitis in children. World J Gastroenterol. 2018;24(43):4870–9. https://doi.org/10.3748/wjg.v24.i43.4870.

Chapter 92
Urinary Tract Infections

Jennifer M. Dunnick and Lindsay Ercole

Case 1 A 10-year-old female is complaining of "pain when she pees". She describes the pain as burning and is now fearful of urinating again. She also has some mild lower abdominal pain. Her symptoms began this morning, and she has never felt pain like this before. You recall that she was out of school with a diarrheal illness for the past few days. Today, she does not have a fever and denies nausea or vomiting.

Urinary tract infections (UTI), both cystitis and pyelonephritis, are common in school aged children, though much less so than in younger children. Among those with urinary symptoms, such as painful urination or increased urinary frequency, 8% of children will have a UTI [1].

92.1 Uncomplicated Cystitis

Due to anatomical factors, school-age females are more likely to suffer from UTIs than males, even those that are uncircumcised [2]. Most commonly, urinary pathogens are enteric in origin, such as *Escherichia coli,* which is responsible for 80–90% of pediatric UTIs. Other common uropathogens include *Enterobacter, Enterococcus* species, and *Klebsiella* [3, 4]. Diarrhea or poor toileting skills, such as wiping back to front, allow migration of stool bacterial into the urinary tract. Constipation can

J. M. Dunnick (✉)
Division of Pediatric Emergency Medicine, Duke University Hospital, Durham, NC, USA
e-mail: jennifer.dunnick@duke.edu

L. Ercole
UPMC Children's Hospital of Pittsburgh, Pittsburgh, PA, USA
e-mail: ercolelj@upmc.edu

R. P. Olympia, J. Brady-Olympia (eds.), *Clinical Considerations in School-based Health*, https://doi.org/10.1007/978-3-031-85765-2_92

also be a precipitating factor, as rectal stool balls can lead to bladder outlet obstruction and incomplete emptying of urine.

Lower urinary symptoms, as described in the case above, are the typical presentation for uncomplicated cystitis. This includes dysuria, urinary frequency or hesitancy, hematuria, new onset urinary incontinence, or suprapubic abdominal pain [5]. Urethritis from sexual activity can also present similarly and should be considered. The presence of fever, vomiting, or flank pain is concerning for complicated cystitis, such as pyelonephritis, rather than cystitis alone.

In additional to bacterial causes of cystitis, viral infections can cause urinary symptoms. Adenovirus is a classic viral pathogen and may be associated with upper respiratory tract symptoms in addition to dysuria and hematuria [6]. History and exam cannot differentiate between bacterial and viral UTIs. Vulvovaginitis, or irritation of the perineum, can also happen in female students and result in dysuria. Therefore, students presenting with urinary symptoms should have a urinalysis performed. Urine culture can also be used to definitively diagnose a UTI, though results will not be available for at least 2 days. Blood tests are not routinely indicated for the diagnosis of cystitis.

92.2 Diagnosis

Clean-void samples are appropriate in this age group, though the importance of properly cleaning with disinfecting wipes prior to providing the sample should be stressed to reduce the likelihood of a contaminated specimen. Pyuria, positive leukocyte esterase (LE), positive nitrite and bacteriuria are indicators of a bacterial UTI. Urine dipstick alone has a sensitivity of 88% and is a reasonable first test, especially in the school setting (Table 92.1). The addition of microscopy will improve the sensitivity of urine testing, though only slightly. The definition of pyuria depends on the type of microscopy performed: ≥5 white blood cells per high power field (WBC/HPF) with automated microscopy and >10 WBC/mm^3 when utilizing enhanced microscopy. If rapid urine testing, either dipstick or urinalysis with microscopy, are negative then culture is not necessary, and the student should not receive antibiotics. If LE and/or nitrite are positive or there is bacteriuria, a urine

Table 92.1 Sensitivity and specificity of leukocyte esterase (LE) and nitrite positive urine dipstick results [7, 10, 11]

Urine dipstick	Sensitivity (%)	Specificity (%)	Management
LE	84	78	+LE (-nitrite): Send microscopy and culture, treatment based on results
Nitrite	50	93	+Nitrite (-LE): Send urine culture, consider empiric treatment with antibiotics
LE + nitrite	72	96	+LE/+nitrite: Send urine culture, empirically treat with antibiotics

culture should be sent, which often requires referral to the child's PCP, urgent care or the emergency department [7–9].

92.3 Treatment

In a well-appearing and otherwise healthy child, pyuria alone should not be treated for a UTI. In this instance, await culture results before initiating antibiotics. If a symptomatic child has bacteriuria, with or without pyuria, and the sample appears uncontaminated, it is reasonable to empirically treat with antibiotics prior to culture results. Asymptomatic bacteriuria should not be treated with antibiotics (unless pregnant), so deferring treatment in the interest of antibiotic stewardship is appropriate [8].

Antibiotic selection should ultimately be determined by local antibiograms describing resistance rates. In general, however, most urinary bacterial pathogens are susceptible to third-generation cephalosporins, such as cefdinir, and resistant to amoxicillin. Resistance is increasing for first-generation cephalosporins and trimethoprim-sulfamethoxale. *E. coli* is responsible for upwards of 90% of UTIs, so being familiar with local treatment recommendations for this bacterium would be beneficial for the care of students with UTIs [4].

Duration of treatment varies with some patient characteristics. For those with uncomplicated cystitis (fever free and no systemic symptoms), oral antibiotics should be given for 5 days. If the UTI is recurrent, consider increasing the duration to 7–10 days [12, 13]. To reduce antibiotic resistance, ensure that students complete the course of antibiotics prescribed.

Case 2 A 12-year-old female was seen at her PCP 4 days ago and diagnosed with a urinary tract infection. She was started on Trimethoprim-sulfamethoxazole. After 3 days of medication, she has now developed fevers. This morning, her teacher grew concerned when she saw her shivering during class. She reports to the school nurse feeling weak and nauseous, though denies any other symptoms.

92.4 Complicated Cystitis

Acute uncomplicated cystitis references an infection of the bladder or lower urinary tract.

Complicated UTI is characterized by extension of the infection to the upper urinary tract and kidneys, including pyelonephritis, or infections in symptomatic patients who are immunosuppressed or have known urinary tract anomalies. Children or adolescents with a UTI and systemic symptoms concerning for early urosepsis would be identified as a complicated UTI [14].

To better explore the risks for complication, the patient history must be further elucidated. Key factors to consider would be a prior history of UTI, organisms cultured, or failure to respond to prior antibiotic therapies. As most UTIs are due to *E. coli*, identification of another organism would warrant concern for complicated UTI [4]. Any patient with prior surgical correction or instrumentation, or those with known renal or urologic anomalies, such as duplicate collecting systems, vesicoureteral reflux, should also raise your suspicion for more serious infection, given the potential for seeding of the upper urinary tract due to anomalous urine flow or stasis [15].

Physical exam will often show an ill appearing child, likely febrile. Children and adolescents with upper urinary tract infections, such as pyelonephritis, often present with nausea, vomiting, and vague abdominal or lower lumbar pain [16]. Urinary frequency, urgency, hematuria or dysuria may also be present, as would also be noted in an uncomplicated UTI. Early vital sign changes include fever and tachycardia, with blood pressures remaining normotensive initially. For sexually active females who present with the symptoms listed above, a pelvic examination should be considered to also evaluate for tenderness during a bimanual exam that could indicate pelvic inflammatory disease.

Urinalysis from a clean void sample is appropriate in school aged children. A urine culture should additionally be obtained at the time of urinalysis, though with results pending several days, initial treatment should not be withheld in a symptomatic patient. Recent studies have shown that urine cultures with greater than 10,000 colony forming units (CFU) have been indicative of a urinary tract infection [17]. For patients who are sexually active, consider obtaining urine studies for gonorrhea and chlamydia at the same time of urinalysis.

Consideration should be taken given the possibility for morbidity among untreated urinary tract infections. Known complications include progressions to pyelonephritis, urosepsis, and renal scarring [18].

92.5 Treatment

Consideration for treatment will depend on the clinical condition of the patient. Patients tolerating oral intake, with minimal signs of systemic infection, can reasonably be treated in the outpatient setting with an oral antibiotic and close follow up in 3–5 days. Antibiotic choices could include a second or third generation cephalosporin, though often these will require dosing three times daily. Twice daily dosing with trimethoprim-sulfamethoxazole (TMP-SMX) could also be considered if available. Escalation of antibiotic therapy should include a duration of at least 10–14 days with close follow up. For patients with worsening symptoms, evaluation in the Emergency Department is appropriate. Patients unable to tolerate oral intake, or those with concerns for worsening systemic findings, including pyelonephritis or abnormal vital sign changes will require inpatient treatment with parental antibiotics such as third generation cephalosporins. Though, considerations for local resistance patterns, prior culture growth, and clinical status of the patient is helpful when titrating parental antibiotic choices [19].

Specific antibiotic regimens should be targeted to any known prior pathogens if patients have a prior history of UTI, local resistance patterns, or institution specific antibiograms. For specific recommendations, see prior section on simple urinary tract infections.

Patients with acute complicated UTI who have mild to moderate symptoms will require initial stabilization, including rehydration and antimicrobial therapy. If the patient is improving following stabilization and early treatment, they may be discharged home to continue oral antimicrobial therapy. Ability to tolerate oral medications should also be considered when discussing a patient's treatment plan.

Given the renal excretion and high bioavailability of most oral antibiotics used to treat cystitis, oral therapy should be considered first line when clinically appropriate. A recent trial of children with pyelonephritis showed no significant treatment failure between oral and parental therapy followed with oral antibiotics [20]. Consideration for imaging should include retroperitoneal ultrasound if the patient's presentation is consistent with pyelonephritis [8].

Case 3 A 15-year-old female with a history of spastic cerebral palsy and neurogenic bladder is presenting with fever for 3 days. She has had a lower abdominal pain, vomiting, and fevers to 39 °C for the last several days. The patient performs bladder catheterizations and reports scant hematuria the last several days.

92.6 Medically Complex Patients

Pediatric patients with complex medical needs may often present with atypical symptoms of UTI, or symptoms that are more vague. A discussion of past medical history and a review of systems is key for any patient, and it remains a critical component of the encounter in a child with medical complexity. Such patients often experience inequities in medical care, and biases may contribute to patient outcomes [21].

A review of systems and history should include any prior bladder or urologic tract instrumentation, surgical correction, home catheter use, changes to urinary and stooling patterns, as well as systemic symptoms. Additionally, patients who have recurrent UTIs may have a history of bladder colonization that has required alternative antibiotic therapies given their individual resistance patterns. Therefore, particular attention should be directed to any prior UTI history and culture growth. Presence of systemic symptoms, such as nausea, vomiting, fevers or temperature instability, altered mental status, or increases to baseline oxygen needs, should warrant prompt review and treatment initiation. Systemic symptoms are concerning for the progression of pathology that could include urosepsis, which carries significant morbidity and mortality without adequate resuscitation [22].

Escalation of care is appropriate, and the emergency department is a reasonable disposition. Diagnosis is made utilizing tools as previously referenced in this chapter, to include a catheterized urine specimen with urinalysis and urine culture. Enteric flora, such as *E. coli*, should be considered as a part of the pathology, as well as any other known prior colonization in complex patients. Local resistance patterns will play a significant role in the treatment for known bacterial colonization in any medically complex patient. Use resistance and susceptibilities from prior cultures to guide therapy.

Medically complex patients may present with findings consistent with sepsis, but often such patients may warrant a careful evaluation for more subtle signs of systemic infection. High risk medical conditions that could predispose patients to systemic infection could include immunocompromised status, asplenia, transplant recipients, prematurity, those with central venous access, known malignancy, or preexisting cardiac conditions. Vital sign changes concerning for sepsis are tachycardia for age, tachypnea, fever, or hypotension. It is important to note that normotension is often seen in early stages of sepsis, so do not be reassured by a lack of hypotension. Physical exam may show a patient with delayed or brisk capillary refill, skin with mottling or petechiae. Mental status changes include depression, irritability, or confusion [23]. For patients with concerns for urosepsis, fluid resuscitation and antibiotic administration remain the mainstays to prevent significant complications [24].

Empiric therapy with a third-generation cephalosporin is indicated unless a recent urine culture with susceptibilities is available to guide care. Prioritization of a Beta-lactam as the first administered antibiotic has been associated with improved outcomes [25]. For patients with prior steroid use or adrenal insufficiency, it is important to recognize that stress dose steroids also aid in the reduction of morbidity and mortality in pediatric patients. Early laboratory values to obtain include appropriate cultures, electrolytes, hepatic function, cortisol, lactate, and coagulation factors [26].

Overall, the care of a medically complex child or adolescent requires careful consideration for additional risk factors given known comorbidities. Early recognition of urinary tract infections and prompt treatment can often reduce the risk for systemic involvement, thus reducing morbidity and mortality.

Extra Credit Points

1. UTIs are more common in females than males and most often due to *E. coli*
2. Uncomplicated cystitis can be treated based on dipstick results with oral antibiotics
3. Lengthen treatment course in complicated cystitis to include 10–14 days.
4. Consider urinary tract sources for infection in medically complex children.
5. Table 92.2 distinguishes uncomplicated versus complicated cystitis, and urinary tract infections in the medically complex student.

Table 92.2 Uncomplicated versus complicated cystitis versus UTI in a medically complex patient

	Presentation	Diagnosis	Treatment
Uncomplicated cystitis	Dysuria, urinary frequency or hesitancy, hematuria	Positive urine dipstick, confirmed by urine culture	Oral antibiotics for 5–10 days Third generation cephalosporin often first-line
Complicated cystitis	Dysuria, fevers, hematuria, abdominal pain in patient with comorbidities	Positive urine dipstick, confirmed by urine culture	Oral antibiotics for 7–14 days. Third generation cephalosporin
Medically complex	Temperature instability, altered mental status, increased respiratory efforts, sepsis	Positive urine dipstick, confirmed by culture	Intravenous antibiotics in the hospital setting

References

1. Shaikh N, Morone NE, Bost JE, Farrell MH. Prevalence of urinary tract infection in childhood: a meta-analysis. Pediatr Infect Dis J. 2008;27:302–8.
2. Edlin RS, Shapiro DJ, Hersh AL, Copp HL. Antibiotic resistance patterns of outpatient pediatric urinary tract infections. J Urol. 2013;190:222–7.
3. Kaufman J, Temple-Smith M, Sanci L. Urinary tract infections in children: an overview of diagnosis and management. BMJ Paediatr open. 2019;3:e000487.
4. Chang SL, Shortliffe LD. Pediatric urinary tract infections. Pediatr Clin N Am. 2006;53:379–400, vi.
5. Azzarone G, Liewehr S, O'Connor K. Cystitis. Pediatr Rev. 2007;28:474–6.
6. Mufson MA, Belshe RB. A review of adenoviruses in the etiology of acute hemorrhagic cystitis. J Urol. 1976;115:191–4.
7. Gorelick MH, Shaw KN. Screening tests for urinary tract infection in children: a meta-analysis. Pediatrics. 1999;104:e54.
8. Mattoo TK, Shaikh N, Nelson CP. Contemporary management of urinary tract infection in children. Pediatrics. 2021;147:e2020012138.
9. Tullus K, Shaikh N. Urinary tract infections in children. Lancet (London, England). 2020;395:1659–68.
10. Shaikh N, Morone NE, Lopez J, Chianese J, Sangvai S, D'Amico F, et al. Does this child have a urinary tract infection? JAMA. 2007;298:2895–904.
11. Urinary tract infection in under 16s: diagnosis and management. NICE guideline. 2022. https://www.nice.org.uk/guidance/ng224/chapter/Recommendations.
12. Afolabi TM, Goodlet KJ, Fairman KA. Association of antibiotic treatment duration with recurrence of uncomplicated urinary tract infection in pediatric patients. Ann Pharmacother. 2020;54:757–66.
13. Fitzgerald A, Mori R, Lakhanpaul M, Tullus K. Antibiotics for treating lower urinary tract infection in children. Cochrane Database Syst Rev. 2012;2012:CD006857.
14. Wagenlehner FME, Bjerklund Johansen TE, Cai T, Koves B, Kranz J, Pilatz A, et al. Epidemiology, definition and treatment of complicated urinary tract infections. Nat Rev Urol. 2020;17:586–600.
15. Heyns CF. Urinary tract infection associated with conditions causing urinary tract obstruction and stasis, excluding urolithiasis and neuropathic bladder. World J Urol. 2012;30:77–83.
16. Hay AD, Sterne JAC, Hood K, Little P, Delaney B, Hollingworth W, et al. Improving the diagnosis and treatment of urinary tract infection in young children in primary care: results from the DUTY prospective diagnostic cohort study. Ann Fam Med. 2016;14:325–36.

17. Shaikh N, Lee S, Krumbeck JA, Kurs-Lasky M. Support for the use of a new cutoff to define a positive urine culture in young children. Pediatrics. 2023;152:e2023061931.
18. Keren R, Shaikh N, Pohl H, Gravens-Mueller L, Ivanova A, Zaoutis L, et al. Risk factors for recurrent urinary tract infection and renal scarring. Pediatrics. 2015;136:e13–21.
19. Chakupurakal R, Ahmed M, Sobithadevi DN, Chinnappan S, Reynolds T. Urinary tract pathogens and resistance pattern. J Clin Pathol. 2010;63:652–4.
20. Baker PC, Nelson DS, Schunk JE. The addition of ceftriaxone to oral therapy does not improve outcome in febrile children with urinary tract infections. Arch Pediatr Adolesc Med. 2001;155:135–9.
21. Kuo DZ, Goudie A, Cohen E, Houtrow A, Agrawal R, Carle AC, et al. Inequities in health care needs for children with medical complexity. Health Aff (Millwood). 2014;33:2190–8.
22. Eisenberg MA, Riggs R, Paul R, Balamuth F, Richardson T, DeSouza HG, et al. Association between the first-hour intravenous fluid volume and mortality in pediatric septic shock. Ann Emerg Med. 2022;80:213–24.
23. Dellinger RP, Levy MM, Rhodes A, Annane D, Gerlach H, Opal SM, et al. Surviving Sepsis Campaign: international guidelines for management of severe sepsis and septic shock, 2012. Intensive Care Med. 2013;39:165–228.
24. Schlapbach LJ, Watson RS, Sorce LR, Argent AC, Menon K, Hall MW, et al. International consensus criteria for pediatric sepsis and septic shock. JAMA. 2024;331:665–74.
25. Amoah J, Klein EY, Chiotos K, Cosgrove SE, Tamma PD. Administration of a β-lactam prior to vancomycin as the first dose of antibiotic therapy improves survival in patients with bloodstream infections. Clin Infect Dis. 2022;75:98–104.
26. Paul R, Niedner M, Riggs R, Richardson T, DeSouza HG, Auletta JJ, et al. Bundled care to reduce sepsis mortality: the Improving Pediatric Sepsis Outcomes (IPSO) Collaborative. Pediatrics. 2023;152:e2022059938.

Chapter 93
Septic Arthritis and Osteomyelitis

Elizabeth Zorovich and Vlad Panaitescu

Case 1 8 year Elliot presents to your office with a painful right leg. He says he visited a family member this weekend and while playing with the dog he was bit on the right knee. The wound was cleaned and dressed. Now, Elliot has pain in his right shin and does not want to bear any weight on the right leg. On exam, the wound is clean and dry and there is normal range of motion of the knee and ankle. Elliot continues to refuse to bear any weight on the leg. What should you do?

Osteomyelitis is one of the most prevalent musculoskeletal infections in children [1] Osteomyelitis is 2.5 times more common in boys and is most common in the first decade of life. The most common bacteria that causes osteomyelitis is *Staphylococcus aureus.* Most cases of osteomyelitis are caused by hematogenous spread. This means the infection is spread by the blood in the circulatory system. Initial bacteremia may occur from a skin lesion, infection or trauma and then spread hematogenously to the bone. Pediatric patients are at a greater risk for developing osteomyelitis than adults for a few anatomical reasons. In pediatric patient there is sluggish blood flow in the metaphyseal capillaries allowing bacteria to lodge in this region. The low pH and oxygen tension around pediatric growth plates also assists in bacterial growth [2]. The evaluation of a pediatric patient with suspected osteomyelitis may be difficult. In contrast to septic arthritis, pediatric patients with osteomyelitis are generally not toxic appearing [3]. Patients may or may not have a fever. A thorough history and physical examination should be performed. The physical examination should include a full sign of vital signs and thorough examination of the site of pain. In particular, physical exam findings that should be noted are redness, warmth, swelling, ability to move the limb and/or bear weight, and any drainage present. If

E. Zorovich (✉) · V. Panaitescu
University of Florida-Jacksonville, Jacksonville, FL, USA
e-mail: elizabeth.zorovich@jax.ufl.edu; vlad.panaitescu@jax.ufl.edu

R. P. Olympia, J. Brady-Olympia (eds.), *Clinical Considerations in School-based Health*, https://doi.org/10.1007/978-3-031-85765-2_93

any of these concerning physical exam findings are present, patient should be referred to an emergency department for further evaluation.

Case 2 8-year Johnny presents to your office with a painful left knee. He says he was playing kickball a few days ago and tried to slide into second base. When he did, he scraped his left knee. Now, the left knee is swollen, red and he can't move it. When you take Johnny's vitals his temperature if 103 F and his heart rate is 140 beat per minute. What do you do?

Septic arthritis is an intra-articular infection. In contrast to osteomyelitis, septic arthritis is relatively rare with peak occurrence in the first 2 years of life. The most common affected joints are the hip and the knee. Septic arthritis can be developed from contagious spread of osteomyelitis and/or can be caused by hematogenous seeding. An upper respiratory infection precedes about 80% of cases [4]. In contrast to osteomyelitis, patients with septic arthritis may be toxic appearing. Some vital signs abnormalities that may be presents are fever, hypotension and tachycardia. On physical exam, the affected joint will have severe pain with passive motion, exhibit localized swelling, effusion tenderness and warmth. When there is concern for septic arthritis of the hip, the Kocher criteria can be used (Table 93.1). This tool helps distinguish septic arthritis from transient synovitis for patients with a painful hip. If all 4 criteria of the Kocher criteria are met, there is a 99% probability the patient has septic arthritis. If you suspect septic arthritis, patient should be sent to the emergency department for an urgent evaluation and further work up [5].

93.1 Case Conclusions

Case 1 Elliot is transported to his local emergency department. Initial x-ray of the right tibia and fibula are normal. Due to persistent pain and concern for osteomyelitis labs are drawn and patient is admitted to this children's hospital for MRI of the tibia. Labs included a complete blood count, inflammatory markers and blood cultures. On MRI there is evidence of osteomyelitis in the tibia and Elliot is started on IV clindamycin. After a few days, Elliot is discharged home with continued clindamycin treatment for 4 weeks.

Table 93.1 Kocher Criteria for assessment of pediatric hip pain

Kocher criteria
Non-weight bearing on affected side
ESR greater than 40 mm/hour
Fever
WBC greater than 12,000

Probability of Pediatric Septic Arthritis of the hip- 4/4 = 99%, 3/4 = 93%, 2/4 = 40%, 1/4 = 3%

Case 2 Johnny is urgently transported to the local emergency department. With high suspicion of septic arthritis, blood cultures and labs are drawn. Labs are concerning for a leukocytosis, and elevated inflammatory markers. X-ray shows slight widening of the knee joint. Orthopedic team is consulted and due to high suspicion of septic arthritis an arthrocentesis is performed. This is when fluid is removed from the joint using a needle and sent to the lab for analysis. The fluid obtained by the orthopedic team is concerning for septic arthritis. Johnny is taken to the operating room with the orthopedic team for an urgent joint wash out. After surgery Johnny stayed in the hospital for a few days of IV clindamycin and discharged home on oral clindamycin for 4 weeks.

Extra Credit Points

1. Table 93.2 highlights the difference in presentation, symptoms, signs and disposition for septic arthritis and osteomyelitis.
2. Table 93.3 lists the most common etiologies, laboratory abnormalities and treatment for septic arthritis and osteomyelitis [6].
3. Septic arthritis and osteomyelitis are caused by hematogenous spread. The affected bone or joint may not be at the original place of trauma or infection.
4. Patient with septic arthritis and osteomyelitis may not be toxic appearing.
5. Risk factors for both septic arthritis and osteomyelitis include immune compromised patients and diabetes. Review patient's medical records and medication list prior to history and physical exam.
6. Septic arthritis is a surgical emergency and requires an urgent referral to the emergency department.
7. When there is concern for septic arthritis and an arthrocentesis is performed, a fluid analysis is done in the lab to determine the white blood cell count and neutrophil percentage of the fluid. This helps the medical team determine the cause of the swelling [7]. Table 93.4 lists the differential diagnosis based off the fluid analysis.

Table 93.2 Characteristics of septic arthritis and osteomyelitis

	Septic arthritis	Osteomyelitis
Vital signs	± Fever	± Fever
Symptoms	Pain in affected joint or extremity, inability to bear weight	Pain in affected joint extremity, inability to bear weight
Signs	Joint is erythematous, swollen, tender to palpation, pain to active and passive range of motion	Pain on active range of motion or palpation of the extremity
Disposition	Referral to emergency department	Referral to emergency department

Table 93.3 Causes, diagnostic criteria and treatment of osteomyelitis and septic arthritis

	Septic arthritis	Osteomyelitis
Etiology	Staphylococcus aureus Group A streptococcus Kingella kingae	Staphylococcus aureus Group A streptococcus Kingella kingae
Most common sites involved	Knee > hip > ankle > other	Femur > tibia > hands and feet > humerus > pelvis
Diagnosis	↑ WBC (70%), CRP (95%), sed rate (90%), (+) Blood culture (40%) Synovial fluid analysis Kocher criteria (Table 93.1)	Leukocytosis, ↑ CRP (95%), ↑ sed rate (90%), (+) blood culture (35–50%), bone aspirate (50–80%) Radionuclide bone scan (80–100%) MRI (92–100%)
Treatment	IV clindamycin or vancomycin (or oxacillin) for 3–4 weeks	IV clindamycin or vancomycin (or oxacillin or ceftriaxone) for 3–6 weeks

Table 93.4 Differential diagnosis based on fluid analysis

Diagnosis	White blood cells (cells/mm^3)	Neutrophils (%)
Normal	<200	10–20
Traumatic effusion	<2000	10–30
Rheumatologic	10,000–50,000	50–80
Septic arthritis	>50,000	>80
Lyme arthritis	15–125,000	>50

References

1. Walter N, Bartle S, Alt V, Rupp M. The epidemiology of osteomyelitis in children. Children. 2021;8(11):1000. https://doi.org/10.3390/children8111000.
2. Yi J, Wood JB, Creech CB, Williams D, Jimenez-Truque N, Yildirim I, Sederdahl B, Daugherty M, Hussaini L, Munye M, Tomashek KM, Focht C, Watson N, Anderson EJ, Thomsen I. Clinical epidemiology and outcomes of Pediatric musculoskeletal infections. J Pediatr. 2021;234:236–244.e2. https://doi.org/10.1016/j.jpeds.2021.03.028. Epub 2021 Mar 24. PMID: 33771580; PMCID: PMC8238832.
3. Stephan AM, Faino A, Caglar D, Klein EJ. Clinical presentation of acute osteomyelitis in the pediatric emergency department. Pediatr Emerg Care. 2022;38(1):e209–13. https://doi.org/10.1097/PEC.0000000000002217.
4. Brown DW, Sheffer BW. Pediatric septic arthritis: an update. Orthop Clin North Am. 2019;50(4):461–70. https://doi.org/10.1016/j.ocl.2019.05.003. Epub 2019 Aug 2
5. Erkilinc M, Gilmore A, Weber M, Mistovich RJ. Current concepts in pediatric septic arthritis. J Am Acad Orthop Surg. 2021;29(5):196–206. https://doi.org/10.5435/JAAOS-D-20-00835.
6. American Academy of Pediatrics. Committee on infectious diseases. Red Book: Report of the committee on infectious diseases. Elk Grove Village: American Academy of Pediatrics; 2021–2024.
7. Saavedra-Lozano J, Falup-Pecurariu O, Faust SN, Girschick H, Hartwig N, Kaplan S, Lorrot M, Mantadakis E, Peltola H, Rojo P, Zaoutis T, LeMair A. Bone and joint infections. Pediatr Infect Dis J. 2017;36(8):788–99.

Part VII
Common Infections in the School Setting

Chapter 94
Infections of the Head and Neck

Robert P. Olympia

Case 1 Samantha, a 16 year old student, presents with bilateral eye discharge after a few days of nasal congestion, cough, and fever. She denies any visual disturbances. She does not wear contact lenses. On examination, she has bilateral conjunctival injection with purulent discharge and bilateral, nontender periorbital edema. She does not have proptosis and has full range of motion of her extraocular muscles. What do you do?

Table 94.1 lists a differential diagnosis of infectious causes of conjunctival injection and periorbital swelling.

Viruses, specifically adenoviruses, cause up to 80% of all infectious conjunctivitis. Conjunctivitis can occur through direct inoculation or respiratory tract droplet spread, and infectivity can be reduced by effective hand hygiene methods. Students with conjunctivitis typically require evaluation by their primary care physician or in an urgent care center. Referral to an ED is recommended if the student has "red flag" symptoms associated with their conjunctivitis, delineated in Table 94.1. Approximately 60% of bacterial conjunctivitis cases are self-limiting and disappear within 1–2 weeks of presentation. Studies have shown that the use of broad-spectrum antibiotics results in a quicker recovery, decrease in disease transmission, and early return to school.

Case 2 Jordan, a 5 year old student, presents with severe right ear pain. You notice that he feels warm and that his right ear appears "pushed out" com-

R. P. Olympia (✉)
Department of Emergency Medicine and Pediatrics, Penn State College of Medicine
Attending Physician, Hershey, PA, USA

Division of Pediatric Emergency Medicine, Department of Emergency Medicine, Penn State
Milton S. Hershey Medical Center, Hershey, PA, USA
e-mail: rolympia@hmc.psu.edu

R. P. Olympia, J. Brady-Olympia (eds.), *Clinical Considerations in School-based Health*, https://doi.org/10.1007/978-3-031-85765-2_94

Table 94.1 Differential diagnosis of infectious causes of conjunctival injection and periorbital swelling

Infection	Clinical presentation	Diagnosis	Treatment
Conjunctivitis	Unilateral or bilateral conjunctival injection and chemosis, clear or purulent discharge, foreign body sensation, tearing, photophobia, concomitant upper respiratory symptoms	Eye culture may distinguish between viral and bacterial (bacterial etiology often associated with more pronounced, thicker and purulent discharge)	Cool compresses, artificial tears, topical antibiotics [1] (for bacterial etiology—trimethoprim-polymyxin B, erythromycin, or ciprofloxacin) Red flags: Consider ED transfer and ophthalmology referral for vision loss, intense eye pain with eye movement, if student wears contacts, visible ulcers/vesicles, trauma related or associated with chemical exposure, intense photophobia, abnormally shaped pupil
Preseptal cellulitis [2]	Periorbital swelling, erythema, and tenderness often associated with local trauma or infection (hordeolum, chalazion)	Clinical diagnosis	Oral antibiotics (cephalexin, clindamycin or trimethoprim sulfamethoxazole)
Orbital cellulitis [2]	Periorbital swelling, erythema, and tenderness associated with fever, proptosis, orbital pain, pain with eye movement, visual loss or abnormal pupillary reactivity	IV contrast CT scan of the orbits (refer to the ED)	Intravenous antibiotics (ampicillin/sulbactam or clindamycin or vancomycin), ± surgical intervention Consultation with ophthalmology and otolaryngology

pared to the left. He also has purulent discharge dripping from his right ear. What do you do?

Table 94.2 lists a differential diagnosis of infectious causes of ear pain.

Mastoiditis is a severe complication of otitis media and occurs when infection invades into the mastoid portion of the temporal bone resulting in an osteitis and subperiosteal abscess. Complications of mastoiditis can include intracranial extension with cranial nerve palsy, meningitis, sigmoid sinus thrombosis, cranial osteomyelitis, as well as subdural empyema and brain abscess. Treatment involves hospitalization for intravenous antibiotics. If there is no improvement despite antibiotics, or if there is bony destruction or an associated abscess, surgical management directed by otolaryngology may be indicated.

Case 3 Hailey, a 13 year old student, presents with severe facial pain and headache. She has been sick for the past week with nasal congestion, cough and daily fevers to 104 °F. You notice thick purulent nasal discharge from both nos-

Table 94.2 Differential diagnosis of infectious causes of ear pain

Infection	Clinical presentation	Diagnosis	Treatment
Otitis media [3]	Ear pain, fever, ear discharge, decreased hearing, headache Bulging tympanic membrane, loss of light reflex, purulent material behind tympanic membrane or purulent material within the ear canal (associated with a perforation or myringotomy tube)	Clinical	Oral antibiotics (amoxicillin, cefdinir, azithromycin, clindamycin; duration varies based on age/symptoms), topical benzocaine Antibiotic ear drops (ofloxacin and ciprofloxacin combined with either hydrocortisone or dexamethasone) for students with myringotomy tubes
Otitis externa	Ear pain, fever, ear discharge, tenderness with pulling pinna, tender periauricular lymph nodes, decreased hearing, headache	Clinical	Antibiotic ear drops (Neomycin, Polymyxin B or Trimethoprim sulfate with Hydrocortisone or ofloxacin and ciprofloxacin combined with either hydrocortisone or dexamethasone) Placement of a wick for severe canal edema
Mastoiditis [4]	Signs of otitis media and displacement of the pinna (rotated forward), tenderness/swelling/erythema over the mastoid	IV contrast CT scan of the temporal bones (refer to the ED)	Intravenous antibiotics (ampicillin/sulbactam or clindamycin), ± surgical intervention including myringotomy

trils. She does not have periorbital swelling, visual disturbances, neck stiffness, or altered mental status. What do you do?

Table 94.3 lists a differential diagnosis of infectious causes of facial pain.

A presumptive diagnosis of bacterial sinusitis should be made in a child/adolescent between the ages of 1 and 18 years presenting with an upper respiratory infection and any of the following additional features: (1) Persistent illness, i.e., nasal discharge (of any quality) or daytime cough or both lasting more than 10 days without improvement, (2) biphasic illness with worsening or new onset of nasal discharge, daytime cough, or fever after initial improvement, or (3) severe onset, i.e., concurrent fever (temperature $\geq$ 39 °C/102.2 °F) and purulent nasal discharge for at least 3 consecutive days. Indications for imaging include suspected orbital or central nervous system involvement, and should not routinely be utilized to differentiate between bacterial sinusitis and viral upper respiratory infection.

Case 4 Josiah, a 10 year old student, presents with significant sore throat and fever. He does not have a "hot potato voice", does not have drooling or difficulty breathing, and does not have limitation to range of motion of his neck. What do you do?

Table 94.4 lists a differential diagnosis of infectious causes of sore throat.

Table 94.3 Differential diagnosis of infectious causes of facial pain

Infection	Clinical presentation	Diagnosis	Treatment
Viral upper respiratory infection (URI)	Fever, nasal congestion/discharge, headache, cough, sneezing, facial pain	Clinical	Supportive care
Sinusitis	Viral URI symptoms >10 days without improvement (fever may not be present, nasal discharge may be clear) Fever >39 °C and purulent nasal discharge for at least 3 days Headache, facial pain, tenderness to palpation over sinuses	Clinical IV contrast CT scan for signs of orbital cellulitis or altered mental status or severe headache (possible meningitis, brain abscess, sinus venous thrombosis)	Oral (amoxicillin, amoxicillin-clavulanate, clindamycin) or intravenous (ampicillin/sulbactam or clindamycin) antibiotics [5] Nasal decongestants, intranasal steroids, saline irrigation
Dental abscess	Fever, facial swelling/pain, dental caries, tooth pain with adjacent gum swelling/tenderness, pain on eating	Clinical	Oral (penicillin, amoxicillin-clavulanate, clindamycin) or intravenous (ampicillin/sulbactam or clindamycin) antibiotics, referral to a dentist

There is no one clinical finding that is specific nor sensitive for streptococcal pharyngitis. For Centor criteria, the risk of Group A beta-hemolytic streptococcal (GABHS) pharyngitis is 1–2.5% (total score of 0), 5–10% (total score of 1), 11–17% (total score of 2), 28–35% (total score of 3), and 51–53% (total score of >4). Recommendations for testing include: total score of 0–1 (no testing is suggested), for a total score of 2–3 (testing is suggested), and for a total score >4 (antibiotic treatment is suggested without testing). Since GABHS testing is considered inexpensive and non-invasive, and because the predictive qualities of the Centor criteria is rather poor, many practitioners will test all students with moderate risk (Centor > 2). GABHS pharyngitis is treated with antibiotics to decrease the risk of Rheumatic fever, and does not decrease duration of symptoms or the risk of post-streptococcal glomerulonephritis and pharyngeal/neck abscesses.

Case 5 Alexis, a 7 year old student, presents with significant right sided neck swelling and pain. She was recently treated for GABHS pharyngitis. The right side of her neck is swollen, erythematous, and tender to palpation. She does not have difficulty swallowing, but has some limitation to the range of motion of her neck. What do you do?

Table 94.5 lists a differential diagnosis of infectious causes of neck swelling and pain.

Table 94.4 Differential diagnosis of infectious causes of sore throat

Infection	Clinical presentation	Diagnosis	Treatment
Group A beta-hemolytic Streptococcal (GABHS) pharyngitis	Sore throat, headache, cough, abdominal pain, nausea/vomiting, scarlatinaform rash (may also present with urticarial or petechiae rash) Circumoral pallor, strawberry tongue, palatal petechiae, exudative pharyngitis, tender cervical lymphadenopathy	Centor criteria: (1) Absence of cough (1 point) (2) Swollen and tender anterior cervical lymphadenopathy (1 point) (3) Temperature >100.4 °F (1 point) (4) Tonsillar exudates or swelling (1 point) (5) Age 3–14 years (1 point) or age 15–44 years (0 points) Rapid strep test, throat culture	Oral (amoxicillin, cephalosporin, azithromycin, clindamycin) or intramuscular antibiotics (Penicillin G Benzathine) [6], supportive care, oral dexamethasone Student is contagious for 24 hours from the initiation of antibiotic therapy
Viral pharyngitis	Similar to GABHS, more likely to have viral URI symptoms (nasal congestion or discharge, sneezing)	Negative testing for GABHS pharyngitis Monospot or EBV titers (see Chap. 101)	Supportive care, oral dexamethasone
Retropharyngeal abscess [7] (less likely seen in students >8 years of age)	Similar to pharyngitis above, moderate sore throat, respiratory distress, hot potato voice, drooling, dehydration, dysphagia, neck stiffness, decreased range of motion of the neck	Soft tissue radiograph of the neck or CT scan of the neck with intravenous contrast	Intravenous antibiotics (ampicillin/sulbactam or clindamycin), ± surgical intervention
Peritonsillar abscess [7]	Similar to pharyngitis above, moderate sore throat (often unilateral), respiratory distress, hot potato voice, drooling, dehydration, dysphagia, decreased range of motion of the neck, trismus, deviation of the uvula away from the affected side	Ultrasound or CT scan of the neck with intravenous contrast	Intravenous antibiotics (ampicillin/sulbactam or clindamycin), drainage

Table 94.5 Differential diagnosis of infectious causes of neck swelling and pain

Infection	Clinical presentation	Diagnosis	Treatment
Cervical lymphadenitis	Unilateral or bilateral neck swelling associated with erythema and tenderness, fever	Clinical	Oral antibiotics (cephalexin, clindamycin or trimethoprim sulfamethoxazole) Needle aspiration or incisional drainage if poor response to oral antibiotics
Deep neck abscess	Similar to cervical lymphadenitis, swelling may be larger, indurated or fluctuant, often associated with difficulty breathing or swallowing or decreased range of motion of the neck	Ultrasound or CT scan of the neck with intravenous contrast	Intravenous antibiotics (ampicillin/sulbactam or clindamycin), ± surgical intervention [8]
Lemierre's syndrome	Fever, signs of pharyngitis, neck pain/swelling/mass Metastatic spread of an oropharyngeal infection along the lateral spaces of the neck with subsequent thrombophlebitis of the internal jugular vein and/or septic emboli	Doppler ultrasound, contrast enhanced CT scan, or MRI/MRV of the neck/brain	Intravenous antibiotics (ampicillin/sulbactam or clindamycin or metronidazole), ± surgical intervention (abscess formation, thrombus formation of the brain/lungs/mediastinum) Anti-coagulation is controversial
Acute parotitis/salivary gland infection	Swelling, pain and erythema over the parotid gland or salivary gland, fever, trismus, pain with mastication	Clinical (often bacterial or viral)	± oral antibiotics (clindamycin, amoxicillin-clavulanate), supportive care, warm massage, sialagogues (sour candies)

Aerobic (*Streptococcus pyogenes, Staphylococcus aureus*, and *H. influenzae*) and anaerobic (*Prevotella, Fusobacterium, and Peptostreptococcus* spp.) organisms are typically associated with deep neck infections in children. Almost 66% of deep neck abscesses contain β-lactamase–producing organisms. Cervical lymph nodes often associated with malignancies are described as located supraclavicular or in the posterior triangle (behind or lateral to the sternocleidomastoid muscle); very rapid increase in size; confluent and matted shape; firm or rubbery consistency; lack of tenderness or warmth; fixated to deep tissues; associated with fever, malaise, weight loss or night sweats (Fig. 94.1).

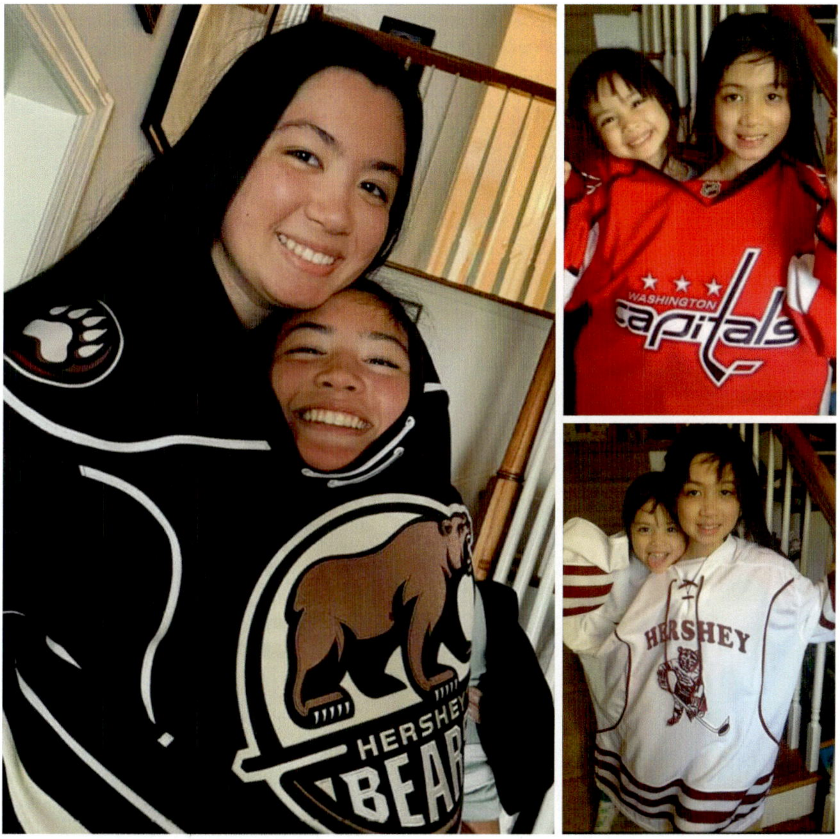

Fig. 94.1 Cute heads and necks repping the Hershey Bears and Washington Capitals hockey teams

Extra Credit Points

1. The evaluation of a student who presents with a possible infection of the head or neck begins with a thorough history and physical examination, focusing on airway, breathing, and circulation.
2. The majority of head and neck infections can be assessed and managed in an urgent care setting or primary care physician's office.
3. Red flags for head and neck infections that require immediate ED referral utilizes the mnemonic "HEAD NECK":

H	Headache (severe)	Retrobulbar (orbital cellulitis), generalized (sinus venous thrombosis associated with sinusitis), facial (dental abscess), or post-auricular (mastoiditis)
E	Eyesight disturbance	Associated with orbital cellulitis (due to involvement of the ocular nerve or extra-ocular muscles)
A	Airway obstruction	"Hot potato voice" or drooling associated with retropharyngeal, peritonsillar, or deep neck abscess
D	Displacement	Of the pinna (mastoiditis) or eye (proptosis associated with orbital cellulitis)
N	Neck stiffness	Meningitis (associated with sinusitis or mastoiditis) or associated with retropharyngeal, peritonsillar, or deep neck abscess
E	Extraocular muscle limitation or pain with extraocular muscle movement	Associated with orbital cellulitis
C	Cyanosis and circulation	Involvement of airway, breathing, and circulation resulting in respiratory compromise (from a retropharyngeal, peritonsillar, or deep neck abscess) or shock (hypoperfusion from sepsis or significant dehydration)
K	Kissing tonsils or displacement of the uvula	Associated with peritonsillar or a deep neck abscess

References

1. Honkila M, Koskela U, Kontiokari T, et al. Effect of topical antibiotics on duration of acute infective conjunctivitis in children: a randomized clinical trial and a systematic review and meta-analysis. JAMA Netw Open. 2022;5(10):e2234459.
2. Williams KJ, Allen RC. Paediatric orbital and periorbital infections. Curr Opin Ophthalmol. 2019;30(5):349–55.
3. Venekamp RP, Sanders SL, Glasziou PP, et al. Antibiotics for acute otitis media in children. Cochrane Database Syst Rev. 2023;11(11):CD000219.
4. Loh R, Phua M, Shaw CKL. Management of paediatric acute mastoiditis: systematic review. J Laryngol Otol. 2018;132(2):96–104.
5. Shaikh N, Hoberman A, Shope TR, et al. Identifying children likely to benefit from antibiotics for acute sinusitis: a randomized clinical trial. JAMA. 2023;330(4):349–58.
6. Hedin K, Thorning S, van Driel ML. Different antibiotic treatments for group A streptococcal pharyngitis. Cochrane Database Syst Rev. 2023;11(11):CD004406.
7. Akhavan M. Ear, nose, throat: beyond pharyngitis: retropharyngeal abscess, peritonsillar abscess, epiglottitis, bacterial tracheitis, and postoperative tonsillectomy. Emerg Med Clin North Am. 2021;39(3):661–75.
8. Demongeot N, Akkari M, Blanchet C, et al. Pediatric deep neck infections: clinical description and analysis of therapeutic management. Arch Pediatr. 2022;29(2):128–32.

Chapter 95
Acute Gastroenteritis—Viral and Bacterial

Sixtine Valdelièvre Herold

Case 1 **Donovan is a 10 year old male who was noted to be somewhat quiet this AM by his teacher. When she checks in, he complains of abdominal pain. She sends Donovan to the nurse, where he promptly has a large episode of nonbilious nonbloody emesis. He has a temperature to 100.6 Fahrenheit. He appears very quiet and lethargic to the school nurse. What should you do next?**

Case 2 **Six teachers in your elementary school have called for substitutes this morning, citing the stomach bug as the culprit. As the day goes on, the school nurse reports multiple visits from kids with vomiting and/or abdominal pain symptoms throughout the day, whom she has sent home. By the end of the day, a few more teachers have had to go home as well, for similar reasons. What do you think is going on?**

Acute gastroenteritis (AGE) is inflammation of the gastrointestinal tract, characterized by a variety of symptoms often including but not limited to nausea, vomiting, diarrhea and abdominal pain. Malaise, fever and muscle pain are often also involved. The shared environment in school settings facilitates the spread of infectious gastroenteritis among students and staff and can lead to substantial academic disruption, arguably contributing to our nation's mental health crisis in kids [1]. Improving hand hygiene and surface disinfection can lead to lower rates of absenteeism in schools [2]. AGE can be caused by a variety of pathogens, frequently divided in bacterial, viral, and parasitic causes. For the purpose of this chapter, we will only cover the most common bacterial and viral causes. While these two etiologies may present similarly, there are some distinctive presentations which may help to discern between the two (Table 95.1).

S. V. Herold (✉)
Boston Children's Hospital, Boston, MA, USA
e-mail: sixtine-pacifique.herold@childrens.harvard.edu

R. P. Olympia, J. Brady-Olympia (eds.), *Clinical Considerations in School-based Health*, https://doi.org/10.1007/978-3-031-85765-2_95

Table 95.1 Typical signs and symptoms of bacterial versus viral causes of gastroenteritis and their potential treatments [3–5]

Agent	Presenting signs and symptoms	Typical treatment(s)
Viral (norovirus, rotavirus, adenovirus, Norwalk virus, astrovirus, and calcivirus)	Typically watery, nonbloody diarrhea. Low-grade fever possible. Usually comes on quickly and lasts 1–3 days. Vomiting may be more common and pronounced than with bacterial causes.	Supportive, focused on hydration (oral rehydration therapy ± ondansetron), followed by IV if former is failed.
Bacterial	Nausea, vomiting, diarrhea (may be watery or bloody) Severe abdominal pain Higher fever. Tends to persist longer than viral causes.	Usually supportive, focused on hydration (first PO, then IV if unsuccessful). See individual rows for specific treatments.
	Bacterial etiologies	
	Salmonella	Only if bacteremia is suspected (immunocompromised or infants <3 months)
	Campylobacter	Antibiotics may be used
	Shigella	If patient displays severe symptoms requiring hospitalizations or is immunocompromised, should use antibiotics
	Shiga toxin-producing E coli	Antibiotics are contraindicated.
	Others (Vibrio, Yersinia, Listeria)	Antibiotics may be used to decrease shedding in Yersinia

Symptoms for both etiologies generally begin for 12–48 hours after a first exposure, and generally last 1–3 days. It is important to remember that each victim is different, and to be cognizant that shedding of the virus and therefore perpetuation of the infection can continue for *up to two weeks* post recovery.

According to the National Outbreak Reporting System (NORS), a voluntary surveillance reporting system of the Center for Disease control, the four major causes of AGE in schools and childcares were responsible for over 32 thousand person-to-person or foodborne outbreaks from 2009 to 2020 [6]. In school cases, the large majority (72%) was attributable to norovirus, while childcares' main culprits were both norovirus (46.6%) and shigella (20.3%) [6] (Table 95.2). Because these stomach bugs are largely spread person to person via fecal-oral route, settings such as schools or child-care centers are the perfect set-up.

Additionally, the second most common route of spread for a pathogen like norovirus is foodborne (Table 95.3), and as nearly all schools in the US have meal programs and cafeterias, this is just another opportunity for possible outbreak sources in schools [7].

Table 95.2 Etiology of school and childcare cases of AGE, from National Outbreak Reporting System [6]

Outbreak etiology	School cases (%)	Childcare cases (%)
Norovirus	72.3%	46.6%
Shigella	2%	20.3%
Escheria	0.2%	3%
Salmonella	0.2%	2.2%
Others/unknown	24.7%	27.8%

Table 95.3 Onset, symptoms, and etiology of food-borne illnesses

Time of onset	Main symptoms	Organism or toxin
1–6 hours	Nausea, vomiting, usually febrile	Staphylococcus aureus
1–6 hours	Nausea, vomiting, afebrile	Bacillus cereus (emetic form)
8–16 hours	Diarrhea, febrile	B. cereus (diarrheal form)
6–24 hours	Foul smelling diarrhea, cramps, afebrile	Clostridium perfringens
16–48 hours	Abdominal cramping, diarrhea, fever	Vibrio cholera, Norwalk virus, Escherichia coli O157:H7, Cryptosporidium spp.
16–72 hours	Bloody diarrhea, fever, abdominal cramping	Salmonella, Shigella, and Campylobacter spp. E. coli
16–72 hours	Bloody diarrhea, fever, pseudoappendicitis, pharyngitis	Yersinia enterocolitica
1–6 weeks	Mucoid diarrhea (fatty stools), abdominal pain, weight loss	Giardia lamblia
12–36 hours	Neurologic manifestations: vertigo, diplopia, areflexia, weakness, difficulty breathing and swallowing, constipation	Clostridium botulinum
14 days	All the above, plus vomiting, rose spots, constipation, abdominal pain, fever, chills, malaise, swollen lymph nodes	Salmonella typhi

95.1 Prevention and Containment of Outbreaks

Whether the etiology of AGE is bacterial or viral, shigella, norovirus, or any other pathogen, ideal management in schools starts with prevention. Handwashing and surface disinfection have been shown to be effective in reducing transmission of AGE [2], translating to a reduction of absenteeism in schools secondary to AGE [8]. While some studies show that hand washing with soap and water is superior in some ways to hand sanitizers, the use of the latter continues to be an effective tool to help curb the spread as they are often more convenient and thus more readily used [9, 10]. Hand sanitizers can be made available throughout a school in key places to encourage use (at entrance of cafeterias, bathrooms, and classrooms). For younger students, routines of hand-washing before entering a classroom and before lunch time can be worked into the day. Child-friendly and playful additions to bathrooms such as musical hand-activated timers can help a young child with appropriate hand washing (Fig. 95.1). Additionally, while schools usually have a safe maximum

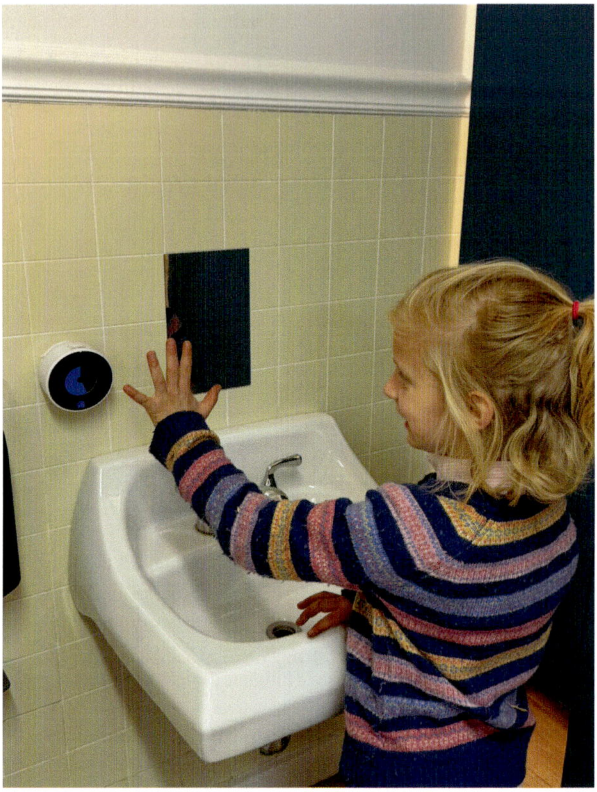

Fig. 95.1 A musical hand-activated timer motivates a 4 year old to keep washing for the full 20 seconds

temperature for water used in hand-washing sinks to avoid burning, there may not be a need for cold water at all, possibly further improving how well little hands are being washed.

95.2 Treatment

The basic standard for treatment of AGE, no matter the etiology, is hydration and gut rest [11]. Complications such as nonketotic hypoglycemia, especially in young children or more severe cases, can occur and the school health professional should be aware of his or her available resources to be prepared for this potential emergency (glucometer vs. needing to call emergency services if this is suspected). Severe dehydration requiring intravenous fluids, age, or underlying chronic medical problems may complicate disposition and require a child to be admitted to a hospital (Table 95.4).

Often, medical professionals will use ondansetron to help with nausea so that a child can rehydrate as the virus passes. A strict return policy after vomiting and/or

Table 95.4 Indications for hospitalization in children with gastroenteritis [12]

Infants <3 months who appear ill (fever, irritability, abdominal distension)
Children with underlying chronic illness (diabetes, renal disease, cardiopulmonary disease, immunodeficiency, gastrointestinal disease, etc.)
Evidence of shock (hypoperfusion) or significant dehydration
Persistent vomiting, especially if bloody or bilious
Severe abdominal pain or distension or concern for a surgical abdomen
Neurologic abnormalities (altered mental status, seizures)
Failure of oral rehydration

diarrheal symptoms should be implemented in all schools or daycare centers (24–48 hours symptom-free prior to return), and some state public health departments, such as California's, have tool kits available to follow and use in the event of an outbreak [13].

95.3 Case Conclusions

Case 1 Donovan's school nurse or health professional should assess if his symptoms are consistent with hypoglycemia and determine next steps (check his sugar if available, and/or call 911). He should be out of school for 24–48 hours based on the school's policy for vomiting and fever.

Case 2 This case illustrates how fast a school can be struck by contagious acute gastroenteritis, to the point of forcing full school closures for a period of decontamination. Communal foods such as candy jars should be eliminated, individually wrapped or provided with utensils.

Extra Credit Points
1. Acute gastroenteritis is usually spread via the person-to-person or foodborne routes, and outbreaks are a common occurrence in schools and childcare settings, making it a contributor to school absenteeism.
2. Prevention methods such as hand hygiene measures and sanitary food preparation practices can help a school with spread of AGE.
3. Schools should have a clear policy on when students and staff may return to school after a vomiting or diarrheal illness to try and curb the spread of acute gastroenteritis.

References

1. Askeland KG, Bøe T, Lundervold AJ, Stormark KM, Hysing M. The association between symptoms of depression and school absence in a population-based study of late adolescents. Front Psychol. 2020;11:1268. https://doi.org/10.3389/fpsyg.2020.01268. PMID: 32655449; PMCID: PMC7325985.
2. Ejemot RI, Ehiri JE, Meremikwu MM, Critchley JA. Hand washing for preventing diarrhoea. Cochrane Database Syst Rev. 2008;1:CD004265.
3. Sattar SBA, Singh S. Bacterial gastroenteritis. [Updated 2023 Aug 8]. In: StatPearls [Internet]. Treasure Island: StatPearls Publishing; 2024. Available from: https://www.ncbi.nlm.nih.gov/books/NBK513295/?utm_source=perplexity.
4. American Academy of Pediatrics. Committee on infectious diseases. In: Red book: report of the committee on infectious diseases. Elk Grove Village: American Academy of Pediatrics; 2021–2024.
5. Fleckenstein JM, Matthew Kuhlmann F, Sheikh A. Acute bacterial gastroenteritis. Gastroenterol Clin N Am. 2021;50(2):283–304. https://doi.org/10.1016/j.gtc.2021.02.002. Epub 2021 Apr 23. PMID: 34024442; PMCID: PMC8793005.
6. Centers for Disease Control and Prevention (CDC). National outbreak reporting system dashboard. Atlanta: U.S. Department of Health and Human Services, CDC. Last accessed 5 Jan 2018. Available from URL: wwwn.cdc.gov/norsdashboard.
7. Mattison CP, Calderwood LE, Marsh ZA, Wikswo ME, Balachandran N, Kambhampati AK, Gleason ME, Lawinger H, Mirza SA. Childcare and school acute gastroenteritis outbreaks: 2009–2020. Pediatrics. 2022;150(5):e2021056002. https://doi.org/10.1542/peds.2021-056002.
8. Sandora TJ, Shih MC, Goldmann DA. Reducing absenteeism from gastrointestinal and respiratory illness in elementary school students: a randomized, controlled trial of an infection-control intervention. Pediatrics. 2008;121(6):e1555–62. https://doi.org/10.1542/peds.2007-2597. PMID: 18519460.
9. Center for Disease Control (CDC). Prevent norovirus. n.d.. https://www.cdc.gov/norovirus/about/prevention.html#:~:text=Hand%20sanitizer%20does%20not%20work,for%20handwashing%2C%20which%20is%20best.
10. Center for Disease Control (CDC). Hand sanitizer use out and about. n.d.. https://www.cdc.gov/handwashing/hand-sanitizer-use.html#:~:text=Although%20alcohol%2Dbased%20hand%20sanitizers,difficile%2C%20as%20well%20as%20chemicals.
11. King CK, Glass R, Bresee JS, Duggan C, Centers for Disease Control and Prevention. Managing acute gastroenteritis among children: oral rehydration, maintenance, and nutritional therapy. MMWR Recomm Rep. 2003;52(RR-16):1–16. PMID: 14627948.
12. CaJacob NJ, Cohen MB. Update on diarrhea. Pediatr Rev. 2016;37(8):313–22.
13. Norovirus toolkit for school and childcare center outbreaks, California Department of Public Health. 2019. www.cdph.ca.gov/Programs/CID/DCDC/CDPH%20Document%20Library/Norovirus-School-Toolkit.pdf.

Chapter 96
Infections of the Skin—Cellulitis, Abscess, Ringworm, Impetigo, Scabies, Molluscum

Katherine Hole and Thuy Ngo

Case 1 8-year-old Lily is sent to the school nurse by her teacher for a rash on her face. Upon examination, the rash is golden-yellow and honey-crusted around her nose. Lily recalls the spots started as small bumps that burst open and then crusted over. The remainder of her skin examination is normal and unaffected. She has no evidence of mouth or throat involvement and she does not have a fever.

Impetigo is often caused by Group A *Streptococcus pyogenes* (GAS) or *Staphylococcus aureus (S. Aureus)* and is a bacterial skin infection resulting in characteristic yellow, crusted lesions. Impetigo is spread by skin-to-skin contact or following a break in the skin (i.e. turf injuries). If the lesions are isolated, they can be treated with topical mupirocin (Bactroban) antibiotic ointment alone. However, if the lesions spread to a larger surface area of the body, they may require oral antibiotics. In some cases, the lesions may progress from papules to vesicles to rapidly enlarging flaccid bullae that rupture clear, yellow fluid easily. This presentation is a classification of impetigo called bullous impetigo. These infections represent a localized infection of *S. Aureus* that produces exfoliative toxin. Bullous impetigo can be treated with topical mupirocin but may require oral antibiotic treatment if the blisters become widespread.

For medical management of impetigo, it is recommended to perform a polymerase chain reaction (PCR) wound culture. If only beta-hemolytic streptococci are detected on culture, oral penicillin or amoxicillin can be prescribed. If the child has risk factors for methicillin resistant *S. aureus* (MRSA) such as close family members in healthcare, previous MRSA infections, immunocompromised status, or if MRSA is detected on culture, then trimethoprim-sulfamethoxazole (TMP-SMX), clindamycin, or doxycycline can be administered orally.

K. Hole (✉) · T. Ngo
Johns Hopkins All Children's Hospital, St. Petersburg, FL, USA
e-mail: khole2@jh.edu; thuy.ngo@jhmi.edu

R. P. Olympia, J. Brady-Olympia (eds.), *Clinical Considerations in School-based Health*, https://doi.org/10.1007/978-3-031-85765-2_96

It is important for students with impetigo to practice good personal hygiene, wound care, wash their hands frequently, and avoid sharing sports equipment. The incubation period between GAS acquisition on healthy skin and development of lesions is a 7- to 10-day period [1]. As outlined by the National Federation of State High School Association (NFHS), athletes with impetigo may return to contact sports when they have completed 72 hours of antibiotic therapy, and all lesions have well-adhering scabs [2]. Affected areas should be covered with a bio-occlusive dressing until complete resolution has occurred. If lesions are draining or there are new lesions within the past 48 hours, athletes should abstain from contact participation.

'Red flag' signs and symptoms include fever greater than 38 °C (100.4 °F), inability to drink, generalized malaise, or intraoral lesions. If present, escalation of medical care in students with an impetigo infection is necessary. Impetigo can seed hematogenous spread of exfoliative toxin producing *S. Aureus* leading to Staphylococcal scalded skin syndrome (SSSS). This is a rapidly progressing infection that starts with skin erythema and sensitivity followed by blister breakdown and widespread skin sloughing. Importantly, there is no mucosal membrane involvement in SSSS. The treatment for SSSS is oral antibiotics. For severe infections in which the child has systemic signs or is unable to tolerate fluids or medication by mouth, intravenous (IV) antibiotics are indicated. Due to the severity of SSSS, transformation and spread of impetigo lesions to multiple areas of the body (typically to the trunk and extremities) warrants evaluation by a healthcare provider to ensure appropriate level of medical management.

Additionally, impetigo infections can lead to cellulitis, abscess formation, and lymphangitis. Cellulitis is distinguished from impetigo by features of swelling, induration, indistinct borders or erythema, and possibly fever. An abscess appears as a fluid-filled area that is warm, fluctuant, and edematous. If these cutaneous infections are colonized with MRSA and not properly treated, they can lead to serious consequences such as bacteremia, septic arthritis, and osteomyelitis. Impetigo can also seed infection to the lymphatic channels leading to acute lymphangitis characterized by fever and tender, erythematous streaks extending proximally from the lesion. Associated lymphadenopathy may be present. Due to the risk of rapid progression of these cutaneous infection complications, cellulitis, abscesses, and suspected lymphangitis should be sent to the child's doctor, urgent care, or emergency department for further evaluation. IV antibiotics are indicated if oral antibiotics fail or in children who are ill-appearing. If MRSA is present, the abscess should have incision and drainage and the athlete may return to practice and competition after 72 hours of treatment, provided the abscess is not actively draining purulent fluid.

Case 1 Resolution The school nurse applies mupirocin ointment to the lesions and calls Lily's mother to discuss impetigo. Her mother is grateful for the update. She will apply the ointment 2–3 times daily at home and see the pediatrician in 2–3 days to ensure the lesions are improving.

Case 2 5-year-old Sierra is brought to the school nurse because she can't stop scratching her hands and wrists. Her hands are erythematous with small bumps in a linear formation between the bases of her fingers. Sierra doesn't remember when this started, but her older brother has similar pruritic bumps on his hands.

Scabies is a mite infection of the skin. The characteristic lesions present as interdigital burrow lines in the web space of the hands and feet. The rash can extend to the flexor wrists, extensor elbows, axillae, umbilicus, and genitalia. The lesions are intensely pruritic and worsen with hot showers or at night as the mites burrow deeper. Scabies is transmitted through skin-to-skin contact and fomite contact on clothes and belongings. The scabies parasite can survive on clothing for up to 4 days without skin contact [3]. Treatment includes the application of topical 5% permethrin lotion to the entire body below the neck (excluding pregnant adolescents). The lotion is left on for 8–14 hours before bathing. The affected child and any close contact family members or friends should undergo topical treatment. It is essential to launder bedding and clothing worn during the 3 days before initiation of therapy in a washer with hot water and dried on a hot setting. Wrestlers are particularly susceptible to scabies. Sparring partners should be evaluated and treated in suspected cases. The itching may persist for weeks due to the natural course of hypersensitivity reactions, this is not an indication of treatment failure.

In contrast, molluscum contagiosum will have a raised, papular appearance that is not pruritic. Molluscum is a viral infection of the skin that has a characteristic flesh-colored dome appearance with an umbilicated "dimpled" center. In children, these are most often found on the face, back, chest, and extremities. Molluscum lesions can also spread through contact, such as sharing towels in the locker room. However, more commonly they are limited to spread on the affected individual from auto inoculation.

Molluscum papules will resolve on their own in 6–12 months, however, medical providers can apply 10% KOH, cryotherapy, or remove the lesions via curette. Return to play guidelines by the National Collegiate Athletic Association (NCAA) and National Athletic Trainers Association (NATA) recommend curettage or cryotherapy removal of lesions before resuming contact competition [4, 5]. Localized lesions may be covered with a gas permeable dressing followed by under wrap and stretch tape.

Case 2 Resolution The school nurse discusses scabies with Sierra's father. She informs him that Sierra does not need to be sent home early from school, as scabies has a low contagion rate within classrooms [6]. She instructs him to purchase permethrin lotion over the counter and apply to both Sierra and her older brother, as well as any household members. He expresses understanding and reiterates how he will wash all bedding and clothes.

Case 3 17-year-old Michael comes to the school nurse at the prompting of his wrestling coach for evaluation of a rash on his left extensor forearm. Michael reports the rash began last week after a wrestling event. His forearm has multiple red, scaling rings with central clearing and a raised border. They are now itchy. He does not have any similar rashes on his scalp or genital region.

Tinea corporis, often referred to as 'ringworm,' is a topical dermatophyte fungal infection. Athletes with skin-to-skin contact in humid environments are most at risk for developing ringworm. First line management for localized infections includes topical antifungals (i.e. Clotrimazole or Terbinafine). For more extensive spread or scalp/nail involvement, oral antifungals (i.e. griseofulvin) may need to be prescribed for 4–6 weeks. Extensive, widespread tinea corporis should raise suspicion for compromised immunity via autoinoculation. Athletes may return to contact sports after a minimum of 72 hours of topical or systemic antifungal therapy [2]. The lesions should be covered with a bio-occlusive dressing during sport activity once the athlete is no longer considered contagious. The NCAA has more stringent guidelines including disqualification of athletes with extensive and active tinea corporis lesions that cannot be covered [4].

Case 3 Resolution Michael expresses understanding and appreciates the recommendations. The school nurse discusses the plan with his guardian. They agree to purchase topical antifungal at the drugstore and monitor for spread or worsening of the rash. They will ensure Michael applies the ointment twice daily until the lesions are completely resolved.

Extra Credit Points

1. Close visual inspection is critical to correctly diagnosing skin infections
2. Rash with associated fever, malaise, or mucous membrane involvement should be triaged to the pediatrician, urgent care provider, or emergency department.
3. Most skin infections can be treated topically, however, if they become widespread, they often require oral medication
4. Majority of athletes with contact-spread skin infections can return to sport competition after 72 hours of treatment with covered lesions that are not actively draining, weeping, or spreading
5. Table 96.1 summarizes features, transmission, treatment, triage, and return to sport for common infection of the skin.

Table 96.1 Features, transmission, treatment, triage, and return to sport for common infection of the skin

	Impetigo	Cellulitis	Lymphangitis	Scabies	Molluscum	Ringworm
Features	Yellow, honey-crusted lesions **Bullous Impetigo:** Papules progress to vesicles and flaccid bullae that easily rupture	**Non-purulent:** Swelling, induration (hardened), erythema **Purulent (Suppurative, Abscess):** Fluid filled, warm, fluctuant, edematous	Erythematous, tender streaks extending proximally from the lesion. Lymphadenopathy may be present	Thin, gray or white, serpiginous burrow lines May have 2–5 mm red-brown nodules	Flesh colored papule with umbilicated center	Erythematous, scaling ring with central clearing and raised border
Transmission	Contact Skin injury	Contact Skin injury Infection spread Fluid drainage if purulent	Spread from existing infection	Contact Fomite contact	Contact Auto inoculation	Contact
Treatment	Topical mupirocin +/– Oral antibiotics if widespread: **Cephalexin** 50 mg/kg/day PO divided every 8 hours (maximum dose 500 mg) **Amoxicillin-Clavulanate (Augmentin)** 25–45 mg/kg/day amoxicillin component divided every 12 hours Typical duration of 7 days.	Oral antibiotics 5 day duration for uncomplicated infection but may be prolonged if unresolved or severe infection IV antibiotics 5–7 days duration if severe infection with systemic symptoms *See below for antibiotic choice (*)*	Oral or IV antibiotics for 5 day duration *See below for antibiotic choice (*)*	Topical 5% permethrin lotion applied for 8–14 hours. Additional applications may be indicated.	Observe for resolution 10% KOH application, curettage, or cryotherapy removal	Topical antifungals (Clotrimazole or terbinafine) for 7 days Oral antifungals for more extensive spread or scalp/nail involvement for 4–6 weeks **Griseofulvin** 10–20 mg/kg/day orally divided BID

(continued)

Table 96.1 (continued)

	Impetigo	Cellulitis	Lymphangitis	Scabies	Molluscum	Ringworm
Triage to pediatrician, urgent care, or emergency department if:	Fever, mucous membrane lesions, surface area affected, spread of lesions from face to trunk and extremities	All cases	All cases	Resistant, recurring cases, or if secondarily infected	Not an urgent condition	Not an urgent condition
Return to contact sport practice and competition following:	Completion of 72 h of antibiotic therapy with scabbed lesions covered No new skin lesions for 48 h and no actively purulent lesions	Completion of 72 h of antibiotic therapy	Completion of 72 h of antibiotic therapy	Completion of permethrin cream application and washing of clothes and bedding, as recommended	Papule removal via curettage or cryotherapy Localized lesions covered with a gas permeable dressing	Minimum of 72 h of topical or systemic antifungal therapy Cover lesions with bio-occlusive dressing once no longer contagious

(*) Antibiotic choice for cellulitis is tailored to the target bacteria. If wound culture PCR is available, it is ideal to collect wound samples prior to antibiotic initiation. MRSA coverage should be considered for patients with history of MRSA infections, immunocompromised status, and close family members in healthcare. Local sensitivities vary by region and clinicians should reference their local antibiogram prior to choosing the antibiotic. Antibiotic choices based on methicillin sensitive staphylococcus aureus (MSSA) or methicillin resistant staphylococcus aureus (MRSA) bacterial cultures [7, 8] are seen in Table 96.2

Table 96.2 MSSA and MRSA antibiotic choices

	MSSA coverage	MRSA coverage
Oral	Cephalexin (25–50 mg/kg/day divided every 8 hours) Amoxicillin-Clavulanate (25–45 mg/kg/day divided every 12 hours)	Sulfamethoxazole and trimethoprim (8 mg/kg/day of TMP component divided every 12 hours) Doxycycline (4.4 mg/kg/day divided every 12 hours)
Intravenous[a]	Oxacillin Cefazolin Clindamycin Ampicillin-sulbactam	Sulfamethoxazole and trimethoprim Clindamycin Vancomycin Daptomycin

[a]Reference your local antibiogram and/or consult infectious disease services for appropriate dosage and monitoring

References

1. Kimberlin DW, Banerjee R, Barnett ED, Lynfield R, Sawyer M. Group A streptococcal infections. In: Red book: 2024–2027 report of the committee on infectious diseases. 33rd ed. American Academy of Pediatrics; 2024. p. 785–98. https://doi.org/10.1542/9781610027373-S3_018_010.
2. National Federation of State High School Association, Sports Medicine Advisory Committee. Sports-related skin infections position statement and guidelines. 2022. https://www.nfhs.org/media/5546437/2022-nfhs-sports-related-skin-infections-position-statement-and-guidelines-final-3-8-22.pdf.
3. Davies HD, Jackson MA, Rice SG, Committee on Infectious Diseases; Council on Sports Medicine and Fitness. Infectious diseases associated with organized sports and outbreak control. Pediatrics. 2017;140(4):e20172477. https://publications.aap.org/pediatrics/article/140/4/e20172477/38139/Infectious-Diseases-Associated-With-Organized.
4. National Collegiate Athletic Association. 2014–2015 NCAA sports medicine handbook; 2014. https://www.ncaapublications.com/productdownloads/MD15.pdf.
5. Zinder SM, Basler RS, Foley J, Scarlata C, Vasily DB. National athletic trainers' association position statement: skin diseases. J Athl Train. 2010;45(4):411–28. https://doi.org/10.4085/1062-6050-45.4.411. https://www.ncbi.nlm.nih.gov/pmc/articles/PMC2902037/.
6. Kimberlin DW, Banerjee R, Barnett ED, Lynfield R, Sawyer M. Scabies. In: Red book: 2024–2027 report of the committee on infectious diseases. 33rd ed. American Academy of Pediatrics; 2024. p. 751–3. https://doi.org/10.1542/9781610027373-S3_018_002.
7. Wible K, Tregnaghi M, Bruss J, Fleishaker D, Naberhuis-Stehouwer S, Hilty M. Linezolid versus cefadroxil in the treatment of skin and skin structure infections in children. Pediatr Infect Dis J. 2003;22(4):315–23. https://doi.org/10.1097/01.inf.0000059403.21440.2c. [PubMed 12690270].
8. Stevens DL, Bisno AL, Chambers HF, et al. Infectious Diseases Society of America. Practice guidelines for the diagnosis and management of skin and soft tissue infections: 2014 update by the Infectious Diseases Society of America. Clin Infect Dis. 2014;59(2):e10–52. [PubMed 24973422].

Chapter 97
Head Lice

Kathryn Italia and Alissa Cerny

Head lice (*Pediculus humanus capitis*) have been persistent pests for millennia and will be for years to come. There are approximately 6–12 million cases of head lice infestations per year in the United States [1] and though head lice are not known to transmit disease or cause serious health problems, cases of head lice account for billions of dollars of healthcare costs and parental lost wages annually [2]. These tiny parasites most commonly infest children ages 3–11 and occur among all socio-economic and demographic groups [3]. Prevalence studies pose challenges with worldwide studies rates ranging from 0% to 61.4% [4]. In one US study, prevalence of children with live lice was 1.6% [5] but other studies have indicated higher rates.

Many myths exist regarding head lice transmission. Lice are not capable of jumping or flying; they crawl and cling to hair strands. Pets do not transmit head lice; lice are specific to humans. Generally, head lice live within one quarter inch of the scalp. Once detached from the scalp, their survival is limited to around 24 hours, though lice eggs (nits) may survive longer. While there has been controversy about the frequency of spread through indirect contact or fomites, most studies indicate that the majority of human lice transmission occurs with direct head-to-head contact.

Children with head lice will often complain of scalp irritation and itchiness. Itching may not develop for 4–6 weeks since it results from sensitization to the louse saliva components. Though lice are not known to be vectors of disease, secondary infections, such as impetigo, may occasionally develop. Additionally, there are rare reports of iron deficiency anemia resulting from severe lice infestations [6].

K. Italia (✉)
Downingtown, PA, USA

A. Cerny
All Star Pediatrics, Exton, PA, USA

R. P. Olympia, J. Brady-Olympia (eds.), *Clinical Considerations in School-based Health*, https://doi.org/10.1007/978-3-031-85765-2_97

Case Study Mary, a 6-year-old child in 1st grade, presents to your office with scalp itching and complaints of a "sore on her head." What should you do to determine whether this child has lice?

Definitive diagnosis of head lice should be made by identifying live lice in the hair. This can be challenging given that the average infested child may have just 10 or fewer live lice present [7]. These elusive creatures tend to avoid light and move swiftly, complicating visual detection. A metal lice comb with minimal space between teeth is preferred over direct visualization. Use of a quality lice comb results in quicker visualization of lice as well as more accurate identification of true infestations compared with visual examination only [8]. The presence of nits alone does not indicate an active lice infestation. Nits within a quarter inch of the scalp are more likely to result in an active infestation but even with that risk factor, only 32% of children with nits alone converted to a case of pediculosis [5]. Nits that are white and further than 1 centimeter from the scalp are rarely viable. Additionally, nits can sometimes be confused with dandruff, debris such as hairspray or dirt, or hair casts.

97.1 School Policies and Prevention

Case Study Continued With gloves and a fine-toothed metal lice comb, you check Mary's hair close to the scalp for nits and live lice. Quickly, you confirm a lice infestation. In talking to Mary, you learn that she lives at home with her parents, her grandparents, her aunt and uncle, and two cousins. One cousin, a 7-year-old girl, shares a room with her, and is in 2nd grade at the same elementary school. What should be your next steps be after diagnosis is made?

In the past, schools served as primary locations for lice diagnosis and screening. Unfortunately, these screening procedures resulted in substantial over-diagnosis of active lice infestations. Consequently, millions of dollars were spent on unnecessary treatments, countless school days were lost, and parental wages suffered in the range of $4–8 billion [2]. Research also showed that school nurse screenings disrupted in-class learning, diverted considerable time away from other school nursing duties, and frequently failed to identify new infestations [9]. Further investigations show that children are more likely to acquire a new lice infestation in their home; the in-school setting is not as likely to be the source of infection [9, 10]. As a result of this data, general school screenings are no longer recommended.

If a child is diagnosed with lice during the school day, experts no longer advocate that the child immediately be sent home from school since it is likely they have been infested with lice for several weeks. Instead, parents or guardians should be notified and the child should be allowed to return to the classroom with instructions to avoid direct head-to-head contact with classmates [11]. It is essential to handle this situation delicately, avoiding any comments or actions that might identify the infested student and therefore cause needless emotional or social distress.

Debates persist regarding the best way to handle notifications of those in contact with a child diagnosed with lice. Some would advocate for in-school screenings of siblings and close contacts [3]. Alternatively, others recommend notifying parents or guardians that their children may have been exposed during school and, therefore, should perform lice checks at home [12]. However, privacy concerns and risk of creating unnecessary anxiety must be carefully considered when implementing any notification policy. The American Academy of Pediatrics suggests each school come up with their own policy based on school specific needs [11]. Flexibility is key, recognizing that different schools face unique circumstances. Most importantly, schools and caregivers should be educated about lice infestations and myths should be dispelled.

Parents and guardians should be informed regarding head lice, diagnosis, and treatment. Though direct head-to-head contact accounts for the majority of head lice transmission, children should be instructed to not share brushes, combs, hats, and pillows with one another. If a child develops scalp itching, parents should be familiar with how to effectively use a lice comb to check for lice.

Case Study Continued You inform Mary that she may return to class but should not have any head-to-head contact with her classmates. Then you call the cousin down to your office and confirm a case of lice with her as well. Next you notify the parents of both children to inform them of the diagnosis. Over the phone, you relay information about treatment as well as send handouts about diagnosis and treatment home with each girl.

97.2 Treatment

Once a diagnosis of head lice has been made, the entire household should be screened and all individuals with an active infestation should be treated, ideally at the same time. Lice medication, also called pediculicide, should be applied with careful attention paid to the instructions. The product should be removed by rinsing hair over a sink rather than in a tub or shower to minimize contact with the skin, and warm water should be used rather than hot in order to limit vasodilation which may increase skin absorption. After application, do not rewash the treated hair for 1–2 days after the pediculicide is removed. Instructions for retreatment depend on the properties of the compound used. Ovicidal products kill both lice and nits and typically only require a single treatment. Non-ovicidal products require a second treatment to treat any recently hatched lice. Because no product is 100% effective, manual removal of nits within 1 cm of the scalp is reasonable following treatment and may also help to reduce social stigma [11]. Cost will also be a consideration in treatment. Some products require multiple applications which should be considered in the total cost of treatment, and certain products cost more than two hundred dollars [13]. Side effects of treatment with pediculicides may include mild itching and

Table 97.1 Topical treatments for head lice

Product	Brand name	Age range	Ovicidal	Instructions for retreatment
Over the counter				
Ivermectin (0.5%) lotion	Sklice	≥ 6 mo	Limited	Single use
Permethrin 1% lotion	Example: Nix	≥ 2 mo	No	9–10 days
Pyrethrins + piperonyl butoxide shampoo	Example: Rid	≥ 24 mo	No	9–10 days
Prescription				
Abametapir (0.74%) lotion	Xeglyze	≥ 6 mo	Yes	Single use
Malathion (0.5%) lotion	Ovide	≥ 6 yr	Limited	7–9 days if live lice are seen after initial treatment
Spinosad (0.9%) suspension	Natroba	≥ 6 mo	Yes	7 days if live lice are seen after initial treatment

burning for several days following treatment and these can be managed with topical corticosteroids and antihistamines.

There is an array of topical pediculicide treatments available as listed in Table 97.1. As of 2016, Permethrin was the most widely used and most studied pediculicide in the United States [14]. Lindane (1%), though still available by prescription, is no longer recommended for use in children given the widespread availability of safer products and significant neurotoxicity risks [11]. Oral ivermectin may be considered for use in patients with infestation that has failed treatment with all other topical agents.

Case Study Continued Mary's mother visits the pharmacy section of their local grocery store that evening. She selects a product based on price and ease of application, buying one container for Mary and one for her cousin. Later that evening, both girls are treated at home.

Treatment failure may be the result of improper application, incorrect diagnosis, reinfestation, or head lice resistance to the product used. Following FDA introduction in the 1980s, these products boasted effectiveness rates as high as 99.2% for permethrin, but decades of use eroded these rates to as low as 25% in a 2009 study [14]. The American Academy of Pediatrics treatment algorithm includes "suspected community pyrethroid resistance" as a guiding factor in selection of a pediculicide [11], but this information is often unavailable. Resistance is also possible with other products. A 2012 review reported cases of malathion resistance in France, Australia, the United Kingdom, and Denmark, though it remains more effective than pyrethroids [15]. Given the risks of resistance, an individual should not be treated more than two or three times with the same product without discussing with a physician as a treatment change may be appropriate.

Families may turn to alternative treatment methods in order to avoid the use of neurotoxic pediculicides. A number of studies have investigated the use of occlusive agents such as dimethicone, petroleum jelly, mayonnaise, butter, and olive oil. One systematic review found that occlusive agents were equally effective or perhaps even superior to neurotoxic pediculicides [16]. Essential oils such as lavender oil and tea tree oil have also been compared to occlusive methods and pediculicides with favorable treatment rates that outperformed pediculicides, but were also associated with higher levels of stinging, dry/flaking scalp, and erythema [17]. As of 2021, the American Academy of Pediatrics Committee on Infectious Diseases considers there to be insufficient data to recommend the use of occlusive agents as effective for the treatment of head lice [18]. The most recent position statement of the American Academy of Pediatrics also recommends against the use of natural herbal products on infants, children and adolescents given the absence of sufficient safety data or FDA regulation [11].

Though head lice are not often spread through shared clothing or other items, the CDC does recommend taking precautions to minimize the risk of transmission. Combs used by the infected person can be disinfected in hot water (130 °F) for five to ten minutes. Clothing, bed sheets, and towels used by the infested person in the two days preceding treatment can be washed at 130 °F and then dried on high heat [1]. Non-washable items that may have been in close contact with lice may be bagged for two weeks. Carpets or furniture may also be vacuumed to prevent spread, though a study published in 2002 indicated very low risk of lice transmission through carpeting [10]. Extensive and painstaking cleaning of a household is not advantageous [11].

97.3 Return to School

Generally, students may return to school immediately following treatment. It is important to note that some nits may remain after an effective pediculicide treatment. As discussed above, nits alone are not an indicator of an active lice infestation and "no nit" policies are not recommended. The AAP suggests that school nurses familiar with head lice can recheck a child privately if requested to do so by the caregiver [11].

Case Study Continued At the request of their parents, Mary and her cousin are called down to the nurse's office for private rescreening after they return to school. No live lice are seen. Their parents are notified and encouraged to follow product guidelines for retreatment and CDC control measures.

Extra Credit Points

1. Nits alone do not indicate an active lice infestation and "no nit" policies are not recommended.
2. Incorrect diagnosis, improper application, reinfestation, or resistance can result in treatment failure. Consult a physician before treating more than 2 or 3 times with the same pediculicide.
3. There is insufficient evidence supporting the use of occlusive agents and botanical agents. These methods are often used by families who wish to avoid neurotoxic pediculicides. Students treated with these methods should be monitored for side effects and treatment failure.

References

1. Center for Disease Control and Prevention. Parasites: lice: head lice. Available at: https://www.cdc.gov/parasites/lice/head/index.html. Accessed 13 Feb 2024.
2. Mumcuoglu KY, Meinking TA, Burkhart CN, Burkhart CG. Head louse infestations: the "no nit" policy and its consequences. Int J Dermatol. 2006;45(8):891–6.
3. Birkemoe T, Heggen Lindstedt H, Ottesen P, Soleng A, Næss Ø, Arne Rukke B. Head lice predictors and infestation dynamics among primary school children in Norway. Fam Pract. 2016;33(1):23–9.
4. Falagas ME, Matthaiou DK, Rafailidis PI, Panos G, Pappas G. Worldwide prevalence of head lice. Emerg Infect Dis. 2008;14(9):1493–4.
5. Williams LK, Reichert A, MacKenzie WR, Hightower AW, Blake PA. Lice, nits, and school policy. Pediatrics. 2001;107(5):1011–5.
6. Guss David A, Mark K, Castillo Edward M. Severe iron deficiency anemia and lice infestation. J Emerg Med. 2011;41(4):362–5.
7. Mumcuoglu KY, Miller J, Gofin R, Adler B, Ben-Ishai F, Almog R, Kafka D, Klaus S. Epidemiological studies on head lice infestation in Israel. I. Parasitological examination of children. Int J Dermatol. 1990 Sep;29(7):502–6.
8. Mumcuoglu KY, Friger M, Ioffe-Uspensky I, Ben-Ishai F, Miller J. Louse comb versus direct visual examination for the diagnosis of head louse infestations. Pediatr Dermatol. 2001;18(1):9–12.
9. Hootman J. Quality improvement projects related to pediculosis management. J Sch Nurs. 2002;18(2):80–6.
10. Speare R, Thomas G, Cahill C. Head lice are not found on floors in primary school classrooms. Aust N Z J Public Health. 2002;26(3):208–11.
11. Nolt D, Moore S, Yan AC, Melnick L, Committee on Infectious Diseases, Committee on Practice and Ambulatory Medicine, Section on Dermatology. Head lice. Pediatrics. 2022;150(4):e2022059282.
12. Cummings CS, Finlay JC, MacDonald NE. Head lice infestations: a clinical update. Paediatr Child Health. 2018;23(1):e18–24.
13. Rubio A. How much does head lice treatment cost. In: Goodrx.com. https://www.goodrx.com/conditions/lice/how-much-lice-treatment-costs. Accessed 20 Mar 2024.
14. Koch E, Clark JM, Cohen B, Meinking TL, Ryan WG, Stevenson A, Yetman R, Yoon KS. Management of head louse infestations in the United States-a literature review. Pediatr Dermatol. 2016 Sep;33(5):466–72.
15. Durand R, Bouvresse S, Berdjane Z, Izri A, Chosidow O, Clark JM. Insecticide resistance in head lice: clinical, parasitological and genetic aspects. Clin Microbiol Infect. 2012;18(4):338–44.
16. Flores-Genuino RNS, Gnilo CMS, Dofitas BL. Occlusive versus neurotoxic agents for topical treatment of head lice infestation: a systematic review and meta-analysis. Pediatr Dermatol. 2020;37(1):86–92.
17. Barker SC, Altman PM. A randomised, assessor blind, parallel group comparative efficacy trial of three products for the treatment of head lice in children--melaleuca oil and lavender oil, pyrethrins and piperonyl butoxide, and a "suffocation" product. BMC Dermatol. 2010;10:6.
18. Kimberlin D, Barnett E, Lynfield R, Sawyer M. Pediculosis capitis (head lice). In: Redbook 2021–2024. Report of the committee on infectious diseases. 32nd ed. American Academy of Pediatrics. Itasca, Illinois.

Chapter 98
Human and Animal Bites

Keanna Chang and John Park

Case 1 5-year-old Samuel is rushed into your office. He was playing whiffle ball with his friends and someone had hit the ball into a backyard neighboring the school. He climbed over the fence to retrieve the ball, and the neighbor's Pitbull bit him over the left eye. He is crying but able to be consoled. You find a 2 cm, jagged, floppy laceration above his left eyebrow with two shallow puncture marks on his left cheek. What is your next course of action?

An estimated 4.5 million dog bites occur each year in the US in adults and children. About 10% of these occur to the face and are least likely to become infected. About 75% of these bites occur to the hand and extremities and have the highest risk of becoming infected. See Table 98.1 for common bacteria associated with dog (as well as cat and human) bites. The most common dog breeds associated with severe bites are German shepherd, Pitbull, Rottweiler, and Doberman due to the size and strength of their jaws [1].

After a thorough history and physical exam, initial management should include hemostasis and irrigation of the wound (Table 98.2). After ensuring adequate analgesia (by mouth or topical/injectable) adequate irrigation can be achieved with water or normal saline in a syringe and should be done on all wounds except deep puncture wounds as foreign or infectious material may be pushed deeper into the wound [2]. The wound should be explored for foreign bodies and injury to deeper tissues. Devitalized tissue may be cut off with sterile scissors or scalpel. Primary closure may increase the risk of infection, so is generally not recommended for wounds except to achieve hemostasis or for those to the face with cosmetic importance and generally lower risk of infection [3]. Tetanus immunoglobulin and tetanus vaccination should be administered if the patient has received fewer than 3 doses of their tetanus vaccine or if the vaccine status is unknown. Tetanus vaccination should

K. Chang · J. Park (✉)
Maria Fareri Children's Hospital at Westchester Medical Center, Valhalla, NY, USA

R. P. Olympia, J. Brady-Olympia (eds.), *Clinical Considerations in School-based Health*, https://doi.org/10.1007/978-3-031-85765-2_98

Table 98.1 Common bacteria associated with dog, cat, and human bites [1, 2]

Source	Aerobes	Anaerobes
Dog	Pasteurella species Staphylococcus aureus Streptococci species Corynebacteria species Neisseria species	Fusobacterium species Bacteroides species Peptostreptococci species Prevotella species
Cat	Pasteurella species Streptococci species Staphylococcus aureus Moraxella species	Fusobacterium species Bacteroides species Prevotella species Propionobacterium species
Human	Streptococci species Staphylococcus aureus Eikenella corrodens Haemophilus species	Fusobacterium species Prevotella species Peptostreptococci species Veilonella species

be administered for any patient who has had over 3 doses of their tetanus vaccine, but their last dose was over 5 years ago [1].

Rabies is a common parental concern in the case of animal bites. The most common animal reservoirs for rabies are bats, raccoons, skunks, and foxes, in decreasing order of prevalence. Dogs make up and even smaller percentage of cases in animals, especially in domesticated dogs as canine vaccination has increased. If the vaccine status of the dog is unknown, or the dog is not available to be observed for 10 days for signs of rabies infection, rabies prophylaxis should be initiated and includes a four-dose series of rabies vaccines and a dose of human rabies immune globulin [1].

Case 2 7-year-old Cathryn presents to your office with a pain in her left hand. She was at her friend's house after school yesterday, and she was trying to pet their cat when bit Cathryn's hand. She washed it out with soap and water and applied a bandage. The wound was fine until the last hour when the pain over the wound has worsened. She is afebrile and does not appear distressed. She has 3 puncture wounds on the pad of her middle finger and it is swollen compared to the others. She has tenderness along her entire finger and cannot fully extend it. What should you do?

All bites have a risk of becoming infected, even after being washed out. Wounds from dog bites have about 20% risk of becoming infected, while data on cat bite infections in children is variable but can be up to 50% of cases, often with relatively rapid onset. Symptoms of an infection typically arise within hours to days and include worsening pain, erythema, and swelling of the affected area. Purulent discharge may or may not be present, and most patients are afebrile [1].

As with any other break in the skin, the most common pathogens are skin flora: staphylococcal and streptococcal species (Table 98.1). A bite wound is more likely than other wounds to be polymicrobial from bacteria present in the saliva of the animal, most notably Pasteurella species, though many other aerobes and anaerobes may be present. Treatment of an infected bite wound should include coverage for all these organisms, most easily achieved with amoxicillin-clavulanate (Augmentin). *A*

Table 98.2 Stepwise approach to a student who has sustained an animal or human bite

History	Animal Type of animal Health of animal Vaccination status of the animal (if known) Attack provoked or unprovoked Patient Immunocompromised (e.g. asplenia, liver disease, cancer, etc.) Tetanus status
Evaluation	Vitals and general appearance Wound characteristics: location, depth, shape, edge approximation Type of wound: puncture, laceration, avulsion Presence of foreign bodies Presence of erythema, edema, purulent discharge, or other signs of infection Neurovascular examination
Analgesia	Analgesia options Oral Topical lidocaine epinephrine tetracaine gel Injectable lidocaine (wound edges vs. nerve block) Consider procedural sedation if Child unable to sit still for duration of procedure Duration of procedure longer than duration of action of anesthetic
Initial management	Irrigate wounds with water or normal saline Do NOT blindly irrigate puncture wounds May require diagnostic imaging to rule out foreign bodies or other injuries Xray to evaluate for fractures Ultrasound to assess for foreign bodies [4] CT scan for deep head bites to assess for intracranial penetration Debridement of devitalized tissue and removal of foreign bodies Wound cultures if evaluation is over 8 hours after the event or if the wound has signs of infection
Wound closure	Early primary closure recommended for wounds of face and neck Primary closure may be considered if NONE of the below are present: Hand injury—consider hand surgeon consult Existing signs of infection More than 8 hours from time of injury Crush injuries Immunocompromised patient Do NOT use subcutaneous sutures, skin glue, or overlapping skin tape Delayed wound closure may be indicated for heavily contaminated wounds [5] Clean, debride, cover with moist dressing Dressing changed daily until reassessment in 3–4 days If no signs of infection present at reassessment, may close wound

(continued)

Table 98.2 (continued)

Prophylaxis	Determine need for rabies and tetanus prophylaxis Most providers advise prophylactic antibiotics for nearly all bite wounds. Amoxicillin-clavulanate (oral) Ampicillin-sulbactam (IV) Extended-spectrum cephalosporin or trimethoprim-sulfamethoxazole PLUS Clindamycin (penicillin allergic patients)
Follow up	Wound inspection within 48 hours to evaluate for evidence of infection
Emergency Department Referral	Bites associated with fractures Bites involving joint capsule, tendon, nerves, vessel disruption Infected bites Cosmetically important wounds Bites associated significant traumatic injuries

helpful mnemonic to remember this is dog-mentin. An appropriate regimen for penicillin allergic patients is a dual therapy with clindamycin AND either a 2nd or 3rd generation cephalosporin or TMP-SMX. All wounds should be reexamined within 24–48 hours to assess for clinical response to antibiotic. Therapy duration depends on wound location and severity and the clinical response. A simple soft tissue infection may be appropriately treated by 7–10 days, while a deeper infection like infections flexor tenosynovitis may require up to 6 weeks of antibiotic therapy [2]. Prophylactic antibiotics may not be indicated for low risk wounds (non-puncture wounds, wounds not involving the hands/feet/face, immunocompetent host), however there is a subset of these patients who may develop an infection if not treated despite being low risk [3].

Case 3 16-year-old Steve presents to your office after sustaining a hand injury in an altercation with another student. He has no complaints besides the after-school detention and pain in his right hand. He has four jagged, sub-centimeter superficial lacerations over his 3rd and 4th MCP joints with one laceration over his 3rd MCP joint that is deeper and about 1 cm long. He has full mobility of his fingers with superficial pain over his wounds but no deeper tenderness to palpation. What should you do?

Clenched fist injuries often occur as "fight bites" when the patient has struck their closed fist against another person's mouth, cutting their knuckles in the process. The most commonly affected joint is the 3rd metacarpophalangeal joint of their dominant hand. These injuries may not look very serious and can be overlooked, but have a high likelihood of infection and other complications. Any skin infection, especially those from bite wounds, has a risk of spreading to deeper infection. The hands and feet are at an increased risk of these complications due to the superficial nature of the tendons and bones, higher risk of contamination, and less robust vasculature [1]. See Table 98.3 for further characterization of complications of bite wounds. Human bites also carry a small risk of transmission of Hepatitis B and C, CMV, herpes, and HIV [1].

Table 98.3 Complications associated with animal and human bite wounds

Complication	Presentation	Disposition	Treatment
Cellulitis [6]	Erythema, swelling, induration, tenderness around break in skin May have fever	Urgent care	PO amoxicillin-clavulanate
Abscess [6]	Erythema, swelling, tenderness, induration around break in skin with central fluctuance May have fever	Urgent care	Incision and drainage PO amoxicillin-clavulanate
Lymphangitis [6, 7]	Linear, erythematous streaks from break in the skin Tender, enlarged regional lymph nodes Fever, chills, malaise	Urgent care	PO amoxicillin-clavulanate
Infectious flexor tenosynovitis [8]	Kanavel signs: Symmetric swelling of entire digit Tenderness along course of tendon sheath Holding digit in semi-flexed position Pain with passive extension of digit	Emergency department	Empiric IV antibiotics Open I&D if no improvement after 48 hours on antibiotics
Osteomyelitis [9]	Pain, edema, erythema, tenderness over affected bone Fever Involved bone may be close to break in skin, or may be far (hematogenous spread)	Emergency department	Surgical debridement Empiric IV antibiotics
Necrotizing fasciitis [6]	Pain out of proportion to physical exam Rapidly progressing infection Cutaneous anesthesia, crepitus, and hemorrhagic/bullous changes over infected area Fever	Emergency department	Surgical debridement Empiric IV antibiotics

Case 4 9-year-old Charlotte is on a field trip to the local park where she and friends are jumping into a pile of leaves. She comes up to you complaining of severe abdominal pain and nausea. She describes a "pinprick" sensation on her left leg that started about an hour ago when she jumped in the leaf pile. On her calf, you see a small red dot with a 0.5 cm area of erythema around it. What organism may have caused the bite and what should you do next?

Black widow spiders are widely distributed. They are identified by their characteristic red hourglass marking on their abdomen. They tend to live in areas with leaf cover or yard debris and their bite typically feels like a pinprick. Crampy muscle spasms may occur within a few hours. Nausea, weakness, sweating, and facial edema may occur. Minor bites should be washed with soap and water and pain can be treated with over the counter analgesics. Bites associated with severe systemic signs may require hospital admission for observation and possible administration of antivenom. Supportive care includes intravenous benzodiazepines for muscle spasms and opioids for pain. If these methods are not effective, antivenom may be given within 48 hours, however risk versus benefit should be considered as the antivenom has been associated with serum sickness. Before treating a bite, if possible it should be determined what organism inflicted the bite, as treatment varies [10]. See Table 98.4 for the clinical presentations associated with different arthropod, insect, or reptile bites or stings.

Table 98.4 Clinical presentations associated with various arthropod, insect, or reptile bites and stings

Organism	Clinical presentation	Management after wound care and tetanus administration	Disposition
Black widow spider bite [10]	Pinprick bite Chest or abdominal muscle spasms Nausea, weakness, sweating, edema	Benzodiazepines Pain control Antivenom if severe systemic signs	Urgent care vs. Emergency department
Brown recluse spider bite [10]	Bites occur indoors Potentially painless bite Tender, erythematous halo around bite that develops central necrosis Hemolysis, coagulopathy, morbilliform rash	Steroids Minor debridement if necrosis	Urgent care vs. Emergency department
Pit viper bite [11]	Hemotoxic 2 fang punctures at site Damaged capillaries cause local swelling, bleeding, and necrosis Systemic signs: edema, weakness, tachycardia, ecchymosis, muscle fasciculations, vomiting Severe systemic signs: DIC, acute renal failure, hypovolemic shock Compartment syndrome and infection are rare	Immobilize extremity May place constriction band to block superficial venous and lymphatic flow but must easily be able to slide 2 fingers under band No benefit from incision and suction Tetanus administration IV fluids Antivenin most effective within 4 hours but may be given within 24 hours after bite Manage ABCs for severe systemic symptoms	Emergency department
Coral snake bite [11]	Neurotoxic Local numbness/minimal pain, ptosis, weakness, diplopia, dysphagia, sweating, salivation, hyporeflexia Severe signs: cranial nerve palsies, respiratory paralysis		ED

(continued)

Table 98.4 (continued)

Organism	Clinical presentation	Management after wound care and tetanus administration	Disposition
Hymenoptera (Bee) sting [12]	Local: pain and swelling around sting, resolves in a few hours Large local reaction: 5–10 cm swelling and erythema, may last a week Anaphylaxis: urticaria, flushing, wheezing, nausea/vomiting/abdominal pain, shock	Remove stinger by scraping, NOT by tweezers OTC analgesics, ice packs, antihistamines Steroids for large local reaction Anaphylaxis: Manage ABCs, epinephrine, steroids, IV fluids	Urgent care vs. Emergency department
Scorpion sting [13]	Pain, erythema, local inflammation, followed by numbness at site Severe symptoms: blurry vision, nystagmus, salivation, vomiting, sweating, bronchoconstriction Cranial nerve or skeletal muscle dysfunction May cause pulmonary edema or cardiogenic shock	OTC analgesics Manage ABCs for severe systemic symptoms Benzodiazepines for muscle spasticity Antivenom if skeletal muscle or cranial nerve dysfunction (may cause serum sickness)	Emergency department

98.1 Case Conclusions

Case 1 Samuel is taken to the local ED where he has his laceration anesthetized, irrigated, and repaired by interrupted, non-absorbable sutures. His puncture wounds (with wound bases visible) are explored for foreign bodies, washed out, and dressed with a bandage. He is discharged with 7 days of amoxicillin-clavulanate and follows up with his pediatrician the next day.

Case 2 Cathryn is taken the ED where she is admitted for ampicillin-sulbactam, she eventually requires drainage/debridement in the OR.

Case 3 Steve is taken to a nearby urgent care where a hand x-ray was normal. His lacerations are irrigated, and he was given prophylactic antibiotics.

Case 4 Charlotte is taken to the local urgent care where her bite is washed with soap and water. She receives acetaminophen which relieves the abdominal pain within an hour and is sent home.

Extra Credit Points

1. Bite wounds are polymicrobial with both aerobic and anaerobic bacteria, so prophylactic or empiric coverage should make sure it covers all these different pathogens.
2. Suturing of bites is generally only recommended for areas of cosmetic importance and should be done with caution as it may increase the risk of infection.
3. Superficial infections associated with bite wounds have risk of spreading to deeper tissues.
4. Bites carry risk of systemic infections as well: tetanus and rabies with animals, and Hepatis B and C, CMV, herpes, and HIV with humans; risk of transmission should be assessed and appropriate post-exposure prophylaxis should be provided.
5. Insects, arthropods, and reptiles may inflict bites or stings that may cause a range of symptoms from local to systemic reactions. Identifying the type of bite is important for determining the correct antivenom to give, but many reactions may be treated with non-specific supportive care.

References

1. Bula-Rudas FJ, Olcott JL. Human and animal bites. Pediatr Rev. 2018;39(10):490–500. https://doi.org/10.1542/pir.2017-0212.
2. Kimberlin DW, Banerjee R, Barnett ED, Lynfield R, Sawyer MH. Bite wounds. In: Red book: 2024–2027 report of the committee on infectious diseases. 33rd ed. Itasca: American Academy of Pediatrics; 2024. p. 202–6. https://doi.org/10.1542/9781610027373-S2_008.
3. Stevens DL, et al. Practice guidelines for the diagnosis and management of skin and soft tissue infections: 2014 update by the Infectious Diseases Society of America. Clin Infect Dis. 2014;59(2):e10–52. https://doi.org/10.1093/cid/ciu296.
4. Chen K-C, Lin AC-M, Chong C-F, Wang T-L. An overview of point-of-care ultrasound for soft tissue and musculoskeletal applications in the emergency department. J Intensive Care. 2016;4:55. https://doi.org/10.1186/s40560-016-0173-0.
5. Nicks BA, Ayello EA, Woo K, Nitzki-George D, Sibbald RG. Acute wound management: revisiting the approach to assessment, irrigation, and closure considerations. Int J Emerg Med. 2010;3(4):399–407. https://doi.org/10.1007/s12245-010-0217-5.
6. Ramakrishnan K, Salinas RC, Higuita NIA. Skin and soft tissue infections. Am Fam Physician. 2015;92(6):474–83.
7. Kano Y, Momose T. Acute lymphangitis. Cleve Clin J Med. 2020;87(3):129–30. https://doi.org/10.3949/ccjm.87a.19095.
8. Chapman T, Ilyas AM. Pyogenic flexor tenosynovitis: evaluation and treatment strategies. J Hand Microsurg. 2019;11(3):121–6. https://doi.org/10.1055/s-0039-1700370.
9. Bury DC, Rogers TS, Dickman MM. Osteomyelitis: diagnosis and treatment. Am Fam Physician. 2021;104(4):395–402.
10. Juckett G. Arthropod bites. Am Fam Physician. 2013;88(12):841–7.
11. Juckett G, Hancox JG. Venomous snakebites in the United States: management review and update. Am Fam Physician. 2002;65(7):1367–75.
12. Booker GM. Insect stings. Pediatr Rev. 2005;26(10):388–9. https://doi.org/10.1542/pir.26-10-388.
13. Shamoon Z, Peterfy RJ, Hammoud S, Khazaeni B. Scorpion toxicity. In: StatPearls. Treasure Island: StatPearls Publishing; 2024. Accessed 31 July 2024. [Online]. Available: http://www.ncbi.nlm.nih.gov/books/NBK430928/.

Chapter 99
Lyme Disease

Marie E. Schwalbe and Robert P. Olympia

Case 1 Jamie is a 5-year-old girl in New Hampshire who presents in June with a Deer tick attached in the left axilla. She denies any symptoms. The tick was not there yesterday. You remove the tick using fine-tipped tweezers, then clean the area with a sterile alcohol swab. The tick does not appear engorged.

99.1 What Are Risk Factors for Deer Tick Bites? [1]

- Living in the northeast or midwestern Unites States (See map of cases at https://www.cdc.gov/lyme/data-research/facts-stats/lyme-disease-case-map.html) [2].
- Spending more time outdoors.
- Living in a wooded area with plentiful wildlife (deer and rodents), which supports the tick life cycle.
- Age 5–15 years or 45–55 years [1].

Proper tick remove is demonstrated in this video by the CDC [3]: https://youtu.be/S4Ny5YJh6Ws

M. E. Schwalbe
Penn State Hershey Medical Center, Hershey, PA, USA
e-mail: mschwalbe@pennstatehealth.psu.edu

R. P. Olympia (✉)
Department of Emergency Medicine and Pediatrics, Penn State College of Medicine Attending Physician, Hershey, PA, USA

Division of Pediatric Emergency Medicine, Department of Emergency Medicine, Penn State Milton S. Hershey Medical Center, Hershey, PA, USA
e-mail: rolympia@hmc.psu.edu

R. P. Olympia, J. Brady-Olympia (eds.), *Clinical Considerations in School-based Health*, https://doi.org/10.1007/978-3-031-85765-2_99

99.1.1 Prognosis

Tick removal and monitoring for the development of symptoms is the preferred method of prophylaxis after a tick bite. However, if the tick bite is high risk (identified as Ixodes, located in an endemic area, estimated to have been attached for >36 hours and/or appears engorged), then a single dose of antibiotics can be given. The sooner you remove the tick the lower the risk of infection. However, there is no minimum time before which the risk of infection is zero [4].

Case 2 Eliza is a 7-year-old girl who presents to clinic in July with a large, 4 cm targetoid rash on her lower abdomen that has been growing in diameter over the past few days. She endorses mild pruritus of the rash and is feeling fatigued. You identify the rash as erythema migrans and diagnose early, localized Lyme disease.

99.2 Erythema Migrans

- Present in 2/3 cases of symptomatic Lyme disease but easily missed if it is in a hard to see location.
- Typically develops within 3–14 days at the site of the tick bite but often the tick bite when unnoticed [5].
- A macular or papular erythematous lesion develops first, which starts small and gradually expands up to several inches in diameter. It may range from erythematous to purplish. It may develop central clearing or a targetoid appearance. The central area may also become vesicular or necrotic [6].
- The rash may be mildly pruritic or be accompanied by paresthesias, or it may not have any local symptoms.
- There may be nonspecific systemic symptoms (fatigue, malaise, headache, myalgias, arthralgias, and lymphadenopathy) [5].
- Eighty percent of cases of Lyme disease present with erythema migrans. In 18% of patients, there will be systemic symptoms without erythema migrans and 2% present with other complications of early, disseminated or late disease [1].

99.2.1 Diagnosis (Table 99.1)

Diagnosis of early localized Lyme disease is via identification of a rash consistent with erythema migrans in an area where Lyme disease is endemic. If a deer tick bite was previously seen, this further supports the diagnosis, but is not necessary to make the diagnosis. No serologic testing is necessary and would likely be falsely negative at this point in the infection.

Table 99.1 Diagnosis of Lyme disease [1, 6]

Sign/Serology	Interpretation	Notes
Erythema migrans	Active Borrelia infection	Serology will likely be negative in the first few weeks of infection
ELISA ➔ Western Blot: <30d after symptom onset, at least two IgM bands are positive, of: 23, 39 or 41 kD	Positive IgM antibodies suggest an active *Borrelia* infection, in the right clinical setting. Negative IgM antibodies in a treated patient indicate no infection or successful treatment of infection and no risk for development of late complications	This test is not helpful is patients have had symptoms for several weeks or if they have signs/symptoms of later stages of Lyme disease. Also, can remain positive for months or years after successful eradication of bacteria. It can provide a false positive result in either situation.
ELISA ➔ Western Blot: >30d after symptom onset, at least five IgG bands are positive, of: 18, 23, 28, 30, 39, 41, 45, 58, 66 or 93 kD	Positive IgG antibodies suggest an ongoing (more than a couple weeks) or resolved *Borrelia* infection, in the right clinical setting.	Can remain positive for months or years after successful eradication of bacteria. IgG Ab to flagella protein are present in 20–50% healthy people, p41 band can be a false positive
Antibodies in the CSF	As above	Account for passive diffusion of antibodies from blood to CSF
Positive PCR	+PCR suggests an ongoing or resolved *Borrelia burgdorferi* DNA may persist in the body after the bacteria have been killed.	Not FDA approved. May be useful for diagnosing Lyme arthritis via testing of the synovial fluid

Currently, any urine testing, CD57 assays, cultures, and other antibody panels are not valid

99.2.2 Prognosis (Table 99.2)

Treatment results in resolution of the rash within several days of starting antibiotics and typically prevents further complications [8].

Case 3 Oliver is a 10-year-old boy living in eastern Pennsylvania and an avid soccer player. He asked to go to the nurse today due to headache. The nurse noticed that he did not appear able to move the right side of his face. Over the phone his parents relate that he has been having headaches for a few days. The school nurse sent him home early [9]**. The next morning, he developed worsened headache, neck stiffness, fever, and fatigue. His pediatrician advised his mother to bring him to the ED due to concern for meningitis and facial nerve palsy. Work-up eventually revealed positive Lyme serology. Upon further questioning, his parents relate that he had a mild febrile illness a few months ago with a target-like rash on his inner thigh.**

Table 99.2 Treatment of Lyme disease

Stage	Signs/Symptoms	Treatment options [7]
Prophylaxis	Attached tick	One dose of Doxycyline at 4.4 mg/kg for children of any age up to a maximum of 200 mg can be used for prophylaxis within 72 hours
Early, localized	Days to weeks after tick bite, erythema migrans may appear on skin at location of tick bite. Often the tick bite was not noticed.	Doxycycline 4.4 mg/kg/day PO divided BID for 10 days (max dose 200 mg/day) or Amoxicillin 50 mg/kg/day PO divided TID for 14 days (max 1500 mg/day) or Cefuroxime 30 mg/kg/day PO divided BID for 14 days (max 1000 mg/day) or Azithromycin 10 mg/kg/day PO daily for 7 days (max 500 mg/dose)
Early, disseminated: Carditis	Carditis can present with syncope, chest pain, shortness of breath, or palpitations. EKG may show heart block.	Doxycycline 4.4 mg/kg/day PO divided BID for 14–21 days (max dose 200 mg/day) or Amoxicillin 50 mg/kg/day PO divided TID for 14–21 days (max 1500 mg/day) or Cefuroxime 30 mg/kg/day PO divided BID for 14–21 days (max 1000 mg/day) or Azithromycin 10 mg/kg/day PO daily for 14–21 days (max 500 mg/dose) or Ceftriaxone 50–75 mg/kg IV every 24 hours for 14–21 days
Early, disseminated: Cranial nerve palsy	Bell's Palsy presents with unilateral facial weakness affecting upper and lower facial muscles.	Doxycycline 4.4 mg/kg/day PO divided BID for 10 days (max dose 200 mg/day)
Early, disseminated: Neuroborreliosis	Meningitis often presents with mild symptoms (such as headache, neck stiffness, or photophobia)	Doxycycline 4.4 mg/kg/day PO divided BID for 14–21 days (max dose 200 mg/day) or Ceftriaxone 50–75 mg/kg IV every 24 hours for 14–21 days or Penicillin G 300,000 U/kg/day IV every 4 hours for 14–21 days

(continued)

Table 99.2 (continued)

Stage	Signs/Symptoms	Treatment options [7]
Late	Months after infection, late Lyme causes a mono- or oligoarticular arthritis mostly affecting large joints such as the knee.	Doxycycline 4.4 mg/kg/day PO divided BID for 28 days (max dose 200 mg/day) or Amoxicillin 50 mg/kg/day PO divided TID for 28 days (max 1500 mg/day) or Cefuroxime 30 mg/kg/day PO divided BID for 28 days (max 1000 mg/day) or Azithromycin 10 mg/kg/day PO daily for 28 days (max 500 mg/dose)
Persistent Lyme arthritis	Persistent arthritis after *first* course of antibiotics.	28-day course of PO antibiotics as above for Lyme arthritis* or 14–28 days of IV ceftriaxone (50–75 mg/kg every 24 hours).* *After this second round of antibiotics, no additional antibiotics are recommended

This is the early, disseminated phase of Lyme disease, which starts days-weeks after initial infections. Bell's palsy and meningitis, if present, occur in this stage, but usually months after initial infection [1]. Lyme disease can also affect other peripheral nerve causes radiculopathies, and in rare cases, cerebellar ataxia or encephalomyelitis [1].

99.3 Clinical Manifestations of Bell's Palsy [10]

- Unilateral facial weakness affecting upper and lower facial muscles
- Drooping of eyebrow and mouth on the affected side

99.4 Clinical Manifestations of Lyme Meningitis [11]

- Symptoms are often mild
- Headache may be present, can be mild—severe
- Other symptoms may include neck stiffness or photophobia

99.4.1 Diagnosis (Table 99.1)

- Clinical

99.4.2 Prognosis (Table 99.2)

Eighty-five percent of patients with facial nerve palsy recover fully in 2 months. Twenty percent have a longer course or recovery and may have lingering symptoms [9]. Treatment prevents additional complications of Lyme disease, but does not reduce time to resolution of facial nerve palsy [7]. Lyme Meningitis is effectively treated by antibiotic therapy [1].

Case 4 Caleb is an otherwise healthy 15-year-old boy scout living in upstate New York who presented to the ED in November after an episode of syncope at school. About 1 month ago, he returned from a camping trip. One week ago, he developed fever and rash. On exam in the ED, he was found to have multiple targetoid lesions consistent with disseminated erythema migrans. EKG revealed second-degree Mobitz type 2 heart block. He has no personal or family history of cardiac conditions. He was admitted to the hospital where work-up revealed positive Lyme serology. EKG showed that the AV block fluctuated frequently at times 1st, 2nd, or even 3rd degree (on the order of hours to days). He was started on Ceftriaxone 50–75 mg/kg IV every 24 hours for 21 days for Lyme carditis [7]**.**

99.5 What Are the Possible Cardiac Complications of Lyme Disease? [12]

- Fluctuating degree of AV block (most common)
- Other arrhythmias
- Myocarditis, pericarditis, endocarditis
- Left ventricular dysfunction
- Cardiomegaly
- Valvular heart disease

99.5.1 Diagnosis (Table 99.1)

In a patient known to have Lyme disease, acquire an EKG if there are symptoms of carditis such as presyncope/syncope, palpitations, shortness of breath, or chest pain [8]. One can consider Lyme on the differential for other patients with unexplained

AV block. It is more likely in patients living in a Lyme endemic area who frequent the outdoors. One should have a high suspicion if there is a history of tick bite, erythema migrans, constitutional symptoms, and/or facial nerve palsy, presenting with heart block or other unexplained cardiac complication as listed above [13].

99.5.2 Prognosis (Table 99.2)

Lyme Carditis can resolve on its own, however treatment shortens the duration of the illness and decreases the risk of additional complications. Symptomatic patients or those with higher degree (2nd or 3rd) AV blocks require hospitalization. Additionally, some patients may require a temporary pacemaker. With treatment, >90% patients recover 1–2 weeks. It is rare that minor conduction abnormalities persists >6 weeks [13].

Case 5 Melanie is an 11-year-old girl living in Minnesota who presented to the clinic after sitting out of gym class due to knee pain, and her right knee was found to be erythematous, edematous, and warm. She denied any specific trauma to that knee. She plays soccer, but the season ended a few weeks ago. Her parents said that she has complained of knee swelling or pain a few times over the winter and fall, but it always seemed to go away on its own. There was no family history of autoimmune or rheumatologic conditions.

99.6 Characteristics of Lyme Arthritis [1, 6]

- Mostly affects large joints (esp. knee)
- Usually a mono- or oligo-arthritis
- Presents with joint swelling with elevated WBC in synovial fluid
  - In contrast, arthralgias *without* arthritis may be present at any stage of Lyme disease
- Usually intermittent (usually lasting weeks at a time) over several years
- Resolves with antibiotics. Rarely, there can be persistent arthritis following successful eradication of *Borrelia burgdorferi*.

99.6.1 Diagnosis (Table 99.1)

Sixty percent of untreated Lyme disease cases will progress to arthritis. Patients with Lyme arthritis may present similarly to patients with septic arthritis. Arthrocentesis can show WBC count >50 × 109 cells/L and elevated inflammatory markers in either condition, but they may be managed differently in the acute setting (septic arthritis requiring surgical management). In school-aged children presenting with acute arthritis, without fever and without profound decreased range of motion of the joint, Lyme should be high on the differential. These features are also more typical of Lyme arthritis than of septic arthritis [14].

99.6.2 Prognosis (Table 99.2)

Arthritis may persist after adequate treatment. A second course of antibiotics is recommended. Persistent arthritis after this course is then treated symptomatically because the organism has been successfully eradicated and no further antibiotics are required or beneficial [7].

Case 6 Kevin is a 17-year-old male with a history of anxiety and depression who is being seen at the nurse's office to take antibiotics for the 6th time this school year. He has a note for the treatment of "chronic Lyme." He has been missing school 3–4 times per month due to symptoms of fatigue and generalized pain. He complains of insomnia and difficulty concentrating in classes. His teachers have noted that he also sometimes walks with a noticeable limp. You recall that Kevin had Lyme arthritis 3 years ago and was treated with doxycycline for 28 days. Symptoms successfully resolved, but he tells you within a couple months he started to feel fatigued with joint pain again. You are surprised and concerned to hear that he has been off and on antibiotics frequently since then.

While symptoms of Lyme disease may last beyond the initial infection, there is no benefit to continued treatment with antibiotics once the initial infection is treated. Due to the nature of the diagnostic testing, results will remain positive for years (IgG and even IgM antibodies can linger), possibly contributing to mismanagement. IgM testing is only helpful in patients with symptoms for <4 weeks.

99.7 Post-treatment Lyme Disease Syndrome (PTLDS)

- Lingering symptoms of mild cognitive impairment, fatigue, depression, myalgias, and arthralgias for at least 6 months following successfully treated Lyme disease
- Responds to symptomatic treatment

99.8 Chronic Lyme

- May have different definitions in different contexts, but often implies that long-term antibiotic treatment is required to treat a chronic *Borrelia* infection, which is not evidence-based and is shown to be harmful due to side effects.

99.9 Recurrent Infection

- Past infection with Borrelia does not provide immunity, so subsequent acute infections should be treated with antibiotics [6].

Extra Credit Points

1. Symptoms of Lyme vary by stage and include erythema migrans, Bell's palsy, meningitis, radiculopathy, heart arrhythmias, and arthritis.
2. Early, localized Lyme disease can be diagnosed without laboratory testing if classic erythema migrans is present, and the region is endemic for Lyme. The patient should be treated with antibiotics.
3. Symptoms of Lyme meningitis can be mild, such as mild headache and/or neck stiffness.
4. Lyme antibodies can remain positive for months after successful eradication of bacteria, so positive serology in the setting of a prior Lyme infection does not necessarily indicate new infection.

References

1. Steere AC, Strle F, Wormser GP, et al. Lyme borreliosis. Nat Rev Dis Primers. 2016;2(1):16090. https://doi.org/10.1038/nrdp.2016.90.
2. Lyme Disease Case Map. U.S. Centers for Disease Control and Prevention. https://www.cdc.gov/lyme/data-research/facts-stats/lyme-disease-case-map.html.
3. How to remove a tick. Center for Disease Control and Prevention. Philadelphia, PA; 2023. Accessed 17 July 2024. https://youtu.be/S4Ny5YJh6Ws.
4. Cook MJ. Lyme borreliosis: a review of data on transmission time after tick attachment. Int J Gen Med. 2015;8:1–8. https://doi.org/10.2147/IJGM.S73791.
5. Zitelli BJ, McIntire SC, Nowalk AJ, Garrison J. Zitelli and Davis' atlas of pediatric physical diagnosis. 8th ed. Elsevier, Inc; 2021.
6. Kimberlin DW, Barnett ED, Lynfield R, Sawyer MH, editors. Red book: 2021–2024 report of the committee on infectious diseases. 32nd ed. American Academy of Pediatrics. Itasca, IL; 2021.
7. Bradley JS. 2024 Nelson's pediatric antimicrobial therapy. 30th ed. American Academy of Pediatrics. Itasca, IL; 2024.
8. Meissner HC, Steere AC. Management of pediatric Lyme disease: updates from 2020 Lyme guidelines. Pediatrics. 2022;149(3):e2021054980. https://doi.org/10.1542/peds.2021-054980.
9. Siwula JM, Mathieu G. Acute onset of facial nerve palsy associated with Lyme disease in a 6 year-old child. Pediatr Dent. 2002;24(6):572–4.

10. Loukas M. The neurologist's dilemma: a comprehensive clinical review of Bell's palsy, with emphasis on current management trends. Med Sci Monit. 2014;20:83–90. https://doi.org/10.12659/MSM.889876.
11. Halperin JJ. Nervous system Lyme disease. Curr Infect Dis Rep. 2015;17(1):445. https://doi.org/10.1007/s11908-014-0445-6.
12. Shen RV, McCarthy CA, Smith RP. Lyme carditis in hospitalized children and adults, a case series. Open Forum Infect Dis. 2021;8(7):ofab140. https://doi.org/10.1093/ofid/ofab140.
13. Radesich C, Del Mestre E, Medo K, et al. Lyme carditis: from pathophysiology to clinical management. Pathogens. 2022;11(5):582. https://doi.org/10.3390/pathogens11050582.
14. Ortiz CD, Barsi J. Differentiating between septic arthritis and Lyme arthritis in the pediatric population. J Pediatr Orthop Soc North Am. 2023;5(3):706. https://doi.org/10.55275/JPOSNA-2023-706.

Chapter 100
Influenza, RSV, and Other Respiratory Viruses

Matthew Demarest and Emily Rose

Case 1 After returning back to school after Winter Break, 7 year old Peter comes into your office with 2 days of fevers, sore throat, runny nose, and dry cough. He has two siblings at home with the same symptoms. He is breathing comfortably on room air and has clear lung sounds. What might explain Peter's symptoms? What can you do to both treat his symptoms and to prevent further spread of infection?

Influenza and Respiratory Syncytial Virus (RSV) are the two most common of the dozens of respiratory viruses. Outbreaks of Flu and RSV occur worldwide, infecting millions of people every year. Cases occur primarily in the Autumn and Winter months, beginning in October and peaking between December and February. Flu and RSV infections continue into late Spring typically ending around May. However, since the COVID-19 pandemic, the timing and duration of seasonal RSV/Flu has become far less predictable [1].

The respiratory viruses are spread from person to person primarily through the transmission of respiratory secretions. This means that sneezing, coughing, and even talking can spread the virus. The virus is often transmitted directly from person to person. However, contaminated objects can also harbor live viruses and spread them to unsuspecting targets when they come into contact. Door handles, phones, and drinks are common culprits for spreading disease. Because children tend to have poor hand hygiene and are always around other children, school-aged children are one of the most common transmitters of Influenza, RSV, and other respiratory viruses. Respiratory viruses can survive for hours on objects and commonly touched

M. Demarest
Los Angeles General Medical Center, Los Angeles, CA, USA

E. Rose (✉)
Los Angeles General Medical Center, Los Angeles, CA, USA

Keck School of Medicine of USC, Los Angeles, CA, USA

R. P. Olympia, J. Brady-Olympia (eds.), *Clinical Considerations in School-based Health*, https://doi.org/10.1007/978-3-031-85765-2_100

surfaces [2]. Frequent hand hygiene and sanitization of surfaces prevents the spread of disease. This is especially important because respiratory viruses are so easily transmissible and because children can be contagious and spread disease before they even develop any symptoms of infection [3–5].

The signs and symptoms of viral respiratory infections vary from case to case. Presentations can be vague. In certain cases, the only symptoms present are fever and fatigue. However, the most common clinical features of respiratory viruses are fevers, headaches, and body aches in addition to both upper and lower respiratory tract involvement (i.e. runny nose, sore throat, cough, and sneezing). Treatment should focus on supportive care. Aggressive oral hydration, acetaminophen, and ibuprofen are mainstays of therapy.

The diagnosis of Influenza, RSV, or other Viral Respiratory infection is a clinical one. The diagnosis is made through history and physical examination. Chest X-Ray and Viral PCR testing are not required to make the diagnosis or to initiate treatment. Patients who are ill-appearing, hypoxic, or at increased risk of serious complications as outlined below may warrant imaging (i.e. chest x-ray) and/or Viral PCR testing. However, the routine use of radiographs and laboratory testing for viral respiratory infections is not recommended.

It is important to note that most children will have 3–6 viral upper respiratory tract infections per year (up to 14/year in younger children in daycare) and that the symptoms often last for 10 days. The typical clinical course in younger children is that symptoms peak on days 2–3 and gradually resolve over 1–14 days. In older children/adolescents, symptoms resolve quicker, often in 5–7 days. Symptoms resolve after 3 weeks in 90% of URIs [6]. Most schools require students to be fever-free for 24 hours prior to returning. This is reasonable as many children with fever are fatigued and require rest while they have a fever. Requiring symptoms to be completely resolved is unrealistic as symptoms can be prolonged and children are often just as infectious prior to illness onset.

Supportive care for viral URIs include maintenance of hydration and rest. Antipyretics (ibuprofen, acetaminophen) help with the discomfort of fever but do not impact the disease course or hasten disease resolution. Over the counter remedies such as antihistamines or cough medicine should not be used in children <4 years due to risks of respiratory depression and associated deaths with use. Antihistamines may be used for symptom control in older children. Nasal saline rinses or spray may be used with little risk. Children older than one year of age may use honey to help with cough (darker, thicker honeys such as buckwheat or blackberry are most effective).

Case 2 11 year old Claire comes into your office after 2 days of fever, dry cough, and sore throat. Despite drinking lots of fluids and resting, she is feeling much worse. She has a history of asthma and has developed difficulty breathing and shortness of breath despite using her inhaler. When you examine her, you see that she is febrile and breathing 30 times per minute. What should you do?

While most cases of Influenza, RSV, and other respiratory viruses are generally benign and self-limiting, complications do occur. Complications from viral respiratory tract infections range from common to rare and severe complications which may require aggressive therapy and hospitalization (Table 100.1).

Table 100.1 Complications of viral upper respiratory tract infections

Complication	Clinical features	Treatment	Disposition
Acute otitis media (AOM)	Fever, ear pain, bulging tympanic membrane, purulent middle ear effusion	Observe or antibiotics if severe pain, fever, or symptoms persist longer than 48 hours.	Primary care provider or urgent care
Acute asthma exacerbation	Tachypnea, shortness of breath, wheezing	Inhaled bronchodilators, systemic steroid	Urgent Care Or Emergency Department
Bacterial pneumonia	Fever, Tachypnea, hypoxia, rales on lung auscultation, infiltrate on chest X-ray	Antibiotics with supplemental oxygen and hospitalization for severe cases	Urgent care or Emergency Department Final disposition: Home with oral antibiotic; Hospital admission if hypoxic or respiratory distress
Bacterial sinusitis	Fever, sinus type headache, serous or purulent nasal discharge	Antibiotics for persistent or severe symptoms	Urgent care or Emergency Department Final disposition: Home with oral antibiotics; Hospital admission if toxic or Complications (e.g. meningitis, cerebral venous thrombosis)
Myocarditis	Chest pain, hypotension, pulmonary edema, persistent tachycardia	Respiratory and cardiopulmonary support	Urgent care or Emergency Department Hospital admission if diagnosed
Myositis	Severe muscle pains and tenderness, and elevated creatinine kinase (CK)	IV hydration, supportive care	Urgent care or Emergency Department Final disposition: Mild influenza associated myositis—h Home with supportive care (i.e. acetaminophen, NSAIDs) Rhabdomyolysis (CK >1500 units/L or 5× the upper normal limits), acute kidney injury, suspected necrotizing infection, or electrolyte abnormalities, require hospital admission
Pleural effusion	Diminished lower lung sounds, persistent fever, chest pain, respiratory distress	IV antibiotics, hospital admission, thoracostomy tube	Emergency Department for hospital admission

While the vast majority of seasonal viral infections are mild, every year thousands of children are hospitalized with Influenza and seasonal Influenza kills dozens of children every year [7]. Unfortunately, certain groups of children are at an increased risk of morbidity and mortality. As a healthcare provider, the treatment of complications as they arise is not adequate. It is critical to identify children who carry a high risk of developing severe complications. A wide range of factors, both social and medical, contribute to a child's risk of developing complications from Influenza and RSV (Table 100.2) [8].

Although most serious illnesses and most deaths are associated with immunocompromised and those with pre-existing medical conditions, approximately half of pediatric hospitalizations for influenza occur in children without any pre-existing medical conditions [9]. In all children, you should monitor for abnormalities concerning for serious disease which should prompt referral to the child to the Emergency Department.

Indications for referral to the Emergency Department:

- Hypoxia
- Shortness of breath or increased rate of breath (tachypnea) while at rest
- Drowsiness or any other persistent change in mental status
- Dehydration with inability to tolerate oral rehydration

The mainstay of treatment for viral respiratory infections is supportive as previously mentioned. However, if Influenza is suspected, antiviral therapy with Oseltamivir (Tamiflu) is recommended if administered within 48 hours of symptom onset. Oseltamivir has been shown to reduce hospitalizations and death from Influenza, especially during severe seasons [7]. Oseltamivir for 5 days is recommended in hospitalized patients, in those with serious complications, or progressive disease. The most common medication side effects include nausea, vomiting, diarrhea, irritability, and headache. Less common potential side effects include Stevens-Johnson Syndrome and Erythema Multiforme.

Prevention remains the cornerstone of reducing morbidity and mortality from seasonal respiratory viruses. Regular hand-sanitization and cleaning of high contact surfaces are the most effective prevention against infection. The Influenza Vaccine is a critical component of public health and prevention of Influenza infections. Vaccination is known to prevent Influenza infections and to reduce the severity of

Table 100.2 Risk factors for complications or severe disease in Influenza and RSV

Category	Example
Racial and ethnic minorities	African-American, Hispanic/Latinos, American Indian, and Alaskan Native
Neuro-developmental disorders	Cerebral palsy, epilepsy, moderate to severe developmental delay, muscular dystrophy, prematurity
Pulmonary disorders	Asthma, cystic fibrosis, congenital lung disease, bronchopulmonary dysplasia
Cardiac disorders	Congenital heart disease, heart transplant, acquired cardiac conditions

infections that do occur. The influenza vaccine is estimated to have prevented more than 4000 hospitalizations in the US last year [7]. Both the American Academy of Pediatrics and the CDC recommend that children receive the vaccine as soon as it becomes available.

Extra Credit Points

1. Influenza, RSV, and other Respiratory Viruses are extremely common. They spread easily from person to person and through contaminated objects to infect millions every Winter causing fevers, headache, cough, sore throat, and runny nose. Using hand sanitizer regularly and wiping down frequently touched surfaces are the most effective prevention strategies.
2. Supportive care for respiratory infections include drinking plenty of fluids, getting extra sleep, cleaning hands frequently (to minimize spread) and covering cough. Antipyretics, antihistamines, nasal saline, and honey may be used to help with symptom control (but do not impact disease resolution).
3. While the vast majority of cases resolve on their own, severe complications (including hospitalization and death) do occur. Be aware of children with pre-existing medical conditions who are at high risk of severe disease.

References

1. Centers for Disease Control. https://www.cdc.gov/flu/about/season/index.html.
2. Hall CB, Walsh EE, Schnabel KC, Long CE, McConnochie KM, Hildreth SW, Anderson LJ. Occurrence of groups A and B of respiratory syncytial virus over 15 years: associated epidemiologic and clinical characteristics in hospitalized and ambulatory children. J Infect Dis. 1990;162(6):1283–90. https://doi.org/10.1093/infdis/162.6.1283. PMID: 2230258.
3. Lau LL, Cowling BJ, Fang VJ, Chan KH, Lau EH, Lipsitch M, Cheng CK, Houck PM, Uyeki TM, Peiris JS, Leung GM. Viral shedding and clinical illness in naturally acquired influenza virus infections. J Infect Dis. 2010;201(10):1509–16. https://doi.org/10.1086/652241. PMID: 20377412; PMCID: PMC3060408.
4. Suess T, Buchholz U, Dupke S, Grunow R, an der Heiden M, Heider A, Biere B, Schweiger B, Haas W, Krause G, Robert Koch Institute Shedding Investigation Group. Shedding and transmission of novel influenza virus A/H1N1 infection in households—Germany, 2009. Am J Epidemiol. 2010;171(11):1157–64. https://doi.org/10.1093/aje/kwq071. Epub 2010 May 3. PMID: 20439308.
5. Ip DKM, Lau LLH, Chan KH, Fang VJ, Leung GM, Peiris MJS, Cowling BJ. The dynamic relationship between clinical symptomatology and viral shedding in naturally acquired seasonal and pandemic influenza virus infections. Clin Infect Dis. 2016;62(4):431–7. https://doi.org/10.1093/cid/civ909. Epub 2015 Oct 30. PMID: 26518469; PMCID: PMC4725380.
6. Pappas DE, Hendley JO, Hayden FG, Winther B. Symptom profile of common colds in school-aged children. Pediatr Infect Dis J. 2008;27(1):8–11. https://doi.org/10.1097/INF.0b013e31814847d9. PMID: 18162930.
7. Committee on Infectious Diseases. Recommendations for prevention and control of influenza in children, 2022–2023. Pediatrics. 2022;150(4):e2022059275. https://doi.org/10.1542/peds.2022-059275. PMID: 36065750.
8. cdc.gov/flu/highrisk/index.htm.

9. Kamidani S, Garg S, Rolfes MA, Campbell AP, Cummings CN, Haston JC, Openo KP, Fawcett E, Chai SJ, Herlihy R, Yousey-Hindes K, Monroe ML, Kim S, Lynfield R, Smelser C, Muse A, Felsen CB, Billing L, Thomas A, Talbot HK, Schaffner W, Risk I, Anderson EJ. Epidemiology, clinical characteristics, and outcomes of influenza-associated hospitalizations in US children over 9 seasons following the 2009 H1N1 pandemic. Clin Infect Dis. 2022;75(11):1930–9. https://doi.org/10.1093/cid/ciac296. PMID: 35438769.

Chapter 101
Infectious Mononucleosis

Leah Kaye

Case 1 A 16-year-old female soccer player complains of sore throat and fatigue for a week. She is febrile to 38.4 C and other vitals are within normal limits. On exam you note anterior and posterior cervical lymphadenopathy, symmetric tonsillar hypertrophy with exudates, palatal petechiae, and a diffuse morbilliform rash. She was treated with amoxicillin 5 days ago after a positive rapid test for group A strep (GAS).

This presentation is suggestive of infectious mononucleosis (IM). IM is a common clinical syndrome caused by the Epstein-Barr Virus (EBV). IM is seen in ages 5–25 years, most commonly among those aged 16–20 years [1]. It is estimated almost the entire population (90%) will be infected with EBV, although many are not aware of having been infected due to the variable presentation of symptoms it can cause [1]. Patients commonly present with sore throat, fever, and fatigue. Posterior cervical lymphadenopathy, palatal petechiae, tonsillar hypertrophy, rash, and tonsillar exudate are common physical exam findings. Splenomegaly is present in a majority of patients [2], but is often not detected on physical exam. A positive test for GAS cannot entirely rule out IM as ~30% of patients with IM also have GAS. Rash is also a common sign in IM, and more common 5–7 days after treatment with a beta-lactam antibiotic such as amoxicillin. She should be seen by her primary care physician.

Testing is not required for a clinical diagnosis, but is recommended for athletes and children involved in physical activities, as it will guide your recommendations for activity. A heterophile antibody test (commonly called monospot) may confirm the diagnosis. This test is approximately 80% sensitive and can be used in children over 4 years of age. False negatives can occur in the first week of illness. The test can stay positive for up to a year after infection so cannot definitively differentiate

L. Kaye (✉)
Penn State College of Medicine, Hershey, PA, USA
e-mail: lkaye@pennstatehealth.psu.edu

R. P. Olympia, J. Brady-Olympia (eds.), *Clinical Considerations in School-based Health*, https://doi.org/10.1007/978-3-031-85765-2_101

between acute and resolved illness, but with a high clinical suspicion for IM it is helpful. A CBC typically shows >50% lymphocytes with >10% atypical lymphocytes [3]. EBV antibody testing (Table 101.1) can be performed if greater sensitivity is needed, or clarity on acute vs resolved infection is needed but requires more involved interpretation.

Does the patient need to be isolated from her classmates?

Transmission is by oral secretions—sneezing, sharing cups/food, or kissing. These activities should be avoided, but total isolation is not necessary. IM has a long incubation period (~30–50 days) so contact tracing is not possible [2, 4].

The patient's mother asks whether steroids or another medication could help her severe sore throat. What do you recommend?

Treatment is supportive, aimed at maintaining hydration and controlling discomfort. Ibuprofen or acetaminophen, throat lozenges/sprays, and salt water gargles can help. Avoid aspirin due to risk of bleeding or thrombocytopenia. Corticosteroids have shown an effect on pain control for up to 12 hours, but the benefit is lost at 2–4 days [2, 5, 6]. Given the risks of corticosteroids, they are typically reserved for airway compromise or for severe pharyngitis; in cases where pain is not well controlled, leading to dehydration from lack of oral intake, a short course of corticosteroids is reasonable [7, 8]. Typical dosing is 0.6 mg/kg orally, with a maximum of 10 mg.

Case 2 A 17-year-old male presents for a follow up visit after his diagnosis of IM. He developed sore throat and posterior lymphadenopathy 2 weeks ago. Today his sore throat is improved, but he endorses fatigue and occasional headaches. His spleen is not palpable on exam. He requests clearance to attend football tryouts in 2 days. What should you do?

This patient cannot return to play for multiple reasons; risk of prolonging symptoms and risk of splenic rupture. Splenic rupture is a relatively rare but feared complication of IM, with splenic injury being the most common cause of death in abdominal trauma among athletes [9]. It is most likely to occur in the first 3–4 weeks of illness, though it has been reported up through 7–10 weeks of illness. IM itself changes the structure of the spleen which increases its risk of rupture, and splenomegaly further increases this risk.

Table 101.1 EBV antibody testing and interpretation of the results

Test name	Timing of positive test	Using these tests together:
EBV VCA (viral capsid antigen) IgM	Positive early in illness Negative by weeks 4–6	+IgM, −IgG = acute IM +IgM, +IgG = acute IM −IgM, +IgG = prolonged IM symptoms (over a month), or prior resolved infection −IgM, +IgG, +EBNA = resolved/old infection
EBV VCA IgG	Peak positive at 2–4 weeks Stays positive for life	
EBNA	Usually negative in early illness Positive at 2–4 months and stays positive for life	

Chronic fatigue syndrome (CFS) may be a complication of IM. It presents with fatigue, daytime sleepiness, and depression. Further research is needed to determine if this is a physiologic reaction vs. psychologic reaction to IM infection. However, there is concern that vigorous exercise before resolution of IM symptoms can prolong the acute symptoms and increase risk of CFS.

Upset about missing football, the patient points out that you told him his spleen feels normal today—so can he play?

Clinical exam assessment of splenomegaly with both percussion and palpation is not sensitive, though it is specific; lack of a palpable spleen on exam does not sufficiently rule out splenomegaly. There are no studies looking at reliability of splenic exam in athletes, but given their typically well-developed abdominal muscles, sensitivity may be even lower in this population.

Ultrasound can accurately determine spleen length. There are available guidelines on normal spleen length. However, these numbers were based on small, non-diverse studies, making them harder to use on an individual basis since you do not know how big your patient's spleen is when he is well [2]. Serial ultrasounds can be useful in showing a decreasing or increasing spleen size, but are not routinely recommended.

The patient wonders when he can return to play if you cannot use your physical exam to follow the size of his spleen. What should you tell him?

There are no evidence-based consensus guidelines on return to play. There is a general consensus in the literature that return to light activity (no contact sports) can occur 3–4 weeks from symptom onset of symptoms have resolved [2, 9]. To return to contact sports, a risk/benefit discussion should be held with the patient and his family. Risk of splenic rupture is relatively low after 4 weeks [2], but still exists; contact sports and Valsalva (such as weightlifting) can increase the risk. However, prolonged absence from sports risks depriving the patient of the physical and mental benefits of the sport. With that understanding, the patient can gradually return to full activities after 4 weeks if he is completely asymptomatic. If symptoms recur as he increases his activity, he will require a longer avoidance of return to play.

Case 3 A 15-year-old female lacrosse player was diagnosed with IM 3 weeks ago. She is overall feeling better and started doing light conditioning. She presents today with left shoulder pain without an inciting injury. What should you do next?

Not all splenic rupture cases involve contact sports; spontaneous rupture or rupture after regular Valsalva have been reported. Sudden left shoulder pain (known as positive Kehr's sign) should raise suspicion for a splenic rupture in a patient 3 weeks from IM diagnosis. Other concerning symptoms would be acute abdominal pain or scapula pain. She needs to be evaluated today. If her vital signs are stable, call her parent/caregiver so they can bring her to an urgent care or emergency department (or her primary care physician if same-day appointments are available). If her vital signs are not stable (elevated heart rate or low blood pressure), call EMS.

Case 4 A 16-year-old male presents to your office and is diagnosed with IM. Last week you had a patient with splenic rupture due to IM and are wondering whether to expect other complications with this patient. How worried should you be?

Complications are relatively rare (5% or less total). Shortness of breath when laying flat should raise concern for worsening oropharyngeal swelling/inflammation—these patients need evaluation to determine if they need corticosteroids. Other rare complications include hemolytic anemia, aplastic anemia, thrombocytopenia, DIC, meningitis, or meningoencephalitis; these will typically present with petechial rash, severe headache or change in mental status, or severe fatigue.

101.1 Future of the Topic

The presentation and diagnosis of IM are well-understood and seen commonly in middle and high-school aged children. Further research and consensus are needed to provide clear, evidence-based guidelines for athletes to protect them from complications and allow them to return to physical activities in a timely manner.

Extra-Credit Points

1. Sore throat, fever, posterior cervical lymphadenopathy, and tonsillar hypertrophy are common in both IM and group A strep pharyngitis; coinfection is present in 30% of cases.
2. Splenomegaly is present in 50–100% of patients so vigorous physical activity should be avoided for all patients for 3–4 weeks from symptom onset.
3. Acute abdominal, shoulder, or scapula pain in a patient with IM is concerning for splenic rupture, and requires emergency evaluation.
4. Patients with IM who have received a beta-lactam (such as amoxicillin or ampicillin) will often develop a rash 3–7 days after starting the medication; this is not a drug allergy.
5. No official guidelines exist for return to sports after IM infection. At the minimum, patients should refrain from sports 3–4 weeks and be asymptomatic before starting a gradual return to play.

References

1. Becker JA, Smith JA. Return to play after infectious mononucleosis. Sports Health. 2014;6:232–8.
2. Putukian M, O'Connor FG, Stricker P, et al. Mononucleosis and athletic participation: an evidence-based subject review. Clin J Sport Med. 2008;18:309–15.
3. Wu Y, Ma S, Zhang L, et al. Clinical manifestations and laboratory results of 61 children with infectious mononucleosis. J Int Med Res. 2020;48(10):0300060520924550.

4. American Academy of Pediatrics. Managing infectious diseases in child care and schools. Elk Grove Village; 2005.
5. Wing A, Villa-Roel C, Yeh, et al. Effectiveness of corticosteroid treatment in acute pharyngitis: a systematic review of the literature. Acad Emerg Med. 2010;17(5):476–83.
6. Swaffield TP, Greene A, Tsai AY, et al. Two cases of splenic injuries in adolescent lacrosse players. J Pediatr Surg Case Rep. 2022;86:102433.
7. Candy B, Hotopf M. Steroids for symptom control in infectious mononucleosis. Cochrane Database Syst Rev. 2006;(3).
8. Shephard RJ. Exercise and the athlete with infectious mononucleosis. Clin J Sport Med. 2017;27:168–78.
9. Bartlett A, Williams R, Hilton M. Splenic rupture in infectious mononucleosis: a systematic review of published case reports. Injury. 2016;47(3):531–8.

Chapter 102
Hepatitis

Dieudonne Nonga

Case 1 Eric is an 11-year-old student who presents to the school nurse's office with extreme fatigue and inability to stay awake in class. You notice that Eric's eyes are yellow, and he complains of mild right upper quadrant abdominal pain. Upon further inquiry, he reveals that his family had just returned from a mission trip out of the country. What are your thoughts?

Hepatitis is the process of inflammation and/or necrosis of liver tissue that can be caused by infection, drugs, toxins, metabolic disorders, and autoimmune disorders. The main etiology of hepatitis in children is from a hepatotropic (liver is the main target organ) or non-hepatotropic (systemic infection with secondary liver injury) viral infection. The common hepatotropic viruses (Table 102.1) are a group of diverse pathogens which comprise a Hepatitis A (HAV), Hepatitis B (HBV), Hepatitis C (HCV), Hepatitis D (HDV) and a Hepatitis E (HEV). More than 500,000 cases of acute viral hepatitis are diagnosed in the US every year; 32% are caused by HAV, 43% by HBV and 21% by HCV. About 4% of hepatitis infections remain unexplained. However, a long list of systemic infections can also include hepatitis as a disease expression, including adenovirus, arbovirus, COVID-19, coxsackievirus, enterovirus, EBV, HSV, HIV, paramyxovirus, Rubella and Varicella zoster virus [1–3].

D. Nonga (✉)
Nationwide Children's Hospital, Columbus, OH, USA
e-mail: dieudonne.nonga@nationwidechildrens.org

R. P. Olympia, J. Brady-Olympia (eds.), *Clinical Considerations in School-based Health*, https://doi.org/10.1007/978-3-031-85765-2_102

Table 102.1 Hepatotropic virus transmission and screening

	Exposure and transmission	Incubation	Testing and screening	Course	Treatment
Hepatitis A	Close person-to-person contact and eating contaminated food or drink.	28 days (range 15–50 days). In children aged <6 years, most (70%) infections are asymptomatic; Among older children and adults, the illness usually lasts <2 months, but ~10–15% of infected people have prolonged or relapsing symptoms over 6–9 months.	Ig M Ab to HAV in serum or HAV RNA in serum or stool indicates acute infection while Ig G Ab to HAV indicates immunity from past infection or vaccination.	Highly contagious but self-limited and provides lifelong immunity, making fulminant and chronic infections rare.	Treatment is symptomatic and supportive. Ig G can provide short-term protection preexposure, and hepatitis A vaccine and IG can provide protection when administered within 2 weeks after exposure.

(continued)

Table 102.1 (continued)

	Exposure and transmission	Incubation	Testing and screening	Course	Treatment
Hepatitis B	Blood, drugs, or sexual contact. The virus can live on objects for 7 days or more.	90 days (range 60–150 days). Most children <5 years of age are asymptomatic when newly infected, whereas 30–50% of newly infected people aged ≥5 years have signs and symptoms [2] Symptoms usually appear 3–4 months after exposure to the virus.	See Table 102.2	Approximately, 90% of HBV-infected infants and 20–25% of those infected before 5 years of age will develop chronic infection, compared with 5% for teens or adults.	Treatment of acute HBV is supportive. Several antiviral medications are available for people with chronic HBV infection.[a]
Hepatitis C	Primarily through exposure of infectious blood, and those who have cleared or have been cured from the virus can be re-infected.	2–12 weeks (range: 2–26 weeks).	Ig G Ab to HCV (HCV IgG) and HCV ribonucleic acid (RNA). Tests can detect viral RNA as early as 1–2 weeks after exposure. to the virus[b]	Many are asymptomatic. Less than half of people who are infected will clear the infection in less than 6 months and most people infected would develop a chronic, lifelong infection that could lead to end stage liver disease and cancer.	Direct-acting antiviral (DAA) treatment is the mainstay therapy for hepatitis C. Starting treatment right away after diagnosis is recommended for all except for pregnant women and children under the age of 3.[c]

(continued)

Table 102.1 (continued)

	Exposure and transmission	Incubation	Testing and screening	Course	Treatment
Hepatitis D	Sexual contact, IV drug use and contact with blood from the open sores of a person who is infected. Can be contracted only by people with hepatitis B infection.	Symptoms usually appear 3–7 weeks after infection with HDV.	A blood test is the only way to confirm HDV infection.	Can occur through an isolation infection in a person with existing hepatitis B infection (superinfection) or a co-infection, at the time a person is infected with hepatitis B virus.	Hepatitis B vaccination prevents both infection against hepatitis B and D viruses. A prescription medication called interferon can help treat some people with hepatitis D
Hepatitis E	Fecal-oral route.	Young children do not usually present with symptoms. If symptoms occur, they usually appear anywhere from 2 to 6 weeks after exposure to HEV.	Ig M Ab	Most people recover fully from hepatitis E without any complications. In rare cases, some people with compromised immune systems develop chronic hepatitis E.	There is no specific treatment for hepatitis E. Most people recover from hepatitis E with rest and supportive management.

[a]Drugs approved for treatment of hepatitis B in children include adefovir dipivoxil and tenofovir alafenamide for 12 years of age and older, entecavir and tenofovir disoproxil fumarate for 2 years of age and older, interferon α-2b for 12 months of age and older, and lamivudine and Peg-IFN alfa-2a for 3 years of age and older

[b]Testing for hepatitis C is recommended for all adults, all pregnant persons, and for anyone with a recent exposure to the virus. Testing is important because safe and effective treatments can cure most people in 8–12 weeks

[c]Treatment is curative in more than 95% of cases, regardless of HCV genotype

102.1 Signs and Symptoms of Hepatitis

Signs and symptoms associated with infection with hepatotropic viruses can range from asymptomatic to fulminant hepatitis that can cause death. Signs and symptoms may include jaundice, discomfort in the upper right abdomen, fever, headache, flu-like symptoms, nasal discharge or congestion, sore throat, and cough. The urine color could become dark and the stool pale. Extrahepatic manifestations such as arthralgia, arthritis, rash, thrombocytopenia, glomerulonephritis, or papular acrodermatitis (Gianotti-Crosti syndrome) may occur early in the disease. Hepatitis B, C and D may cause chronic liver disease, with a risk for the development of cirrhosis and liver cancer. Fulminant hepatitis occurs in a small proportion of children infected with hepatitis A or B viruses.

Table 102.2 Interpretation of serologic test results for hepatitis B virus infection [1–4]

Clinical state	HBsAg	Total Anti-HBs	Total Anti-HBc	Action
Chronic infection	Positive	Negative	Positive	Needs direct care[a]
Acute infection	Positive	Negative	Positive (HBc IgM)	Needs direct care[a]
Resolved infection	Negative	Positive	Positive	Counseling, reassurance
Immune	Negative	Positive[b]	Negative	Reassurance
Susceptible (never infected and no evidence of immunization)	Negative	Negative	Negative	Vaccinate
Isolated core antibody[c]	Negative	Negative	Positive	Depends on situation

[a]Direct care includes a physical examination and laboratory evaluation for liver transaminase, hepatitis B virus DNA, and hepatitis B e antigen

[b]An anti-HBs titer of ≥10 mIU/mL correlates with protection only after a documented, complete hepatitis B vaccine series

[c]If false-positive results are suspected, repeat testing. If results are from past infection or passive transfer to infants born to HBsAg-positive mother, no specific action is needed. If results could indicate occult hepatitis B virus infection, inform patient of risks from future chemotherapy, immunosuppression, or hepatitis C virus infection antiviral therapy, and consider checking hepatitis B virus DNA

Children infected with non-hepatotropic viruses can show symptoms including jaundice and markedly increased liver transaminase levels requiring hospitalization. Abdominal pain, nausea, vomiting, fatigue and fevers can precede hepatitis. Most children recover, but in few cases, the disease can progress to severe liver injury.

102.2 Diagnostic Testing

The biochemical profile of acute hepatitis may reveal elevated alanine aminotransferase (ALT) and aspartate aminotransferase (AST), reflecting parenchymal inflammation. Alkaline phosphatase and total and conjugated bilirubin indicate the degree of cholestasis due to hepatocellular and bile duct damage. Prothrombin time is a good predictor of hepatocellular damage and the progression of fulminant liver failure. Resolution of hyperbilirubinemia and normalization of transaminases takes 6–8 weeks.

102.3 Management and Prevention of Hepatitis

Management of acute hepatitis is symptomatic and supportive, including adequate rest, hydration, and nutrition. Hospitalization is indicated for children with severe vomiting and dehydration, prolonged prothrombin time, or signs of hepatic encephalopathy. Treatment of chronic HBV and HCV infection is growing, and new antiviral drugs are being discovered. The decision to administer therapy is based on the patient's age, viral genotype, and degree of viral infection. Table 102.3 discusses immunization for hepatotropic viruses.

Case 2 Emma is a 14-year-old student with a history of chronic liver failure who presents with fever and chills, fatigue, body aches, and abdominal distension toward the end of the school day. Her vital signs demonstrate a temperature of 103 °F, heart rate of 160 beats per minute, respiratory rate of 24 breaths

Table 102.3 Immunizations for hepatotropic viruses [4]

	Immunizations
Hepatitis A	Two doses of the hepatitis A vaccine are recommended for children, between 12 and 23 months of age, unvaccinated children, and adolescents between age 12 and 18 and all people with increased risk factors[a]. **For catch up vaccination:** The second dose at least 6 months after the first dose. Unvaccinated age 12 months or older, traveling to or working in countries with high or intermediate endemic hepatitis A, should receive 1 dose of hepatitis A, as soon as travel is considered. **Immunizations**
Hepatitis B	3 doses of the hepatitis B vaccine are recommended for children as the best way to protect against the hepatitis B. The first dose is to be given shortly after birth, for babies that weight more than 2 g. For babies that weigh less than 2 g, the first dose should be given at month of chronological age, or at hospital discharge, whichever comes first. **For catch up vaccination:** If started late, the second dose should be given at least 4 weeks after the first dose The third dose should be given at least 8 weeks after the second dose and 16 weeks after the first dose. Post-vaccination serology testing and revaccination is recommended for people on dialysis or immunocompromised if anti-HBs <10 mlU/mL.
Hepatitis C	There is no vaccination for hepatitis C. The best way to prevent contracting hepatitis C is to avoid behaviors that can spread the disease like sharing or reusing needles or other personal items that might come into contact with infected blood.
Hepatitis D	Although there is no hepatitis D vaccine, getting hepatitis B vaccine also protects you from hepatitis D.
Hepatitis E	No vaccine is available in the US to protect against hepatitis E. Travelers to areas of the world with poor sanitation are at greatest risk for hepatitis E. In the US and other countries where hepatitis E is not common, people have gotten sick with hepatitis E after eating raw or undercooked pork, venison (deer), wild boar meat and shellfish.

[a]International travelers, men who have sex with men, homelessness, people whose jobs increase the risk of exposure and people who anticipate close personal contact with an international adoptee

Table 102.4 Signs and Symptoms in acute on chronic liver failure (ACLF)

	Signs and laboratory findings	Disposition	Treatment
Spontaneous bacterial peritonitis	Abdominal pain, fevers, nausea, vomiting and fatigue in a child with ascites	Refer to emergency department	Requires antibiotics and supportive care
Cholangitis	Right upper quadrant pain, jaundice with or without itching and intermittent fevers in a child that has a history of a procedure involving the biliary tree.	Refer to the emergency department	Requires antibiotics and supportive care
Pneumonia	Fever, chest pain or shortness of breath in a child that is on an immunosuppressive medication after a liver transplant	Refer to the emergency department	Requires antibiotics and supportive care and may require immunosuppressive or prophylactic medications adjustment.
Septic shock	High fevers, lethargy, jaundice, abdominal pain, other systemic symptoms	Refer to the emergency department	Requires antibiotics, supportive and often intensive care

per minute, and a blood pressure of 80/45. Capillary refill is prolonged (>5 seconds) with cool extremities and a weak, thready pulse. Her abdomen is distended and very tender to palpation throughout. What should you do?

Students with chronic liver disease are at risk for acute-on-chronic liver failure (ACLF), presenting with significant bacterial infections, such as spontaneous bacterial peritonitis, cholangitis, pneumonia and severe sepsis/shock (Table 102.4), increasing the risk for morbidity and mortality [5]. Early recognition and transfer to an emergency department is critical.

Case 3 Rose is a 17-year-old student with a history of depression who presents to your office with persistent vomiting and diffuse abdominal pain. She admits to you that she ingested a bottle of Tylenol the previous evening with the intent to end her life. What should you do?

Non-infectious causes of hepatitis are described in Table 102.5.

102.4 Case Conclusions

Case 1 Eric was referred to your emergency department were laboratory testing revealed elevated liver function values and a non-surgical abdomen. He was fluid resuscitated and discharged home. The following week he was diagnosed with Hepatitis A by immunologic testing. He was managed conservatively with supportive care and recovered well. He has had no recurrent symptoms of liver disease.

Case 2 Emma is presenting with signs and symptoms of septic shock and possible spontaneous bacterial peritonitis, with fever, significant hypoperfusion, fever, and

Table 102.5 Noninfectious causes of hepatitis

Etiology	Examples	Signs, symptoms and laboratory findings	Disposition	Treatment
Hemolytic diseases	Sickle cell anemia Glucose-6-phosphate dehydrogenase deficiency (G6PD)	Jaundice, fatigue, elevated transaminases and mostly indirect bilirubin	Refer to Emergency room for evaluation Or close follow up with pediatrician if mild symptoms or asymptomatic.	Avoidance of triggers Hydration, blood transfusion
Metabolic disorders	Hypothyroidism, alpha one antitrypsin deficiency, Wilson disease, fructosemia, galactosemia, tyrosinemia, mitochondrial disorders	Jaundice, fatigue, abdominal pain, elevated transaminases and bilirubin, can lead to acute liver failure	Refer to Hepatologist or Emergency department for evaluation	Supportive, avoidance of triggers, chelation, in some cases, liver transplant
Anatomic abnormalities	Biliary atresia, choledochoal cysts	Marked jaundice, pale stools, abdomen distension, anemia, elevated transaminases	Refer to Hepatologist or Emergency department for evaluation	Surgery repair and/or liver transplant
Malignancy	Hepatic adenoma, hepatoblastoma, hepatocellular carcinoma	Can be asymptomatic early or presents with abdominal distension or pain, jaundice and/or fatigue, elevated transaminases, bilirubin and alpha fetoprotein	Refer to Hepatologist or Emergency department for evaluation	Ablation, embolization, chemotherapy Surgical excision and/or liver transplant
Gallstones or gallbladder disease	Stones in the gallbladder or in the biliary tree, sometimes with inflamed gallbladder wall	Right upper quadrant pain, jaundice, nausea, vomiting, with or without fever	Refer to Emergency department for evaluation or close follow up with pediatrician if mild symptoms or asymptomatic.	Elective surveillance, pain control, antibiotics or surgery

(continued)

Table 102.5 (continued)

Etiology	Examples	Signs, symptoms and laboratory findings	Disposition	Treatment
Medications/ toxins	Tylenol, anti-epileptics, anti-depressants, mushrooms	Nausea, vomiting, abdominal pain, jaundice, fatigue, can lead to acute liver failure	Refer to Emergency department for evaluation	Detoxification, supportive care, removal of trigger, rarely liver transplant
Inflammation	Celiac disease, autoimmune hepatitis, graft versus host disease, hemophagocytic syndrome	Jaundice, abdominal pain, diarrhea, Elevated transaminases, acute liver failure	Refer to Hepatologist	Avoid triggers, treat primary disease, anti-inflammatory

abdominal pain/distension. This is likely acute-on-chronic liver failure, and requires prompt transfer to your nearest emergency department for stabilization, intravenous fluids and vasopressors, and antibiotics. She is ultimately transferred to the intensive care unit and improves over time.

Case 3 Rose was transported to the emergency department where she was found to have elevated transaminases and acetaminophen levels in her blood. She was started on N-acetylcysteine (NAC). On day two of admission, she became mentally altered and her transaminases significantly increased from presentation, requiring management in the intensive care unit. On day four of admission, her liver function tests and transaminases started improving, was transferred back to the inpatient ward, and ultimately discharged on day 7 to an inpatient psychiatric hospital for management of her mental health.

Extra Credit Points

1. Signs and symptoms associated with infectious hepatitis can range from asymptomatic to fulminant hepatitis, and may include jaundice, discomfort in the upper right abdomen, fever, headache, flu-like symptoms, nasal discharge or congestion, sore throat, and cough.
2. Students with chronic liver disease are at risk for acute-on-chronic liver failure (ACLF), presenting with significant bacterial infections, such as spontaneous bacterial peritonitis, cholangitis, pneumonia and severe sepsis/shock
3. Non-infectious causes of hepatitis include hemolytic disease, metabolic disorders, anatomic abnormalities, malignancy, gallbladder disease, toxin/mediations, and inflammatory processes.
4. For the initial assessment of suspected liver disease in school children, pertinent points to derive from history include:

   (a) Onset of Jaundice or symptoms
   (b) Perceived changes in mental status

(c) Constitutional symptoms, including fever
(d) Careful medication history and timeline of ingestion if suspected
(e) Travel and exposures
(f) Previous and family history

References

1. Jensen KM, Balistreri FW. Viral hepatitis. In: Behrman RE, Kliegman RM, Jenson HB, editors. Nelson textbook of pediatrics. 21st ed. Philadelphia: Saunders; 2019. p. 2106–19.
2. Rizzetto M. Viral hepatitis. In: Bircher J, Benhamou JP, McIntyre N, Rizzetto M, Rodes J, editors. Oxford textbook of clinical hepatology. 2nd ed. New York: Oxford University Press; 1999. p. 827–70.
3. Antala S, Diamond T, Kociolek LK, et al. Severe hepatitis in pediatric coronavirus disease 2019. J Pediatr Gastroenterol Nutr. 2022;74(5):631–5.
4. Centers for Disease Control and Prevention. Viral hepatitis surveillance — United States, 2022. Atlanta: US Department of Health and Human Services, Centers for Disease Control and Prevention; 2022. https://www.cdc.gov/hepatitis/statistics/2022surveillance/hepatitis-c/table-3.8.htm.
5. Fernández J, Acevedo J, Wiest R, Gustot T, Amoros A, Deulofeu C, Reverter E, Martínez J, Saliba F, Jalan R, Welzel T, Pavesi M, Hernández-Tejero M, Ginès P, Arroyo V, European Foundation for the Study of Chronic Liver Failure. Bacterial and fungal infections in acute-on-chronic liver failure: prevalence, characteristics and impact on prognosis. Gut. 2018;67(10):1870–80.

Chapter 103
Varicella and Herpes Simplex

Andrea Riley and Alice I. Sato

Case 1 An 8-year-old boy is sent to the health office by his teacher. He says he doesn't feel good and is itching the skin on his torso. You put on a surgical mask and gloves to assess him and check his vital signs. His temperature is 100.4 on a forehead thermometer reading, other vital signs are normal. You examine his skin and see the appearance of a number of red bumps, half of which are vesicular, or blister-like. The area around them is also red, possibly from scratching. He is very tired and says that he was at a family reunion by a lake a few days ago and the mosquitoes really got him. What do you do?

The National Federation of State High School Associations (NFHS) encourages school staff to think about three things when evaluating a skin condition: its location, any activities or hobbies the student participates in, and identifying possible symptoms [1]. We recommend also checking vaccination status. Asking about illnesses in household members or asking about recent travel may also provide information that could help the school staff.

Case 1 *Continued*
- Ask about activity: He says he likes sports, and that he plays soccer after school. No contact sports.
- Ask about any pain or tingling sensations: He says it hurts where he has been itching.
- Check his immunization status: You log in to your school's record system and see that he has a waiver in place and has not received the varicella vaccine.

A. Riley
Children's Nebraska, Omaha, NE, USA
e-mail: anriley@childrensnebraska.org

A. I. Sato (✉)
The University of Nebraska Medical Center, Omaha, NE, USA
e-mail: alice.sato@unmc.edu

R. P. Olympia, J. Brady-Olympia (eds.), *Clinical Considerations in School-based Health*, https://doi.org/10.1007/978-3-031-85765-2_103

Differential diagnosis: You are aware of the risk of insect bites, and you see that he does have mosquito bites on his arms and legs. You consider multiple causes of rash with vesicles (Table 103.1). However, with the fever, fatigue, and vesicles on his trunk, plus his unvaccinated status, you suspect his symptoms are caused by a virus and could be varicella. You also wonder if he has had chickenpox in the past and that is why he is not vaccinated, but you do not see records showing this.

Table 103.1 Common pediatric vesicular rashes

		Clinical signs and symptoms	Diagnosis	Treatment	Disposition
Varicella-related					
	Primary chickenpox	Fever for 1–2 days followed by rash that turns into itchy, fluid-filled blisters that scab over. Lesions appear in waves. Usually all crusted over by 10 days.	PCR test used to diagnose VZV DNA from vesicular swabs.	Acetaminophen may be used for fever. Do not use aspirin or ibuprofen due to risk of Reye syndrome. Antiviral medication may be recommended for those over 12.	Direct the student to their primary care physician for testing if chickenpox is suspected. Chickenpox is a reportable disease in many states. Primary disease is spread both by respiratory route (through the air) and by contact, so need to notify at risk staff and students promptly.
	Shingles	Painful, itchy, or tingly rash consisting of blisters that scab over in 7–10 days. Rash is unilateral (either on the left or right side of face or body) and in a band (dermatome). Pain may precede rash and may persist.	Healthcare providers may diagnose based on distinctive rash or symptoms. May be confirmed by PCR testing of lesions for VZV.	Antiviral medications can shorten the length and severity, best to take as soon as the rash appears. Pain relievers also may be used.	Direct student to their primary care physician. Spread by contact with skin lesions so should be covered and not touched.

(continued)

Table 103.1 (continued)

		Clinical signs and symptoms	Diagnosis	Treatment	Disposition
HSV-related					
	Cold sore	Painful fluid-filled lesions around lips and in mouth. May have fever if first infection.	Diagnosed by appearance. May be confirmed by PCR testing for HSV.	May need antiviral medication if severe or if subject is an immuno-compromised patient.	Child may go home; emphasize good hygiene; no sharing of toys, utensils, or personal articles. Should be urgently referred to ED or ophthalmologist if there is eye involvement. See provider if this is his/her first cold sore. Treatment not necessary with recurrent cold sores.
	Herpetic whitlow	Fluid-filled blisters on fingers or thumb seen in young children arising from spread of HSV-1 from mouth (cold sores) to fingers. Usually occurs at same time as oral lesions.	Diagnosed by appearance. May be confirmed by PCR testing for HSV.	Blisters will go away on their own, no treatment necessary unless superinfection or immuno-compromised.	Child may go home; emphasize good hygiene; no sharing of toys, utensils, or personal articles.
	Herpes gladiatorum	Fluid filled blisters on the face, neck, extremities or trunk spread by skin-to-skin contact.	Diagnosed by appearance. May be confirmed by PCR testing for HSV.	May need antiviral medication if severe or if subject is an immuno-compromised patient.	Direct student to their primary care physician.

(continued)

Table 103.1 (continued)

		Clinical signs and symptoms	Diagnosis	Treatment	Disposition
	Eczema herpeticum	Widespread skin involvement by HSV infection of skin of persons with eczema or other dermatitis. Clusters of fluid-filled blisters most often on face and neck, generally red but can also be purple or black.	Diagnosed by appearance. May be confirmed by PCR testing for HSV.	Antiviral medication may be given orally or intravenously, depending on severity.	Direct student to their primary care physician. If large areas of skin involved, may need to be seen in ED.
Other infectious rashes					
	Impetigo	Rash around the mouth, nose, hands, or forearms of children that is usually crusted with small fluid-filled blisters. These blisters burst easily, leaving small red sore areas which then develop yellow or tan crust.	Diagnosed by appearance. May have bacterial cultures sent by provider.	Treated by topical or oral antibiotics.	Direct student to their primary care physician.

(continued)

Table 103.1 (continued)

		Clinical signs and symptoms	Diagnosis	Treatment	Disposition
	Hand foot and mouth disease	Fever, sore throat, rash (red spots and painful blisters) inside the mouth and on palms of hands and soles of feet. Rarely can cause skin rash (eczema coxsackium) that mimics eczema herpeticum in persons with eczema.	Diagnosed by appearance. May be confirmed by PCR testing for enteroviruses.	Supportive care. At risk for bacterial superinfection that may need antibiotics.	Direct student to their primary care physician.
Non-infectious rashes					
	Chigger (mite) bites	Small itchy bumps that may appear like pimples, vesicles or small hives. Usually in clusters around the waist, ankles or skin folds. On penis may cause itching, swelling and dysuria (summer penile syndrome).	History of suspicious exposure and physical exam findings.	Scrub skin with soap and water to remove any chiggers still attached to skin. Avoid scratching; cutting nails short may help prevent damage. Cool compresses, calamine lotion (not to face or genitals) for comfort. May need antihistamines.	Refer to medical provider if: • appears superinfected • itching severe, not well controlled • symptoms of summer penile syndrome

(continued)

Table 103.1 (continued)

		Clinical signs and symptoms	Diagnosis	Treatment	Disposition
	Poison ivy rash or other allergic contact dermatitis	Develops usually 1–2 days after skin exposed to an allergen. Often on a limited area of exposed skin and may be linear and well demarcated. Often pruritic. May have local swelling. Lesions may ooze and become crusty.	History of suspicious exposure and physical exam findings. Patch testing may be performed to confirm inciting agent.	Avoid scratching; cutting nails short may help prevent damage. Cool compresses, calamine lotion (not to face or genitals) for comfort. May need antihistamines or topical corticosteroids.	Refer to medical provider if: • diagnosis uncertain (especially if accompanied by fever) • large amount of skin involved • involves face or genitals • appears superinfected or otherwise worsening despite home methods
	Contact dermatitis, irritant	Reaction to skin damage caused by exposure to irritants causing physical or chemical damage to skin (e.g. detergents, bleach, solvents), including over-washing of hands. Redness, swelling of involved area. Ranges from chapping and drying or fissuring of skin to vesicles or bullae in more severe cases. Pain, burning or stinging sensation may be more prominent than pruritis.	History of suspicious exposure and physical exam findings.	Moisturizers and emollients to decrease irritation and restore skin barrier function. Avoidance of inciting agent, protective measures (e.g. vinyl gloves) as needed. Topical corticosteroids may be needed; steroid potency selected based on severity and location of rash.	Refer to medical provider if: • diagnosis uncertain (especially if accompanied by fever) • large amount of skin involved • involves face or genitals • bullae, denuded areas of skin, and/or severe pain appears superinfected or otherwise worsening

These conditions may present with vesicles (small fluid-filled lesions) or progress to bullae (large blister-like lesions)

Children who have had chickenpox in the past may later get shingles (herpes zoster) resulting in a vesicular rash in a band (following a dermatome) on one side of the body accompanied by itching, tingling, or pain [2]. You check his skin again and see that the vesicles and rash are evenly distributed on both sides of his body, so this is probably not shingles. Lesions on his back also seem to have halos of redness without appearing to have been scratched.

Case 1 Continued *You contact the child's mother. She states that he was itching this morning but she did not notice any blisters, just the raised bumps she attributed to bug bites. She confirmed that he has not been vaccinated for varicella and has not had chickenpox in the past. You ask about siblings and the mom says that he has a 2-year-old sister who attends childcare but is currently home with a fever. Mom states that she will be there to pick him up soon but will have to take his little sister with her so she is not left alone. What do you do?*

- You instruct the child's mother not to enter the school building with the sibling, but to call when she gets to the school and you will bring her son out to meet her (you do not want to potentially expose any other students or staff members). You tell her that this is important because you are concerned that he might have chickenpox so the sibling might be affected as well, and to call the child's doctor right away. You ask her to let her daughter's childcare center know about your concerns. You tell her you will call her tomorrow to follow up.
- You tell the child to try his best to avoid scratching his skin, as that can lead to a secondary bacterial infection.
- Primary chickenpox (unlike zoster) is also spread through the air, not just touching lesions. If he is willing to put on a mask, you provide him with one. You increase ventilation in the health office by opening a window or turning on a HEPA air filtration machine.
- After the child leaves you instruct his teacher to also increase ventilation in her classroom. Then you clean and disinfect the areas in the health office and classroom he may have touched [3].

Case 1 Continued *The child's mother calls later that afternoon and tells you that he and his little sister have chickenpox. You are concerned because his homeroom teacher is pregnant. What do you do?*

- Inform the school principal that there was a confirmed case of chickenpox in the building. Notification must be made to unvaccinated students and staff members, pregnant women, and parents of immunocompromised children. You do not have to exclude any contacts from school unless they develop symptoms [3].
- You tell the student's pregnant teacher about this exposure. She is fully vaccinated and follows up with her doctor's office per your advice.
- You also tell your principal that you will be contacting the local health department both to inform them (as reporting chickenpox is mandatory in your state), and to follow any instructions they may have. Most states report varicella cases

to the National Notifiable Diseases Surveillance System (NNDSS) via the National Electronic Disease Surveillance System (NEDSS).
- The local health department helps you craft a letter to parents of immunocompromised students, which is sent out by you and your principal.

Case 1 Conclusion *You check your state regulations, health department guidance, and school policy to follow up with the child's mother to tell her that he may return to school when all lesions are crusted or scabbed over, he has not had a fever in 24 hours (without the use of medication), and he feels good enough to participate in class* [3]. *She tells you that she was notified from her daughter's childcare provider that there was another child at the center who had chickenpox, and that is how he was exposed.*

The diagnosis of primary chickenpox is made clinically based on fever and a pruritic, vesicular rash, often with small halos of erythema around it (sometimes described as "dewdrops on a rose petal"). Lesions appear in waves over 2–4 days, evolving from small red bumps to thin-walled blisters (vesicles) that easily break open then scab over. Lesions at different stages will be present at the same time, and the whole process generally ends in 10 days. In vaccinated children there may be fewer lesions and milder symptoms overall. In persons who have been previously infected and/or immunized, reactivation of zoster involves vesicular lesions often preceded by pain in the nerve root distribution (dermatome) involving only one side of the body or face. Pain may be quite severe and may occur both before and after the appearance of rash.

Case 2 A 16-year-old boy was sent to the health office after complaining to his gym teacher about painful sores on his shoulders and neck. You don a surgical mask and gloves (best practice with unknown rashes) and take his vital signs. He has a fever of 101.0. He says he has a headache and sore throat and feels like he's getting sick. You assess the areas on his neck and shoulders and see clusters of fluid-filled blisters. You also notice swollen lymph nodes on his neck. What do you do?

- Ask about activity: The student is on the wrestling team, they are mid-season right now.
- Ask about pain or tingling: He says the lesions feel tingly but not very painful or itchy.
- Ask about travel: he says he has not been out of state, but he travels frequently in state with his wrestling team. His last wrestling meet was a week ago in a town nearby.
- Check his immunization status: he is fully immunized.
- Differential diagnosis: a rash with clear vesicles could be due to a variety of causes, including contact dermatitis, impetigo, or shingles [4]. Because it is accompanied by headache, fever, and sore throat, you suspect a viral or bacterial cause. You know that wrestlers are at risk for skin infections such as MRSA, impetigo, ringworm, or herpes gladiatorum [5]. You do not see any of the vesi-

cles crusted over, leaving yellow or orange crusts characteristic of impetigo. You also have seen the larger pus-filled bumps of MRSA on other students and this does not look anything like it.

Case 2 Continued *You call the student's father to come pick him up, stating that the student has headache, sore throat, and a fever. You ask the father if he has noticed any sores on the child. He says he left for work early this morning without seeing his son and hadn't noticed anything yesterday. You ask if anyone else in the household is sick or has any fluid-filled blisters, and he says that your patient has a younger brother and older sister but neither of them were sick. What do you do?*

- While you wait for the student's father to arrive, you call the wrestling coach to come to the health office immediately. You show him the rash on the student and ask if any other wrestlers have anything like that. He is not aware of any, but as an experienced wrestling coach he identifies it as herpes gladiatorum, which is what you had suspected. He tells you that he checks student athletes for undiagnosed rashes, blisters, or sores on exposed areas of the body and around the eyes and mouth before practice or competition, and excludes any students found to have lesions.
- The student's father comes to the health office while the wrestling coach is still there. You both talk to him about the likelihood of herpes gladiatorum and instruct him to go to a doctor for confirmation, giving him a medical release form for the doctor to fill out.

Case 2 Continued *The student's father calls the wrestling coach and says that it is in fact herpes gladiatorum, and asks him how long his son has to stay out of wrestling. The coach calls you to confer. What advice do you have for him?*

- You check with your state school activities association's guidance. They have on their website a position statement from the National Federation of State High School Associations Sports Medicine Advisory Committee (SMAC) [5]. It gives the following guidance, which you relay to the coach:
  - "For a primary infection (first episode of Herpes Gladiatorum), wrestlers should be treated and not allowed to practice or compete for a minimum of 10 days.
  - If general body signs and symptoms like fever and swollen lymph nodes are present, that minimum period of treatment should be extended to 14 days.
  - If antivirals are not used, the infected participant may return to full contact wrestling only after all lesions are well-healed with well-adhered scabs, there has been no new vesicle formation in the preceding 72 hours, and there are no swollen lymph nodes near the affected area."

Case 2 Continued *The coach now asks you and the school custodian how to clean the wrestling mats so that no one else will be exposed. What do you tell him?*

Herpes gladiatorum is generally transmitted via skin-to-skin contact or contact with saliva. Although it is not generally transmitted by contact with contaminated surfaces such as wrestling mats [6], good infection control practices are still important. You advise them to clean and disinfect mats using an EPA-approved disinfectant effective against the herpes simplex virus, such as bleach. Per the Minnesota Department of Health [7]:

- The proper bleach concentration to disinfect wrestling mats is 800 ppm, or ¼ cup bleach mixed with 1 gallon of water. Mats should be washed after every practice session or competition.
- Locker rooms and shower areas should be cleaned and disinfected with this bleach solution.
- Mop heads and cleaning cloths should be laundered daily using regular detergent and hot water, and dried on high heat setting.

Case 2 Continued *You are invited to speak to the wrestling team about herpes gladiatorum. What do you tell them they can do to prevent skin infections?*

- Emphasize good personal hygiene [8]:
  - Proper handwashing is the best way to prevent the spread of this and a variety of illnesses.
  - Shower after every practice or meet. Use a new clean towel to dry off. Towels should be washed and dried on high heat.
  - Do not share soap, towels, or any other personal articles with anyone else.
  - Keep headgear clean by wiping down with a disinfectant wipe daily.
- Educate them on the importance of reporting skin abnormalities immediately to the coach.

Case 2 Conclusion *You locate fact sheets that you send home with the wrestlers and encourage their parents to contact you with any questions. You work with your administration and coaches to write a standard procedure for cleaning and disinfecting athletic equipment, including wrestling mats. You request all coaches be trained on identifying skin infections.*

103.1 Additional Resources for School Health Providers and Coaches

National Federation of State High School Associations (NFHS) Resources:

- NFHS General Guidelines For Sports Hygiene, Skin Infections And Communicable Diseases https://nfhs.org/media/5546438/2022-nfhs-general-guidelines-for-sports-hygiene-skin-infections-and-communicable-diseases-final-3-8-22.pdf
- NFHS Sports-Related Skin Infections Position Statement and Guidelines: https://www.nfhs.org/media/5546437/2022-nfhs-sports-related-skin-infections-position-statement-and-guidelines-final-3-8-22.pdf

Minnesota Department of Health Resources:

- Herpes Gladiatorum infection: https://www.health.state.mn.us/diseases/herpes/glad.html#NaN
- Infectious Diseases in Childcare and Schools Manual; Section 3—Infection Control Recommendations For School Athletic Programs https://www.hennepin.us/childcaremanual#Sec3

Children's Nebraska and Nebraska AAP

- The Nebraska Infection Control in Education (NICE) Book: Chickenpox, Herpes Simplex, Herpes Zoster https://online.flippingbook.com/view/558804203/

Extra Credit Points

1. Vesicular rashes on children may be caused by viruses such as herpes simplex, or varicella. These rashes may be difficult to distinguish from one another, and medical attention is necessary. Check vaccination status and ask about accompanying symptoms, pain, tingling, or itching as well as asking about the student's activities and exposures.
2. School staff, especially coaching staff, should familiarize themselves with common skin infections and how to prevent them.
3. School nurses and administrators need to actively communicate the importance of vaccination to prevent illnesses and outbreaks (also see Chap. 8)

References

1. Communicable Skin Infections.; NFHS Course (free, registration required): https://nfhslearn.com/courses/communicable-skin-infections.
2. CDC. Chickenpox (Varicella). https://www.cdc.gov/chickenpox/about/index.html.
3. The Nebraska Infection Control in Education (NICE) Book: Chickenpox, herpes simplex, herpes zoster. https://online.flippingbook.com/view/558804203/.
4. Vesicular rash: what it is, how it's treated, and more (webmd.com).
5. NFHS sports-related skin infections position statement and guidelines: https://www.nfhs.org/media/5546437/2022-nfhs-sports-related-skin-infections-position-statement-and-guidelines-final-3-8-22.pdf.
6. Minnesota herpes gladiatorum provider fact sheet. herpes-gladiatorum-provider-2023 (mc-379cbd4e-be3f-43d7-8383-5433-cdn-endpoint.azureedge.net).
7. MN Dept of Health. Herpes gladiatorum Infection - MN Dept. of Health (state.mn.us).
8. Pennsylvania HG Fact Sheet Herpes Gladitorum.pdf (pa.gov).

Part VIII
Sports Medicine and Traumatic Injuries

Chapter 104
The Pre-participation Physical Examination

Makenna Brezitski and Joseph Andrie

Participation in youth sports has rapidly expanded in recent years. It is estimated that almost eight million students at the high school level participated in youth sports in the 2022–2023 academic year [1]. Participation in sport and physical exertion at all levels places increased physiologic stress on the body. It is necessary to ensure the health of each athlete is assessed prior to participation in organized physical activity. The pre-participation examination (PPE) is intended to be a screening examination to identify health-related contraindications to participation in sport. It can be done either within the student's medical home, such as their primary care physician's office, or can be done as part of a mass screening event in a school setting. The pre-participation exam recommendations date back to 1992, when five medical organizations published a consensus statement outlining the examination and its importance [2]. In its nascent form, the exam was essentially a routine physical exam aimed toward identifying individuals at risk of sudden cardiac death. Since its inception, the PPE has evolved into many different algorithms, formats and requirements.

In today's world, the PPE has evolved in a number of directions and has a very diverse profile nationally. All states in the United States require a PPE for participation in interscholastic athletics with the exception of Vermont [3]. Components of the exam vary significantly but the general concepts remain the same: screening for cardiac and pulmonary disease. Much of the screening occurs through the history-taking part of the exam, most importantly a personal or family history of cardiac disease. The ultimate goal of the exam is to prevent sudden cardiac death among young athletes. Within the school setting, the responsibility for ensuring each student has completed a PPE falls within the job description of the athletic trainer. However, athletic trainers commonly consult with the school nurse to help with

M. Brezitski · J. Andrie (✉)
Penn State Milton S. Hershey Medical Center, Hershey, PA, USA
e-mail: mbrezitski@pennstatehealth.psu.edu; jandrie@pennstatehealth.psu.edu

R. P. Olympia, J. Brady-Olympia (eds.), *Clinical Considerations in School-based Health*, https://doi.org/10.1007/978-3-031-85765-2_104

coordination and planning of a mass PPE event. Each state typically has specific documentation that must be completed, both by the parent or guardian of each student as well as a clinician. The type of clinician who can complete the form has evolved over the years, and is now inclusive of not only physicians and advanced practice providers, but also chiropractors and dentists in some states. It is vital to know the PPE policy in the state where you practice.

Case 1 As the school nurse, you have been asked to assist with planning and implementation of a mass PPE event at your high school. What factors should be taken into consideration when approaching this event? What factors influence medical eligibility for participation in sport?

104.1 Personal Medical History

The most important role of the PPE is to identify and evaluate for any potential underlying cardiac condition in the athlete. Typically, the form required by the state athletic association will include a questionnaire addressing the relevant medical history. However, it is important to be aware of some of the key factors in medical eligibility. The most important questions for the examiner to ask are highlighted in Table 104.1.

Diagnoses of hypertrophic cardiomyopathy (HCM), arrhythmias, and other cardiac structural abnormalities have been considered a risk factor of sudden cardiac death (SCD) in sports [4]. Therefore, it is important to recognize if the athlete has any previously diagnosed health conditions, including cardiac, pulmonary, neurologic, or metabolic disorders [5, 6]. If the answer to this question is 'yes,' it is necessary to clarify if the conditions have been or are currently being cared for by a physician and if so, the treating physician will need to provide clearance for the athlete.

Table 104.1 A brief screen for cardiac conditions would include the following questions

Are you able to keep up with your teammates during exercise?
Have you ever passed out or felt as though you might pass out from exercise?
Do you feel like your heart skips a beat with exercise?
Do you regularly experience chest pain during exercise that forces you to stop?
Any one in your family have a history of a heart condition before the age of 50?
Any one in your family pass away for an unknown reason?

In addition to medical conditions, the examiner will want to be aware of any previous injuries or surgeries. A previous injury is the biggest risk factor for a repeat injury [6]. Knowledge of past concussions is also vital [7, 8]. Male students should be asked about testicular pain and female students should be asked about the regularity of their menstruation [9]. Mental health history and current concerns are also important to discuss to ensure proper support and treatment is provided if needed [8].

104.2 Family History

Knowledge of the family history of the athlete can uncover possible risk factors for sudden cardiac death. A family member with of any of the below warrants further evaluation by the athlete's primary care physician or a cardiologist [6, 9]:

- Cardiac disease related death or sudden cardiac death before age 50 years
- Arrhythmia, unexplained syncope, unexplained seizures
- Genetic disorders:
  - Cardiac structural disorder (HCM, dilated cardiomyopathy, arrhythmogenic right ventricular cardiomyopathy)
  - Cardiac conduction abnormalities (Brugada, long-QT syndrome)
  - Connective tissue disorder (Marfan syndrome, Ehlers-Danlos syndrome)
  - Blood cell disorders (sickle cell disease, sickle cell trait)

104.3 What Should Be Focused on in the Physical Exam?

The goal of a preparticipation physical exam is to assess for abnormalities that may potentially be fatal while participating in vigorous activities, such as cardiac abnormalities [9]. Most pre-participation physical examinations also include an assessment of other large organ systems and a general musculoskeletal exam (Table 104.2).

Table 104.2 Physical exam components

Vitals	Heart rate and blood pressure, Body Mass Index, consider vision screen
Cardiac	Auscultation of the heart both supine and standing positions OR with and without use of Valsalva maneuver. Evaluate for symmetric radial and dorsalis pedis pulses.
Pulmonary	Lung auscultation in anterior and posterior lung fields
Abdomen	Palpation in 4 quadrants and assessment for hepatomegaly or splenomegaly
Musculoskeletal	Brief Screening Examination including from cervical spine range of motion assessment of gait as well as range of motion and strength testing of the shoulder, elbow, wrist, and fingers. Having the athlete perform a "duck walk" is a sufficient general assessment of the lower extremities as well as with toe and heel walking [6].

Abnormalities in the physical exam, especially when they correspond with symptoms during exercise, should result in evaluation by the athlete's primary care physician or a specialist.

104.4 What Is the Format of the PPE?

There are many variations of the PPE. Some are paper forms from the school district or state athletic association and others are included in pediatricians well child checks. These exams are typically repeated yearly.

It is recommended that the exam be conducted by a physician, physician assistant, or nurse practitioner who has appropriate training in preparticipation exam [7]. Flow is typically history taking then targeted physical exam followed by anticipatory guidance and counseling. It may be beneficial to have a history form outlining the above questions completed by athlete and guardian prior to exam; the clinician can then review the form with the athlete, ultimately increasing efficiency [8].

104.5 What Are Best Practices for the PPE in the School Health Setting?

As outlined in this chapter there is significant variation in how the PPE is employed, the components and even the setting in which it is performed. We would like to conclude this chapter by outlining best practices for performing the PPE in the School Health setting. These best practices do not apply to completion of the PPE in a clinician office, but rather at a mass participation event held at a school.

104.6 Environment

Typically, the performing of physicals is either held in a gymnasium or the office of the school nurse. Multiple examination stations are spread throughout the physical space and adjoining spaces. Each examination space includes a folding table or exam table and two chairs. Examination space should be kept as quiet as possible with at least 10 feet between examination stations. Individuals waiting in line should be in a physical space separated by a door to decrease noise pollution.

104.7 Resources

The event should include at least one physician with specific training in pre-participation examinations, such as a primary care physician, pediatrician or primary care sports medicine physician. Ideally, the event would include the school physician or team physician, if applicable. Additional clinicians include advanced practice providers, residents or medical students. At least 1 nurse, ideally more to assist with obtaining vital signs and answering questions about the form. The athletic trainer at the school would ideally help with flow and answer questions. Students should come with the parent/guardian portion of the form already completed.

104.8 Organization

Each clinician should have their own physical examination station. A separate check-in station to ensure students have the appropriate documentation signed by their parent or guardian should be present at the entrance. The pathway for each student to rotate between stations should be clearly marked.

104.9 Timing

According to the American Academy of Pediatrics, the PPE should be completed at least 6 weeks from the start of practice or competitive play. Depending on the number of clinicians, staff and volunteers, the mass physical event may be able to accommodate 10–15 students per 15 minutes. Students can sign-up ahead of the event into designated time-slots or be permitted to be 'walk-ins' during a pre-determined timeframe.

104.10 Follow-Up

Any student who is not deemed to be fully medically cleared to participation will require follow-up with their primary care provider. This should be communicated to the student's parent or guardian on the day of determination. If they do not have a primary care provider, a social worker from the school can be included to assist with arranging the recommended medical follow-up.

Case 2 During the PPE at your school, a student athlete is deemed to be "not cleared" for participation in sports. What are the next steps to consider with this athlete's care? How to approach medical ineligibility?

It is the clinician's responsibility to place the athlete's health, well-being, and best interest at the forefront of medical eligibility decisions [5]. The Americans with Disabilities Act and the Rehabilitation Act notes that an "otherwise qualified individual" may participate in sport so long as their physical impairment does not alter their capacity to do so; they also leave space for individual institutions to put forth their own requirements for eligibility [5]. It is overall recommended that team physicians and/or general practitioners/pediatricians, in conjunction with the athlete and other medical specialties, deem medical eligibility [4].

Eligibility for sport participation occurs on a spectrum and is often not a yes or no answer. Forms of eligibility may include eligible with restriction, eligible or not eligible with recommendation of further treatment, not eligible for specific activities and not eligible for any activity. If an athlete has new underlying conditions or uncontrolled chronic diseases, they should be evaluated by a specialist prior to sports initiation. For example, those with uncontrolled asthma not controlled by medications, should first be evaluated by a pulmonologist. Those with controlled and stable asthma do not necessarily warrant pulmonology consultation [9].

104.11 What Is the Current State of Evidence Regarding the PPE?

The overall research validating the utility and format of the PPE is limited [8], though all associations and governing bodies agree that having a preparticipation physical exam is important. There are no formal regulations set forth by the National College Athletic Association (NCAA) or National Federation of High Schools about eligibility requirements [5]. Without a clearly recognized standard-format from a national organization, significant heterogeneity has emerged on a state-by-state and organization-by-organization stand point. Using EKG as a screening tool in a preparticipation physical exam is controversial and highly debated. It should certainly be considered in athletes with red flags in personal or family history or abnormal cardiac physical exams and may be a recommended screening tool for certain governing bodies [4, 9].

Extra Credit Points

1. The main objective of the pre-participation physical exam is to screen for any student athletes who may be at increased risk of sudden cardiac death based on personal and family history and physical examination findings.
2. In order to be successful and provide the best care of the student-athlete, the PPE must include a collaborative inter disciplinary group of clinicians and volunteers.
3. Screening with an electrocardiogram is not necessary for clearance for sport in most states, however, determination of further cardiac work-up must be individualized to each student-athlete.

References

1. Associations NFoHS. High school participation survey archive. https://www.nfhs.org/sports-resource-content/high-school-participation-survey-archive.
2. Stumph JM, Marie S, Justin. The preparticipation physical evaluation. Am Fam Physician. 2024;103(9):539–46.
3. Pediatrics AAo. PPE: Preparticipation Physical Evaluation state policy database. https://www.aap.org/en/patient-care/preparticipation-physical-evaluation/.
4. Petek BJ, Baggish AL. Pre-participation cardiovascular screening in young competitive athletes. Curr Emerg Hosp Med Rep. 2020;8(3). https://doi.org/10.1007/s40138-020-00214-5.
5. Maron MS, Mitten M, Borchers J, Rowin EJ, Maron BJ. Medical and legal determinants of sports eligibility for young competitive athletes with cardiovascular disease. brief-report 2023-8-29. 2023.
6. Carek SM, Edenfield KM, Carek PJ. Preparticipation evaluation. Prim Care. 2020;47:1. https://doi.org/10.1016/j.pop.2019.10.001.
7. Maloy W, Schroeder J, Rhodehouse B. Athlete preparticipation physical evaluation. Sports Med Arthrosc Rev. 2021;29(4). https://doi.org/10.1097/JSA.0000000000000330.
8. Pediatrics AAo. Preparticipation physical evaluation. 5th ed. https://www.aap.org/en/catalog/categories/sports-medicine-and-orthopaedics/preparticipation-physical-evaluation-5th-edition-paperback/
9. Turska-Kmieć A, Neunhaeuserer D, Mazur A, et al. Sport activities for children and adolescents: the Position of the European Academy of Paediatrics and the European Confederation of Primary Care Paediatricians 2023-Part 1. Pre-participation physical evaluation in young athletes. Front Pediatr. 2023;11. https://doi.org/10.3389/fped.2023.1125958.

Chapter 105
Sudden Cardiac Arrest and AEDs

Matthew Turner and Jeff Lubin

Case 1 An 11-year old boy comes to your office for a routine school physical. He endorses a brief episode of near-syncope several weeks ago that spontaneously resolved.

Sudden cardiac arrest (SCA) is a public health threat in the United States that appears to be increasing [1]. Unfortunately, SCA can progress to sudden cardiac death (SCD) within minutes if not properly treated [1]. While SCD is rare in children [2], its poor outcomes make it imperative to properly screen and assess for this potentially devastating complication.

Since the typical child spends 14% of the year in school [1], school nurses should have a thorough, consistent approach to screening students for potential SCA. Nurses should ensure that their facilities have an effective emergency action plan in place, centered on quick identification of SCA, immediate initiation of CPR, and rapid placement and use of automated external defibrillators (AEDs).

105.1 SCA Causes

SCA can be generally attributed to three primary causes: structural/functional defects of the heart, electrical abnormalities of the heart, and miscellaneous etiologies, ranging from medication and drug use [1] to traumatic mechanisms such as commotio cordis [3]. However, up to 40% of SCA patients may have no explanatory diagnosis found at all [4].

Structural defects include hypertrophic cardiomyopathy (HCM), the most frequently identified cause of SCD, identified in up to 20% of confirmed cases of SCA

M. Turner (✉) · J. Lubin
Penn State Milton S. Hershey Medical Center, Hershey, PA, USA
e-mail: mturner7@pennstatehealth.psu.edu; jlubin@pennstatehealth.psu.edu

R. P. Olympia, J. Brady-Olympia (eds.), *Clinical Considerations in School-based Health*, https://doi.org/10.1007/978-3-031-85765-2_105

[3, 5]. It may develop at any age and has a presentation that ranges from exertional fatigue to no symptoms at all. Most commonly, it presents after age 10 and is often associated with a systolic ejection murmur at the right upper sternal border [3]. Coronary artery anomalies are the second most common cause of SCA and include a wide range of underlying pathologies, such as Kawasaki disease and anomalous origin of the coronaries [3]. HCM appears to be more common in college athletes, presenting about half of all cases of SCA and SCD, while coronary artery anomalies are more common in younger patients, often around middle-school years [5]. Other structural defects include Marfan syndrome, dilated cardiomyopathy, restrictive cardiomyopathy, myocarditis, congenital heart defects, and valvular defects [1].

Electrical abnormalities of the heart constitute the second group. These channelopathies are due to abnormal conduction of electrical signals throughout the heart, and often present with a benign physical exam [3]. Common abnormalities include Long QT Syndrome (LQTS), Short QT Syndrome (SQTS), Wolff-Parkinson-White syndrome (WPW), Brugada syndrome, and heart block [3].

The third group includes SCA due to prescription medications. Psychotropic medications—including antidepressants, antipsychotics, opioids, benzodiazepines, and non- benzodiazepine hypnotics—may increase the risk of SCA, although research into this area is ongoing [6]. Anti-epileptic medications, as well as a history of severe epilepsy, also appear to increase the risk of SCD [7]. The use of stimulants, such as ADHD medications and pseudoephedrine found in over-the-counter medications, has been suggested to increase the risk of SCA as well, particularly in the setting of an upper respiratory tract infection [8]. Other causes include commotio cordis, due to blunt thoracic trauma typically sustained from blows to the chest from baseballs, softballs, and hockey pucks. The mechanical energy from this blow is enough to alter the heart's electrical stability, sending the patient into ventricular fibrillation that is usually fatal unless immediate life-saving measures are taken [9].

105.2 SCA Screening

Screening for SCA risk should be done uniformly in compliance with recommendations made by the American Heart Association. Unfortunately, recent studies suggest that less than half of high school athletic organizations fully comply with AHA recommendations [10].

Students should be assessed for signs and symptoms indicative of an underlying abnormality that may develop into SCA. Symptoms include severe fatigue with exercise, wheezing, dizziness, chest pain, syncope, palpitations, and dyspnea. Occult chest pain may present in patients with structural abnormalities, but is rare in patients with electrical abnormalities, who are more likely to present with a history of seizure or presyncope/syncope due to undiagnosed arrhythmias [1].

However, signs and symptoms alone are not sufficient for screening; the vast majority of SCA victims have no documented warning symptoms [10]. Symptoms that are noticed may be generalized and nonspecific, particularly in children under the age of 10 and in student athletes, and may be discounted by family members and medical personnel [1, 3]. As students may develop signs and symptoms concerning for SCA after initial screening is done, it is recommended that both students and family be provided education on potential warning signs [10]. It is important to remember that the severity of symptoms does *not* reflect the potential risk of SCD because even minor-appearing symptoms may be indicative of a potentially fatal disease process [11]. A list of any precipitating factors to these symptoms, as well as a medication list, should be gathered as part of the screening process [11].

Many cases of SCA, including HCM and many of the channelopathies, have a strong genetic component [1]. A detailed and comprehensive family history should be gathered as part of the screening process, including a family history of premature and unexpected sudden death, congenital deafness (associated with LQTS), syncope, seizures, and drowning [1]. A history of SIDS or repetitive pregnancy losses in the family may also indicate an inherited cardiac channelopathy [11]. We recommend the screening questions shown in Table 105.1 [1]. If any of these risk factors is present, the child should refrain from athletics until a full cardiovascular assessment can be done. In their 2019 guidelines for sports assessments, the American Academy of Pediatrics (AAP) recommends that this cardiovascular assessment be performed with a cardiologist if possible, with possible tests including ECG, echocardiography, stress ECG, and possibly more advanced imaging [12].

The physical exam should assess for any signs of cardiac murmurs, gallops, or additional heart sounds that may indicate a structural abnormality such as HCM or another etiology [3]. Providers should also simultaneously palpate the radial and femoral artery pulses—any delay in femoral pulses may indicate coarctation of the aorta [12]. Patients should also be assessed for signs of Marfan syndrome and have their brachial blood pressure assessed while in a calm state in a seated position [12].

The use of ECG in screening for children at risk for SCA remains a highly controversial topic. Their efficacy in routine screening is unclear—one study of 8 student athletes that died from SCD found that 6 of them had had prior unremarkable ECGs [12]. The AAP and the American Medical Society for Sports Medicine recommend that ECGs be done only on the basis of several factors: athletes at higher risk of SCA due to personal or family history, the ability of the provider to accurately interpret ECG readings, and the local resources available to ensure a proper follow-up with cardiology services is conducted in a timely manner [12]. Any facilities that do add the ECG to the normal sports examination should use only the most current criteria and ensure that all providers are capable of properly interpreting ECG findings to minimize cost and potential false-positive findings [12].

Ultimately, any temporary or permanent sports ban should be made in consultation with a cardiologist, preferably one with experience with student athletes [12].

Table 105.1 Pediatric sudden cardiac death risk assessment form [1]

Patient history questions: Tell me about any of these in your child...	Yes	No
Has your child fainted, had an unexplained seizure, or passed out during or after exercise, emotion, or startle (such as doorbells, alarm clocks, ringing telephones)?		
Has your child ever had extreme shortness of breath and/or discomfort, pain, or pressure in his or her chest during exercise?		
Has your child had extreme fatigue associated with exercise (different from other children)?		
Has a doctor ever ordered a test for your child's heart?		
Has your child ever been diagnosed with an unexplained seizure disorder? Or exercise-induced asthma not well controlled with medication?		
Family history questions: Tell me about any of these in your family...		
Are there any family members who had a sudden, unexpected, unexplained death before age 50 (including SIDS, car crash, drowning, others) or near-drowning?		
Are there any family members who died suddenly of "heart problems" before age 50?		
Are there any family members who have had unexplained fainting or seizures?		
Are there any relatives with certain conditions, such as:		
Enlarged heart: HCM		
Dilated cardiomyopathy		
Heart rhythm problems: LQTS		
Short QT syndrome		
Brugada syndrome		
Catecholaminergic ventricular tachycardia		
Arrhythmogenic right ventricular cardiomyopathy		
Marfan syndrome (aortic rupture)		
Heart attack, age 50 or younger		
Pacemaker or implanted defibrillator		
Deaf at birth (congenital deafness)		
Please explain more about any "yes" answers here:		
Parent signature:		
Physician signature:		
Date:		

105.3 AEDs

Case 2 A 16-year-old athlete has suddenly gone limp and unresponsive at a sporting event. Initial assessment shows no normal breathing and no pulse.

A 2014 survey of public school nurses revealed that 32% of nurses lacked confidence in their ability to respond to SCA [13]. We strongly recommend familiarity and repeated training with the Pediatric Basic Life Support Algorithm for Healthcare Providers algorithm published by the American Heart Association to develop confidence and a rapid response. School providers should also be intimately familiar with the automated external defibrillator (AED), a device that is under their responsibility on the majority of campuses [13]. The presence of an AED program at a school is tied with a significant decrease in mortality for victims of SCA [13].

AEDs are portable devices that both detect and treat life-threatening arrhythmias such as ventricular tachycardia and ventricular fibrillation [14]. Special pediatric pads are available for children aged 1–8 years [14]. As the third step in the AHA chain of survival—immediate recognition of cardiac arrest, early CPR, and rapid defibrillation—AEDs are the standard of care in treating SCA [14].

Providers should be trained in the use of AEDs; these machines should also be stored in a safe, easily accessible area, and undergo monthly checks of their battery life and system integrity [14]. The pads, which have a shelf-life of approximately 2 years, should be routinely replaced [14]. Regardless of the location in the school, an AED should be available to the victim within 5 minutes of arrest [14]. We recommend routine drills to increase teamwork and support among school staff; prior training during these high-stress events can be invaluable source of strength and confidence [13]. Videos demonstrating the use of an AED may be found on the AHA website at https://newsroom.heart.org/multimedia/animation-video/cpr-and-aeds-9749/aeds [15].

In cases of SCA, CPR should be initiated immediately, following AHA guidelines. The 9-1-1 system should be activated and the AED should be brought to the patient as quickly as possible. After the pads are applied, if the machine detects a shockable rhythm, a shock should be delivered. CPR should be continued if the machine does not recommend a shock; further instructions on when to pause for rhythm analysis should be followed when prompted by the AED [14]. This should be continued until EMS arrives or until the patient is otherwise able to be moved to a higher level of care [13].

105.4 Case Conclusions

Case 1 A full history and exam are done and an EKG is obtained. Because the patient's ECG has an abnormal QT prolongation, he is referred to a local pediatric cardiologist for further evaluation and workup.

Case 2 CPR is immediately initiated, and EMS is activated. An AED is brought to the child and applied within 5 minutes. A shock is advised and is delivered to the patient. At the time of EMS arrival, the patient has achieved return of spontaneous circulation. EMS assumes patient care and transports the patient to the hospital.

SCA is a rare occurrence that can be devastating in the school setting. We recommend that school nurses follow a comprehensive screening protocol based on symptoms, prior family history, a physical exam, and ECG whenever possible. In the event of SCA occurring in the school, nurses should have an emergency action plan in place that includes the immediate initiation of CPR and use of an AED.

Extra-Credit Points

1. Include personal and family history in screening for SCA
2. Include an ECG in screening for SCA, whenever possible
3. AEDs significantly decrease mortality from SCA and should be used as soon as possible
4. Having an emergency action plan in place that is drilled regularly will results in the best outcomes from SCA

References

1. Campell R, Berger S, Ackerman M, et al. Pediatric sudden cardiac arrest. Pediatrics. 2012;129(4):e1094–102.
2. Ackerman M, Atkins DL, Triedman JK. Sudden cardiac death in the young. Circulation. 2016;133(10):1006–26.
3. Scheller RL, Johnson L, Lorts A, et al. Sudden cardiac arrest in pediatrics. Pediatr Emerg Care. 2016;32(9):630–6.
4. Robinson JA, LaPage MJ, Atallah J, et al. Outcomes of pediatric patients with defibrillators following initial presentation with sudden cardiac arrest. Circ Arrhythm Electrophysiol. 2021;14(2):e008517.
5. Peterson DF, Kucera K, Thomas LC, et al. Aetiology and incidence of sudden cardiac arrest and death in young competitive athletes in the USA: a 4-year prospective study. Br J Sports Med. 2021;55(21):1196–203.
6. Allan KS, Morrison LJ, Pinter A, et al. Unexpected high prevalence of cardiovascular disease risk factors and psychiatric disease among young people with sudden cardiac arrest. J Am Heart Assoc. 2019;8(2):e010330.
7. Bardai A, Blom MT, Van Noord C, et al. Sudden cardiac death is associated both with epilepsy and with use of antiepileptic medications. Heart. 2015;101(1):17–22.
8. Alapati S, Strobel N, Hashmi S, et al. Sudden unexplained cardiac arrest in apparently healthy children: a single-center experience. Pediatr Cardiol. 2013;34:639–45.
9. Maron BJ, Estes NM III. Commotio cordis. N Engl J Med. 2010;362(10):917–27.
10. Drezner JA, O'Connor FG, Harmon KG, et al. AMSSM position statement on cardiovascular preparticipation screening in athletes: current evidence, knowledge gaps, recommendations and future directions. Br J Sports Med. 2017;51(3):153–67.
11. Al-Khatib SM, Stevenson WG, Ackerman MJ, et al. 2017 AHA/ACC/HRS guideline for management of patients with ventricular arrhythmias and the prevention of sudden cardiac death: a report of the American College of Cardiology/American Heart Association Task Force on Clinical Practice Guidelines and the Heart Rhythm Society. J Am Coll Cardiol. 2018;72(14):e91–220.
12. Bernhardt DT, Roberts WO, editors. PPE preparticipation physical evaluation. 5th ed. Itasca: American Academy of Pediatrics; 2019.
13. Boudreaux S, Broussard L. School nurses' perceived barriers and perceptual influences when implementing AED programs. J Sch Nurs. 2020;36(3):187–92.
14. Link MS, Myerburg RJ, Estes NM. Eligibility and disqualification recommendations for competitive athletes with cardiovascular abnormalities: task force 12: emergency action plans, resuscitation, cardiopulmonary resuscitation, and automated external defibrillators: a scientific statement from the American Heart Association and American College of Cardiology. J Am Coll Cardiol. 2015;66(21):2434–8.
15. AEDs. The American Heart Association. https://newsroom.heart.org/multimedia/animation-video/cpr-and-aeds-9749/aeds. Accessed 7 Apr 2024.

Chapter 106
General Concepts in Nutrition and Exercise

Jeremy Swisher and Laura Lintner

Case 1 9-year-old Michael visits your office complaining of fatigue and difficulty concentrating in class. His diet primarily consists of processed snacks and sugary drinks. What should you do?

Nutrition is foundational to the health and well-being of children, impacting their growth, development, and cognitive function. The American Academy of Pediatrics (AAP) recommends a balanced diet that includes carbohydrates, proteins, and fats in appropriate proportions for children. The evaluation of a child's nutritional status should involve a thorough dietary assessment, focusing on the intake of macronutrients and micronutrients. Children should consume a diet rich in fruits, vegetables, whole grains, lean proteins, and healthy fats. Encouraging Michael to reduce his intake of processed foods and increase his consumption of nutrient-dense foods can improve his energy levels and cognitive function. Referral to a registered dietitian may be beneficial for personalized nutrition counseling. School Lunch Reform has been a well-studied program for decades. There is evidence to support good outcomes for those children who have access to school lunch programs [1–4].

J. Swisher
Wake Forest University School of Medicine, Winston-Salem, NC, USA

L. Lintner (✉)
Wake Forest Baptist Medical Center, Winston-Salem, NC, USA
e-mail: llintner@wakehealth.edu

R. P. Olympia, J. Brady-Olympia (eds.), *Clinical Considerations in School-based Health*, https://doi.org/10.1007/978-3-031-85765-2_106

106.1 Benefits of Proper Nutrition

We can agree that Michael's diet does not sound well-balanced. The evidence shows us that this will likely not only affect his physical health, but also his mental health and possibly lead to poorer physical and cognitive performance into adulthood. Establishing these habits early also lowers his long-term risk of obesity, diabetes, and heart disease.

106.2 Limitations in Data and Need for More Knowledge

There has been significant work done in infancy and early childhood nutrition. However, school-age nutrition has received a lower level of scientific attention. It is unclear why this is the case, but potentially due to the misconception that early deficits in development cannot be overcome [1].

106.3 Important Growth Period

Puberty occurs in the middle of school-age years, thus including several points of change in somatic and brain development, which directly affect behavior. Bone mineral content (BMC), which expresses the strength of bones, accrues at peak velocities between 11.5 and 13.5 years. Optimizing nutrition, including protein, calcium, and vitamin D can positively impact this development and potentially decrease the risk of fractures later in life. As for the brain, the specific cortices that process input and generate behaviors develop at peak velocities between 5 and 15 years of age. All of this growth and development comes with a high energy cost and it is imperative that these needs are met by nutritional intake to ensure optimal change [1]. According to a study published in "Pediatrics", the interplay between genes and the environment begins at conception and extends through middle childhood. Children raised with adequate care, nutrition, and disease protection thrive compared to those raised in conditions of poverty. Children with limited access to proper nutrition are at risk for negative health outcomes and social outcomes throughout their lives [2].

106.4 Specific Recommendations for School-Aged Children

To best help Michael and children in a similar place, we need to know what the current recommendations are for the ideal nutrient intake. There are many ways to evaluate and encourage a healthy diet including the 5 food groups or assessment of

Table 106.1 Specific macro and micro-nutrient information

Nutrient	Description	Recommended advice
Macronutrients		
Carbohydrates	Main source of energy for the body; found in grains, fruits, vegetables, and dairy products.	Choose complex carbohydrates (whole grains, fruits, vegetables) over simple sugars for sustained energy levels. Maintain a balanced intake throughout the day.
Proteins	Essential for growth, repair, and maintenance of body tissues; found in meat, poultry, fish, beans, and nuts.	Incorporate lean protein sources into meals (chicken, turkey, fish, legumes) for muscle development and repair. Aim for a balanced intake throughout the day.
Fats	Provide energy, support cell growth and hormone function, protect organs, and help the body absorb nutrients; found in oils, nuts.	Focus on healthy fats (monounsaturated and polyunsaturated) found in nuts, seeds, avocados, and fatty fish. Limit intake of saturated and trans fats.
Micronutrients		
Vitamins	Essential for various physiological functions, including immune function, vision, and bone health.	Consume a variety of fruits, vegetables, and whole grains to ensure adequate intake of vitamins (A, C, D, E, K) and minerals.
Minerals	Important for bone health, muscle function, nerve transmission, and fluid balance.	Include sources of calcium (dairy, leafy greens), iron (red meat, beans, fortified cereals), and potassium (bananas, potatoes) in the diet.
Fiber	Important for digestive health, helps maintain bowel regularity, and may reduce the risk of chronic diseases.	Choose fiber-rich foods such as whole grains, fruits, vegetables, beans, and legumes. Aim for a variety of sources to meet daily fiber needs.
Water	Essential for hydration, nutrient transport, temperature regulation, and overall bodily functions.	Drink an adequate amount of water throughout the day, aiming for at least 8 cups (64 ounces) daily for children and more for adolescents and active individuals.

macro and micronutrient intake (Table 106.1). Healthychildren.org, a product of the American Academy of Pediatrics (AAP) provides valuable information regarding this topic.

106.5 The 5 Food Groups

One of the best recommendations is that children should be eating a variety of foods from the five major food groups, since each supplies important nutrients.

Vegetables: 3–5 servings per day (1 cup of raw, leafy vegetables, ½ cup of other vegetables)

Fruits: 2–4 servings per day (½ cup sliced fruit, medium-size whole fruit)

Bread, Cereal, or Pasta: 6–11 servings per day (1 slice of bread, ½ cup rice/pasta, 1 oz cereal)
Protein Foods: 2–3 servings per day (2–3 oz lean meat, poultry, or fish; ½ cup cooked beans, 1 egg)
Dairy Products: 2–3 servings per day (1 cup milk or yogurt, 1.5 oz cheese)

106.6 Macronutrients

Protein is required for growth and proper function of the body such as building new tissues and producing antibodies to help fight infection. Humans require fats to provide essential fatty acids for metabolism, blood clotting, and vitamin absorption. Fats should take up less than 30% of the calories in a child's diet, but it is important to include them for proper development and hormone function. Carbohydrates are a source of quick energy. They are necessary for important metabolic processes and so that other macronutrients can be utilized to their fullest potential [3, 4].

106.7 Case 1 Conclusion

The most important thing we can do for Michael is to educate him on all types of foods and the importance of a balanced diet. Since he is only 9 years old, his family should be intimately involved in this discussion. We can describe food as a fuel for his body and brain to grow and develop in the healthiest way, so that he may do the activities that he loves to do. If Michael presents in a school-based setting, we can encourage the availability of balanced food groups in the classroom and cafeteria. His case is all too common. We can continue to work towards education on proper nutrition and access for all children to a healthy diet.

Case 2 15-year-old Anna participates in softball and desires to improve her performance on the field. She asks about starting a strength training program, but doesn't have previous experience. What guidance do you provide?

Youth strength training can be safe and beneficial when performed appropriately under qualified supervision. The American Academy of Pediatrics (AAP) recommends incorporating strength training exercises for children and adolescents to improve muscular strength, endurance, and overall physical fitness.

106.8 Importance of Youth Strength Training

Strength training isn't just for professional athletes; it's for everyone, including adolescents like Anna. Youth strength training offers a myriad of benefits, such as:

1. **Improved Performance**: Strength training enhances muscular strength, power, and endurance, translating to better performance on the softball field. Anna can throw harder, run faster, and hit with more power.
2. **Injury Prevention**: Strengthening muscles, tendons, and ligaments reduces the risk of sports-related injuries, such as sprains, strains, and fractures. By building a robust musculoskeletal system, Anna can withstand the demands of her sport more effectively.
3. **Enhanced Body Composition**: Strength training helps increase lean muscle mass and reduce body fat percentage. This not only improves Anna's physique but also boosts her metabolism and overall health.
4. **Increased Bone Density**: Adolescence is a critical period for bone development. Weight-bearing exercises like strength training stimulate bone growth, reducing the risk for fractures as well as protect against osteoporosis later in life.
5. **Boosted Confidence**: Achieving strength and fitness goals can significantly enhance self-esteem and confidence, both on and off the field. Anna will feel more empowered and capable of tackling challenges.

106.9 Safety Considerations

Safety is paramount in youth strength training to prevent injuries and ensure long-term success. Here are some essential safety considerations for Anna's program:

1. **Proper Technique**: Emphasize the importance of maintaining proper form throughout each exercise to avoid strain or injury. Start with lighter weights or resistance and focus on mastering the technique with full range of motion before progressing to heavier loads.
2. **Supervision and Instruction**: Anna should perform strength training exercises under the supervision of a qualified coach or instructor who can provide feedback on technique and ensure safety.
3. **Warm-Up and Cool-Down**: Begin each session with a dynamic warm-up to increase blood flow to the muscles and prepare the body for exercise. Likewise, conclude with a thorough cool-down consisting of stretching to aid in muscle recovery and flexibility.
4. **Progression**: Gradually increase the intensity, volume, and complexity of Anna's workouts over time to promote continuous improvement while minimizing the risk of overtraining or injury.
5. **Rest and Recovery**: Allow adequate rest periods between workouts to facilitate muscle repair and growth. Encourage Anna to listen to her body and prioritize rest days as needed.

As per the AAP guidelines, it is advised to incorporate rest periods into a youth athlete's training regimen (Table 106.2), ensuring at least 1–2 days off per week from competitive athletics, sport-specific training, and practice. This rest time is crucial for both physical recovery and psychological rejuvenation. Moreover,

Table 106.2 Youth strength training exercises

Exercise	Muscle groups worked	Recommended sets and reps	Pearls
Bodyweight squats	Quadriceps, hamstrings, glutes, core	2–3 sets of 10–12 reps	Ensure proper knee alignment over toes. Start with body weight and gradually add resistance.
Lunges	Quadriceps, hamstrings, glutes, core	2–3 sets of 10–12 reps per leg	Maintain an upright posture and engage core muscles. Perform controlled movements to prevent knee instability.
Push-ups	Chest, shoulders, triceps, core	2–3 sets of 8–15 reps	Keep hands slightly wider than shoulder-width apart. Maintain a straight line from head to heels throughout the movement.
Resistance band rows	Upper back (latissimus dorsi, rhomboids, rear deltoids)	2–3 sets of 10–12 reps	Keep shoulders relaxed and retract shoulder blades during the pulling motion. Use a sturdy anchor point for the resistance band.
Planks	Core (abdominals, obliques, lower back)	2–3 sets of 20–30 seconds hold	Maintain a neutral spine alignment, avoiding sagging or arching. Engage glutes and core muscles to stabilize the body. Progress with longer seconds hold as tolerated.

maintaining adequate fluid and caloric intake is essential to fuel exercise, support competition, facilitate recovery, and promote overall growth and development. Neglecting proper nutrition and hydration can lead to under-recovery and undernourishment, increasing the risk of overtraining, injuries, and susceptibility to illnesses, particularly in athletes engaged in high-volume training regimens [5–9].

106.10 Case 2 Conclusion

As Anna embarks on her strength training journey, she experiences improvements in her softball performance, including enhanced speed, agility, and throwing power. Through consistent training and proper guidance, Anna not only reduces her risk of injury but also builds confidence in her abilities on the field. Her case underscores the transformative impact of youth strength training on athletic performance and overall well-being.

Extra Credit Points

1. Nutritional Support: In addition to strength training, emphasize the importance of proper nutrition in supporting Anna's athletic endeavors. Encourage a balanced diet rich in lean proteins, complex carbohydrates, healthy fats, and micronutrients to fuel her workouts, promote muscle recovery, and optimize performance on the softball field.

2. Mind-Body Connection: Highlight the significance of mindfulness and mental well-being in Anna's strength training journey. Incorporating techniques such as visualization, goal setting, and stress management can help her develop a positive mindset, enhance focus, and overcome challenges both in training and competition.
3. Long-Term Development: Emphasize the long-term perspective of youth strength training, focusing on gradual progress, injury prevention, and overall physical literacy. By instilling healthy habits and a lifelong love for fitness, Anna can enjoy sustained athletic success and improved health outcomes well beyond her adolescent years.
4. Meeting Children where they are on Exercise and Nutrition: Encourage the child in what they are currently doing and offer additional advice on a balanced diet and appropriate exercise to improve health and development.

References

1. Saavedra J, Prentice A. Nutrition in school-age children: a rationale for revisting priorities. Nutr Rev. 2023;81(7):823–43.
2. John CC, Black MM, Nelson CA 3rd. Neurodevelopment: the impact of nutrition and inflammation during early to middle childhood in low-resource settings. Pediatrics. 2017;139(S1):S59–71.
3. HealthyChildren.org, American Academy of Pediatrics Committee on Nutrition. 2021.
4. Lunborg P, et al. Long-term effects of childhood nutrition: evidence from a school lunch reform. Rev Econ Stud. 2022;89:876–908.
5. Brenner JS, American Academy of Pediatrics Council on Sports Medicine and Fitness. Overuse injuries, overtraining, and burnout in child and adolescent athletes. Pediatrics. 2007;119(6):1242–5.
6. Petrie HJ, Stover EA, Horswill CA. Nutritional concerns for the child and adolescent competitor. Nutrition. 2004;20(7–8):620–31.
7. Solomon ML, Weiss Kelly AK. Approach to the underperforming athlete. Pediatr Ann. 2016;45(3):e91–6.
8. Solomon ML, Briskin SM, Sabatina N, Steinhoff JE. The pediatric endurance athlete. Curr Sports Med Rep. 2017;16(6):428–34.
9. Lloyd RS, Faigenbaum AD, Stone MH, et al. Position statement on youth resistance training: the 2014 International Consensus. Br J Sports Med. 2014;48(7):498–505.

Chapter 107
Mental Health Issues in Young Athletes

Ashley K. Sturts and Jessica F. Butts

Case 1 **Gary is a 16-year-old naturally talented multi-sport athlete currently playing basketball. While he does not struggle with generalized anxiety, he has noticed that before games he feels nervous and fearful with physical symptoms such as heart racing, muscle tightness and difficulty focusing. As a result, while he can land 90% of his shots in practice and recreational play, his shooting percentage is much lower in the competition setting. As his symptoms have progressed, his competition performance has continued to decline. This has affected him to the point that he no longer enjoys playing and is thinking about quitting the team.**

Gary's symptoms are consistent with "performance anxiety," also known as "state anxiety." State anxiety is a subtype of social anxiety disorder, as classified by the 5th version of Diagnostic and Statistical Manual of Mental Disorders (DSM-5). In the setting of athletic performance, this anxiety is often triggered by fear of failure, fear of social judgement, or perceived negative consequences of an athletic performance. Extrinsic factors which may contribute to this are judgement from coaches or teammates, crowd effects, athletic endeavors which involve an athlete being judged, or ambiguous scoring procedures [1]. The Sport Anxiety Scale-2 may help evaluate for anxiety in sport performance settings [2]. While validity is variable across school-age athletes, this tool may be a good starting point for providers to assess for performance-based state anxiety. Distinguishing between state/performance anxiety and generalized anxiety/panic is important and informs the development of successful treatment plans (Chap. 68).

In the setting of sports performance, anxiety can hinder or enhance athletic performance depending on the athlete's emotional response to the anxiety and the athletic task. As it is normal for many athletes to experience pre-competition state

A. K. Sturts · J. F. Butts (✉)
Penn State Hershey Medical Center, Hershey, PA, USA
e-mail: asturts1@pennstatehealth.psu.edu

R. P. Olympia, J. Brady-Olympia (eds.), *Clinical Considerations in School-based Health*, https://doi.org/10.1007/978-3-031-85765-2_107

anxiety which does not otherwise affect their daily life, primary pharmacologic prevention of anxiety (SSRIs) may not be the best initial intervention. As-needed anxiolytics for performance (such as buspirone, beta-blockers or benzodiazepines) are also rarely indicated and may affect athletic performance [3].

Cognitive behavioral therapy (CBT) is the primary intervention for the treatment of performance anxiety. There are some psychologists who specialize in sports psychology and competition-related state anxiety. It is also important to emphasize other good health habits such as regular physical activity, optimizing sleep and sleep hygiene, encouraging adequate nutrition and mindfulness training.

Case 2a (Overtraining) Elizabeth is a 16-year-old female who plays soccer for both her high school team and a local club travel team. She has been playing soccer as a single year-round sport since she was 8 years old. She has spent her life looking up to her 20-year-old sister who is a starter for a successful NCAA Division 1 soccer team. Her goal is to follow in her sister's footsteps. To achieve this, Elizabeth had been increasing her training intensity with her club team optional practices during the high school season. She has noticed recently that she is not lifting as much or running as fast as she used to. She feels sluggish during the school day and falls asleep during her classes. She needs to stay up late at night to keep up with her schoolwork. She had been feeling increasingly stressed to maintain her previous 4.0 GPA to impress college coaches when the next NCAA recruitment season starts. Unfortunately, due to her decreasing performance on field, she was also removed from her position as a starting midfielder this week.

Elizabeth is displaying a pattern of symptoms concerning for "overtraining syndrome." This is a diagnosis of exclusion for an athlete experiencing long term decrease in performance accompanied by psychological and/or physiological symptoms that develop secondary to accumulation of training and life stressors [4]. A hallmark of this diagnosis is that there is no improvement after 2 weeks of rest. For the young athlete, consider a workup to rule out drug use, anemia, infection, hypothyroidism, diabetes, and adrenal disorder. Careful consideration for disordered eating and confounding mental health diagnoses, such as depression, must be considered as well [4].

Diagnosing overtraining syndrome can be difficult given the lack of objective biomarkers for definitive diagnosis. If available, training logs can help to see practice patterns and their time course related to decreased performance. Specialized mood screeners have been validated for use in athletics: Recovery-Stress Questionnaire for Athletes (RESTQ-Sport) and Profile of Mood States (POMS 2,) [4]. However due the costs associated with the above validated questionnaires, we may recommend PHQ-9 and GAD-7 for simple and readily available mental health screeners.

If a diagnosis of overtraining syndrome is suspected, prolonged rest which can vary from weeks to months depending on the individual athlete is the hallmark of treatment. Consideration for referral to a psychologist may be beneficial if comorbid mood disorders develop, commonly anxiety and/or depression. SSRIs and

SNRIs have shown benefit to address concomitant mood symptoms and speed recovery. There is an increased risk for hyponatremia and overheating with these medications, particularly in athletes—so careful consideration of the risks versus benefits for the individual athlete is necessary.

Case 2b (Psychological Response to Injury) Elizabeth continued to push to improve her athletic performance. She also opted out of the club team's "ACL prevention program" instead focusing on additional strength training on her own. Unfortunately, in the first game of the state tournament in her junior year, she suffered a complete tear of her ACL. She is now 6 months following a complete repair, knowing that it could take her 9–12 months to fully return to competitive soccer. She is feeling increased pressure to return to training as soon as possible for her teammates. She feels stressed that she may not achieve her goal of playing NCAA Division I soccer if she does not get back to training soon. She misses being at practice with her teammates. She worries if she will ever get back to being the high achieving soccer player she once was.

There are inherent psychological stressors in youth athletics that can increase risk for injury including sport specialization, lack of rest periods, over training, and improper coaching [5]. For the youth athlete, sport related injuries can be a major life stressor. An athlete's "psychological response to injury" is often related to the stressors in their life and their response to stressors. Elizabeth displays many of the psychological risk factors for a less successful recovery: young, female, limited experience with injury, negative emotion, and perception of isolation [6].

Often, physical recovery and psychological recovery do not occur on the same timeline. The clinician must maintain a high level of suspicion for cognitive, emotional, and behavioral responses that could delay overall recovery [5]. Even after full physical recovery, these can be indicators that the young athlete is not ready for a full return to sport. Psychological recovery can be aided by social support from their team, brief solution-based counseling, and stress management techniques such as imagery, goal setting and relaxation.

Referral to sport psychologist if symptoms of co-morbid mood disorders arise, in-office motivational interviewing, and encouragement to stay integrated with team events may all be next steps the clinician can take if there is concern for a slowed psychological recovery.

Extra Credit Points

1. Performance anxiety is common but may be disruptive to sports performance. CBT (cognitive behavioral therapy) is the preferred primary intervention.
2. Overtraining syndrome is a diagnosis of exclusion but when suspected requires a prolonged period of rest, greater than 2 weeks in duration.
3. Injury is a major life stressor for young athletes. Multi-disciplinary care including patient, coach, physician and psychologist are often needed for successful return to sport.

References

1. Chang CJ, Putukian M, Aerni G, Diamond AB, Eugene S, Ingram YM, Reardon CL, Wolanin AT. Mental health issues and psychological factors in athletes: detection, management, effect on performance, and prevention: American Medical Society for Sports Medicine Position Statement. Clin J Sport Med. 2020;30(2):e61–87. https://doi.org/10.1097/JSM.0000000000000817.
2. Smith RE, Smoll FL, Cumming SP, et al. Measurement of multidimensional sport performance anxiety in children and adults: the Sport Anxiety Scale-2. J Sport Exerc Psychol. 2006;28:479–501.
3. Powell DH. Treating individuals with debilitating performance anxiety: an introduction. J Clin Psychol. 2004;60:801–8. https://doi.org/10.1002/jclp.20038.
4. Carfagno DG, Hendrix JC 3rd. Overtraining syndrome in the athlete: current clinical practice. Curr Sports Med Rep. 2014;13(1):45–51. https://doi.org/10.1249/JSR.0000000000000027.
5. Wiese-Bjornstal DM. Psychology and socioculture affect injury risk, response, and recovery in high-intensity athletes: a consensus statement. Scand J Med Sci Sports. 2010;20:103–11. https://doi.org/10.1111/j.1600-0838.2010.01195.x.
6. Forsdyke D, Smith A, Jones M, et al. Psychosocial factors associated with outcomes of sports injury rehabilitation in competitive athletes: a mixed studies systematic review. Br J Sports Med. 2016;50:537–44.

Chapter 108
Performance Enhancing Substances

Ellen M. Benitah Bulbarelli and Greta L. S. Bires

Case 1 **Mario is a 17-year-old male football player presenting with persistent nausea, vomiting, abdominal pain, and diarrhea. He reported tiredness and a metallic taste in his mouth. Vital signs: Afebrile, BP 152/96, HR 99 bpm, RR 18, O_2 sat 98% on room air. He appears fatigued, with mild abdominal distension and diffusely tender, with generalized muscle weakness. Three weeks prior he started taking a dietary supplement to enhance energy and immune function, purchased from a local health food store.**

Case 2 **Lester is a 16-year-old boy, presented with severe acne, change in behavior, now being aggressive toward his classmates, insomnia, and increased muscle mass and muscle pain. Vital signs showed BP 162/96 mmHg and HR 90 bpm. He began testosterone 6 months ago, obtained online and dosages recommended by bodybuilding forums.**

A performance-enhancing substance (PES) is any compound consumed to improve appearance or athletic performance [1]. This includes substances that boost strength, power, speed, or endurance, modify body weight or composition, or enhance performance by influencing behavior, alertness, or pain perception. Doping is defined as the use of prohibited medications, drugs or treatments by athletes with the intention of improving athletic performance [2]. The World Anti-Doping Agency (WADA) defines PESs as meeting two out of three of the following criteria: enhances performance, represents a health risk, and/or violates the spirit of the sport [1]. Examples of PESs include legal or illegal pharmacological agents used at higher than recommended doses or without medical necessity such as stimulants, diet pills, diuretics, laxatives, products to increase muscle mass, agents to improve oxygen delivery [3].

E. M. Benitah Bulbarelli (✉) · G. L. S. Bires
Einstein Healthcare Network, Philadelphia, PA, USA
e-mail: Greta.Bires@jefferson.edu

R. P. Olympia, J. Brady-Olympia (eds.), *Clinical Considerations in School-based Health*, https://doi.org/10.1007/978-3-031-85765-2_108

PES use has become increasingly common in children and adolescents with increased access through internet suppliers and continued spread [3]. For most young athletes, using PESs doesn't provide much benefit compared to the natural gains from puberty and a good diet and training routine [3]. Sports participation, body dissatisfaction, higher Body Mass Index (BMI), training in a commercial gym and exposure to appearance-focused media all correlate with PES use [3].

Some prescription medications are also labelled performance enhancing substances, but when used as directed are necessary for underlying medical conditions in the athlete such as methylphenidate for attention deficit hyperactive disorder. Having documentation from the student's physician of the diagnosed medical condition and prescription is key along with a therapeutic use exemption on file for regulated sports like the NCAA. To see a list of regulated medications, refer to the WADA International Standard Prohibited List which is published every year.

Dietary supplements are among the most used PESs in adolescents and generally found being sold over the counter [3]. The Food and Drug Administration (FDA) defines dietary supplements as products containing a dietary ingredient taken by mouth. There is mixed data on the benefits of supplements in sports. Many dietary supplements are allowed in sports, omitted from the WADA prohibited list. Supplements though are not evaluated or approved by the FDA before being sold. Consequently, contaminated supplements are sold and can be dangerous to consumers or contain illegal PESs. Although companies are required to test ingredients, these tests are not standardized and may not detect contaminants. There have been reports of protein supplements showing contamination with a significant number of heavy metals, anabolic steroids and stimulants [3]. There is also concern that initial use of safe over-the-counter PESs may increase the risk of future anabolic steroid use and additional risky behaviors, with younger users particularly at risk of using multiple substances.

Overall, the FDA struggles to prevent the sale of dangerous supplements, highlighting the importance of consumer awareness and caution. The National Sanitation Foundation (NSF) certified for sport program provides guidelines regarding supplement use and is recommended by many professional athletic organizations to help athletes and coaches make safer decisions when choosing sport supplements. A list of specific supplements certified for sports can be found at https://www.nsfsport.com/certified-products.

Anabolic Androgenic Steroids (AASs) are prohibited by WADA, but a commonly used performance enhancing substance (Table 108.1). AASs increase lean body mass and decrease fat, overall increasing muscle mass and strength. Clinicians may suspect abuse of androgens in adolescents that present with behavior problems. Other situations that may suggest exogenous androgen use would be in athletes that compete in sports or activities in which excess androgens are perceived as improving performance such as football or weightlifting. Lab findings such as the high hematocrit, undetectably low luteinizing hormone, and low sex-hormone binding globulin may be present.

AAS, also known as prohormones, can lead to severe side effects like hypogonadism, infertility in men, and acute liver toxicity. It is vital that school-based

Table 108.1 Examples of anabolic androgenic steroids

Performance enhancing substance	Desired effect	Short-term and long-term side effect
Anabolic-androgenic steroids Testosterone (Depo-testosterone) Nandrolone (Deca-durabolin) Methandrostenolone (Dianabol) Oxymetholone (Anadrol) Stanozolol (Winstrol) Trenbolone (Finaplix) Veterinary use—cows Boldenone (Equipoise) Veterinary use—horses	Preserving muscle mass Preventing muscle breakdown Increased fat-free mass Increased muscle strength Muscle hypertrophy Increased number of muscle fibers Speed Agility [4]	**Acne:** Increase sebum production leading to clogged pores and acne (face, chest, and back). **Baldness:** Hair loss, by increasing dihydrotestosterone (DHT). **Breast development** **Deepening voice** **Liver damage:** Steroids metabolized in the liver can cause liver damage, including tumors and cysts, potentially requiring liver transplants in severe cases. **Cardiovascular problems:** Hypertension, high cholesterol levels, myocardial infarction, strokes, heart failure, and arrhythmias. **Kidney damage:** Overload and enlarge the kidneys, leading to kidney damage, stones, and failure. **Infertility:** Anabolic steroids can disrupt hormone production, leading to infertility in both men (reduced testosterone, sperm count, and motility) and women (disrupted menstrual cycle). **Increased cancer risk:** Anabolic steroids have been linked to liver, kidney, and prostate cancers. **Genito-urinary:** Accelerated puberty in youth, infertility, benign prostate hypertrophy, impotence **Musculoskeletal:** Tendon ruptures, premature closure of growth plates **Psychological:** Mania, agression, psychosis, addiction, and dépression [5]

practitioners can identify the use of performance-enhancing substances (PES) and recognize their side effects (Table 108.2). No standardized screen has been developed, but some signs may include aggressive behavior, obsession with appearance and performance, depression, or alcohol use. Specific symptoms that should be screened for include weight changes, sleeplessness, racing heart, headaches, and changes in memory or alcohol use. Additional signs include changes in resting heart rate or blood pressure along with aggression, isolation, drop in school performance, and body and muscle dysmorphia. This ability is crucial for timely intervention, allowing practitioners to discuss concerns with parents and advise scheduling an appointment with a primary care provider to ensure the student receives appropriate care.

108.1 Education and Prevention

Education and prevention of PES use among school students is vital for fostering a healthy, fair, and ethical sports environment (Table 108.3).

Table 108.2 Common performance enhancing substances: desired effects and side effects

Performance enhancing substance	Desired effect	Side effect
Anabolic-androgenic Steroids DHEA Testosterone Androstenedione	Increase muscle mass, speed, agility	Acne Hepatic dysfunction Hypogonadism Breast development Amenorrhea Deepening voice Organ enlargement Lipid profile changes Mania Aggression Premature closure of growth plates Myocardial infarction Atherosclerosis
Stimulants Dextromethorphan Ephedrine	Increased alertness Improve endurance Improve anaerobic performance Improve reaction time	Addiction Hypertension Tachycardia/arrythmias Heart attack Headaches Tremors Insomnia Anxiety/panic attacks Aggression Psychosis
Diuretics Acetazolamide Furosemide Hydrochlorothiazide Spironolactone	Weight loss Dilute steroid use	Dehydration Muscle cramps Kidney failure
Growth Hormone	Increase bone growth Increase muscle strength and fat-free mass Increased strength, power, and aerobic performance Increased respiratory muscle strength	Hyperglycemia Insulin resistance Edema Myalgias, arthralgia Gynecomastia Cardiovascular disease Intracranial hypertension
Epo stimulating agents	Enhanced oxygen delivery Increase aerobic power Increase physical exercise tolerance	Heart attack Stroke Deep venous thrombosis Pulmonary embolism

It is recommended to begin education in early adolescence and before use of PESs, focusing on behavior change education and teaching the value of competing within one's own physical limitations. It is thought that prevention efforts directed at avoidance of adverse consequences of PES use are likely to be less effective than those focused on lack of benefit of PESs to users [1]. One could collaborate with coaches and teachers to create educational programming, preferably implemented

Table 108.3 American Academy of Pediatrics (AAP) recommendations

1. Discourage PES use	Strongly discourage the use of performance-enhancing substances for athletic or other purposes.
2. Parental involvement	Parents should firmly oppose PES use and ensure coaches are informed about the adverse health effects.
3. Organizational proactivity	Schools and sports organizations should actively discourage PES use through policies and educational materials.
4. Positive interventions	Develop positive interventions promoting substance-free competition, emphasizing sound nutrition and training.
5. Educational programs	Implement educational interventions that encourage open discussions about PES use and fair competition.
6. Coaching practices	Coaches should promote healthy nutrition and training, stand against cheating, and avoid a "win-at-all-costs" mindset.
7. Inquiry practices	Inquire about PES use similarly to tobacco, alcohol, or other substance abuse, maintaining patient confidentiality.
8. Medical information	Provide unbiased medical information to athletes admitting PES use, including benefits, adverse effects, and risks.
9. Motivational exploration	Explore motivations and associated high-risk behaviors in athletes using PESs, offering safer alternatives for fitness goals.
10. Reinforce nonuse	Support nonusers' decisions and maintain open communication about PES use.
11. Promote safe activity	Health professionals should promote safe sports participation, offering information on exercise, nutrition, and injury prevention.

before students reach high school. Once PES use has begun, the approach should shift towards motivational interviewing (MI) to help individuals find their own reasons for change through collaboration, evocation, and respecting autonomy. It uses techniques like open-ended questions, affirmations, reflective listening, and summarizing. MI involves engaging, focusing, evoking, and planning to support positive behavioral changes. MI is more effective than education, scare tactics, or random drug testing [1]. Healthcare providers should direct patients and families to reliable resources for accurate information on PESs. If one is not as experienced with managing the effects of certain PESs then reach out to local health departments for drug treatment advice or refer to substance use professionals as needed. Through comprehensive education, supportive programs, and strict enforcement, schools can help students make informed choices and prioritize their health and integrity over short-term gains.

108.2 Case Resolution

Case 1 Mario was sent to the emergency department where he was diagnosed with acute arsenic intoxication due to contamination in the dietary supplement. Clinicians should always inquire about supplement use and maintain a high index of suspicion for supplement-related toxicity. Advise the use of only supplements certified for sports by the National Sanitation Foundation (NSF) to reduce risk.

Case 2 Lester was sent to his primary care physician. He had elevated AST and ALT, creatinine, and LDL, and decreased HDL. Hormone panel showed elevated testosterone, suppressed LH and FSH, and elevated estradiol. Abdominal ultrasound indicated mild hepatic steatosis and echocardiogram revealed mild left ventricular hypertrophy. This case illustrates severe complications from AAS use, including dermatological, psychological, cardiovascular, and endocrine issues.

Extra Credit Points

1. A performance enhancing substance is any compound consumed for the purpose of improving appearance or athletic performance.
2. Recognizing signs of PES use and the potential adverse effects are critical for intervention and protection of students.
3. Early education before PES use is key in preventing PES use while motivational interviewing is useful for treating those who already engage in PES use.

References

1. Siegmund LA. Appearance and performance enhancing drugs and substances: the role of the school nurse. NASN Sch Nurse. 2022;37(5):263–9. https://doi.org/10.1177/1942602X221093938.
2. Pope HG, Wood RI, Rogol A, Nyberg F, Bowers L, Bhasin S. Adverse health consequences of performance-enhancing drugs: an Endocrine Society scientific statement. Endocr Rev. 2014;35(3):341–75. https://doi.org/10.1210/er.2013-1058.
3. LaBotz M, Griesemer BA, Council on Sports Medicine and Fitness, et al. Use of performance-enhancing substances. Pediatrics. 2016;138(1):e20161300. https://doi.org/10.1542/peds.2016-1300.
4. Dandoy C, Gereige RS. Performance-enhancing drugs. Pediatr Rev. 2012;33(6):265–71; quiz 271–2. PMID: 22659257; PMCID: PMC4528343. https://doi.org/10.1542/pir.33-6-265.
5. Mantri S, Agarwal S, Jaiswal A, Yelne S, Prasad R, Wanjari MB. Bodybuilding: a comprehensive review of performance-enhancing substance use and public health implications. Cureus. 2023;15(7):e41600. https://doi.org/10.7759/cureus.41600. PMID: 37559855; PMCID: PMC10409494.

Chapter 109
Concussion

Michael Osterholt and Natalie Ronshaugen

Case 1 An 8-year-old boy falls from the monkey bars flat on his back and hits his head on the ground. He does not lose consciousness. He cries immediately. Once he is calmed down, he describes a headache and nausea.

A concussion is a traumatic brain injury caused by a direct blow to the head, neck or body resulting in a force being transmitted to the brain. This initiates a complex cascade resulting in an energy mismatch which leads to symptoms. Signs and symptoms may present immediately or evolve over minutes to hours. No abnormality is seen on standard neuroimaging. Clinical signs and symptoms cannot be explained by another diagnosis [1].

Concussion remains a clinical diagnosis made by carefully synthesizing history and physical exam findings as the injury evolves. Diagnosis and management should be performed by trained healthcare professionals. Sports related concussion grading is no longer recommended (i.e. simple vs. complex or mild, moderate, severe) as it has very little prognostic value. Multiple fluid based and imaging biomarkers are currently being studied and do have promise, particularly for diagnosis and prognosis. These are still largely used in research and are not yet clinically widely used or available [1].

Knowing the symptoms and their associated implications on a child's well-being can help guide accommodation and management. Symptoms can be classified into five domains of function (Table 109.1) [2].

The Center for Disease Control (CDC) publishes a Concussion Signs and Symptoms Check list for initial evaluation of concussion at the school [3]. It

M. Osterholt
University of Nebraska Medical Center, Omaha, NE, USA

N. Ronshaugen (✉)
Children's Nebraska, Omaha, NE, USA
e-mail: nronshaugen@childrensnebraska.org

R. P. Olympia, J. Brady-Olympia (eds.), *Clinical Considerations in School-based Health*, https://doi.org/10.1007/978-3-031-85765-2_109

Table 109.1 Concussion symptoms

Somatic
Headache, doesn't feel right, nausea/vomiting, neck pain, light sensitivity, and noise sensitivity
Vestibular and ocular
Vision problems, hearing problems, balance problems, and dizziness
Cognitive
Confusion, "brain fog", difficulty concentrating or remembering, answering slowly, repeating questions, loss of consciousness
Emotional
Irritable, sad, nervous or anxious, more emotionally labile
Sleep
Changes in sleep patterns, fatigue, feeling slowed down

Table created by the authors

includes a symptom checklist, a list of "Danger signs", and can help build a plan for next steps in treatment:

https://www.cdc.gov/heads-up/media/pdfs/schools/tbi_schools_checklist_508-a.pdf?CDC_AAref_Val=https://www.cdc.gov/headsup/pdfs/schools/TBI_schools_checklist_508-a.pdf

Return to Learn is the process of transitioning back to the classroom following concussion. Often a multidisciplinary team of stakeholders is involved for successful management. Early return to school should be promoted and is not considered dangerous. Students should return to school as soon as they can tolerate it even if they still have symptoms. Not all individuals will require a return to learn protocol and often individuals return to full participation quickly. However, for some, a graded return may be necessary focusing on essential classes as tolerated and slowly increasing time at school and cognitive load [1, 4]. School accommodations should be individualized and tailored to symptom burden and deficits. Table 109.2 offers suggestions for possible accommodations based on symptom burden [4, 5].

109.1 Concussion Team

Many schools develop a concussion team. The build of the team depends in part on each school's resources but often includes the school nurse, athletic trainer, school counselor, teacher representative, and coach. When possible, concussion cases should be discussed among the team and a return to learn and safe return to play program for each individual student with concussion should be established. When a multi-team approach is not possible, a school nurse or principal can progress students through return to learn based on symptom tolerance, however, full return to contact play should not occur until the student is released by a concussion health

Table 109.2 School accommodations samples

Slow to finish work, difficulty concentrating	Extra time to finish assignments or tests. Condensed or shortened assignments. Allow breaks during school as needed. Consider limiting essays in favor of multiple choice.
Light sensitivity, sound sensitivity	Print off work instead of doing it on tablet. Lunch in a quiet room. Allow to walk to next class early to avoid crowds. Use of a hat during school to limit light exposure.
Severe headaches	Allow to take medication at school as needed. Allow breaks during school as needed (may need to schedule breaks for younger students). Shortened school days.
Emotional lability	Allow breaks during school as needed. Access to a school psychologist if available. Reassurance. Ensure safety against self-harm.
Sleep disturbance	Encourage regular wake time. Encourage minimizing napping when able and if nap necessary, help plan for one around class time. May need shortened class days with a goal of slowly increasing them.
Prolonged symptoms	Consider implementing a 504 plan.

Table created by the authors

care provider, i.e. a primary care provider, sports medicine physician, or in some states, an athletic trainer [4] (Fig. 109.1).

Case 2 During football practice a 15-year-old boy is tackled to the ground. He was seen stumbling off the field and has a bloody nose but states he feels fine now.

As stated previously, prompt diagnosis of a concussion is imperative for positive long-term outcomes. Prompt removal of a player from competition should be done if there is suspicion of concussion. Signs or symptoms that require immediate removal include suspected loss of consciousness, gross motor instability, confusion, blank or vacant look, amnesia, behavioral changes, seizure, or even a high-risk impact [1].

Concussion assessment should be done in a distraction free environment. The Consensus Statement on Concussion in Sport: the 6th International Conference on Concussion in Sport provides comprehensive assessment tools which help with diagnosis (Table 109.3). The four tools include the SCAT6 (ages 13+) and the Child-SCAT6 (ages 8–12), which can be used within the first 72 hours after injury. The SCOAT6 and Child SCOAT6 can be used for follow-up in the office setting after 72 hours [1].

These tools assist healthcare providers in the evaluation of concussion but are not intended to be used in isolation for making the diagnosis. The primary endpoint is to determine the probability an athlete has a concussion. If concussion is deemed

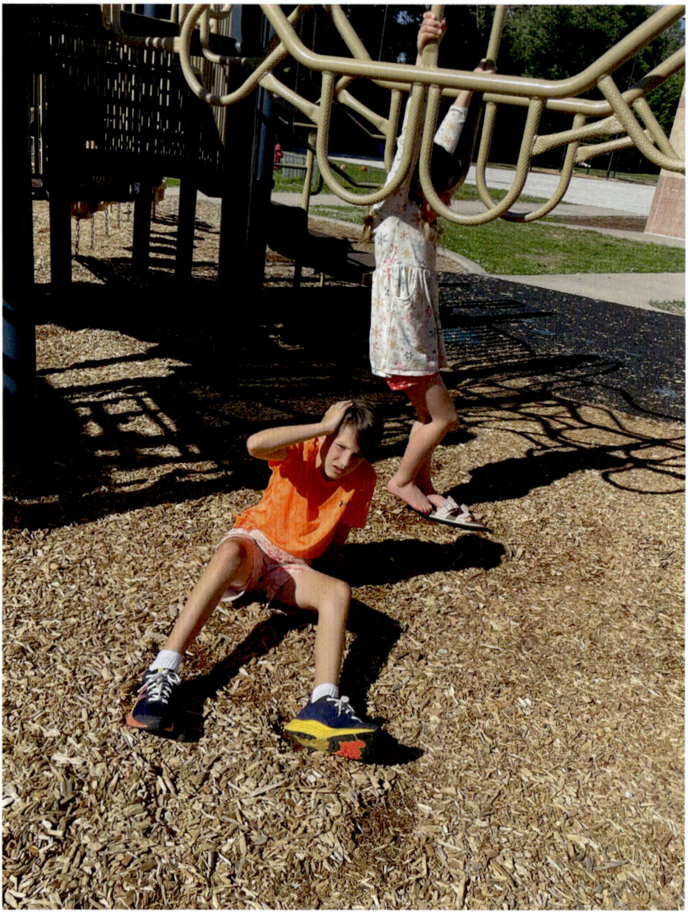

Fig. 109.1 Concussion is a common playground injury. Swift diagnosis and appropriate management can aid recovery and minimize long-term effects

unlikely, continued participation should be safe. If a probable or confirmed concussion is diagnosed, the athlete should be removed from play with no same day return to play. Immediate steps include (1) Notifying parents (2) Recommending rest (3) Limit screen use until symptoms comfortably allow it (4) Acetaminophen or NSAIDs for pain relief (5) Counseling on red flag symptoms discussed in case 3. Athletes with suspected concussion should then follow-up with a health-care provider trained in concussion prior to returning to competition or any contact practices [1].

Following concussion diagnosis, prior evidence recommended complete physical and cognitive rest or "Cocooning," which was found to lead to prolonged symptoms and poor outcomes. Current guidelines recommend rest for the first 24–48 hours promoting activities of daily living. From there, athletes are encouraged to return to

Table 109.3 Concussion comprehensive assessment tools

Links to the SCAT and SCOAT forms can be found below [6–9]:
SCAT6—https://bjsm.bmj.com/content/bjsports/57/11/622.full.pdf
Child SCAT6—https://bjsm.bmj.com/content/bjsports/57/11/636.full.pdf
SCOAT6—https://completeconcussions.com/wp-content/uploads/2023/06/SCOAT6.pdf
Child SCOAT6—https://bjsm.bmj.com/content/bjsports/57/11/672.full.pdf

Table 109.4 Return-to-Sport (RTS) strategy

Exercise step	Functional exercise each step	Goal of each step
1. Symptom limited activity	Daily activities that do not exacerbate symptoms (i.e. walking).	Gradual reintroduction to work/school.
2. Aerobic exercise 55–75% max heart rate	Stationary cycling, walking, or jogging at a slow to medium pace.	Increase heart rate.
3. Individual sports specific exercise	Sports specific training in a controlled environment without other athletes (i.e. Running, change of direction, agility, individual training drills). Light resistance training.	Add movement and change of direction.
Steps 4–6 should not begin until all concussion symptoms have resolved and medical clearance has occurred.		
4. Non contact training drills	Higher intensity exercise. More challenging training drills, (i.e. Passing drills, multiplayer training). Can integrate into a team environment as long as drills are non-contact.	Resume usual intensity of exercise, coordination, and increased thinking.
5. Full contact practice	Participation in normal training activities.	Restore confidence and assess function skills by coaching staff.
6. Full return to sport	Normal activity with no limitations	

Table created by the authors

early physical activity including walking and stationary bike. Trained providers can prescribe sub-symptom threshold exercise which is a graded exercise return that does not exacerbate symptoms above a specific level. Determining return to play should be performed by a healthcare provider trained in concussion management. The return to play protocol is a 6 step progression (Table 109.4). Each step takes at least 24 hours. It is important to know that athletes should not advance to stage 4 prior to return-to-learn and resolution of symptoms [1].

109.2 Neurocognitive Testing

When accessible, neurocognitive test batteries may be useful for evaluating Sport Related Concussion and sequelae. Testing is particularly helpful when it can be compared to a baselines or community norms. Computer based testing can also be helpful when looking at reaction speed. Neurocognitive testing should be used with the broader clinical context in mind and not in isolation. Baseline testing in younger athletes is of minimal benefit due to rapid neurocognitive developmental changes [1].

109.3 When to Refer

A sports medicine physician can be a great resource for any sports related concussion. Reasons to refer include but are not limited to those seen in Table 109.5.

109.4 Retirement from Sport

Retirement is an unpleasant discussion for any athlete but can be particularly challenging for concussion. Athletes with multiple concussions, concussions with severe symptoms or that limit their ability to return to the classroom, warrant further discussion about retirement. Retirement conversations ideally should be multidisciplinary and should include parents as well as health care professionals well versed in concussion or sports medicine. Discussions should include psychosocial components and weigh potential detriment of removing the athlete from sport. All students should be encouraged to continue physical activity even if contact or collisions sports are discouraged [1].

Table 109.5 Reasons to refer to a Sports Medicine Physician

Severe concussion symptoms
Symptoms lasting more than 4 weeks
Highly competitive athletes
A history of multiple concussions
Concern that retirement from sport is of benefit

Table created by the authors

Table 109.6 Red flags [5]

Neck pain or tenderness
Seizure or convulsion
Double vision
Loss of consciousness
Weakness or tingling/burning in more than 1 arm or in the legs
Deteriorating conscious state
Vomiting
Severe or increasing headache
Increasingly restless, agitated, or combative
GCS <15
Visible deformity of the skull

Table created by the authors

Case 3 A 10-year-old girl is playing soccer in PE class and collides with the goal post. She is noted to have loss of consciousness for a few seconds associated with rhythmic jerking movements. When she regains consciousness she vomits once, is sleepy, but can tell you her name and where she is.

Understanding when to seek immediate medical evaluation is crucial. Initial on-field evaluation should be assessment of the "ABCs": airway, breathing, and circulation. If an athlete remains unconscious a cervical spine injury should be suspected and managed with cervical spine immobilization and prompt transport. If the athlete regains consciousness, the athlete's cervical spine can be assessed as well as any red flag symptoms. Any of the red flags above (Table 109.6), should prompt immediate medical assessment and transport to a hospital or medical center for further evaluation. In the case above, she has evidence of seizure like activity and vomiting with documented loss of consciousness [1].

109.5 Case Conclusions

Case 1 The 8-year-old who fell off the monkey bars had immediate signs concerning for concussion. His parents were notified, and he was seen by her primary care provider that day. Once diagnosis of concussion was established, the multidisciplinary team at his school developed a return to learn plan for him based on his symptoms. At his elementary school, the team consisted of the school nurse, principal, and school counselor.

Case 2 The 15-year-old football player with a bloody nose and stumbling was immediately evaluated by his school athletic trainer, who was on the sideline. While the athlete noted that he "felt fine", his initial stumbling was concerning to the athletic trainer. His bloody nose was treated, and he was pulled from play until half-time, when he was further evaluated in a quiet space using the SCAT6 form. He struggled with balance testing and had developed a headache. He had no red flag symptoms. He was seen by a sports medicine physician the next Monday who agreed that he had a concussion. His school concussion team was made up of his athletic trainer, school nurse, school counselor, and his football coach. He started both return to learn and return to play protocols and eventually returned without restrictions to both.

Case 3 10-year-old soccer player collided with a goal post and developed seizure-like activity. The PE teacher stayed with the injured student and sent another student to fetch the school nurse. EMS was contacted and she was transported to the emergency department for further assessment due to her red flag symptoms.

Extra Credit Points

1. Concussion is a functional and not a structural diagnosis. It is not visualized on any imaging but produces clinical findings which can be recognized early after injury.
2. Early return to school should be encouraged for students with a concussion but some students may need individualized accommodations to help with class work and symptom management.
3. Athletes who sustain a concussion should be pulled from play immediately. A graded return to play protocol should be used to guide their return to sports.
4. Aerobic exercise should be encouraged for any athlete or student experiencing a concussion. Research has found aerobic exercise that does not increase symptoms, is safe and may shorten symptom duration.
5. On the field (or playground) assessment should include ABCs (airway, breathing, circulation) and assessment for Red Flags that would prompt immediate medical assessment and transport to a hospital or medical center.

References

1. Patricios JS, Schneider KJ, Dvorak J, et al. Consensus statement on concussion in sport: the 6th International Conference on Concussion in Sport–Amsterdam, October 2022. Br J Sports Med. 2023;57:695–711.
2. Halstead ME, Walter KD, Moffatt K, Council on Sports Medicine and Fitness, LaBella CR, Alison Brooks M, Canty G, Diamond AB, Hennrikus W, Logan K, Nemeth BA, Brooke Pengel K, Peterson AR, Stricker PR. Sport-related concussion in children and adolescents. Pediatrics. 2018;142(6):e20183074. https://doi.org/10.1542/peds.2018-3074.
3. Center for Disease Control (CDC). HEADS UP to schools: online concussion training for school professionals. https://www.cdc.gov/heads-up/training/school-professionals.html. Accessed 29 July 2024.
4. Halstead ME, McAvoy K, Devore CD, Carl R, Lee M, Logan K, Council on Sports Medicine and Fitness, Council on School Health, Brenner JS, Demorest RA, Halstead ME, Weiss Kelly AK, Koutures CG, LaBella CR, LaBotz M, Loud KJ, Moffatt KA, Alison Brooks M, Martin SS,

Guinn-Jones M. Returning to learning following a concussion. Pediatrics. 2013;132(5):948–57. https://doi.org/10.1542/peds.2013-2867.
5. Harmon KG, Clugston JR, Dec K, et al. American Medical Society for Sports Medicine position statement on concussion in sport. Br J Sports Med. 2019;53:213–25.
6. Patricios JS, Schneider KJ, Dvorak J, et al. Sport Concussion Assessment Tool 6 (SCAT6). Br J Sports Med. 2023;57:622–31.
7. Patricios JS, Schneider KJ, Dvorak J, et al. Child SCAT6. Br J Sports Med. 2023;57:636–47.
8. Patricios JS, Schneider KJ, Dvorak J, et al. Sport Concussion Office Assessment Tool 6 (SCOAT6). Br J Sports Med. 2023;57:651–67.
9. Patricios JS, Schneider KJ, Dvorak J, et al. Child SCOAT6. Br J Sports Med. 2023;57:672–88.

Chapter 110
Eye and Facial Injuries

Bradley Lauck and Jill Sylvester

110.1 Facial Trauma

Case 1 **8-year-old Lilly presents with a bleeding lip after falling at recess. She tripped over a loose paving stone while playing tag, falling face-first onto the ground. Upon examination, she is crying, and you observe a superficial laceration of her lower lip, with active bleeding and tissue swelling. Her teeth appear to be intact, with no trauma inside the mouth. What should you do?**

Case 2 **At the end of a seated group activity, 11-year-old Maya is accidentally struck in the face by her classmate's elbow as they stand up from the floor. Maya instinctively brings her hand to her face and feels warm blood flowing from her nose. In your clinic, you instruct Maya to tilt her head slightly forward and keep her nostrils pinched to control the bleeding. No bony deformities are visualized. As the bleeding stops, you examine her nares and notice an erythematous, asymmetric nasal septum that is tender to palpation. What should you do?**

Facial injuries occur more frequently in children than in adults and carry significant morbidity, while only accounting for 4.6% of total pediatric trauma [1]. Most pediatric facial trauma is caused by motor vehicle crashes, assaults, and accidental injuries such as falls. The history and presentation are crucial to understanding how these injuries should be triaged. Table 110.1 reviews some of the more common facial injuries encountered in a school-based setting, signs and symptoms seen at initial presentation, and suggestions for management.

B. Lauck · J. Sylvester (✉)
University of North Carolina School of Medicine, Chapel Hill, NC, USA
e-mail: bradley_lauck@med.unc.edu; jillian_sylvester@med.unc.edu

R. P. Olympia, J. Brady-Olympia (eds.), *Clinical Considerations in School-based Health*, https://doi.org/10.1007/978-3-031-85765-2_110

Table 110.1 Facial injuries in children and adolescents

Injury	Initial presentation	Disposition and treatment
Lip laceration	Bleeding from the mouth with visible laceration on the surface of the lip Secondary evaluation needed to look for underlying dental or facial injuries and/or concussion	*Transfer to ED if:* Transfer to Urgent Care (UC) is appropriate for simple lacerations requiring repair where provider is uncomfortable with closure More complex laceration repairs should be sent to the ED. Heavy bleeding or if unable to achieve hemostasis after 15 minutes Patient will not be cooperative with repair (may require sedation) *Management:* Rinse and remove debris Apply firm, direct pressure Through-and-through lacerations or deep lacerations that involve the orbicularis oris muscle require laceration repair In repair, it is critical that vermillion border is well-aligned for best cosmetic outcome Anesthesia with regional nerve block for optimal wound closure Consider tetanus prophylaxis if cut with a rusty object.
Tongue laceration	Bleeding from the mouth with visible laceration on the tongue Secondary evaluation needed to look for underlying dental or facial injuries and/or concussion	*Transfer to ED if:* Transfer to Urgent Care (UC) is appropriate for simple lacerations requiring repair where provider is uncomfortable with closure More complex laceration repairs should be sent to the ED. Heavy bleeding or if unable to achieve hemostasis after 15 minutes Patient will not be cooperative with repair (may require sedation) Heavy bleeding or if unable to achieve hemostasis after 15 minutes *Management:* Rinse and remove debris Apply firm, direct pressure Avulsion or partial amputation Persistent bleeding Problematic configurations (e.g., the lacerations are bisecting, gaping, u-shaped, or include large flaps) Wound size >2 cm (smaller, if involving a split in the tip of the tongue)

(continued)

Table 110.1 (continued)

Injury	Initial presentation	Disposition and treatment
Scalp laceration	Bleeding from the scalp may present with Dark/matted hair from bleeding Tenderness to palpation "Throbbing" sensation Secondary evaluation for underlying bony injury and/or concussion recommended	*Transfer to Urgent Care if:* Cut with rusty object (tetanus prophylaxis needed) Superficial lacerations where provider is uncomfortable with laceration closure *Transfer to ED if:* Brisk bleeding or inability to achieve hemostasis Deeper lacerations exposing bone Signs of severe closed head injury (neurologic deficits, confusion, recurrent vomiting, etc.) *Management*: Rinse and remove debris and apply firm, direct pressure Wound closure CT scan without IV contrast recommended in deep lacerations if there is concern for skull fracture
Facial bone fractures (zygomatic, frontal, or mandibular bones)	Typically occurs from direct trauma to the fractured bone. May present with pain swelling, gross deformity, epistaxis, loss of ability to open and close mouth	EMS activation to the ED CT without IV contrast ENT or Plastic Surgery consultation If bleeding, control with elevation of the head and applying gentle pressure while protecting the cervical spine Minimally displaced, stable fractures are usually treated nonoperatively. Unstable fractures require urgent surgical consultation
Orbital fracture	Typical mechanism involves blunt trauma to the orbit by an object bigger than orbit (baseball, shoulder, etc.). Symptoms include Diplopia Loss of extraocular movement Periorbital hypoesthesia Enophthalmos (sunken eye)	Transfer to ED for further imaging with CT without IV contrast of orbits and further management *Management* Ophthalmology consultation Avoid Valsalva, blowing nose, sneezing, etc. Typically, non-operative management with activity restriction Surgery can be indicated with persistent diplopia, enophthalmos, or in lateral or downward gaze restriction
Nasal fracture	Typically occurs from direct, blunt trauma to the nose Severe epistaxis Swelling Bony deformity may not be evident until swelling improves Periorbital ecchymosis Difficulty with breathing through nose	Non-displaced fractures can be managed without transfer. Refer to ED if persistent epistaxis or gross displacement. X-rays are not necessary for isolated fractures and rarely helpful [2] Nonoperative management preferred for fractures without deformity Closed or open reduction in cases where realignment is needed Needs close evaluation for septal hematoma

(continued)

Table 110.1 (continued)

Injury	Initial presentation	Disposition and treatment
Epistaxis	Nosebleeds can occur from dry air, colds, allergies, or objects into the nose, but can be present in trauma Bleeding from one or both nostrils Bad taste in the mouth Blood in cough or spit Swallowing draining blood down throat can cause nausea	*Refer to ED if:* Bleeding does not slow for 30 minutes with direct pressure and/or nasal packing Posterior nasal bleed is suspected *Management*: Direct pressure via pinching the nostrils, lean forward Can use anterior nasal packing if bleeding continues Refractory cases can be treated with topical or oral tranexamic acid (TXA) [3] In trauma, evaluate for septal hematoma
Septal hematoma	These are almost always the result of facial trauma. Symptoms include Midline septal swelling upon examination Nasal airway obstruction Nasal tenderness Epistaxis If untreated, there is risk of septal abscess and "saddle nose" deformity.	*Transfer to UC/ED if:* Transfer to UC if provider is uncomfortable with hematoma evacuation and there are no signs or symptoms of systemic infection If ENT is accessible, can contact for direct referral for definitive management Refer to ED if displaying signs of systemic infection *Management* Hematoma drainage with nasal packing. Antibiotics are recommended after drainage CT is often obtained in patients with signs of systemic infection to rule out abscess
Auricular hematoma	Common in contact sports such as wrestling and rugby Loss of auricular landmarks Edema Erythema If left untreated, can result in permanent deformity known as "cauliflower ear"	Depending on provider comfort level, these can be incised and drained in-office. Transfer to UC vs ED if provider is uncomfortable with procedure Cotton dental rolls are secured via sutures on both sides of the ear to prevent re-accumulation of fluid Arrange for an ENT follow up for definitive management

Abbreviations: *CT* computed tomography, *ED* emergency department, *EMS* Emergency Medical Services, *ENT* ear, nose, and throat, *IV* intravenous, *XR* radiography

Many of these common facial injuries in children can present on a spectrum of severity. Disposition is dependent upon the severity of the injury, stability of the patient, and the providers level of comfort and experience with this condition. However, there are certain red flags that should trigger emergency department (ED) transport including gross bony deformity, significant swelling, and heavy or refractory bleeding. In the setting of facial trauma, providers should evaluate for concussion. Signs of closed head trauma, such as neurologic deficits, prolonged loss of consciousness, severe or progressing headache, vomiting, or seizure should prompt immediate referral to the ED.

110.2 Orbital Trauma

Case 3 8-year-old John is brought to clinic by his teacher after a classmate threw a pencil that struck him in his right eye, causing bleeding. His right pupil appears misshapen like a teardrop, and the surrounding conjunctiva is red. His vision in the right eye is 20/200, left eye is 20/20. He does not wear glasses or contact lenses. What do you do?

Case 4 9-year-old Julie comes to the nurse's office complaining of right eye pain and sensitivity to light. She was playing tag outside when she felt a sudden pain and a gritty feeling in her eye. She is blinking frequently, and her right eye appears red and teary. Her vision is 20/20, pupils are equal and reactive, and her extraocular movements are intact, but uncomfortable. You evert her eyelid and find a small piece of debris that is easily removed with a cotton-tipped applicator.

Ocular trauma is the #1 cause of non-congenital blindness in children and accounts for approximately 10% of all pediatric ED visits annually. Boys are affected approximately four times more often than girls, with incidence peaking at ages 11–15 [4]. Most ocular injuries occur from direct impact, either blunt or penetrating. Examinations can be difficult due to patient cooperation and ability to evaluate visual acuity, particularly in young children.

The assessment of ocular trauma begins with careful collection of the child's history of present illness, their ophthalmologic history, and the presence of other medical conditions that may affect outcomes in ocular injury. Specifically, providers should inquire about patient's sickle cell trait status and any conditions that may increase their risk of bleeding. Crucial components of the eye exam are discussed in Table 110.2.

Table 110.2 Evaluation of an injured eye

Visual acuity: test vision using their glasses, if applicable. The use of Snellen chart or age-appropriate validated chart is recommended
Inspection: evaluate for anisocoria, pupillary defects, areas of erythema, or the presence of foreign bodies/obvious trauma
Visual assessment of the eye: Pupillary assessment Extra-ocular movements Visual field confrontation Light reflex assessment Penlight assessment of anterior chamber Red reflex test
External examination: Presence of periorbital ecchymosis, erythema, or presence of proptosis? Tenderness to palpation of the orbital rim or palpable bony step-offs? Is facial sensation in-tact along nerves V1, V2, and V3?

The American Academy of Ophthalmology details some of these maneuvers in their Guide to the Bedside Adult Eye Exam: https://www.youtube.com/watch?v=xsTz9x5EFuI

A review of the most common ocular injuries in school-age children is presented in Table 110.3 [5]. When management dictates protection of the injured eye, an eye shield can be applied to the orbital bones and affixed with medical tape. If an eye shield is unavailable, a Styrofoam cup can instead be used, affixed over the eye and secured to the periorbital bones with medical tape. Pressure dressings are contraindicated if there is concern for a globe rupture.

Non-accidental trauma should always be considered in ocular trauma [5]. Specifically, conditions causing periorbital ecchymosis, eyelid trauma, retinal detachment, dislocated lens, or orbital fracture should prompt further questioning. A careful history is imperative to help identify possible child abuse. Mandatory reporters should report all suspected of non-accidental trauma as directed by their local institutions.

Athletes are considered functionally monocular when their best corrected vision is worse than 20/40. These athletes require eye protection for all sports and should be restricted from combat sports like boxing, wrestling, or martial arts due to the risk of injury to their stronger eye [6]. The American Academy of Pediatrics recommends eye protection be used for all participants in high-risk sports, namely those including small, fast projectiles (shooting sports, paintball); sports using hard projectiles or sticks (baseball/softball, cricket, hockey, lacrosse, squash); or those sports that involve intentional injury (boxing, martial arts) [6].

Table 110.3 Ocular injuries in children and adolescents

Injury	Initial presentation	Disposition and treatment
Corneal abrasion	Significant pain and photosensitivity Blepharospasm Best diagnosed via fluorescein stain and evaluation under cobalt blue light. May be associated with foreign body, particularly if fluorescein pattern is linear	Treatment is symptomatic control. Transport or escalation of care is not typically needed An antibiotic ointment or antibiotic eye drops should be applied until the abrasion has healed and the patient is asymptomatic. Ointment is preferred as it also acts as a lubricant Follow-up in clinic is recommended in 72 hours if not feeling improved, as it may suggest foreign body, corneal ulcer, or alternative diagnosis Do not wear contact lenses until symptoms have fully resolved
Foreign body	Acute onset pain Foreign body sensation Photophobia On exam, visual acuity is unaffected, normal pupil and extraocular exam Carefully inspect with eyelid inversion to locate foreign bodies	Transfer to UC or ED if unable to remove foreign body or if uncomfortable. Transfer to ED if foreign body is suspected but not localized *Management:* Superficial foreign bodies may be removed using cotton tipped applicator Topical anesthetic can be helpful for patient comfort Requires evaluation for corneal abrasion after removal Ophthalmology follow-up recommended
Hyphema	Occurs after blunt or perforating trauma to eye Can report acute, painless vision loss On exam, there is blood in anterior chamber. A fluid level occurs between cornea and iris	ASAP transfer to ED Ophthalmology consultation Place eye shield, avoid NSAIDs Maintain head of bed >30° *Management:* Hospital admission is rare but can be needed for severe cases, such as blood covering >50% of anterior chamber, severely increased intraocular pressure, or in the setting of coagulopathy or sickle cell disease or trait. Close interval follow-up with ophthalmology for several days Patients with sickle cell disease or trait are at increased risk of vision loss

(continued)

Table 110.3 (continued)

Injury	Initial presentation	Disposition and treatment
Chemical injury	Typically presents with significant pain. Mild burns can cause conjunctival inflammation and mild corneal erosions Severe injury may show corneal opacification	Immediate irrigation with 0.9% normal saline or water while activating EMS to transfer to ED Remove contact lenses before irrigating Irrigation should continue for at least 30 minutes or until 2 L of fluid has been used. More severe cases can require more extensive irrigation
Open globe rupture	Occur with penetrating or blunt trauma followed by sudden vision changes and ocular pain On exam, the pupil appears irregularly shaped. Vision typically impaired. There is often conjunctival erythema or 360-degree sub-conjunctival hemorrhage, also known as an "8-ball eye"	Activate EMS, emergent transfer to ED Upon diagnosis, stop exam, activate EMS, and place eye shield *Management* Urgent ophthalmology consultation CT scan of the orbits Surgical correction Increased risk of permanent vison loss
Eyelid laceration	Often occurs after being struck in the closed eye by an object Careful examination of the eyelid and underlying eye is critical to ensure secondary injuries are not missed	Transfer to ED if laceration involves the lid margin, canaliculus or lacrimal duct drainage system, or if full thickness reaching the ocular musculature and orbital fat. Ophthalmology consult needed for these repairs Superficial lacerations can be repaired in-office or at an UC depending on comfort level of provider. If uncomfortable, refer to the ED for primary repair.

110.3 Case Conclusions

Case 1 You rinse Lilly's laceration and hold pressure on her wound to stop the bleeding. The size of the laceration necessitates suture repair for proper healing and optimal cosmetic outcome. Depending on provider comfort, this laceration can be repaired in your clinic, with close attention to ensuring the vermillion border repair is even. If uncomfortable with repair, she should be transferred a higher level of care to maximize the cosmetic outcome.

Case 2 Maya's anterior epistaxis was managed well in the clinic. However, her septal hematoma requires further care. With parental consent, you take Maya to the nearby urgent care, where the staff physician drains the hematoma and packs her nares. She is discharged with antibiotics and a referral for close-interval ENT follow-up.

Case 3 John's exam is concerning for a globe rupture. You stop your exam, activate EMS, and cover his right eye with an eye shield or Styrofoam cup affixed with tape to orbital bone. EMS transfers him to the ED for emergent ophthalmology consultation and CT scan of the orbits.

Case 4 After removing the foreign body, you find a corneal abrasion using fluorescein stain. You prescribe ophthalmic erythromycin for 7 days and recommend her parents give her oral analgesics for pain. You instruct her to avoid contact lenses until symptoms have fully resolved.

Extra Credit Points

1. In nasal trauma, it is critical to evaluate for septal hematoma. Missed septal hematomas pose risk of infection and cartilage loss, resulting in a permanent "saddle nose" deformity.
2. Repair of lip lacerations require precise alignment of the vermillion border for optimal cosmetic outcome. Anesthetizing the laceration with nerve blocks rather than local injection helps to avoid distortion of normal tissues for optimal repair.
3. Globe ruptures area a true medical emergency. Upon diagnosing a globe rupture, apply an eye shield to the affected eye and transport directly to the Emergency Department. Delays of care increase the risk of permanent vision loss.

References

1. Nawar EW, Niska RW, Xu J. National Hospital Ambulatory Medical Care Survey: 2005 emergency department survey. Atlanta: Center for Disease Control and Prevention, National Center for Health Statistics; 2007.
2. Arnstead N, Chan Y, Kilty S, Ganeshathasan R, Rahmani A, Monteiro E, Rhinology Subspecialty Group of the Canadian Society of Otolaryngology – Head & Neck Surgery. Choosing wisely Canada rhinology recommendations. J Otolaryngol Head Neck Surg. 2020;49(1):10.
3. Joseph J, Martinez-Devesa P, Bellorini J, Burton MJ. Tranexamic acid for patients with nasal haemorrhage (epistaxis). Cochrane Database Syst Rev. 2018;(12):CD004328. https://doi.org/10.1002/14651858.CD004328.pub3.
4. Abbott J, Shah P. The epidemiology and etiology of pediatric ocular trauma. Surv Ophthalmol. 2013;58(5):476–85.
5. Romaniuk VM. Ocular trauma and other catastrophes. Emerg Med Clin North Am. 2013;31(2):399–411.
6. Bernhardt DT, Roberts WO, editors. PPE: preparticipation physical evaluation. 5th ed. American Academy of Pediatrics; 2019. Itasca, IL.

Chapter 111
Dental Injuries

Christina Kim and Douglas Comeau

Organized sports and recreational activities have grown in popularity for children and adolescents. In 2019, it was estimated that more than 44 million US children participated in organized sport teams and recreational activities [1]. Participation in some of these activities can create an increase in risk for traumatic dental injuries (TDIs) as a result of falls, collisions, and contact with sports equipment.

111.1 Tooth Anatomy

The tooth is made up of the enamel, dentin and pulp. The hard-outer surface is the enamel which is followed by the dentin, and then the pulp, which has the neurovascular structures for the tooth. The crown is the portion of the tooth above the gum line and the root is the portion of the tooth below the gum line. Periodontal ligaments hold the tooth with the gum socket. Damage to the dentin will often result in sensitivities to temperature and pressure. Injury involving the pulp will demonstrate a bleeding spot [2]. Avulsion or displacement of a tooth from the socket indicates disruption of the periodontal ligaments. Teeth can be identified by orientation within the oral cavity, either along the maxillary or mandibular arch, and positioning along the arch (central incisor, lateral incisor, cuspid, bicuspid, and molars) [3].

Case 1 A 6-year-old girl falls from a slide on the playground and presents with bleeding in her mouth. Upon examination, there is an absence of a lower central incisor.

C. Kim (✉) · D. Comeau
Boston College, Chestnut Hill, MA, USA
e-mail: kimfsq@bc.edu; comeaudo@bc.edu

R. P. Olympia, J. Brady-Olympia (eds.), *Clinical Considerations in School-based Health*, https://doi.org/10.1007/978-3-031-85765-2_111

Falls are the most common mechanism for traumatic dental injury (TDI) in children <7 years old and in children ages 7–12 years old [1]. TDIs in children <7 years old are most likely associated with playground equipment [1]. As a result of this child's fall, the tooth has avulsed and is completely out of the socket. Once the child is approached, it is important to evaluate for the location of the lost tooth. The mouth should be thoroughly examined and a knee-to-knee examination (which can be viewed in the following video https://tinyurl.com/kneetokneeexamination) may be helpful [4]. Avulsed teeth can sometimes be embedded in the lip, cheek, tongue, ingested or aspirated [4]. If an avulsed tooth cannot be found and the child is having difficulty breathing or other respiratory symptoms, the child should be evaluated in the Emergency Department [4]. Children begin to lose their primary teeth at 6 years old until age 12 [5]. As for the tooth in this case, avulsed primary teeth should not be replanted. Follow up with the child's dentist is recommended for radiographs for definitive displacement of the involved tooth. It is recommended that the child have a softer diet to avoid traumatizing the injured tissue, brushing teeth after each meal with a soft brush, and cleaning with topical chlorhexidine gluconate twice a day for 1 week [6].

Case 2 An 8-year-old girl runs across the base while playing tee-ball and she trips and falls, landing on her chin. Once the child is calmed down, you are able to inspect her mouth and observe an intact midline crack involving the enamel only across the upper central incisor.

Tables 111.1 and 111.2 discuss common dental injuries and guidelines for primary teeth fracture.

Radiographs are strongly recommended for accurate and complete diagnosis with every effort to minimize a child's exposure to radiation. There is no evidence to support use of systemic antibiotics for luxation injuries in primary dentition. Antibiotic use may be warranted if there is concomitant soft tissue injury or if surgical intervention is pursued. A tetanus booster may be required if there is environmental contamination has occurred. Patients should be educated on avoiding further traumatization to the injured teeth while eating by incorporating softer foods into

Table 111.1 Ellis and Davey classification of tooth fractures [7]

Classification	Description
Class I	Simple crown fracture with little or no dentin damage
Class II	Extensive crown fracture with loss of dentin but no damage to pulp
Class III	Extensive crown fracture with considerable amount of dentin loss and pulp exposure
Class IV	Tooth is devitalized by trauma with or without loss of tooth structure
Class V	Teeth are lost due to trauma
Class VI	Root fracture with or without loss of the crown structure
Class VII	Displacement of tooth without root or crown fracture
Class VIII	Complete crown fracture
Class IX	Traumatic injuries of primary teeth

Table 111.2 Guidelines for primary teeth fractures [3, 8]

Type of fracture	Symptoms and clinical findings	Follow up
Enamel fracture Involves enamel	Roughness along the incisal edge of the tooth crown	Referral to dentist can be delayed up to 24 hours
Enamel-dentin fracture (no pulp exposure) Involves only enamel and dentin	Presents as thin white tooth enamel surrounding underlying yellow layer of dentin Sensitivity to air, cold or touch Missing tooth fragments should be investigated. If found, placed in milk or saline, or Hank's solution	Referral to dentist can be delayed up to 24 hours
Complicated crown fracture Involves enamel, dentin and pulp is visible	Fracture of enamel and dentin with exposure of pulp +/− hemorrhage Acute pain Missing tooth fragments should be investigated. If found, placed in milk or saline, or Hank's solution	Immediate referral to dentist
Crown-root fracture Fracture involves enamel, dentin and root +/− pulp exposure Result of direct trauma	May find loose but attached fragments of tooth Acute pain, sensitivity to air, touch, or cold, mobility within socket	Immediate referral to dentist
Root fracture Fracture involves dentin, pulp, cementum and root Result of direct trauma	Increased mobility or displacement of fragment of tooth, discoloration, tenderness, gingival bleeding	Immediate referral to dentist
Alveolar fracture Fracture involves alveolar bone and may extend to adjacent bone	Pain, increased mobility, malocclusion, dislocation of several other teeth, gingival hematoma	Immediate referral to dentist

the diet. In addition, parents should clean the affected area with a soft brush or cotton swab with chlorhexidine gluconate mouth rinse twice a day for 1 week [4].

Case 3 A 16-year-old male playing ice hockey during a game gets hit in the mouth by an opponent's hockey stick resulting in avulsion of lateral incisor and canine.

Most children have 28 of their permanent teeth by age 13 [5]. Avulsion of permanent teeth occur in 0.5–16% of all dental injuries [9]. Rates of dental injury are higher in competition than in practice [10]. Adolescents aged 13–17 years old are more likely to sustain an injury by being "struck" by something [1]. Once an avulsed tooth is identified, the tooth should be picked up by the crown and there should be extreme caution to avoid injury to the root. If there is debris on the tooth, it can be rinsed gently in milk, saline or the patient's saliva in order to replant the tooth [9]. Replantation of the tooth must be attempted within 5 minutes. Once the tooth is in proper position, the child should bite down on gauze or a napkin to hold the tooth in place and should be transported to dentist or Emergency Department immediately.

If the affected tooth cannot be replanted appropriately, the tooth can be stored in Hank's Balanced Salt Solution, low-fat milk, saline or saliva [3]. Water may be used as a last resort in order to prevent desiccation of the tooth. Systemic antibiotics are recommended after avulsion and replantation of an avulsed tooth due to contamination by bacteria in the oral cavity. Preferred antibiotics are amoxicillin or penicillin with weight and age-based dosing. Tetracyclines or doxycycline are not recommended under the age of 12 years old. Athletes should be advised to avoid participation in contact sports until cleared by their dentist, follow a soft diet up to 2 weeks, brush their teeth with a soft toothbrush after meals, use chlorhexidine mouth rinse twice a day for 2 weeks [9].

Case 4 A 14-year-old female playing basketball sustains an opponent's elbow to her mouth. Upon examination, there is an upper lip laceration and loss of the lower half of her central incisor. Bleeding is controlled with direct pressure using gauze and the missing fragment is located and placed in low fat milk for transport.

Table 111.3 demonstrates guidelines for the management of permanent teeth fracture.

Plain film radiographs are necessary to make a complete diagnosis. Initial radiographs are also helpful to provide a baseline, especially if serial examinations are warranted. In addition, cone beam computerized tomography (CBCT) provides in-depth visualization of TDIs, especially root fractures, crown-root fractures, and lateral luxations. The location, extent, and direction of the fracture can be identified using CBCT. Tetanus booster may be required if environmental contamination has occurred [11].

Case 5 15 year-old male jumps up for a header during his soccer match when an opposing player's head hits him in the jaw while up in the air. Your patient lands on his feet but is holding his mouth due to some bleeding. Evaluation on the sideline demonstrates that his lower central incisor is partially displaced out if its socket and the tooth appear to be elongated.

Table 111.4 demonstrates guidelines for the displacement of permanent teeth.

There is limited use of systemic antibiotics in emergency management of luxation injuries. Antibiotics are to be used at the discretion of the clinician related to other soft tissue injuries or if surgical intervention is warranted. If environmental contamination has occurred during injury, then tetanus booster is recommended. Patients and parents should be advised to avoid injuring the affected tooth/teeth, avoid participation in activity until cleared by dentist, brush with a soft tooth brush after meals, and rinse with chlorhexidine gluconate twice a day for 1 week [11].

Case 6 A 15-year-old female lacrosse player is running down the field during a transition play when she is struck in the jaw with an opponent's lacrosse stick. Due to pain, she asks to be evaluated. Upon evaluation, she takes out her mouthguard and there is no damage to her dentition, just soreness to her temporo-mandibular joint. She is cleared to return to the game as tolerated.

Table 111.3 Guidelines for permanent teeth fractures [11]

Type of fracture	Symptoms and clinical findings	Follow up
Enamel fracture Incomplete fracture of the enamel without loss of tooth structure	Partial loss of enamel without signs of exposed dentin No pain with palpation Normal mobility Coarseness along edge of tooth	Referral to dentist can be delayed up to 24 hours
Uncomplicated crown fracture (enamel-only fracture) Fracture involving enamel only without structural loss	Loss of enamel without visibility of dentin Normal mobility Missing fragments should be found	Immediate referral to dentist
Complicated crown fracture (Enamel-dentin fracture with pulp exposure) Involves enamel and dentin +/− pulp involvement	Fracture of enamel and dentin with exposure of pulp +/− hemorrhage Acute pain Sensitivity to temperature, air, foods Missing tooth fragments should be investigated. If found, placed in appropriate solution	Immediate referral to dentist
Crown-root fracture Fracture involves enamel, dentin and root +/− pulp exposure Result of direct trauma	May find loose but attached fragments of tooth Acute pain, sensitivity to air, touch, or cold, mobility within socket Tender to percussion	Referral to dentist within 24 hours
Root fracture Fracture involves dentin, pulp, cementum and root Result of direct trauma	Increased mobility or displacement of fragment of tooth, discoloration, tenderness, gingival bleeding Tenderness to percussion From bloody gingival tissue	Immediate referral to dentist
Alveolar fracture Fracture involves alveolar bone	Pain, increased mobility, malocclusion, dislocation of several other teeth, gingival hematoma	Immediate referral to dentist

When mouthguards are worn by athletes, studies demonstrate that there is a reduction in dental injuries. The mouth guard absorbs shock to reduce jaw and teeth fractures, provides soft tissue protection for lip and oral lacerations, and gives support to spaces where teeth are absent [2]. The American Academy of Pediatric Dentistry (AAPD), the American Dental Association (ADA) and the Academy for Sports Dentistry (ASD) recommend wearing a properly fitted mouthguard when participating in sports. Currently, the National Federation of State High School Associations recommends mouthguards for the following sports: field hockey, ice hockey, football, and lacrosse. If a wrestler has orthodontic appliances, then a mouthguard is also recommended [10].

Case 7 A 16 year-old-male baseball player is fielding a baseball when the baseball takes an unexpected bounce and hits him in the mouth. Upon examination, the athlete has braces and you notice that there is some bleeding along his upper lip. After irrigation with tap water, you notice that a bracket is loose and the baseball has broken a metallic wire on his braces.

Table 111.4 Guidelines for displacement of permanent teeth [11, 12]

Type of displacement	Clinical findings and symptoms	Follow up
Concussion Injury to the structures that support the tooth	Tender tooth without displacement Normal mobility, no bleeding Tenderness to percussion	Can delay referral to dentist for several days Not a true dental emergency
Subluxation Injury to periodontal tissues	Tender tooth with increased mobility No displacement, +/− gingival bleeding Pain with biting, loose tooth sensation	Referral to dentist within 24 hours
Lateral luxation Injury to periodontal ligament and alveolar bone fractures	Laterally displaced tooth with the crown in a palatal direction +/− fracture or compression of alveolar socket wall or facial bone Tooth will be immobile at apex Occlusion may occur Pain, temperature insensitivity, fixed tooth in new position	Immediate referral to dentist
Extrusive luxation Injury to periodontal ligament	Partial displacement of tooth out of its socket Tooth may seem elongated, very mobile Occlusion may occur	Immediate referral to dentist
Intrusive luxation Fracture of alveolar bone which causes the tooth to move up into the socket Most severe dental injury	Tooth displaced into alveolar bone Tooth has completely or nearly disappeared into socket	Immediate referral to dentist Do not attempt to pull back

Fixed dental appliances such as braces are at an increased risk for damage in athletes who participate in sports who do not utilize mouthguards. These athletes are at risk of sustaining dental traumatic injuries which may include loosening of brackets and disruption of orthodontic wires [13]. The use of a custom-made or mouth-formed mouthguard is recommended for athletes playing contact sport with braces [14]. Temporary treatment can be performed for the athlete so that an orthodontic appointment can be made the next day. If a bracket is loose and flush with the tooth, then the bracket may be left as is. If a bracket falls, then the bracket can be removed with tweezers. If a metallic wire is broken and is causing soft tissue trauma or pain, the wire can be pushed back with a small eraser on the back of a pencil or orthodontic relief wax can be applied to the end of the wire [15].

School health providers should follow the following Dental First Aid Steps [6] when dealing with a student who has sustained dental trauma, and ensure that their school has dental specific first aid supplies (Table 111.5).

1. Keep calm
2. Clean bleeding wounds with saline solution (0.9%) or tap water

Table 111.5 Dental specific first aid supplies [3]

Adhesive tape	Biohazard bags
Cotton rolls	Cotton-tip applicators
Dental floss	Elastic bandage
Extra mouth guards	Gauze
Gloves	Tongue depressors
Mirror	Tooth culture medium (Hank's Balanced Salt Solution)
Orthodontic relief wax	Tweezers

3. Control and stop bleeding by applying pressure with cotton
4. If skin and soft tissue injuries occur, refer to Emergency Department or Urgent Care
5. If there are dental injuries, refer to Pediatric Dentist if available. If the dentist is unavailable and the child is anxious or in pain and unable to tolerate first aid, then seek treatment in the Emergency Department. Or, if the provider is uncomfortable providing first aid, then refer to the Emergency Department

Extra Credit Points
1. Avulsed primary teeth should never be replanted
2. Fragments and avulsed teeth should be placed in an appropriate medium such as Hank's Balanced Salt Solution, saliva, or low-fat milk
3. Mouth guard use decreases orofacial and dental injury when worn correctly

References

1. Montero E, Kistamgari S, Chounthirath T, et al. Pediatric sports- and recreation-related dental injuries treated in US emergency departments. Clin Pediatr. 2019;58(11–12):1262–70.
2. Young EJ, Macias CR, Stephens L. Common dental injury management in athletes. Sports Health. 2015;7(3):250–5. https://doi.org/10.1177/1941738113486077.
3. Gould TE, Piland SG, Ranalli D, et al. National athletic trainer's association position statement; preventing and managing sport-related dental and oral injuries. J Athl Train. 2016;51(19):821–39. https://doi.org/10.4095/1062-6050-51.8.01.
4. Day PF, Flores MT, O'Connell AC, et al. International Association of Dental Traumatology guidelines for the management of traumatic dental injuries: 3. Injuries in the primary dentition. Dent Traumatol. 2020;36:343–59.
5. Tooth eruption. J Am Dent Assoc. 2006;137(1):127. https://doi.org/10.14219/jada.archive.2006.0031.
6. Flores MT. Traumatic injuries in the primary dentition. Dent Traumatol. 2002;18:287–98.
7. Gupta M, Das D, Soodan K, et al. Dental injuries in patients associated with fracture of facial bones. Oral Maxillofac Surg. 2019;23:63–9. https://doi.org/10.1007/s10006-019-00743-8.
8. Abbott PV. Diagnosis and management of transverse root fractures. Dent Traumatol. 2019;35:333–47. https://doi.org/10.1111/edt.12482.
9. Fouad AF, Abbott PV, Tsilingaridis G, et al. International Association of Dental Traumatology guidelines for the management of tramatic dental injures: 2. Avulsion of permanent teeth. Dent Traumatol. 2020;36:331–42. https://doi.org/10.1111/edt.12573.

10. Azadani EN, Peng J, Townsend JA, Collins CL. Traumatic dental injuries in high school athletics in the United States of America from 2005 to 2020. Dent Traumatol. 2023;39:109–18. https://doi.org/10.1111/edt.12800.
11. Bourguignon C, Cohenca N, Lauridsen E, et al. International Association of Dental Traumatology guidelines for the management of traumatic dental injuries: 1. Fractures and luxations. Dent Traumatol. 2020;36:314–30. https://doi.org/10.1111/edt.12578.
12. Tooth luxation: symptoms, causes, and treatment. Cleveland Clinic. Accessed 29 May 2024. https://my.clevelandclinic.org/health/diseases/21770-tooth-luxation.
13. Chowdhury RU, Churei H, Tanabe G, Yoshida Y, et al. Useful design of custom-made mouthguard for athletes undergoing orthodontic treatment with brackets and wires. J Dent Sci. 2022;17:308–15. https://doi.org/10.1016/j.jds.2021.03.010.
14. Kalra A, Harrington C, Minhas G, Papageorgiou SN, et al. Wearability and preference of mouthguard during sport in patients undergoing orthodontic treatment with fixed appliances: a randomized clinical trial. Eur J Orthod. 2022;44(1):101–9. https://doi.org/10.1093/ejo/cjab062.
15. Caprioglio A, Pizzetti GB, Zecca PA, Fastuca R, et al. Management of orthodontic emergencies during 2019-NCOV. Prog Orthod. 2020;21:10. https://doi.org/10.1186/s40510-020-00310-y.

Chapter 112
Cervical Spine Injuries

Joshua Glasser

Case 1 **A 13 year old student suffers an accidental head to head collision while playing touch football during PE class. He lost consciousness for 10 seconds after the collision. He reports pain in the back of his neck as well as tingling and decreased sensation to his arms and legs. He is otherwise conscious and alert, breathing comfortably, and has no signs of other injury.**

Case 2 **A 5 year old student climbed on his desk to hang a project high on the wall. He slipped and fell. He did not lose consciousness, but is holding his neck turned to the right and says he cannot move. He is conscious and alert, breathing comfortably, and has no signs of other injury.**

Case 3 **A 17 year old student driver was struck by a car moving 25 miles per hour while pulling out of the parking lot to drive to her driver's education course. She was wearing her seat belt and did not lose consciousness. She reports mild neck pain more prominently on the right side of the neck. She is conscious and alert, breathing comfortably, and has no signs of other injury.**

Cervical spine injuries are uncommon in children and occur in 1–2% of children with significant blunt trauma with the majority of injuries occurring in adolescents. Motor vehicle collisions are the most common cause of cervical spine injuries. Falls are a common cause in children under 8 years of age. Sports related injuries are common in children over 8 years of age with the most common mechanisms being diving and football. Inflicted trauma or child abuse is also a potential cause of cervical spine injury [1].

The cervical spine is the upper portion of the spine between the shoulders and the base of the skull. There are seven cervical vertebrae, numbered C1–C7. The fulcrum

J. Glasser (✉)
Penn State Hershey Medical Center, Hershey, PA, USA
e-mail: jglasser@pennstatehealth.psu.edu

R. P. Olympia, J. Brady-Olympia (eds.), *Clinical Considerations in School-based Health*, https://doi.org/10.1007/978-3-031-85765-2_112

of movement in the cervical spine is at C2–C3 vertebrae and in infants and children, reaches C4–C5 in children 5–6 years of age, and reaches C5–6 in children 8 years of age and above. These levels define the most common sites of injury in each of these age groups [2].

With respect to the mechanism by which children sustain cervical spine injury, common mechanisms include falls from height or dives, particularly if there is an axial-loading mechanism; sports injuries with head-on collision or "spearing" motions; impact of heavy objects on the head; and "clothesline" type injuries. Motor vehicle collisions are perhaps the most common cause of cervical spine injuries, particularly those involving high speeds. Any child who has suffered multiple traumatic injuries, particularly trauma to the head and face or upper torso should be assumed to have a cervical spine injury. Ultimately, knowledge of the mechanism of injury is critical to making an informed risk assessment.

112.1 Examination of a Student with a Potential Cervical Spine Injury

Evaluation of the cervical spine goes hand in hand with evaluation of mental status including pupillary response, Glasgow coma scale, and motor and sensory function of the extremities. While midline neck pain is the most obvious potential feature of a cervical spine injury, any neck pain should be regarded as a possible sign of cervical spine injury by school based personnel. Patients who are "guarding" or self-limiting neck movement should not be encouraged to move. Torticollis or neck muscle spasm may be seen and patients demonstrating this should likewise not be moved. Abnormal motor or sensory examination, altered mental status, abnormal reflexes, clonus, age-inappropriate incontinence, or autonomic instability (unexplained changes in blood pressure with flushing or sweating) are all possible signs of cervical spine injury. Notably, in any patient with altered mental status, cervical spine injury cannot be reliably ruled out without imaging.

When there is concern for significant cervical spine injury, close attention must be paid to hemodynamics (heart rate, blood pressure, and perfusion) as these patents may develop neurogenic shock. Neurogenic shock occurs soon after injury and is characterized by hypotension and bradycardia (or an inappropriately normal heart rate in severe injury) owing to the loss of vagal tone in the cardiovascular system. Cutaneous vasodilation occurs which leads to warm skin and widened pulse pressure. Of note, other causes of hypotension, such as uncontrolled hemorrhage should also be considered though typically such patients would exhibit reflect tachycardia. Additionally, Neurogenic shock is frequently mislabeled as spinal shock, a term which in fact refers to reversible impairment (often with complete paralysis and areflexia) in spinal cord function below the level of the injury. This phenomenon may recover with some improvement in function over a period of days following an injury. Table 112.1 describes common pediatric cervical spine injuries.

Table 112.1 Common pediatric cervical spine injuries

Condition	Mechanism	Signs/Symptoms	Treatment
Cervical spine vertebrae fracture	Axial load, hyperextension, hyperflexion	Severe pain, midline tenderness, inability to move the neck, numbness/tingling/paresthesia with associated cord injury	Immediate immobilization with long term immobilization +/− surgery
Spinal cord injury	Axial load, hyperextension, hyperflexion.	Any injury associated with numbness, tingling, paresthesia or with hemodynamic instability should be considered a potential cord injury. Pattern may follow specific injury but treatment outside the hospital is the same	Immediate immobilization with long term immobilization +/− surgery
Atlantoaxial subluxation	Potentiated by inflammatory, infectious, or connective tissue disorders followed by minor trauma causing ligament injury or dens fracture. Trisomy 21 places children at high risk	Pain followed by neurologic symptoms if there is cord damage or damage to vertebral vasculature	Immediate immobilization in position of comfort +/− surgery
Spinal cord injury without radiographic abnormality (SCIWORA)	Similar mechanism to fracture but without bony injury on imaging (rare now that MRIs are more commonly available in hospital)	Severe pain, inability to move the neck, numbness/tingling/paresthesia	Immediate immobilization with long term immobilization +/− surgery
Ligamentous injury	Axial load, hyperextension, hyperflexion	Severe pain, midline tenderness, inability to move the neck. May appear less severe than fracture. Numbness/tingling/paresthesia with associated cord injury	Immediate immobilization with long term immobilization +/− surgery
Torticollis	May be traumatic or atraumatic associated with pharyngitis or subtle trauma	Inability to move the neck, tenderness lateral with palpable muscle spasm rather than midline tenderness. No neurologic findings unless associated with trauma	**If traumatic:** Immediate immobilization in position of comfort **If atraumatic:** May trial anti-inflammatory medications and warm compresses
"Stinger"	Stretch or compression or cervical nerve roots from athletic injury	Burning or stinging pain radiating from the neck to the shoulder/hand, numbness and weakness following injury	Immobilization in cases of numbness and weakness but may ultimately recover quickly

ID: 10722273 S: 0005 PS1000-1 TS: 155x235 Pg: 925/1144 BS: 220x251 H: 3 T: 13 PB

112.2 Clearance of the Cervical Spine

Clearance of the cervical spine refers to the clinical assessment that a cervical spine injury is not present based on history and physical examination obviating the need for immobilization and imaging. There are important limitations to evidence in the pediatric literature to guide clearance even among hospital personnel, and there is likewise limited evidence for clearance by prehospital personnel (Emergency Medical Technicians and Paramedics). This reasonably extends to school-based medical personnel who should not undertake this evaluation in the school based setting without significant training and experience.

The most recent data guiding clearance versus injury was developed by the Pediatric Emergency Care and Research Network in 2024. Over 22,000 children 0–17 years of age presenting to trauma centers with known or suspected blunt trauma were enrolled. Four high risk factors for cervical spine trauma were identified: Glasgow coma scale of 3–8, unresponsiveness, abnormal airway, breathing or circulation, or any abnormal neurologic exam including paresthesia, numbness, or weakness. Five additional risk factors: any altered mental status, report of neck pain, substantial torso injury, substantial head injury, and posterior cervical spine tenderness were identified. Absence of all of these risk factors suggested a patient may be clinically cleared of concern for cervical spine injury with 0.2% having any cervical spine injury. Notably, these patients were examined by a trauma team [3].

Other commonly used rules include the NEXUS Criteria in which a patient without focal neurological defect, midline spinal tenderness, altered level of consciousness or intoxication, or distracting injury could be cleared clinically with a sensitivity of 99.6% though very few patients under 8 years of age were included in the study therefore limiting the applicability of the criteria in younger children [4]. The Canadian Cervical Spine Rule suggests that patients without high risk injury and without paresthesias who meet any low risk criteria: ambulation after injury, seated position at evaluation, delayed onset of neck pain, absence of midline tenderness, or involvement in low speed motor vehicle collision, those who can rotate their neck 45° in either direction may be clinically cleared without imaging. The list of high risk injuries is relatively extensive and this rule applies in limited fashion to children, so caution should be used applying this rule without experience with the supporting literature [5].

112.3 Cervical Spine Immobilization

When immobilizing the cervical spine, if cervical collars are available, choose the longest collar that does not extend the neck. There is no significant difference in efficacy between one and two piece collars. When using two piece collars, the front of the collar should be placed first.

If a spine board is available, the cervical spine can be immobilized with either the addition of a collar or by placing a rolled towel on each side of the patient's head secured by tape over the chin and forehead. Foam blocks can also be used in place of rolled towels. Use caution in placing very young children on spine boards as the board may position their head and neck in a flexed position contributing to airway compromise. If no such materials are available, the child should be left in a position of comfort or immobility as long as it is safe to do so until emergency personnel with appropriate equipment arrive.

If a child with suspected cervical spine injury must be moved, cervical spine stability should be ensured by one rescuer standing at the patient's head with one hand on each side of the neck. Hands should extend down to the patient's shoulder and the head and neck should be gripped with the hands and forearms to prevent movement. Multiple people should assist in moving the child to avoid extraneous movement. In patients with a cervical spine injury, the incidence of a second non-contiguous spinal injury is up to 20%, so it is reasonable to ensure immobilization of the entire spine with the use of a spine board in cases of suspected injury [6].

In children wearing football or hockey uniforms, the National Athletic trainer's association has released a position statement recommending an all-or-nothing approach of removing all of a child's uniform pieces or transferring them to care with their uniform intact [7]. If helmets and pads are removed, this should be accomplished with multiple people to avoid extraneous movement.

112.4 Transfer of Care

All children who have suspected cervical spine injury require activation of EMS services and transfer to the emergency department, preferably a trauma center. While for patients without significant risk factors or exam abnormalities, plain radiographs may be sufficient to rule out injury, the imaging capabilities of urgent care centers are widely variable. Therefore, there is little role in urgent care centers in the further management of patients with suspected cervical spine injury if any risk factors suggesting a need for imaging are present. For higher risk patients, computed tomography (most commonly used for bony injury) or magnetic resonance imaging (most commonly used for spinal cord and ligament injury in absence of bony injury) may be required.

112.5 Special Populations

Consider that children with certain chronic medical conditions including Down's syndrome, Klippel-Feil Syndrome, cerebral palsy, neurofibromatosis, juvenile rheumatoid arthritis, Morquio Disease, and Larsen syndrome all may have greater baseline instability in the cervical spine and may therefore be more likely to sustain significant injury with minor trauma to the head and neck [8].

ID: 10722273 S: 0005 PS1000-1 TS: 155x235 Pg: 927/1144 BS: 220x251 H: 3 T: 13 PB

112.6 Care After an Injury

Students who return to school with a cervical collar after injury, for example those who have suffered fractures, vertebral ligament injury, or spinal cord injury, typically wear the collar for 6–8 weeks or more. Collars may cause skin irritation or injury. Skin should be kept clean, dry, and cool. If a collar needs to be removed to clean or dry skin it should be done with the child sitting or lying down and should not be done by the child [9]. Children can do basic activities of daily living while in a collar including walking, using a computer, and riding in a car. They cannot participate in sports, running, or rough play without the approval of a physician.

112.7 Case Conclusions

Case 1 This 13 year old student is at high risk for cervical spine injury given the mechanism of injury and his symptoms. He was not moved, but was able to be placed in a cervical collar. EMS was activated immediately and transported the child in full spinal precautions. He was found to have a fracture which required surgery, but made a full recovery.

Case 2 This 5 year old by demonstrates a clearly concerning exam sign given his unwillingness to move his neck. EMS was immediately activated who transported him in his position of comfort on a backboard with foam blocks and tape so as not to force him to move his neck. He was found to have atlantoaxial subluxation but made a full recovery.

Case 3 This 17 year old girl is at low risk for suffering a cervical spine injury. Nevertheless, there is no clear rule by which school-based personnel can determine that she is completely without injury. She was immobilized and transported to the emergency department where she ultimately had negative imaging and no injury.

Extra Credit Points

1. Cervical spine injuries are rare but potentially devastating
2. Suspect cervical spine injury in any injured child who complains of neck pain, difficulty moving the neck, or who complains of weakness or loss of sensation after an injury. Take steps to safely immobilize the neck.
3. Injuries caused by diving or other axial load or clothesline type injuries are the most likely to result in cervical spine injury. High speed motor vehicle collisions are also very concerning.
4. Any injured child with altered mental status or intoxication should be immobilized after significant trauma as any evaluation of their cervical spine will be unreliable.

References

1. Mohseni S, Talving P, Branco BC, Chan LS, Lustenberger T, Inaba K, Bass M, Demetriades D. Effect of age on cervical spine injury in pediatric population: a National Trauma Data Bank review. J Pediatr Surg. 2011;46(9):1771–6. https://doi.org/10.1016/j.jpedsurg.2011.03.007. PMID: 21929988.
2. Shaw KN, Bachur RG, editors. Fleisher & Ludwig's textbook of pediatric emergency medicine. 7th ed. Wolters Kluwer, Philadelphia, PA. 2016.
3. PECARN prediction rule for cervical spine imaging of children presenting to the emergency department with blunt trauma: a multicentre prospective observational study. Lancet Child Adolesc Health. 2024;8(7):482–90. https://doi.org/10.1016/S2352-4642(24)00104-4. Epub 2024 Jun 4. PMID: 38843852; PMCID: PMC11261431.
4. Hoffman JR, Mower WR, Wolfson AB, Todd KH, Zucker MI. Validity of a set of clinical criteria to rule out injury to the cervical spine in patients with blunt trauma. National Emergency X-Radiography Utilization Study Group. N Engl J Med. 2000;343(2):94–9. https://doi.org/10.1056/NEJM200007133430203. Erratum in: N Engl J Med 2001 Feb 8;344(6):464. PMID: 10891516.
5. Stiell IG, Wells GA, Vandemheen KL, Clement CM, Lesiuk H, De Maio VJ, Laupacis A, Schull M, McKnight RD, Verbeek R, Brison R, Cass D, Dreyer J, Eisenhauer MA, Greenberg GH, MacPhail I, Morrison L, Reardon M, Worthington J. The Canadian C-spine rule for radiography in alert and stable trauma patients. JAMA. 2001;286(15):1841–8. https://doi.org/10.1001/jama.286.15.1841. PMID: 11597285.
6. Miller CP, Brubacher JW, Biswas D, Lawrence BD, Whang PG, Grauer JN. The incidence of noncontiguous spinal fractures and other traumatic injuries associated with cervical spine fractures: a 10-year experience at an academic medical center. Spine (Phila Pa 1976). 2011;36(19):1532–40. https://doi.org/10.1097/BRS.0b013e3181f550a6. PMID: 21242872.
7. Swartz EE, Boden BP, Courson RW, Decoster LC, Horodyski M, Norkus SA, Rehberg RS, Waninger KN. National athletic trainers' association position statement: acute management of the cervical spine-injured athlete. J Athl Train. 2009;44(3):306–31. https://doi.org/10.4085/1062-6050-44.3.306. PMID: 19478836; PMCID: PMC2681208.
8. Webber-Jones JE, Thomas CA, Bordeaux RE Jr. The management and prevention of rigid cervical collar complications. Orthop Nurs. 2002;21(4):19–25; quiz 25–7. PMID: 12224182. https://doi.org/10.1097/00006416-200207000-00004.
9. Ghanem I, El Hage S, Rachkidi R, Kharrat K, Dagher F, Kreichati G. Pediatric cervical spine instability. J Child Orthop. 2008;2(2):71–84. https://doi.org/10.1007/s11832-008-0092-2. Epub 2008 Mar 4. PMID: 19308585; PMCID: PMC2656787.

Chapter 113
Traumatic Injuries to the Chest

Madelyn Olympia and Robert P. Olympia

Case 1 While making a TikTok video during homeroom, 9 year old Michael presents to your office after sustaining a chest injury. While standing on his desk, he attempts to jump to the adjacent desk, slips and falls, landing directly on his chest upon the chair below. He is crying, complains of significant chest pain and trouble breathing. His heart rate and respiratory rate are elevated for age, and you notice a large linear bruise that crosses his anterior chest. What should you do?

Thoracic injuries in children account for less than one-tenth of all pediatric trauma-related injuries but comprise 14% of pediatric trauma-related deaths [1]. Most chest injuries result from falls and motor vehicle crashes. The complaint chest wall of a child can make the evaluation of patients more challenging, as there can be significant intra-thoracic injury with little or no external signs of trauma.

The evaluation of a child who has sustained thoracic trauma includes a thorough history and physical examination, focusing on airway, breathing, and circulation. Recognize that 70% of children with intra-thoracic injury may have normal vital signs, so disposition (Emergency Medical Services (EMS) activation to an Emergency Department (ED), or referral to an urgent care center or primary care provider) should be based on your differential diagnosis (Table 113.1).

M. Olympia
Harrisburg Christian School, Harrisburg, PA, USA
e-mail: Madelyn.olympia@csagh.org

R. P. Olympia (✉)
Department of Emergency Medicine and Pediatrics, Penn State College of Medicine
Attending Physician, Hershey, PA, USA

Division of Pediatric Emergency Medicine, Department of Emergency Medicine, Penn State Milton S. Hershey Medical Center, Hershey, PA, USA
e-mail: rolympia@hmc.psu.edu

R. P. Olympia, J. Brady-Olympia (eds.), *Clinical Considerations in School-based Health*, https://doi.org/10.1007/978-3-031-85765-2_113

Table 113.1 Thoracic injuries in children

	Initial presentation	Disposition and treatment
Chest contusion	Mild chest tenderness and bruising None to mild SOB	Refer to urgent care center or primary care provider Anti-inflammatories
Rib fracture	Moderate to severe chest tenderness Moderate to significant SOB In younger children, intra-thoracic injuries may be associated with rib fractures due to the high impact mechanism	Refer to urgent care center or ED for CXR or CT scan Anti-inflammatories
Pulmonary contusion	Often present without external indicators of chest wall injury or rib fractures Chest wall tenderness and bruising Hemoptysis Tachypnea Hypoxia Decreased BS	EMS activation to the ED CXR has sensitivity rates of 65–97% While most pulmonary contusions heal within 1 week, 20% will develop pneumonia and 30% will require intubation and mechanical ventilation
Pneumothorax/ Hemothorax	Chest wall tenderness or crepitus Tachypnea Hypoxia Decreased BS Dullness to percussion	EMS activation to the ED Small pneumothorax (<20%): oxygen and observation Large pneumothorax/hemothorax: tube thoracostomy or pigtail catheter placement Blood transfusions
Tension pneumothorax	As per pneumothorax/ hemothorax PLUS: Jugular venous distention Displaced cardiac apex Contralateral tracheal deviation Shock	EMS activation to the ED CXR Needle decompression Tube thoracostomy or pigtail catheter placement
Pneumomediastinum	Mild chest pain Mild SOB Crepitus of the anterior chest or neck May be associated with tracheobronchial or esophageal injuries	Refer to urgent care or ED if symptoms for CXR
Tracheobronchial injury	Chest wall tenderness or crepitus Tachypnea Hypoxia Stridor Hoarse voice Difficulty swallowing	EMS activation to the ED CT scan Operative treatment

(continued)

Table 113.1 (continued)

	Initial presentation	Disposition and treatment
Esophageal injury	Chest wall tenderness or crepitus Tachypnea Hypoxia	EMS activation to the ED Esophagram or esophagoscopy Operative treatment

Abbreviations: *BS* breath sounds, *CT* chest tomography, *CXR* chest radiography, *ED* emergency department, *EMS* Emergency Medical Services, *SOB* shortness of breath

Table 113.2 Predictors of thoracic injury in children

	Holmes et al. (2002) [2]	McNamara et al. (2016) [3]	Weerdenburg et al. (2019) [4]
Study specifics	Prospective Single institution Age < 16 years N = 986	Retrospective Single institution Age < 18 years N = 166	Retrospective Trauma registry Age < 17 years N = 493
Predictors of thoracic injury			
Vital signs and GCS	Elevated adjusted RR Low systolic BP GCS < 15	Oxygen saturation < 93% GCS < 15	Oxygen saturation < 95% BP < 5th percentile
Symptoms		Syncope or dizziness	Chest pain
Chest findings	Abnormal results on thoracic examination (erythema, abrasions, contusions, lacerations, crepitus, or tenderness of the anterior or posterior thorax) Abnormal chest auscultation (BS decreased or absent, or crackles/rhonchi)		Abnormal thoracic symptoms and signs (chest tenderness, abrasions or bruising over anterior or posterior aspect of thorax) Abnormal chest auscultation (crackles, rhonchi, or decreased/absent breath sounds)
Other injuries related to mechanism of injury	Femur fracture	Cervical spine tenderness Thoraco-lumbar-sacral spine tenderness Abdominal/pelvic tenderness	Femur fracture

Abbreviations: *BP* blood pressure, *BS* breath sounds, *GCS* Glasgow Coma Score, *RR* respiratory rate

Several studies have examined predictors of intra-thoracic injuries in children following blunt chest trauma (Table 113.2), although a prospective, multi-institutional study has yet to be performed and published.

Advanced Trauma Life Support (ATLS) guidelines currently recommend a CXR in all pediatric blunt trauma patients [5]. Although the sensitivity of CXR in detecting intra-thoracic injury was recently reported to be 58% [6], thoracic CT scan may identify occult injuries that do not require surgical intervention while increasing radiation dose exposure. CT scans of the chest should be considered in a pediatric patient who sustains blunt chest trauma with abnormal vital signs, stable patients sustaining high-energy trauma, and patients with a concern for aortic or cardiac injury. Studies have shown that ultrasound is effective in the diagnosis of pleural and pericardial effusions, pneumothorax/hemothorax, rib fractures, and pulmonary contusions in children who have sustained blunt chest trauma.

Case 2 While pitching during a softball game, 15 year old Anna is struck by a hit softball that bounces once before striking her in the chest. She falls to the ground, but is not unconscious. She complaints of significant chest pain, trouble breathing, and dizziness. Her heart is racing, but she is able to speak in short phrases. What do you do?

Pediatric patients who sustain significant chest trauma should be evaluated in an ED for possible blunt cardiac injury (BCI), especially those who complain of significant chest pain, palpitations, shortness of breath, or dizziness/lightheadedness. Although the incidence of BCI was recently reported to be <0.2%, the associated mortality rate was 26% [7]. Recent literature has shown a correlation between pulmonary contusions and hemothorax with BCI [7]. Clinical features of BCI include new onset arrhythmias (70% of children with BCI), new murmurs, hypotension, narrow pulse pressure, muffled heart tones, and jugular vein distention. A 12-lead EKG and serum troponin should be performed in any patient suspected of having a BCI; normal studies effectively rules out BCI, and stable, asymptomatic patients may be discharged from the ED. Children with an abnormal EKG (arrhythmia, ST changes, ischemia, and heart block), abnormal cardiac enzymes, or low cardiac output/cardiogenic shock should be admitted to telemetry.

In youth sports, commotio cordis, the second leading cause of death (second to hypertrophic cardiomyopathy), may occur after a high impact force to the chest, leading to unresponsiveness and ventricular fibrillation. Variables that increase the risk of developing commotio cordis include: age (peak incidence between 11 and 19 years), sex (male—95% of cases), mechanism (being struck by a small projectile with a dense core propelled at a high velocity ~ 40 mph—baseball, lacrosse ball, hockey puck), and genetic susceptibility. The pathophysiology of the commotio cordis involves impact during a narrow window of repolarization (10–20 milliseconds prior to the peak of the T-wave) leading to ventricular fibrillation. Subsequent symptoms include instantaneous collapse or brief lightheadedness before losing consciousness. On-the-field resuscitation has been successful in up to 60% of cases, most likely due to improved awareness and the availability of automated external defibrillators (AEDs) at sporting events and schools (Fig. 113.1).

113.1 Case Conclusions

Case 1 Michael is transported to his local ED. Although his initial CXR was normal, he was subsequently hospitalized due to persistent tachypnea and chest pain. A CT scan of the chest was performed on Day #2 due to hypoxia, demonstrating small

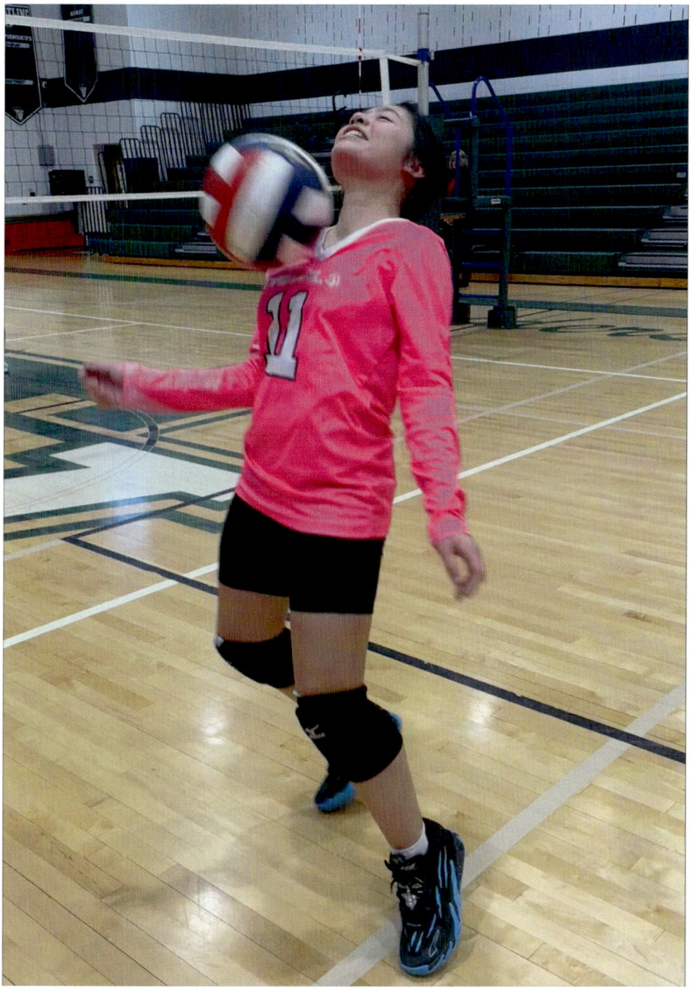

Fig. 113.1 Madelyn Olympia attempting to avoid blunt chest trauma during a volleyball game

bilateral pulmonary contusions not requiring surgical intervention. His EKG and serum troponin were normal (rule out BCI), and he was discharged after 1 week without complications.

Case 2 Anna is transported to her local ED. A CXR, EKG, and serum troponin were ordered and normal. Her chest pain, shortness of breath and dizziness improved with intravenous fluids and anti-inflammatories, and she was discharged from the ED following a 6 hours observation period.

Table 113.3 delineates the CHEST mnemonic which may help school health care providers determine disposition of a student following blunt chest trauma.

Table 113.3 CHEST mnemonic to determine immediate transfer to an Emergency Department (developed by authors)

C	Complaint of chest pain	Significant complaints of chest pain
H	Hypotension	A systolic blood pressure less than: 70 + 2 (age in years) for children aged 4–8 years <90 for children greater than 9 years of age
E	Ecchymosis of the chest	Immediate bruising following impact may indicate significant impact to the chest
S	Shortness of breath or syncope	Shortness of breath (tachypnea or hypoxia) Syncope (including near syncope or dizziness or palpitations)
T	Traumatic mechanism	A higher impact to the chest is more concerning for an intra-thoracic injury

Extra Credit Points

1. Due to the elasticity and chest wall compliance of a child, consider intra-thoracic injuries based on the mechanism of injury and presenting symptoms, regardless of whether there are external signs of injury to the chest wall. Pulmonary contusions often present without rib fractures.
2. CT scans of the chest rarely change management when occult injuries detected on CT are not found on initial CXR.
3. Obtain an EKG and serum troponin in patients with pulmonary contusions or a hemothorax. Recent literature has demonstrated a correlation between these intra-thoracic injuries and BCI.
4. Remember the mnemonic "CHEST" when considering disposition of a pediatric patients following blunt chest trauma.

References

1. Goodwin G, Bengio M, Ryckeley CB, et al. Emergency department management of pediatric blunt thoracic injuries. Pediatr Emerg Med Pract. 2023;20(Suppl 11):1–30.
2. Holmes JF, Sokolove PE, Brant WE, et al. A clinical decision rule for identifying children with thoracic injuries after blunt torso trauma. Ann Emerg Med. 2002;39(5):492–9.
3. McNamara C, Mironova I, Lehman, et al. Predictors of intrathoracic injury after blunt torso trauma in children presenting to an emergency department as trauma activations. J Emerg Med. 2017;52(6):793–800.
4. Weerdenburg KD, Wales PW, Stephens D, et al. Predicting thoracic injury in children with multitrauma. Pediatr Emerg Care. 2019;35(5):330–4.
5. Subcommittee on Advanced Trauma Life Support (ATLS) of the American College of Surgeons (ACS), Committee on Trauma. Pediatric trauma. In: ATLS advanced trauma life support student course manual. 10th ed. Chicago; 2018. p. 186–209.
6. Ugalde IT, Prater S, Cardenas-Turanzas M, et al. Chest x-ray vs. computed tomography of the chest in pediatric blunt trauma. J Pediatr Surg. 2021;56(5):1039–46.
7. Emigh B, Grigorian A, Dilday J, et al. Risk factors and outcomes in pediatric blunt cardiac injuries. Pediatr Surg Int. 2023;39(1):195.

Chapter 114
Traumatic Injuries to the Abdomen

Charles Webb and Ryunosuke Hisatomi

Case 1 While riding his bicycle to school, 12-year-old William presents to your office after sustaining an abdominal injury. He explained that he attempted to abruptly stop his bicycle on a curb, and the handlebar struck him in the abdomen, causing him to fall over. He complains of significant right-sided abdominal pain and nausea. You notice a small bruise located in his upper right abdomen and tenderness on palpation. What should you do?

Blunt abdominal trauma is the third most prevalent cause of traumatic fatalities among pediatric patients, following head and chest injuries [1]. Approximately 8–12% of all patients experiencing blunt trauma sustain intra-abdominal injuries. The primary mechanism for such injuries is direct blunt-force trauma, commonly resulting from motor vehicle collisions, bicycle accidents, falls, sports related incidents, or nonaccidental trauma. The spleen and liver are the organs most frequently affected, followed by the kidney, small bowel, and pancreas [2].

The initial management of abdominal trauma patients prioritizes rapid stabilization and the identification of life-threatening injuries. For hemodynamically unstable individuals or those with significant abdominal trauma, activating emergency medical services (EMS) for transportation to the closest emergency department (ED) is crucial. In cases of hemodynamic stability, conducting a thorough history and physical examination is essential to detect any suspected intra-abdominal injury. Children with intra-abdominal injury may exhibit limited findings shortly after the injury. One should maintain a low threshold for activating EMS to prevent delayed diagnosis and treatment. Refer to Table 114.1 for major intra-abdominal injuries and their associated symptoms and signs.

Several studies have examined predictors of intra-abdominal injuries in children following blunt abdomen trauma (Table 114.2).

C. Webb (✉) · R. Hisatomi
LSU Health Science Center Shreveport, Shreveport, LA, USA
e-mail: charles.webb@lsuhs.edu; ryunosuke.hisatomi@lsuhs.edu

R. P. Olympia, J. Brady-Olympia (eds.), *Clinical Considerations in School-based Health*, https://doi.org/10.1007/978-3-031-85765-2_114

Table 114.1 Abdominal injuries in children (Differential diagnosis)

	Symptoms	Physical examination
Spleen injury	LUQ abdominal and left shoulder pain (Kehr's sign) Nausea and vomiting Shock [a]Enlargement of the spleen (e.g., due to infectious mononucleosis) makes the spleen more susceptible to injury	LUQ tenderness Bruising over the left side of the abdomen (Grey Turner's sign) Abdominal distension Peritoneal signs (e.g., abdominal rigidity, guarding, or rebound on palpation)
Liver injury	RUQ pain and right shoulder pain Nausea and vomiting Shock	RUQ tenderness Bruising over the right side of the abdomen or around the umbilicus (Cullen's sign) Abdominal distension Peritoneal signs
Pancreatic injury	Epigastric pain with potential radiation to the back Nausea and vomiting Fever Shock	Epigastric tenderness Bruising to the upper abdomen Abdominal distension Peritoneal signs
Gastrointestinal injury	Abdominal pain Nausea and vomiting Shock	Abdominal tenderness Bruising over the abdominal wall Abdominal distension Peritoneal signs Absent bowel sounds
Kidney injury	Flank pain Abdominal pain Nausea and vomiting Gross hematuria Fever [a]Shock	Tenderness to palpation, palpable mass, bruising in the flank Abdominal distension

Abbreviations: *LUQ* left upper quadrant, *RUQ* right upper quadrant
[a]Signs/symptoms of shock: Hypotension, tachypnea, tachycardia, pale skin, dizziness, and light-headedness

Handlebar injuries can result in significant abdominal trauma, with over one-third of cases necessitating surgical intervention. The presence of abdominal pain, vomiting, fever, or a circular imprint on the chest or abdomen should prompt further evaluation [6]. However, handlebar injuries, particularly those involving the bowel and pancreas (e.g., gastrointestinal tract perforations, duodenal hematomas, and pancreatic pseudocysts), may have delayed presentations, which could manifest a few days to weeks after the injury [7].Laboratory tests, including a complete blood count (CBC), comprehensive metabolic panel (CMP), and pancreatic enzymes, urinalysis are particularly valuable for evaluating intra-abdominal injury. Specifically, AST levels greater than 200 IU/L or ALT levels greater than 125 IU/L should raise suspicion of liver injury. While amylase and lipase levels may not reliably indicate acute pancreatic or other intra-abdominal organ injuries, they serve as valuable benchmarks for tracking the progression of pancreatic complications. Gross blood

Table 114.2 Predictors of abdominal injury in children

	Holmes et al. (2002) [3]	Holmes et al. (2013) [4]	Adelgais et al. (2014) [5]
Study specifics	Prospective Single institution Age < 16 years N = 1095	Prospective Multi-institution Median age of 11.1 years N = 12,044	Prospective Multi-institution Age < 18 years N = 12,044
Predictors of abdominal injury		If none of the 7 findings listed below are present, the risk is very low	
Vital signs and GCS	Low systolic BP	GCS score greater than 13	
Symptoms		No complaints of abdominal pain No vomiting	
Abdominal findings	Abdominal tenderness	No evidence of abdominal wall trauma or [a]seat belt sign No abdominal tenderness No evidence of thoracic wall trauma No decreased BS	Peritoneal irritation Abdominal distension Any abdominal tenderness Bowel sounds absent
Other injuries related to mechanism of injury	Femur fracture		
Labs	AST > 200 U/L or ALT > 125 U/L Hct < 30% Urinalysis > 5 RBCs per HPF		
Definition of IAI	An injury was documented to the spleen, liver, pancreas, kidney, adrenal glands, or gastrointestinal tract	Clinically important IAI: IAI undergoing acute intervention (therapeutic laparotomy, angiographic embolization, blood transfusion, or intravenous fluid for ≥2 nights)	Clinically important IAI: IAI undergoing acute intervention (therapeutic laparotomy, angiographic embolization, blood transfusion, or intravenous fluid for ≥2 nights)

Abbreviations: *BP* blood pressure, *BS* breath sounds, *GCS* Glasgow Coma Score, *AST* aspartate aminotransferase, *ALT* Alanine Aminotransferase, *RBC* red blood cell, *Hct* hematocrit, *HPF* high-powered field, *IAI* intra-abdominal injury

[a]Ecchymosis and/or abraded skin in the distribution of a seatbelt extending across the abdomen after a motor vehicle accident

on urinalysis is suggestive of injury to the genitourinary system, including the bladder, kidneys, and ureters [8]. Computed tomography (CT) remains the gold standard for diagnosing abdominal injuries in hemodynamically stable patients. Patients who are hemodynamically unstable with suspected abdominal injury should undergo immediate surgery. Focused abdominal sonography for trauma (FAST) has become an integral part of the initial trauma evaluation due to its speed, noninvasiveness, and absence of radiation exposure. Recent publications have shown that the FAST exam should not be used as the sole screening tool to rule out intra-abdominal injuries, but it may be used in conjunction with physical examination and laboratory findings [9].

Case 2 While defending a shot during a soccer game, 11-year-old goalkeeper, Emily is struck by the opponent's cleat. She complains of significant abdominal pain in the left upper quadrant of the abdomen and the left rib cage, along with nausea. She is not capable of returning to the game. What do you do?

Abdominal injuries are rare in sports, but when they do occur, it is important to recognize the warning signs of potentially life-threatening intra-abdominal injuries. According to data from the National Pediatric Trauma Registry, abdominal injuries due to contact sports were identified in only 0.56% of patients. The most frequently involved sports were football, hockey, baseball, soccer, and basketball. The spleen is the most commonly injured organ, followed by the kidney and the liver [10].

Splenic injuries often present with left upper quadrant or generalized abdominal pain, potentially radiating to the left shoulder due to diaphragmatic or phrenic nerve irritation (Kehr's sign). Signs of peritoneal irritation or hypovolemic shock should also raise suspicion for hemoperitoneum secondary to splenic injury. However, physical examination and laboratory data are often nonspecific, particularly in pediatric patients, who usually have greater hemodynamic reserve than adults [11]. Pediatric patients who sustain significant abdominal trauma should undergo evaluation in an emergency department for possible intra-abdominal injury.

For hemodynamically stable children with traumatic intra-abdominal injury, nonoperative management has increasingly become the standard of care over the last few decades and is associated with decreased morbidity and mortality [9]. Children showing any signs of hemodynamic instability or requiring volume resuscitation should be admitted to an ICU for continuous monitoring. Patients with stable vital signs and physical examination or laboratory findings suggestive of acute intra-abdominal injury can be safely monitored on a pediatric ward. In both settings, patients should undergo serial abdominal examinations to assess clinical worsening and the need for subsequent intervention [1].

114.1 Case Conclusions

Case 1 *William is transported to his local ED. Upon arrival, he was hemodynamically stable. Physical examination revealed intense localized pain in the right upper quadrant. Laboratory studies showed AST 255 U/L and ALT 205 U/L, with Hb and Hct within normal range. A contrast-enhanced abdominal CT scan identified hepatic lacerations within the right lobe, without signs of active bleeding, corresponding to a grade III injury on the organ injury scale of the American Association for the Surgery of Trauma (AAST), not requiring surgical intervention. The patient* *was admitted to the hospital and remained hemodynamically stable throughout his stay and had stable laboratory parameters. He was discharged on day 5 with a good clinical status.*

Case 2 *Emily is transported to her local ED. All laboratory tests were normal. FAST revealed mild hemorrhage in the abdominal cavity. A contrast-enhanced abdominal CT scan showed a laceration of the spleen classified as a grade IV splenic injury according to the AAST, with secondary mild free fluid into the peritoneal cavity.* She underwent nonoperative management due to her hemodynamic stability and the isolated spleen lesion. She was closely monitored for hemodynamic parameters and pain control. *She was discharged on day 7 with a good clinical status.* She engaged in light activity for the first 3 weeks, gradually increasing her activity level as tolerated. She resumed full activity, including contact, after 3 months [12].

Table 114.3 delineates the ABDOMEN mnemonic which may assist school healthcare providers in identifying intra-abdominal injury in a student following blunt abdominal trauma

Extra Credit Points

1. Children with significant traumatic mechanisms or signs should be suspected of intra-abdominal injury, especially if they are hemodynamically unstable. Blunt abdominal trauma, being the leading cause of initially undetected fatal injuries, may lack external signs [1]. You should maintain a lower threshold for activating EMS to prevent delayed treatment.
2. CT scan is widely regarded as the gold standard for assessing blunt abdominal trauma. However, recent literature has shown that FAST, when combined with physical examination and laboratory findings, serves as an effective screening tool for intra-abdominal injuries in children after blunt abdominal trauma [9].

Table 114.3 ABDOMEN mnemonic to determine immediate transfer to an Emergency Department

A	Absent bowel sounds	This may indicate ileus, peritonitis, bowel ischemia
B	Bruising	Immediate bruising following impact may indicate significant impact to the abdomen (e.g., Grey Turner's sign, Cullen's sign)
D	Distension of the abdomen	Blood, fluid, intestinal perforation, or acute gastric distension
O	Overwhelming tenderness	This may indicate injury to the organ directly beneath the tender point
M	Mechanism of trauma	A higher impact to the abdomen is more concerning for an intra-abdominal injury
E	Elicited peritoneal signs	These signs include abdominal rigidity, guarding, or rebound on palpation. May indicate peritonitis, visceral perforation, or solid organ rupture
N	Nausea/vomiting	This may indicate underlying organ damage, bleeding, or peritonitis

Developed by authors

3. Most solid organ abdominal injuries are managed non-surgically. Patients are often admitted to the hospital and undergo serial abdominal examinations to assess clinical worsening and the need for subsequent intervention.
4. Remember the mnemonic "ABDOMEN" to identify intra-abdominal injury in a pediatric patient following blunt abdominal trauma.

References

1. Kuas C, Acar N, Ozakin E, et al. The diagnostic value of laboratory tests in detecting solid organ injuries in pediatric patients with blunt abdominal trauma. Am J Emerg Med. 2022;57:133–7. https://doi.org/10.1016/j.ajem.2022.04.039. Epub 2022 May 1. PMID: 35576793.
2. Mikrogianakis A, Grant V. The kids are alright: pediatric trauma pearls. Emerg Med Clin North Am. 2018;36(1):237–57. https://doi.org/10.1016/j.emc.2017.08.015. PMID: 29132580.
3. Holmes JF, Sokolove PE, Brant WE, Palchak MJ, Vance CW, Owings JT, Kuppermann N. Identification of children with intra-abdominal injuries after blunt trauma. Ann Emerg Med. 2002;39(5):500–9. https://doi.org/10.1067/mem.2002.122900. PMID: 11973557.
4. Holmes JF, Lillis K, Monroe D, et al., Pediatric Emergency Care Applied Research Network (PECARN). Identifying children at very low risk of clinically important blunt abdominal injuries. Ann Emerg Med. 2013;62(2):107–116.e2. https://doi.org/10.1016/j.annemergmed.2012.11.009. Epub 2013 Feb 1. PMID: 23375510.
5. Adelgais KM, Kuppermann N, Kooistra J, et al. Intra-Abdominal Injury Study Group of the Pediatric Emergency Care Applied Research Network (PECARN). Accuracy of the abdominal examination for identifying children with blunt intra-abdominal injuries. J Pediatr. 2014;165(6):1230–1235.e5. https://doi.org/10.1016/j.jpeds.2014.08.014. Epub 2014 Sep 27. PMID: 25266346.
6. Cheung R, Shukla M, Akers KG, et al. Bicycle handlebar injuries - a systematic review of pediatric chest and abdominal injuries. Am J Emerg Med. 2022;51:13–21. https://doi.org/10.1016/j.ajem.2021.09.043. Epub 2021 Sep 28. PMID: 34649007.
7. Lam JP, Eunson GJ, Munro FD, Orr JD. Delayed presentation of handlebar injuries in children. BMJ. 2001;322(7297):1288–9. https://doi.org/10.1136/bmj.322.7297.1288. PMID: 11375234; PMCID: PMC1120385.
8. Kenefake ME, Swarm M, Walthall J. Nuances in pediatric trauma. Emerg Med Clin North Am. 2013;31(3):627–52. https://doi.org/10.1016/j.emc.2013.04.004. Epub 2013 Jun 27. PMID: 23915597.
9. Schonfeld D, Lee LK. Blunt abdominal trauma in children. Curr Opin Pediatr. 2012;24(3):314–8. https://doi.org/10.1097/MOP.0b013e328352de97. PMID: 22450250.
10. Schacherer N, Miller J, Petronis K. Pediatric blunt abdominal trauma in the emergency department: evidence-based management techniques. Pediatr Emerg Med Pract. 2014;11(10):1–23; quiz 23–4. Update in: Pediatr Emerg Med Pract. 2020 Jan 15;17(Suppl 1):1–59. PMID: 25928975.
11. Lynn KN, Werder GM, Callaghan RM, et al. Pediatric blunt splenic trauma: a comprehensive review. Pediatr Radiol. 2009;39:904–16. https://doi.org/10.1007/s00247-009-1336-0.
12. Juyia RF, Kerr HA. Return to play after liver and spleen trauma. Sports Health. 2014;6(3):239–45. https://doi.org/10.1177/1941738114528468. PMID: 24790694; PMCID: PMC4000477.

Chapter 115
The Acutely Injured Shoulder, Elbow, and Wrist

Andrew Wilkinson and Peter H. Seidenberg

Case 1 During a middle school football game, 12-year-old Matthew experiences sudden left shoulder pain after being tackled and landing directly on the affected shoulder. Upon initial evaluation on the sideline, he is supporting his left arm with his uninjured arm and has pain with decreased range of motion in all directions. Brachial and radial pulses are palpable in his left upper extremity, and there are no changes in sensation. What is the next step?

Table 115.1 describes common shoulder injuries in children and adolescents. Matthew's mechanism of injury and initial presentation is most consistent with an anterior shoulder dislocation. The next steps in treatment would include presentation to an urgent care facility or emergency department for closed reduction of the affected shoulder. Imaging with x-rays may be obtained if there are any further concerns for a fracture. The patient and family should be educated on the injury, and that he will be more likely to experience recurrent dislocations and shoulder instability.

Shoulder dislocations are commonly seen in older pediatric patients, with 20% of all dislocations occurring in people less than 20 years of age. A dislocation may occur when there is direct force applied to the shoulder, most commonly anterior. Mechanism of injury (MOI) is blunt force or trauma, such as landing directly on the shoulder when falling. It is also more prevalent in athletes competing in overhead throwing sports [1]. The patient would present with pain overlying the affected shoulder, with decreased range of motion in all directions. The shoulder may appear foreshortened with loss of normal convex contour. It is important to first assess for any neurovascular compromise, such as decreased sensation or strength. The axillary nerve may be affected, which would cause changes in muscle strength and

A. Wilkinson · P. H. Seidenberg (✉)
LSU Health Shreveport School of Medicine, Shreveport, LA, USA
e-mail: alw001@lsuhs.edu; peter.seidenberg@lsuhs.edu

R. P. Olympia, J. Brady-Olympia (eds.), *Clinical Considerations in School-based Health*, https://doi.org/10.1007/978-3-031-85765-2_115

Table 115.1 Shoulder injuries of the pediatric population

Injury	Common age group	Mechanism of injury	Presentation	Imaging	Treatment
Shoulder dislocation	Older pediatric patients. Fractures are more common in younger pediatric patients. Common in athletes competing in overhead throwing sports.	Direct force applied to the shoulder, landing directly on shoulder when falling.	Pain overlying the affected shoulder, with decreased range of motion in all directions. The shoulder may appear foreshortened with loss of normal convex contour. The axillary nerve may be affected, which would cause changes in muscle strength and sensation of the deltoid muscle.	X-rays will be the initial imaging of choice. MRI may be used if there is a need for further evaluation. Imaging may display abnormalities such as Bankart and Hill-Sachs lesions as discussed above.	Initial management includes closed reduction of the shoulder, which may require presentation to an urgent care facility or emergency department for sedation if the reduction is delayed. Conservative management vs Orthopedic intervention depending on if a fracture or neurovascular compromise is present.
Clavicle fracture [3]	More common in the older pediatric age group, greater than 10 years of age.	May occur with blunt trauma of force to the clavicle. Most often occurring as the result of a fall.	The patient will present with significant shoulder pain and decreased range of motion in all planes secondary to pain. They often support the affected arm with uninjured one.	X-ray will be the initial imaging of choice for evaluation. Additional imaging is not routinely needed.	Initial management includes placing the patient in a sling. Further evaluation in an urgent care facility or emergency room is recommended, as some of these injuries may require surgery. Indications for emergent Orthopedic evaluation include open fracture, tented skin, displaced fracture with risk of non-union, significantly anteriorly and posteriorly displaced medial third and lateral third clavicle fractures, and concerns for pneumothorax or neurovascular compromise. Uncomplicated clavicle fractures typically heal in 6–8 weeks.

Rotator cuff tear/ tendonitis [4]	These injuries are more common in the older pediatric population due to increased participation in contact sports and sports involving repetitive overhead arm movements	Rotator cuff injuries may be caused by repetitive overhead movements, and less commonly direct contact or force applied to the shoulder.	A patient may present with tenderness to palpation of the subacromial space and posteriorly over the rotator cuff tendons. The patient often has limited ROM due to pain. Most rotator cuff injuries involve the supraspinatus, which is responsible for shoulder abduction.	Imaging modalities initially include x-ray and may progress to ultrasound or MRI for further evaluation.	Initial treatment may involve presentation to a clinic or urgent care facility for further evaluation, as these injuries may require further imaging. Indications for imaging may include decreased ROM, gross deformity, bruising, swelling, and concerns for a tear.
Rotator cuff tear [4]	Rotator cuff injuries are more common in the older pediatric population due to increased participation in contact sports and sports involving repetitive overhead arm movements	Repetitive overhead movements, and less commonly direct contact or force applied to the shoulder.	A patient may present with tenderness to palpation of the subacromial space and posteriorly over the rotator cuff tendons. The patient often has limited ROM due to pain. Most rotator cuff injuries involve the supraspinatus, which is responsible for shoulder abduction. Physical exam signs for a tear include a positive drop-arm test. For this test, a patient will have their arms out to the side with 90° of shoulder flexion and their thumbs pointed down. Pressure is then applied to the upper extremities. A positive test is displayed if a patient is unable to keep their shoulder flexed at 90°, resulting in a "drop" of the affected arm.	Imaging modalities initially include x-ray and may progress to ultrasound or MRI for further evaluation.	Initial treatment may involve presentation to a clinic or urgent care facility for further evaluation, as these injuries may require further imaging. Indications for imaging may include decreased ROM, gross deformity, bruising, swelling, and concerns for a tear. It is important to note that rotator cuff tears are uncommon in the pediatric population but may be present in the setting of a shoulder dislocation.

(continued)

Table 115.1 (continued)

Injury	Common age group	Mechanism of injury	Presentation	Imaging	Treatment
Little league shoulder (proximal humeral epiphysiolysis) [5]	This injury is most commonly seen in adolescents, especially those playing sports with overhead movements/ throwing.	Repetitive overhead movement or throwing. Patients may have a history of previous shoulder or elbow injury.	A patient may present with generalized shoulder pain with overhead movements and throwing, along with pain and swelling located over the lateral aspect of the proximal humerus.	X-ray is the initial imaging of choice, and may be normal or display a wide proximal humeral physis. Point-of-care ultrasound may also be used in the clinic setting.	Rest is the goal standard of treatment, with these injuries typically requiring 3–6 months of rest from the overhead activity. A gradual return to activity is recommended.
Acromioclavicular joint separation (shoulder sprain) [6]	AC joint injuries are overall uncommon in pediatric patients, but may be more common in adolescents or patients involved in sports.	This type of injury will be caused by direct force to the shoulder or a FOOSH injury.	A patient may present with pain and swelling of the AC join, along with visible deformities of the shoulder in some cases. The patient may be using the non-affected arm to support the injured arm.	X-ray is the initial imaging of choice, with MRI or CT being used if inconclusive findings.	Treatment may be based on the degree of separation, ranging I-VI. Non-operative treatment includes rest, ice, heat, NSAIDs, short duration of a sling. Surgery may be indicate if there is any associated fracture, dislocation, or soft tissue impingement.

sensation of the deltoid muscle. Pulses should also be examined, including brachial and radial. Initial management includes closed reduction of the shoulder, which may require presentation to an urgent care facility or emergency department for sedation if the reduction is delayed. X-rays may be obtained at that time if there is concern for fracture. There are two different deformities that may be appreciated on imaging. A Bankart lesion is an injury to the glenoid labrum that may occur after a shoulder dislocation or repeated subluxations. This could ultimately lead to labrum-glenoid partial detachment at the antero-inferior aspect. These lesions may be present with or without a glenoid fracture. A Hill-Sachs deformity is a lesion caused by a shoulder dislocation that leads to a humeral head injury at the poster-lateral aspect [2]. Patients with shoulder dislocations with subsequent fractures on imaging will require an Orthopedic referral. For uncomplicated shoulder dislocations, patients may be referred to Sports Medicine for further follow-up. Uncomplicated dislocations may be managed conservatively, along with patient education. It is important to note that these patients will also be predisposed to recurrent dislocation and instability. The following link demonstrates different anteriorly dislocated shoulder reduction methods. https://emergencycarebc.ca/clinical_resource/anterior-shoulder-dislocation-reduction-methods/

Case 2 Tyler, a 10-year-old student in 5th grade, is playing with his school friends during recess. While running, he trips after stepping in a hole and falls forward with his arms in front of him. He immediately experiences pain around his right elbow and upper arm. He then goes to his teachers. At this time, his right elbow has become red, painful, and swollen. He has decreased range of motion of his right arm due to pain. His upper extremity pulses appear to be intact, and there are no changes in sensation of his upper extremities. What do you do?

Table 115.2 describes common elbow injuries in children and adolescents. Tyler's injury is suspicious and concerning for a supracondylar humerus fracture. Initial management should involve evaluation for any neurovascular compromise, should as diminished pulses or decreased sensation. He should be brought to an urgent care facility or emergency department. X-ray imaging will determine if operative or non-operative treatment is needed. If non-operative, treatment may involve casting of the affected arm. A sling may also be used to assist with support. If operative management is indicated, an Orthopedic referral is needed.

Supracondylar Humerus Fractures are the most common elbow fracture in the pediatric population. It is typically caused by a FOOSH (fall on outstretched arm). There will be a painful and swollen elbow, bruising, and possibly a visible deformity. ROM is often decreased. Neurovascular injury should immediately be ruled out. Be sure to check for sensation, numbness/tingling, and motor strength [7]. Check upper extremity pulses including brachial and radial. It is important to examine for any color or temperature changes between the affected and non-affected arm, as this could warrant urgent evaluation for vascular compromise. X-ray imaging will determine the next steps, either operative vs. non-operative management. Indications for surgery may include fractures with risk of nonunion, displacement,

Table 115.2 Elbow injuries of the pediatric population

Injury	Common age group	Mechanism of injury	Presentation	Imaging	Treatment
Supracondylar humerus fracture	These fractures are more common in younger pediatric patients, less than 10 years of age.	This is typically caused by a FOOSH (fall on outstretched arm).	There will be a painful and swollen elbow, bruising, and possibly a visible deformity. ROM is often decreased.	X-ray imaging will be the initial imaging modality and will determine the next steps, either operative vs. non-operative management.	Indications for surgery may include fractures with risk of nonunion, displacement, or neurovascular compromise. Volkmann's contracture, or Volkmann's ischemic contracture, is a possible complication that may result from this injury as listed above. Non-operative treatment may include casting with or without a sling.
Little league elbow (medial epicondyle apophysitis) [10]	More common among adolescent athletes (more commonly baseball players).	Repetitive overhead/ overhand motions such as throwing, swinging a racket.	The patient will have pain at the medial epicondyle made worse with valgus stress. Different exam maneuvers using valgus torque with flexion/ extension of the elbow may reproduce pain.	X-ray imaging is the initial imaging choice. Point-of-care ultrasound may also be used in the clinical setting.	Treatment mainly involves complete rest of the affected arm for approximately 4–6 weeks. Conservative management with ice, heat, NSAIDs may be used. Physical therapy and strengthening exercises may be used once returning to activity. Medial epicondyle avulsion fracture is a common complication, and can commonly be treated with casting, splinting, and bracing. Instability and displacement may require Orthopedic intervention.

Elbow dislocation [11]	These injuries are overall uncommon in the pediatric population, but are most commonly seen in the adolescent age group.	This type of injury is usually the result of FOOSH (fall on outstretched hand). Posterior dislocations are the most common, resulting from a FOSSH injury with the elbow extended.	The patient will present with pain and decreased range of motion of the affected elbow. There may also be a visible deformity, such as a shortened appearance of the affected upper extremity.	X-ray imaging is the initial imaging f choice to evaluate for any associate fracture.	Treatment involves presentation to an urgent care facility or emergency department for closed reduction of the dislocation. Imaging may be used to evaluate for any associated fractures. Immobilization with casting/bracing may be used, followed by early active range of motion exercises. Operative management may be indicated if there is neurovascular compromise, open injury, or persistent instability.
Radial head fracture [12, 13]	This type of injury occurs most commonly in pre-teen aged pediatric patients.	These fractures are caused by FOOSH, direct trauma, or force to the affected elbow	The patient presents with pain, swelling, bruising, and limited ROM (pronation, supination) of the affected elbow. The proximal radius will be tender to palpation.	Imaging with x-ray is the initial imaging modality, and is required to determine next steps.	Further treatment includes immobilization, closed reduction, or possibly even surgery. Indications for surgery include displacement, angulation, or decreased ROM due to mechanical block. Depending on the type of radial head fracture, healing may take a few days up to 6–12 weeks. Be sure to assess neurovascular status, which if compromised, requires urgent referral to Orthopedics.

or neurovascular compromise. Volkmann's contracture, or Volkmann's ischemic contracture, is a possible complication that may result from this injury. It is caused by lack of blood flow to the forearm muscles, and results in a permanent flexion of the hand and fingers. This gives the hand and forearm a "claw-like" appearance [8]. Because of the higher risk for complications, these injuries should be managed with orthopedic consultation. Of note, these fractures can be divided into flexion type fractures and extension type fractures, with extension being much more common. The Gartland classification system further divides the extension type fractures into three sub-types. Type I fractures are classified as un-displaced transverse fractures. Type II fractures are posteriorly displaced fractures. Type III fractures are classified as oblique fractures with severe displacement and rotation [9].

Case 3 Alex is an 8-year-old on her elementary school's girls basketball team. During practice one evening, she begins having immediate left wrist pain after falling on the court while diving for a loose ball. She fell forward with both hands outstretched towards the ball on the court. Her left wrist is tender and has limited range of motion of her wrist due to the pain. There is mild swelling, but no bruising, warmth, or erythema. There are no signs or symptoms of neurovascular compromise. What do you do next?

Table 115.3 describes common wrist injuries in children and adolescents. Alex's presentation and mechanism of injury is consistent with a wrist sprain. As there is only mild swelling with no obvious physical deformities, routine imaging is not needed. Initial treatment may be conservative with wrist splinting or bracing. Without any concerns for complications, Alex may be seen her Pediatrician or an urgent care facility for splinting or bracing. Depending on the severity of the sprain, healing time may take 1–8 weeks. If wrist tenderness or decreased range of motion persist, further evaluation with imaging may be required.

Wrist sprains often involves stretching or tearing of the ligaments in the wrist. Mechanism of injury is bending, twisting, or FOOSH. The patient presents with pain, swelling, and decreased ROM secondary to pain. These injuries can be classified as mild, moderate, and severe, depending on the degree of stretching or tearing of the ligaments. Treatment involves immobilization with a wrist splint or prefabricated brace. Imaging is not routinely needed unless there are concerns for a fracture, such as carpal bone tenderness, persistent pain and swelling despite immobilization, and loss of ROM. Imaging modalities include x-ray (first line), CT, and MRI arthrogram. Healing time depends on severity of sprain and may take anywhere from 1 to 8 weeks [14]. Surgery may be indicated for complete ligament tears, especially in the scapholunate ligament.

Table 115.3 Wrist fractures of the pediatric population

Injury	Common age group	Mechanism of injury	Presentation	Imaging	Treatment
Distal radius buckle (Torus) fracture [15]	Most common in pediatrics aged 7–12 years	FOOSH injury, falling on outstretched arm; increased axial load	Pain, bruising, swelling, decreased ROM; observe for any gross deformity or neurovascular compromise	X-ray initially, be sure to obtain imaging of contralateral extremity as well; may display "buckling" of cortex of radius	If fracture is stable, will require splinting/ casting for 2–3 weeks
Colles fracture (distal radius fracture with dorsal displacement and comminution) [16]	Adolescents, pediatrics around age of puberty	FOOSH injury, falling with hand/wrist in dorsiflexion	Pain, bruising, swelling, decreased ROM, dorsiflexion deformity due to fracture displacement; observe for gross deformity and neurovascular compromise	X-ray is best initial imaging modality; CT may be used for further evaluation if surgery is indicated; MRI may be used to further evaluate for ligament or soft tissue damage	Non-operative management includes closed reduction, immobilization, and splinting/ casting for up to 6 weeks; surgery is indicated for extraarticular fractures, unstable fractures (LaFontaine criteria), progressive loss of reduction, neurovascular compromise
Monteggia fracture—ulnar fracture with radial head dislocation [17]	These fractures are more common in younger pediatric patients, less than 10 years of age.	The most common mechanism of injury is FOOSH.	Pain and swelling at the elbow and forearm, along with decreased range of motion. It is important to evaluate for any gross deformities or neurovascular compromise.	X-ray is the initial imaging of choice. Additional imaging is not routinely needed. It is important to obtain views of both the elbow and forearm.	Closed reduction and immobilization with casting is the preferred initial treatment. Operative management may be indicated if there is failure with closed reduction, instability, or neurovascular compromise.

(continued)

Table 115.3 (continued)

Injury	Common age group	Mechanism of injury	Presentation	Imaging	Treatment
Galeazzi fracture—radial fracture with distal radioulnar dislocation [18]	This type of injury is most commonly seen in pre-teens and adolescents.	These fractures are most commonly associated with FOOSH injuries.	A patient may present with pain and swelling of the forearm or wrist, along with decreased range of motion. A visible deformity may be present.	X-ray is the initial imaging of choice, with further imaging not routinely indicated. CT may be used to identify radioulnar joint dislocation.	The preferred method of treatment is closed reduction and immobilization with casting. Operative management may be indicated with failed closed reduction, degree of radioulnar disruption, or neurovascular compromise.

Extra Credit Points

1. Have an understanding of the basic exam maneuvers, including: inspection, palpation, active/passive range of motion, and special exams. Understand how to properly perform special exams such as the drop arm test, and what specific findings you are looking for.
2. As many of these injuries can present very similarly, understand how to properly differentiate and diagnose each one. An example would be the many different injuries that can result from a FOOSH injury. Utilizing physical exam maneuvers, and detailed histories can help narrow down differential diagnoses. A great example would be differentiating Galeazzi and Monteggia fractures.
3. Be sure to have a basic understanding of when a pediatric patient should be conservatively managed versus being evaluated in an emergency department. Conservative management with an urgent care facility or PCP may be appropriate if there are little to no concerns for a fracture, no visible deformities, no neurovascular compromise, no restricted range of motion due to mechanical block, and no concerns for compartment syndrome. Emergency department evaluation is warranted if there are concerns for fractures, open fractures, neurovascular compromise, decreased range of motion due to mechanical block, concerns for compartment syndrome, or if closed reduction is needed and unable to be performed remotely.

References

1. Longo UG, et al. Epidemiology of paediatric shoulder dislocation: a nationwide study in Italy from 2001 to 2014. Int J Environ Res Public Health. 2020; U.S. National Library of Medicine. www.ncbi.nlm.nih.gov/pmc/articles/PMC7215533/.
2. Morganti-Kossmann AC. Bankart and Hill-Sachs lesions of the shoulder joint. Lex Medicus, 2023. https://lexmedicus.com.au/bankart-and-hill-sachs-lesions-of-the-shoulder-joint/.
3. Clavicle Fractures. Johns Hopkins Medicine. 2021. www.hopkinsmedicine.org/health/conditions-and-diseases/clavicle-fractures.
4. Perez JR, et al. Rotator cuff tears in the pediatric population: comparing findings on arthroscopic evaluation to pre-operative magnetic resonance imaging. J Clin Orthop Trauma. 2018; U.S. National Library of Medicine. www.ncbi.nlm.nih.gov/pmc/articles/PMC5883904/.
5. Casadei K. Proximal humeral epiphysiolysis. In: StatPearls [Internet]; 2023. https://www.ncbi.nlm.nih.gov/books/NBK534301/#article-43405.s6.
6. Wahal N, Kendirci AS, Abondano C, Tauber M, Martetschläger F. Acromioclavicular joint lesions in adolescents-A systematic review and treatment guidelines. J Clin Med. 2023. https://www.ncbi.nlm.nih.gov/pmc/articles/PMC10488848/.
7. Hope N. Supracondylar humerus fractures. In: StatPearls [Internet]. U.S. National Library of Medicine; 2023. www.ncbi.nlm.nih.gov/books/NBK560933/.
8. Mirza TM. Volkmann contracture. In: StatPearls [Internet]. U.S. National Library of Medicine; 2023. www.ncbi.nlm.nih.gov/books/NBK557754/.
9. Shah M, Agashe MV. Supracondylar humerus fractures: classification based treatment algorithms. Indian J Orthop. 2020. https://www.ncbi.nlm.nih.gov/pmc/articles/PMC7851217/.
10. Hodge C. Medial epicondyle apophysitis (little league elbow). In: StatPearls [Internet]. U.S. National Library of Medicine; 2023. www.ncbi.nlm.nih.gov/books/NBK570592/#article-131176.s6.
11. Lewallen L, et al. Pediatric elbow dislocations and associated fractures. Children (Basel). 2023;10(6):993. https://doi.org/10.3390/children10060993. Accessed 25 Feb 2024.
12. Macken AA, et al. Diagnosis, treatment and complications of radial head and neck fractures in the pediatric patient. World J Orthop. 2022. U.S. National Library of Medicine. www.ncbi.nlm.nih.gov/pmc/articles/PMC8935328/.
13. Radial Head Fractures of the Elbow - Orthoinfo - Aaos. OrthoInfo. orthoinfo.aaos.org/en/diseases%2D%2Dconditions/radial-head-fractures-of-the-elbow. Accessed 16 May 2024.
14. Linkin J. Wrist sprains. The Pediatric Orthopedic Center, 5 June 2023. pediatricorthopedics.com/wrist-sprains/.
15. Asokan A. Pediatric torus buckle fracture. In: StatPearls [Internet]. U.S. National Library of Medicine; 2023. www.ncbi.nlm.nih.gov/books/NBK560634/.
16. Summers K. Colles fracture. In: StatPearls [Internet]. U.S. National Library of Medicine; 2023. www.ncbi.nlm.nih.gov/books/NBK553071/.
17. He JP, et al. Comparison of treatment methods for pediatric Monteggia fracture. Medicine. 2019;98(2):e13942. https://doi.org/10.1097/md.0000000000013942. Accessed 12 Feb 2024.
18. Eberl R, et al. Galeazzi lesions in children and adolescents: treatment and outcome. Clin Orthop Relat Res. 2008;466(7):1705–9. https://doi.org/10.1007/s11999-008-0268-6. Accessed 18 Sept 2019.

Chapter 116
The Acutely Injured Hip, Knee, and Ankle

Jeremy Swisher and Kimberly Burbank

Case 1 During a routine soccer practice, a 13-year-old boy, Noah, experiences a sudden onset of left hip pain after performing a jumping drill. He reports persistent discomfort in the left hip and has a noticeable limp. Over the next few weeks, Noah's parents observe a subtle change in his gait, with the left leg appearing slightly externally rotated. On examination, there is limited internal rotation of the left hip, pain with passive motion, and a leg length discrepancy. What do you do?

Hip pain is one of the most common complaints that pediatric orthopedic surgeons and pediatricians encounter in the clinic setting [1]. Often, children will have progressive worsening of pain around the groin (may also present with anterior or medial thigh pain and knee pain) with associated changes in gait or refusal to bear weight. The pain can often be exacerbated by physical activity. Table 116.1 discusses common hip injuries in the pediatric athlete.

The assessment should initially focus on a clinical history, including a description of the pain, trauma, or mechanism of injury, mechanical symptoms (i.e. popping, clicking, catching, snapping), systemic symptoms (i.e. fevers, night sweats), and neurological symptoms (i.e. weakness, neuropathy, altered sensation). In the field, the physical exam should be focused on assessing the patient for gait abnormality, deformity around the pelvis or hip, swelling, erythema, weakness, and tenderness to palpation over the groin, lower back, and upper leg. Special tests, including FABER (Flexion, Abduction, External Rotation), FADIR (Flexion, Adduction, Internal Rotation), Trendelenburg, or Ober, can be useful, but often may be difficult in the setting of acute injury. Diagnostic imaging is often required for definitive diagnosis [1, 2].

J. Swisher (✉) · K. Burbank
Wake Forest University School of Medicine, Winston-Salem, NC, USA

R. P. Olympia, J. Brady-Olympia (eds.), *Clinical Considerations in School-based Health*, https://doi.org/10.1007/978-3-031-85765-2_116

Table 116.1 Common Hip Injuries in the Pediatric Athlete

Diagnosis	Clinical Pearls	Disposition	Treatment
Slipped Capital Femoral Epiphysis (SCFE)	Typically occurs during growth spurts. Presents with hip or groin pain, limp, and limited internal rotation. High risk in overweight or obese pediatric athletes. The classic X-ray finding in slipped capital femoral epiphysis (SCFE) is the "ice cream scoop" sign or the absence of the intersecting Klein line between the femoral head and neck.	Referral to Orthopedics	Urgent orthopedic evaluation Non-weight bearing or limited weight-bearing on affected leg Surgical fixation
Transient Synovitis	Often follows an upper respiratory infection. Presents with hip pain, limp, and limited range of motion. X-rays are usually normal, and symptoms resolve spontaneously. Ultrasound may show a small joint effusion.	Referral to PCP or Sports Medicine	Symptom management (rest, analgesics) Follow-up as needed
Legg-Calvé-Perthes Disease	Avascular necrosis of the femoral head in children. Presents with insidious onset of hip or groin pain and limp. X-rays can be normal early, but may show fragmentation of the femoral head. MRI is more sensitive in the early stages.	Referral to Orthopedics	Observation Physical therapy Possible surgical intervention in severe cases
Hip Joint Effusion (Septic or Aseptic)	Septic effusion may present with fever and systemic symptoms. Aseptic effusion may follow trauma or be associated with inflammatory conditions. Aspiration is diagnostic and may be necessary for evaluation. Kocher Criteria can be used to distinguish septic arthritis from transient synovitis and includes non-weightbearing status, fever, elevated ESR and WBC.	Referral to ED if concerned for septic effusion Referral to PCP if there is low concern for septic effusion	Joint aspiration and culture in septic cases Treatment of underlying cause (e.g., antibiotics for septic effusion, anti-inflammatory for aseptic effusion)
Labral Tear	Often related to sports or activities with repetitive hip motions. Presents with groin pain, clicking, or locking sensations. Magnetic resonance arthrography (MRA) is a sensitive diagnostic tool and is preferred over standard MRI.	Referral to Orthopedics or Sports Medicine	Physical therapy Possible arthroscopic surgery

(continued)

Table 116.1 (continued)

Diagnosis	Clinical Pearls	Disposition	Treatment
Inguinal Hernia	More common in boys; may present with a bulge in the groin. Pain may be exacerbated with physical activity or straining. Physical examination and imaging confirm the diagnosis.	Referral to PCP or Urgent Care	Surgical repair
Apophysitis of the pelvis	Localized pain, swelling, and limited ROM. X-rays may show widening of the apophyseal growth center or displacement in severe cases. MRI may be considered in cases with unclear X-ray findings, significant soft tissue injury, or persistent pain despite conservative management.	Referral to PCP or Sports Medicine	Rest and activity modification Symptom management (analgesics, ice) Physical therapy Return to play typically occurs within 4 to 8 weeks.
Pelvic Avulsion Fracture	Commonly occurs in adolescent athletes during sports involving sudden acceleration or deceleration (e.g., sprinting, jumping). Presents with acute onset of localized pain at the site of the avulsion (e.g., anterior superior iliac spine, ischial tuberosity). X-rays may show a small bony fragment displaced from the main bone, but MRI can provide more detailed information.	Referral to PCP or Sports Medicine	Symptom management Physical therapy NSAIDs

Case 2 Hannah, a 14-year-old female basketball player, jumps for a rebound during her eighth-grade basketball practice. As she lands, she feels her right knee buckle and give out. She also reports hearing loud, popping sounds as she landed. She is only able to bear minimal weight and describes feeling unstable on her right leg. Examination reveals immediate swelling to the area. She is guarding significantly secondary to discomfort, so it is difficult to obtain an accurate Lachman's and anterior drawer test on the sideline. However, you do feel some laxity compared to her left knee. What are your next steps?

Participation in organized sports among children and adolescents in the United States is widespread, with an estimated 60 million youngsters engaging in various athletic activities annually. The knee stands out as one of the most frequently injured body parts, with an estimated 2.5 million sports-related injuries occurring in adolescents in the US each year (Table 116.2). These injuries often lead to substantial time loss from physical activity and sports participation and may necessitate surgical intervention. The most frequent traumatic knee injuries involve the cruciate and collateral ligaments, menisci, and patella. Overuse injuries commonly reported include Osgood-Schlatter disease, Sinding-Larsen-Johansson syndrome, patellofemoral pain syndrome, and various forms of tendonitis. Female athletes face a considerably higher risk of ACL injury, with a risk magnitude of 2–8 times greater than that of their male counterparts [3].

In the field, initial assessment should focus on the mechanism of injury, presence of pain, swelling, deformity, and the ability to bear weight. Specific tests such as the Lachman's or anterior drawer test may be challenging to perform accurately due to guarding and pain. However, observing for asymmetry, joint laxity, and assessing for any obvious deformity can provide valuable diagnostic clues. If feasible, immobilization with a splint or knee brace and elevation of the affected limb can help reduce pain and swelling until further evaluation by a healthcare provider. Patients presenting with suspected knee injuries, especially those associated with significant swelling, instability, or inability to bear weight, should be promptly referred for further evaluation, including imaging studies such as MRI. Urgent orthopedic consultation may be warranted for suspected ACL tears or patellar dislocations. Patients with less severe symptoms may benefit from conservative management strategies such as protection, rest, ice, compression, and elevation (PRICE) before further evaluation by a healthcare provider.

Case 3 During a friendly basketball game at the local park, 16-year-old Alex attempts a quick change of direction and feels a sudden twist in his left ankle. He falls to the ground in pain and notices immediate swelling. Alex is unable to bear weight on the affected ankle and experiences significant discomfort with any attempt to move it. What do you do?

Ankle fractures are prevalent among children and adolescents, particularly older children and teenagers, with a higher incidence in boys than girls (Table 116.3). They represent approximately 5% of all fractures and 15–20% of all physeal injuries in this age group, making them the most common pediatric lower-limb physeal injury. Most ankle fractures occur due to sports injuries or low-energy trauma, such as those encountered in basketball, soccer, or inline skating. In fact, they account for up to 40% of all fractures in skeletally immature athletes. Fractures involving the distal tibial physis pose a significant risk of complications, including premature physeal arrest, angular deformity, and articular incongruity, with reported growth arrest rates of up to 66.7%. Conversely, distal fibular physeal fractures are associated with a relatively lower risk of long-term complications.

In the field, initial assessment should focus on assessing the mechanism of injury, presence of pain, swelling, deformity, and the ability to bear weight. Performing specific tests such as the Thompson test for suspected Achilles tendon injuries or evaluating for tenderness along the ankle ligaments can provide valuable diagnostic

Table 116.2 Common Knee Injuries in the Adolescent

Diagnosis	Clinical Pearls	Disposition	Treatment
Patellofemoral Pain Syndrome (PFPS)	Common cause of anterior knee pain in pediatric athletes. Aggravated by activities such as squatting, running, or prolonged sitting (theater sign). Tenderness around the patella with no significant swelling.	Referral to PCP or Sports Medicine	Activity modification Quadriceps strengthening exercises Physical therapy
Osgood-Schlatter Disease	Traction apophysitis at the tibial tubercle. Occurs in pediatric athletes during growth spurts, especially in sports involving jumping or running. Presents with anterior knee pain and a visible, tender bump below the knee.	Referral to PCP or Sports Medicine	Activity modification Symptom management (rest, ice, NSAIDs) Quadriceps and hamstring stretching
Meniscal Tear	Often related to twisting or direct trauma. Presents with joint line tenderness and swelling. May present with mechanical symptoms such as locking or catching, which more often require surgery if present. Positive McMurray's or Thessaly test may indicate a meniscal injury.	Referral to Orthopedics	RICE protocol (Rest, Ice, Compression, Elevation) Physical therapy Arthroscopic surgery (for severe cases)
Anterior Cruciate Ligament (ACL) Injury	Common in sports with sudden stops or changes in direction. Often described as a "pop" at the time of injury. Presents with immediate pain, swelling, and instability. Positive Lachman's and anterior drawer tests suggest ACL injury.	Referral to Orthopedics	RICE protocol (Rest, Ice, Compression, Elevation) Physical therapy Surgical reconstruction (for complete tears)
Patellar Tendonitis (Jumper's Knee)	Overuse injury common in sports involving jumping. Presents with anterior knee pain, especially during activities. Tenderness over the inferior pole of the patella.	Referral to PCP or Sports Medicine	Activity modification Quadriceps and hamstring stretching Eccentric strengthening exercises

(continued)

Table 116.2 (continued)

Diagnosis	Clinical Pearls	Disposition	Treatment
Infection (Septic Arthritis or Osteomyelitis)	May present with fever, local swelling, and systemic symptoms. Joint aspiration is diagnostic for septic arthritis. Elevated CRP and ESR are often present. Imaging studies, including MRI, help identify osteomyelitis.	Referral to ED or PCP	Joint aspiration and culture (for septic arthritis) Antibiotic therapy (for septic arthritis) Surgical debridement and antibiotic therapy (for osteomyelitis)
Ligamentous Sprain (e.g., MCL or LCL)	Often results from a direct blow or forceful twisting of the knee. Presents with pain, swelling, and tenderness along the affected ligament. Stress testing may reveal laxity in the involved ligament.	Referral to PCP or Sports Medicine	RICE protocol (Rest, Ice, Compression, Elevation) Physical therapy Bracing (for stability)
Sinding-Larsen Johansson Syndrome	Apophysitis of the inferior pole of the patella. Typically seen during growth spurts. Presents with localized anterior knee pain, especially with jumping or kneeling.	Referral to PCP or Sports Medicine	Activity modification Symptom management (rest, ice, NSAIDs) Quadriceps stretching and strengthening exercises
Osteochondritis Dissecans	A condition where a fragment of bone and cartilage becomes detached from the joint surface. Commonly affects the knee joint, particularly the femoral condyles. Presents with deep, aching joint pain, swelling, and decreased range of motion. May present with locking of the knee if a fragment is loose. Xray findings may include a detached piece of bone and cartilage in the joint space	Referral to Orthopedics	Activity modification Non-weight bearing or limited weight-bearing on affected joint Physical therapy Surgical intervention (for unstable or large lesions)
Patellar Subluxation	Partial displacement of the patella from its normal position within the femoral groove. Often occurs due to an imbalance in muscle strength or anatomical factors such as trochlear dysplasia. Presents with anterior knee pain, instability, and a feeling of the knee giving way.	Referral to PCP or Sports Medicine	Activity modification Quadriceps and hip abductor strengthening exercises Patellar bracing or taping

Table 116.3 Common Ankle Injuries in the Pediatric Athlete

Diagnosis	Clinical Pearls	Disposition	Treatment
Ankle Sprain (Inversion/ Eversion)	Common cause of acute ankle pain, often related to sports or missteps. Pain, swelling, and bruising localized to the affected ligaments. Grading based on ligament injury severity (Grade I to III). **Grade I:** Mild stretch of the ligament **Grade II:** Partial tear of the ligament **Grade III:** Complete tear of the ligament	Referral to PCP or Sports Medicine	RICE protocol (Rest, Ice, Compression, Elevation) **Grade I**: Supportive care, ankle bracing, and early mobilization **Grade II**: Immobilization (boot or cast) and physical therapy **Grade III**: Surgical intervention (for severe tears)
Achilles Tendon Rupture	May occur during forceful push-off or sudden dorsiflexion of the ankle. Sudden onset of severe pain, swelling, and a palpable gap in the tendon. Thompson test: absence of plantarflexion on squeezing the calf.	Referral to Orthopedics	Surgical repair (for complete tears) Non-surgical: Immobilization (boot or cast) and physical therapy
Peroneal Tendonitis or Subluxation	Repetitive ankle inversion can lead to peroneal tendon injuries. Pain, swelling, and a snapping sensation over the lateral ankle. MRI or ultrasound helps visualize tendon abnormalities and subluxations.	Referral to PCP or Sports Medicine	RICE protocol (Rest, Ice, Compression, Elevation) NSAIDs or corticosteroid injections (for inflammation) Physical therapy

(continued)

Table 116.3 (continued)

Diagnosis	Clinical Pearls	Disposition	Treatment
Fracture	May result from trauma or repetitive stress. Tenderness, swelling, and possible deformity over the affected bone. X-rays are essential for diagnosing fractures; MRI for soft tissue injuries. Use Ottawa ankle rules—https://www.mdcalc.com/calc/1670/ottawa-ankle-rule	Referral to Orthopedics or ED	Immobilization (splint, cast, or boot) Surgical intervention (for displaced fractures)
Syndesmotic (High Ankle) Sprain	Occurs with external rotation or dorsiflexion injuries. Tenderness over the anterior aspect of the ankle, above the joint line. Positive squeeze test or external rotation stress test.	Referral to Orthopedics	RICE protocol (Rest, Ice, Compression, Elevation) Immobilization (boot or cast) Physical therapy
Talar Dome Osteochondral Lesion	Often results from trauma or repetitive microtrauma. Presents with chronic ankle pain, especially with weight-bearing. Imaging studies, including MRI or CT, help visualize the lesion.	Referral to Orthopedics	Activity modification NSAIDs or corticosteroid injections (for inflammation) Surgical intervention (for unstable lesions)
Septic Arthritis	Uncommon but may occur after penetrating trauma or systemic infection. Presents with severe pain, swelling, and systemic symptoms. Fever is not always present. Joint aspiration is diagnostic for septic arthritis.	Referral to ED or PCP	Joint aspiration and culture (for diagnosis) Antibiotic therapy (for bacterial infections) Surgical debridement (for severe cases)

clues. However, definitive diagnosis often requires clinical examination supplemented by imaging studies, particularly in cases of suspected fractures or soft tissue injuries.

Patients presenting with severe pain, inability to bear weight, significant swelling, or suspected fractures should be promptly referred for further evaluation, including imaging studies such as X-rays. Urgent orthopedic consultation may be warranted for suspected Achilles tendon ruptures, high ankle sprains, or fractures requiring immediate intervention. Patients with less severe symptoms may benefit from conservative management strategies such as protection, rest, ice, compression, and elevation (PRICE) before further evaluation by a healthcare provider.

116.1 Case Conclusions

Case 1 In Noah's case, the constellation of symptoms, including sudden onset left hip pain following physical activity, persistent discomfort, altered gait, and limited internal rotation, raises suspicion for slipped capital femoral epiphysis (SCFE), a potentially serious hip condition. SCFE is an important hip disorder in adolescents, can be more often during growth spurts, and requires prompt recognition and intervention to prevent complications such as avascular necrosis and hip deformity.

Given Noah's presentation, an urgent referral to a pediatric orthopedic specialist for further evaluation and management is warranted. Imaging studies, such as X-rays, are essential for confirming the diagnosis of SCFE and assessing the severity of slippage. Treatment typically involves surgical stabilization of the femoral head to prevent further displacement and preserve hip function [1, 2].

Case 2 Hannah's mechanism of injury, reported symptoms, and physical exam are most consistent with a torn anterior cruciate ligament (ACL). Given the high suspicion of an ACL tear, Hannah should be urgently referred to orthopedic surgery for further imaging and evaluation. If there is any concern for other pathology or fractures, the patient should be referred to the emergency department for further evaluation and coordination of care. Definitive management often involves ACL reconstruction and at least 6 months of rehabilitation following surgery.

Case 3 Based on the mechanism of injury and clinical presentation, Alex likely sustained a Weber A distal fibular fracture, an important injury seen in adolescents involved in sports activities. Immediate management involves immobilization, ice application, and elevation to reduce swelling and pain. Additionally, weight-bearing as tolerated (WBAT) in a walking-controlled ankle motion (CAM) boot can be initiated to promote early mobility and prevent stiffness. However, further evaluation, including a thorough clinical examination and possibly imaging studies such as X-rays, are crucial to confirm the diagnosis and assess the fracture's stability. Non-operative management with WBAT in a CAM boot is often effective for stable Weber A fractures, but close monitoring of symptoms and periodic follow-up appointments are essential to ensure proper healing and functional recovery. Typically, patients with stable Weber A distal fibular fractures can gradually increase weight-bearing over the course of several weeks while wearing the boot. However, specific weight-bearing instructions may vary depending on the patient's pain tolerance and fracture stability, as determined by clinical evaluation and initial imaging studies [4].

Extra Credit Points

1. Utilize a combination of clinical examination techniques such as palpation, range of motion assessment, and specific tests like the Thompson test for Achilles tendon injuries or Lachman's test for ACL tears. Imaging modalities, including

X-rays, MRI, or ultrasound, play a crucial role in confirming diagnoses, particularly for fractures or soft tissue injuries.
2. It is essential to be aware of the diverse range of conditions that can present with similar symptoms. For example, hip pain in children may stem from conditions like slipped capital femoral epiphysis (SCFE), transient synovitis, Legg-Calvé-Perthes disease, or even inguinal hernias. Knee injuries can include patellofemoral pain syndrome (PFPS), meniscal tears, and ACL injuries. Ankle injuries may involve sprains, tendon injuries, fractures, or syndesmotic sprains.
3. The Ottawa ankle rules include bony tenderness along distal 6 cm of the posterior edge of the lateral malleolus, distal 6 cm of the posterior edge of the medial malleolus, base of the fifth metatarsal, and navicular, or inability to bear weight both immediately after injury and for 4 steps during the initial evaluation. These can be used to determine the need for ankle or foot x-rays.
4. The guidelines below can help guide your decision on sending patients to the ER or an Urgent Care:

Immediate ER Referral

- Suspected fractures with significant deformity or inability to bear weight immediately after injury.
- Suspected septic arthritis with severe joint pain, swelling, and systemic symptoms.

Appropriate for Urgent Care Center

- Suspected sprains, strains, or minor fractures without significant deformity or inability to bear weight.
- Suspected tendonitis or tendon injuries presenting with localized pain, swelling, and tenderness over the affected area.
- Suspected ligamentous injuries with localized pain, swelling, and tenderness along the affected ligament, without signs of severe instability.
- Suspected non-septic joint effusion or bursitis with localized swelling and limited range of motion, particularly if traumatic or associated with inflammatory conditions.
- Suspected non-urgent musculoskeletal conditions like patellofemoral pain syndrome, transient synovitis, or minor ligamentous sprains with stable joint function.

References

1. Yagdiran A, Zarghooni K, Semler JO, Eysel P. Hip pain in children. Dtsch Arztebl Int. 2020;117(5):72–82. PMID: 32070474; PMCID: PMC7054595.
2. Houghton KM. Review for the generalist: evaluation of pediatric hip pain. Pediatr Rheumatol Online J. 2009;7:10. PMID: 19450281; PMCID: PMC2686695.

3. Butler LS, Janosky JJ, Sugimoto D. Pediatric and adolescent knee injuries: risk factors and preventive strategies. Clin Sports Med. 2022;41(4):799–820. https://doi.org/10.1016/j.csm.2022.05.011.
4. Steiger C, De Marco G, Cuérel C, Tabard-Fougère A, Chargui M, Dayer R, Ceroni D. A retrospective epidemiological cohort study of ankle fractures in children and teenagers. J Child Orthop. 2023;17(4):348–53.

Chapter 117
Hand and Foot Injuries

Avani Chopra and Olivia Waldron

117.1 Hand and Finger Injuries

Hand and finger injuries are the most commonly injured body parts in children. Such injuries are more common in boys than girls. Injury mechanisms range from crush injuries to sports-related fractures. Typically, children between 1 and 5 years old often sustain fingertip injuries while teenagers are more likely to sustain hand fractures [1].

The evaluation of a hand and finger injury includes a thorough history and a detailed hand exam assessing the neurovasculature (finger/fingertip perfusion and sensation), range of motion, tendons and soft tissues. Additional care should be taken to determine hand dominance and age of the patient as this can affect treatment choice [2]. Differential diagnosis of finger (Table 117.1) and hand (Table 117.2) injuries based on presentation and examination can lead to the disposition of the injured student. In general, most significant finger and hand injuries require Emergency Department (ED) management in the acute phase, and then long term management with a hand specialist to ensure proper healing and functionality.

Concomitant fractures are common with nail bed and fingertip injuries. Tuft fractures are the most common fracture associated with injuries that cause subungual hematomas [3]. A tuft fracture is a distal phalanx fracture from a crush injury. These injuries must be evaluated with both the bony and soft tissue/nail bed components considered together. Often antibiotics will be used due to the open nature of the fracture as well as splinting or surgical intervention. Disposition to the ED when fractures are suspected is imperative [9, 10].

A. Chopra (✉) · O. Waldron
Penn State College of Medicine, Hershey, PA, USA
e-mail: owaldron@pennstatehealth.psu.edu

R. P. Olympia, J. Brady-Olympia (eds.), *Clinical Considerations in School-based Health*, https://doi.org/10.1007/978-3-031-85765-2_117

Table 117.1 Finger Injuries in Children [3–8]

Diagnosis	Initial Presentation and Exam	Acute Disposition and Treatment
Case #1: Nail Bed Laceration and/or Avulsion	Crush mechanism (i.e. hand/fingertip stuck in a door jamb) Partial or complete removal of nail plate from the nail bed with surrounding pain and soft tissue loss Nail abnormality with or without underlying subungual hematoma	Disposition: ED for x-ray to rule out underlying fracture and suture repair with need for possible nail removal Nails that are displaced from underneath the eponychial fold need to be replaced to ensure regrowth of the nail
Case #2: Finger Dislocation	Most commonly the MC joint Pain and swelling over affected joint with visible deformity	Disposition: ED or urgent care Closed reduction with splinting Dislocations associated with fractures require hand surgery consultation
Case #3: Gamekeeper's Thumb/Skier's Thumb	Acute or chronic injury of the ulnar collateral ligament (strain or tear) leading to weakened grasp or pinching ability of the thumb Hyperextension and forced abduction of MCP joint Pain, swelling and laxity of the MCP joint Worsening of pain with extension	Disposition: ED or urgent care Requires an X-ray to rule out fracture Treatment involves splinting with a thumb spica Surgical intervention may be necessary
Case #4: Finger Sprain	Partial ligamentous tear Pain without significant laxity Lateral stress test shows pain without lateral opening	Disposition: Follow up with PCP or urgent care Immobilize with a finger splint

Case #5: Pyogenic Tenosynovitis	Puncture wound ➔ bacterial inoculation that spreads to nearby tendon sheath
	Kanavel Signs:
	  Affected finger held in a flexed position at rest
	  Tenderness along the tendon sheath
	  Pain with passive extension of the affected finger
	  Fusiform swelling
	Skin injury (i.e. abrasions, puncture wound)
		Disposition: ED
		Often requires surgical intervention for washout and debridement and intravenous antibiotics

(continued)

Table 117.1 (continued)

Diagnosis	Initial Presentation and Exam	Acute Disposition and Treatment
Subungual hematoma	Discoloration of the nail bed with throbbing pain	Disposition: Urgent care or ED for significant subungual hematomas (>50% of the nail or moderate pain) for X-ray of the finger (to rule out underlying fracture), trephination of the nail, and/or removal of the nail to identify a nail bed laceration
Seymour Fracture	Associated displaced distal phalanx fractures with overlying nail bed lacerations Visible open fracture Pain, swelling and bruising to finger tip *See Nail Bed Laceration/ avulsion above*	Disposition: ED Treatment varies but often includes washout (due to high risk of infection), and surgical fixation
Fingertip Amputation	Crush or degloving injury Avulsion of the pulp of the fingertip with or without nail bed involvement or underlying bony involvement	Disposition: ED for surgical intervention
Tuft Fractures	Associated with crush injuries Pain to the fingertip Can have associated subungual hematoma or nail bed laceration	Disposition: ED or urgent care Immobilization or reduction depending upon bony involvement; management of concomitant subungual hematoma and soft tissue repair
Jersey Finger	Named for a finger getting caught in a jersey of another player creating a pull on the tendon Avulsion of FDP from the distal phalanx	Disposition: ED or urgent care Surgical tendon repair required
Mallet Finger	Sudden DIP joint flexion (ex: jamming against an incoming ball) Partial or complete avulsion of extensor tendon from the insertion point on the distal phalanx Inability to extend the distal phalanx and associated pain	Disposition: ED or urgent care Splinting of the digit with the DIP in extension Surgery rarely necessary

Abbreviations: *DIP* Distal interphalangeal, *ED* Emergency department, *FDP* Flexor digitorum proundus, *MC* Metacarpal, *MCP* Metacarpophalangeal, *PCP* Primary care provider

Table 117.2 Hand Injuries in Children [3, 4]

Diagnosis	Initial Presentation and Exam	Disposition and Treatment
Case #6: Scaphoid Fracture	Fall on outstretched hand Anatomic snuff box tenderness Positive Watson Test (tenderness with pressure at the distal scaphoid tubercle while moving the wrist from ulnar to radiation deviation)	Disposition: ED Requires a wrist X-ray with a scaphoid view due to risk of avascular necrosis in the setting of proximal scaphoid fractures
Case #7: Boxer Fracture	Direct trauma to fourth or fifth metacarpal (ex: punching a wall, getting hit with a bat) Bruising and pain over lateral hand Loss of knuckle prominences Can be associated with skin injury (i.e. fight bite)	Disposition: ED Managed with closed reduction and immobilization in a splint If skin injury from a tooth ➔ can lead to a septic joint therefore antibiotics recommended
Case #8: Metacarpal Fracture	Direct trauma to metacarpal (MC) Can affect the head, shaft, or base Pain, swelling and bruising to affected metacarpal	Disposition: ED Treatment depends upon the degree of fracture displacement ➔ closed or open reduction with immobilization Thumb MC fractures must have the carpometacarpal joint evaluated

Abbreviations: *MC* Metacarpal

117.1.1 Finger Injury Cases

Case #1 7-year-old Jacob was rushing to class when he got his hand caught in between the door as he was entering his math class. He begins to cry and complains of pain to his whole hand but specifically his index finger. The teacher notices blood to multiple fingertips. After evaluating Jacob, you see discoloration of the nailbed with a small laceration to the tip of his index finger with associated pain. What other injury may you be worried about? How should you manage these? What are your next steps in evaluating Jacob?

Case #2 11-year-old Jason was playing basketball in gym class when he jammed his index finger into the ball and felt a popping sensation immediately followed by pain. While examining him, you notice that he cannot extend the distal interphalangeal (DIP) joint of his index finger and there is a visible deformity. What is your differential diagnosis?

Case #3 14-year-old Oliver went on a trip with the ski club at school. While skiing, he fell forward while holding his ski pole and felt his thumb get pulled backward during the fall. He complains of pain at rest. On exam, he has localized pain to the first metacarpophalangeal (MCP) joint with laxity of the joint in abduction.

Case #4 8-year-old José was playing dodgeball when he notices pain to his middle finger. On exam, he has pain with active and passive motion of the middle finger. There is no significant deformity. Upon performing a lateral stress test, he has pain but no lateral opening.

Case #5 12-year-old Alexis plays on the schools soccer team. During the championship game a few days ago, her right hand was stepped on by another player's cleat. She presents today with increasing pain in her small finger and redness that is spreading up her hand. On exam, she has pain with passive extension of her small finger and her small finger is in a flexed position at rest. There is tenderness along the tendon sheath and diffuse swelling to the finger.

117.1.2 Hand Injury Cases

Case #6 7-year-old Makayla is playing kickball in gym class. While running she falls and catches herself on her outstretched hands. On exam, she complains of pain to the lateral aspect of her left hand and thumb. She has anatomic snuff box tenderness. When the Watson test is performed, she has pain when moving her wrist ulnarly to radially.

Case 7 13-year-old Jeremy becomes angry with another student and punches his locker. He complains of pain over the dorsum of his hand. On exam, you notice bruising to his small finger with associated pain with passive and active motion.

Case 8 16-year-old Eric accidentally hits his hand with a baseball bat during a game. He has pain to his right ring finger and notices significant swelling of his finger. There is bruising and he has trouble flexing his finger into a fist. What are your differential diagnoses?

117.2 Foot and Toe Injuries

Taking a focused history is crucial when assessing foot injuries in school-aged children (Table 117.3). Begin by inquiring about the onset of pain, distinguishing whether it is acute or chronic, and clarify the context of the pain. Identify the exact location of the pain—whether it is in the toes, heel, top or bottom of the foot, or on the medial or lateral side. Assess their ability to bear weight on the affected foot, whether they can walk with full weight, partial weight, or not at all [20].

Table 117.3 Foot and Toe Injuries in Children [11–19]

Diagnosis	History	Physical Exam	Disposition and Treatment
Case 1: Plantar Fasciitis	Sub-acute onset [6] Plantar heel pain that increases with activity Typically occurs at start of sport season	Tenderness over anteromedial aspect of the heel with the foot in dorsiflexion [7]	Refer to primary care provider Activity modification Ice massage Arch supports Fascial and heel-cord stretching and strengthening Orthotics (controversial)
Case 2: Iselin's disease (Apophysitis of the fifth metatarsal)	Pain along the lateral aspect of the foot with increased activity	Tenderness and swelling over base of fifth metatarsal Pain increases with resisted eversion, extreme dorsiflexion, and plantar flexion of the foot	Refer to primary care provider Activity modification Ice NSAIDs Stretching regularly Strengthening exercises Casting or immobilization (if severe)
Case 3: Acute fracture of fifth metatarsal	Acute onset following sudden foot inversion injury Unable to bear full weight	Swelling Bruising or erythema over lateral foot Tenderness over fracture site along lateral foot	Ottawa rules: XRs indicated if (1) pain in midfoot and (2) bone tenderness at base of fifth MT, bone tenderness at navicular bone, or inability to bear weight for four steps Immobilize with CAM boot or cast Activity restriction Surgical fixation (if severe)
Case 4: Sever's disease (Calcaneal apophysitis)	Heel pain that increases with activity, particularly running and jumping	Localized tenderness of the posterior heel at the insertion of the Achilles tendon Heel-cord tightness Weakness of the ankle dorsiflexors Pain reproduced with heel squeeze	Refer to primary care provider Activity modification Ice NSAIDs Shoe inserts Supervised heel cord stretching and strengthening of dorsiflexors

(continued)

Table 117.3 (continued)

Diagnosis	History	Physical Exam	Disposition and Treatment
Case 5: Lisfranc fracture (Tarsometatarsal fracture/ dislocation due to traumatic disruption between medial cuneiform and base of the second metatarsal)	Acute onset following crush injury or forced plantarflexion and abduction of fixed foot Unable to bear full weight Pain at the midfoot	Swelling (risk of compartment syndrome with severe swelling) Bruising over plantar aspect of medial longitudinal arch	Refer to ED for XR and monitoring for compartment syndrome Immobilize with cast Activity restriction Surgical fixation (if severe)
Case 6: Metatarsal stress fractures	Pain initially occurs only with activity, but may progress to pain at rest Presents as insidious, progressively worsening pain Associated with sudden increase in training volume or intensity or changing type of sports	Localized tenderness at the fracture site Full range of motion at joint Normal muscle power and bulk	Refer to primary care provider or urgent care center Activity modification or restriction (depends on severity) Immobilize with CAM boot or cast
Case 7: Snowboarder's fracture (Fracture of the lateral process of talus)	Associated with fall from a height or other high-energy mechanism	Swelling and tenderness anterior to lateral malleolus Pain with inversion	Refer to ED or urgent care center for XR Immobilization with cast Surgical fixation (if severe)
Case 8: Phalangeal fracture	Typically associated with objects falling on to the foot or stubbing a toe	Swelling and bruising over the affected toe Localized tenderness	Tape the injured toe to the neighboring toe ("buddy taping") If open injury, refer to urgent care or ED for irrigation and debridement

Abbreviations: *NSAIDs* nonsteroidal anti-inflammatory drugs, *ED* emergency department, *XR* radiograph, *CAM* controlled ankle movement, *MT* metatarsal

Performing a thorough physical exam will help refine your diagnosis of foot injuries. Begin by inspecting the foot for visible signs such as bruising or swelling, as this may indicate a bony injury or ligament tear [11]. Palpate each region of the foot individually and palpate specific bony structures that are weaker in children relative to the ligaments and tendons [11]. These structures include the proximal fifth metatarsal, the malleoli, and the tarsal navicular. Assess for pain or weakness with various movements, including wiggling the toes, everting or inverting the foot, and pointing the foot up or down. Additionally, observe the patient walk and watch for a limp.

After diagnosing the problem, it is crucial to generate an appropriate management plan for the patient. If a fracture is suspected, refer the patient to the ED for possible x-rays. Similarly, deep open wounds or nail bed injuries should prompt an ED referral due to the potential need for thorough cleaning and antibiotic treatment [17]. These injuries are unlikely to improve with rest alone. Conversely, other injuries, typically overuse injuries, can be managed conservatively. In such cases, self-management is appropriate, as the long-term prognosis is generally favorable.

117.2.1 Foot and Toe Injury Cases

Case #1 Sarah is a 10-year-old presenting with heel pain that has been worsening over the past 2 weeks. She reports the pain is most severe when she takes her first steps in the morning or after sitting for a long period. Upon examination, there is no swelling or bruising.

Case #2 Jenna is a 12-year-old presenting with persistent pain on the outer side of her foot, specifically around the base of the fifth metatarsal. The pain has increased over the last 3 weeks, especially after soccer practice. On examination, there is localized tenderness at the growth plate of the fifth metatarsal, but no swelling or redness.

Case #3 Mackenzie is a 13-year-old presenting with sudden pain and swelling on the outer side of her foot after tripping and falling during a soccer game. She reports immediate pain at the time of injury and is unable to bear weight on the affected foot. On examination, there is noticeable swelling and bruising over the lateral foot.

Case #4 Ryan is an 11-year-old presenting with heel pain that has developed gradually over the past few months. He reports the pain is worse during and after physical activities such as running and jumping, but improves with rest. On examination, there is tenderness at the back of the heel, but no significant swelling or bruising.

Case #5 Marcus is a 14-year-old presenting with sharp pain and swelling in his midfoot following a fall during a basketball game. He reports the pain worsened when he tried to stand and walk. He has noticeable bruising on the top of his foot and difficulty bearing weight.

Case #6 James is a 15-year-old presenting with diffuse pain in the forefoot that has gradually worsened over the last month. He mentions the pain flares up during long-distance running and subsides with rest. There are no signs of acute trauma, but he reports a feeling of "aching" that doesn't completely go away. Examination reveals tenderness along the length of his second metatarsal, with no obvious swelling or redness.

Case #7 Tyler is a 13-year-old who presents with acute ankle pain following a fall while attempting a jump on his skateboard. He describes the pain as sharp and localized to the outside of his ankle. Tyler reports hearing a "pop" at the time of injury and now has difficulty bearing weight. There is noticeable swelling and tenderness around the lateral aspect of his ankle.

Case #8 Jessica, a 10-year-old gymnast, presents with acute pain in her right little toe after accidentally stubbing it against a balance beam during practice. She describes the pain as intense and throbbing, localized at the tip of her toe. Upon examination, there is noticeable bruising and tenderness at the distal phalanx of her little toe.

Extra Credit Points

1. Focused History: Inquire about the onset, mechanism of injury and exact location of pain, as well as any swelling and the child's ability to move the affected extremity or bear weight on the affected foot.
2. Thorough Physical Examination: Inspect for visible signs, palpate each region individually, compare with the uninjured finger, hand or foot, and assess pain or weakness with various movements.
3. Appropriate Management: Refer to the ED for suspected fractures or deep open wounds, and manage overuse injuries conservatively with self-management strategies.

References

1. Liao JCY, Chong AKS. Pediatric hand and wrist fractures. Clin Plast Surg. 2019;46(3):425–36. https://doi.org/10.1016/j.cps.2019.02.012.
2. Sullivan MA, Cogan CJ, Adkinson JM. Pediatric hand injuries. Plast Surg Nurs. 2016;36(3):114–20. https://doi.org/10.1097/PSN.0000000000000145.
3. Fastle R, Bothner J. Subungal hematoma. In: UpToDate. Wolters Kluwer.
4. Brown D, Adidharma W, Hespe G. Michigan manual of plastic surgery. 3rd ed. Wolters Kluwer; 2023.

5. Hartley RL, Lam J, Kinlin C, et al. Surgical and nonsurgical pediatric hand fractures: a cohort study. Plast Reconstr Surg Glob Open. 2020;8(3):e2703. https://doi.org/10.1097/GOX.0000000000002703.
6. Kiely AL, Nolan GS, Cooper LRL. The optimal management of Seymour fractures in children and adolescents: a systematic review protocol. Syst Rev. 2020;9(1):150. https://doi.org/10.1186/s13643-020-01407-5.
7. Brusalis CM, Thibaudeau S, Carrigan RB, Lin IC, Chang B, Shah AS. Clinical characteristics of pyogenic flexor tenosynovitis in pediatric patients. J Hand Surg Am. 2017;42(5):388.e1–5. https://doi.org/10.1016/j.jhsa.2017.02.007.
8. Pulos N, Kakar S. Hand and wrist injuries. Clin Sports Med. 2018;37(2):217–43. https://doi.org/10.1016/j.csm.2017.12.004.
9. Yorlets RR, Busa K, Eberlin KR, et al. Fingertip injuries in children: epidemiology, financial burden, and implications for prevention. Hand (New York, N,Y). 2017;12(4):342–7. https://doi.org/10.1177/1558944716670139.
10. Kilincoglu V, Gonder N, Demir IH, Acikgoz I, Karsli B. Fixation of open, unstable tuft fractures in toddlers and preschool-aged children using a 25-gauge hypodermic needle. J Pediatr Orthop B. 2022;31(5):486–92. https://doi.org/10.1097/BPB.0000000000000920.
11. Pommering TL, Kluchurosky L, Hall SL. Ankle and foot injuries in pediatric and adult athletes. Prim Care. 2005;32(1):133–61. https://doi.org/10.1016/j.pop.2004.11.003.
12. Green A. The pediatric foot and ankle. Pediatr Clin N Am. 2020;67(1):169–83. https://doi.org/10.1016/j.pcl.2019.09.007.
13. Davis WA, Yagnik GP. In-Season management of acute and subacute sports foot injuries. Foot Ankle Clin. 2021;26(1):187–203. https://doi.org/10.1016/j.fcl.2020.12.001.
14. Kishan TV, Mekala A, Bonala N, Sri PB. Iselin's disease: traction apophysitis of the fifth metatarsal base, a rare cause of lateral foot pain. Med J Armed Forces India. 2016;72(3):299–301. https://doi.org/10.1016/j.mjafi.2015.06.015.
15. Roche AJ, Calder JDF. Treatment and return to sport following a Jones fracture of the fifth metatarsal: a systematic review. Knee Surg Sports Traumatol Arthrosc. 2013;21(6):1307–15. https://doi.org/10.1007/s00167-012-2138-8.
16. Christopher NC, Congeni J. Overuse injuries in the pediatric athlete: evaluation, initial management, and strategies for prevention. Clin Pediatr Emerg Med. 2002;3(2):118–28. https://doi.org/10.1053/epem.2002.126514.
17. Gill LA, Klingele KE. Management of foot and ankle injuries in pediatric and adolescent athletes: a narrative review. ORR. 2018;10:19–30. https://doi.org/10.2147/ORR.S129990.
18. Leibner ED, Simanovsky N, Abu-Sneinah K, Nyska M, Porat S. Fractures of the lateral process of the Talus in children. J Pediatr Orthop B. 2001;10(1):68–72.
19. Ribbans WJ, Natarajan R, Alavala S. Pediatric foot fractures. Clin Orthop Relat Res. 2005;432:107–15. https://doi.org/10.1097/01.blo.0000156451.40395.fc.
20. Houghton KM. Review for the generalist: evaluation of pediatric foot and ankle pain. Pediatr Rheumatol. 2008;6(1):6. https://doi.org/10.1186/1546-0096-6-6.

Chapter 118
Overuse Injuries in School Athletes

Robert T. Tisherman and Jennifer M. Dunnick

In this chapter we will focus on overuse injuries in the student athlete at the high school and collegiate level. There are an abundance of overuse injuries which can be secondary to poor mechanics during sport, increased training intensity, or renewal of training after a prolonged pause, such as summer or winter breaks. These overuse injuries are often insidious in onset and can take weeks to months to finally diagnose and treat. Prompt recognition of these injuries can improve overall health of your students and reduce the amount of time until they can return to normal sports and activities.

We will focus on each of these injuries in terms of their typical history, physical examination findings, management, and prevention. Presentations with chronic overuse injuries can vary, but we will discuss the most common presentations (Table 118.1).

Case 1 12-year-old male basketball player presents with 2 months of worsening anterior knee pain along his patellar tendon distally. Pain is worse when going up and down steps and when he tries to jump. His mother has given him intermittent ibuprofen, and this improves his pain. He has noticed swelling over the lower portion of his patella over the last 2 months.

118.1 Tendinitis

Tendinitis is the most common overuse injury seen across all age groups and in all sports. During training activities and sports, the muscles and tendons in our bodies constantly undergo micro-injuries, which are healed during rest periods. When this

R. T. Tisherman (✉) · J. M. Dunnick
Duke University Hospital, Durham, NC, USA
e-mail: Robert.tisherman@duke.edu; Jennifer.dunnick@duke.edu

R. P. Olympia, J. Brady-Olympia (eds.), *Clinical Considerations in School-based Health*, https://doi.org/10.1007/978-3-031-85765-2_118

Table 118.1 Summary of common overuse injuries seen in adolescent and college-level athletes by body location. Where applicable, the most common sport associated with each injury is noted

Body Location	Injuries (*most common sports if applicable*)
Shoulder	Rotator cuff tendinitis Subacromial or internal Impingement Little League shoulder (*baseball*)
Elbow	Medial ulnar collateral ligament injury (*baseball*) Little League elbow (*baseball*) Medial epicondylitis/"Golfer's elbow" Lateral epicondylitis/"Tennis elbow"
Hip	Femoral neck stress fracture (*running*) Labral tear
Knee	Osgood-Schlatter's/Tibial tubercle apophysitis "Shin splints" (*running*) Tibial stress fractures (*running*) Patellar tendinitis Quadriceps tendinitis Patellofemoral syndrome
Foot and Ankle	Navicular Stress fracture (*basketball, dance*) Fifth metatarsal fracture (*basketball*) Calcaneal stress fracture (*running*) Peroneal tendinitis Anterior Ankle Impingement (*football*) Sever's Disease/Achilles tendinitis

healing response is unable to keep up with the training, or the healing response leads to pathologic tissue that does not function as well as native tissue, pain and dysfunction can occur. These overuse injuries often go under-managed for weeks to months and can result in significant pain and dysfunction in students. As students reach periods of growth in their early teenage years, they can be at particularly high risk for tendinitis around the knee and ankle.

Management of tendinitis consists of resting the affected extremity with supplemental use of non-steroidal anti-inflammatories (NSAIDs), ice, stretching, and heat as tolerated. Cryotherapy (ice packs, gel packs, cold water immersion) can help with recovery by reducing inflammation and swelling through local tissue vasoconstriction. There is strong evidence that both eccentric and heavy slow resistance exercises can improve symptoms and allow for return to normal activity [1]. It is important to keep the student out of competition, or other activities which can repeat the microtrauma to the tendon, until their symptoms have begun to resolve. Once symptoms abate, progressive return to play can be attempted.

Case 2 ***14-year-old female cross-country running presents with 4 weeks of worsening groin pain. She was increasing her distance and trying to lose weight to improve her times just prior to the pain starting. Initially, pain was only when she would go further than 4 miles, but now is hurting even with walking. She has pain with passive internal and external rotation of her hip while sitting.***

118.2 Stress Fractures

The lower extremity is more prone to stress fractures as it is weight bearing. Stress fractures of the upper extremities are extremely rare but can occur in the wrist and at the elbow.

118.3 Femoral Neck Fractures

Femoral neck stress fractures are one of the most clinically significant overuse injuries that can lead to permanent disability in students. These are most commonly seen in long distance runners but can occur in any student who does repetitive running activities. Classically, they have been described in younger individuals who have chronic energy deficits secondary to malnutrition, eating disorders, or overtraining. There should be a high index of concern for this in any athlete who presents with new onset or worsening hip pain. Initially, patients will typically only complain of pain while they are running. They may even be able to note the distance they can run before they feel the pain. As the stress fracture progresses, patients may notice that they even have pain with walking. Typical presentations of this include primarily groin pain and as the stress fracture becomes worse, patients can feel pain with even passive internal and external rotation of their hip. Plain x-rays will often miss femoral neck stress fractures unless there is a sclerotic reaction to the fracture. If there is a high suspicion, MRI is the gold standard and should be utilized in almost all cases.

Management of suspected femoral neck stress fractures is complex. If a student is complaining of progressive groin pain, especially if present with low-energy activities such as walking, they should be made non-weight bearing with crutches and referred to an orthopaedic surgeon for immediate evaluation.

118.4 Tibial Stress Fractures and Medial Tibial Stress Syndrome ("Shin Splints")

Similar to femoral neck stress fractures, tibial stress fractures are common in runners after increasing their distance or changing the intensity of their workout routine. These can present with worsening shin pain. This can be clouded as there is very little difference in initial presentation between what is colloquially called "shin splints", also known as medial tibial stress syndrome, and a developing tibial stress fracture. True fractures through the tibia are very rare, but they can happen and are associated with significant morbidity. Shin splints, on the other hand, are an overuse injury which is caused by repetitive pulling of the anterior tibialis muscle against the periosteum of the anterior tibia. The location of the pain is often overlapping.

Students will typically present with tenderness palpation over their anterior tibia as well as some swelling of the area for both conditions. This pain is often responsive to activity modification and NSAIDs.

Initial management should be evaluation with radiographs. If there is concern for a tibial stress fracture on x-rays, MRI or CT can be used to further evaluate this.

Cessation of running is the mainstay of management for both conditions. Often, patients will need to be kept out of running for a period of 2–4 weeks as these symptoms begin to resolve. Students should work on stretching of their anterior tibialis with plantar flexion of the ankle to alleviate some of the pain and stress along the anterior tibialis periosteum. If there is beaking or a periosteal stress reaction seen on radiographs or advanced imaging, a physician should be consulted to determine if this may need surgical intervention or can continue to be managed non-operatively.

118.5 Foot and Ankle Stress Fractures

Stress fractures of the foot and ankle are extremely common injuries which occur in all sports and can be due to overuse in almost any position of any sport. The most common stress fractures seen in the foot and ankle are fifth metatarsal fractures and navicular fractures, but stress fractures of the calcaneus and metatarsals are all possible and should be included in the differential of foot pain in an overuse situation.

118.6 Navicular Fractures

Navicular stress fractures are seen commonly in gymnasts and cheerleaders who have particularly high needs for flexibility of their feet due to the nature of their sports. They can also be seen in basketball and football players due to the repetitive ankle flexion they undergo. Pain is typically over the dorsum of the foot, slightly medial to the midline and is worse with forced forefoot inversion on physical examination.

118.6.1 Fifth Metatarsal Fractures

Fifth metatarsal fractures are common injuries seen across all sports, presenting either as acute injuries or chronic overuse from overloading the lateral edge of the foot in patients with a high foot arch. Stress fractures of the fifth metatarsal present with pain over the lateral edge of the foot with palpation and during ambulation. There may be focal swelling over the lateral edge of the foot as well.

For most foot stress fractures, immobilization in a boot for a period of 2 weeks should be initial management and then progressive mobilization if pain has resolved. If pain returns, a longer period of immobilization or non-weight bearing may be necessary. In rare cases, due to poor blood supply to the body of the navicular bone and fifth metatarsal, surgery may be necessary to stabilize the navicular and aid in healing. Due to the chronic nature of these injuries and the poor blood supply to the fifth metatarsal, they often require invasive intervention in the form of injections or surgery to promote healing. Any students with a history of fifth metatarsal stress fractures should have appropriate footwear with lateral posting inserts or orthotics to prevent overloading of the lateral compartment [2].

Case 3 ***14-year-old male baseball player presents with progressive shoulder pain in his pitching arm. He is a starting pitcher for the school team and plays on a U-16 travel team. He practices 5–6 days per week, sometimes twice per day, and has been pitching 4–5 innings at least twice a week. He gets mild relief from ibuprofen, but he has noticed his pitch velocity is decreasing and his pain is getting worse.***

118.7 Little League Shoulder

"Little League" shoulder is a unique entity seen in baseball players, especially with the increasing prevalence early sports specialization. "Little League" shoulder involves injury to the growth plate due to repetitive strain from pitching. This will typically present as decreased pitch speed and slowly evolve into worsening shoulder pain, most often along the anterior or lateral shoulder. Students are most at risk for this during their accelerated high steel growth stages, between the ages of 11 and 16 years old.

Plain radiographs may show lateral widening of the growth plate, but this can also be subtle and may require comparison films of the contralateral arm. Physical examination will often reveal loss of internal rotation, what is called glenohumeral internal rotation deficit (GIRD), which occurs in most baseball pitchers. This loss of internal rotation is evaluation with the arm in 90 degrees of abduction and should be compared to the contralateral arm.

If there is concern for "Little League" shoulder or confirmation of widening on radiographs, initial management should consist of a period of rest until pain is resolved. Students can slowly resume normal activities if they remain painless. Interventions such as strict pitch counts have helped with the long-term prevention of this disease. However, many patients are on multiple teams, including school and traveling teams, which do not always communicate with one another. Coaches are often unaware that their player is exceeding what has been determined to be safe. After a period of rest, the students can be slowly advanced into a return to pitching. Students with this injury should also have their pitching biomechanics evaluated by a trainer or physical therapy, as this may contribute to the development of this disease process in the first place. If ignored, continued throwing can lead to a fracture through the growth plate of the proximal humerus, so prompt evaluation is necessary. This condition typically resolves as the patient reaches skeletal maturity, at approximately 15 or 16 years of age [3].

118.8 "Little League" Elbow/Ulnar Collateral Ligament Injury of the Elbow

Baseball pitchers place extreme valgus stress on the elbows during pitching and are at increased risk for overuse injuries of the ulnar-sided soft tissue structures. The ulnar collateral ligament (UCL) is the primary restraint to valgus stress of the elbow and repetitive stress seen in younger pitchers can lead to tears of the UCL or injury to the growth plate. Again, pitch count maximums have been implemented in an attempt to protect players from these type of overuse injuries, but these do not prevent all injuries [4]. During pitching, the elbow can see five times the pitchers body weight of force. This repetitive trauma can cause attrition of the ligament or stress across the growth plate. Students typically present with pain along their medial elbow, as well as loss of pitch speed. They will feel this most during the cocking phase at the very top of their pitch, when the valgus moment is maximum. Plain radiographs should be used for initial evaluation and may show widening of the medial epicondylar physis, where the UCL inserts, but are often normal. Diagnosis is primarily based on physical examination findings of tenderness along the medial aspect of the elbow, worse with valgus motion.

Management of "Little League" elbow is similar to "Little League" shoulder: pitching rest can be used for initial management with a progressive return to pitching and maintaining strict counts. In patients with recurrent symptoms, surgery with UCL reconstruction may be necessary, also known as the "Tommy John" procedure. If trying non-operative management, rest for 3 months and progressive return to sports has been shown to successfully allow around 42% of athletes to return to throwing [5]. Alternatively, with reconstruction, return to sport rates of 80–90% have been cited [5].

118.9 Modern Treatment Modalities

Non-operative management strategies for musculoskeletal injuries and overuse injuries have evolved in the last two decades to include advanced rehabilitation strategies and injection options. Orthobiologics is a broad term for injections of the patient's own adipose-derived mesenchymal stem cells, embryonal stem cells, or the patient's blood products (platelet-rich plasma (PRP), e.g.) for the purposes of concentrating cytokines and anti-inflammatory products in the area that is affected.

PRP has been used widely to treat tendinitis with varied results and is typically an out-of-pocket cost to patients. The use of adipose-derived stem cells, embryonic stem cells, and platelet-rich plasma injections in overuse injuries is controversial and the literature is varied as to their efficacy [6].

Rehabilitation of overuse injuries in complex and joint-dependent, but there are general principles which can improve muscle recovery and function. Protocols focusing on eccentric exercises (lengthening the muscle under tension) improve muscle strength and rehabilitation faster than concentric exercises (shortening the muscle under tension). Heavy, slow resistance training is another modality commonly used in tendinitis because it promotes remodeling of the tendon. Heavy, slow resistance uses sub-maximal weight (approximately 70–80% of maximum weight) with a low number of repetitions (6–8) at a much slower pace than most exercises (6–8 seconds per repetition is commonly used). This keeps the tendon fibers under load for a longer period of time and does not rely on the elastic properties of the tendon, which are loaded at higher speeds [1].

Adjunct therapeutic options for students with tendon and muscle pain from overuse injuries include cold immersion, shockwave therapy and kinesio taping. Cold-water or ice-bath immersion have both been shown to improve muscle recovery after workouts through reducing inflammation and delayed-onset muscle soreness through vasoconstriction. Extracorporeal shockwave therapy utilizes a machine that creates a forceful soundwave transdermally, which leads to increased local cytokine release and tendon remodeling. It has been shown to improve pain with Achilles tendinitis, plantar fasciitis, and lateral epicondylitis, but its use in other conditions is currently under-studied [7]. Kinesio taping, or KT, is a frequently used technique. Flexible taping around joints provides stability and increases athletes' proprioception abilities. There is moderate evidence that it improves ankle stability and may improve symptoms related to shoulder tendinitis, but the evidence is inconclusive for its effects on pain and stability across most overuse injuries [8].

118.10 Prevention Strategies

There are multiple intrinsic and extrinsic factors which place students at risk for injury. Intrinsic factors, such as gender, abnormally high or low body mass index, and certain anatomic variants, can increase student's risk for developing overuse injuries, but these are mostly non-modifiable. All teams should employ prevention strategies for overuse injuries that focus on extrinsic factors, such as repetitive loading without adequate change to recover, muscle imbalances, or poor biomechanics. Pitch-counts in baseball and softball have been shown to reduce the rates of shoulder injury in pitchers and should be counted across all teams that students play on. For running sports, hip strengthening programs and assessment of running biomechanics may reduce rates for medial tibia stress syndrome, patellofemoral pain, and patellar tendinitis. Students who are at risk for stress fractures are those who have a chronic calorie deficit, whether due to an eating disorder or overtraining. Monitoring students for calories deficits and providing appropriate dietary education is essential to reduce the risk for stress fracture development. Amenorrhea may be an additional sign of chronic caloric deficit in female students and should be asked about during health assessments. Overall, prevention of all overuse injuries is possible and mitigation efforts can improve student health and wellbeing.

Extra Credit Points

1. Most overuse injuries can be managed with rest and a progressive return to sport, but some injuries should not be ignored—including progressive hip pain or shin pain
2. Sport- and position-specific injuries are common and therapy is tailored to the specific muscle groups involved
3. Anti-inflammatory medications and ice have been shown to have synergistic effects on pain relief and promoting return to normal activities

References

1. Lim HY, Wong SH. Effects of isometric, eccentric, or heavy slow resistance exercises on pain and function in individuals with patellar tendinopathy: a systematic review. Physiother Res Int. 2018;23(4):e1721. https://doi.org/10.1002/pri.1721.
2. Patel KA, Christopher ZK, Hubbard CE, O'Malley MJ. Stress fractures of the fifth metatarsal in athletes. J Am Acad Orthop Surg. 2021;29(12):507–17. https://doi.org/10.5435/JAAOS-D-20-01060.
3. Bednar ED, Kay J, Memon M, Simunovic N, Purcell L, Ayeni OR. Diagnosis and management of little league shoulder: a systematic review. Orthop J Sport Med. 2021;9(7):23259671211017564. https://doi.org/10.1177/23259671211017563.
4. Reiman MP, Walker MD, Peters S, Kilborn E, Thigpen CA, Garrigues GE. Risk factors for ulnar collateral ligament injury in professional and amateur baseball players: a systematic review with meta-analysis. J Shoulder Elb Surg. 2019;28(1):186–95. https://doi.org/10.1016/j.jse.2018.08.018.
5. Zaremski JL, Vincent KR, Vincent HK. Elbow ulnar collateral ligament: injury, treatment options, and recovery in overhead throwing athletes. Curr Sports Med Rep. 2019;18(9):338–45. https://doi.org/10.1249/JSR.0000000000000629.
6. Mautner K, Gottschalk M, Boden SD, Akard A, Bae WC, Black L, et al. Cell-based versus corticosteroid injections for knee pain in osteoarthritis: a randomized phase 3 trial. Nat Med. 2023;29(12):3120–6. https://doi.org/10.1038/s41591-023-02632-w.
7. Auersperg V, Trieb K. Extracorporeal shock wave therapy: an update. EFORT Open Rev. 2020;5(10):584–92. https://doi.org/10.1302/2058-5241.5.190067.
8. Biz C, Nicoletti P, Tomasin M, Bragazzi NL, Di Rubbo G, Ruggieri P. Is kinesio taping effective for sport performance and ankle function of athletes with Chronic Ankle Instability (CAI)? A systematic review and meta-analysis. Medicina (Kaunas). 2022;58(5) https://doi.org/10.3390/medicina58050620.

Chapter 119
Back Injuries and Pain

Kiran Mullur, Matthew Waldrop, and Chris Nelson

Case 1 Following lacrosse practice, 12-year-old Madison presents to your office with back pain. She has been complaining of low back pain for almost 7 weeks that gets worse with activity. She does not remember a specific inciting event. She denies radiating symptoms, weakness, loss of bowel or bladder control, or constitutional symptoms. Her vital signs are normal. What should you do?

Pediatric back pain is much more common than previously assumed, with a lifetime prevalence of 40% in patients ≤18 years old [1, 2] and 4.8% of kids aged 8–16 identified as having chronic back pain [1, 3]. In pediatric and adolescent patients, back pain is associated with both overuse and inadequate conditioning [1, 4–7]. Specifically, sports such as football, basketball, and soccer that involve twisting, extension, and axial loading of the spine increase risk of back pain [1, 5, 8]. The diagnosis of pediatric back pain can be challenging, often with overlapping symptoms and uncertain time frames. Many cases are due to idiopathic mechanical causes [1]. The evaluation of a child complaining of back pain without an acute injury includes a thorough history and physical examination, focusing on timeline of symptoms, associated symptoms, identifying common risk factors, and evaluating for sensorineural deficits. These will ultimately guide next steps in the management of various pathologies known to cause back pain in pediatric and adolescent patients (Table 119.1).

In an effort to decrease unnecessary radiation exposure in pediatric patients, the American College of Radiology recommends delaying imaging unless the patient experiences neurologic deficits, nighttime pain, symptoms radiating to extremities, or symptoms lasting ≥4 weeks [9, 23]. If any of those criteria are met, plain AP and lateral radiographs should be obtained without oblique or spot views as they add further unnecessary radiation exposure [9, 24, 25].

K. Mullur (✉) · M. Waldrop · C. Nelson
Wake Forest University School of Medicine, Winston-Salem, NC, USA
e-mail: kmullur@wakehealth.edu; mdwaldro@wakehealth.edu; chmnelso@wakehealth.edu

R. P. Olympia, J. Brady-Olympia (eds.), *Clinical Considerations in School-based Health*, https://doi.org/10.1007/978-3-031-85765-2_119

Table 119.1 Chronic Back Pain in Pediatric and Adolescent Patients [9]

	Initial presentation	Disposition and treatment
Spondylolysis	Pain & decreased ROM with lumbar extension +/− LE radiation + hamstring tightness [10] + Stork Test (balance on one leg & extend spine) [11]	XR [12] Rest & PT: 90% resolve [10, 13] Bracing only if constant pain [13–16] MRI if no improvement or concern for stress fracture [12] Surgery last resort [12]
Scoliosis	Progressive constant pain Associated deformity of spine Symptoms develop in 2–3% adolescents [17]	Full spine XR Spine surgeon referral if [18]: (a) <12 years-old (b) Significant pain (c) Progressive disease (d) Structural defects (e) Cobb angle >20 degrees
Inflammatory Spondyloarthropathy	Polyarthritis Uveitis Morning stiffness SI joint TTP	XR Labs: HLA-B27, RF, ESR, CRP Referral to Pediatric Rheumatology
Iliac Crest Apophysitis	Most from 12 to 17 years-old RFs: tight hip & thigh muscles TTP along iliac crest Progressive pain with activity	POCUS with tenderness to sono-palpation Rest, ice, PRN NSAIDs PT
Scheuermann Kyphosis	Poor & rigid posture Does not improve with extension or supine [19] Upper back pain worse at end of day, relieved by rest	XR Reassurance & PT MRI if no improvement If pain or affects breathing, consider surgery [20, 21] Pain improves with age [22]
Chronic Widespread Pain (ex: Fibromyalgia)	Most common >9 years-old Pain not limited to back 3+ months of generalized pain & TTP Fatigue Light, sound & smell sensitivity	Multidisciplinary treatment: (a) Education (b) Exercise (c) Cognitive Behavior Therapy Consider medications: TCA

Abbreviations: *ROM* range of motion, *LE* lower extremity, *XR* X-ray, *PT* physical therapy, *MRI* magnetic resonance imaging, *SI* sacroiliac, *TTP* tenderness to palpation, *RF* rheumatoid factor, *ESR* erythrocyte sedimentation rate, *CRP* C-reactive protein, *RFs* risk factors, *POCUS* point of care ultrasound, *PRN* as needed, *NSAID* non-steroidal anti-inflammatory drug, *TCA* tricyclic antidepressant

Figure 119.1 outlines an algorithm that may help school healthcare providers determine next steps for a student presenting with back pain, including the need for imaging studies.

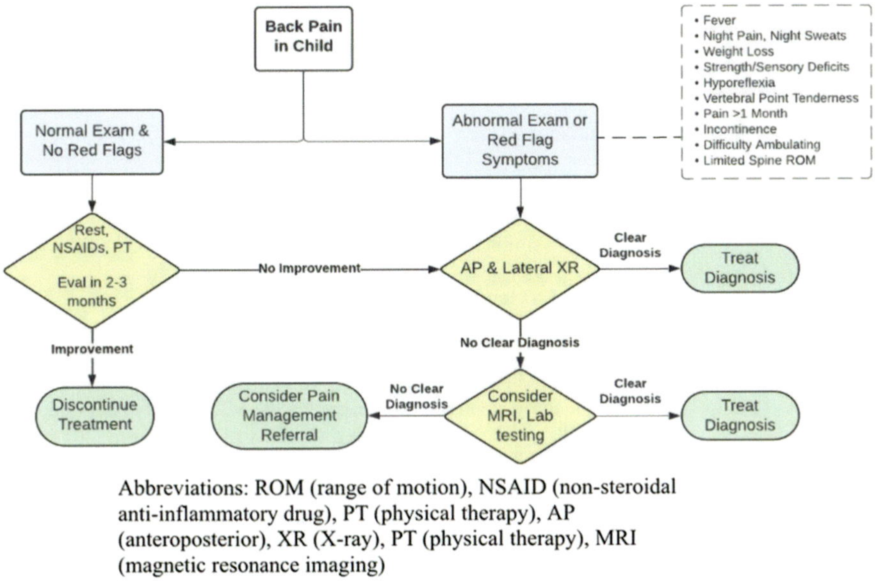

Fig. 119.1 Algorithm for the evaluation of a student with back pain [9]

Case 2 Your presence is requested on the playground to evaluate 8-year-old Jerome, who sustained a back injury while playing two-hand-touch football during recess. While he was running with the ball, he was pushed into a nearby picnic table, and his back directly impacted the side of the wooden table. He is crying, complains of significant back pain and left leg numbness. His vital signs are stable and within normal limits. What should you do?

While acute thoracolumbar injuries are not as common as cervical spine injuries, they can still be dangerous. Pediatric bones are more compressible and elastic than adult bones. Therefore, trauma does not lead to direct bony injury as often. Because of their immature skeletal systems, pediatric patients can have an increased risk of severe nerve injury, especially from birth to 9-years-old [26–29]. Injuries in the thoracolumbar region are also at higher risk of gastrointestinal system injuries [26, 30], so it is important to take acute back injuries very seriously.

With acute back pain in pediatric patients, spinal cord injuries are the first and most important etiology to rule out. The mechanism of injury often leads to a consideration of spinal cord injury. The patient should be encouraged to stay in current position, while orientation, sensation, and strength questions are asked. Following that, a brief neuromuscular exam should be performed on bilateral upper and lower extremities. Sensorineural deficits heighten concern for spinal cord injury and the patient should be transported immediately to the emergency department for trauma survey and spinal survey. Only 30–40% of pediatric patients with spinal cord injuries have abnormal findings on X-ray [26, 31–33], so if suspicion is high and X-ray is negative, they should undergo CT scan followed by MRI [26, 34]. In these

Table 119.2 Acute Back Pain in Pediatric and Adolescent Patients [9]

Diagnosis	Initial presentation	Disposition and treatment
Paraspinous Muscle Strain	Pain lateral to spine +/− TTP Without radiation to UE/LE	No imaging needed Rest & PT Resolves in a few weeks [35]
Herniated Disk	LBP with radiation to LE Pain worse with Valsalva + SLR [36], + slump test [37] Reduced ROM w/ lumbar flexion	XR [38] Rest & PT MRI if no improvement at 6 weeks [37] Consider surgery as last resort
Apophyseal Ring Fracture	LBP with radiation to LE Pain worse with Valsalva RF's: axial loading, central obesity [39, 40]	XR often negative Rest, PT—if no improvement: CT can detect, but MRI usually better due improved visibility of nerve tissue [40] Consider surgery as last resort
Vertebral Fracture	Midline bony point TTP Radiation to UE/LE UE/LE weakness & numbness Hyporeflexia possible	EMS activation to the ED Spinal precautions Urgent XR & MRI Stat orthopedic surgery consult
Neoplasm/Tumor/Infection	Fever Worsening of pain at night Night sweats Weight loss Other generalized symptoms	EMS activation to the ED Urgent XR & MRI Stat neurosurgery & oncology consults

Abbreviations: *TTP* tenderness to palpation, *UE* upper extremity, *LE* lower extremity, *PT* physical therapy, *LBP* low back pain, *SLR* straight leg raise, *ROM* range of motion, *XR* X-ray, *MRI* magnetic resonance imaging, *RF* risk factor, *EMS* emergency medical services, *ED* emergency department

scenarios, the benefit of early identification of a spinal cord injury far outweighs the risk of additional radiation to pediatric patients. Following the initial evaluation and exclusion of spinal cord injury, a more complete history and physical exam can be performed to evaluate other causes of acute back pain in the pediatric population (Table 119.2).

119.1 Case Conclusions

Case 1 *You performed a physical exam on Madison, which revealed pain with lumbar spine extension, and pain with stork test. While performing a negative straight leg raise test, you also noted she had tight hamstring muscles. You ordered AP and Lateral Lumbar Spine X-rays which showed L5 spondylolysis. You advised her to rest and sent her to physical therapy. Symptoms resolved, and she gradually returned to full participation over the next 5 months.*

Case 2 *You performed a physical exam on Jerome, where you noted decreased strength, sensation, and reflexes in his left leg. He was taken to the emergency department by EMS. Stat X-ray revealed nondisplaced fractures of L3 and L4 vertebrae. Stat MRI revealed no acute spinal cord compression, and he was diagnosed with a transient nerve injury with moderate improvement of symptoms within hours. Orthopedic surgery was consulted, he was treated nonoperatively, symptoms resolved, and he returned to his previous state of activity following a period of relative immobilization.*

Extra Credit Points

1. A majority of back pain in pediatric patients is benign in nature and will resolve with relative rest and physical therapy. Lack of response to conservative treatment warrants exploration of alternative diagnoses.
2. To avoid missing more malignant causes of back pain, counsel students and families on "red flag symptoms" and return precautions, such as fevers, night sweats, numbness, weakness, and loss of bowel or bladder control.
3. Limit unnecessary radiation exposure by delaying imaging unless the patient experiences neurologic deficits, nighttime pain, symptoms radiating to extremities, or symptoms lasting ≥4 weeks.
4. If there is any concern for a spinal cord injury, minimize patient movement, and call EMS for transport to the ED for a full trauma and spine survey.

References

1. Lamb M, Brenner JS. Back pain in children and adolescents. Pediatr Rev. 2020;41(11):557–69. https://doi.org/10.1542/pir.2019-0051.
2. Calvo-Muñoz I, Gómez-Conesa A, Sánchez-Meca J. Prevalence of low back pain in children and adolescents: a meta-analysis. BMC Pediatr. 2013;13:14. https://doi.org/10.1186/1471-2431-13-14. PMID: 23351394; PMCID: PMC3571904.
3. Huguet A, Miró J. The severity of chronic pediatric pain: an epidemiological study. J Pain. 2008;9(3):226–36. https://doi.org/10.1016/j.jpain.2007.10.015. Epub 2007 Dec 21.
4. Taimela S, Kujala UM, Salminen JJ, Viljanen T. The prevalence of low back pain among children and adolescents: a nationwide, cohort-based questionnaire survey in Finland. Spine. 1997;22(10):1132–6.
5. Jones GT, Macfarlane GJ. Epidemiology of low back pain in children and adolescents. Arch Dis Child. 2005;90(3):312–6.
6. MacDonald J, Stuart E, Rodenberg R. Musculoskeletal low back pain in school-aged children: a review. JAMA Pediatr. 2017;171(3):280–7.
7. Sato T, Ito T, Hirano T, et al. Low back pain in childhood and adolescence: assessment of sports activities. Eur Spine J. 2011;20(1):94–9.
8. Haus BM, Micheli LJ. Back pain in the pediatric and adolescent athlete. Clin Sports Med. 2012;31(3):423–40.
9. Achar S, Yamanaka J. Back pain in children and adolescents. Am Fam Physician. 2020;102(1):19–28.
10. Sato M, Mase Y, Sairyo K. Active stretching for lower extremity muscle tightness in pediatric patients with lumbar spondylolysis. J Med Investig. 2017;64(1.2):136–9.

11. Stork Test (2024, March 10). Physiopedia. Retrieved 22:14, 29 May 2024.
12. Bouras T, Korovessis P. Management of spondylolysis and low-grade spondylolisthesis in fine athletes. A comprehensive review. Eur J Orthop Surg Traumatol. 2015;25(suppl 1):S167–75.
13. Klein G, Mehlman CT, McCarty M. Nonoperative treatment of spondylolysis and grade I spondylolisthesis in children and young adults: a meta-analysis of observational studies. J Pediatr Orthop. 2009;29(2):146–56.
14. Virkki E, Holstila M, Mattila K, et al. Radiographic outcomes of immobilization using Boston brace for pediatric spondylolysis [published online January 1, 2020]. Scand J Surg. Accessed 20 April 2020. https://journals.sagepub.com/doi/full/10.1177/1457496919896998.
15. Panteliadis P, Nagra NS, Edwards KL, et al. Athletic population with spondylolysis: review of outcomes following surgical repair or conservative management. Global Spine J. 2016;6(6):615–25.
16. Wheatley BM, Nappo KE, Christensen DL, et al. Effect of NSAIDs on bone healing rates: a meta-analysis. J Am Acad Orthop Surg. 2019;27(7):e330–6.
17. Teles AR, Ocay DD, Bin Shebreen A, et al. Evidence of impaired pain modulation in adolescents with idiopathic scoliosis and chronic back pain. Spine J. 2019;19(4):677–86.
18. Kuznia AL, Hernandez AK, Lee LU. Adolescent idiopathic scoliosis: common questions and answers. Am Fam Physician. 2020;101(1):19–23. Accessed 6 May 2020. https://www.aafp.org/afp/2020/0101/p19.html.
19. Horn SR, Poorman GW, Tishelman JC, et al. Trends in treatment of Scheuermann kyphosis: a study of 1,070 cases from 2003 to 2012. Spine Deform. 2019;7(1):100–6.
20. Tsirikos AI, Jain AK. Scheuermann's kyphosis; current controversies. J Bone Joint Surg Br. 2011;93(7):857–64.
21. Lorente A, Barrios C, Lorente R, et al. Severe hyperkyphosis reduces the aerobic capacity and maximal exercise tolerance in patients with Scheuermann disease. Spine J. 2019;19(2):330–8.
22. Huq S, Ehresman J, Cottrill E, et al. Treatment approaches for Scheuermann kyphosis: a systematic review of historic and current management. J Neurosurg Spine. 2020;32(2):235–47.
23. Booth TN, Iyer RS, Falcone RA, et al. Expert panel on pediatric imaging. ACR appropriateness criteria: back pain—child. J Am Coll Radiol. 2017;14(5S):S13–24.
24. Calloni SF, Huisman TA, Poretti A, et al. Back pain and scoliosis in children: when to image, what to consider. Neuroradiol J. 2017;30(5):393–404.
25. Tofte JN, CarlLee TL, Holte AJ, et al. Imaging pediatric spondylolysis: a systematic review. Spine (Phila Pa 1976). 2017;42(10):777–82.
26. Slotkin JR, Lu Y, Wood KB. Thoracolumbar spinal trauma in children. Neurosurg Clin N Am. 2007;18(4):621–30. https://doi.org/10.1016/j.nec.2007.07.003. PMID: 17991587.
27. Hamilton MG, Myles ST. Pediatric spinal injury: review of 174 hospital admissions. J Neurosurg. 1992;77:700–4.
28. Carreon LY, Glassman SD, Campbell MJ. Pediatric spine fractures: a review of 137 hospital admissions. J Spinal Disord Tech. 2004;17:477–82.
29. Vitale MG, et al. Epidemiology of pediatric spinal cord injury in the United States: years 1997 and 2000. J Pediatr Orthop. 2006;26:745–9.
30. Cirak B, et al. Spinal injuries in children. J Pediatr Surg. 2004;39:607–12.
31. Buldini B, et al. Spinal cord injury without radiographic abnormalities. Eur J Pediatr. 2006;165:108–11.
32. Launay F, Leet AI, Sponseller PD. Pediatric spinal cord injury without radiographic abnormality: a meta-analysis. Clin Orthop Relat Res. 2005;433:166–70.
33. Pang D. Spinal cord injury without radiographic abnormality in children, 2 decades later. Neurosurgery. 2004;55:1325–42.
34. Dias MS. Traumatic brain and spinal cord injury. Pediatr Clin N Am. 2004;51:271–30.
35. Yang S, Werner BC, Singla A, et al. Low back pain in adolescents: a 1-year analysis of eventual diagnoses. J Pediatr Orthop. 2017;37(5):344–7.
36. Straight Leg Raise Test (2023, March 21). Physiopedia. Retrieved 22:25 29 May 2024.

37. Cahill KS, Dunn I, Gunnarsson T, et al. Lumbar microdiscectomy in pediatric patients: a large single-institution series. J Neurosurg Spine. 2010;12(2):165–70.
38. Lavelle WF, Bianco A, Mason R, et al. Pediatric disk herniation. J Am Acad Orthop Surg. 2011;19(11):649–56.
39. Ginsburg GM, Bassett GS. Back pain in children and adolescents: evaluation and differential diagnosis. J Am Acad Orthop Surg. 1997;5(2):67–78.
40. Yen CH, Chan SK, Ho YF, Mak KH. Posterior lumbar apophyseal ring fractures in adolescents: a report of four cases. J Orthop Surg (Hong Kong). 2009;17(1):85–9.

Chapter 120
Environmental Emergencies

Neil Sparks and Matthew Waldrop

Environmental emergencies encompass several conditions, many of which are specific to a school's location. As such, planning and preparation are key to a successful response. School health providers should perform periodic assessments of their location to identify environmental threats and update existing policies, procedures, and emergency action plans. Reviews of each Emergency Action Plan (EAP) should include key personnel and identify areas of strengths and weaknesses. Locations should also be regularly assessed to ensure the proper equipment is available and functional. In addition, outside resources such as local emergency departments (ED) and emergency medical services (EMS) should be identified. Relevant staff and school leaders should be educated on environmental threats and periodic simulations and rehearsals should be performed. Communication networks and back-up procedures should be in place and readily available. Medical staff should also be aware of special populations within their schools who may require additional resources, such as people with disabilities, pre-existing injuries, or limited mobility. Providers should also ensure support and recovery resources are available following an emergency

Case 1 You are working in a school-based health clinic on a sunny Friday morning. The outdoor school field day is planned for the afternoon, but storms are expected. Your vice principal asks what they should do if they hear thunder or see lightning.

Lightning is a significant health threat, especially in the southeastern United States during June, July, and August [1, 2]. Injury and death primarily occur from ground current where the energy travels outward along the ground away from a strike, rather than a direct lightning strike to the body [3]. Cardiac arrest is the most

N. Sparks (✉) · M. Waldrop
Wake Forest University School of Medicine, Winston-Salem, NC, USA
e-mail: nsparks@wakehealth.edu; mdwaldro@wakehealth.edu

R. P. Olympia, J. Brady-Olympia (eds.), *Clinical Considerations in School-based Health*, https://doi.org/10.1007/978-3-031-85765-2_120

common cause of death but other injuries impacting the nervous system, eyes, and skin do occur [3]. In fact, lightning causes more life-long debilitating injuries than it kills [3, 4]. Most lightning strikes occur within 10 miles of a thunderstorm; however, strikes can occur up to 50 miles away [4]. As such, no place outdoors is safe near a thunderstorm. Education using slogans such as "when thunder roars, go indoors" or safety posters from the National Weather Service can be helpful [5, 6]. The lightning emergency response plan is delineated in Table 120.1.

Case 2 You're assisting a high school pre-health immersion program when someone starts yelling that a football player collapsed during practice. It's August and the temperature is 95 F. You arrive at the field and see an athlete who appears flushed, confused, and emotional. He can stand but needs assistance.

Heat stroke is a life-threatening emergency. Preparation and a rapid response focused on cooling are critical to saving lives. From 2006 to 2010 3332 deaths were attributed to heat stroke and these deaths are expected to almost triple between 2030 and 2050 due to climate change [7, 8]. Heat stroke is the most severe type of heat illness and a life threatening medical emergency (Tables 120.2 and 120.3). Heat cramps and heat exhaustion are non-emergent forms of heat illness and do not necessarily proceed heat stroke but still require early recognition and prompt medical

Table 120.1 Lightning Emergency Response [3–5]

Injury Background	Death from cardiac arrest Long term morbidity from secondary injuries

Preparation/ Planning	EAP in place
	<u>Identify lightning safe buildings</u>
	  Fully enclosed building or hard-topped vehicle
	  Pavilions, trees, sheds, and tents ARE NOT lightening safe
	Automatic External Defibrillators available
	Educate school personnel and students on lightning safety
	  "When Thunder Roars Go Indoors"
	  Do not contact electric outlets, plumbing, corded phones
	  Stay away from doors, windows, concrete floors

Emergency Response	Keys to lightning safety:
	  Thunder or lightning within 6 miles is a significant threat
	  Lightning Observed: 30:30 Rule—When you see lightning count the time until you hear thunder. If that is 30 secs or less the thunderstorm is close enough to be dangerous.
	  Thunder Heard Only: Seek shelter immediately.
	Wait 30 minutes after last observable sign of lightning and thunder
	Emergency Strike response:
	  Watch for follow-up strikes and respond only when safe.
	  Move victim(s) to lightning safe locations
	  Activate EAP, call 911
	  Primary assessment, assess airway, breathing, circulation
	  Skin findings such as a fern pattern (Lichtenberg figures) may indicate a strike victim
	  All victims should be transported to an Emergency Department

Table 120.2 Heat Stroke Emergency Response [7–14]

Injury Background	Central nervous system dysfunction + Core temperature > 105 F Risk of death if not quickly identified and rapid cooling initiated Risk of long-term consequences (neurologic, renal, hepatic, cardiovascular, respiratory, musculoskeletal, hematologic, endocrine, gastrointestinal)
Preparation/ Planning	Heat illness-specific EAP in place Monitor WetBulb Globe Temperate (WBGT) using National Weather Service or similar service for your area Adjust activity based on WBGT (Table 120.3) Encourage hydration, conditioning, and acclimation to the heat Equipment at locations: rectal thermometer, water tub, water source, ice Educate students/athletes and staff Protocols to closely monitor athletes before during and after training
Emergency Response	Remove all equipment and excess clothing Rectal temperature preferred, tape to leg for continuous monitoring Place in ice-water immersion tub and begin rapid cooling. Circulate water. If immersion not possible move to cool area and use cold wet towels, ice, etc. Activate EAP, call 911 Goal: cool rapidly within 30 minutes Monitor vital signs and keep water < 60 F, circulate water and ice **Do not transport until core temperature is** < **102 F** if core temp is available If unable to obtain core temperature do not use alternate methods Heat stroke victims need physician clearance before returning to sports

Table 120.3 Example of WetBulb Globe Temperature (WBGT) activity guidelines. (Adapted from the Georgia High School Association and used with permission)

WBGT Index (Fahrenheit)	Athletic activity guideline
< 80 degrees	Unlimited activity with primary cautions for new or unconditioned athletes or extreme exertion; schedule mandatory rest/water breaks (5 minute water/rest break every 30 minutes)
80–84.9 degrees	Normal practice for athletes; closely monitor new or unconditioned athletes and all athletes during extreme exertion. Schedule mandatory rest/water breaks (5 minute water/rest breaks every 25 minutes)
85–87.9 degrees	New or unconditioned athletes should have reduced intensity practice and modifications in clothing. Well-conditioned athletes should have more frequent rest breaks and hydration as well as cautious monitoring for symptoms of heat illness. Schedule frequent mandatory rest/water breaks (5 minute water/rest breaks every 20 minutes). Have cold or ice immersion pool on site for practice.
88–89.9 degrees	All athletes must be under constant observation and supervision. Remove pads and equipment. Schedule frequent mandatory rest/water breaks (5 minute water/rest breaks every 15 minutes). Have cold or ice immersion pool on site for practice.
Greater than 90 degrees	Suspend practice/must include mandatory breaks as directed by gameday administrator during contest.

treatment. The key phrase to remember regarding heat stroke is "**cool first, transport second**," [9]. This concept can be an area of conflict in emergency situations. Specifically, heat stroke differs from most emergency situations, as transporting prior to cooling can delay temperature correction, increase complications, and increase risk of death [10]. Different types and responses to heat-related illness are further addressed in Table 120.4.

Case 3 A middle school student presents to your school health clinic in January with concerns for "cold hands." She waited an hour in 20-degree F weather for the bus, and when it did not come, she walked 1 mile to school. She is dressed in a light jacket, dress, athletic shoes, and is not wearing gloves or a hat. Her hands are red, tender, and cool to the touch. Sensation and capillary refill are normal.

Cold injuries are classified as accidental hypothermia, frostnip, freezing cold injuries (FCI), and non-freezing cold injuries (NFCI) [15–18]. Accidental hypothermia occurs when the core temperature decreases to less than 95 F risking hypothermic cardiac arrest [15]. Treatment of accidental hypothermia focuses on rapid warmth and supportive care (Table 120.5) [15]. Frostnip is a self-limited superficial cold injury associated with discomfort and pallor. Frostnip may proceed FCI but symptoms resolve with rewarming [16]. FCI, also known as frostbite, is on a spectrum from superficial to deep based on the degree of tissue injury. Treatment of FCI emphasizes rapid rewarming only if refreezing is not possible, otherwise focuses on moving to a warm area and protecting the affected area (Table 120.6) [16, 17]. NFCI, formerly known as trench foot, results from prolonged exposure to cold and wet environments that don't quite reach freezing threshold. Treatment of NFCI

Table 120.4 Heat-related Illness Types, Signs/Symptoms, and Response [9]

Heat Cramps	Painful **cramps**, especially in **legs** **Flushed**, sweaty skin Move to a cool place, rest, discontinue exertional activity Gentle stretching cramping muscles Replace sweaty clothes with dry clean clothes, fan skin Consume cold beverage containing salt and sugar
Heat Exhaustion	**Pale**, sweaty skin, painful cramps Usually, **T** > **100.4 F** GI symptoms (nausea, vomiting, diarrhea) Headache, fatigue, weakness, lightheadedness/presyncope, anxiety Move to a cool place, rest, discontinue exertional activity Gentle stretching cramping muscles Replace sweaty clothes with dry clean clothes, fan skin Consume cold beverage containing salt and sugar If no improvement, take to ED for evaluation
Heat Stroke	**Warm, dry skin** **T** > **105 F (core temp)**, tachycardic CNS disturbances (confusion, agitation, lethargy, coma, seizures, death) GI symptoms (nausea, vomiting, diarrhea, anorexia) To do: As outlined in Table 120.2

Table 120.5 Accidental Hypothermia Emergency Response [15, 16]

Injury Background	Drop in core temperature < 95 F, poses risk of cardiac arrest Symptoms progress in severity as core temperature decreases. Use symptoms to estimate core temperature Mild: Alert + shivering without mental changes = 89.6 F to 95 F Moderate: Mental status changes + shivering = 82.4 F to 89.6 F Severe/Profound: Unconscious = < 82.4 F
Preparation/Planning	Monitor weather (temperature, wind chill, precipitation) Cold-Injury EAP in place Educate on proper clothing, hydration, nutrition, and awareness Contingencies for cancelling outdoor activities for extreme weather Closer monitoring of athletes before, during, and after training
Emergency Response	Activate EAP, call 911 Remove from cold and initiate warming Remove wet and tight clothing, cover with blankets head to toe Warm liquids ok if alert Monitor and reassess until EMS arrives.

Table 120.6 Freezing Cold Injuries and Non-Freezing Cold Injuries Signs/Symptoms and Response [16–18]

Frostnip and Freezing Cold Injury	Signs and Symptoms and Classification: Frostnip: Skin red, purple, white patches. Cold, sore, pain. No blisters Superficial: Pins and needles sensation. Skin blisters, peeling in patches Deep: Numbness. Skin firm and black. To do: Move to a warm protected area if possible If refreezing not possible: **warm water immersion** (98.6–102 F) until skin red/purple and soft—approximately 30 minutes If re-freezing is possible, do not actively warm. Frostnip symptoms should resolve with rewarming. If symptoms persist or there are signs of a FCI seek emergent medical care. Protect the area (e.g. dressings, non-weight bearing) until assessed **DO NOT:** Rub area, use hot water bottles, heaters, or hair dryers
Non-Freezing Cold Injury	Signs and Symptoms: Numbness, tingling, erythema, edema, blistering To do: move to warm area, remove wet clothing, **passive** re-warming **DO NOT:** Warm water immerse or actively rewarm. May worsen injury

focuses on removing wet clothing and passively warming the affected area (Table 120.6) [17, 18]. Many cold injuries can be prevented by weather awareness, proper clothing, education on risks of cold injury, and limiting exposure to cold.

120.1 Case Conclusions

Case 1 You take the proper precautions, and everyone is safely inside when thunderstorms hit the area.

Case 2 You activate your heat-illness EAP and call 911. The rectal thermometer reads 105.5 F and he is immersed in a cold tub. When EMS arrives, his temperature has decreased to 101.9 F and he is transported to the ED. He suffers no complications and weeks later you clear him to return to sports.

Case 3 You diagnose Frostnip. You immerse her fingers in warm water and all symptoms resolve. You ensure she stays inside for recess and recheck before dismissal. She remains asymptomatic and well.

Extra Credit Points

1. Three of the most common emergencies include heat-related illness, cold-related illness, and lightning-related emergencies. Other environmental emergencies include high altitude, carbon monoxide poisoning, animal bites/stings, allergic reactions, earthquakes, and fires/burns.
2. Lightning can strike up to 50 miles from its parent thunderstorm. Be aware of local weather and seek shelter when risk for lightning strike is present.
3. Cool first, transport second is the most important takeaway regarding heat stroke.
4. Not all cold-related injuries are treated with rapid rewarming.
5. In NFCI's, rapid rewarming can worsen symptoms.

References

1. Vagasky C, Holle R, Murphy MJ, et al. How much lightning actually strikes the United States? Bull Am Meteorol Soc. 2024:E749–59. https://doi.org/10.1175/BAMS-D-22-0241.1.
2. Jensenius J (2020) A detailed analysis of lightning deaths in the United States from 2006 through 2019. National Weather Service. https://www.weather.gov/media/safety/Analysis06-19.pdf. Accessed 5 May 2024.
3. Jensen JD, Thurman J, Vincent AL (2023) Lightning injuries. In: StatPearls [Internet]. Treasure Island (FL): StatPearls Publishing. Available from: https://www.ncbi.nlm.nih.gov/books/NBK441920/. Accessed 9 May 2024.
4. Frequently Asked Questions (2023) National oceanic and atmospheric administration. https://www.noaa.gov/jetstream/lightning/frequently-asked-questions. Accessed 5 May 2024.
5. Lightening safety brochure. National Weather Service lightening safety for you and your family. https://www.weather.gov/media/safety/Lightning-Brochure18.pdf. Accessed 5 May 2024.
6. Lightening safety poster. National Weather Service. https://www.weather.gov/safety/lightning-posters. Accessed 9 May 2024.
7. Berko J, Ingram D, Saha S, Parker J. Deaths attributed to heat, cold, and other weather events in the United States, 2006-2010. Natl Health Stat Rep. 2014;76:1–15.
8. Jacobsen A, Khiew Y, Duffy E, et al. Climate change and the prevention of cardiovascular disease. Am J Prev Cardiol. 2022;12:100391. https://doi.org/10.1016/j.ajpc.2022.100391.
9. "When Treating Athletes for Heat Stroke, Cool First, Transport Second" Loyola Med; 2018.
10. Monseau A, Hurlburt G, Balcik B, et al. Status of US emergency medical service protocols regarding pre-transfer cooling for exertional heat stroke. Cureus. 2021;13(11):e19505. https://doi.org/10.7759/cureus.19505.
11. Morris A, Patel G Heat stroke [Updated 2023 Feb 13]. In: StatPearls [Internet]. Treasure Island (FL): StatPearls Publishing; 2024. Available from: https://www.ncbi.nlm.nih.gov/books/NBK537135. Accessed 9 May 2024.

12. Gauer R, Meyers B. Heat-related illnesses. Am Fam Physician. 2019;99(8):482–9.
13. Prevention of heat illness. In: North Carolina High School Athletic Association, Inc. 2022-2023 Handbook. https://www.nchsaa.org/wp-content/uploads/2023/05/NCHSAAHandbook2022-2023FinalJan2023.pdf. Accessed 9 May 2024.
14. Heat stroke treatment. Korey Stringer Institute, 5 Aug 2019. https://ksi.uconn.edu/emergency-conditions/heat-illnesses/exertional-heat-stroke/heat-stroke-treatment/pdf. Accessed 9 May 2024.
15. Dow J, Giesbrecht GG, Danzl DF, et al. Wilderness Medical Society clinical practice guidelines for the out-of-hospital evaluation and treatment of accidental hypothermia: 2019 update. Wilderness Environ Med. 2019;30(4S):S47–69. https://doi.org/10.1016/j.wem.2019.10.002.
16. Rathjen NA, Shahbodaghi SD, Brown JA. Hypothermia and cold weather injuries. Am Fam Physician. 2019;100(11):680–6.
17. McIntosh SE, Freer L, Grissom CK, et al. Wilderness medical society clinical practice guidelines for the prevention and treatment of frostbite: 2019 update. Wilderness Environ Med. 2019;30(4S):S19–32. https://doi.org/10.1016/j.wem.2019.05.002.
18. Zafren K. Nonfreezing cold injury (Trench Foot). Int J Environ Res Public Health. 2021;18(19):10482. https://doi.org/10.3390/ijerph181910482.

Chapter 121
Infectious Diseases and the Athlete

Sarah Meyers, Jeffrey Campbell, and Sandra Schumacher

There are many potential ways for infections to be transmitted during sports participation, including airborne spread, droplets, and physical contact; some microbes may be spread by more than one of these routes. Airborne infections are transmitted by infectious agents that are typically extremely small at <5 microns and remain viable and suspended in the air over long distances. Those with a potential airborne infection should be treated away from others and ideally in a negative pressure room. Droplet infections are transmitted by large respiratory droplets and do not travel more than 3–6 feet. Direct skin to skin involvement can cause infectious spread via the contact route. Additionally, it is possible for microbes to infect individuals outside these usual forms of transmission, such as from contaminated water encountered during swimming.

Case #1 Andy is a high school sophomore on the wrestling team. His coach noticed a red rash on his left upper thigh and sent him to you for further evaluation. Andy tells you that he first noticed a small "bump" on his groin and didn't think much of it but now has developed a larger red rash. He denies any fevers or chills. Upon evaluation, you see a 4 × 6 inch erythematous rash on his left upper inner thigh with clearly defined borders. He then shows you the "bump" on his groin suggestive of a small, tender lymph node. Andy asks, "Can I go back to practice?" What would you do?

Students who play sports involving skin-to-skin contact, such as wrestling, are at risk of developing skin and soft tissue infections. Traumatic breaks in the skin can

---

S. Meyers · J. Campbell
Boston Medical Center, Boston, MA, USA
e-mail: sarah.meyers@bmc.org; jeffrey.campbell@bmc.org

S. Schumacher (✉)
Boston Children's Hospital, Boston, MA, USA
e-mail: sandra.schumacher@childrens.harvard.edu

R. P. Olympia, J. Brady-Olympia (eds.), *Clinical Considerations in School-based Health*, https://doi.org/10.1007/978-3-031-85765-2_121

facilitate introduction of infectious organisms [1]. *Staphylococcus aureus* is a common bacterial cause of skin and soft tissue infections, including pustules, abscesses, and cellulitis. The school-based provider should evaluate size, depth, and extent of the skin/soft tissue involvement, as well as signs of systemic infection, such as fevers or chills [2]. Methicillin-resistant Staph aureus (MRSA) is becoming increasingly prevalent in community settings, and many asymptomatic high school athletes are colonized with MRSA [1]. Herpes gladiatorum, caused by herpes simplex virus 1, is also common among athletes who play contact sports. It presents as a vesicular (fluid-filled) rash on an erythematous base and is highly contagious [2]. These athletes are also at risk of fungal infections, such as tinea corporis and tinea capitis (located on the body and the scalp, respectively), otherwise known as "ringworm".

Prevention of skin and soft tissue infections among athletes who play contact sports involves regular skin checks, routine cleaning of all shared equipment (such as mats) with disinfectant, avoidance of sharing personal items like towels, and encouraging players to shower with soap and hot water after every practice and competition [2]. For athletes with Staphylococcal infections, including MRSA, the Centers for Disease Control and Prevention (CDC) recommends at least 3 days of oral antibiotics prior to return to play (RTP) [3]. Given the highly contagious nature of herpes infection, it is recommended that athletes with herpes gladiatorum who play sports with skin-to-skin contact should avoid practice and competition for at least 10 days [2]. The CDC recommends completing 3 days of oral or topical antifungal therapy prior to RTP for individuals with tinea corporis, and 14 days of oral antifungals prior to RTP for tinea capitis [3]. The school-based provider has an important role to play in timely recognition of skin and soft tissue infections in young athletes, and prompt recognition and initiation of appropriate antimicrobial therapy will ensure a timely return to their sport.

Case 2 Eric is a 15-year-old cross-country runner who comes to your office with headache, muscle pain, and nausea that began earlier this morning. You find that he is febrile and has a non-pruritic maculopapular rash on his trunk. He participated in a race through the woods in South Carolina 2 weeks ago and tells you that he found an engorged tick in his hair a few days later. What are the potential diagnoses?

Athletes who participate in outdoor sports are at risk for a variety of tick-borne infections. In this case, Eric has Human Ehrlichiosis, typically caused by the intracellular bacteria *Ehrlichia chafeensis*, which usually presents with fever, malaise, nausea, and occasionally with a maculopapular rash. *Ehrlichia* species and the related *Anaplasma phagocytophilum* are usually transmitted through the bites of infected lone star (*Amblyomma americanum)* and blacklegged (*Ixodes scapularis*) ticks [4]. *Ehrlichia* and *Anaplasma*, along with other tick-borne bacteria, parasites, and viruses, commonly infect children who spend time outside or who live with outdoor pets. The most common tick-borne illness in the United States is Lyme Disease (caused by the bacteria *Borrelia burgdorferi*), but the epidemiology of tick-borne illness varies by region (Table 121.1), by season, and by the types of activities that children engage in that expose them to ticks [5].

Table 121.1 Common Pathogens Transmitted by Ticks in the United States

Disease	Pathogen	Early symptoms	Typical geographic range
Lyme Disease	*Borrelia burgdorferi*	Target rash (single or many), fever, headache, arthritis	Northeast, Midwest
Ehrlichiosis	*Ehrlichia* species	Fever, chills, malaise, nausea, maculopapular rash	Northeast, Midwest, South
Anaplasmosis	*Anaplasma phagocytophilum*	Fever, chills, malaise, nausea, maculopapular rash	Northeast, Midwest
Babesiosis	*Babesia microti*	Fever, malaise, headache, nausea, fatigue	Northeast, Midwest
Rocky Mountain Spotted Fever	*Rickettsia rickettsii*	Fever, myalgias, headache, abdominal pain, petechial rash (late finding)	Northeast, Midwest, South
Tularemia	*Francisella tularensis*	Most common form in children is local maculopapular/ulcerating rash with regional lymphadenopathy (ulceroglandular form)	Northeast, Midwest

Several tick-borne infections can quickly progress to severe illnesses, and rapid initiation of antibiotics—often prior to confirming a diagnosis—can be lifesaving. It is particularly important to recognize early symptoms of Rocky Mountain Spotted Fever (RMSF, caused by *Rickettsia rickettsii*). Initial symptoms of RMSF include high fevers, myalgia, headache, malaise, and abdominal symptoms [6]. Importantly, the classic petechial RMSF rash usually does not appear until 2–4 days after symptom onset, and about 10% of patients with RMSF do not have this classic rash at all [6].

Prevention of tick-borne illnesses primarily relies upon preventing tick bites or removing ticks promptly after they bite. Children who participate in sports taking place in tick habitats (e.g., wooded areas, fields with long grasses, or with animals) should be encouraged to use insect repellants. They should also check for ticks daily after participating in sports in tick habitats and should shower soon after being outdoors to identify and remove ticks that have not yet embedded.

Case 3 Ann is a 12-year-old volleyball player who developed a low-grade fever and a mild cough today. Her coach smartly advised her not to play because she was sick, despite Ann wanting to play in the championship game. In addition to coughing, Ann developed coryza (rhinorrhea) and conjunctivitis and had white spots with a bluish center (Koplik spots) in her mouth. She then developed a rash of red spots that spread from her head to the rest of her body. Unfortunately, Ann never had the MMR vaccine due to parental choice and had recently traveled to India where the prevalence of measles is much higher than in the US. What are the most important next steps?

Being near others, particularly in an enclosed area such as a gym, is a way of acquiring an infection spread by droplets such as influenza, but also pathogens spread via the airborne route such as measles. In Ann's case, the 3 C's of cough, coryza, conjunctivitis along with Koplik spots, a much less common but pathognomonic sign, suggest measles.

Measles is caused by a virus only seen in humans and is highly contagious. The incubation period is typically 8–12 days. Individuals are contagious from 4 days before the rash through 4 days after the appearance of the rash. Measles can be prevented with the MMR vaccine, which is recommended at 12–15 months of age with the second dose given at 4–6 years old. This vaccine should be administered to teenagers and adults if not given in childhood. One dose of the MMR vaccine is about 93% effective and two doses are about 97% effective at preventing measles. Treatment of measles is usually symptomatic, although vitamin A has been associated with decreased morbidity and mortality in resource-limited countries [7, 8].

121.1 Case Conclusions

Case 1 Andy is transported to the local emergency department, where he undergoes incision and drainage of the abscess and is started on cephalexin. He returns to school. However, his rash continues to spread beyond the marked borders, so he returns to your office. You refer him to his primary care doctor who checks the culture obtained in the emergency department and notes he has a MRSA infection so is switched to clindamycin which covers his MRSA isolate, and the cephalexin is stopped. Over the next couple days, his symptoms begin to improve.

Case 2 You refer Eric to the emergency department, where he promptly is given doxycycline and is hospitalized. Laboratory testing shows leukopenia and thrombocytopenia. A blood PCR for Ehrlichia chaffeensis returns positive. Fever abates after 2 days. Eric ultimately completes a 10-day course of doxycycline.

Case 3 Ann slowly improves with supportive cares at home. There is no specific antiviral therapy, although ribavirin and vitamin A may be considered with severe illness. Some may develop a bacterial infection such as pneumonia as a complication of measles, but Ann does not. The department of public health is notified to assist with outbreak control. Fortunately, all of Ann's other contacts are properly vaccinated and no one else becomes ill with measles, further emphasizing the importance of vaccination for this preventable disease. After Ann recovers, she and her family agree to the administration of vaccinations, including MMR.

Extra Credit Points

1. MRSA colonization is common in students who participate in sports involving skin-to-skin contact, such as wrestling, and thus MRSA coverage should be

considered in formulating an antibiotic plan for skin and soft tissue infections in these student-athletes.

2. Tick-borne illness should be considered in students with consistent symptoms (fever, rash, etc.) who participate in outdoor activities in endemic areas, even if a tick is not visualized on exam.
3. Remember to consider the vaccination status of student-athletes, and do not assume all have been vaccinated according to the standard CDC vaccine schedule because some parents obtain religious or personal exemptions.

References

1. Armento A, VanBaak K, Mayer SW, Dahab KS, Vidal A. Sports medicine. In: Bunik M, Hay WW, Levin MJ, Abzug MJ, editors. Current diagnosis & treatment: pediatrics. New York: McGraw-Hill Education; 2022. p. 26e.
2. Selected issues for the adolescent athlete and the team physician: a consensus statement. Med Sci Sports Exerc. 2008;40(11):1997–2012. https://doi.org/10.1249/MSS.0b013e31818acdcb.
3. Bultas MW, Brueggemann EM, Daily H. Common skin infections in high school athletes and the role of the school nurse. NASN Sch Nurse. 2023;38(6):285–91. https://doi.org/10.1177/1942602X231199768.
4. Choi E, Pyzocha NJ, Maurer DM. Tick-borne illnesses. Curr Sports Med Rep. 2016;15(2):98–104. https://doi.org/10.1249/jsr.0000000000000238.
5. Centers for Disease Control and Prevention. Tickborne diseases of the United States. Accessed online at: https://www.cdc.gov/ticks/tickbornediseases/index.html. Last accessed 29 March 2024.
6. Bryant KA, Marshall GS. Clinical manifestations of tick-borne infections in children. Clin Diagn Lab Immunol. 2000;7(4):523–7. https://doi.org/10.1128/CDLI.7.4.523-527.2000.
7. Davies HD, Jackson MA, Rice SG, Committee On Infectious D, Council On Sports M, Fitness. Infectious diseases associated with organized sports and outbreak control. Pediatrics. 2017;140(4) https://doi.org/10.1542/peds.2017-2477.
8. Centers for Disease Control and Prevention. Measles (Rubeola). Accessed online at https://www.cdc.gov/measles/index.html. Last accessed 28 March 2024.

Chapter 122
National Standards for Physical Education

Jack Keeley and Laura Lintner

Case #1 You are a school physician and you have been asked to review the current state of physical education for the schools in your district. How do you start?

Case #2 A high school student with cerebral palsy has transferred to your school. What resources can you use to effectively incorporate this student into your physical education curriculum?

Physical education has been considered one of the key aspects of a well-rounded education for millennia. Some of the earliest proponents of incorporating physical training into overall education, the ancient Greeks, placed significant emphasis on the concept of "dualism", or the simultaneous pursuit of both academic and physical excellence [1]. The concept of incorporating physical fitness as an integral educational component waxed and waned in prevalence over following periods of history, with de-emphasis of the material during the Middle Ages, followed by a re-emergence of focus on physical training during the Renaissance. Closer to home, physical education emerged as a designated field of study in American education during the 1800s, with physical education pioneer Luther Halsey Gulick referring to it as the "new profession" in 1885 [2]. While the components of organized physical education have greatly evolved since that time, a particularly formative period occurred in the 1950s–60s during the years of the Eisenhower and Kennedy presidencies [3]. Fearful that America's youth were becoming less physically fit, President Kennedy created the White House committee on Health and Fitness, which developed and disseminated a PE fitness curriculum [4]. These seminal efforts laid the foundation for the present physical education standards and programs available to American physical educators today.

J. Keeley · L. Lintner (✉)
Wake Forest Baptist Medical Center, Winston-Salem, NC, USA
e-mail: jkeeley@wakehealth.edu; llintner@wakehealth.edu

R. P. Olympia, J. Brady-Olympia (eds.), *Clinical Considerations in School-based Health*, https://doi.org/10.1007/978-3-031-85765-2_122

Before discussing the currently available national physical education standards, it is helpful to consider why this field of education is of such pressing importance to present day educators and clinicians. As is frequently mentioned in both mainstream news outlets and research journals alike, America has found itself entrenched in a pediatric obesity epidemic [5]. At the time of a Mayo Clinic data review shortly before the COVID-19 pandemic, one in three U.S. children were found to be overweight or obese, with corresponding increases in the pediatric prevalence of chronic disease such as type 2 diabetes, hypertension, obstructive sleep apnea, and fatty liver disease [6]. These grim findings have only been exacerbated post-pandemic, with recent studies noting that the rate of BMI increase among U.S pediatric populations doubled over the course of the COVID-19 pandemic [7].

The national standards for physical education are a helpful resource for educators and school-based clinicians alike as they attempt to combat these troubling pediatric health trends. These national standards are housed in the guidelines published by SHAPE (Society of Health and Physical Educators) America, a non-profit organization founded in 1885 and originally known as the American Alliance for Health, Physical Education, and Recreation [8]. SHAPE America is recognized by the CDC as the standard-maker for U.S. physical education [9]. The updated 2024 National physical education standards are separated into four distinct categories with accompanying rationales as outlined in Table 122.1 [10]:

Each individual standard is further subdivided into an extensive list of measurable goals by grade grouping, with these subdivisions divided into grades PreK-2, Grades 3–5, Grades 6–8, and Grades 9–12. While the details of these expansive grade-grouped goals are beyond the scope of this overview (and are readily available for review on the SHAPE America website at https://www.shapeameria.org, Table 122.2 demonstrates a practical, quick reference list of materials, sporting equipment, and/or facilities required to fully address each grade level set of standards.

In addition to the SHAPE America standards, there are also resources available for assessing students' current overall state of physical fitness in an objective, standardized manner. The most preeminent of these resources is the Presidential Youth Fitness Test. Originally created in 1966, the Youth fitness test has gone through multiple evolutions over its lifespan [11]. The most recent iteration of this standardized Presidential Youth Fitness Test exists as part of the larger Presidential Youth Fitness Program, formed in 2012 in conjunction with SHAPE America. The testing component of the Presidential Youth Fitness Program is broken up into two age group-based categories: the PYFP Fitness Club for grades K-3, and the Presidential Youth Fitness Award for grades 4–12. The PYFP Fitness Club is designed to orient and educate younger students on the components of the Fitnessgram test (which comprises the test categories for the Grade 4–12 Presidential Youth Fitness Award). While access to the specific Fitnessgram testing components and associated testing result software requires purchase ($549 per the Fitnessgram website), information regarding the general components of these tests is readily available. Table 122.3 demonstrates an overview of the three main Fitnessgram categories with an accompanying description of each.

Table 122.1 2024 National physical education standards

2024 National Physical Education Standards	Accompanying Rationale
1. Develops a variety of motor skills	"Through learning experiences in physical education, the student develops motor skills across a variety of environments. Motor skills are a foundational part of child development and support the movements of everyday life. The development of motor skills contributes to an individual's physical literacy journey."
2. Applies knowledge related to movement and fitness concepts	"Through learning experiences in physical education, the student uses their knowledge of movement concepts, tactics, and strategies across a variety of environments. This knowledge helps the student become a more versatile and efficient mover. Additionally, the student applies knowledge of health-related and skill-related fitness to enhance their overall well-being. The application of knowledge related to various forms of movement contributes to an individual's physical literacy journey."
3. Develops social skills through movement.	"Through learning experiences in physical education, students develop the social skills necessary to exhibit empathy and respect for others and foster and maintain relationships. In addition, students develop skills for communication, leadership, cultural awareness, and conflict resolution in a variety of physical activity settings."
4. Develops personal skills, identifies personal benefits of movement, and chooses to engage in physical activity.	"Through learning experiences in physical education, the student develops an understanding of how movement is personally beneficial and subsequently chooses to participate in physical activities that are personally meaningful (e.g., activities that offer social interaction, cultural connection, exploration, choice, self-expression, appropriate levels of challenge, and added health benefits). The student develops personal skills including goal setting, identifying strengths, and reflection to enhance their physical literacy journey."

For patients with intellectual or physical disabilities that make administration of the FitnessGram test difficult, a helpful resource is the Brockport Physical Fitness Test, which provides extensive protocols for activity modification to accommodate students' varied intellectual and physical baselines [12].

Extra Credit Points

1. Current national PE standards are housed in the guidelines published by SHAPE (Society of Health and Physical Educators) America
2. The resources and sports equipment required to fully address the SHAPE national standards are low cost and readily attainable for schools of varying sizes and budgets
3. The Fitnessgram test provides a standardized, objective battery to measure students' overall level of physical fitness. The Brockport Physical Fitness Test is a helpful resource for accommodation of students with different intellectual and physical capabilities than their peers

Table 122.2 Recommended materials, sporting equipment, and facilities

Grade Level Grouping	Required Physical Education Materials
PreK-Grade 2	Balls well suited for bouncing/rolling, catching/throwing, and dribbling with feet (e.g. soccer ball) "short handled" implement (e.g. tennis racquet or ping pong paddle) and "long handled implement" (e.g. hockey stick or golf club) jumping rope age-appropriate setting for demonstration of water safety and swimming skills
Grades 3–5	Area suitable for "chasing and fleeing activities" (aka tag, capture the flag, etc.) "short handled" implement (e.g. tennis racquet or ping pong paddle) and "long handled implement" (e.g. hockey stick or golf club) jumping rope Balls well suited for rolling, throwing/catching, dribbling with both feet AND hands (e.g. soccer ball/basketball), and serving (e.g. volleyball) age-appropriate setting for demonstration of water safety and swimming skills
Grades 6–8	"short handled" implement (e.g. tennis racquet or ping pong paddle) and "long handled implement" (e.g. hockey stick or golf club) baseball and/or softball (or other ball amenable to pitching) volleyball tennis/pickleball/ping pong equipment (or other such equipment amenable to volley-related games using hand-held implement)
Grades 9–12	setting for demonstration of water safety and swimming skills While there are no other specific types of sports equipment required to meet the standards for these grade levels, ongoing reinforcement of skills taught at previous grade levels is certainly beneficial

Table 122.3 Fitnessgram categories

Fitnessgram Category	Components
Aerobic Capacity	PACER (Progressive Aerobic Cardiovascular Endurance Run) One-Mile Run One-Mile Walk
Muscular Strength	Abdominal strength and endurance Trunk extensor strength and flexibility Upper body strength and endurance Flexibility
Body Composition	BMI Body Fat Percentage

References

1. de Habyarimana JD, Tugirumukiza E, Zhou K. Physical education and sports: a backbone of the entire community in the twenty-first century. Int J Environ Res Public Health. 2022;19:7296.
2. Guedes C. Physical education and physical activity: a historical perspective. Combating Obesity in K-12 Learners. Education Resources Information Center; 2007.
3. Physical Education Programs, history & importance - playgrounds, rubber mulch and surfacing. Accessed 27 April 2024.
4. The Federal Government takes on Physical Fitness. John F. Kennedy Presidential Library and Museum. https://www.jfklibrary.org/learn/about-jfk/jfk-in-history/physical-fitness.

5. Kelly AS, Kumar S. Review of childhood obesity: from epidemiology, etiology, and comorbidities to clinical assessment and treatment. Mayo Clinic proceedings. Accessed 26 April 2024. https://pubmed.ncbi.nlm.nih.gov/28065514/.
6. Ibid.
7. Lange SJ, Kompaniyets L, Freedman DS, et al. Longitudinal trends in body mass index before and during the COVID-19 pandemic among persons aged 2-19 years - United States, 2018-2020. MMWR. Morbidity and mortality weekly report. 2021.
8. Kennard J. The history of physical education. JSTOR; 1977.
9. Physical Education and physical activity. Centers for Disease Control and Prevention. 2023. Accessed 26 April 2024. https://www.cdc.gov/healthyschools/physicalactivity/index.htm.
10. What Is Physical Education. Accessed 26 April 2024. https://www.shapeamerica.org/publications/resources/teachingtools/teachertoolbox/What_Is_Physical_Education.aspx.
11. Presidential Youth Fitness Program. Accessed 26 April 2024. https://health.gov/our-work/nutrition-physical-activity/presidents-council/programs-awards/presidential-youth-fitness-program.
12. Winnick JP, Short FX. Brockport physical fitness test manual: a health-related assessment for youngsters with disabilities. Human Kinetics; 2014.

Chapter 123
Miscellaneous Sport-Specific Injuries and Conditions

Sophie Baron and Jodi Brady-Olympia

Case 1 A 15-year-old female gymnast is currently training hard for the upcoming State Gymnastics Championships, perfecting her floor routine by training daily. Over the past 2 months, she has been experiencing increasing lower back pain that has made it difficult for her to complete her sessions. Out of sheer determination to succeed, she has been training through this. However, over the past week she has been experiencing increasing hamstring tightness and a new tingling sensation radiating into her left leg and foot. Nervous that this could affect her ability to perform at the Championships, she presents to your office with the hope to find some immediate relief. What should you do?

Sports specialization has been most recently defined in the literature as "intentional and focused participation in a single sport for a majority of the year [8+ months] that restricts opportunities for engagement in other sports and activities" [1]. As youth sports have become increasingly professionalized, many athletes are expected to participate on multiple teams and train intensively for long hours from a young age in order to reach elite or professional status in a single sport (Fig. 123.1). However, most recent evidence shows that early specialization has been associated with increased risk of injury, compromised growth and maturity, social isolation, burnout, and in most cases with decreased athletic performance and ultimate potential [2]. In most cases, later adolescent specialization, as opposed to childhood specialization, has been linked with higher levels of elite success [3], meaning that there

S. Baron
Penn State Children's Hospital, Hershey, PA, USA
e-mail: sbaron1@pennstatehealth.psu.edu

J. Brady-Olympia (✉)
Department of Pediatrics Penn State, College of Medicine Attending Physician,
Division of Adolescent Medicine, Department of Pediatrics,
Penn State Children's Hospital, Hershey, PA, USA
e-mail: jbradyolympia@pennstatehealth.psu.edu

R. P. Olympia, J. Brady-Olympia (eds.), *Clinical Considerations in School-based Health*, https://doi.org/10.1007/978-3-031-85765-2_123

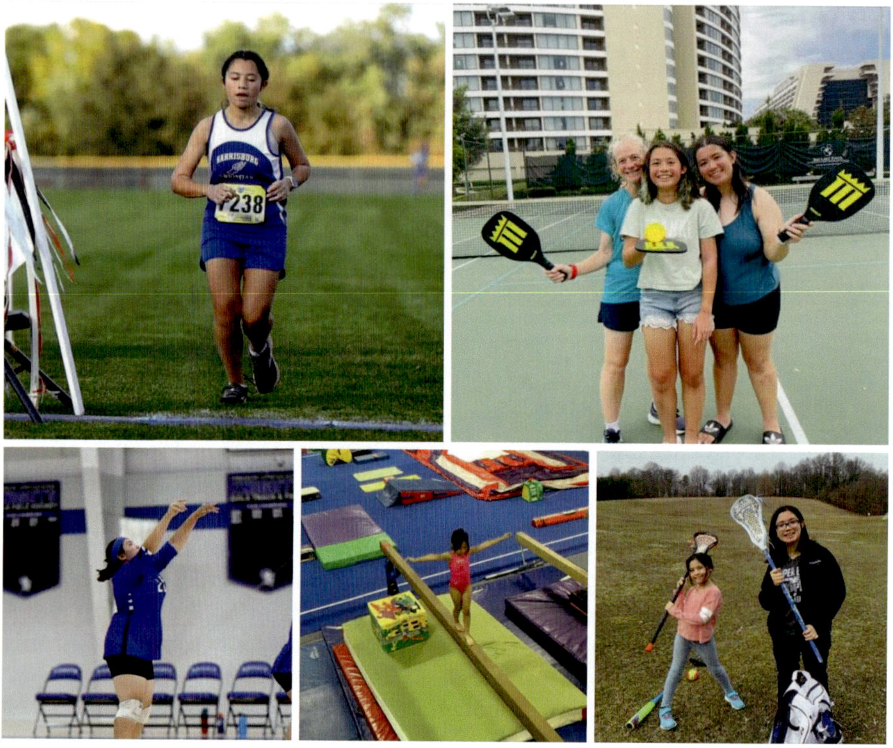

Fig. 123.1 Participation in different sports is important to the development of young athletes

is benefit to early multi-sport participation. However, this pattern is not always true, particularly for sports where peak performance is often met before full physical maturation, such as in gymnastics, dance, figure skating, swimming, and diving [1, 4].

In these early specialization sports, there are additional risks to consider, particularly surrounding overtraining and overuse injuries on the still-developing body. Overuse injuries occur due to repetitive microtrauma to specific muscles, joints, and tendons that are utilized during sport-specific maneuvers, without sufficient time for recovery. Children are at increased risk of sustaining these types of injuries given their less stress-tolerant bones as well as increased vulnerability at the growing apophyses and epiphyses [5]. The risk is often highest during periods of rapid growth (i.e. around early adolescence).

For example, repetitive hyperextension and axial loading of the spine in gymnasts can lead to predictable back injuries such as spondylolysis, a stress fracture of the pars interarticularis of the lumbar vertebrae. Studies have shown rates of spondylolysis up to 30% in adolescent athletes compared to the 3–10% in the general population [6]. Furthermore, skeletal immaturity has proven to be a risk factor for progression to spondylolisthesis, which involves slippage of the vertebrae and more serious injury [7]. As a medical provider taking care of young athletes, it is important to be aware of some of these common overuse injuries that might occur more frequently in specific sports and to know when they may be treated conservatively versus when they may need further evaluation (Table 123.1). Any of these injuries can lead to decreased athletic performance and time away from play.

Table 123.1 Common overuse injuries associated with specific sports

Sport	Common injuries	History and common symptoms	Evaluation
Gymnastics	Spondylolysis	Hx: repetitive axial loading and back hyperextension Sx: lower back pain for > 2 weeks, hamstring tightness	Lumbar radiograph; may require CT/MRI for leg numbness or weakness indicating possible progression to spondylolisthesis
	Gymnast's wrist (distal radius epiphysitis)	Hx: repetitive axial loading to the wrist (seen in young gymnasts with open growth plates) Sx: radial-sided wrist tenderness and swelling (may be chronic in nature), pain with wrist hyperextension	Wrist radiograph; MRI should be obtained in all patients with chronic/refractory symptoms or with neurovascular compromise (there is a risk of concomitant scaphoid fracture)
Dance/ Cheer	Sever's Disease (calcaneal apophysitis)	Hx: repetitive jumping/ running (seen in young athletes with open growth plates) Sx: pain in the heel (at Achilles insertion), heel stiffness, limping, pain reproducible with compression of the calcaneus and standing on tiptoes (Sever's sign)	Normally a clinical diagnosis; foot radiograph may be useful to exclude other traumas; MRI or US can help detect retrocalcaneal bursitis
	Dancers Tendinopathy (flexor hallicus longus tendinopathy)	Hx: dancing en pointe position Sx: pain posterior and inferior to the medial malleolus, trapping/locking of the great toe	Normally a clinical diagnosis; lateral radiographs may be used to differentiate from posterior impingement; MRI or US can distinguish from tendon tear
Wrestling	Concussion	Hx: direct blow to head, face, or neck (+/− LOC) Sx: headache, confusion, amnesia, nausea, vomiting, drowsiness	Normally a clinical diagnosis; CT is indicated for complicated concussions according to PECARN algorithms[a]
	Cervical Sprain or Strain	Hx: sudden impact of head with the mat or opponent Sx: pain with head/neck movement, muscle spasms, headache	Normally a clinical diagnosis; consider radiograph or CT if there is concern for fracture or midline tenderness

(continued)

Table 123.1 (continued)

Sport	Common injuries	History and common symptoms	Evaluation
Tennis	Tennis Elbow (lateral epicondylitis)	Hx: repetitive wrist extension (e.g. backhand with poor form) Sx: pain or burning in the lateral elbow, forearm weakness, decreased grip strength, worse with wrist extension	Normally a clinical diagnosis; consider MRI/CT for clicking or locking or for numbness
Golf	Golfer's elbow (medial epicondylitis)	Hx: repetitive valgus stress or a traumatic blow Sx: pain over medial elbow worse with forearm motion, gripping, and throwing	Normally a clinical diagnosis; consider MRI/CT for clicking or locking or for numbness
Volleyball	Runner's knee or Jumper's knee (patellofemoral pain syndrome)	Hx: insidious onset after repetitive jumping or running; more common in females Sx: anterior knee pain felt around the kneecap, worse with walking up an incline or squatting, "popping" while walking up steps (note that swelling and erythema are not typically seen)	Normally a clinical diagnosis; consider radiographs after 1–2 months of failed conservative management
	Mallet Finger (extensor avulsion fracture or distal extensor tendon rupture)	Hx: forced flexion of the fingertip at the DIP joint due to impact with the ball Sx: pain and swelling around the DIP joint, the tip of the finger is bent and cannot be straightened without the assistance of the other hand	Normally a clinical diagnosis; plain radiograph may help distinguish an avulsion fracture from tendon rupture
Skiing	Ski Thumb (ulnar collateral ligament tear)	Hx: forced abduction of thumb MCP joint after a fall Sx: pain, bruising, swelling at the base of the thumb or the web between thumb and index finger, laxity with valgus stress	Hand radiograph to help rule out avulsion fracture; MRI confirms diagnosis if needed

(continued)

Table 123.1 (continued)

Sport	Common injuries	History and common symptoms	Evaluation
Figure Skating	Retrocalcaneal Bursitis	Hx: tight or poorly-fitted skates causing pressure on the posterior heel Sx: pain and swelling at the back of the heel, worse on tiptoes	Normally a clinical diagnosis; radiograph may help exclude other trauma
	Lace/Skate Bite (tibialis anterior tendinopathy)	Hx: poorly fitted skate Sx: anterior ankle pain and inflammation, worse with dorsiflexion and inversion	Normally a clinical diagnosis; imaging is not typically recommended
Ice Hockey	Osgood-Schlatter Disease (proximal tibial apophysitis)	Hx: repetitive squatting or jumping, most common in adolescent males Sx: anterior knee (over tibial tuberosity) pain worsened with jumping or squatting	Normally a clinical diagnosis; consider radiograph after 1 to 2 months of conservative therapy to rule out other diagnoses (e.g. osteochondritis dissecans)
	Shoulder Instability	Hx: history of high-speed collisions and possible prior shoulder dislocation Sx: shoulder pain, clicking, "dead arm" with throwing motion, increased ROM	Consider MRI to rule out other trauma such as labral tear
Swimming	Swimmer's shoulder (rotator cuff tendinopathy)	Hx: repetitive freestyle or butterfly stroke Sx: point tenderness over antero-lateral shoulder, impaired shoulder strength or range of motion, difficulty finding comfortable sleep position	Start with shoulder radiographs; may require more advanced imaging (e.g. MRI) for neurovascular compromise, severe weakness or restricted range of motion of the shoulder, or shoulder instability
	Swimmer's knee (most commonly MCL sprain)	Hx: frequent breaststroke swimming, repetitive valgus stress Sx: medial knee pain, swelling, restricted ROM, weakness or instability in severe cases	Consider MRI to distinguish from medial meniscal tear if pain is not improving with conservative therapy

(continued)

Table 123.1 (continued)

Sport	Common injuries	History and common symptoms	Evaluation
Rowing	De Quervain's Tenosynovitis	Hx: repetitive rowing motion, especially in cold weather (early Spring) Sx: pain, swelling, crepitus at the base of the thumb which extends into the forearm with grasping or extension of the thumb	Normally a clinical diagnosis; imaging is not typically recommended

Abbreviations: *Hx* History, *Sx* symptoms, *PE* physical exam, *LOC* loss of consciousness, *DIP* distal interphalangeal, *MCP* metacarpophalangeal, *ROM* range of motion, *MCL* medial collateral ligament

[a]The PECARN (Pediatric Emergency Care Applied Research Network) pediatric head injury algorithm is a validated tool that predicts clinically important traumatic brain injury (defined as death, intubation, neurosurgical intervention, and hospitalization for greater than 2 days due to the head injury) in children and adolescents who present with mild head injury.

Students who present with mild head injury should be evaluated in an emergency department for a possible CT scan of the head if they present with *any of the following 7 predictors*: Glasgow Coma Score (GCS) < 14; signs of altered mental status (agitation, somnolence, repetitive questioning, slow to respond to verbal communication); signs of basilar skull fracture; history of loss of consciousness; history of vomiting; severe mechanism of injury (motor vehicle crash with patient ejection or death of another passenger, rollover, pedestrian or bicyclist without helmet struck by a motorized vehicle, fall > 5 feet, head struck by high velocity object); or severe headache [8]

Case 2 A 17-year-old male swimmer recently increased his training regimen, now training over 15 hours and swimming over 50 km per week, attempting to shave off time in the freestyle event. He has been experiencing a deep aching in his shoulder during and after his sessions that has more recently been keeping him up at night. He maintains full range of motion of his shoulder but notices the peak of pain occurs as he is reaching during the freestyle stroke. He notes that his dad has recently received corticosteroid injections in his shoulder for similar aching pains, which brought him quick relief, and is wondering if he should also try this. What should you do?

In addition to being able to recognize common sports-specific injuries, it is important to focus on proper prevention and management of injuries before they become more problematic with longer-lasting effects. Although most overuse injuries last for less than 3 weeks, duration of symptoms can be highly variable and could lead to ultimate career-ending consequences [9]. Prevention strategies are aimed at finding a balance between repetitive stress and recovery. Common strategies include advancing training loads by no more than 10–20% each week, promoting age-appropriate training, allowing 2–3 months off from each sport each year, and optimizing recovery time (e.g. encouraging proper hydration, nutrition, and sleep) [10]. Furthermore, there is evidence that incorporating increased variation in training regimens and promoting cross-training can decrease injury risk. This may occur due to the effects of decreasing stress from the body structures typically involved, allowing time for recovery, and shifting the biomechanical load to be more well-balanced. One example of this can be seen with "swimmer's shoulder," which describes pain and dysfunction of the shoulder complex mainly referring to multiple tendinopathies. Joint overload and muscular imbalances due to overtraining particular muscle and tendon groups leads to impingement at the joint. However, studies have shown that incorporating endurance and strength training of the core muscle groups and lower limbs, as well as increased dry-land exercises, can decrease this overload and injury burden [11].

Case 3 A 10-year-old boy recently joined a local ski racing team and has been eagerly hitting the slopes every day. While he was skiing down a steep incline last week, he caught an edge and lost control, falling forward onto his hands. He remembers a sharp pain shoot through his thumb as he landed on his ski pole, forcing the thumb backwards. He now has pain and swelling at the base of his thumb and reports that he has been dropping objects all week. He comes to you for advice.

For driven athletes, time away from play due to injury is often very difficult. However, most of the injuries listed in Table 123.1 are primarily treated with R.I.C.E. therapy (rest, ice, compression with braces/wraps/tapes, elevation), non-steroidal anti-inflammatory medications, cross training, and physical therapy (focusing on strengthening surrounding structures). In many cases, radiographs are the first-line imaging techniques utilized, however plain radiographs are of limited use in the evaluation of soft tissues. As a general rule, if pain or disability is not improving after 6–8 weeks with conservative therapy, more advanced imaging (MRI) and management may be required, including surgical interventions. In cases with more severe initial presentation, such as symptoms of numbness, tingling, weakness, and/or deformity, sending the athlete to an emergency department for immediate imaging may be necessary as there may be a higher risk of cartilaginous, ligamentous, or nerve injury.

123.1 Case Conclusions

Case 1 On physical examination, you discover that the dedicated gymnast has moderate tenderness to palpation over the L5 vertebrae as well as pain reproducible with lumbar extension. Furthermore, she has a positive straight-leg test and 4/5 strength with extension of the toes of her left foot. You send her for a spinal radiograph, which reveals a bilateral pars interarticularis defect with evidence of mild 25% slippage. She is referred to spinal surgeon who performs an MRI revealing a low-grade spondylolisthesis injury at L5. She unfortunately has to miss the Championships during her recovery period, but after 3 months of rest followed by physical therapy, as well as improvement on subsequent imaging, she is able to slowly return to competition.

Case 2 On exam, he has point tenderness over the greater tuberosity and anterior acromion, intact neurovascular exam, and full range of motion of the shoulder with pain elicited by the Hawkin's test and Jobe's test (empty can test). You suspect that he may be experiencing "swimmer's shoulder," more specifically a supraspinatus tendinopathy. You recommend against imaging and corticosteroid injection at this time and suggest starting with more conservative measures such as ice, NSAIDs, increasing dry-land training, and appropriate core and external rotator strengthening exercises. After a few weeks of including some variation in his training, he feels significantly better and beats his own personal best time at his next swim meet.

Case 3 On your exam, you note swelling and bruising at the base of the thumb. When you apply valgus stress to the thumb, you note increased laxity compared to the other thumb (laxity > 20 degrees). You decide to send him for a hand radiograph to rule out a possible avulsion fracture, however imaging is unrevealing. Suspecting an ulnar collateral ligament tear, you recommend R.I.C.E. therapy, immobilization with a thumb spica splint, and physical therapy. Despite these measures, he reports persistent pain and weakness after 6 weeks, at which time you refer him to a hand surgeon to evaluate for possible surgical repair.

Extra Credit Points

1. Early sports specialization has become more common, leading to increased risk of injury in youth athletes, and does not often correlate with progression to elite athletic status.
2. Overuse injuries occur due to repetitive microtrauma on growing structures without proper recovery, and often occur in predictable patterns depending on sport-specific maneuvers.
3. Healthcare providers should be aware of common patterns of injury that occur in specific sports in order to better guide prevention and minimize long-term risk.
4. Increasing variation in training regimens, including cross-training, has been shown to decrease injury burden in young athletes.
5. In general, failure of conservative therapy after 6–8 weeks, or severe initial presentation (e.g. numbness, weakness, deformity) are indications for more advanced imaging and management.

References

1. Bell DR, Snedden TR, Biese KM, et al. Consensus definition of sport specialization in youth athletes using a Delphi approach. J Athl Train. 2021;56(11):1239–51.
2. McLellan M, Allahabadi S, Pandya NK. Youth sports specialization and its effect on professional, elite, and olympic athlete performance, career longevity, and injury rates: a systematic review. Orthop J Sports Med. 2022;10(11):23259671221129594.
3. Jayanthi N, Pinkham C, Dugas L, Patrick B, LaBella C. Sports specialization in young athletes: evidence-based recommendations. Sports Health. 2013;5(3):251–7. https://doi.org/10.1177/1941738112464626.

4. Malina RM. Early sport specialization: roots, effectiveness, risks. Curr Sports Med Rep. 2010;9(6):364–71.
5. DiFiori JP, Benjamin HJ, Brenner JS, et al. Overuse injuries and burnout in youth sports: a position statement from the American Medical Society for Sports Medicine. Br J Sports Med. 2014;48(4):287–8. https://doi.org/10.1136/bjsports-2013-093299.
6. Selhorst M, Fischer A, MacDonald J. Prevalence of spondylolysis in symptomatic adolescent athletes: an assessment of sport risk in nonelite athletes. Clin J Sport Med. 2019;29(5):421–5. https://doi.org/10.1097/JSM.0000000000000546.
7. Mohile NV, Kuczmarski AS, Lee D, et al. Spondylolysis and isthmic spondylolisthesis: a guide to diagnosis and management. J Am Board Fam Med. 2022;35(6):1204–16. https://doi.org/10.3122/jabfm.2022.220130R1.
8. Kuppermann N, Holmes JF, Dayan PS, et al. Identification of children at very low risk of clinically-important brain injuries after head trauma: a prospective cohort study. Lancet. 2009;374(9696):1160–70.
9. Schroeder AN, Comstock RD, Collins CL, Everhart J, Flanigan D, Best TM. Epidemiology of overuse injuries among high-school athletes in the United States. J Pediatr. 2015;166(3):600–6. https://doi.org/10.1016/j.jpeds.2014.09.037.
10. Brenner JS, Watson A. Overuse injuries, overtraining, and burnout in young athletes. Pediatrics. 2016;138(3):e20162148.
11. Bak K. The practical management of swimmer's painful shoulder: etiology, diagnosis and treatment. Clin J Sport Med. 2010;20(5):386–90.

Chapter 124
Running Injuries

Makenna Brezitski and Matthew Silvis

Case 1 17 y/o female runner increases her running distance per week from 20 to 40 miles. She now has pain over her distal medial tibia. Pain initially occurred at the end of her runs only. Now she is experiencing pain during regular ambulation. You note focal pain in this location and recommend she see her primary care provider to obtain x-rays.

The number of high school cross country runners has doubled over the past 4 decades with a subsequent 30–40% increase in running related injuries (RRIs). This equates to ~200,000 adolescent runners experiencing a RRI/year [1]. Risk factors for adolescent RRIs include: high level of sport specialization (75% greater risk of RRI than low specialization), lower cadence (<170 steps/minute), poor sleep quality, oligo/amenorrhea, history of RRI (50% greater odds of sustaining a second RRI), female sex, no variability in mileage across a training cycle, and large increases in mileage (>10 miles/week).

M. Brezitski (✉)
Penn State Milton S. Hershey Medical Center, Hershey, PA, USA
e-mail: mbrezitski@pennstatehealth.psu.edu

M. Silvis
Penn State Health, Hershey, PA, USA
e-mail: msilvis@pennstatehealth.psu.edu

R. P. Olympia, J. Brady-Olympia (eds.), *Clinical Considerations in School-based Health*, https://doi.org/10.1007/978-3-031-85765-2_124

124.1 Evaluation of the Adolescent Runner

When seeing an injured adolescent runner, it is important to ask specific questions about their running background and injury details. A targeted physical evaluation should also be completed for determination of the type of injury. In an adolescent runner, the most common injuries are of the lower extremity (Table 124.1).

History taking:

- How and when did the injury happen?
- Where is the pain? How intense? We often ask adolescents to point with one finger to the location of maximal discomfort for better injury localization and differential diagnosis.
  - Shin injuries are common and account for up to 40% of adolescent RRIs [5]
- Does the pain occur constantly or with certain activities/movements?
- Do they play an organized sport? Or are they a recreational runner?

Table 124.1 Common Adolescent Running Injuries

Condition	Key Characteristics	Key Exam Findings	Management & Next steps
Patellofemoral pain syndrome	Thought to be related to imbalance of muscle strength (vastus medialis obliquus) and hamstring/ quadricep flexibility [2] Generalized anterior knee pain Inciting event is usually increased activity Worse with sitting for long periods of time Often worse with squatting or going down stairs [2]	Tenderness of the patella facets with associated poor patella mobility/tilt Valgus knee movement with single-leg squat [2]	Decrease activity to nonpainful activities for first 2–3 weeks; critical to avoid deep knee bends NSAIDs and icing as needed Patellar taping or knee bands are sometimes beneficial Physical therapy is the mainstay of treatment to strengthen hip and knee and improve flexibility [2]
IT band friction syndrome	Often consequence of tightness/increased tone in the IT band, leading to friction against the lateral femoral condyle [3] Lateral knee pain with associated snapping Usually begins after period of increased activity	Pain over lateral femoral condyle [2] May have pain at insertion site of Gerdy's tubercle (lateral condyle of tibia) Ober test often shows tightness of the IT band Weak hip abductors	Decrease activity to nonpainful activities NSAIDs and icing as needed Foam rolling [3] Physical therapy to stretch the IT band and strengthen/stabilize hip abductors

(continued)

Table 124.1 (continued)

Condition	Key Characteristics	Key Exam Findings	Management & Next steps
Medial tibial stress syndrome (MTSS or "shin splints")	Suspected to be related to underlying tibial overload resulting in microdamage and periostitis [4] Diffuse pain over the distal/medial portion of the tibia exacerbated by exercise Paresthesias and swelling are not typical	Tenderness to palpation of the posteromedial tibial border for at least 5 cm [4] Diagnosis is unlikely if pain is not reproducible	Important to set expectations with runners; may take several weeks to be able to run with minimal pain and up to 12 months for healing [4] Decrease running load by ~50% to achieve at most mild pain with activity [4] Evaluate running shoes to determine if need replaced X-ray to exclude stress fracture Consider referral to specialist for consideration of MRI to differentiate between shin splints and stress fracture if exam/x-ray is equivocal [5]
Stress Fractures	Result from increased load on bone, often from rapidly increasing and repetitive training load [5] Pain localizes to area of fracture, commonly tibia and metatarsals Also occur in femur and fibula May be associated with Relative Energy Deficiency in Sport (RED-S) where low energy availability reduces resilience of the underlying bone [5] Recurrent stress fractures require further evaluation including detailed training history, gait analysis, and nutritional evaluation.	Tenderness over the distal posteromedial tibial border for less than 5 cm [4] Positive Hop test	X-ray as initial imaging modality (callus formation can be seen on radiographs after 2–3 weeks) Consider MRI for grading of severity (Grade 1–4) which can help guide the recommended rest period [4] Crutches often used initially if pain with regular ambulation Ensure adequate vitamin D and calcium intake Recommend close follow up with primary provider, especially if there is concern for malnutrition or lack of menstrual cycles [5]

(continued)

Table 124.1 (continued)

Condition	Key Characteristics	Key Exam Findings	Management & Next steps
Chronic exertional compartment syndrome (CECS)	Swelling of muscle compartments with exercise, increasing compartment pressure resulting in pain, paresthesias, and/or weakness Most common in the anterior compartment of the leg, followed by lateral Severe pain, burning/tingling, tightness of the area that begins soon after activity is initiated at a reproducible distance [6] Quickly resolves with rest	Tightness or tenderness of the area just after exercise May have decreased sensation and/or weakness	Intramuscular compartment pressure testing by a specialist can confirm the diagnosis [6] 3–6 months of conservative measures while continuing low impact activities Physical therapy, NSAIDs, massage Progressive return to running program Fasciotomy (removing the tissue that covers muscles) can be considered for refractory cases [6]

- How frequent and what distances are their runs?
- Have they recently increased the frequency or distance of their runs?
- What is the running terrain? Are they running on a treadmill? Track? Flat road? Trail?
- Have they had a running injury before? If so, what was it?
- Do they have other medical conditions such as asthma, low bone density, or eating disorders?
- For girls who have undergone menarche, are they still getting their menses regularly?****In our clinical practice, ~75% of RRIs are related to training errors with an additional 15–20% related to underlying running gait/biomechanics and 5–10% related to inadequate nutrition***

  Targeted physical exam:

- Inspection: Are there any cuts, open areas, bleeding? Is there obvious swelling, bruising, or deformity of the area?
- Palpation: Is it tender to touch? If so, where does it hurt? Are there bony abnormalities?
- Movement (range of motion): Is range of motion preserved and comparable to the non-injured, contralateral side? Is there a locking, clicking, catching sensation that would raise suspicion for intra articular involvement?
- Strength: Are they able to put weight/pressure on the affected area? Can they walk? Run? Is strength symmetric bilaterally?

- Special tests:
  - Ober test for IT band tightness: positioned on unaffected side with knees flexed to 90°. The affected hip is moved into extension and adduction from flexion and abduction. Positive test if there is pain/clicking/tightness over IT band.
    - https://youtu.be/Amjv6FzDeLE?si=EQNHNJwlrFIzOet_
  - Noble test for IT band tightness: palpate lateral femoral condyle and extend knee. Positive test if there is pain or clicking over the lateral femoral condyle.
    - https://youtu.be/PmUGl7ryQOo?si=tOLSudLh1whmfmXm
  - Hop test for stress fracture: hop on affected leg. Positive if pain is reproduced and localized over the area of concern.
    - https://youtu.be/IyVrcXaJptQ?si=z5D0UHNMpAXw4JzE

Case 2 A 16-year-old male cross-country runner presents to you with anterior knee pain for the last several weeks. He typically runs about 25 miles per week and gets about 6 hours of sleep per night. Exam reveals tenderness of the patella facets and significantly worn soles of his running shoes.

124.2 Running Injury Prevention

As school-based clinicians and providers we can help prevent injuries in our adolescent runners. In addition to running patterns and practices, lifestyle may also impact risk for running injuries.

- Running/training Factors
  - Lower extremity strength: muscle endurance and hip strength are essential for long distance running [7]; decreased abductor strength is often associated with IT band friction syndrome [7]
    - Preventative measure: suggest athletes incorporate strength/weight training into their training regimen; focus should be on hip strength, namely strengthening the abductor muscles for pelvic stability.
  - Training distance and intensity: higher weekly miles (> 40 miles/week) or an abrupt increase in intensity/mileage is associated with running related injuries [7, 8]; increasing weekly distance by greater than 30% significantly increases risk [8]
    - Preventative measure: increase weekly distance by no more than 10%/week to decrease risk of running related injuries [8]
  - Running shoes [9]:

    - Every time a runner buys running shoes, they should have their feet sized as their feet may not be the same size. Runners should also buy running shoes at the end of the day when their feet are maximally swollen (½ inch of space is ideal between toes and shoe).
    - Runners should purchase neutral shoes without motion control or stability components. These components interfere with normal foot motion during weight bearing. Running shoes should also have minimal heel to toe drop (</= 6 mm) to allow for normal loading support during each gait cycle.
    - Running shoes should be light in weight. Without shoes, the cost of leg swing = 20% cost of running. For every 100 g increase in shoe mass, the metabolic cost of running increases by 1%.
    - Foot shape/arch height are not good indicators of what kind of running shoe to buy. Runners should avoid advice given after someone in a running store has watched them run as gait/foot motion are very different between walking and running.
    - Runners should change their running shoes every 350 miles. Shoe aging is influenced by runner weight, speed, foot strike, and type of running surface. If wear patterns on shoes reveal the sole layers underneath, need replaced!

- Lifestyle Factors
  - Sleep: Fatigue and decreased nightly sleep may impact runner's performance and place them at risk for running related injuries. It also decreases the essential bodily recovery time [7]
    - Preventative measure: adequate nightly sleep for which we recommend 8–10 hours per night.
  - Nutrition: Poor nutrition, especially athletes with the intention to lose weight, is a large predictor of running related injury as it can result in lower available energy (RED-S), contributing to decreased bone density [7]
    - Preventative measure: adequate daily calories, accounting for energy expenditure with running; sufficient vitamin D and calcium intake; supervision, rest, and nutrition counseling for athletes where disordered eating or intentional weight loss is suspected.
- Pedestrian Safety [10]
  - Runner versus vehicle collisions are relatively rare but the result can be catastrophic.
    - As cross-country participation has increased over the past 4 decades, pedestrian fatalities have also increased.
  - Nearly all pedestrian fatalities occur at a location other than a sidewalk.
  - Pedestrian safety measures for high school runners should include the following:

- Run while facing traffic
- Cross streets at intersections within cross walks
- Avoid running in the dark
  - Many incidents occur in early AM or later afternoon/early PM.
  - Wear bright and reflective clothing on limbs (wrists/ankles) not just torso.
- Establish runner safety measures as part of school emergency action plans.

124.3 Case Conclusions

Case 1 X-ray shows callus formation over the tibia. She is diagnosed with a stress fracture. She is recommended to rest and avoid strenuous activities for 4–6 weeks. She uses crutches initially until she is able to ambulate without pain. She takes a daily calcium and vitamin D supplement as recommended by her primary care provider. She maintains her fitness with stationary cycling and swimming and slowly returns to running over the next several weeks. She is encouraged to increase her weekly mileage by <10 miles week to reduce her risk for running related injuries. She is grateful to be at her baseline mileage and participates in her running season 12 weeks later.

Case 2 You diagnose him with patellofemoral pain syndrome. You recommend he decrease to nonpainful activities for 2–3 weeks, being careful to avoid deep knee bends. He works with a physical therapist on hip and knee strengthening. He is encouraged to obtain new running shoes given the significant wear and tear from his mileage. You also discuss basic sleep hygiene techniques focused on obtaining at least 8 hours of sleep nightly.

Extra Credit Points

1. Running-related injuries are common among adolescent athletes, especially with increased participating in running-involved sports.
2. A detailed history focused on common training errors accompanied by a focused physical examination and supplemental imaging can lead to the correct diagnosis in the majority of runners with common diagnoses being patellofemoral pain syndrome, IT band syndrome, "shin splints", stress fractures, and exertional compartment syndrome.
3. Most running related injuries will benefit from physical therapy. When injuries are not improving as expected, athletes should be referred to a sports medicine physician. If there is an extremity deformity after trauma, significant bleeding or suspected neurovascular compromise, athletes should be sent to the emergency department for evaluation.

4. Running related injury prevention may by optimized by focusing on a runner's lower extremity strength and mobility, sleep and nutrition. Nutritionist referral may be beneficial in athletes with disordered eating to ensure adequate caloric intake.
5. Educating about selecting and replacement of running shoes can help prevent injury.
6. All runners should be educated on running safety and emergency action planning to prevent catastrophic collisions with motor vehicles.

References

1. Joachim MR, Kuik ML, Krabak BJ, Kraus EM, Rauh MJ, Heiderscheit BC. Risk factors for running-related injury in high school and collegiate cross-country runners: a systematic review. J Orthop Sports Phys Ther. 2024;54:1–132.
2. Lintner LJ, Swisher J, Sitton ZE. Childhood and adolescent sports-related overuse injuries. Am Fam Phys. 2023;108(6):544–53.
3. Friede MC, Klauser A, Fink C, Csapo R. Stiffness of the iliotibial band and associated muscles in runner's knee: assessing the effects of physiotherapy through ultrasound shear wave elastography. Phys Ther Sport. 2020;45:126–34.
4. Milgrom C, Zloczower E, Fleischmann C, et al. Medial tibial stress fracture diagnosis and treatment guidelines. J Sci Med Sport. 2021;24:526–30.
5. De Jong Lempke AF, Stracciolini A, Willwerth SB, et al. Clinical assessment, treatment, and referral trends for adolescent runners seeking care at an injured runners' clinic. J Pediatr Rehabil Med. 2023:1–13.
6. Velasco TO, Leggit JC. Chronic exertional compartment syndrome: a clinical update. Curr Sports Med Rep. 2020;19:347–52.
7. De Jong Lempke AF, Whitney KE, Collins SE, d'Hemecourt PA, Meehan WP. Intrinsic and extrinsic factors contributing to running-related lower limb injuries among adolescent runners. J Sports Sci. 2022;40:2468–74.
8. Vincent H, Vincent K. Evaluation of the injured runner. In: Harrast M, editor. Clinical care of the runner. Elsevier; 2020. p. 19–26.
9. Vincent H, Vincent K. Selecting running shoes. 2014. Accessed 15 May 2024. https://www.acsm.org/docs/default-source/files-for-resource-library/running-shoes.pdf?sfvrsn=6123deef_2.
10. Shore E, De Long R, Powell E, et al. Pedestrian safety among high school runners: a case series. Sports Health. 2023;15:633–7.

Chapter 125
Special Considerations in the Young Female Athlete

Jodi Brady-Olympia

Over the decades, and particularly since the passage of Title IX, the number of girls participating in high school sports has increased significantly, from 24.2% in 1973 to 42.9% in 2018 [1] (Fig. 125.1). In addition, the number of sports that girls participate in has widened, with the most recent additions including wrestling and ice hockey [1]. With the increase in the number of female students participating in a wider variety of sports, typical injury patterns are more commonly seen in females than males [2].

Case 1 Lilly is a ninth grader who has participated in soccer since elementary school and hopes to play on the varsity team next year. She comes into the clinic concerned about a teammate who recently had an anterior cruciate ligament (ACL) injury. She read that this type of injury is more common among female athletes and is concerned about her risk for a similar injury. One of her coaches had talked to the team about exercises for strength and conditioning. Lilly is wondering if there are any exercises she could do to decrease her risk of an ACL injury.

The incidence of non-contact ACL injuries are higher among females than males. This increased risk may be due to an increased Q-angle in women (the angle created by the quadriceps muscle and patellar tendon), hormonal fluctuations during menstrual cycles that can impact the elasticity of collagen within the knee, landing techniques (women are more likely to land with straighter knees and less core engagement), muscle mass (women generally have less muscle mass about their knees, which leads to less stability), and range of motion of the knee .

J. Brady-Olympia (✉)
Department of Pediatrics Penn State, College of Medicine Attending Physician, Division of Adolescent Medicine, Department of Pediatrics, Penn State Children's Hospital, Hershey, PA, USA
e-mail: jbradyolympia@pennstatehealth.psu.edu

R. P. Olympia, J. Brady-Olympia (eds.), *Clinical Considerations in School-based Health*, https://doi.org/10.1007/978-3-031-85765-2_125

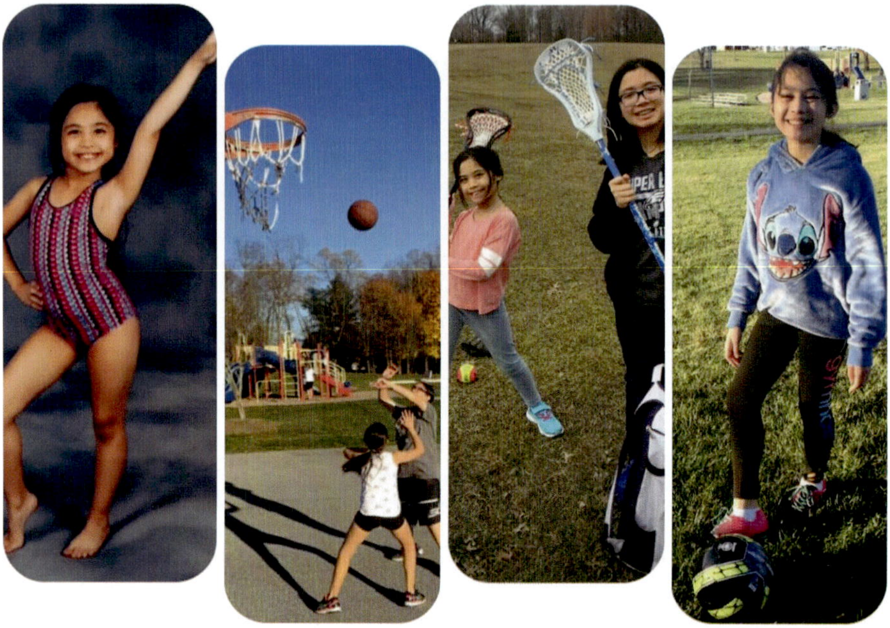

Fig. 125.1 "Courage, sacrifice, determination, commitment, toughness, heart, talent, guts. That's what little girls are made of; the heck with sugar and spice." Bethany Hamilton (American surfer and author)

ACL injuries are seen more commonly with cutting, twisting, and pivoting movements [3]. When comparing sports where adolescent males and females both participate such as basketball, soccer, and lacrosse, the rate of ACL injury was higher among female than male adolescent athletes (Relative Risk 1.28 in lacrosse to 3.10 in soccer and 4.14 in basketball) [4]. When comparing ACL injuries among different sports, ACL injuries were more commonly seen in soccer and gymnastics [4]. Given the increased risk for ACL injuries among females, there have been programs developed over the years which aim to decrease athletes' risk of injury [3]. Ramirez et al. performed a systematic review looking at the incidence of ACL rupture in athletes who participated in a neuromuscular training programs compared with athletes who did not and found there was a higher incidence of ACL rupture in athletes, particularly soccer players, who did not participate in these types of programs [5]. It is important to identify athletes who are at increased risk for these injuries, based on the sports they participate in and the maneuvers (such as cutting, twisting and pivoting movements) that make up that sport, to guide them towards neuromuscular training programs to decrease the risk for ACL injuries.

With this information regarding the risk of ACL injuries among adolescent female soccer players and the benefit of neuromuscular training programs, you suggest that Lily speak to her parents about signing up for a neuromuscular training program through a local physical therapist who specializes in pediatric athletes.

Case 2 Bella, a 14-year-old high school freshman, comes to the clinic with a complaint of right knee pain that started about 2 weeks ago. She joined the cross-country team and has been running about 30 minutes a day at practice. She denies any history of trauma to her right knee, denying any recent falls or twisting of the knee. She also denies any redness or swelling. The pain seemed to start gradually but now increases when she is running. She also says it bothers her when she stands up after sitting in class for a while and when she goes up and down stairs. She remembers that she had a similar pain in the left knee at the end of the last track season, but it got better over the summer; however, she didn't really run or do much exercise over the summer.

As you are talking with Bella, you recall her story is like many other adolescent females you have seen over the years. Her history, particularly discomfort after sitting, pain with climbing stairs and lack of trauma history is consistent with Patellofemoral pain syndrome; however, it is crucial to obtain a full history and perform a thorough physical exam. On examination she has tenderness just below the patella and denies any joint line tenderness. There is no effusion or laxity, and she has full range of motion. You also do a complete hip exam which is unremarkable. When evaluating knee pain in children and adolescents it is also important to consider hip pathology as patients with hip injuries or pathology such as Slipped Capital Femoral Epiphysis (SCFE) syndrome can also present with knee pain [2]. Treatment of Patellofemoral pain syndrome may include the use of NSAIDs (Nonsteroidal anti-inflammatory drugs), exercises to strengthen the hip and knee joints, orthotics and/or referral to physical therapy. For Bella, you refer her to a pediatric physical therapist in the community, who suggests strength training, NSAIDs, and gradual return to sport as her symptoms improve.

Table 125.1 describes several injuries and conditions seen more commonly in adolescent females.

Case 3 Hannah, a 17-year-old cross country runner, comes in with a complaint of left shin pain which has been gradually getting worse over the past 2 weeks. Initially it only hurt after running, but recently she experiences pain even when she is walking around after her practices. She says she has had a good season and consistently placed high or won all her meets. She has been training harder lately with the hope of qualifying for states and has been strength training and doing an extra workout in the morning. She has also been making "healthy" changes in her diet, eating more fruits and vegetables and more protein, but doesn't think she is eating less than her usual diet. She denies wanting to lose weight or having body dissatisfaction. In general, she says she has been feeling well although a little more fatigued, which she attributes to getting up early to work out and being up late studying. When you ask about her periods, she says they were light during the preseason workouts, but she has not gotten her period in almost 3 months, although says she is not concerned and comments it is "normal" for runners. She says this has happened in the past during her track and cross-country seasons and has also happened with other runners she knows. With her last menstrual period being about 3 months ago, you obtain a

Table 125.1 Injuries/conditions seen more commonly in adolescent females [2, 3, 6]

Injury	Examples of sports	History	Examination	Management
Patellofemoral pain syndrome	Running, biking, basketball, jumping	Gradual onset without acute injury Pain with climbing stairs, running, jumping pain after prolonged sitting	Tenderness around patella + grind test	NSAID, strengthening exercises/Physical therapy, Orthotics/arch supports
Patellofemoral instability[a]/Patellar subluxation/dislocation	Girls' gymnastics, girls' soccer	Internal rotation of femur when foot is planted	+tenderness around patella +apprehension test	Referral orthopedics Consider referral to emergency department
Anterior Cruciate Ligament tear	Basketball, gymnastics, soccer, lacrosse and skiing	Pivot on planted foot Knee hyperextension	+swelling/effusion +inability to weight bear +Lachman test	Xray/ MRI Referral to orthopedics or emergency department
Shoulder injury—glenohumeral/multidirectional instability [7]	Swimming, softball, tennis, volleyball, gymnastics	Often related to overuse or overload [3]	+ sulcus sign + apprehension test	Strength and conditioning exercises/physical therapy consider referral to orthopedics if neurological deficit, decreased range of motion or not improving with physical therapy

[a]in sex-comparable sports- i.e. girls soccer > boys' soccer [6]

urine sample for pregnancy testing which is negative. Given her complaint of increasing shin pain for 2 weeks and oligomenorrhea, you also refer her to a sports medicine physician to evaluate for a stress fracture. She comes back to see you the following week to tell you that she had an MRI which showed a stress fracture and is very upset that she was told she cannot run.

Amenorrhea or irregular periods in an athlete should not be considered "normal" (Chap. 128). In addition, while she denies body image concern or intentionally restricting her intake for weight loss purposes (Chap. 75), it is likely that she may not be properly "fueling" her body for the amount and intensity of exercise she is engaging in. Hannah's case raises concern for what has been termed the Female Athlete Triad, which includes low energy availability (which may or may not include disordered eating), menstrual dysfunction, and decreased bone density [8]. When the term was first coined by the Task Force on Women's Issues of the American College of Sports Medicine in 1992, all three components of the triad were required for diagnosis—osteoporosis, amenorrhea, and disordered eating [8];

however, in 2007 this definition was broadened to include of a spectrum of presentations. This expanded definition allowed the inclusion of athletes who did not meet the original strict inclusion criteria but were still at risk for the complications that can result from inadequate energy availability [9].

While the Female Athlete Triad has been researched and written about over the years, more recently there has been increasing evidence for similar impact of decreased energy availability in males as well as seen with decreased testosterone levels or decreased bone density [10]. In 2014, the International Olympic Committee introduced the term Relative Energy Deficiency in Sport (REDs) to emphasize the role that low energy availability has on the body and the fact that this can be seen in both males and females [11].

It is important to identify students who meet the criteria for the diagnosis of REDS or any of the components of the Female Athlete Triad and refer them to a multidisciplinary team that may include an adolescent medicine or sports medicine physician, a dietician, and a psychologist/behavioral health practitioner for evaluation and treatment [12]. Treatment would include restoring energy balance and increasing nutritional intake to meet energy expenditure resulting in resumption of menses [8, 12]. The dietician can provide guidance to ensure there is adequate intake of micro and macro nutrients including vitamin D and calcium.

As illustrated in the case above, athletes may not be aware that irregular menses or amenorrhea are problematic or may choose not to share that information with their coaches or medical providers. While this should be discussed during the preparticipation physical and routine well care visit, the significance of irregular menses or amenorrhea may be overlooked or underappreciated. Nose-Ogura, et al. looked at elite female athletes in their 20s and noted a correlation between low bone mineral density and history of amenorrhea during their teenage years [13]. Studies have shown that parents, athletes, coaches, and training staff may not be aware of the resulting consequences of REDS or aware of the 3 facets of the "Female Athlete Triad"; and therefore, education should be provided to the recognition of these disorders [11].

Extra Credit Points

1. ACL injuries are seen more commonly among female athletes compared with male athletes. Studies have shown that the risk of ACL rupture is higher in athletes who do not participate in neuromuscular training programs.
2. The preparticipation physical examination is an important opportunity to identify areas of previous injury and provide education about the need for strength training, stretching, or activity modification.
3. Amenorrhea in female athletes should serve as a red flag to delve into a deeper discussion about risk factors leading to Relative Energy Deficiency, and therefore should include a thorough menstrual history, dietary history, and training history.

References

1. Tanaka MJ, LiBrizzi CL, Rivenburgh DW, Jones LC. Changes in U.S. girls' participation in high school sports: implications for injury awareness. Phys Sportsmed. 2021;49(4):450–4. https://doi.org/10.1080/00913847.2020.1852861. Epub 2020 Dec 10.
2. Coleman N. Sports injuries. Pediatr Rev. 2019;40(6):278–90. https://doi.org/10.1542/pir.2018-0221.
3. Female athlete issues for the team physician: a consensus statement—2017 update. Med Sci Sports Exerc 2018;50(5):1113–1122. https://doi.org/10.1249/MSS.0000000000001603.
4. Bram JT, Magee LC, Mehta NN, Patel NM, Ganley TJ. Anterior cruciate ligament injury incidence in adolescent athletes: a systematic review and meta-analysis. Am J Sports Med. 2021;49(7):1962–72. https://doi.org/10.1177/0363546520959619. Epub 2020 Oct 22.
5. Ramirez RN, Baldwin K, Franklin CCD. Prevention of anterior cruciate ligament rupture in female athletes: a systematic review. JBJS Rev. 2014;2(9):e3. https://doi.org/10.2106/JBJS.RVW.M.00129.
6. Mitchell J, Magnussen RA, Collins CL, Currie DW, Best TM, Comstock RD, Flanigan DC. Epidemiology of patellofemoral instability injuries among high school athletes in the United States. Am J Sports Med. 2015;43(7):1676–82. https://doi.org/10.1177/0363546515577786. Epub 2015 Apr 21.
7. Wessel LE, Eliasberg CD, Bowen E, Sutton KM. Shoulder and elbow pathology in the female athlete: sex-specific considerations. J Shoulder Elb Surg. 2021;30(5):977–85. https://doi.org/10.1016/j.jse.2020.10.020.
8. Maya J, Misra M. The female athlete triad: review of current literature. Curr Opin Endocrinol Diabetes Obes. 2022;29(1):44–51. https://doi.org/10.1097/MED.0000000000000690.
9. Matzkin E, Curry EJ, Whitlock K. Female athlete triad: past, present, and future. J Am Acad Orthop Surg. 2015;23(7):424–32. https://doi.org/10.5435/JAAOS-D-14-0016800000000690.
10. Tenforde AS, Barrack MT, Nattiv A, Fredericson M. Parallels with the female athlete triad in male athletes. Sports Med. 2016;46(2):171–82. https://doi.org/10.1007/s40279-015-0411-y.
11. Mountjoy M, Ackerman KE, Bailey DM, et al. International Olympic Committee's (IOC) consensus statement on Relative Energy Deficiency in Sport (REDs) [published correction appears in Br J Sports Med. 2024 Feb 7;58(3):e4. https://doi.org/10.1136/bjsports-2023-106994corr1]. Br J Sports Med. 2023;57(17):1073–97. https://doi.org/10.1136/bjsports-2023-106994.
12. Grabia M, Perkowski J, Socha K, Markiewicz-Żukowska R. Female athlete triad and relative energy deficiency in sport (REDs): nutritional management. Nutrients. 2024;16(3):359. Published 2024 Jan 25. https://doi.org/10.3390/nu16030359.
13. Nose-Ogura S, Yoshino O, Dohi M, Kigawa M, Harada M, Kawahara T, Osuga Y, Saito S. Low bone mineral density in elite female athletes with a history of secondary amenorrhea in their teens. Clin J Sport Med. 2020;30(3):245–50. https://doi.org/10.1097/JSM.0000000000000571.

Part IX
Topics in Adolescent Medicine

Chapter 126
Legal Issues in Caring for the Adolescent Student—Consent and Privacy

Kristen Reilly and Ashley Ebersole

Case 1 **Maria is a 16-year-old female who comes to your office asking about getting tested for sexually transmitted infections. She had sex for the first time a few weeks ago with her age-matched boyfriend without a condom. She has taken an at-home pregnancy test, which was negative, and has had a menstrual period since it happened. Though she has no symptoms, she wants to be tested to be safe. Her mother knows that she has a boyfriend, but Maria doesn't want her to know that she's sexually active.**

Case 2 **Sam is a 15-year-old male who comes to your office for a sports physical. You complete a comprehensive social history, and Sam discloses that he has started smoking cannabis a few times a month. He has never tried any other drugs, and he has never been in a car when people were drinking or using drugs. He smokes at his friend's house and does not buy it himself. He has never really thought about cutting back.**

Case 3 **Jaylin is a 14-year-old female who comes into your office for on-going headaches. In talking with her, she reveals that she has been feeling depressed for a while and is having thoughts of hurting herself. She has never been diagnosed with any mental health issue nor has she ever received therapy or counseling. She has not discussed how she has been feeling with her mother.**

K. Reilly (✉)
Division of Adolescent and Transition Medicine, Cincinnati Children's Hospital Medical Center, Cincinnati, OH, USA
e-mail: Kristen.Reilly@cchmc.org

A. Ebersole
Nationwide Children's Hospital, Columbus, OH, USA
e-mail: Ashley.Ebersole@nationwidechildrens.org

R. P. Olympia, J. Brady-Olympia (eds.), *Clinical Considerations in School-based Health*, https://doi.org/10.1007/978-3-031-85765-2_126

126.1 Consent

Generally, the law requires parents or guardians to consent before medical care can be provided to a minor. However, all 50 states have enacted statutes allowing minors to consent to their health care in certain circumstances. Care may be provided in emergencies without prior consent, though guardians must be notified immediately. Furthermore, there are categories of minors that are allowed to consent to their health care and specific health services that minors can consent to (Table 126.1).

Though most states allow minors to provide consent to some aspects of their health care, state laws are highly variable and, unfortunately, do not always align with established best practices. Healthcare providers should consult the relevant laws in their state (Table 126.2). Though state laws can vary considerably for minor consent for sexual and reproductive care, there is federal legislation that makes confidential reproductive health services available for free or at low cost to all people, including adolescents, in every state known as The Title X Family Planning Program (Title X). It is implemented through competitively awarded grants to a diverse network of public and private nonprofit health and community-based clinics, including Planned Parenthood [2].

Table 126.1 Common Exceptions to Parental Consent

Specific health care services minors can provide consent for in certain states	Groups of minors able to provide consent to their health care in certain states
Emergency situations Contraceptive care Pregnancy-related care Diagnosis and treatment of sexually transmitted infections, including HIV and AIDS Counseling and treatment for mental health issues Counseling and treatment of substance use Examination and treatment related to sexual assault	Emancipated minors[a] Minors living apart from their parents Married minors Minors in the armed services Minors who are parents High school graduates Minors who have attained a certain age "Mature minors" who are explicitly authorized by statute to consent for care in a few states

[a]Someone who has been legally deemed an adult by a court in his or her state of residence

Table 126.2 Resources on Laws Related to Minor Consent

Resources on Minor Consent	
Guttmacher Institute https://www.guttmacher.org/state-policy/explore/minors-access-contraceptive-services	Up to date state by state summary of contraceptive care available to minors
Guttmacher Institute https://www.guttmacher.org/state-policy/explore/minors-access-sti-services	Up to date state by state summary of testing and treatment of STI
National Center for Youth Law Minor Consent Laws: A State-by-State Summary https://teenhealthlaw.org/resources-for-other-u-s-states/	Summary of state adolescent consent laws
Sharko et al. [1]	Summary of state adolescent consent laws

126.2 Confidentiality

Confidentiality refers to the "agreement between the patient and health care provider that information discussed during or after the encounter will not be shared with others without the explicit permission of the patient" [3]. In most (but not all) states, confidentiality is tied to consent, meaning that when a patient consents to care, it is the duty of the provider to maintain confidentiality. It is crucial to be aware of laws in your state, as some states do allow (but do not compel) healthcare providers to inform parents if their children consent to care.

Confidential health care is important for adolescents as it increases their willingness to disclose risky health behaviors and increases the likelihood of returning for care [4]. Moreover, adolescents will avoid care if privacy cannot be maintained [5]. A study of adolescent females accessing Planned Parenthood services found that if mandatory parental notification for contraceptives went into effect, 47% would stop using *all* Planned Parenthood services, including STI testing and treatment, pregnancy testing, contraception, health examination and HIV testing and treatment and additional 12% would change the services they received. However, only 1% reported they would stop having sex [6]. Connecting adolescents to needed health care services such as reproductive care or substance use treatment depends on open communication with providers about sensitive health issues, and maintaining confidentiality is a critical aspect of this.

126.3 Setting the Stage of Confidential Adolescent Health Care

When providers explicitly discuss confidentiality, adolescents are more likely to openly discuss sensitive issues with clinicians and return for future care [7]. Table 126.3 provides tips on introducing the topic of confidentiality and privacy to

Table 126.3 Tips to Lay Groundwork for Confidentiality [8]

Tips	Example Language
Introduce the concept of confidentiality early before it is most needed.	It is a privilege to take care of *name of child.* To best do that, I would like to spend some time one-on-one with your child. This helps them develop necessary skills for becoming an adult. What we talk about together is confidential, or private. This information goes into the medical record, and may be used by medical people, like doctors and nurses, to take care of you. I will not share this information with anyone else, without your permission. I mean it. I may encourage you to talk to your parents, but that would be up to you. There are, however, a couple circumstances that would require me by law to break our agreement of confidentiality: If someone were hurting you If you were going to hurt someone If your life or health was in danger
Be clear on purpose of confidentiality	
Note exceptions to confidentiality	
Reassure that goal is not to create secrecy	
Reiterate your willingness to discuss health-related issues with both patient and parent	

Table 126.4 Potential Unintended Confidentiality Breaches

Breaches	What Providers Can Do
Diagnoses and medications may appear on after visit summaries	Create a sensitive after visit summary that does not include confidential health care (i.e. STI testing or medications)
Insurance companies will send an explanation of benefits to the policy holder, often the guardian, of health services received	Warn your patient that this may be mailed to their home or refer to clinic where minors can receive low cost, confidential care such as a Title X facility
Pharmacies often call the guardian when prescriptions are available to be picked up	Warn your patient of this so that they are aware
Paper charts may be inappropriately accessed	Store paper charts in locked cabinet within a locked room

patients and their parents and Table 126.4 describes potential unintended confidentiality breaches.

126.4 Legal Considerations in School-Based Health

The laws related to consent to treatment for adolescent patients remain the same when services are provided in a school setting. However, different confidentiality rules may apply. In most medical settings, confidentiality is protected by the Health Insurance Portability and Accountability Act (HIPAA), which created national

Table 126.5 Tips for Optimizing Privacy in a School Setting

Hang white noise machines outside of exam room to minimize sound transfer
Use a designated, private bathroom for medical care in the clinic space
Complete registration for medical visits in a separate location from other school activities
Provide treatment for STIs in clinic to avoid accidental disclosure of sensitive information at pharmacies or through insurance authorizations
If clinic space is used for other school activities, make sure patient health information is stored securely at the end of clinic session
Educate school personnel including administrators, teachers and staff about confidentiality, including not asking students why they are at the school clinic

standards to protect sensitive patient health information from being disclosed without the patient's consent or knowledge [9]. However, health records that are directly related to a student and maintained by an educational agency (such as a school district) or institution (such as a public elementary, secondary school, or postsecondary school such as a college or university) are protected under The Family Educational Rights and Privacy Act (FERPA) [10]. This law prohibits schools from disclosing personally identifiable information (PII) from students' education records without consent. It also allows parents full access to their child's educational records, including potentially sensitive health information. Notably, health records of students 18 and older are protected. The federal government has provided some guidance on which confidentiality rules apply: health records maintained by a person or entity that provides health services to students under contract with the school or otherwise under direct control, such as a school nurse, are subject to FERPA and, therefore, accessible by parents [11]. However, outside parties that provide healthcare services directly to students, including on school premises, but are not employed by or under contract with the school are subject to HIPAA confidentiality rules [11]. Therefore, providers in the school setting must understand which confidentiality rules apply depending on how health care is administered within the school. Table 126.5 provides recommendations for maintaining privacy in a school setting.

126.5 Electronic Medical Record

The electronic medical record is another aspect of healthcare delivery where confidentiality can be inadvertently breached. The twenty-first Century Cures Act was passed in 2020 to increase patient access to their electronic health information. This law includes the Final Rule, which gives patients and, in the case of minors, their guardians access to their medical information electronically [12]. This has raised unique challenges for healthcare providers of adolescent patients because parents may be able to access sensitive health information in the electronic health portal. In general, the Final Rule prohibits information blocking, which interferes with patient access or use of electronic health information. The law, however, does provide exceptions to information sharing. The two most relevant to adolescent confidentiality are the "Privacy Exemption" which allows information blocking to comply with established state and federal laws that allow minor patients to consent for medical care and therefore compel confidentiality, and the "Preventing Harm Exception" which allows information blocking if there is a reasonable belief that it will reduce the risk of harm to the patient. Providers should document sensitive health information in a separate private note that can be appropriately blocked to maintain confidentiality.

126.6 Case Conclusions

Case 1 Regardless of medical testing or treatment provided to Maria, she should be counseled on how to reduce her risk. The most effective way to prevent pregnancy and sexually transmitted infections is abstinence. However, patients who are sexually active should be counseled on barrier methods such as condoms to reduce the risk of infection and on various methods of contraception to prevent pregnancy, even if you are unable to provide this care. Be familiar with local Title X Family Planning Clinics such as Planned Parenthood and refer patients to these clinics if needed. If you can provide reproductive health care, such as contraception and/or STI testing and treatment, understand the laws regarding minor consent in your state and if parental consent is needed. As a reminder, all 50 states explicitly allow minors to consent to STI services, though some states require the minor to be a certain age (e.g., 12, 14 or 16).

Case 2 In a non-stigmatizing, compassionate manner, Sam should be provided information on the health and psychosocial risks of cannabis use. This information should be documented in a separate note that can be blocked from parental access. If you suspect a substance use disorder, refer Sam to appropriate treatment. Review the consent laws in your state to determine if a parent would need to provide consent for this. Most states allow minors to consent for substance use treatment, 15 states have minimum age requirements [1].

Case 3 Though most states allow for adolescents to consent to mental health treatment, situations in which the patient's safety is in danger necessitate involving parents or guardians. In this scenario, confidentiality would have to be breached to protect the adolescent. As the provider, you should inform Jaylin that you must tell her mother so that it is not a surprise to her, and you can even do this together. Given the acuity of her thoughts of self-harm, she should be evaluated by a mental health specialist or at the local psychiatric crisis department or emergency department.

Extra Credit Points

1. Review the minor consent and confidentiality laws in your state. Laws vary widely and do not always reflect established best practices.
2. Familiarize yourself with local resources that can offer free, confidential care to adolescent patients (i.e. health department, Title X clinics, Planned Parenthood, local providers specializing in adolescent medicine)
3. Introduce the concept of confidentiality early to your patients and their parents.
4. Take steps to make your clinic space a safe and private environment.

References

1. Sharko M, et al. State-by-State variability in adolescent privacy laws. Pediatrics. 2022;149(6) https://doi.org/10.1542/peds.2021-053458.
2. OASH. Title X Family Planning Program.
3. Lerand SJ. Consent and confidentiality. In: Adolescent medicine today: a guide to caring for the adolescent patient. World Scientific; 2012. p. 651–66.
4. Cheng TL, et al. Confidentiality in health care: a survey of knowledge, perceptions, and attitudes among high school students. JAMA. 1993;269(11):1404–7.
5. Fuentes L, et al. Adolescents' and young adults' reports of barriers to confidential health care and receipt of contraceptive services. J Adolescent Health. 2018;62(1):36–43.
6. Reddy DM, Fleming R, Swain C. Effect of mandatory parental notification on adolescent girls' use of sexual health care services. JAMA. 2002;288(6):710–4.
7. Ford CA, et al. Influence of physician confidentiality assurances on adolescents' willingness to disclose information and seek future health care. A randomized controlled trial. JAMA. 1997;278(12):1029–34.
8. Berlan ED. Adolescent consent and confidentiality in the 21st century, in Nationwide Children's Hospital Pediatric Grand Rounds. Columbus; 2022.
9. CDC. Health Insurance Portability and Accountability Act of 1996 (HIPAA). 2022 4/10/2024; Available from: https://www.cdc.gov/phlp/publications/topic/hipaa.html#:~:text=The%20Health%20Insurance%20Portability%20and,the%20patient's%20consent%20or%20knowledge.
10. CDC. Family Educational Rights and Privacy Act (FERPA). 2022 4/10/2024; Available from: https://www.cdc.gov/phlp/publications/topic/ferpa.html.
11. HHS. FAQ 514 Does FERPA or HIPAA apply to elementary or secondary school student health records maintained by a health care provider that is not employed by a school? 2008; Available from: https://www.hhs.gov/guidance/document/faq-514-does-ferpa-or-hipaa-apply-elementary-or-secondary-school-student-health-records.
12. Cures Act Final Rule Information Blocking Exceptions. The Office of the National Coordinator for Health Information Technology.

Chapter 127
Breast Health and Disorders

Jessica Santucci and Theodore Miller

Case 1 13-year-old Stacy notices that many of her friends wear sports bras to gym class, and she begins to wonder why she has not started to develop breasts yet. Her mom has mentioned that all of Stacy's sisters were "late bloomers," but Stacy does not want to seem like an outlier amongst her peers. She presents to your school-based health clinic and asks "Am I weird?" What are your next steps?

Early education regarding breast health has been shown to improve female adolescent attitudes towards engaging in positive breast habits [1]. However, openly discussing breast health is often seen as taboo, leaving adolescents in the dark about what constitutes "normal" pubertal development. Pubertal development varies by age, sex, ethnicity, and environment. Tanner Staging was developed to objectively classify secondary sex characteristics of children and adolescents to promptly detect developmental abnormalities. One component of Tanner staging involves breast development, also known as thelarche, as well as increased sex hormone production, referred to as gonadarche. Tanner Stage 1 is considered pre-pubertal, and it continues until Tanner Stage 5, which is synonymous with obtaining the size and shape of adult breasts (Fig. 127.1) [2].

Reaching Tanner Stage 2 before the age of 8 in females and 9 in males is termed "precocious puberty" and warrants further evaluation. Causes of precocious puberty include congenital adrenal hyperplasia (CAH), exogenous testosterone administration, or adrenal adenomas. Idiopathic precocious puberty is also becoming increasingly more common in Westernized countries. In contrast, lack of thelarche by the age of 13 in females is concerning for delayed puberty. Common causes of delayed puberty include growth hormone deficiencies, hypothyroidism, malnutrition, craniopharyngiomas, genetic syndromes, and chronic illnesses.

J. Santucci (✉) · T. Miller
Penn State College of Medicine, Hershey, PA, USA
e-mail: jsantucci@pennstatehealth.psu.edu; tmiller51@pennstatehealth.psu.edu

R. P. Olympia, J. Brady-Olympia (eds.), *Clinical Considerations in School-based Health*, https://doi.org/10.1007/978-3-031-85765-2_127

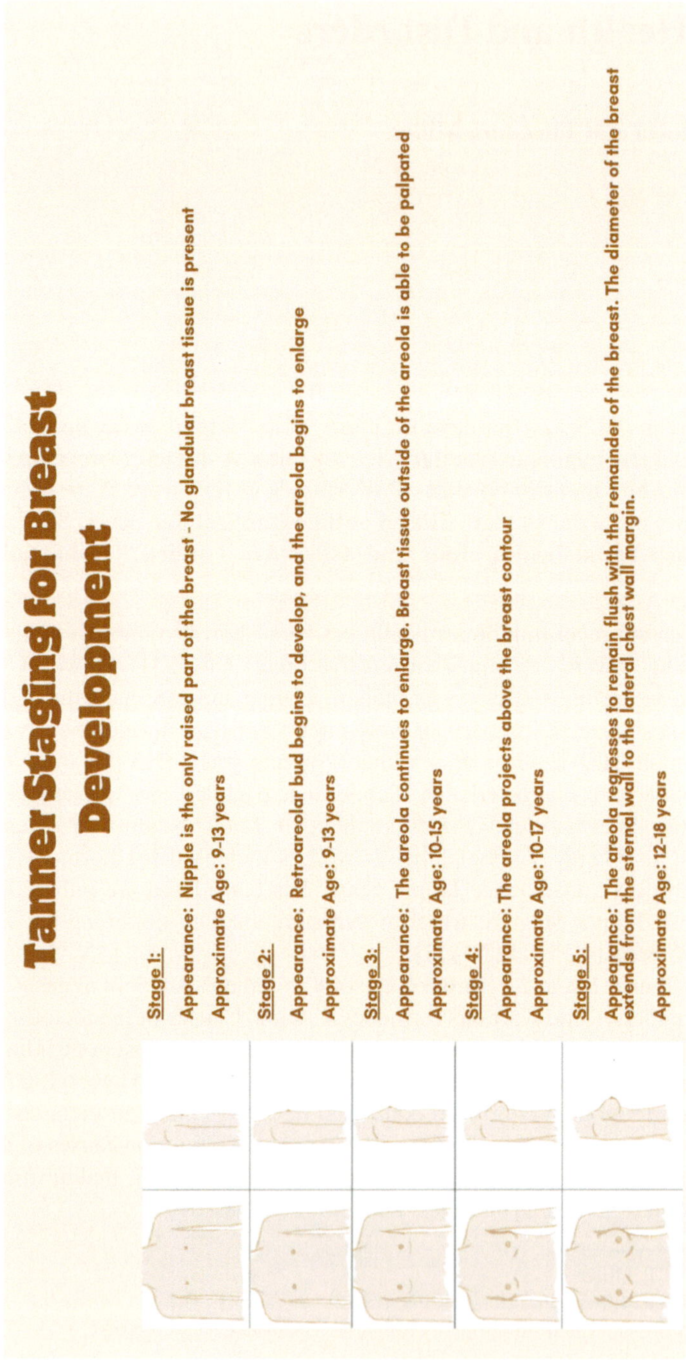

Fig. 127.1 Phases of Tanner Staging

Case 2 14-year-old Emily arrives at the nurse's office complaining of a few small, tender, bilateral breast "lumps" that she noticed a couple of days ago while showering. She has a history of irregular periods and started taking birth control several months ago. She starts crying and tells you her friend's mother was just diagnosed with breast cancer. She is now worried she may have cancer." What are your next steps?

Breast disease is rarely malignant in adolescents, with most newly discovered masses being benign, such as fibroadenomas. Other common sources of breast masses are listed in Table 127.1 [3–5]. Proper assessment and management of

Table 127.1 Etiology of Breast Masses in Adolescents [3, 4]

Cause	Etiology	Clinical/exam	Treatment
Fibroadenoma	Idiopathic; correlated with increased estrogen (i.e. pregnancy, OCP)	Well Circumscribed, Non-tender, mobile, rubbery Usually slow growing	Follow clinically - most regress over months Ultrasound if >5 cm, rapid growth If atypical appearance or symptomatic, refer for biopsy Differentiate from phyllodes tumor
Fibrocystic Changes	Cyclical changes Associated with menstrual cycle	Diffuse nodularity Tender breasts	Follow clinically, reassurance Supportive care - warm compresses, NSAIDs for pain control, +/- oral contraceptive pills, supportive bra
Breast Cyst	Ductal ectasia, Montgomery tubercles or lymphatic malformations	Well circumscribed, round, firm or fluctuant, mobile	Repeated clinical exam Ultrasound if persistent or enlarging. May require aspiration and biopsy
Phyllodes Tumor	Originate from periductal stromal cells Range from benign to malignant	Oval, well circumscribed Often >5 cm, rapidly growing, cystic	Biopsy necessary for diagnosis and determination if benign or malignant
Mastitis/ Abscess	Most common bacteria: S. aureus, S. pyogenes, enterococcus, pseudomonas	Swollen, tender, erythematous Fluctuance if abscess	Warm compress Antibiotics May require incision/ drainage if no response to antibiotics [5]
Breast Cancer	Primary breast cancer is rare (80% juvenile secretary carcinoma) Secondary/metastatic more common than primary: (i.e. lymphomas, rhabdomyosarcoma, neuroblastoma)	Painless, hard, irregular mass	

Table 127.2 Clinical findings warranting additional history and evaluation

Factors	Exam finding
Nipple/Breast Changes	Discharge (white/cloudy), retraction, new onset nipple inversion, breast asymmetry
Mass Characteristics	Firm consistency, fixed to underlying tissue, indeterminate borders, non-tender mass, consistently increasing size (does not fluctuate with the menstrual cycle)
Lymphadenopathy	Enlarged axillary masses
Skin Changes	Peau d'orange (skin dimpling), inflammation/redness

adolescents' breast health should include a thorough evaluation of prominent risk factors, history findings, and physical presentation.

Any palpable breast mass necessitates a thorough workup regardless of age or presenting risk factors [3, 4]. Risk factors for the development of breast cancer include family history of BRCA gene mutations, personal history of cancer, radiation to the chest, smoking, or alcohol consumption [4, 5]. Table 127.2 highlights more serious concerns, including signs that may suggest need for further history and evaluation.

Low clinical suspicion for malignancy allows for conservative management with observation and follow-up examinations after 1–2 months. Breast ultrasounds are preferred as a first-line diagnostic tool for all unidentified breast masses in children and adolescents. Resolution of the mass requires no further management, yet persistent masses should be referred to a pediatric gynecologist or breast surgeon.

Case 3 Thirteen-year-old Bryce has noticed over time that while his friends have flat chests and some have chest hair, he has instead developed breast tissue. He comes to the school nurse's office reporting how he has become more self-conscious and is bothered by feeling different from his friends. He asks the school nurse "is something wrong with me?" What are your next steps?

Gynecomastia is the enlargement of male breast tissue resulting from an imbalance between estrogen and androgens. In obese adolescent males, one of the most common causes is the increased conversion of androgens to estrogen in peripheral adipose tissue due to elevated aromatase activity. This process is often exacerbated during puberty when hormonal fluctuations are prevalent. Often, gynecomastia is physiologic and resolves as puberty progresses. However, it can also be associated with some prescription medications as well as illicit and recreational drugs, such as marijuana or anabolic steroids [6]. Other causes of gynecomastia include adrenal or pituitary disorders, primary hypogonadism, testicular tumors, Klinefelter Syndrome, and idiopathic factors.

The presentation can vary, appearing symmetrically or asymmetrically based on its underlying cause. Bilateral gynecomastia often suggests a physiological or systemic origin, while unilateral occurrence raises concerns about a localized tumor or idiopathic factors. Gynecomastia may cause tenderness in the region around the areola. Even beyond the physiological symptoms, the psychological impacts can be profound amongst adolescents striving to conform to peer norms. This can potentially lead to social challenges like bullying or feelings of marginalization within their social circles [6].

In most cases, gynecomastia is managed with reassurance and monitoring. If obesity is identified as a contributing factor, lifestyle modifications, including increased exercise and a balanced diet, may be recommended. For persistent cases that significantly impair daily functioning, treatment options may include aromatase inhibitors or selective estrogen receptor modulators (SERMs) to reduce estrogen production. Additionally, individuals with body image concerns, particularly during early adolescence, may be referred for counseling to receive psychosocial support.

Case 4 Leah is a 17-year-old female with a history of a mood disorder who comes into the health clinic appearing anxious and asks to talk with you in private. She says she recently noticed a white discharge coming from her breasts. She was looking online for information, saw pregnancy can cause a milky discharge, and is concerned she may be pregnant. You ask her to come back to a more private location where you can talk with her alone. On further history, she had sex with her boyfriend once, 3–4 months ago. She says it was consensual, and they used a condom. She noted the discharge about a month ago. Her periods have been irregular with her last period being 2 months ago. She also started a new medication, risperidone, about 3 months ago. She denies any breast trauma, redness, or pain, as well as any frequent headaches, visual changes, or fatigue.

While nipple discharge is uncommon in children and adolescents, galactorrhea is one of the most common causes of nipple discharge [5, 7]. A complete history should be obtained, as noted above, including menstrual, sexual, and medication history, as well as a complete physical exam, including breast evaluation. The adolescent should also be asked if the discharge is spontaneous or provoked and if it is bilateral or unilateral. A systemic process is more likely to produce bilateral discharge, while unilateral discharge is suggestive of a localized process, such as intraductal papillomas. Prolactin levels should be measured in the early morning hours, about 1–2 hours after waking [7]. Elevated prolactin levels are seen in pregnancy, and elevated prolactin levels can also cause amenorrhea or menstrual irregularities, so it is important to evaluate for pregnancy. Medications are another relatively common cause of elevated prolactin, most often seen with first- and second-generation antipsychotics, such as risperidone or haloperidol. In addition, other medications such as metoclopramide or methyldopa have been reported to cause elevated prolactin [8]. Other causes of elevated prolactin include hypothyroidism, chest wall trauma, and pituitary adenomas. With pituitary adenomas, prolactin levels are over 100–200 ng/ml. Smaller microadenomas may not have levels as high [7].

127.1 Case Conclusions

Case 1 Stacy was ultimately seen by her pediatrician out of concern for delayed puberty, where her Tanner Staging, bloodwork, and karyotyping were assessed. Given her family history of delayed puberty, lack of other presenting symptoms, and lab abnormalities, Stacy was determined to have a constitutional delay of puberty. She progressed to Tanner Stage 2 by the age of 14 and has been following a non-concerning pubertal developmental curve since.

Case 2 Emily was asked more questions by the nurse provider to get a better understanding of the patient's nipple discharge, contraceptive use, family history, and mass characteristics. Upon further questioning, Emily's pain correlated with the timing of her menstrual cycle, and she had no nipple discharge. Physical exam revealed firm, movable lumps that were consistent with benign bilateral fibrocystic breast changes. Emily was instructed to return if she noticed any new breast masses or changes in visual appearance.

Case 3 Upon further evaluation, it was determined that Bryce was severely overweight for his height and age. Additionally, his brother confided in him that he also experienced enlarged breast tissue during his pre-pubescent years. After a discussion with the nurse, Bryce committed to eating a balanced diet that was rich in fruits, vegetables, and protein. Subsequently, he experienced a growth spurt alongside significant weight loss, which led to a gradual improvement in his gynecomastia. Bryce was advised to follow-up with his primary care physician if he noticed any breast asymmetry or new masses.

Case 4 After examining Leah, you have her give a urine sample for a pregnancy test, which was negative; she was then referred to the adolescent medicine clinic. At the clinic, the physician ordered lab work, which included a prolactin level, thyroid function tests, basic chemistry panel (including blood urea nitrogen and creatinine). Her prolactin level returned at 50 ng/ml. Her thyroid stimulating hormone and thyroxine level (free T4) were both within normal range. Leah stopped in to clinic to tell you her psychiatrist plans to meet with her and her parents to discuss other possible medication options and repeat the prolactin levels in a month.

Extra Credit Points

1. It is important to practice both sensitivity and scrutiny when handling intimate topics such as breast health.
2. While breast cancer is exceedingly rare in children and adolescents, certain features when performing clinical exams, taking family histories, or having personal histories of cancer or chest wall irradiation warrant further history and evaluation.

3. It is not common for males to develop glandular breast tissue, termed gynecomastia, during adolescence due to an imbalance between estrogen and testosterone levels. Gynecomastia typically resolves when hormone levels stabilize after puberty.
4. Nipple discharge is uncommon in adolescents. Adolescents with nipple discharge, should be undergo a thorough history and physical and be referred to a gynecologist experienced with adolescents, pediatric endocrinologist, or adolescent medicine physician.

References

1. Marcell AV, et al. Sexual and reproductive health care services in the pediatric setting. Pediatrics. 2017;140(5):e20172858. https://doi.org/10.1542/peds.2017-2858.
2. De Sanctis V, et al. Methods for rating sexual development in girls. Pediatr Endocrinol Rev: PER. 2016;14(1):27–32. https://doi.org/10.17458/PER.2016.SESEEM.MethodsforRating.
3. Szar M, Dendy CB, Hillenbrand K. Breast conditions (disorders) in children. Pediatr Rev. 2023;44(11):665–7. https://doi.org/10.1542/pir.2022-005534.
4. Adekeye A, et al. Pediatric and adolescent breast conditions: a review. J Pediatr Adolesc Gynecol. 2023;36(1):5–13. https://doi.org/10.1016/j.jpag.2022.11.001.
5. Mareti E, Vatopoulou A, Spyropoulou GA, Papanastasiou A, Pratilas GC, Liberis A, Hatzipantelis E, Dinas K. Breast disorders in adolescence: a review of the literature. Breast Care (Basel). 2021;16(2):149–55. https://doi.org/10.1159/000511924. Epub 2020 Nov 30. PMID: 34012369; PMCID: PMC8114041.
6. Young CC, et al. Psychosocial correlates of idiopathic gynecomastia in young males: preliminary findings from a mixed-methods study. J Adolesc Health. 2017;60(2) https://doi.org/10.1016/j.jadohealth.2016.10.069.
7. Matalliotakis M, Koliarakis I, Matalliotaki C, Trivli A, Hatzidaki E. Clinical manifestations, evaluation and management of hyperprolactinemia in adolescent and young girls: a brief review. Acta Biomed. 2019;90(1):149–57. https://doi.org/10.23750/abm.v90i1.8142. PMID: 30889169; PMCID: PMC6502148.
8. Golshan M. Nipple discharge. In: Chen W, editor. UpToDate. 2024. Retrieved 23 Nov 2024, from https://www.uptodate.com/contents/nipple-discharge/contributors.

Chapter 128
Menstrual Disorders

Jennifer Kosoy Shook

From menarche (the onset of the first menstrual period) to each subsequent menstrual cycle, adolescent girls may experience a range of physical and emotional symptoms accompanying these experiences. The American College of Obstetricians and Gynecologists (ACOG) and the American Academy of Pediatrics (AAP) both consider the menstrual cycle to be a vital sign [1], indicating the importance of the menstrual pattern and presentation for overall health. Adolescents typically have cycles lasting 21–45 days with 3–7 days of bleeding [1]. It is important to take a detailed menstrual history, including age of menarche, usual pattern and flow, and date of last menstrual period. Sometimes teenagers get confused and may think periods are not "regular" if they do not occur on the same date each month so it is helpful to let them know about this wide range of normal cycles. This chapter will discuss some cases of when periods may not appear as normal and some ways to help students coming to the school-based health center with various presentations of menstrual concerns.

Case 1 Samantha is a 14-year-old that comes in to the health center asking for a menstrual pad. She mentions she has been bleeding for 10 days and already went through all five pads she brought with her today. She is worried she is going to bleed onto her clothes, which would be extremely embarrassing. She looks a little pale to you, and you are worried about the heavy bleeding she is describing so you decide to ask her some more questions rather than just point her to the basket of menstrual hygiene products that you keep available for students. Why might this be happening to Samantha, and what should you do?

Abnormal uterine bleeding (AUB), an umbrella term that encompasses irregularity in menstrual timing and bleeding flow, is relatively common in teenagers, and

J. K. Shook (✉)
Penn State Children's Hospital, Hershey, PA, USA
e-mail: jshook1@pennstatehealth.psu.edu

R. P. Olympia, J. Brady-Olympia (eds.), *Clinical Considerations in School-based Health*, https://doi.org/10.1007/978-3-031-85765-2_128

there are several potential causes. It is important to identify situations requiring urgent or timely intervention and evaluate for anemia or hypovolemic shock. The International Federation of Gynecology and Obstetrics (FIGO) created the acronym PALM-COEIN to help in the evaluation of AUB, with the first part being structural causes that are rare in adolescents, and the second part being non-structural causes, which are most likely in this age group. PALM-COEIN stands for polyp, adenomyosis, leiomyoma, malignancy and hyperplasia, coagulopathy, ovulatory dysfunction, endometrial, iatrogenic, and not yet classified [2]. This chapter will focus more on the non-structural causes as these are more common in adolescents. Table 128.1 displays the COEIN causes of AUB.

Ovulatory dysfunction accounts for 90% of AUB in adolescents and is therefore the most common etiology [1]. This includes anovulation, which is most frequently due to an immature hypothalamic-pituitary-ovarian axis and may be normal for the first 2 years after menarche. In these cases, there is no ovulation thus no formation of the corpus luteum. Estrogen is still present, which leads to proliferation of the endometrium, but there is insufficient progesterone to stabilize the endometrium, which can lead to unpredictable or heavy menstrual bleeding. This is a diagnosis of

Table 128.1 Nonstructural causes of AUB

Cause of Amenorrhea	Presenting Signs and Symptoms	Diagnosis	Treatment
Coagulopathy	Heavy menstrual bleeding Bleeding from other sources (e.g. nosebleeds, dental bleeding)	Lab evaluation: complete blood count, iron studies, ferritin, prothrombin time, partial thromboplastin time, fibrinogen, von Willebrand panel	Stop the bleeding: hormonal, tranexamic acid Desmopressin in von Willebrand disease Treat anemia if present
Ovulatory Dysfunction	Anovulatory cycles- irregular and heavy bleeding	Luteinizing hormone, follicle stimulating hormone, estradiol, prolactin, free and total testosterone, sex hormone binding globulin, dehydroepiandrosterone sulfate, thyroid stimulating hormone	Stop the bleeding: hormonal, tranexamic acid Treat anemia if present
Endometrial Cause	Pelvic pain Abnormal bleeding Vaginal discharge	Pelvic exam Sexually transmitted infection screening	Antibiotics
Iatrogenic	Irregular bleeding	Evaluate medication use	Reassurance Consider stopping or changing the medication
Not Classified	Pregnancy Trauma Foreign bodies	Thorough history Pelvic exam +/− imaging	Management of underlying cause

exclusion. Second most common in adolescents is a coagulopathy. Heavy periods beginning with menarche may be the first presentation of a bleeding disorder. These may include von Willebrand disease, thrombocytopenia, and other platelet or clotting factor issues. Additional important common causes of AUB include pregnancy, sexually transmitted infections, genital trauma, foreign bodies, and medications such as exogenous hormones, anticoagulants, and some psychotropic medications [1].

When you evaluate Samantha, you notice that in addition to being pale, she is also mildly tachycardic. This is a patient that should be seen urgently for labs to evaluate for anemia. If you have the ability to do so in your school-based health center, you should check a complete blood count and a pregnancy test to start with. If you cannot do these on site, she should be sent to an urgent care or emergency department. Additional lab testing should include ferritin if there is a concern for iron deficiency, prothrombin time, activated partial thromboplastin time, fibrinogen, von Willebrand factor antigen and activity, and factor VIII. Sexually active teenagers should also be screened for gonorrhea and chlamydia. Other causes of AUB might be thyroid disease or polycystic ovarian syndrome (Table 128.2) so she may need other labs for those work-ups, as well.

If Samantha is anemic, she will possibly need a transfusion or an iron infusion or oral iron depending on the severity. It will also be important acutely to stop the bleeding, which is usually done with hormonal treatment of estrogen and/or progesterone but may also be done with nonhormonal options, such as oral tranexamic acid. Treatment is usually oral, but estrogen may be given intravenously if the patient is not able to tolerate oral treatment.

Case 2 Madison, a 15-year-old student at your school, presents with concern that she has not had her period in 6 months. She had menarche at 13 years old, and her periods were previously regular. She is surprised this has happened because she knows she cannot be pregnant! When chatting with her other friends on the field hockey team, they all have their period so she feels very alone and worried, although she is also glad she doesn't have to worry about cramps or heavy bleeding during field hockey games like they do!

Primary amenorrhea is when someone who is expected to have periods has not yet reached menarche. The median age of menarche is between 12 and 13 years old. This usually occurs 2–3 years following thelarche (breast budding), which is the first step of pubertal development for girls. Primary amenorrhea should be considered if an adolescent is 15 years old and has not yet reached menarche or if it has been more than 3 years since thelarche. Secondary amenorrhea is seen when someone has previously been having periods, and then they stop having periods for at least 3 months. We know their bodies are capable of having periods since they have had them in the past. A good history will help elicit why this may be happening. The most common cause of secondary amenorrhea is pregnancy so remember to rule this out! Table 128.2 shows some other possible causes of amenorrhea.

There are other causes to consider, as well, but a good history together with laboratory evaluation of hormones can help to narrow down a differential. Lab work-up

Table 128.2 Possible causes of amenorrhea and some distinguishing features of each [3]

Cause of Amenorrhea	Presenting Signs and Symptoms	Diagnosis	Treatment
Eating Disorder	Weight loss Caloric restriction Possibly excessive exercise, purging, or laxative or diuretic abuse	Hypogonadotropic hypogonadism along with meeting eating disorder criteria from the Diagnostic and Statistical Manual Disorders-5	Weight restoration
Relative Energy Deficiency in Sport (RED-S)	Increased energy expenditure relative to caloric intake	Hypogonadotropic hypogonadism along with triad of amenorrhea, insufficient caloric intake, and low bone density	Increased caloric intake
Hyperprolactinemia	+/− galactorrhea Delayed pubertal development	Elevated prolactin	Dopamine agonist is first line May require surgical resection
Polycystic Ovarian Syndrome (PCOS)	Acne Hirsutism +/− overweight or obese May have acanthosis nigricans due to insulin resistance	Clinical or biochemical evidence of hyperandrogenism	Lifestyle modifications (improved nutrition and physical activity) Hormonal contraceptives Spironolactone (antiandrogen) Metformin
Primary Ovarian Insufficiency	Hot flashes Bone density loss May have normal pubertal development May have features of Turner Syndrome (45, X0)	Elevated FSH with low estradiol (hypergonadotropic hypogonadism) Karyotype Pelvic ultrasound	Estrogen replacement (transdermal or transvaginal) with cyclic progesterone

(continued)

Table 128.2 (continued)

Cause of Amenorrhea	Presenting Signs and Symptoms	Diagnosis	Treatment
Thyroid Disease	Hypothyroidism: weight gain, cold intolerance, constipation, bradycardia, depressed mood, galactorrhea Hyperthyroidism: weight loss, heat intolerance, anxiety, palpitations	TSH, Free T4 No mid-cycle LH peak in hyperthyroidism	Treat the underlying thyroid disorder
Non-classic Congenital Adrenal Hyperplasia	May present similarly to PCOS with hyperandrogenism and oligomenorrhea or amenorrhea	Early morning (7:30 to 8:00 am) 21-hydroxyprogesterone to screen Adrenocorticotropic hormone (ACTH) Stimulation Test to confirm	Combined hormonal oral contraceptive pills Antiandrogens (spironolactone) May need glucocorticoids

for amenorrhea may include luteinizing hormone, follicle stimulating hormone, estradiol, prolactin, free and total testosterone, sex hormone binding globulin, dehydroepiandrosterone sulfate (DHEA-S), thyroid stimulating hormone, and 21-hydroxyprogesterone. It is important to figure out a cause to help counsel on or prevent against risks that may happen with each. For example, in malnutrition from an eating disorder or RED-S, a low estrogen state may lead to low bone density, which can be prevented by ensuring improved nutrition and weight restoration. Another example is in untreated PCOS where endometrial hyperplasia from unopposed estrogen may lead to endometrial carcinoma. After ruling out pregnancy and talking more with Madison about signs and symptoms she may be experiencing, sending her for labs is the next best step for her management. She later updates you that her physician diagnosed her with RED-S. She is working closely with her physician, along with a dietitian, to help make sure she is able to get in all the proper nutrition she needs in order to safely continue with field hockey. It would be important to closely monitor her weight and menstrual status until stabilized.

Case 3 You are working in the school-based health clinic when Abigail, a 16-year-old student who frequently comes to see you for "cramps," comes in with complaint of cramps and vomiting. She finds it very hard to sit through class due to the pain and is hoping to be able to lie down in the clinic. Is there anything else you can offer her?

Dysmenorrhea can be very disruptive to adolescent girls; some studies have shown that it is the leading cause of short-term absences from school [4]. Equipping them with tools such as medications or non-pharmacological treatments such as heating pads to manage their dysmenorrhea will allow them to participate in their usual daily activities without letting their periods dictate what they can do. There are two types of dysmenorrhea: primary and secondary. Primary dysmenorrhea is cramping at the time of or right before the period but is not due to another condition. Secondary dysmenorrhea is due to an underlying pelvic condition, such as endometriosis, but presents similarly. Secondary dysmenorrhea should be considered if someone is not improving from typical treatments, such as non-steroidal anti-inflammatory drugs, hormonal regulation of periods, or supportive care.

Since the pathogenesis of dysmenorrhea involves prostaglandin release, it makes sense that a great treatment is the use of a non-steroidal anti-inflammatory drug (NSAID) since NSAIDs block prostaglandin synthesis. If your health center is able to dispense medications, providing an NSAID, such as ibuprofen or naproxen, to Abigail could hopefully help with her pain. NSAIDs are first line medication for dysmenorrhea, and acetaminophen is not as effective for it. You should also advise Abigail for the future that using NSAIDs will work best when taken right when her menses begins, rather than waiting for the cramps to get bad. Many teenagers prefer to wait to take medication to see if they can get by without taking anything, but, by then, there is more release of prostaglandins so pain medication may be less effective. Additionally, some adolescents may need additional pain control, and they may benefit from using hormonal regulation of periods to prevent endometrial proliferation [4]. Any of the hormonal contraception methods may also be used for treatment of dysmenorrhea. If you are able to prescribe in your health center, these can be good additional treatments. If not, you can also refer a student to be seen in their primary care physician's office to further discuss options. Adolescent medicine physicians, along with pediatric and adolescent gynecologists, are also highly skilled in offering this care.

Treating painful periods is extremely important due to the frequency of missed school days and other life events. Pain control is vital for Abigail to fully participate in day-to-day life, including sitting in class.

In the cases above of Samantha, Madison, and Abigail, they are all experiencing common menstrual disorders of the adolescent population. Whether periods are heavy, absent, or painful, these can all be distressing to students. Proper management including evaluation and treatment can alleviate medical risks and improve overall quality of life.

Extra Credit Points

1. When evaluating someone with AUB, in addition to considering work-up for different causes, it is important to also assess a complete blood count as losing too much blood during a menstrual cycle can lead to anemia.
2. The number one cause of secondary amenorrhea is pregnancy so remember to rule this out.
3. Dysmenorrhea can be disruptive to daily lives during menses and is a major cause of missed school days.
4. You should direct adolescents with very heavy bleeding leading to filling a menstrual pad or tampon in less than 1 hour or any signs of anemia to an emergency department. Most other menstrual disorders can be best cared for in an outpa-

tient setting, such as in adolescent medicine or pediatric and adolescent gynecology offices.

References

1. Kabra R, Fisher M. Abnormal uterine bleeding in adolescents. Curr Probl Pediatr Adolesc Health Care. 2022;52(5):101185.
2. Munro MG, Critchley HOD, Broder MS, Fraser IS. FIGO classification system (PALM-COEIN) for causes of abnormal uterine bleeding in nongravid women of reproductive age. Int J Gynecol Obstet. 2011;113:3–13.
3. Kerns J, Itriyeva K, Fisher M. Etiology and management of amenorrhea in adolescent and young adult women. Curr Probl Pediatr Adolesc Health Care. 2022;52(5):101184.
4. Gutman G, Nunez AT, Fisher M. Dysmenorrhea in adolescents. Curr Probl Pediatr Adolesc Health Care. 2022;52(5):101186.

Chapter 129
Sexually Transmitted Infections

Isabel Hendrickson and Leighton Reed

Approximately 30% of U.S. teenagers report being sexually active, yet only 5% are tested for sexually transmitted infections (STIs) annually. STIs often go unreported by teenagers, which may suggest why 15 to 24-year-olds represent 50% of all newly acquired STI's annually [1]. STIs can be asymptomatic or present with vague symptoms that mimic other conditions. STIs may cause serious and long-term effects if untreated.

Case 1 16-year-old Robbie is sent to the school nurse by his teacher for a rash on his hands. The rash is not itchy nor painful and has been present for several weeks. Robbie has also been feeling tired in his classes and has occasional body aches, but he denies cough or cold symptoms. When you ask about other skin problems, he discloses that last month he had a "cold sore" on his penis that is starting to go away. It has not caused him any pain or urinary problems, and he has never had a "cold sore" in the past. He denies penile discharge. You counsel him on confidentiality and inquire about sexual history. He discloses to you that a few months ago he was sexually active with multiple female partners at different times, and he was not using protection. You visualize reddish brown, maculopapular lesions symmetrical distributed to bilateral palms that are not painful to palpation.

Syphilis cases in the U.S. have increased by 80% since 2018 [2]. Syphilis is called "the great imitator" because it tends to have subtle, nonspecific symptoms that develop over weeks to years and can easily go unnoticed. In Case #1, the adolescent presents with a rash on the palms of the hands that is not bothersome. He also has some other symptoms (fatigue, body aches) and recalls a painless genital sore (Table 129.1). The first typical symptom of primary syphilis is the painless

I. Hendrickson (✉) · L. Reed
Johns Hopkins All Children's Hospital, St. Petersburg, FL, USA
e-mail: ihefner1@jhmi.edu; LReed26@jhmi.edu

R. P. Olympia, J. Brady-Olympia (eds.), *Clinical Considerations in School-based Health*, https://doi.org/10.1007/978-3-031-85765-2_129

Table 129.1 Differential diagnosis for genital ulcers

Disease	Clinical presentation	Diagnosis	Treatment
Herpes Simplex Virus (*HSV*)	Single or multiple vesicles that rupture and form shallow, painful ulcers over an erythematous base	DNA polymerase chain reaction (PCR) Lesion culture Serologic testing (IgM, IgG)	Primary Acyclovir 400 mg PO TID for 7–10 days, OR Acyclovir 200 mg PO 5×/day for 7–10 days, OR Valacyclovir 1 g PO BID for 7–10 days OR Famciclovir 250 mg PO TID for 7–10 days.
Syphilis (*Treponema pallidum*)	Chancre: painless, papule eroding to an indurated ulcer	Non treponemal test: Venereal Disease Research Lab (VDRL) or Rapid plasma reagin (RPR) Treponemal test: Fluorescent Treponemal antibody absorption (FTA-ABS)	Primary syphilis: Benzathine Penicillin G 2.4 million units IM × 1 dose
Lymphogranuloma venereum (*C. trachomatis* L1, L2, L3)	Painless genital papule or ulcer associated with tender suppurative inguinal adenopathy (buboes)	Clinical + positive serology	Doxycycline 100 mg PO BID × 21 days OR
Chancroid (*Haemophius ducreyi*)	Superficial, painful ulcer(s) with an erythematous base; associated with unilateral painful adenopathy (buboes)	Clinical Often difficult to obtain culture or PCR becoming a diagnosis of exclusion	Azithromycin 1 g PO × 1 OR Ceftriaxone 250 mg IM × 1 OR Ciprofloxacin 500 mg PO BID × 3 days OR Erythromycin base 500 mg PO TID × 7 days.
Granuloma Inguinale	One or more painless ulcers that become friable with rolled margins	Visualization of dark-staining Donovan bodies on tissue crush preparation or biopsy	Azithromycin 1 g PO once weekly for 3 weeks and all lesions completely heal

chancre, which is an ulceration on the skin usually in the area of sexual contact. The chancre goes away after several weeks, during which time the symptoms of secondary syphilis begin: flu-like symptoms such as fever, fatigue, body aches, and rash develop. The rash is notable for its location, as very few other conditions will cause a rash on the palms and soles of the feet. These symptoms may resolve, and the patient can have months to years without symptoms before developing serious neurologic problems associated with tertiary syphilis such as decreased vision, hearing loss, tabes dorsalis and general paresis [2, 3]. Diagnostic testing can be done in a doctor's office or health department, and treatment of early syphilis with antibiotics is curative. The gold standard antibiotic is Penicillin G given at different intervals pending the staging of disease.

Most STI's begin with mild symptoms that a teen may not recognize as abnormal. Rashes, skin lesions, painful urination or penile/vaginal discharge are all symptoms that a teen may not recognize as abnormal, so they may present weeks to months after their symptoms started.

Risk for STI's is highest in those who do not use barrier protection (i.e. condoms) and those who have multiple sexual partners. However, it is important to know that ALL sexually active youth are at high risk for STI's, regardless of their practices. Therefore, healthcare professionals should keep a high index of suspicion and low threshold for referral to a diagnostic testing center (such as the local Health Department, certain urgent care centers, or a child's primary care office) when evaluating sexually active adolescents.

Case Continued The school nurse thanks Robbie for disclosing his history and shows appreciation that he trusts her with this information. She refers Robbie to the local Health Department, and the following week he receives same day testing and treatment for syphilis.

Case 2 17-year-old Sarah comes to the school-based health clinic at the direction of the school counselor. She tearfully disclosed to the school counselor that she recently developed thick malodorous vaginal discharge and is concerned that she has an STI. In the clinic, she has no tenderness to palpation of her abdomen and vital signs are all within normal limits. The pediatrician decides to perform a pelvic examination demonstrating punctate hemorrhages on the vaginal mucosa and confirms the presence of thick, green-yellow discharge. There was no cervical motion tenderness. Nucleic acid amplification test (NAAT) for Trichomoniasis is positive. She received treatment with Metronidazole with resolution of symptoms. However, 3 weeks later she came back to the clinic with the same symptoms. She has only been sexually active with the same partner. Her partner has no symptoms and is accusing her of having sex with other partners. She wants to know if the previous treatment failed.

The differential diagnosis for vaginal discharge is broad (Table 129.2). Important history to obtain when evaluating vaginal discharge includes duration of discharge, odor, pruritus, pain, color of discharge, abdominal pain and systemic symptoms

Table 129.2 Differential diagnosis of vaginal discharge

Disease	Clinical presentation	Diagnosis	Treatment
Bacterial vaginosis	Thin, homogenous, grey-white vaginal discharge Pruritus "Fishy" odor	Amsel criteria At least three of following: Clue cells (on at least 20% of epithelial cells) pH > 4.5 + whiff -amine test (fishy odor) Homogenous thin, gray/white vaginal discharge, adheres to vaginal walls Various NAATs available	Metronidazole 500 mg PO BID × 7 days, OR Metronidazole gel 0.75% 1 applicator (5 g) intravaginal daily × 5 days, OR Clindamycin cream 2% 1 applicator (5 g) intravaginal QHS × 7 days
Vulvovaginal candidiasis (*C. albicans*)	Pruritus, dysuria, dyspareunia, thick white "cottage cheese" vaginal discharge	Vulvar/vaginal erythema/edema with satellite lesions or fissures, whitish discharge pH < 4.5 KOH prep: pseudohyphae or blastospores	Clotrimazole 1% cream 5 g intravaginal daily × 7–14 days, OR Clotrimazole 2% cream 5 g intravaginal daily × 3 days Miconazole, Tioconazole, Butoconazole, Teraconazole, and Fluconazole are treatment alternatives with varying administration lengths and routes
Trichomonas (*T. vaginalis*)	Pruritus, dysuria, dyspareunia, lower abdominal pain, post coital bleeding Vaginal discharge—malodorous, greenish yellow, frothy Vulvar irritation	Wet prep motile trichomonads KOH is malodorous pH > 4.5 Nucleic acid amplification tests (NAAT) Rapid Antigen Test—OSOM TV DNA Probe - Affirm™ VP III	Metronidazole 2 g PO × 1 dose OR Tinidazole 2 g PO × 1, OR Metronidazole 500 mg PO BID × 7 days
Cervicitis (*C. trachomatis, N. gonorrhoeae*)	Vaginal discharge, abnormal bleeding or dysuria Physical examination: Friable cervix, erythema, discharge from cervical os, and cervical petechiae	Nucleic acid amplification tests (NAAT)	Azithromycin 1 g PO × 1, OR Doxycycline 100 mg PO BID × 7 days PLUS Ceftriaxone 250 mg IM × 1 dose, OR Cefixime 800 mg PO × 1

such as fever. In addition, vaginitis may present with urinary tract infections as well, so be sure to inquire about urinary symptoms and systemic symptoms consistent with pyelonephritis (fever, chills, nausea/vomiting, flank pain). This history and your physical exam should help delineate a more targeted work up and rule more concerning possibilities such as PID. This patient was diagnosed with trichomonas via NAAT. If NAAT is not available, microscopy of motile trichomonads on wet mount is also diagnostic [4]. However, Sarah's concern about a recurring STI after receiving treatment presents an opportunity to discuss prevention of STI's and the role for partner treatment.

The only way to guarantee prevention of an STI is to practice total abstinence from sexual activity. However, sexually active teens should use barrier methods (male or female condoms) to decrease the risk of STI transmission. The CDC found that 52% of sexually active teens report consistent use of condoms [1]. Having condoms available and educating teens on their proper use can help encourage them to follow safe sex practices. It is important for teens to understand that non-barrier methods of contraceptives (oral contraceptives, intrauterine devices or implants, the depo shot, and birth control rings) will decrease the risk of pregnancy, but they do not reduce STI transmission risk.

When discussing STIs with teens, information should be conveyed as factual and non-judgmental. The stigma surrounding STIs can cause the teen to feel shame and fear. It is important to recognize that males are often asymptomatic for STIs, and therefore females often feel they are to blame when they develop symptoms. Sarah expresses concern that she is unable to clear this infection, and she is sad that her partner thinks she is getting it from other people. However, it is likely that her partner has the same infection himself but is asymptomatic. Many STIs can be passed back and forth between monogamous partners if one does not seek treatment.

Case Continued The pediatrician praises Sarah for taking responsibility for her sexual health and seeking treatment when she has abnormal symptoms. The pediatrician encourages Sarah to talk to her partner about getting tested and treated, and Sarah is educated on the use of barrier methods to prevent STI transmission.

Case 3 14-year-old Karla comes to the school nurse to get a menstrual pad and ibuprofen. She states that she has had some light vaginal bleeding and cramping for the past 2 weeks, and this week she has been feeling nauseous and "flu-ish". Upon further discussion, she reveals that she had her period 2 weeks ago but has continued to have cramping and spotting, and these symptoms are getting worse. She has not had any pain with urination, vaginal discharge, urinary urgency or increased urinary frequency. She discloses that she last had unprotected sexual intercourse with a male partner 2 months ago. You take her temperature, and she has a fever of 101.5 °F. After taking the ibuprofen, she still has a cramping pain in her left and right lower abdomen.

Karla has symptoms concerning for Pelvic Inflammatory Disease (PID). PID occurs in females and is most often caused by gonorrhea or chlamydia infections that have gone untreated. These bacterial infections spread to the uterus, fallopian tubes, and/or ovaries and cause worsening symptoms as the infection spreads. Symptoms can be mild or severe, and cases can go undetected for weeks to months. PID often presents with lower abdominal pain, and may be associated with pain with intercourse, intermenstrual spotting or prolonged menses, nausea and vomiting. Vaginal discharge is not always associated with PID. Patients can start to have flu-like symptoms and fevers. PID requires treatment with antibiotics to prevent abscess formation, scarring, and worsening infection in the abdomen. Broad antibiotic coverage is recommended with the first line option of ceftriaxone, doxycycline, and metronidazole for coverage of gonorrhea, chlamydia, gram negative bacteria and anaerobes [5]. In serious cases, the teen may require hospitalization for treatment. Reasons for hospitalization include abscess formation, failure of treatment of oral antibiotics, pregnancy, or systemic symptoms concerning for severe illness [6]. Females who are suspected to have PID should be referred to an Emergency Department, as this can affect future fertility or even be life-threatening if left untreated. Table 129.3 reviews STI complications for various genitourinary structures.

Case 4 Gerald is a 16-year-old male who mentioned to his trusted coach that he recently noticed a new "bump" on his penis. The coach recommended Gerald see the school clinic for evaluation. He has been sexually active with two partners and does not use protection. He denies any systemic symptoms, pain, dysuria, or penile discharge. On examination, there is a single 5 mm broad-based, "flesh colored" lesion with a cauliflower-like appearance at the base of the penis. No other lesions are noted. Gerald shares that he has become very concerned that he has cancer and wants to know the next steps for diagnosis.

This lesion is consistent with condyloma acuminata (anogenital warts) which is associated with human papillomavirus (HPV). The diagnosis is clinical based on the appearance of the lesion. It is very unlikely to be malignant, but a biopsy can be obtained if there are any concerning features on examination such as ulceration, bleeding, or atypical pigmentation. Gerald should also be screened for other STIs at this time. Imiquimod, podophyllotoxin, and interferons are topical treatment options that can be self-administered. If there are vaginal lesions or failure to previous treatment options, trichloroacetic acid and bichloroacetic acid may be considered but are caustic acids requiring application by a health care provider [7, 8]. More importantly, Gerald should be counseled to start the HPV vaccination series. There are multiple approved vaccinations. However, Gardasil 9 provides protection against HPV types 6, 11, 16, 18, 31, 33, 45, 52, and 58. This series covers > 90% of genital warts and approximately 80% of cervical cancers. Additionally, vaccination reduces the risk of anal cancer [7].

Table 129.3 STI involvement of various genitourinary structures

Disease	Clinical presentation	Diagnosis	Treatment
Pelvic Inflammatory Disease	Wide spectrum of presentation Cardinal symptom is lower abdominal pain Cervical motion, uterine, or adnexal tenderness on pelvic exam Purulent endocervical discharge	Diagnosis is clinical Should undergo screening for pregnancy and STIs specifically Chlamydia and Gonorrhea Low threshold to treat	Ceftriaxone 1 g IV Q24H PLUS Doxycycline 100 mg PO or IV Q12H PLUS Metronidazole 500 mg PO or IV Q12H, OR, Cefotetan 2 g IV Q12H PLUS Doxycycline 100 mg PO or IV Q12H, OR, Cefoxitin 2 g IV Q6H PLUS Doxycycline 100 mg PO or IV Q12H
Urethritis	Dysuria and penile discharge Some are asymptomatic	NAAT for Chlamydia and Gonorrhea Urine Culture, urethral swab and urinalysis Confirmed by presence of one of the following: Purulent urethral discharge Urethral swab Gram stain suggestive of urethritis +Leukocyte esterase or > 9 WBC/hpf on UA	If gonococcal, Ceftriaxone 500 mg IM × 1 If chlamydia, Doxycycline 100 mg BID × 7 days
Epididymitis	Unilateral testicular pain and tenderness Swelling of the testicle + Cremasteric reflex	Testicular torsion is a medical emergency with a similar presentation. US assessing blood flow should be obtained. Screen for Chlamydia and Gonorrhea	Ceftriaxone 500 mg IM × 1 PLUS Doxycycline 100 mg PO BID × 7 days
Cervicitis	Vaginal discharge, abnormal bleeding or dysuria Physical examination: Friable cervix, erythema, discharge from cervical os, and cervical petechiae	Nucleic acid amplification tests (NAAT)	Azithromycin 1 g PO × 1, OR Doxycycline 100 mg PO BID × 7 days PLUS Ceftriaxone 250 mg IM × 1 dose, OR Cefixime 800 mg PO × 1

(continued)

Table 129.3 (continued)

Disease	Clinical presentation	Diagnosis	Treatment
Perihepatitis (Fitz-Hugh-Curtis)	Right upper quadrant abdominal pain typically in the setting of PID	Clinical diagnosis +/– elevated aminotransferases	Treat underlying PID
Tubo-ovarian Abscess	Typically, PID that doesn't respond to treatment. Symptoms may worsen despite appropriate antimicrobial coverage	Pelvic US or CT	Treat underlying PID May consider surgical drainage

129.1 Assessment & Screening for STIs

When asking a teen about their sexual history, consider the following "5 P's" from the CDC to help guide your discussion [9]. Open the conversation by asking permission: "I need to ask some more specific questions about sexual activity to better understand if you are at risk for sexually transmitted infections or STIs. Would that be OK?"

1. **Partners**: Is the person sexually active with others?

"Are you currently having sex of any kind—oral, vaginal, or anal—with anyone? How many partners have you had in the past several months?"

2. **Practices**: Are they having oral, vaginal, and/or anal sex?

"Different tests are used for the different body parts people use to have sex. What kinds of sexual contact do you have, or have you had? What parts of your body are involved when you have sex?"

3. **Protection**: Are they using methods to prevent STIs (condoms, diaphragm, dental dam)?

"If you use prevention tools, what methods do you use? Do you use this method every time, or only sometimes?"

4. **Past History**: Has the person ever been tested, diagnosed, and/or treated for an STI?

"Have you been diagnosed with an STI in the past? When? Did you receive treatment? Has your current or former partner ever been diagnosed with an STI?"

5. **Pregnancy**: What is the person's method for preventing pregnancy?

"Are you or your partner using contraception or practicing any form of birth control? How important is it to you to prevent pregnancy?"

All sexually active teenagers should be encouraged to seek STI testing annually. If an adolescent has any symptoms suspected for STI, they should be referred to a facility for testing. Any STI symptoms that also present with abdominal pain or fever should be referred to an urgent care or emergency room for evaluation of PID. Most STI's can be cured but the teen's partner will also require treatment for the STI, to prevent recurrence. The HPV vaccine prevents sexually active people from getting cancer-causing strains of HPV. It should be recommended to all teens. Abstinence is the only guaranteed way to prevent STIs. However, sexually active teens can decrease their risk of acquiring STIs by using barrier methods such as condoms, diaphragms, and dental dams.

Extra Credit Points

1. Obtaining a sexual history (and menstrual history in biologic females) can be helpful in determining risk for STIs. However, this should be done in a non-judgmental manner, and teens should be encouraged to talk to their healthcare provider.
2. Any pelvic or abdominal symptoms associated with fever should be promptly evaluated in an emergency department.
3. STI symptoms can be very mild, and males are often asymptomatic.
4. All 50 states and D.C. have laws (as of 2024) that allow minors to request STI testing and treatment without consent from a guardian. Note, however, that confidentiality laws differ by state. So any teen may seek testing and treatment, however it is not always guaranteed they can keep this information from their parent. Title X funded health centers (such as Planned Parenthood) provide confidential and affordable access to contraceptive services and STI testing and treatment.

References

1. Division of Adolescent and School Health, National Center for Chronic Disease Prevention and Health Promotion. (n.d.). Youth risk behavior survey data summary & trends report. https://www.cdc.gov/healthyyouth/data/yrbs/pdf/yrbs_data-summary-trends_report2023_508.pdf.
2. Neurosyphilis, ocular syphilis, & otosyphilis. Syphilis. 2024. https://www.cdc.gov/syphilis/hcp/neurosyphilis-ocular-syphilis-otosyphilis/index.html.
3. What is Syphilis? | Syphilis Infection. (n.d.). Planned parenthood. https://www.plannedparenthood.org/learn/stds-hiv-safer-sex/syphilis.
4. What is trichomoniasis? & how do you get it? Planned Parenthood. https://www.plannedparenthood.org/learn/stds-hiv-safer-sex/trichomoniasis.
5. Centers for Disease Control and Prevention. Pelvic inflammatory disease (PID) - STI treatment guidelines. Centers for Disease Control and Prevention. 2022. https://www.cdc.gov/std/treatment-guidelines/pid.htm.

6. Workowski KA, Bachmann LH, Chan PA, et al. Sexually transmitted infections treatment guidelines, 2021. MMWR Recomm Rep. 2021;70:1.
7. Human papillomavirus (HPV) infection - STI treatment guidelines. https://www.cdc.gov/std/treatment-guidelines/anogenital-warts.htm.
8. HPV vaccination: what everyone should know | CDC. https://www.cdc.gov/vaccines/vpd/hpv/public/index.html.
9. Centers for Disease Control and Prevention. How do I discuss sexual health with patients? Centers for Disease Control and Prevention. 2023. https://www.cdc.gov/hiv/clinicians/screening/sexual-health.html#:~:text=The%20following%20questions%20correspond%20with,of%20STIs%2C%20and%20Pregnancy%20Intention.

Chapter 130
Contraception

Jennifer Kosoy Shook

Correct and consistent use of contraception, or birth control, plays an important role in decreasing the risk of unplanned pregnancies among adolescents. Contraception can be split into groups based on type of hormones used, such as combined estrogen and progesterone or progesterone-only. They can also be split into short-acting or long-acting. There are several methods for patients to choose from, and the best choice is most dependent on what each individual patient feels is the right choice for them in terms of comfort, memory to use and ease of use, and acceptability of risks and side effects. There may be medical contraindications, but most healthy teenagers should be able to safely use most of the available options. The Centers for Disease Control and Prevention (CDC) publishes a list of Medical Eligibility Criteria, which is available both on their website (https://www.cdc.gov/reproductivehealth/contraception/pdf/summary-chart-us-medical-eligibility-criteria_508tagged.pdf) and as a free mobile phone application and can be a helpful tool in determining medical conditions that may be associated with risk of use of certain contraceptive methods [1]. Although it is up to each individual patient what method they would choose to use, the American Academy of Pediatrics, Society for Adolescent Health and Medicine, and the American College of Obstetrics and Gynecology all recommend long-acting reversible contraception (LARCs) as these are most effective and also don't require patients remembering to do anything on their end in terms of adherence [2]. Table 130.1 shows contraceptive methods along with their effectiveness, benefits, and risks. It is important to remember to counsel adolescents that no matter which method they choose, they should also be encouraged to use condoms consistently as no method is 100% effective, and no methods prevent against sexually transmitted infections.

J. K. Shook (✉)
Penn State Children's Hospital, Hershey, PA, USA
e-mail: Jshook1@pennstatehealth.psu.edu

R. P. Olympia, J. Brady-Olympia (eds.), *Clinical Considerations in School-based Health*, https://doi.org/10.1007/978-3-031-85765-2_130

Table 130.1 Percentage of women becoming pregnant with each contraceptive method in the first year of use [3], along with risks and benefits of each method

Method	Typical Use[a]	Perfect Use[b]	Benefits	Risks/Complications
No method	85%	85%	No side effects	Unplanned pregnancy
Withdrawal method	22%	4%	No side effects	Unplanned pregnancy
Male condom	18%	2%	Sexually transmitted infection (STI) prevention	Reaction for those that are latex-allergic (are also available in latex-free versions) Must have available at time of sexual activity
Female condom	21%	5%	STI prevention Latex-free	Must have available at time of sexual activity
Oral contraceptive pill	9%	0.3%	Predictable, shorter, and lighter menses May improve cramps May improve acne Protection against endometrial and ovarian cancer	Venous thromboembolism Breakthrough bleeding, headaches, nausea, breast tenderness (these all usually improve by the second or third month) Must remember to use at a consistent time daily
Contraceptive vaginal ring	9%	0.3%	Predictable, shorter, and lighter menses May improve cramps May improve acne Protection against endometrial and ovarian cancer Do not have to remember to do something daily	Venous thromboembolism Breakthrough bleeding, headaches, nausea, breast tenderness (these all usually improve by the second or third month)
Contraceptive patch	9%	0.3%	Predictable, shorter, and lighter menses May improve cramps May improve acne Protection against endometrial and ovarian cancer Do not have to remember to do something daily	Breakthrough bleeding, headaches, nausea, breast tenderness (these all usually improve by the second or third month) Venous thromboembolism Skin irritation May not be private if not placed on clothing-covered skin

(continued)

Table 130.1 (continued)

Method	Typical Use[a]	Perfect Use[b]	Benefits	Risks/Complications
Progestin injection	6%	0.2%	Easy to use	Unpredictable bleeding pattern Increase in appetite which may lead to weight gain Loss of bone mineral density Must remember to get injection every 11–13 weeks
Contraceptive implant	0.05%	0.05%	Easy to use Do not have to do anything once it is placed The most effective method of contraception	Unpredictable bleeding pattern with higher chance of unscheduled bleeding Risk of infection on insertion Risk of migration of implant
Levonorgestrel intrauterine device	0.2%	0.2%	Easy to use Do not have to do anything once it is placed Higher chance of becoming amenorrheic (seen as a benefit by many but not all adolescents)	Unpredictable bleeding pattern Risk of infection of insertion Risk of uterine perforation Risk of expulsion
Copper intrauterine device	0.8%	0.6%	No hormonal side effects Easy to use Do not have to do anything once it is placed	Unpredictable bleeding pattern with higher chance of having heavier bleeding with increased cramping Risk of infection of insertion Risk of uterine perforation Risk of expulsion

[a]Typical Use is when a method is used by regular people in their day-to-day life, which may include variation

[b]Perfect Use is when a method is used exactly as instructed without variation, such as in a clinical trial

Many of the same hormonal methods used for contraception may also be used in treatment of various menstrual disorders, such as dysmenorrhea, irregular menses, abnormal uterine bleeding, and polycystic ovarian syndrome. Other non-contraceptive benefits may include improvement in acne and hirsutism and possible prevention of ovarian cysts.

While open communication between parents and adolescents is encouraged, teenagers' ability to consent for contraception without the knowledge or permission by their parents varies by state. It is important to check your state laws before prescribing as these may also be changed at any time. Currently, twenty-seven states plus the District of Columbia allow teenagers to consent for contraception, although some may be at a certain age, such as 12 or 14 years old. Nineteen states allow only certain categories of teenagers to consent, such as those that are married, pregnant, or considered mature minors. Four states do not have any law regarding this [4].

Case 1 Ellyn, a 14-year-old student at your school, presents to the clinic because she has started to have spotting. She has been on an oral contraceptive pill for a few months, but she forgot to take a couple doses this weekend when she was away at a basketball tournament. She is very worried she may be pregnant as she has never had bleeding in the middle of the pack before. How would you counsel Ellyn?

There are three methods of contraception that are formulated with both estrogen and progesterone. These methods generally give patients predictable menstrual periods and may also help menses to be shorter, lighter, and less painful. There may also be other benefits experienced, such as improvement with acne or hirsutism. The combined hormonal contraceptive methods include a pill, a patch, or a ring.

Oral contraceptive pills are an effective method for someone who is able to be reliable with taking a daily pill, which should be taken at the same time daily. There are combined pills with estrogen and progesterone, which may be more effective and have a little more time leeway for daily use. There are also progesterone-only pills, sometimes called the "mini-pill," which require being stricter with taking at the exact same time every day, which can be challenging for adolescents. However, the progesterone-only pill could be a good option for someone with a contraindication to estrogen (Table 130.2) but who still would prefer to be on a pill method. The combined pill has 3 weeks of hormonal pills and 1 week of placebo pills. The progesterone-only pill does not have a placebo week. The combined hormonal transdermal patch works similarly but is a good option for someone who does not want to take a daily pill. One patch is applied weekly for 3 weeks, and then there is

Table 130.2 Some medical conditions where estrogen use would be a contraindication or not recommended. More details can be found in the CDC's Medical Eligibility Criteria list [1]

Unacceptable Health Risk	Risk Thought to Outweigh Benefit
Breast cancer	Symptomatic gallbladder disease
Severe cirrhosis or liver disease	Certain medications that may interfere, such as some anticonvulsants
History of venous thromboembolism/stroke	
Prolonged immobilization such as following major surgery	
Diabetes mellitus with vascular disease	
Migraines with aura	
Uncontrolled hypertension	
Ischemic heart disease	
Known clotting disorders	
Systemic lupus erythematosus with positive or unknown antiphospholipid antibodies	
Complicated valvular heart disease	
Complicated solid organ transplant	

a patch-free week, which is when a withdrawal bleed would typically take place. Likewise, the combined hormonal ring is another good option for someone who does not want to take a daily pill but likes the idea of a monthly withdrawal bleed. The ring is placed vaginally and remains for 3 weeks, and then it is removed for one ring-free week.

Side effects for estrogen-containing methods are broken down into symptoms that may be intolerable but not dangerous and then those that may be signs for something dangerous. The potential intolerable side effects include headaches, nausea, breast tenderness, and irregular bleeding. These usually get better by the second or third month of use but may persist for some people who may then prefer to try a different method. If someone is not reliable using their pill, patch, or ring, they may also have breakthrough bleeding or experience some of these side effects when they restart taking it. For Ellyn in the case, it is possible that she is having bleeding due to missing pills. However, it would also be important to do a pregnancy test to rule out pregnancy as a possibility for her recent spotting, especially if she is unreliably using her pill. The more severe side effect, which is generally rare in young, healthy patients, is a blood clot. There is a useful mnemonic that physicians, healthcare providers, and patients may use, which is ACHES (Table 130.3), and can be used to remember possible signs of a clot. For progesterone-only methods, the main side effect is unpredictable bleeding, which may include spotting or irregular bleeding or may include amenorrhea. Some progesterones may also increase acne or hirsutism, or may be associated with headaches, nausea, or mood changes.

Case 2 Danielle is a 16-year-old student at the school where you work. Danielle is currently using the birth control shot but has a hard time making it to her appointments in the correct follow-up window. She would like an alternative option that is long-lasting as she previously was not good with remembering to use a daily pill, and she thinks she wouldn't remember to use a patch or ring. She wants an option that will be easy and very effective as she is currently in a sexual relationship with her boyfriend of 2 years. What would you recommend for Danielle?

Depot medroxyprogesterone acetate (DMPA) is the shot that Danielle is currently using. This is given intramuscularly or subcutaneously every 11 to 13 weeks and is a reliable form of birth control if users are receiving it in that time window. A helpful tool to avoid miscounting weeks is to utilize a perpetual calendar, which gives the return timeframe based on the day the injection is administered. One

Table 130.3 ACHES mnemonic for signs of a blood clot

Mnemonic Letter	Possible Blood Clot Sign
A	Abdominal pain
C	Chest pain
H	Headaches
E	Eyes (vision changes)
S	Severe leg pain

example is the Depo-Provera perpetual calendar, which can be found at: https://sa1s3.patientpop.com/assets/docs/25323.pdf [5]. Users of DMPA may have irregular bleeding or may experience amenorrhea. There are some associated side effects of weight gain (due to increased appetite) and a potential loss of bone mineral density.

A long-acting reversible contraception (LARC) would be a good option for someone like Danielle who would like a longer-lasting option that requires little effort by the user. The implant and the intrauterine device (IUD) are also both more than 99% effective at preventing pregnancy so are most effective as compared to other methods when accounting for typical use. The implant is the most effective contraception option and is good for 3 years in place in the upper arm. These are generally placed by adolescent medicine physicians or gynecologists and can also be placed by some general pediatricians or family medicine physicians if they have the additional training for this procedure. One side effect which may cause patients to want it removed sooner than 3 years is the risk of unscheduled bleeding so this should be counseled on before placing the device as some girls may be unbothered by this, but for others the chance of this would be a no-go. There are several IUD options available. There are levonorgestrel IUDs, which come in different dosages, and depending on the dose, can be good for 3–8 years. A non-hormonal option is a copper IUD, which is effective for 10 years. IUDs are generally very well tolerated over their course but may be associated with cramping at the time of placement. The pain can be ameliorated by pre-treating with an anti-inflammatory pain medication, use of numbing medications for insertion, or insertion under sedation. Hormonal IUD users may find a side effect of lighter to no periods, which is a benefit for some girls. The copper IUD may be associated with increased menstrual bleeding and cramping but is a great option for someone who desires contraception but has a contraindication to a hormonal method, which can be found in the CDC's medical eligibility criteria list [1].

Case 3 You are working in the school-based health center when Reese, a 15-year-old girl, presents in a panic. She had sex yesterday after school, and her boyfriend did not use a condom because they forgot. She does not desire pregnancy at this time and wants to know if there is anything you can do.

Emergency contraception can help prevent pregnancy if taken as soon as possible within 120 hours (5 days) of unprotected sexual intercourse. There are a few options that Reese can choose from. One oral option is a levonorgestrel 1.5 mg pill. This is not the most effective of the options, but it is the easiest to obtain as it can be purchased over-the-counter. It also may not work as well in individuals more than 165 pounds [6]. The other oral option is ulipristal acetate 30 mg. This is more effective over the 120 hours than levonorgestrel is as levonorgestrel efficacy drops quicker after 72 hours [7]. Ulipristal acetate may not work as well in patients greater than 194 pounds [6], but would be a better option than levonorgestrel for those that are 165 to 194 pounds. A prescription is required for ulipristal acetate. Copper and levonorgestrel IUDs are the most effective forms of emergency contraception if placed within 120 hours. These can also then be kept in place for contraception going forward if desired. Having emergency contraception available in a school-based health center can be very helpful for adolescents to obtain as soon as possible. The American Academy of Pediatrics policy statement on school-based health centers states that providing emergency contraception in school-based health centers can improve access to reproductive health services [8]. It is also great if condoms can be provided so that students have easy access to get them and thus may be more likely to use them if they're readily available. Additionally, all sexually active adolescents should have screening for sexually transmitted infections, such as chlamydia, gonorrhea, human immunodeficiency virus (HIV), and syphilis.

In summary, there are many options for adolescents to choose from when deciding on a contraception method. There are also emergency contraception options available. The best method to use is the one that the adolescent chooses for herself, but it is also important to know that if someone is not completely satisfied with the option they choose, they can easily switch to an alternative if they would like. Preventing teenage pregnancy can help improve morbidity and mortality in teenagers and can best be achieved by partnering together with adolescent patients to discuss risks and benefits of each option, as well as managing side effect expectations.

Extra Credit Points

1. The CDC's medical eligibility criteria is a good reference for categorized risks of using various contraceptive options in those that have certain medical conditions.
2. Combined hormonal contraception options give a predictable period, and they may be shorter, lighter, and with less cramping.
3. LARCs are a top recommendation in teenagers because they are most effective and also require little to no effort for adherence.
4. Emergency contraception options work best right away but may be used within 120 hours of unprotected sexual intercourse.

References

1. Centers for Disease Control and Prevention. Summary chart of U.S. medical eligibility criteria for contraceptive use. 2020. https://www.cdc.gov/reproductivehealth/contraception/pdf/summary-chart-us-medical-eligibility-criteria_508tagged.pdf.
2. Robbins CL, Ott MA. Contraception options and provision to adolescents. Minerva Pediatr. 2017;69(5):403–14.
3. Centers for Disease Control and Prevention. Morbidity and Mortality Weekly Report Appendix D: Contraceptive Effectiveness. 2014. https://www.cdc.gov/mmwr/preview/mmwrhtml/rr6304a5.htm.
4. Guttmacher. An overview of consent to reproductive health services by young people. 2023. https://www.guttmacher.org/state-policy/explore/overview-minors-consent-law.

5. Depo-Provera perpetual calendar. 1999. https://sa1s3.patientpop.com/assets/docs/25323.pdf.
6. Bedsider. Explore birth control options: emergency contraception. https://www.bedsider.org/birth-control/emergency_contraception.
7. Teal S, Edelman A. Contraception selection, effectiveness, and adverse effects: a review. JAMA. 2021;326(24):2507–18.
8. Kjolhede C, Lee AC, Council on School Health, et al. School-based health centers and pediatric practice. Pediatrics. 2021;145(4):e2021053758.

Chapter 131
Teenage Pregnancy

Mina Cunningham

Case 1 A 16 year old high school sophomore approaches the school nurse's office with a look of discomfort. She hesitantly reports that she's been experiencing nausea every morning for the past 2 weeks. Additionally, she confides that she missed her period, which was due over 3 weeks ago. After ensuring privacy, the nurse conducts a thorough assessment, asking about her past medical history, recent activities, and emotional state. Recognizing the potential implications of these symptoms, the provider gently broaches the subject of a pregnancy test and discusses the next steps, emphasizing confidentiality and support throughout the process.

The above student has reported amenorrhea and morning sickness. Other symptoms of early pregnancy may include tender or tingling breasts, fatigue, increased urine frequency, and abdominal bloating. The likelihood doubles if the patient believes they could be pregnant. On a physical exam one might also palpate a more globus uterus, and depending on gestational weeks may or may not be limited to the pelvis [1]. Given her history, there is a higher chance this student might be pregnant. Obtaining the first day of her last menstrual period (LMP) is paramount for determining gestational age and estimated due date (EDD). This can be calculated by Naegele's Rule. Traditionally, an EDD is calculated based on a 280-day (40-week) pregnancy length and works best for women with regular 28-day menstrual cycles [2]. It involves adding 7 days to the first day of the last menstrual period (LMP) and then subtracting 3 months. The resulting date is adjusted to fall on the same day of the week as the LMP in the following year. For example, a LMP of January 1st would result in an EDD of October 7th, (assuming January 1st was on a Monday in this case). It's important to note that this is an estimation, and menstrual cycle variability can influence accuracy. Ultrasound measurements during early pregnancy

M. Cunningham (✉)
St. Louis University Southwest IL Family Medicine, O'Fallon, IL, USA

R. P. Olympia, J. Brady-Olympia (eds.), *Clinical Considerations in School-based Health*, https://doi.org/10.1007/978-3-031-85765-2_131

can provide a more precise EDD for those with unsure LMP dates or irregular menses. Additionally, various online calculators and pregnancy wheels offer alternative methods for estimating due dates (Table 131.1).

A positive urine pregnancy test indicates the need for further assessment. Ultrasound confirmation is essential to confirm intrauterine pregnancy and should be performed by a qualified healthcare professional as soon as possible. In collaboration with the patient, you can explore options for establishing prenatal care. This could involve their pediatrician, an obstetrical provider, or utilizing your facility's referral network. Developing a trusting relationship is crucial. While parental support is often beneficial, the student may not be comfortable disclosing the pregnancy at home. Your primary focus should be on guiding them towards safe and appropriate prenatal care, recognizing that most pregnant adolescents choose to continue the pregnancy [3].

Before you send this patient off with your recommendations for care providers, you'll want to address her main concern: morning sickness. This particular nausea and vomiting in pregnancy can strike at any time of day. Fortunately, several strategies can help alleviate its unpleasant symptoms. Dietary modifications are a great first step. Opting for frequent, small meals of bland, easily digestible carbohydrates like toast, crackers, or rice can settle the stomach. Ginger, either consumed fresh, in tea form, or as lozenges, has shown promise in reducing nausea. Staying hydrated is essential; sipping fluids throughout the day is recommended, with water and clear broths being excellent options. Proper hydration also helps prevent constipation, which frequently accompanies nausea and vomiting. Identifying and avoiding triggers, like strong smells or greasy foods, can also be helpful. Consider acupressure with wrist bands that place pressure on the P6 (Negan's point) [4].

According to ACOG [4], first line treatments include:

- Vitamin B6 (pyridoxine) 10–25 mg orally 3–4 times daily
- Doxylamine 12.5–25 mg may be taken in combination with B6 or alone according to severity of symptoms.
- OR, B6 10 mg/doxylamine 10 mg combination: 2 tablets at bedtime initially, then increasing to additional AM and noon dose. Max 4 tablets

Table 131.1 Some examples of online calculators to determine estimated due date

Online EDD Calculators	Phone Applications for Download
https://perinatology.com/calculators/Due-Date.htm https://americanpregnancy.org/resources/pregnancy-calculator/	Obstetric Calculator App IPhone: https://apps.apple.com/us/app/obstetrics-calculator/id1564764019 Android: https://play.google.com/store/apps/details?id=com.Alefrei.ObstetricCalculator&hl=en_US Gestational Age App Iphone: https://apps.apple.com/us/app/gestational-age-babys-age/id1536304956?platform=iphone Android: https://play.google.com/store/apps/details?id=com.danproductions.medical.gestational_age&hl=en_US

- OR B6 20 mg/doxylamine 20 mg combination: 1 tablet at bedtime initially then add on AM dose as needed. Max 2 tablets.

If symptoms persist one may add dimenhydrinate, diphenhydramine, prochlorperazine, or promethazine. Third line options for persistent nausea and vomiting include metoclopramide, ondansetron, promethazine, and trimethobenzamide. If dehydration is suspected, IV fluid replacement should occur and the patient should be directed to the Emergency Department to receive this care. Additional labs should be ordered to evaluate for urine ketones and electrolytes, kidney function, and liver function.

A helpful clinically validated tool employed by healthcare professionals to quantify the severity of nausea and vomiting of pregnancy (NVP) is the Pregnancy-Unique Quantification of Emesis (PUQE) scoring system [5]. It focuses on three core symptoms: nausea duration, vomiting frequency, and retching episodes, assigning a point value to each based on their occurrence within a specific timeframe (Table 131.2).

Total PUQE Score Add the points from each category to determine your overall PUQE score:

- 6 or less = Mild NVP
- 7–12 = Moderate NVP
- 13 or greater = severe NVP (Hyperemesis Gravidarum)

This stratification guides the selection of appropriate management strategies. For mild NVP, the PUQE score might indicate the need for dietary modifications. Conversely, a high score suggestive of severe NVP (Hyperemesis Gravidarum) would warrant more aggressive interventions, potentially including medication or hospitalization. Additionally, the PUQE score can be employed serially to monitor a patient's response to treatment and gauge the efficacy of implemented interventions.

However, it's crucial to acknowledge that the PUQE score serves as an adjunct to clinical expertise, not a definitive diagnostic tool in isolation. A specific score shouldn't be solely relied upon to predict a particular clinical course, as individual experiences with NVP can vary significantly. Pregnant women experiencing NVP, especially those with moderate to severe symptoms or substantial disruption to daily activities, should consult a healthcare professional. Through a comprehensive clinical evaluation that incorporates the PUQE score alongside other relevant findings,

Table 131.2 PUQE scoring system for Nausea and vomiting of pregnancy [5]

Symptom	1 point	2 points	3 points	4 points	5 points
Nausea Duration (Hours/day)	None	1 or less	2–3	4–6	>6
Vomiting Frequency (Times/day)	None	1–2	3–4	5–6	>7
Retching Frequency (Times/day)	None	1–2	3–4	5–6	>7

healthcare providers can formulate personalized treatment plans and optimize maternal and fetal well-being throughout pregnancy.

Case 2 A 17 year old student reports to the school nurse office complaining of lower abdominal pain. She is in her second trimester of pregnancy, approximately 26 weeks along. The pain started a few hours ago and has been intermittent. She describes the pain as cramp-like and located mainly in the lower abdomen. The student denies any recent trauma, urinary symptoms, or changes in bowel habits. She has been attending her prenatal visits but missed her last appointment due to transportation issues.

After you obtain normal vital signs, you inquire about any additional symptoms. She denies any nausea, vomiting, fever, vaginal bleeding or discharge, or recent sexual intercourse. She admits to feeling anxious about the cramping and does not know what the signs of labor might be. Her anatomy scan was completed, and she was told everything looked normal. You ask if her pain radiates anywhere, and she admits to a sharp, left-sided pain that goes to her vagina. You have her lie supine on your table for a physical exam. Bowel sounds are present and reactive. Fundal height is 26 cm. The abdomen is soft, and non-tender in all quadrants. You assess fetal heart tones of 143 beats per minute with your handheld Doppler. Satisfied with your exam, you ask the student to give you a midstream urine sample. When she returns, you give her a glass of water to drink and have her rest with a warm pack for her cramping. Your point of care urinalysis is negative for leukocyte esterase or nitrates. At this point, you feel pretty confident the student is experiencing round ligament pain. You ask the student if she feels comfortable calling her obstetric provider to make another appointment. The office can fit her in right after school. She is able to coordinate transportation and agrees to make this office visit.

The round ligaments are two support structures that help to keep the uterus in place. Arising from the upper corners of the uterus, the round ligaments stretch downwards to connect with the labia majora and mons pubis. As the uterus enlarges to accommodate the growing fetus, the round ligaments naturally stretch and elongate. This physiological process can occasionally induce cramping or sharp pain in the lower abdomen or groin region. The discomfort is often exacerbated by sudden movements, coughing, or laughing.

Fortunately, round ligament pain is typically considered a benign consequence of pregnancy. Conservative management strategies are recommended for this discomfort. Rest periods, application of warm compresses, and the use of maternity support belts can provide effective relief. Gentle stretching exercises may also be beneficial. In some cases, acetaminophen can be used for pain relief, adhering to recommended dosages for age and weight. To minimize the occurrence of round ligament pain, it is advisable to avoid sudden movements, prolonged standing, and heavy lifting [6]. By adhering to these preventive measures and employing conservative management techniques, pregnant adolescents can effectively manage this common pregnancy discomfort.

In the management of round ligament pain, it is crucial to maintain a high index of suspicion for potential complications. While conservative measures are often effective, prompt referral to a prenatal care provider or emergency department is warranted in specific scenarios. Other differential diagnoses for abdominal pain in the second trimester include obstetric and non-obstetric causes. A common list included below [7] is not fully comprehensive (Table 131.3).

Case 3 A 15 year old student visits the school physician with concerns of vaginal bleeding. She is 32 weeks pregnant and mentions it started this morning. The bleeding is not heavy but has persisted for a few hours. She denies any recent trauma, sexual intercourse, or physical exertion that could explain the bleeding. She has also been attending her prenatal appointments regularly and has had a relatively uncomplicated pregnancy so far.

You ask her to quantify the amount of bleeding. She shows you a picture from her phone. It is most consistent with light bleeding, as less than half the pad is saturated.

- Spotting is bleeding that only leaves a few drops of blood on underwear. Technically does not require a liner or pad, but if worn would be very scant with less than a quarter covered.
- Light bleeding means the pad is saturated by less than half
- Moderate bleeding is when the pad is saturated by more than half in a few hours
- Heavy bleeding is when the pad is completely saturated by blood within an hour or less, with possible overflow onto underwear. There is frequent need to change the pad.

She is reporting associated lower abdominal cramping while you take her vital signs. Her blood pressure is 124/78, pulse 106, and temperature 97.7 °F. You have her recline on your table, and perform a physical exam. You note her abdomen is soft, nontender with fundal height of 31 cm. She denies any dysuria, increased urine frequency, or unusual vaginal discharge. You have an ultrasound Doppler and find fetal heart tones at a rate of 136 beats per minute. She confirms feeling fetal movement. You check her pulse again, which is now 94, confirming there is no hypovolemic shock or signs of hypoperfusion. She does not have prenatal records with her, but she recalls that her blood type is not negative.

Preterm labor occurs when regular contractions cause cervical dilation prior to 37 weeks gestation. This is of significant concern, as adolescent pregnancy has an increased risk of preterm labor, with the highest risk in those under 16 years of age [8, 9]. Several factors can increase the risk of preterm labor, including a history of preterm delivery, as well as tobacco use, alcohol consumption, drug use, and inconsistent prenatal care [10].

To effectively assess and manage vaginal bleeding in pregnant adolescents, prioritizing the possibility of preterm labor is crucial. Serial vaginal exams with sterile speculums and potential cultures may be necessary to rule out infections. Given these needs, referral to the Emergency Department or OB labor and triage unit is recommended for further evaluation. Additionally, Rh-negative patients require Rhogam administration, which is typically available at higher levels of care. Table 131.4 summarizes other common causes of vaginal bleeding during

Table 131.3 Obstetric and Non-obstetric Causes of Abdominal Pain in Pregnancy

Braxton Hicks Contractions	Common in second and third trimester Symptoms: irregular contractions only causing discomfort Not progressive, relieved with position change, hydration
Round Ligament Pain	Abdominal pain caused by stretching round ligaments. Common in second trimester Symptoms: sharp or cramping pain, often on one side or lower abdomen. Physiologically benign. Conservative management.
Placental Abruption	Premature separation of placenta from uterus Symptoms: severe uterine tenderness, abdominal pain, and vaginal bleeding Medical emergency, requires immediate attention/referral
Preterm Labor	Labor before 37 weeks gestation Symptoms: regular contractions, lower back pain, pelvic pressure, or changes in vaginal discharge Urgent: requires immediate medical attention
Ectopic pregnancy	Implantation outside the uterus Symptoms: severe unilateral abdominal pain, vaginal bleeding, dizziness, or shoulder pain Medical emergency: mostly encountered in first trimester
Preeclamspia	Pregnancy complication characterized by high blood pressures (>140/(and/or) >90) and signs of damage to other organ systems, such as the liver and kidneys Symptoms: severe headache, visual disturbances, proteinuria, right upper quadrant (RUQ) or epigastric pain Urgent: requires immediate medical attention to prevent progression to eclampsia.
Acute Fatty Liver of Pregnancy	Rare, but serious condition characterized by accumulation of fat in the liver Symptoms: RUQ pain, nausea, vomiting, jaundice, or malaise Urgent: requires immediate medical attention
Urinary Tract Infection	Infection of urinary system Symptoms: dysuria, urgency, increased urinary frequency, lower abdominal pain Could increase risk of preterm labor or lead to more serious infection if left untreated leading to maternal or fetal morbidity
Appendicitis	Inflammation of the appendix Symptoms: right lower quadrant pain (RLQ), nausea, vomiting, fever. Pain might be diffuse first before localizing to RLQ Urgent: should seek medical attention to rule out infectious process or need for surgical interventions
Gallstones	Stones or "sludge" in the gallbladder Symptoms: RUQ pain, nausea and/or vomiting especially after eating fatty meals. Pain may radiate to the back or shoulder. Urgent: may be difficult to rule out in a school setting. Consider referral for further work up.
Constipation	Difficulty passing stools Symptoms: crampy, colicky abdominal pain Relief after bowel movement

Table 131.4 Common causes of vaginal bleeding during pregnancy [11–13]

<20 weeks	Abortion—bleeding accompanied by cramping or low back pain with or without passage of fetal tissue depending on type of miscarriage Ectopic pregnancy—bleeding with sharp, unilateral abdominal pain, dizziness or shoulder pain Trophoblastic disease (Molar pregnancy)—bleeding from abnormal pregnancy of non-viable egg Implantation bleeding—spotting or light bleeding when fertilized egg attaches to uterine lining
>20 weeks	Placenta abruption—typically painful bleeding due to premature separation of the placenta Placenta previa—painless bleeding from placenta covering or very near cervix Vasa previa—fetal blood vessels running near or crossing over cervix Preterm labor—mild bleeding due to cervical change Infection—vaginitis or cervicitis causing bleeding

pregnancy. By prioritizing preterm labor evaluation and ensuring prompt referral, you can significantly contribute to managing risks associated with bleeding and potential preterm birth in this adolescent population.

131.1 Case Conclusion

In managing pregnant teens with common pregnancy-related issues, timely assessment and appropriate interventions are essential. For nausea and vomiting in early pregnancy, initial management involved ensuring hydration, using PUQE scoring to determine severity, and recommending antiemetics and dietary adjustments. In the case of abdominal pain in the second trimester, thorough evaluation ruled out serious conditions such as preeclampsia and placental abruption, with comfort measures provided and referral for further medical evaluation. For vaginal bleeding in the third trimester, assessing the bleeding's amount and nature, monitoring vital signs, and promptly referring to the emergency room to rule out preterm labor were critical. These cases highlight the importance of early recognition, supportive care, and timely referral to ensure the health and safety of both mother and baby.

Extra Credit Points

1. Early recognition and referral: Always consider pregnancy in a teen presenting with nausea, vomiting, vaginal bleeding, or abdominal pain.
2. PUQE Scoring system: Use this clinically validated tool to help you assess severity of nausea and vomiting in pregnancy. This can help determine further intervention.
3. Common Causes of Abdominal Pain in Pregnancy: Consider round ligament pain, constipation, urinary tract infection, and other gastrointestinal issues. Be vigilant for serious conditions like preeclampsia, placental abruption, or appendicitis.

4. Vaginal Bleeding Red Flags: Prioritize the assessment of ectopic pregnancy, placenta abruption, placenta previa. Immediate referral for anyone with signs of shock.
5. Emotional support and reassurance: Provide a supportive environment to those that may be feeling anxiety about their symptoms. Provide reassurance when appropriate.

References

1. Bastian LA. Is this patient pregnant? JAMA. 1997;278(7):586. https://doi.org/10.1001/jama.1997.03550070078042.
2. Lawson GW. Naegele's rule and the length of pregnancy - a review. Aust N Z J Obstet Gynaecol. 2021;61(2):177–82.
3. Maddow-Zimet I, Kost K. Pregnancies, births and abortions in the United States, 1973–2017: national and state trends by age. Accessed 31 May 2024. https://www.guttmacher.org/report/pregnancies-births-abortions-in-united-states-1973-2017.
4. Committee on Practice Bulletins-Obstetrics. ACOG practice bulletin no. 189: nausea and vomiting of pregnancy. Obstet Gynecol. 2018;131(1):e15–30.
5. Koren G, Piwko C, Ahn E, et al. Validation studies of the Pregnancy Unique-Quantification of Emesis (PUQE) scores. J Obstet Gynaecol. 2005;25(3):241–4.
6. Chaudhry SR, Chaudhry K. Anatomy, abdomen and pelvis: uterus round ligament. In: StatPearls. StatPearls Publishing; 2023.
7. Gregory DS, Wu V, Tuladhar P. The pregnant patient: managing common acute medical problems. Am Fam Physician. 2018;98(9):595–602.
8. Perez MJ, Chang JJ, Temming LA, et al. Driving factors of preterm birth risk in adolescents. AJP Rep. 2020;10(3):e247–52.
9. Fleming N, O'Driscoll T, Becker G, Spitzer RF, CANPAGO Committee. Adolescent pregnancy guidelines. J Obstet Gynaecol Can. 2015;37(8):740–56.
10. Weismiller DG. Preterm labor. Am Fam Physician. 1999;59(3):593–602.
11. Sakornbut E, Leeman L, Fontaine P. Late pregnancy bleeding. Am Fam Physician. 2007;75(8):1199–206.
12. Francois K, Foley M. Antepartum and postpartum hemorrhage. In: Gabbe's obstetrics: normal and problem pregnancies. 8th ed. Saunders; 2020. p. 123–36.
13. Deutchman M, Tubay AT, Turok D. First trimester bleeding. Am Fam Physician. 2009;79(11):985–94.

Chapter 132
Sexual Education for Youth

Natasha Ramsey and Elizabeth M. Alderman

Case 1 **Jessica is a 16 year old who has been feeling sick. She has been having breast tenderness and nausea. She came to the clinic to get some medication for nausea. After reviewing the confidentiality laws in your state, and upon further questioning she tells you she had vaginal sex without a condom a few weeks ago. She has not had a period in 2 months but says that her periods are not regular and thought it might be due to stress because she has been studying for her tests. You explain to her that missed periods can be a sign of early pregnancy in addition to her other symptoms. She had no idea because she never talked about sex at home and has only learned about abstinence in school. You provide options counseling to her and review sexual health information with her while awaiting the test results. Her pregnancy test is negative, and she is relieved. You provide her with some credible online resources to learn more about sexual health.**

Case 2 **Nataly is 14 years old and when she got her first period at age 12, she did not know why she was bleeding. She thought she cut herself and did not tell anyone. She finally discussed it with her mother and although she learned about periods last year in health class, still had so many questions and was embarrassed to discuss it with anyone. She feels comfortable with you and wants to discuss more about periods. Although her school does not make period products readily available, the school clinic provides menstrual products, so she stops by the clinic to grab some. Upon further discussion you find out that**

N. Ramsey (✉)
Montefiore Medical Group, Bronx, NY, USA
e-mail: naramsey@montefiore.org

E. M. Alderman
The Children's Hospital at Montefiore, Bronx, NY, USA
e-mail: ealderma@montefiore.org

R. P. Olympia, J. Brady-Olympia (eds.), *Clinical Considerations in School-based Health*, https://doi.org/10.1007/978-3-031-85765-2_132

she has been feeling lightheaded and dizzy. She tells you she has been on her period for 6 weeks. Sometimes her clothes and bed sheets even get stained. She has missed several days from school because of menstrual cramps, feeling fatigued and embarrassment around being on her period.

Sexuality is an important aspect of the human experience. While sexual activity is a large part of sexuality, sexuality encompasses physiological changes, attraction, pleasure, and much more. Sexuality is a fundamental part of human development for children and adolescents across the world and in the United States. During adolescence, many young people are exploring their sexuality, are building intimate relationships and may be engaging in a range of sexual behaviors. Adolescents and young adults require evidence-based, medically accurate, comprehensive and non-judgmental services and information that promotes sexual development, reproductive health, and overall health throughout their lives.

Data from the Center for Disease Control (CDC) shows that adolescents are delaying initiation of sex compared to previous years. In 2021 only 30% of high school students had ever had sexual intercourse [1]. However, based on a report by the Guttmacher Institute, most adolescents will have sex by the time they are young adults: 93% of 25 year olds have had sex [2]. These sexual behaviors including anal and oral sex may result in adverse health outcomes, such as unintended pregnancy and sexually transmitted infections (STI). Recent data has shown that adolescents continue to experience high rates of STIs, but lower rates of unintended pregnancy. Adolescents are at a higher risk for STIs due to both biological and behavioral factors. The CDC reports that in 2020, adolescents aged 13–24 accounted for 20% of all new HIV diagnoses in the United States [1]. More than half of the 20 million STIs reported were among adolescents aged 15–24 [1]. Increased rates of STIs may be related to decreased condom use, with the percentage of sexually active adolescents decreasing from 2011 to 2021. In 2021, only 52% of currently sexually active high school students used a condom the last time they had sexual intercourse compared to 60% in 2011 [1].

A positive trend is that the use of other forms of contraception has increased. Approximately 30% of sexually active adolescents used hormonal methods such as birth control pills and intrauterine devices (IUDs) during their last sexual intercourse [1]. Subsequently, the teen birth rate in the United States has significantly declined, dropping by 4% from 2018 to 2019, and by 73% from 1991 to 2019 [1]. This decline in the teen birth rate has been attributed to improved access to contraceptive methods and better sexual education programs. As per the WHO, sexuality education equips children and adolescents with the knowledge, attitudes, values and skills that help them to advocate for their health, make responsible choices and understand and protect the rights of others, develop respectful social and sexual relationships [3]. Table 132.1 describes a brief history of sexual education history.

Today, the landscape of sexual health education in the United States remains varied, with significant differences in implementation and content across states and school districts. There are different models for sexual health education the main two being abstinence only sexual health education and comprehensive sex ed.

Table 132.1 History of Sexual health education

Early 1900s	Sexual health education started in response to public health concerns such as STIs. The American Social Hygiene Association was founded in 1914 and emphasized the dangers of premarital sex and promoting abstinence.
1920s and 1930s	Sexual health education was introduced in public schools. Content was restricted to biology and hygiene, avoiding explicit discussions of sexual behavior. Planned Parenthood Federation of America was formed in 1942, which advocated for more comprehensive sexual education.
1940s and 1950s	In 1953, the American Medical Association (AMA) and the National Education Association (NEA) jointly published "Sexual health education in Schools," advocating for educational programs that included information on human reproduction, anatomy, and the consequences of sexual activity. Resistance from conservative and religious groups limited the scope and implementation of sexual health education programs.
1960s and 1970s	The sexual revolution brought more openness and discussion about sexuality. The federal Office of Adolescent Health was established in 1978. The rise of the AIDS epidemic in the 1980s shifted the focus toward disease prevention. There was clash between proponents of comprehensive sexual health education and advocates of abstinence-only education. The Reagan administration was in support of conservative political groups and policies.
1970s and 1980s	Federal funding for abstinence-only programs increased significantly with the passage of the Adolescent Family Life Act (1981) which allocated substantial funds to abstinence-only education.
2000's	Research showed that comprehensive sexual education programs were superior to abstinence-only programs. The Obama administration's Teen Pregnancy Prevention Program (TPPP), established in 2010, funded evidence-based sexual health education programs The American Academy of Pediatrics publishes clinical report on Sexual health education for Children and Adolescents [16]

Source: https://cdn.plannedparenthood.org/uploads/filer_public/da/67/da67fd5d-631d-438a-85e8-a446d90fd1e3/20170209_sexed_d04_1.pdf [4]

Abstinence-only programs focus primarily on promoting abstinence from sexual activity until marriage, often excluding information on contraception and safe sex practices and have been shown to be less effective compared to comprehensive sexual health education. Comprehensive sexual health education programs provide thorough, evidence-based information includes information about abstinence as well as contraception, healthy relationships, consent, and sexual orientation and are more effective in reducing risky behaviors among adolescents. Efforts continue to promote more inclusive and comprehensive approaches that address the needs of all students, including LGBTQ+ youth and those with diverse backgrounds and experiences [5].

Sexual health education in the United States varies widely by state, school district, and even by who delivers the education, leading to significant differences in the content and quality of the education provided to students. The requirements for sexual health education are determined at the state level. Some states mandate comprehensive sexual health education that covers a wide range of topics. Other states either do not require sexual health education at all or require it only to focus on abstinence. Currently, 38 states and the District of Columbia mandate sexual health education and/or HIV education. Of those, only 18 states require program content to be medically accurate [6]. In addition, many states allow parents to opt their children out of sexual health education classes if they do not want them to participate. Some states have opt-in policies, where students are only included in sexual health education if parents explicitly consent. 35 states and DC allow parents the option to remove their child from instruction [6]. The content of sexual health education curricula can vary greatly with some programs include topics such as STIs, contraception, gender identity, sexual orientation, and consent, while others may not address these topics at all. The inclusion of these topics can be influenced by local community values and politics.

132.1 Defining Comprehensive Sexual Health Education

Comprehensive sexual health education includes teaching about all aspects of human sexuality. Based on expert consensus, comprehensive sexual health education programs have several common elements (Table 132.2) [7]. These programs utilize medically accurate and evidence-based content that employ developmentally appropriate information can be modified for youth with disabilities, contain learning strategies, teaching methods, and materials and provide basic knowledge in 6 key topics areas [7].

Sexual health education programs should start with an early foundation and continue building on that foundation in a developmentally appropriate way across all grade levels. It is recommended that comprehensive sexual health education should occur across the child developmental spectrum and should begin at early ages, as young as 4 and continue throughout childhood, adolescence, and adulthood [8].

Table 132.2 Comprehensive sexual health education elements [7]

Human development, including topics such as anatomy, puberty, sexual orientation, and gender identity.	Relationships, including families, friendships, intimate relationships, marriage, and raising children.	Personal skills, such as understanding values, effective communication, decision making, negotiation, assertiveness, and how to seek help.
Sexual behavior, including abstinence, masturbation, shared sexual behavior, pleasure from sex, and sexual dysfunction across the lifespan.	Sexual health, including contraception, pregnancy, prenatal care, abortion, STIs, HIV and AIDS, sexual abuse, assault, and violence.	Society and culture, including gender roles, diversity, and the intersection of sexuality and the law, religion, media, and the arts.
Other topics include Interpersonal relationships, violence prevention, reproductive coercion, refusal skills/accepting rejection, reproductive rights, cyber solicitation/bullying, consent		

Children can understand concepts related to gender, bodies, and relationships which are pertinent parts of sexual health education [8]. In addition, sexual health education is most effective when it begins before sexual activity so that adolescents are equip with the information needed to protect themselves. Based on data from the CDC, by the age of 18, most teenagers have received formal sexual health education (96% of female and 97% of male teenagers) [9].

Comprehensive sexual health education has been shown to positively impact adolescents' sexual behaviors, leading to safer sex practices and reduced rates of STIs and teen pregnancies. Significant evidence exists that abstinence only programs are not effective at achieving their goal of delaying the start of sexual intercourse until marriage, while comprehensive sexuality education programs do have favorable outcomes on delaying coitarche and other measures. A 2012 meta-analysis by the Centers for Disease Control and Prevention reviewed the efficacy of 66 comprehensive programs and 23 abstinence programs. The comprehensive programs showed improvements in self-reported onset of and current sexual activity, use of protection (condoms and/or hormonal contraceptive methods), frequency of protected and unprotected sexual activity, number of sexual partners, and rates of STIs and pregnancy [10]. The abstinence only programs showed no change in rates of abstinence, sexual behaviors, or other sexual health outcomes such as pregnancy and sexually transmitted infections. Additionally, findings from the US government's own program evaluation showed that participants in abstinence only until marriage (AOUM) programs had no higher rates of abstinence than control groups, and if sexually active, had comparable behaviors to control groups, including number of partners and age at coitarche [11]. Comprehensive sexuality education is supported by the American Academy of Pediatrics; the Society for Adolescent Health and Medicine; the American College of Obstetricians and Gynecologists; the American Medical Association; the American Public Health Association; the Health and Medicine Division of the National Academies of Science, Engineering, and Medicine (formerly the Institute of Medicine); and the National Education Association [4, 12–16].

Comprehensive programs showed improvements in self-reported onset of and current sexual activity, use of protection (condoms and/or hormonal contraceptive methods), frequency of protected and unprotected sexual activity, number of sexual partners, and rates of STIs and pregnancy [10]. Further, comprehensive sexuality education in schools has also been associated with improved academic achievement and attendance [17]. Students who participated in a comprehensive sexual health education program in public schools delayed their sexual debut more effectively than their peers who received limited or no sexual health education [18]. Another systematic review of three decades of research found that comprehensive sexual health education in schools is effective in reducing rates of teen pregnancies and sexually transmitted infections (STIs). These programs also help delay the onset of sexual activity and increase the use of contraceptives among teens who are sexually active and significantly reduce the incidence of teen pregnancies by promoting responsible sexual behaviors and increasing contraceptive use [19]. By addressing topics such as mutual consent, recognizing and preventing sexual coercion, and maintaining healthy boundaries, comprehensive sexual education helps prevent sexual violence and promotes healthier interpersonal relationships among adolescents [19]. Furthermore, interventions that involve a multi-component approach—integrating education, community involvement, and health services—tend to have a more significant impact on adolescents' knowledge and behaviors [19].

132.2 Current Challenges

While there have been positive trends in the reduction of adolescent sexual activity and improved contraceptive use, challenges remain in ensuring consistent and comprehensive sexual education across the U.S. There are disparities in the type and quality of sexual health education provided across different states and school districts, which affects adolescents' knowledge and behaviors regarding sexual health. There are also notable disparities in sexual health outcomes based on race, ethnicity, and socioeconomic status, indicating a need for more targeted and inclusive sexual health education programs [19]. Misinformation about sexual health and contraception remains a significant barrier, underscoring the need for accurate and comprehensive education. Stigma around discussing sexual health can prevent adolescents from seeking the information and services they need. There are also significant disparities in access to reproductive health services based on socioeconomic status, race, and geographic location. Rural and low-income adolescents often face greater barriers to accessing comprehensive sexual health education and reproductive healthcare [19].

While sexual health education is typically associated with schools, comprehensive sexual health education can be delivered in many other settings including the home/family, clinical practices, community or faith-based organizations, and online or on social media. Parents and caregivers can serve as the primary source for sexual health education for their children and can teach fundamental information about development, puberty, gender, and relationships as well as skills and values. However, not all adolescents receive sexual health education at home and for those that do, many factors impact the receipt of sexual health education, including parent/caregiver knowledge, comfort, communication skills, beliefs, culture, social norms, as well as relationship with parent (s). Those students who are not receiving formal education in school or at home, may benefit from sexual health education in other spaces. Reputable online spaces can also minimize stigma and can allow for more youth to access high quality sexual health education on their own terms. This is especially important for youth that lack access to formal comprehensive sexual health education at home or school. Sample websites include https://www.sexetc.org, http://www.advocatesforyouth.org, https://www.bedsider.org, https://www.teenhealth.org, https://www.youngwomenshealth.org, https://www.youngmenshealthsite.org.

132.3 School Based Health and the Role of Sexual Health Education and Reproductive Health Services

Pediatricians can provide education about sexuality that can supplement the education children and adolescents receive at school or at home [11]. Pediatric health clinicians such as school-based health providers are uniquely positioned to provide sexual health education to children and adolescents in a longitudinal manner. While parents and caregivers at home can be a valuable source of sexuality education and information, lack of knowledge, comfort, and communication skills are all potential barriers for home education on this topic to reliably occur. Health care providers can play a critical role in sexuality education by delivering medically accurate and developmentally appropriate information in the health care setting. Healthcare providers can also help to facilitate discussion about sexuality between adolescents and their parents. In addition to providing counseling and education, school-based health providers can provide access to reproductive health-related services such as STI screening and treatment, pregnancy testing and counseling, referral to safe and legal abortion services, referral to prenatal care, emergency contraception, contraceptive options including LARC's, mental health support, care and support for adolescent who experience sexual assault. The AAP has resources for providers regarding care of the adolescent after sexual assault [2]. Moreover, school-based health providers can be resources to the school and school board in developing sexual health education curricula and communication with parents and other community members at meetings through educational programs.

The evidence overwhelmingly supports the benefits of comprehensive sexual health education. By delaying sexual initiation, reducing teen pregnancy and STI rates, promoting consent and healthy relationships, and adopting an inclusive approach, comprehensive sexual education significantly contributes to the overall well-being of adolescents. It is imperative that policymakers, educators, and health care providers continue to advocate for and implement comprehensive sexual health education programs to ensure that young people are equipped with the knowledge and skills necessary for healthy and informed decision-making.

Extra Credit Points

1. Comprehensive sexual health education has been shown to positively impact adolescents' sexual health, leading to safer sex practices and reduced rates of STIs and teen pregnancies.
2. Abstinence only programs are not effective at achieving their goal of delaying the start of sexual intercourse until marriage.
3. The type of sexual health education in the United States varies widely by state, school district, and by who delivers the education, leading to differences in the content and quality of the education provided to students.
4. Pediatric health clinicians such as school-based health providers are uniquely positioned to provide education about sexuality that can supplement the education children and adolescents receive at school or at home.

References

1. Centers for Disease Control and Prevention. Youth risk behavior survey data summary & trends report: 2011-2021. Atlanta: US Department of Health and Human Services; 2023. Available from: https://www.cdc.gov/healthyyouth/data/yrbs/pdf/YRBS_Data-Summary-Trends_Report2023_508.pdf.
2. Guttmacher Institute. American teens' sexual and reproductive health. Guttmacher Institute. Available from: https://www.guttmacher.org/fact-sheet/american-teens-sexual-and-reproductive-health.
3. World Health Organization. Comprehensive sexuality education. Available from: https://www.who.int/news-room/questions-and-answers/item/comprehensive-sexuality-education.
4. American College of Obstetricians and Gynecologists. Comprehensive sexuality education. ACOG. https://www.acog.org/advocacy/policy-priorities/adolescent-health/comprehensive-sexuality-education. Accessed 5 Aug 2024.
5. American Academy of Pediatrics. The importance of access to comprehensive sexual health education. Available from: https://www.aap.org/en/patient-care/adolescent-sexual-health/equitable-access-to-sexual-and-reproductive-health-care-for-all-youth/the-importance-of-access-to-comprehensive-sex-education/.
6. Guttmacher Institute. Sex and HIV education. Guttmacher Institute. Available from: https://www.guttmacher.org/state-policy/explore/sex-and-hiv-education.
7. SIECUS. The Guidelines. Available from: https://siecus.org/resource/the-guidelines/.
8. Meyer S, et al. Comprehensive sexuality education and the development of adolescents. J Adolesc Health. 2020;67(2):218–26. Available from: https://pubmed.ncbi.nlm.nih.gov/22341164/.
9. Centers for Disease Control and Prevention. Data Brief No. 44. Available from: https://www.cdc.gov/nchs/products/databriefs/db44.htm.
10. Kirby D. The impact of sexual health education on the sexual behavior of young people. J Adolesc Health. 2011;48(4):321–9. Available from: https://pubmed.ncbi.nlm.nih.gov/22341164/.
11. Santelli JS, et al. Abortion and public health. Am J Public Health. 2017;107(1):158–60. Available from: https://pubmed.ncbi.nlm.nih.gov/28842065/.
12. American Academy of Pediatrics. Sexuality education for children and adolescents. Pediatrics. 2016;138(2):e20161348. Available from: https://publications.aap.org/pediatrics/article/138/2/e20161348/52508/Sexuality-Education-for-Children-and-Adolescents?autologincheck=redirected.
13. Goldfarb ES, Lieberman LD. Three decades of research: the case for comprehensive sex education. J Adolesc Health. 2021;68(1):13–27. https://doi.org/10.1016/j.jadohealth.2020.07.036. Epub 2020 Oct 12. PMID: 33059958.
14. American Medical Association. Sexuality education, sexual violence prevention, abstinence, and distribution of condoms in schools H-170.968. AMA. https://policysearch.ama-assn.org/policyfinder/detail/Sexuality%.
15. American Public Health Association. Sexuality education as part of a comprehensive health education program in K to 12 schools. APHA. https://www.apha.org/policies-and-advocacy/public-health-policy-statements/policy-database/2015/01/23/09/37/sexuality-education-as-part-of-a-comprehensive-health-education-program-in-k-to-12-schools. Accessed 5 Aug 2024.
16. National Academies of Sciences, Engineering, and Medicine. Sexually transmitted infections: adopting a sexual health paradigm. Washington, DC: The National Academies Press; 2021. https://doi.org/10.17226/25955.
17. Advocates for Youth. Comprehensive sexual health education and academic success. Advocates for Youth. 2019. Available from: https://advocatesforyouth.org/wp-content/uploads/2019/09/comprehensive_sex_education_and_academic_success.pdf.

18. Ponsford R, et al. Comprehensive sexual health education and its impact on adolescent sexual health. BMC Public Health. 2021;21:11388. Available from: https://bmcpublichealth.biomedcentral.com/articles/10.1186/s12889-021-11388-2.
19. Wiley DC, Wilson KL. Comprehensive sexual health education and reproductive health outcomes. BMC Women's Health. 2024;24:2963. Available from: https://bmcwomenshealth.biomedcentral.com/articles/10.1186/s12905-024-02963-x.

Chapter 133
Social Media

Abigail Olympia and Jodi Brady-Olympia

Social media is defined by the Oxford Dictionary as "websites and applications that enable users to create and share content or to participate in social networking" [1]. Although this definition includes applications geared toward messaging and networking, social media is generally thought of as applications made for sharing pictures, videos, and messages with the public. A few of the most popular forms of social media include TikTok, Instagram, Facebook, Snapchat, X (formerly known as Twitter), and YouTube (Table 133.1). In addition, online gaming platforms commonly used by students such as Fortnight or Minecraft also provide opportunities for social networking [2].

The usage of social media by young children and adolescents is worldwide, with platforms such as TikTok and YouTube being some of the most widely used forms of social media (Fig. 133.1). According to data from the Pew Research Center, approximately 90% of adolescents over the age of 13 years use social media regularly [3]. The increase in social media use has created new opportunities for students to communicate with others, learn more about the world, and express their feelings, while also introducing challenges regarding exposure to inappropriate content on the internet, cyberbullying, and mental health struggles affected by social media [4].

A. Olympia
Messiah University, Mechanicsburg, PA, USA
e-mail: Abigail.olympia@csagh.org

J. Brady-Olympia (✉)
Department of Pediatrics Penn State, College of Medicine Attending Physician, Division of Adolescent Medicine, Department of Pediatrics, Penn State Children's Hospital, Hershey, PA, USA
e-mail: jbradyolympia@pennstatehealth.psu.edu

R. P. Olympia, J. Brady-Olympia (eds.), *Clinical Considerations in School-based Health*, https://doi.org/10.1007/978-3-031-85765-2_133

Table 133.1 Examples of Popular Social Media Platforms

YouTube	YouTube is a global video-sharing platform where users can upload and view videos of various topics such as entertainment, personal vlogs, or education.
TikTok	TikTok is a platform that allows users to create, view, and share short-form videos, often featuring popular music, unique dances, comedy, and creative editing effects.
Instagram	Instagram is a platform focused on photo and video sharing, allowing users to post content, follow others, and engage through likes, comments, and direct messages.
Facebook	Similar to Instagram, Facebook is a platform that enables users to connect, share, and communicate through posts, photos, videos, and messages with friends, family members, and communities made for specific topics.
X (previously Twitter)	X is a platform that allows users to post and interact with short messages, share media content, and follow other users or celebrities to stay updated on news and trends.
Snapchat	Snapchat is a multimedia messaging platform that allows users to send photos, videos, and messages that disappear 24 hours after being viewed by the recipient.
Discord	Discord is a communication platform designed for creating communities, where its users can interact through messages, voice, and video channels.
Other	Reddit, Pinterest, WhatsApp, Twitch, Tumblr, BeReal, Threads, Kik, Skype

For younger children between the ages of 5 and 12 years, social media is less prevalent than it is for adolescents. Rather than being used for social interactions with others, social media is more commonly used as entertainment for younger children [2]. However, its influence is still seen at these early ages, as children are introduced to social media platforms through family devices and child-friendly applications directed toward this age group, such as YouTube Kids. As a result of this early exposure, these young children grow up with social media being a major part of their social fabric [2].

This chapter aims to provide an overview of the impact social media has on students between the ages of 5 and 18 years, as well as highlight the positive and negative traits that social media entails for its users. By examining the different aspects associated with social media, we seek to offer insights into how school nurses and providers can navigate this new and complex area of the internet to support the healthy growth of young students in a connected world.

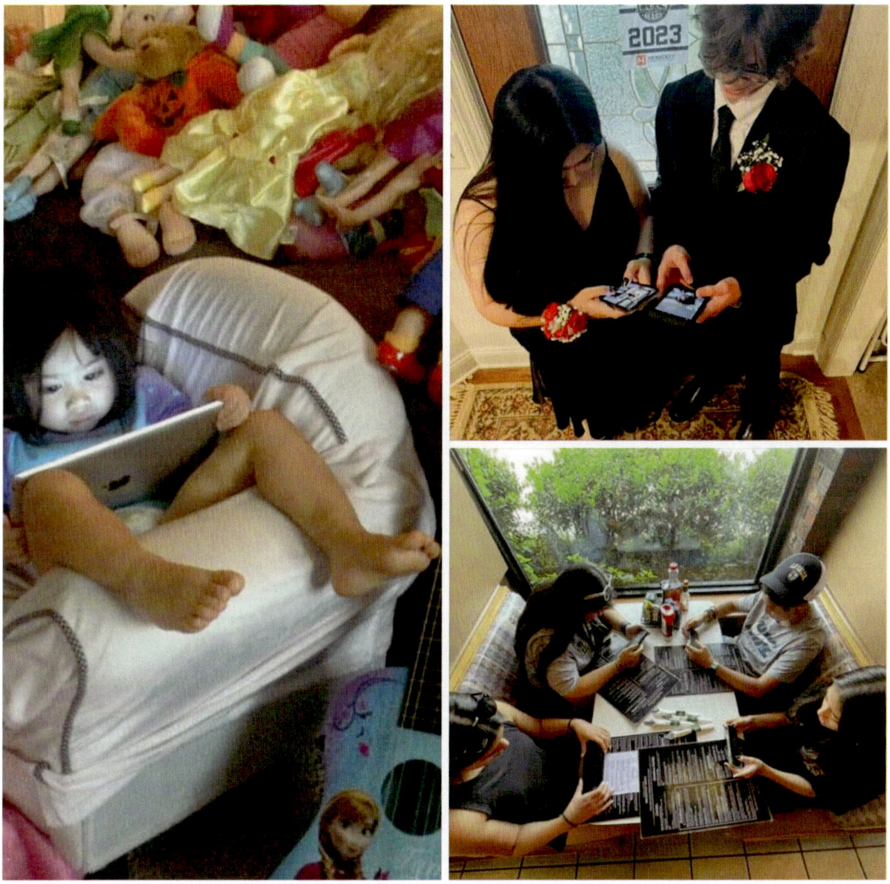

Fig. 133.1 Social media encompasses the lives of children and adolescents

133.1 The Uses of Social Media

While social media use is widespread among children and adolescents, opinions about its positive and negative impact vary. Challenges in interpreting studies looking at the impact of social media use as "negative" or "positive" result from lack of clarity in terms of what is considered social media use, time spent on social media and the type of social media [2, 5, 6].

133.1.1 Positive Uses

1. **Advocacy for Social Issues:** With the wide range of social media, a student can bring advocacy for any social issue that he or she strongly believes in. Additionally, students can learn more about the current social issues in the world through posts from other people.

2. **Connectivity and Communication with Others:** Social media allows students to share their adventures, questions, and stories with their friends, family, or the public. On the other hand, students can stay connected with their friends and family by viewing their posts. Additionally, many social media platforms include a messaging feature, allowing students to communicate with their friends and family [6].
3. **Collaboration on Group Projects:** Group projects are common in schools, so social media can act as a form of communication for the project. For students who may not want to share their personal phone numbers with classmates, messaging platforms such as Snapchat, Discord, or WhatsApp can act as a substitution.
4. **Emotional Support:** Many students go through hard times throughout school. With social media, students can find other people who have or are going through the same issues or create a support group. With the support of others, students may find it easier to get through hard times [6].
5. **Meeting New People:** Although talking to strangers on the internet is not always safe, social media allows students to build social connections with peers with similar interests, backgrounds or beliefs and help with identity formation and social support. For students who may have a hard time creating relationships with their classmates, a new friend on the internet can allow the student to improve their social skills and find others who are like them [7]. Social media can also be a platform for identity development and social support for adolescents from stigmatized or minority communities, such as LGTBQ+ youth [6, 8].
6. **Real-Time Updates:** For students who are interested in sports, singers or bands, or content creators, social media allows them to receive real-time updates about their interests ranging from scores from a football game to the schedule for a band's tour. Additionally, students can use social media to send updates regarding school events using accounts dedicated to student councils, clubs, or sports teams.
7. **Self-Expression:** Social media allows students to be open about who they truly are. By customizing their profiles or posting their interests, students can share their lives with others [6].

133.1.2 Negative Effects

1. **Addiction**: While there are numerous benefits of internet use, internet use can become problematic or addictive [9]. With access to unlimited videos and posts, students may start to become addicted to social media. With no social media restriction, it is easy for students to spend hours on social media without noticing their increasing screen time, thus allowing social media time to replace other crucial areas of their lives such as sleep, nutrition and in person socialization [6].
2. **Cyberbullying:** Students who have public accounts on social media may be more susceptible to cyberbullying from other students at school or even strang-

ers. However, even students with private accounts may be victims of cyberbullying if they are not cautious when accepting friend requests. While social media may offer a platform communicate with other minority youth, it may also leave them susceptible to cyberbullying [6, 7].

3. **Mental Health Concerns:** Studies looking at the effect of mental health have shown a range of results, raised concerns that social media can affect mental health in negative ways. Students may compare themselves with models or others that they see on social media and feel negatively about themselves as a result [4]. There has also been concern raised for an association between Fear of Missing out (FOMO) and mental health with adolescents feeling pressure to post and respond to their peers on social media [6].
4. **Privacy Concerns:** Despite its positive purpose, many adults with negative intentions use social media to prey on students. For example, predators and scammers may try to reach out to students with the intention of receiving the student's personal information. Social media may also be used for sexual exploitation of minors, both for online use, sexting or in person exploitation [2].

133.2 What Age Is Social Media For?

Social media is commonly aimed toward students ages 12 years and older; however, some applications are made for students ages 17 years and older. For example, Instagram is rated safe for ages 12 years and older while X is rated safe for ages 17 years and older. Some applications are made specifically for younger children to ensure that they will have a safe experience while using the social media platform. For example, YouTube Kids is rated safe for children ages 4 years and older. The suggested age for each social media platform is typically written on the download page to allow parents and users to know what the application's content may be like. In many cases, the application will ask for the user's date of birth during the setup process to confirm that the application is safe for the user. The American Academy of Pediatrics site, Social media and Youth Mental Health Center of Excellence, also lists recommended ages for many common social media applications as well as provides information about changing settings on the apps including privacy settings and age restricted content [10]

133.3 Case Studies

Case 1 Issac (age 12 years) downloads Instagram to post about his trip to Florida. He chooses to keep his account public to allow his family and friends to find his account easily; however, several bullies from his school find his account and comment insults regarding his appearance in his posts. Issac views these comments and begins to feel depressed about his looks.

Resolution Case 1 Despite wanting easy accessibility to his account, Issac should change his Instagram account to a private account, preventing strangers and bullies from being able to view his content. In the future, Issac should only give out his username to trusted friends and family members.

Case 2 Casey (age 14 years) downloads Snapchat to communicate with friends. She receives a friend request from a guy named Fred; not knowing if he is a student at her school, she accepts the request. Fred messages Casey and begins a conversation with her, asking friendly questions at first. After some time, Fred begins to ask questions related to personal and private information regarding Casey's life. Casey deletes Snapchat and continues to worry about other people having information about her and has been having trouble sleeping.

Resolution Case 2 If Casey decides to download Snapchat again in the future, she should take precautions by only accepting friend requests from people that she knows personally. If she is unsure if the account belongs to someone she knows, she should either ask the person face-to-face or ignore the request completely.

Case 3 Kelly (age 16 years) moves to a new state during the summer and does not know anyone from her new school. She decides to download Instagram to engage with her new community and classmates. With the use of Instagram, she finds accounts dedicated to the school's different clubs and learns more about what exciting opportunities she will have when school starts in the fall.

Providers in the school-based health setting can build rapport and educate the students they interact with on a daily basis. It is essential that they are educated on the potential risks as well as potential benefits of social media so they can in turn provide guidance to their students and families. Pediatricians who receive training on social media counseling and incorporate the counseling into their visit with adolescents can impact the behaviors of the adolescents [11].

School based health care providers can educate parents and students about the impact of social media on mental health and encourage open communication about the sites they are viewing and social media habits. Many parents are unaware of their child's social media use and have not discussed social media use with their child or adolescent [11].

It is important that parents ensure there is balance between social media use and other areas of their child's life including ensuring adequate time for sleep, schoolwork, meals and other social interactions and relationships. Parents should be aware of the sites that their child is accessing and engage in discussion about the child's social media use, including discussion of cyberbullying, online solicitation, and privacy and safety. It is also important to place time constraints on their use and promote screen free time such as during meals, schoolwork and before bed. In addition, modeling proper social media use is crucial. The American Academy of Pediatrics has resources to guide clinicians as well as parents and caregivers as they navigate social media use among children and adolescents. Their site contains many resources such as "The 5 Cs of Media Use" which can be used to help guide parents and caregivers as they oversee their children's and teens use of social media [12]. This tool encourages parents and caregivers to consider their child, the content they are interacting with, their reaction to the content, balancing social media use and their communication with their children and teens regarding social media.

Extra Credit Points

1. School based health providers should encourage open communication about social media use between parents and adolescents.
2. It is crucial to set limits for social media use, ensuring adolescents use is not encroaching on other essential activities of life and development including age-appropriate sleep needs, nutrition, schoolwork and development of social skills and friendships.
3. It is essential that school staff, as well as parents and guardians, model appropriate social media use skills.

References

1. Oxford English Dictionary, s.v. "social media (n.)," September 2024. https://doi.org/10.1093/OED/5718206998.
2. Hill DL. Social media: anticipatory guidance. Pediatr Rev. 2020;41(3):112–9. https://doi.org/10.1542/pir.2018-0236.
3. Social media use among US teens, by demographic traits. Pew Research Center.
4. Karim F, Oyewande AA, Abdalla LF, Chaudhry Ehsanullah R, Khan S. Social media use and its connection to mental health: a systematic review. Cureus. 2020;12(6):e8627. https://doi.org/10.7759/cureus.8627. PMID: 32685296; PMCID: PMC7364393.
5. Valkenburg PM, Meier A, Beyens I. Social media use and its impact on adolescent mental health: an umbrella review of the evidence. Curr Opin Psychol. 2022;44:58–68. https://doi.org/10.1016/j.copsyc.2021.08.017. Epub 2021 Aug 18.
6. Weigle PE, Shafi RMA. Social media and youth mental health. Curr Psychiatry Rep. 2024;26(1):1–8. https://doi.org/10.1007/s11920-023-01478-w. Epub 2023 Dec 16.
7. Office of the Surgeon General (OSG). Social media and youth mental health: The U.S. Surgeon General's Advisory [Internet]. Washington (DC): US Department of Health and Human Services; 2023.
8. Craig SL, Eaton AD, McInroy LB, Leung VWY, Krishnan S. Can social media participation enhance LGBTQ+ youth well-being? Development of the social media benefits scale. Social Media + Society. 2021;7(1) https://doi.org/10.1177/2056305121988931.
9. Jolliff AF, Moreno MA. #TechAddicted: understanding problematic internet use in adolescents. Pediatr Rev. 2020;41(10):554–5. https://doi.org/10.1542/pir.2019-0249.
10. American Academy of Pediatrics. Center of Excellence on Social Media and Youth Mental Health. Available at https://www.aap.org/en/patient-care/media-and-children/center-of-excellence-on-social-media-and-youth-mental-health/glossary-of-digital-media-platforms/. Accessed on 25 Nov 2024.
11. Moreno MA, Klein JD, Kaseeska K, Gorzkowski J, Harris D, Davis J, Gotlieb E, Wasserman R. A cluster randomized controlled trial of a primary care provider-delivered social media counseling intervention. J Adolesc Health. 2023;73(5):924–30. https://doi.org/10.1016/j.jadohealth.2023.06.007. Epub 2023 Aug 12. PMID: 37578406; PMCID: PMC10592061.
12. American Academy of Pediatrics. Center of Excellence on Social Media and Youth Mental Health. Available at https://www.aap.org/en/patient-care/media-and-children/center-of-excellence-on-soical-media-and-youth-mental-health. Accessed 25 Nov 2024.

Chapter 134
Vaping/Nicotine, Cannabis, and Inhalant Use

Corey McBrayer and Sheryl Ryan

Case 1 Thad, a 15-year-old male, is being evaluated in a school-based health clinic for acute cough. The medical student obtaining the history discovers that he is vaping one pod daily of 5% nicotine 'juice.' The student is curious about negative effects of vaping and if treatment is necessary for this amount of nicotine use.

Nicotine use is prevalent amongst adolescents (Table 134.1). Ninety percent of adults that currently use nicotine products did so prior to age 18. Since their introduction into the US in 2010, vape products have risen in popularity and have overtaken cigarettes and other forms of nicotine consumption. In fact, 10% of high schoolers have used a vape product in the past 30 days compared to 1–2% that have used either cigarettes or smokeless tobacco, such as snus [2].

Vapor products range widely from small, flash drive-like devices to devices that resemble other items such as highlighters, pens, small video game consoles, among others.

There are short- and long-term risks associated with nicotine use (Tables 134.2 and 134.3). While vaping is considered a risk mitigation strategy within the adult addiction world (as compared to cigarettes), this is not the case with adolescents whose brains are particularly susceptible to negative developmental effects of all substances, including nicotine. Vaping can lead to marijuana or other substance use as well as other tobacco products [4].

The American Academy of Pediatrics (AAP) has an excellent guide for the treatment of nicotine use in adolescents [6]. They recommend Ask-Counsel-Treat with each patient and include screening tools to determine level of nicotine dependence. It is important to use the DSM V TR to determine whether the patient has a use disorder and classify it as mild, moderate, or severe, depending on the number of

C. McBrayer (✉) · S. Ryan
Penn State Health Medical Center, Hershey, PA, USA
e-mail: cmcbrayer@pennstatehealth.psu.edu; sryan4@pennstatehealth.psu.edu

R. P. Olympia, J. Brady-Olympia (eds.), *Clinical Considerations in School-based Health*, https://doi.org/10.1007/978-3-031-85765-2_134

Table 134.1 Types of nicotine products

Vapor	See Fig. 134.1; vapes can be modified for greater effect: such as 'dripping' (e-cigarettes heat liquid into a vapor, which the user inhales and then exhales in a larger puffy cloud, giving a stronger sensation in the throat and making the flavors taste better)
Cigarettes	About 1.5 mg nicotine absorbed per cigarette
Nicotine pouches or loose-leaf oral tobacco	Snus, chewing tobacco, dip, snuff
Hookah	Electronic or tobacco smoke bubbled through water
Pipe, cigar, cigarillos	Less common amongst adolescents

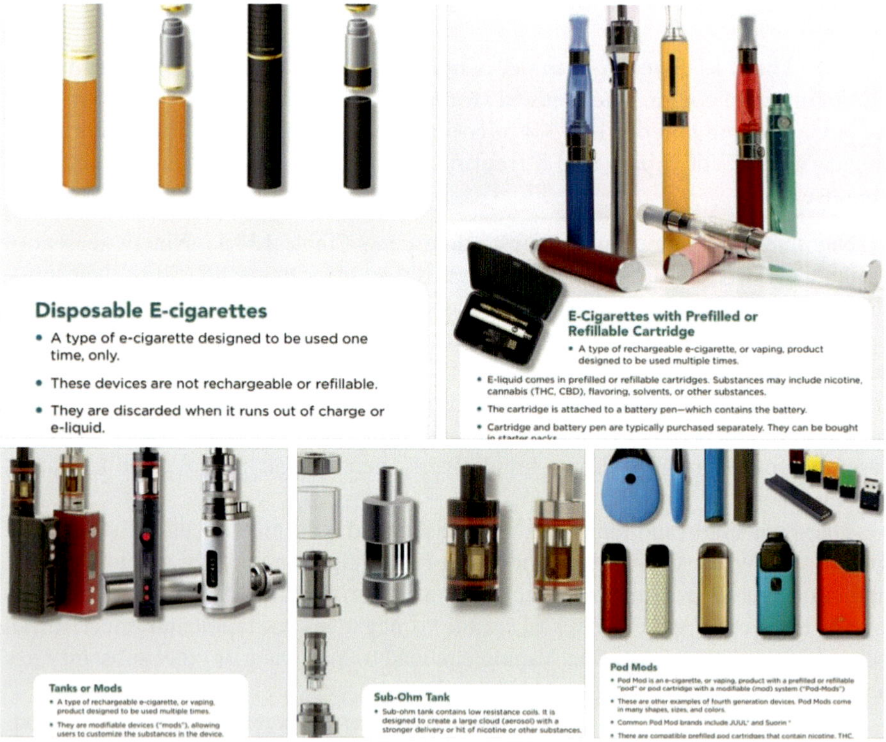

Fig. 134.1 Types of Vape Devices [1]. (Adapted from: E-cigarette, or vaping, products visual dictionary. 2019. https://stacks.cdc.gov/view/cdc/103783)

Table 134.2 Short-term risks associated with nicotine use [3]

Overdose (tachycardia, tremors, tachypnea, death)	Primarily seen with young children drinking flavored vape 'juice'
Vape-associated lung injury (respiratory distress, chest pain, generally associated with vaping THC with nicotine)	Mostly associated with vaping marijuana, though cases exist with nicotine-only vapes
Asthma exacerbation	Vaping, smoking, hookah
Oral mucosal injury	Vape malfunction, pouched tobacco irritation
Burns	Combustible tobacco products (e.g. cigarette, pipe, etc)
Insomnia	Affects circadian rhythm
Weight loss	Nicotine suppresses appetite
Neonatal outcomes	Low birth weight, neurocognitive effects

Table 134.3 Long-term risks associated with nicotine use [3–5]

Toxin exposure (carcinogens)	Vaping: toluene, propylene glycol, aldehydes, acetone; metals such as nickel, lead, copper, chromium Combustible: >500 compounds, including tar, CO, hydrogen cyanide, metals mentioned above
Developmental delay	Affects working memory, attention, learning, the reward center; stunts frontal lobe development
Cancer	Throat and mouth, lung, bladder, stomach
Endocrine issues	Metabolic syndrome (such as type 2 diabetes), thyroid disease
Poor wound healing	Surgeon may request cessation prior to elective surgery or after emergency surgery

criteria reported (see Table 134.4). For a mild use disorder, motivational interviewing in the office or with a clinician specializing in adolescent substance use may be effective in encouraging the teen to change their behavior around vaping. Motivational interviewing involves discovering 'change talk' with the adolescent-motivations they have for change-and then guiding them in a 10–15 minute visit towards aligning their actions with their goals and core beliefs. Cognitive Behavioral Therapy (CBT) is sometimes employed as well. CBT employs skills for saying no to substances, combating urges, and coping with life occurrences, among others. Contingency management is well studied in adolescent substance use. It involves positive enforcement via rewards for specific behaviors (i.e. participating in therapy, negative urine drug screens, etc.). It can be paired with other modalities for better compliance but should not be the only treatment method, as it is not sustainable over time [3].

There are no medications that are FDA approved to treat those under the age of 17 with a nicotine use disorder. However, with moderate and severe nicotine use disorders the AAP recommends consideration of pharmacotherapy along with the therapy modalities mentioned above (Table 134.5).

Table 134.4 DSM V criteria for substance use disorders [7]
Must meet at least two criteria in a 12-month period for an active substance use disorder diagnosis

Impaired Control	Use in larger amounts/for longer time periods Persistent desire or unsuccessful efforts to cut down or control use Excess time spent obtaining, using or recovering Craving or a strong desire or urge
Social Impairment	Failure to fulfill major role obligations at work, school or home Continued use despite recurrent social or interpersonal problems Important social, occupational or recreational activities reduced or given up
Risky Use of Substance	Recurrent use in physically hazardous situations Continued use despite knowledge of medical or psychological problems resulting from use
Pharmacological Criteria	Tolerance—requiring higher amounts to achieve effects or diminishing effects with continued use same amount Withdrawal—having withdrawal symptoms or using to relieve or avoid withdrawal symptoms

Mild: 2–3 criteria, Moderate 4–5 Criteria, Severe 6+ criteria

Table 134.5 Pharmacologic treatment of nicotine use disorder [3]

Nicotine replacement therapy	18+, off-label use in younger adolescent; Use long-acting patch <u>with</u> short-acting such as gum, lozenge, nasal spray. Both are recommended together; short-acting helps with intermittent cravings.	Patch: 7 mg-just a few puffs; 14 mg-½ pod/day; 21 or more mg-1+ pod per day Short-acting: 2 mg if initiates nicotine use >30 minutes after waking, 4 mg if starts <30 minutes after waking
Varenicline	For ages 17+	Ramp up to 1 mg BID for 3 months, can extend to 6 months
Bupropion	18+, off-label in younger adolescents	SR formulation; 150–300 mg BID for 3 months; can extend to 12 months

Case 2 Jenna is a 15 Year old sophomore who was recently found to be intoxicated at school, and has since reported to the school nurse that she has been using cannabis almost daily for the past several months. She vapes THC extract using a vape pen, and reports that it helps her with her anxiety at school and with sleep at night. She is reluctant to reduce her use for fear of her anxiety worsening.

Marijuana is currently the most commonly use illicit substance by teenagers. Data from the 2023 National Monitoring the Future Study found that 29% of 12 graders, 18% of 10 graders, and 78% of eighth graders used marijuana in the last year [8]. Thus, given these numbers of students using cannabis products, it will be very common for school personnel to see students in both middle and high school

Table 134.6 Types of Cannabis products

Name	Form
Flower	Refers to bud of the marijuana plant. It is the smoked form, used rolled as "joints" or in a glass device.
Cannabis Concentrate	Highly potent products that may be sold as liquid used for dabbing or vaporizing using a device
Tinctures	Alcohol based products that are taken sublingually. Can be added to food
Edibles	Ingestible marijuana products, foods or drinks infused with cannabis flower or concentrate such as gummies, brownies, or tea
Topicals	Cannabis infused creams/lotions applied to skin

Table 134.7 Acute effects of Cannabis

Intoxication: Euphoria, relaxation/sedation, change in pain sensation, distortion of sensory perception, thought and time distortion
Delayed motor coordination, slowed reaction to stimuli
Increased heart rate; decreased blood pressure
Excessive vomiting- generally with heavy use
Cough, blood-shot eyes
Hallucinations, paranoia, anxiety, psychosis- can be rarely seen as toxic reaction
Memory impairment

coming to school intoxicated from marijuana or experiencing its short or long-term effects.

Table 134.6 lists the more commonly available forms of cannabis products. It is important to remember that the cannabis products available today are much more potent than those available even a decade or two ago. The concentration of the psychoactive substance in the cannabis plant, THC or delta-9-tetrahydrocannabinol, was previously about 4–5%; species grown now have up to 18–20% THC [9]. Concentrates currently available can contain up to 70–80% THC.

Although there are more than 200 compounds in the marijuana plant, many of which are biologically active, THC causes the euphoria that students seek. Table 134.7 lists the acute effects seen with cannabis intoxication; Table 134.8 lists longer-term effects that can be seen with regular and/or heavy use. Some of the long-term effects may not be reversible and can have significant health consequences [10].

The cannabis hyperemesis syndrome is a specific constellation of symptoms that are occasionally seen with regular, heavy use, and may be more common when highly potent forms of marijuana are used. The presenting symptoms are intractable vomiting, often associated with dehydration [11]. While there are no completely effective treatments for this, other than abstinence from all cannabis products, some symptomatic relief is reported with hot showers, and capsaicin products administered to the lower abdomen (where solar plexus is located).

Table 134.8 Effects of regular use and long-term use

Regular Use	Long Term Use
Dependence develops in 1 of 6 teens who regularly use	Short term memory impairment that is long lasting
Psychotic symptoms and disorders, anxiety in heavy users: Especially with family history of psychosis-represents increased vulnerability	Likely permanent cognitive impairment and loss of IQ in adolescents who begin use at an early age and continue heavy use into late adolescence
Chronic bronchitis and impaired respiratory status	Impaired educational attainment; Amotivational syndrome
50–90% more car accidents when also used with alcohol	Unclear association with respiratory illness
Higher rates of use tobacco and other drugs	Higher rates of schizophrenia, anxiety and mood disorders
Cannabis hyperemesis syndrome Cannabis Use Disorder (mild, moderate or severe disorder using DSM criteria—see Table 134.4)	Neurocognitive deficits associated with executive functioning and memory/learning [10]

With regular, heavy use, a teen can develop Cannabis Use Disorder, which is an addiction to the THC in cannabis; using the DSM criteria, the cannabis use disorder can be mild (2–3 criteria), moderate (4–5 criteria) or severe (6+ criteria) (see Table 134.4). They may also experience withdrawal symptoms when trying to cut back or stop use, such as irritability, anorexia, depression, malaise and difficulty sleeping.

When evaluating a student with regular or problematic marijuana use, ask about the teen's use pattern and whether the teen is using the cannabis to alleviate symptoms such as anxiety, depression, or sleep difficulties. Using the DSM 5 Criteria can help determine whether the student has experienced any negative effects or functioning (Table 134.4). With mild cannabis use disorder (CUD), using motivational interviewing to assist that teen in changing their behavior is the first line of treatment, as there are no medications that are highly effective to treat CUD. With moderate or severe CUD, referral for further assessment or treatment is indicated. Engaging the parents at this point will also facilitate that student getting the help that they need, especially when the adolescent does not see their cannabis use as problematic.

Case 3 Fenn, a 13-year-old nonbinary student, has been failing classes after previously experiencing no academic issues. One teacher notes that Fenn seems to doze off in class and no longer cares much about the material. On exam, you note a faint, papular rash around the mouth as well as silver coloring under the nose. How would you approach an initial conversation with this student?

Close to 10% of those over the age of 12 have tried an inhalant at least once [12], with a slightly higher prevalence in adolescent females. See Table 134.9 for types of inhalants. Signs of use include rash, chemical burns/frostbite, and/or paint over the lower face, smell of gasoline or other volatile chemical, decreased academic

Table 134.9 Examples of types of inhalants and where they are found [3, 12]

Type	Examples	Common places found
Volatile Alkyl Nitrites	'poppers,' such as amyl nitrite	Room deodorizers
Nitrous Oxide	'laughing gas,' 'whippets'	Whipped cream cans, Homemade whipped cream chargers
Solvents, fuels, and anesthetics	Butane, halothane, toluene, etc.	Paint thinner, lighter fluid, adhesive

Table 134.10 Risks associated with inhalant use [3]

Death (sudden sniffing death syndrome)
Demyelination (lead in gasoline for example)
Neurotoxicity (atrophy)
Development of other use disorders
Mood disorders
Eye, nose, mouth irritation
Lung inflammation
Hepatitis (metabolism in the liver)
Renal tubular acidosis (toluene)

performance. Intoxication is short-lived and includes uncoordinated gait, slurred speech, headache, unconsciousness. Generally, these effects have passed prior to evaluation due to their rapid clearance from the body [3, 12].

Inhalant use can have significant health consequences and be a predictor for future substance use (Table 134.10). Thus, it is important to identify inhalant use, as even a single use can result in fatal arrhythmia.

There are no FDA approved or off-label medications for inhalant use disorder. The focus is on either family-based or individual therapy along with motivational interviewing. As with nicotine use, contingency management to aid in engagement can be useful. [3]

Extra Credit Points

1. Nicotine, cannabis, and inhalants impair adolescent brain development
2. Cannabis is a very commonly used substance by adolescents
3. It is important to recognize and treat use disorders; early intervention is key

References

1. E-cigarette, or vaping, products visual dictionary. 2019. https://stacks.cdc.gov/view/cdc/103783.
2. Youth and tobacco use. CDC. https://www.cdc.gov/tobacco/data_statistics/fact_sheets/youth_data/tobacco_use/index.htm.
3. Miller S, Fiellin D, Rosenthal R, Saitz R. The ASAM principles of addiction medicine. 6th ed. Wolters Kluwer; 2019.

4. Dinardo P, Rome ES. Vaping: the new wave of nicotine addiction. Cleve Clin J Med. 2019;86(12):789–98. https://doi.org/10.3949/ccjm.86a.19118.
5. Rose JJ, Krishnan-Sarin S, Exil VJ, et al. Cardiopulmonary impact of electronic cigarettes and vaping products: a scientific statement from the American Heart Association. Circulation. 2023;148(8):703–28. https://doi.org/10.1161/cir.0000000000001160.
6. AAP reference https://downloads.aap.org/AAP/PDF/AAP_Youth_Tobacco_Cessation_Considerations_for_Clinicians.pdf.
7. American Psychiatric Association, editor. Diagnostic and statistical manual of mental disorders. 5rd ed. Washington D.C.: American Psychiatric Association; 2022.
8. Miech RA, Johnston LD, et al. National survey results on drug use & secondary school students. https://www.monitoringthefuture.org/up-content/uploads/2023/12/mtf2023.pdf.
9. Chandra S, Radwan MM, Majumdar CG, et al. New trends in cannabis potency in USA and Europe during the last decade (2008–2017). Eur Arch Psychiatry Clin Neurosci. 269(1):5–15. https://doi.org/10.1007/s00406-019-00983-5.
10. Hammond CJ, Chaney A, Hendrickson B, et al. Cannabis use among US adolescents in the era of marijuana legalization: a review of changing use patterns, comorbidity and health correlates. Int Rev Psychaitry. 2020;32(3):221–34. https://doi.org/10.1080/09540261.2020.1713056.
11. Venkatesan T, Levinthal DJ, Li BUK, et al. ROle of Cannabis use: cyclic vomiting syndrome vs cannabinoid hyperemesis syndrome. Neurogastroenterol Motil. 2019;31(Suppl 2):e13606. https://doi.org/10.1111/nmo.13606.
12. Radparvar S. The clinical assessment & treatment of inhalant abuse. Perm J. 2023;27(2):99. https://doi.org/10.7812/tpp/22.164.

Index

R. P. Olympia, J. Brady-Olympia (eds.), *Clinical Considerations in School-based Health*, https://doi.org/10.1007/978-3-031-85765-2

E

I

W

Y

GPSR Compliance

The European Union's (EU) General Product Safety Regulation (GPSR) is a set of rules that requires consumer products to be safe and our obligations to ensure this.

If you have any concerns about our products, you can contact us on ProductSafety@springernature.com

In case Publisher is established outside the EU, the EU authorized representative is:

Springer Nature Customer Service Center GmbH
Europaplatz 3
69115 Heidelberg, Germany

Batch number: 10722273

Printed by Printforce, the Netherlands